ICD-9-CM Coding

THEORY AND PRACTICE

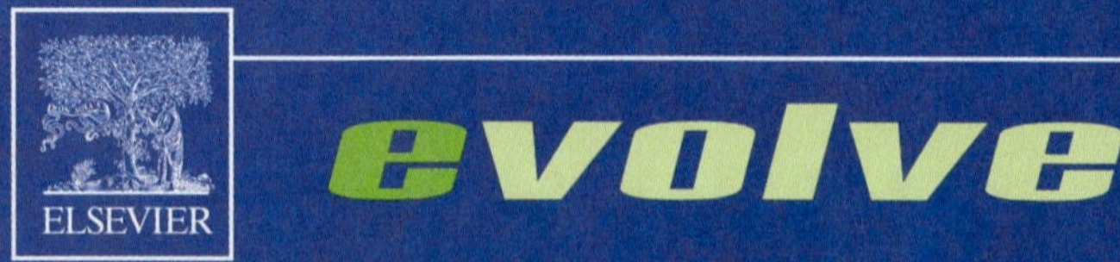

To access your Student Learning Resources, visit:

http://evolve.elsevier.com/lovaasen/icd/

Evolve® Student Learning Resources for ***ICD-9-CM Coding: Theory and Practice*** offers the following features:

- **Content Updates**
  The latest content updates from the authors of the textbook to keep you current with recent developments in this area of study.
- **Reimbursement Updates**
  The latest reimbursement updates to keep you current as the reimbursement system evolves.
- **WebLinks**
  Check out this list of websites chosen to supplement the content of the textbook.

http://evolve.elsevier.com/lovaasen/icd/

Karla R. Lovaasen, RHIA, CCS, CCS-P

Coding and Consulting Services
Abingdon, Maryland

Jennifer Schwerdtfeger, BS, RHIT, CCS, CPC, CPC-H

Partner, Auditing & Coding Experts, LLC
Crofton, Maryland

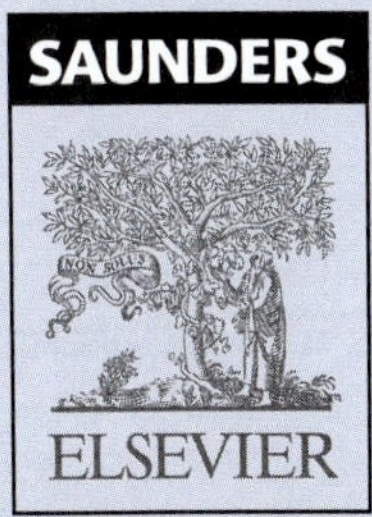

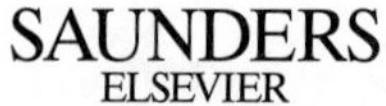

SAUNDERS
ELSEVIER

11830 Westline Industrial Drive
St. Louis, Missouri 63146

ICD-9-CM Coding: Theory and Practice, 2009 edition ISBN: 978-1-4160-5881-6

Notice

Knowledge and best practice in this field are constantly changing. As new research and experience broaden our knowledge, changes in practice, treatment and drug therapy may become necessary or appropriate. Readers are advised to check the most current information provided (i) on procedures featured or (ii) by the manufacturer of each product to be administered, to verify the recommended dose or formula, the method and duration of administration, and contraindications. It is the responsibility of the practitioner, relying on their own experience and knowledge of the patient, to make diagnoses, to determine dosages and the best treatment for each individual patient, and to take all appropriate safety precautions. To the fullest extent of the law, neither the Publisher nor the Authors assume any liability for any injury and/or damage to persons or property arising out of or related to any use of the material contained in this book.

The Publisher

Library of Congress Cataloging-in-Publication Data
Lovaasen, Karla R.
ICD-9-CM coding : theory and practice / Karla R. Lovaasen, Jennifer Schwerdtfeger.—2009 ed.
p. ; cm.
Includes bibliographical references and index.
ISBN 978-1-4160-5881-6 (pbk. : alk. paper) 1. Nosology—Code numbers. I. Schwerdtfeger, Jennifer. II. International classification of diseases, 9th revision, clinical modification. III. Title.
[DNLM: 1. Disease—classification. 2. Forms and Records Control—methods. 3. International Classification of Diseases. WB 15 L896i 2009]
RB115.L68 2009
616.001′2—dc22

2008018553

Vice President, Health Professions: Andrew M. Allen
Executive Editor: Susan Cole
Developmental Editor: Beth LoGiudice
Publishing Services Manager: Patricia Tannian
Project Manager: Claire Kramer
Design Direction: Teresa McBryan

Printed in the United States of America

Last digit is the print number: 9 8 7 6 5 4 3 2 1

To my husband John, who has more faith in me than I have in myself.
You are the best!

To my children and grandchildren for their ongoing support.

Karla

To the memory of my father, Philip Carter, for his endless prodding
of me to complete this text.

To my husband, children, and grandchildren for sharing me
with the world of publishing.

Jenny

Reviewers

Dorine Bennett, MBA, RHIA
Associate Professor and Health Information Management Programs Director
Dakota State University
Madison, South Dakota

Marie T. Conde, MPA, RHIA, RHIT, CCS
Program Director and Instructor
City College of San Francisco
San Francisco, California

Melanie Endicott, MBA/HCM, RHIA, CCS, CCS-P
HIM Program Director
Spokane Community College
Spokane, Washington

Dawn Jackson, MAEd, RHIA, CCS-P
Associate Professor
Eastern Kentucky University
Richmond, Kentucky

Alice Jaramillo, RHIT, CCS, CPC-H
Health Information Management Compliance Specialist, Adjunct Faculty
San Juan Regional Medical Center, San Juan College
Farmington, New Mexico

MariBeth Lane, BS, RHIA
Health Information Technology Program Director
Northwest Iowa Community College
Sheldon, Iowa

Sherri Mallett, Med, RHIA, CCS-P
Health Information Management Program Chairperson
Cincinnati State Technical and Community College
Cincinnati, Ohio

Christina Merle, RHIA
Assistant Professor, Health Information Management
Arkansas Tech University
Russellville, Arkansas

Jody Smith, PhD, RHIA, FAHIMA
Chair, Department of Health Informatics and Information Management
Saint Louis University
St. Louis, Missouri

Leona Thomas, MHS, RHIA
Former Chairperson of the Department of Health Information Administration
Chicago State University
Willowbrook, Illinois

Foreword

It is an honor to have an opportunity to share with you my thoughts and feelings about *ICD-9-Coding: Theory and Practice.*

Karla and Jennifer have taken the mystery out of ICD-9-CM coding by preparing a user-friendly book that meets the needs of not only the student but also the busy instructors. The approach taken by the authors is straightforward, clear, concise, and complete. This book contains the latest in coding assignment and covers a wide variety of coding applications by the use of exercises within the text and the accompanying workbook. The use of color illustrations and photographs further enhances the book and will keep the reader interested.

This is the definitive ICD-9-CM coding text!

Carol J. Buck
Author/Instructor

Preface

Authoritatively referenced and easy to use for teaching, *ICD-9-CM Coding: Theory and Practice* is the first inpatient coding resource designed with instructors and students in mind. This comprehensive guide presents reliable coverage of all three ICD-9-CM volumes in a systematic, straightforward format that guides students through the inpatient coding process. With clear examples, challenging review questions, and outstanding instructor support, this innovative resource is not only a valuable coding tool but also a time-saving teaching tool!

ICD-9-CM Coding: Theory and Practice is intended for those who are learning to code, as well as experienced professionals who wish to have a reference and refresher. Unlike other books in this area, *ICD-9-CM Coding: Theory and Practice* sets out to (1) help students understand why coding is essential and necessary, (2) understand the basics of the health record, and (3) fully understand the rules, guidelines, and functions of ICD-9-CM coding. This book can be used in medical insurance, billing, and coding educational programs; in health information management programs; and as a useful reference to practitioners in the field.

ORGANIZATION

The organization of *ICD-9-CM: Theory and Practice* follows the most logical way to learn this material. The early chapters focus on history, the health record as the foundation for coding, and the *Official Guidelines for Coding and Reporting.* A coder must have a basic understanding of this foundational content before moving on to more complicated material. Specifically, Chapter 4 covers the basic steps of ICD-9-CM coding and the correct process for locating codes in the ICD-9-CM manual, whereas Chapter 7 is devoted entirely to reimbursement and the role that ICD-9-CM plays in reimbursement methodologies.

Chapters 8 through 25 cover each chapter of the ICD-9-CM code book but do not conform to the order of the ICD-9-CM code book chapters. These chapters are sequenced in this book for the following reasons. The assignment of codes for signs, symptoms, infectious diseases, and V and E codes may be applied to all chapters in the ICD-9-CM code book; therefore these are the first coding chapters in this book. The next set of chapters is shorter and perhaps easier for an inexperienced coder to learn. The next several chapters are more complex, and the coding is more difficult. As the semester progresses, it may be necessary to spend less time on the chapters at the end of the text. Therefore the latter chapters include less complex information and material that could be covered more quickly. Each of these chapters follows a very specific template that will help students learn and instructors teach this complex material, beginning with the corresponding coding guidelines from the *ICD-9-CM Official Guidelines for Coding and Reporting.* This reinforces the importance of the guidelines in accurate code assignment. Following this is a section on anatomy and physiology, with full-color illustrations of the body system discussed in the chapter. This allows for more informed decision making when selecting the correct code, and also provides an important review of anatomy and physiology. Key disease conditions are covered and illustrated with examples. References to the *AHA Coding Clinic ® for ICD-9-CM* appear throughout each of the coding chapters. *Coding Clinic* is the authority on ICD-9-CM coding, and these references confirm the validity of the content and give students practice using additional information and resources.

Within each coding chapter is a separate list of V Codes. V codes are used in all sections of the ICD-9-CM code book, and this list gives students, instructors, and practitioners easy reference to the correct V codes for each section.

Featured in select chapters are common medications and treatment for the related disease conditions. It is important to become familiar with common medications to identify chronic illnesses that may be documented in the health record.

Procedures are another important section of the coding chapters. Common and complex procedures relating to the diagnoses are covered in this section using Volume 3 of the ICD-9-CM code book.

Finally, each coding chapter has a section on documentation and MS-DRG assignment. This feature brings together all of the steps of ICD-9-CM coding for optimum reimbursement, supported by documentation in the health record.

Chapter 26 completes the picture of facility coding by covering ICD-9-CM coding for outpatient facility services. Most healthcare facilities today treat patients on both an inpatient and an outpatient basis. Coders may be required to code both types of services, and it is important for students to understand the differences.

Finally, Chapter 27 covers the future of diagnosis and procedure coding: ICD-10-CM, and ICD-10-PCS.

DISTINCTIVE FEATURES

- Logical chapter organization. No other coding textbook is organized like *ICD-9-CM Coding: Theory and Practice!* The hierarchical arrangement of chapters makes learning and teaching easy.
- Full-color design with illustrations. This helps important content such as anatomy and physiology stand out and come alive and provides visual reinforcement of key concepts.
- References to *AHA Coding Clinic ® for ICD-9-CM.* These references verify accuracy and point students to direct citations in *Coding Clinic*, the definitive publication on ICD-9-CM coding.
- Numerous and varied exercises within each chapter. These exercises break the chapter into manageable segments and help students gauge learning while reinforcing important concepts.

ADDITIONAL RESOURCES

Get the most out of your course with these additional learning and teaching resources.

- Student Workbook. Apply the textbook content and prepare for employment with this study guide! The workbook contains:
  - Application activities that give students hands-on practice applying ICD-9-CM coding to actual health records.
  - Case studies that illustrate common scenarios students will encounter on the job.
- TEACH Instructor Resources. TEACH is the complete curriculum manual, giving instructors everything necessary to enhance an ICD-9-CM course and save time!
  - **Lesson plans** tie together related content in the textbook, workbook, and lecture outlines and reduce preparation time.
  - **Lecture outlines** presented in PowerPoint guide instructors through class presentations.
  - **Complete answer keys** for every review and test bank question enable fast, efficient student assessment.
  - **Bound-in CD** helps prepare exams instantly with chapter-specific test banks presented in ExamView.
- Evolve Learning Resources. This companion website contains links to industry updates, reimbursement updates, and important news. The Evolve course management system gives instructors the flexibility of posting course components online.

Acknowledgments

This book was developed to better meet the needs of coding educators, students, and coding professionals.

There are several people who deserve special thanks for their efforts in making this text possible.

Susan Cole, Executive Editor, for never giving up hope.

Beth LoGiudice, Developmental Editor, for assisting us with the publishing process and the development of the manuscripts.

Claire Kramer, Project Manager, for directing the production process of our book.

A special thanks to **Judy Hayes** for her ongoing support and encouragement. Also, thanks to **Louise Thompson** and **Michelle McClister** for their assistance and support of this textbook.

Thanks to all our colleagues who participated in coding discussions and debates about coding issues.

Thanks to **Carol Buck** for her advice and encouragement during this project.

The authors and publisher would like to acknowledge and thank the contributors to the TEACH Instructor Resources and all the textbook reviewers for their constructive comments.

Contents

ICD-9-CM Coding

THEORY AND PRACTICE

CHAPTER 1

The Rationale for and History of Coding

CHAPTER OUTLINE

LEARNING OBJECTIVES

- Describe the application of coding
- Define nomenclature and classification
- Identify the historical timeline of coding
- Describe different coding organizations and credentials
- Recognize the importance of the Standards of Ethical Coding
- Define compliance as it relates to coding
- Explain confidentiality as it applies to coding

ABBREVIATIONS

AAPC American Academy of Professional Coders

AHA American Hospital Association

AHIMA American Health Information Management Association

CCA Certified Coding Associate

CCS Certified Coding Specialist

CCS-P Certified Coding Specialist—Physician Based

CEUs continuing education units

CMS Centers for Medicare and Medicaid Services

CPC Certified Professional Coder

CPC-H Certified Professional Coder—Hospital Based

CPT *Current Procedural Terminology*

DRGs diagnosis-related groups

HIPAA Health Insurance Portability and Accountability Act

ICD-9-CM *International Classification of Diseases, 9th Revision, Clinical Modification*

MS-DRG Medicare Severity diagnosis-related group

NCHS National Center for Health Statistics

OIG Office of the Inspector General

RHIA Registered Health Information Administrator

RHIT Registered Health Information Technician

SNOMED Systematized Nomenclature of Medicine

WHO World Health Organization

BACKGROUND OF CODING

What Is Coding and What Are Its Applications?

As a student in this field, you will often be asked these questions. Why does one study this subject? What type of work does a "coder" do? Basically, medical coding consists of translating **diagnoses** and **procedures** into numbers for the purpose of statistically capturing data. This process is done for us every day in all aspects of daily life. If you buy a banana at the grocery store, the cash register captures that banana as a number, which, in turn, provides data on the number of bananas sold in that store or by that grocery chain; it also yields data of importance to the store on replenishing their inventory, details regarding what time of year the greatest number of bananas are sold, and so forth.

Translation of a disease and/or a procedure into an ICD-9 code is not as simple as it may seem. This process requires a thorough knowledge of anatomy and physiology, disease processes, medical **terminology**, laboratory values, pharmacology, surgical procedures, and, last but not least, a myriad of coding rules and guidelines. Diseases and procedures are translated into a coding system known as the *International Classification of Diseases, 9th Revision, Clinical Modification* (ICD-9-CM). This **classification** system has been used worldwide and has been clinically modified for the United States.

Coded data are used for many purposes. Prior to the advent of diagnosis-related groups (DRGs), which are used by Medicare and other payers as the basis for hospital **reimbursement** (payment), coding was used for research and planning. A healthcare provider or facility could use these data to find out how many cases of appendicitis were treated in a year. This information could be used by a healthcare facility in decisions about the possible purchase of more equipment, the addition of an operating room, the hiring of additional staff, or by the provider to gain additional skills. Since the implementation of DRGs—now known as MS-DRGs—coded data are also used for reimbursement purposes, and they are increasingly used for risk management and quality improvement, as well as in nursing clinical pathways. Coded data were important from the start, but use of these data for reimbursement has elevated the importance of accurate coding to new heights.

Capture of health data through ICD-9 and ICD-10 codes that are used worldwide has proved useful for the study of patterns of disease, disease epidemics, causes of mortality, and treatment modalities. Without the use of a classification system, comparison of data would be impossible.

Nomenclature and Classification

A nomenclature and a classification of diseases are required for development of a coding system. A **nomenclature** is a system of names that are used as preferred terminology, in this case, for diseases and procedures. Often, diseases in different areas of the country or in different countries are identified by dissimilar terminology, which makes the capture of comparative statistical data next to impossible. For example, another name for "amyotrophic lateral sclerosis" is "Lou Gehrig's disease," which is also known as a "motor neuron disease." Nomenclatures of disease were first developed in the United States around 1928. The Systematized Nomenclature of Medicine (SNOMED), published by the College of American Pathologists, is the most up-to-date system in current use.

Classification systems group together similar items for easy storage and retrieval. Within a classification system, items are arranged into groups according to specific criteria. The history of classification systems goes back as far as Hippocrates. During the 17th century, London Bills of Mortality represented the first attempts of scientists to gather statistical data on disease. The ICD-9-CM classification system is a closed system that comprises diseases, injuries, surgeries, and procedures. In a closed classification system a disease, condition, or procedure can only be classified in one place.

HISTORY OF CODING

ICD-9-CM is the coding classification system that is currently in use in the United States. This classification system dates back to Bertillon's Classification of Causes of Death, which was developed in 1893. This system was adopted by the United States in 1898 under the recommendation of the American Public Health Association. System revisions were scheduled to take place every 10 years, and the classification was maintained by the World Health Organization (WHO). Revisions became known as the International Classification of Causes of Death. Over the years, this system has been changed to allow its use not only in mortality reporting but in morbidity reporting as well. Since its inception, this classification has been revised 10 times. The Clinical Modification (CM) was developed in 1977 by the United States to more accurately capture morbidity data for study within the United States, as well as information on operative and diagnostic procedures that were not included in the original publication of ICD. ICD-9-CM, a publication of the U.S. Department of Health and Human Services, consists of three volumes.

Currently, many countries are using ICD-10, which was published in 1993 by the WHO. ICD-10 will also be clinically modified for use in the United States, although an implementation date has not yet been determined. The adoption of ICD-10-CM is subject to government legislation, with the requirement for a 2-year notice of date of implementation. ICD-10 is an alphanumeric system as opposed to the mostly numeric ICD-9. Because ICD-10 will be very different from the ICD-9 that is currently in place, implementation will most likely take time. Please refer to Chapter 27 in this book for additional details on ICD-10.

ICD-9-CM may be updated biannually in April and October. Updates contain additional codes, revised codes, and codes that are deleted. These updates are published in the *Federal Register* (the official daily publication for rules, proposed rules, and notices of U.S. federal agencies and organizations) as a proposed rule and then as a final rule. They are available at the Centers for Medicare and Medicaid Services (CMS) website (www.cms.hhs.gov). It is of the utmost importance that code books and coding software (**encoder**) be updated to ensure that coding is accurate and to facilitate accurate reimbursement.

Maintenance of ICD-9-CM is the responsibility of the National Center for Health Statistics (NCHS), CMS, the American Hospital Association (AHA), and the American Health Information Management Association (AHIMA), which are also known as the Cooperating Parties. Many publications provide coding advice and information, but only one publication is official. This publication, *AHA Coding Clinic for ICD-9-CM* (referred to as *Coding Clinic*), which is published quarterly by the AHA, provides coding advice and guidelines that have been approved by the Cooperating Parties and must be followed by coders.

Coding Clinic references will be used throughout the text with specific issue information provided, such as 2002:4Q:p126-130. This reference alerts the student of information contained in the fourth quarter 2002 issue and the associated page numbers. *Coding Clinic* has publications dating back to 1985. Unless superseded or clarified by additional *Coding Clinic* references, the original publication of any advice remains in effect. Although reference may be made to advice in an issue from 1994, this may be the most current advice available. A date of 1994 for a given source does not mean that the publication is outdated.

CODING ORGANIZATIONS AND CREDENTIALS

Coders come from a variety of educational backgrounds. Many coders have attended 4-year college programs in Health Information Administration; others have completed 2-year college programs in Health Information Technology. Some community colleges offer programs geared only to medical coding. Whatever their background, most coders take certification examinations to earn **credentials** and become members of a professional organization. Many employers include a requirement for certification as part of their coding job description.

Coders can work in a variety of settings; most often, they are employed by hospitals, physician offices, outpatient surgical centers, long-term care facilities, and insurance

companies. It is predicted that the demand for coding professionals will far exceed the number of coders in the workforce.

The two most well-known professional associations for coders are AHIMA (www.ahima.org) and the American Academy of Professional Coders (AAPC) (www.aapc.com). Both of these organizations offer a variety of coding credentials. AHIMA, which has been in existence for over 75 years, has undergone several name changes along the way to keep up with the ever-changing technological skills, educational requirements, and roles of its members. It boasts a membership of over 50,000. Traditionally, this organization has provided support for facility coders, but in recent years, it has expanded to include coders who provide services in physician's offices and outpatient settings. AHIMA offers the following credentials:

CCA Certified Coding Associate
CCS Certified Coding Specialist
CCS-P Certified Coding Specialist—Physician Based
RHIT Registered Health Information Technician
RHIA Registered Health Information Administrator

AAPC has 44,000 credentialed members and was started in 1981. It was founded to assist coders in providing services to physicians and offers the following credentials:

CPC Certified Professional Coder
CPC-H Certified Professional Coder—Hospital
CPC-P Certified Professional Coder—Payer
CPC-A Certified Professional Coder—Apprentice
CPC-H-A Certified Professional Coder—Hospital Apprentice
CPC-P-A Certified Professional Coder—Payer Apprentice

To obtain credentials from either organization, a coder must sit for a certification examination and complete college coursework in several areas such as medical terminology and anatomy and physiology. To maintain their credentials, coders must earn continuing education units (CEUs). The number of CEUs required is dependent on the credential(s) of the coder (Table 1-1).

Table 1-1. Credentials and Continuing Education Unit Requirements

Credential	Organization Offering Credential	Education Required	CEUs Required per 2-Year Cycle
CCA	AHIMA	High school diploma or equivalent	20
CCS	AHIMA	High school diploma or equivalent	20
CCS-P	AHIMA	High school diploma or equivalent	20
RHIT	AHIMA	2-Year degree in accredited HIM program	20
RHIA	AHIMA	4-Year degree in accredited HIM program	30
CPC	AAPC	High school diploma or equivalent and 2 years coding experience	36
CPC-H	AAPC	High school diploma or equivalent and 2 years coding experience	36
CPC-P	AAPC	High school diploma or equivalent and 2 years coding experience	36
CPC-A	AAPC	High school diploma or equivalent	36
CPC-H-A	AAPC	High school diploma or equivalent	36
CPC-P-A	AAPC	High school diploma or equivalent	36

CODING ETHICS

Along with providing credentials, both AHIMA and AAPC have set standards for Coding **Ethics**, which are reprinted in Figures 1-1 and 1-2. Members of these organizations are expected to abide by these coding standards. A coder who is asked to disregard a guideline to facilitate payment should decline on the basis of these standards, by which coders are bound.

AHIMA's Standards of Ethical Coding

1. Coding professionals are expected to support the importance of accurate, complete, and consistent coding practices for the production of quality healthcare data.
2. Coding professionals in all healthcare settings should adhere to the ICD-9-CM (International Classification of Diseases, 9th revision, Clinical Modification) coding conventions, official coding guidelines approved by the cooperating Parties, the CPT (Current Procedural Terminology) rules established by the American Medical Association, and any other official coding rules and guidelines established for use with mandated standard code sets. Selection and sequencing of diagnoses and procedures must meet the definitions of required data sets for applicable healthcare settings.
3. Coding professionals should use their skills, their knowledge of currently mandated coding and classification systems, and official resources to select the appropriate diagnostic and procedural codes.
4. Coding professionals should only assign and report codes that are clearly and consistently supported by physician documentation in the health record.
5. Coding professionals should consult physicians for clarification and additional documentation prior to code assignment when there is conflicting or ambiguous data in the health record.
6. Coding professionals should not change codes or the narratives of codes on the billing abstract so that meanings are misrepresented. Diagnoses or procedures should not be inappropriately included or excluded because payment or insurance policy coverage requirements will be affected. When individual payer policies conflict with official coding rules and guidelines, these policies should be obtained in writing whenever possible. Reasonable efforts should be made to educate the payer on proper coding practices in order to influence a change in the payer's policy.
7. Coding professionals, as members of the healthcare team, should assist and educate physicians and other clinicians by advocating proper documentation practices, further specificity, and resequencing or inclusion of diagnoses or procedures when needed to more accurately reflect the acuity, severity, and the occurrence of events.
8. Coding professionals should participate in the development of institutional coding policies and should ensure that coding policies complement, not conflict with, official coding rules and guidelines.
9. Coding professionals should maintain and continually enhance their coding skills, as they have a professional responsibility to stay abreast of changes in codes, coding guidelines, and regulations.
10. Coding professionals should strive for optimal payment to which the facility is legally entitled, remembering that it is unethical and illegal to maximize payment by means that contradict regulatory guidelines.

Figure 1-1. AHIMA's Standards of Ethical Coding.

COMPLIANCE

Compliance is defined as "acting according to certain accepted standards or, in simple terms, abiding by the rules." In health care, this requires following the rules and guidelines as set forth by the government through Medicare and Medicaid and all professional organizations to which a facility or provider may belong or is participating with, and following the policies and procedures of that organization.

Compliance officers and programs are found in many industries. It wasn't until after the passage of the Health Insurance Portability and Accountability Act of 1996 (HIPAA) that compliance officers became a standard presence in healthcare facilities. HIPAA gave additional funding to the U.S. Department of Health and Human Services, the Office of the Inspector General (OIG), and the U.S. Department of Justice to increase penalties for healthcare fraud and abuse. Ongoing investigations in healthcare institutions across the United States are exploring violations of the False Claim Act and other laws.

As explained in an article by Joette Hanna that appeared in the *Journal of AHIMA*, entitled "Constructing a Coding Compliance Plan,"[1] several steps must be taken if a coding

AAPC's Code of Ethical Standards

Members of the American Academy of Professional Coders shall be dedicated to providing the highest standard of professional coding and billing services to employers, clients and patients. Behavior of the American Academy of Professional Coders members must be exemplary.

American Academy of Professional Coders members shall maintain the highest standard of personal and professional conduct. Members shall respect the rights of patients, clients, employers and all other colleagues.

Members shall use only legal and ethical means in all professional dealings, and shall refuse to cooperate with or condone by silence, the actions of those who engage in fraudulent, deceptive or illegal acts.

Members shall respect the laws and regulations of the land, and uphold the mission statement of the American Academy of Professional Coders.

Mission Statement

- Establish and maintain professional, ethical and educational standards for professional coders
- Provide a national certification and credentialing process
- Support the national and local membership by providing educational products and opportunities to network
- Increase and promote national recognition and awareness of professional coding

Members shall pursue excellence through continuing education in all areas applicable to their profession.

Members shall strive to maintain and enhance the dignity, status, competence and standards of coding for professional services.

Members shall not exploit professional relationships with patients, employees, clients or employers for personal gain.

Above all else, we will commit to recognizing the intrinsic worth of each member.

This Code of Ethical Standards for members of the American Academy of Professional Coders strives to promote and maintain the highest standard of professional service and conduct among its members. Adherence to these standards assures public confidence in the integrity and service of professional coders who are members of the American Academy of Professional Coders. Failure to adhere to these standards may result in the loss of credentials and membership with the American Academy of Professional Coders.

Figure 1-2. AAPC's Code of Ethical Standards.

department wishes to ensure that it is in compliance. Coding departments must do the following:

- Abide by AHIMA's Standards of Ethical Coding
- Develop coding policies and procedures
- Develop a working relationship with the billing department
- Develop a coding compliance work plan
- Conduct coding audits
- Develop an action plan based on audit results

Likewise, a practice brief published by AHIMA in 2001, entitled "Developing a Coding Compliance Policy Document,"[2] states that the following bulleted items should be included in a coding compliance plan:

- Policy statement regarding the commitment of the organization to correct assignment and reporting of codes
- The Official Coding Guidelines used by the facility
- The people responsible for code assignment
- What needs to be done when clinical information is not clear enough to assign codes
- If there are payer-specific guidelines, where these may be found
- A procedure for correcting codes that have been assigned incorrectly
- Plan for education on areas of risk as identified by audits

- Identification of essential coding resources that are available and to be used by coding professionals
- Procedure for coding new and/or unusual diagnoses or procedures
- A policy for which procedures will be reported
- Procedure for resolving coding/documentation disputes with physicians
- Procedure for processing claim rejections
- Procedure for handling requests for coding amendments
- Policy that requires coders to have available coding manuals and not just encoder
- Process for review of coding on those records coded with incomplete documentation

CONFIDENTIALITY

Employees in a healthcare setting must be aware of the confidentiality of the information that is all around them. When they take the Hippocratic Oath, physicians swear to maintain patient confidentiality. Likewise, in the Patient Bill of Rights as prepared by the AHA, the patient's right to privacy is stated. The Code of Ethics of the AHIMA also addresses confidentiality when it says, "Members will promote and protect the confidentiality and security of health records and information."

Coders must read a patient's personal medical information before they can code the encounter and/or patient admission. It is important that this information not be shared with anyone, including other employees, unless they have a legitimate need to know to perform their job; patient information should never be discussed in a place where any visitor could overhear.

CHAPTER REVIEW EXERCISE

Write the correct answer(s) in the space(s) provided.

1. What does a coder do?

   ____

2. What coding system is currently used in the United States for inpatient coding?

   ____

3. What does the CM of ICD-9-CM stand for?

   ____

4. List three uses for coded data.
   1. ______________________________
   2. ______________________________
   3. ______________________________

5. What payment system does Medicare use for facility reimbursement?

   ____

6. Describe the difference between a nomenclature and a classification system.

   ____

7. What nomenclature of disease is used in the United States?

   ____

8. Define a closed classification system.

   ____

9. When was the International Classification of Diseases first adopted by the United States?

   ____

10. When and how often is this system (ICD-9-CM) updated?

    ____

11. What four groups constitute the Cooperating Parties?
    1. ______________________________
    2. ______________________________
    3. ______________________________
    4. ______________________________

12. Who publishes official coding advice and guidance?

    ____

13. What organizations award coding credentials?

    ____

14. What is another word that is used in the industry for "following the rules"?

    ____

15. If you were coding a neighbor's record, would it be okay for you to tell your other neighbors the reason the patient was hospitalized?

    ____

16. What does HIPAA stand for?

    ____

CHAPTER GLOSSARY

Classification: grouping together of items as for storage and retrieval.

Compliance: adherence to accepted standards.

Credential: degree, certificate, or award that recognizes a course of study taken in a specific field and that acknowledges the competency required.

Diagnosis: identification of a disease through signs, symptoms, and tests.

Encoder: computer software system that facilitates code selection.

Ethics: moral standard.

Federal Register: the official daily publication for rules, proposed rules, and notices of U.S. federal agencies and organizations.

Nomenclature: system of names that are used as the preferred terminology.

Procedure: a diagnostic or therapeutic process performed on a patient.

Reimbursement: the manner in which a hospital is paid for services.

Terminology: words and phrases that apply to a particular field.

CHAPTER 2

The Health Record as the Foundation of Coding

CHAPTER OUTLINE

LEARNING OBJECTIVES

- Explain the purpose of the various forms or reports found in a health record
- Define "principal diagnosis"
- Define "principal procedure"
- Identify reasons for assigning codes for other diagnoses
- List the basic guidelines for reporting diagnoses/procedures
- Identify types of documentation acceptable for assigning codes
- Explain the physician query process

ABBREVIATIONS

AHQA American Health Quality Association

BPH benign prostatic hypertrophy

CBC complete blood count

CC chief complaint

CMS Centers for Medicare and Medicaid Services

CPT *Current Procedural Terminology*

COPD chronic obstructive pulmonary disease

DOB date of birth

ED Emergency Department

EEG electroencephalogram

EGD esophagogastroduodenoscopy

EKG electrocardiogram

ER Emergency Room

GERD gastroesophageal reflux disease

H&P history and physical

HPI history of present illness

ICD-9-CM *International Classification of Diseases, 9th Revision, Clinical Modification*

ICU intensive care unit

MAR medication administration record

MRA magnetic resonance angiography

MRI magnetic resonance imaging

MS-DRGs Medicare Severity diagnosis-related groups

MVP mitral valve prolapse

NPI National Provider Identifier

OP note operative note

ABBREVIATIONS—*cont'd*

SOAP Subjective/Objective/Assessment/Plan

TJC The Joint Commission

TPR temperature, pulse, and respiration

UHDDS Uniform Hospital Discharge Data Set

UPIN Unique Physician Identification Number

UTI urinary tract infection

THE HEALTH RECORD

A health record must be maintained for every individual who is assessed or treated. Although Edna Huffman's classic *Health Information Management*[1] book is no longer in print, her definition of the purpose and use of a health record still holds true today. She states "The main purpose of the medical record is to accurately and adequately document a patient's life and health history, including past and present illnesses and treatments, with emphasis on the events affecting the patient during the current episode of care." Huffman goes on to say, "The medical record must be compiled in a timely manner and contain sufficient data to identify the patient, support the diagnosis or reason for health care encounter, justify the treatment and accurately document the results." According to Abdelhak's *Heath Information: Management of a Strategic Resource,*[2] the health record serves five purposes:

1. Describes the patient's health history
2. Serves as a method for clinicians to communicate regarding the plan of care for the patients
3. Serves as a legal document of care and services provided
4. Serves as a source of data
5. Serves as a resource for healthcare practitioner education

The patient's health record in today's environment may be maintained in several formats or **hybrids**. The traditional health record consists of **documentation** on paper prepared by **healthcare providers** that describes the condition of the patient and the plan and course of treatment. As the world advances through electronic forms of documentation, paper notes become more and more obsolete. Most health records are currently in a state of transition. Some paper documentation and some transcribed or electronically stored documentation may be available. Some facilities have actually achieved a predominantly electronic health record. One of the advantages of storing the record electronically is that many users are able to access the record at the same time. Whether in electronic, paper, or hybrid form, documentation serves as the basis of a health record.

The Centers for Medicare and Medicaid Services (CMS) has provided physicians with *General Principles of Medical Record Documentation.*[3]

- Medical records should be complete and legible.
- The documentation of each patient encounter should include:
  - Reason for encounter and relevant history
  - Physical examination findings and prior diagnostic test results
  - Assessment, clinical impression, and diagnosis
  - Plan for care
- Date and legible identity of the observer
- The rationale for ordering diagnostic and ancillary services (if not documented, should be easily inferred)
- Past and present diagnoses should be accessible for treating and/or consulting physician.
- Appropriate health risk factors should be identified.
- Patient's progress, response to changes in treatment, and revision of diagnosis should be documented.
- *Current Procedural Terminology* (CPT) and *International Classification of Diseases, 9th Revision, Clinical Modification* (ICD-9-CM) codes reported on health insurance claim forms should be supported by documentation in the medical record.

SECTIONS OF THE HEALTH RECORD

Every facility has its own policies and procedures regarding the organization of the health record. Records will differ slightly depending upon the course of the patient's condition and treatment. If a record were to be organized similarly to a novel that tells a story, the elements discussed in the next sections would be included.

Administrative Data

- Demographic
- Personal data
- Consents

Information contained in this section will facilitate identification of the patient. Some of the UHDDS data elements included are personal identification, date of birth, sex, race, residence, admit date, and discharge date. See Figure 2-1.

Clinical Data

Inpatient records may be organized in a reverse chronological order. The discharge summary may be found at the beginning of the record.

- Emergency Room record (when applicable) (see Figure 2-2)
- Admission history and physical (see Figure 2-3)
- Physician orders (see Figure 2-4)
- Progress notes recorded by healthcare providers (see Figure 2-6, *A* and *B*)
- Anesthesia forms (when applicable) (see Figure 2-9)
- Operative report (when applicable) (see Figure 2-10)
- Recovery Room notes (when applicable)
- Consultations (when applicable)
- Laboratory test results (when applicable) (see Figure 2-8)
- Radiology report (when applicable) (see Figure 2-11)
- Miscellaneous ancillary reports (when applicable)
- Discharge summary (see Figure 2-12)

Data are collected from the health record as mandated by governmental and nongovernmental agencies. The Joint Commission (TJC) places data requirements and time frames for documentation within the health record. The federal government and state licensing agencies may have similar requirements. Medical staff bylaws often include these documentation requirements. In 1974, the Uniform Hospital Discharge Data Set (UHDDS) mandated that hospitals must report a common core of data. Since that time, the requirements have been revised and will continue to change as necessary. The UHDDS required data elements are listed in Figure 2-1.

Emergency Room Record

The Emergency Room record is a mini health record. It contains a **chief complaint (CC)**, which is the reason, in the patient's own words, for presentation to the hospital. It contains a history, physical examination, laboratory results, radiology reports (if applicable), plan of care, physician orders, and documentation of any procedures performed. Last but not least, it contains a list of working diagnoses and information on the disposition of the patient. See Figure 2-2 for a sample of an ED (Emergency Department, or also called ER for Emergency Room) record.

Admission History and Physical Examination

Admission history and physical documentation normally contains the following elements:

- Chief complaint (CC)
- History of the present illness (HPI)

Uniform Hospital Discharge Data Set

01. **Personal identification**
02. **Date of birth (month, day, and year)**
03. **Sex**
04. **Race and ethnicity**
05. **Residence (usual residence, full address, and zip code [nine-digit zip code, if available])**
06. **Hospital identification number**
    Three options are given for this institutional number, with the Medicare provider number as the recommended choice. The federal tax identification number of the American Hospital Association number is preferred to creating a new number.
07. **Admission date (month, day, and year)**
08. **Type of admission (scheduled or unscheduled)**
09. **Discharge date (month, day, and year)**
10. **Attending physician identification (NPI)**
11. **Operating physician identification (NPI)**
12. **Principal diagnosis**
    The condition established after study to be chiefly responsible for occasioning the admission of the patient to the hospital for care.
13. **Other diagnoses**
    All conditions that coexist at the time of admission of that develop subsequently that affect the treatment received and/or the length of stay. Diagnoses that relate to an earlier episode and have no bearing on the current hospital stay are excluded.
14. **Qualifier for other diagnoses**
    A qualifier is given for each diagnosis coded under "other diagnoses" to indicate whether the onset of the diagnosis preceded or followed admission to the hospital. The option "uncertain" is permitted.
15. **External cause-of-injury code**
    Hospitals should complete this item whenever there is a diagnosis of an injury, poisoning, or adverse effect.
16. **Birth weight of neonate**
17. **Procedures and dates**
    a. All significant procedures are to be reported. A significant procedure is one that (1) is surgical in nature, (2) carries a procedural risk, (3) carries an anesthetic risk, or (4) requires specialized training.
    b. The date of each significant procedure must be reported.
    c. When multiple procedures are reported, the principal procedure is designated. The principal procedure is one that was performed for definitive treatment rather than one performed for diagnostic or explanatory purposes or was necessary to take care of a complication. If two procedures appear to be principal, then the one most related to the principal diagnosis is selected as the principal procedures.
    d. The UPIN of the person performing the principal procedure must be reported.
18. **Disposition of the patient**
    a. Discharged home (not to home health service)
    b. Discharged to acute care hospital
    c. Discharged to nursing facility
    d. Discharged to home to be under the care of a home health service
    e. Discharged to other health care facility
    f. Left against medical advice
    g. Alive, other; or alive, not stated
    h. Died
19. **Patient's expected source of payment**
    a. Primary source
    b. Other source
20. **Total charges**
    List all charges billed by the hospital for this hospitalization. Professional charges for individual patient care by physicians are excluded.

Figure 2-1. Uniform Hospital Discharge Date Set elements.

- Past medical history
- Family medical history
- Social history
- **Review of systems**
- Physical examination
- Impression/Assessment
- Plan

See Figure 2-3 for an example of a history and physical form (H&P).

Text continued on p. 19

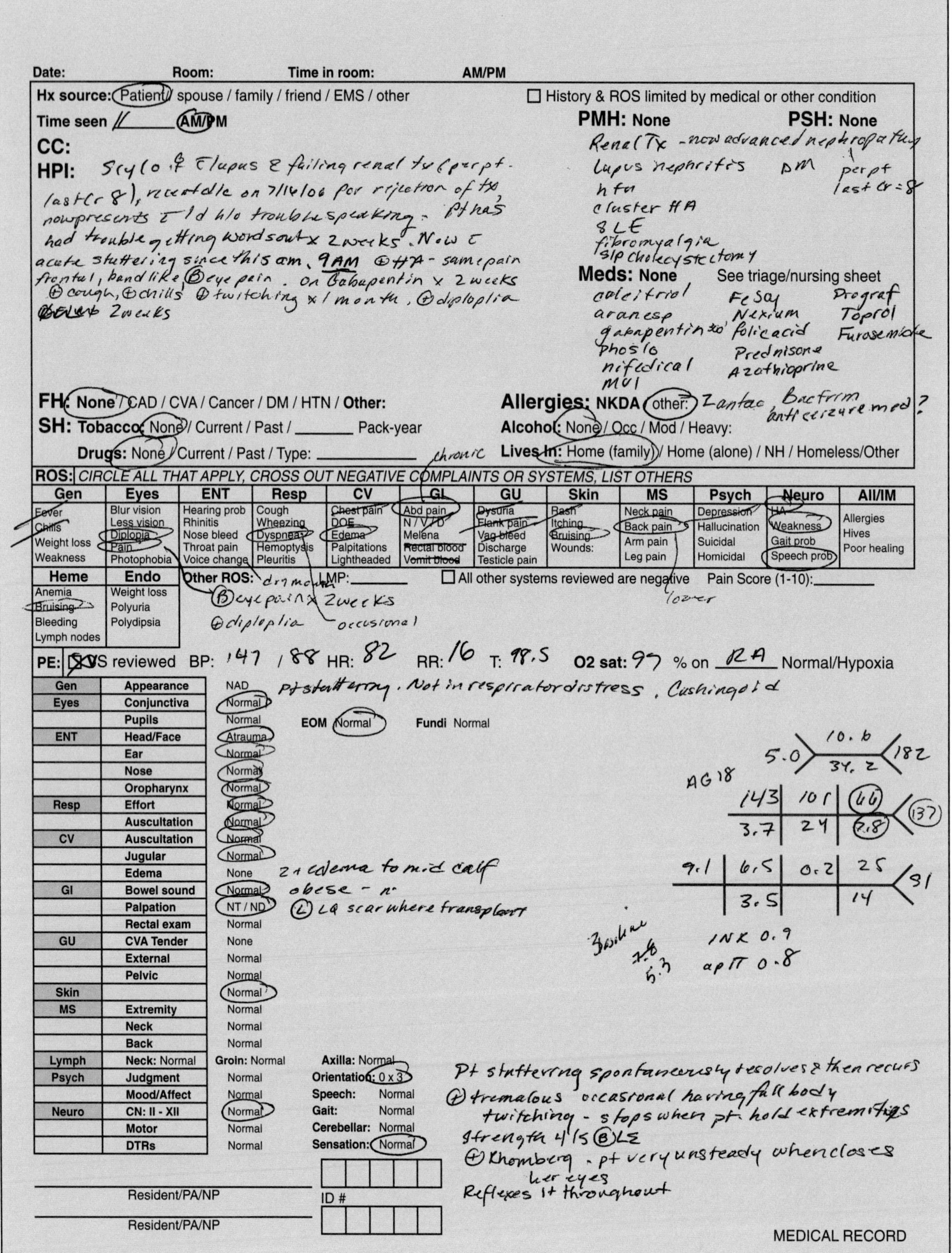

Date: Room: Time in room: AM/PM

Hx source: (Patient) / spouse / family / friend / EMS / other ☐ History & ROS limited by medical or other condition

Time seen ______ (AM)/PM

CC:

HPI: 56 y/o ♀ c lupus & failing renal tx (perpt last Cr 8), recent adm on 7/14/06 for rejection of tx, now presents c c/o h/o trouble speaking. Pt has had trouble getting words out x 2 weeks. Now c acute stuttering since this am, 9 AM ⊕ HA - same pain frontal, band like ⓑ eye pain. On Gabapentin x 2 weeks ⊖ cough, ⊕ chills ⊕ twitching x 1 month, ⊕ diplopia x 2 weeks

PMH: None — Renal Tx - now advanced nephropathy, Lupus nephritis, DM, perpt last Cr = 8, HTN, cluster HA, SLE, fibromyalgia, s/p cholecystectomy

PSH: None

Meds: None See triage/nursing sheet — calcitriol, FeSO4, Prograf, aranesp, Nexium, Toprol, gabapentin, folic acid, Furosemide, Phoslo, Prednisone, nifedical, Azathioprine, MVI

FH: (None) / CAD / CVA / Cancer / DM / HTN / Other:

Allergies: NKDA (other:) Zantac, Bactrim, anti seizure med?

SH: Tobacco: (None) / Current / Past / ______ Pack-year

Alcohol: (None) / Occ / Mod / Heavy:

Drugs: (None) / Current / Past / Type: ______ chronic

Lives In: (Home (family)) / Home (alone) / NH / Homeless/Other

ROS: CIRCLE ALL THAT APPLY, CROSS OUT NEGATIVE COMPLAINTS OR SYSTEMS, LIST OTHERS

Gen	Eyes	ENT	Resp	CV	GI	GU	Skin	MS	Psych	Neuro	All/IM
Fever	Blur vision	Hearing prob	Cough	Chest pain	(Abd pain)	Dysuria	Rash	Neck pain	Depression	HA	Allergies
Chills	Less vision	Rhinitis	Wheezing	DOE	N/V/D	Flank pain	Itching	(Back pain)	Hallucination	(Weakness)	Hives
Weight loss	(Diplopia)	Nose bleed	(Dyspnea)	(Edema)	Melena	Vag bleed	Bruising	Arm pain	Suicidal	Gait prob	Poor healing
Weakness	(Pain)	Throat pain	Hemoptysis	Palpitations	Rectal blood	Discharge	Wounds:	Leg pain	Homicidal	(Speech prob)	
	Photophobia	Voice change	Pleuritis	Lightheaded	Vomit blood	Testicle pain					

Heme	Endo
Anemia	Weight loss
Bruising	Polyuria
Bleeding	Polydipsia
Lymph nodes	

Other ROS: dry mouth, ⓑ eye pain x 2 weeks, ⊕ diplopia - occasional LMP: ______ ☐ All other systems reviewed are negative — lower Pain Score (1-10): ______

PE: ☒ VS reviewed BP: 147/88 HR: 82 RR: 16 T: 98.5 O2 sat: 97 % on RA Normal/Hypoxia

Gen	Appearance	NAD	Pt stuttering. Not in respiratory distress, Cushingoid
Eyes	Conjunctiva	(Normal)	
	Pupils	Normal	EOM (Normal) Fundi Normal
ENT	Head/Face	(Atrauma)	
	Ear	(Normal)	
	Nose	(Normal)	
	Oropharynx	(Normal)	
Resp	Effort	(Normal)	
	Auscultation	(Normal)	
CV	Auscultation	(Normal)	
	Jugular	(Normal)	
	Edema	None	2+ edema to mid calf
GI	Bowel sound	(Normal)	obese - n
	Palpation	(NT/ND)	Ⓛ LQ scar where transplant
	Rectal exam	Normal	
GU	CVA Tender	None	
	External	Normal	
	Pelvic	Normal	
Skin		(Normal)	
MS	Extremity	Normal	
	Neck	Normal	
	Back	Normal	
Lymph	Neck: Normal	Groin: Normal	Axilla: Normal
Psych	Judgment	Normal	Orientation: (0 x 3)
	Mood/Affect	Normal	Speech: Normal
Neuro	CN: II - XII	(Normal)	Gait: Normal
	Motor	Normal	Cerebellar: Normal
	DTRs	Normal	Sensation: (Normal)

Labs: 5.0 > 10.6 / 34.2 < 182; AG 18; 143 | 101 | 66 / 3.7 | 24 | 7.8 < 137; 9.1 | 6.5 | 0.2 | 25 / 3.5 | 14 < 31; INR 0.9; apTT 0.8

Pt stuttering spontaneously resolves & then recurs. ⊕ tremulous occasional having full body twitching - stops when pt hold extremities. Strength 4/5 ⓑ LE. ⊕ Rhomberg. pt very unsteady when closes her eyes. Reflexes 1+ throughout

Resident/PA/NP

ID #

Resident/PA/NP

MEDICAL RECORD

Figure 2-2. Emergency Room record.

Continued

MEDICAL DECISION MAKING

Differential Dx:

1. Stroke
2. uremia
3. infection
4. drug side effect

PLAN

Head CT
labs

1745
Renal (XW) 39842 called. will come to eval.

- [x] Discussed history, plan or diagnosis with other provider.
- [x] Prior medical records reviewed.
- [x] Nursing / EMS notes reviewed.
- [ ] The patient was given: *IM / IV* medications or *IV fluids.*
- [ ] Patient referred for further care.

Radiology Results: ☐ ED interpretation ☐ Discussed with Radiologist

CT - No CT evidence of acute ischemia

EKG/Rhythm: NSR / Arrythmia: ______

ATTENDING PHYSICIAN NOTE: Time seen: 11 00 AM / (PM)

☐ I was present with the resident/midlevel during the patient's history and physical and discussed their management with the resident. I have reviewed the resident's note above and agree with the documented findings and plan of care.

☑ I saw and evaluated the patient. I reviewed the resident/midlevel's note above and agree, in addition to/except that:

Additional findings:

s/p Renal Tx

c̄ word finding difficulty

⊖ tPA

→ CT

Procedure / Progress Note: Time:______ AM / PM **Consult:**______ Called:______ AM / PM

No acute neurological pathology
Pt accepted to medicine for uremia

Provider: ______

Procedures: Central Venous / Intubation / LP / Suture / Chest tube / Nasal Pack / Sedation / Splint / I&D / Other: ______

Diagnosis:

1. Uremia
2. ______
3. ______
4. ______
5. ______
6. ______

☐ **See procedure documentation**

☐ **See additional documentation**

Critical Care Time: ______ minutes

Dispo: Discharge / (Admit) / Transfer / AMA

Condition: Stable / (Good) / Fair / Serious / Expired

Admission/Transfer Location: ______

Discharge time: ______ AM / PM Date:

Attendings: ______

MEDICAL RECORD

Figure 2-2, cont'd Emergency Room record.

ADMISSION NOTE

M.D.: Pager:

Date: Time:

Chief Complaint:
twitching

History of Present Illness:
This Is a 51 year old woman with a history of lupus, lupus nephritis, and cadaveric renal transplant in 2000 who now presents with 2 weeks of worsening twitching. The patient describes starting neurontin for headaches approximately 3 weeks ago. She subsequently noted first subtle twitching of an extremity or her face. The movements have progressed to include difficulty speaking, dysarthria ("I couldn't say what I was thinking") and difficulty walking.

The patient has also noticed worsening fatigue, a change in her skin ("It's ashy") and worsening edema (including LE and peri-orbital).

On Friday the patient called the transplant nurse who recommended she come to the Emergency room. There, she was seen by neuro, who felt most of her symptoms were most likely related to worsening renal failure with gabapentin. They also noted b/l ptosis and findings suggestive of a peripheral neuropathy.

The patient reports no improvement in symptoms since arrival.

ED Course:
As above.

Primary MD:

Emergency Contact:

Code Status:

Review of Systems: (circled) positive; ~~ABC~~ negative

Constitutional:
~~Fevers,~~ ~~Chills,~~ ~~Night Sweats,~~ (Fatigue) Weight Loss, Weight Gain, Heat Intolerance, Cold Intolerance

Neuro:
(Headache) ~~Seizures,~~ ~~Syncope,~~ ~~Lightheaded,~~ ~~Vertigo,~~ ~~Dizziness,~~ ~~Tremor,~~ ~~Weakness,~~ ~~Numbness,~~ ~~Tingling~~

HEENT:
~~Vision change,~~ (Diplopia) Cataracts, Glaucoma, Hearing Loss, Tinnitus, Sinusitis, ~~Sore Throat,~~ Polydipsia, Lymphadenopathy

CV:
~~Chest Pain,~~ ~~Palpitations,~~ ~~Orthopnea,~~ PND Claudication, Exercise Intolerance

Respiratory:
~~SOB,~~ Pleuritic Pain, Wheezing, ~~Cough~~ ~~Sputum,~~ Hemoptysis

GI:
~~Abdominal Pain,~~ ~~Nausea,~~ ~~Vomiting,~~ ~~Diarrhea,~~ ~~Constipation,~~ Jaundice, ~~Melena,~~ BRBPR, Dysphagia, Odynophagia, Reflux, Hematemesis

GU:
~~Dysuria,~~ Frequency, Urgency, Hesitancy, Incontinence, Hematuria, polyuria
LMP ________________

Skin/Skeletal:
(Rashes) (Bruising) Joint Stiffness/Pain, Myalgias

Psych:
~~Depression,~~ Mood Changes, SI, HI, Plan

X All other systems negative

Figure 2-3. History and physical.

Continued

M.D.: Pager:

Date: Time:

Past Medical History:
Lupus diagnosed 1991, h/o lupus arthritis and muscle pain
- No prior lupus involvement in brain
- No recent flairs

Social History:

Tobacco: none

Alcohol: none

Illicits: none

Residence: lives with daughter

Occupation: owned her own hair salon, now not working

Family: son and daughter in area

Other:

Allergies:
Zantac –> decreased muscle tone

Medications:
Imuran 150mg po qd
Prednisone 10mg po qd
Prograf 4mg po bid
nexium 40mg po qd
stresstab + zinc
folate 1mg po qd
Fe 300mg po tid
Toprol XL 100mg po qd
Calcitriol 0.5mg po q.o.d.
PhosLo 2 tab po TID
Aranesp 100 q.o.week
Lasix 40mg po bid
Clonidine 0.1mg po bid

Family History:
Mo - Kidney stones
No lupus, no renal failure

T_c afeb / T_m	HR 72	BP 140/80
RR 20 / Pain 0	SaO_2 98%	FiO_2 None
Wt	I/O	Dexi / Stool

Figure 2-3, cont'd History and physical.

ADMISSION NOTE

M.D.: Pager:

Date: Time:

General:	Pleasant, NAD. Periodic jerking movements of large muscles, small muscles, and facial muscles	**Affect:**	full
HEENT:	B/L ptosis, no scleral icterus. MM sl dry. OP clear.		
Neck:	Neck supple. No LAD.		
Chest:	CTA B/L	**Skin:**	dry
Heart:	RR, soft SM at LUSB	**Vasc:**	
Abd:	Soft, full. BSNA. No ascites		
Ext:	Warm, + edema	**Joints:**	no effusion or erythema
GU/Rectal:	deferred		

Neuro:

Mental Status: attentive, oriented

Cranial Nerves: intact

Sensation:

Motor: grossly intact. sustained clonus b/l

Coordination:

Reflexes

RDW: 15.4% MCV: 87.7 FL

WBC	5030 #/cu mm
Hgb	10.6 G/DL
HCT	34.2%
Plat	182 K/CU MM

11:25 2006/08/18

Na	143 MEQ/L
Cl	101 MEQ/L
BUN	66 MG/DL
K	3.7 MEQ/L
CO_2	24 mEq/L
Cr	7.8 MG/DL
Glu	137⁻ MG/DL

11:25 2006/08/18

Ca	9.1 MG/DL
TP	6.5 G/DL
TB	0.2 MG/DL
AST	25 U/L
Mg	
Alb	3.5 G/DL
DB	
ALT	14 U/L
AlkP	51 U/L

11:25 2006/08/18

L 28.6% M 5.8% N 62.6% E 2.4% B 0.6%

11:25 2006/08/18

PT 9.4 SECONDS INR: 0.9* APTT: 23.9 SECONDS APTTr: 0.8 PAT/NORM

11:25 2006/08/18

EKG:
NSR

Chest XR:
obesity, otherwise clear

Figure 2-3, cont'd History and physical.

Continued

ADMISSION NOTE

M.D.: Pager:

Date: Time:

Radiographic Data:

Impression
51 year old woman with worsening renal failure and muscle twitching.

Plan:
1. Neuro-Muscle twitching is likely due to uremia in the setting of worsened renal function. Suspect contribution of gabapentin, which can cause twitching and is correlated in time. Plan is to start dialysis Monday. Continue prograf (can stop monday per renal).
2. Renal-Continue prograf, nephrovite, phoslo. Renal diet. Renal has seen patient.
3. Rheum-Continue Imuran. No evidence of acute flair, but check ESR & CRP. Continue prednisone.
4. HTN-Continue clonidine, toprol, nifedipine qd.
5. Dispo-See PMD.

DVT Prophylaxis? heparin 5000 units sq bid, stop Sun for dialysis Monday

1. 332.0: Trembling paralysis

2. 586: Renal failure, unspecified

3. 401.9: HTN [Hypertension]

4. 710.0: Lupus nephritis

Date:

Figure 2-3, cont'd History and physical.

Physician Orders

This is the area of the record in which the attending **physician**, as well as physician **consultants**, gives directives to the house staff and to nursing and ancillary services. Physician orders are dated, timed, and signed and become part of the record. Verbal orders by physicians are guided by medical staff regulations. See Figure 2-4 for an example of handwritten physician orders and Figure 2-5 for an electronic physician order.

Progress Notes

Progress notes are a record of the course of a patient's hospital care. They are usually written by the attending physician (see Figure 2-6, *A*). Academic medical centers may have notes written by medical students, interns, and residents, as well as attending physicians and consultants. Some facilities have integrated progress notes, which allow individuals from several disciplines to write in the same area of the record. An integrated progress note may include notes written by dietitians, physical therapists, respiratory therapists, and nurses.

Progress notes written by the attending physician are recorded on a daily basis; the frequency of such note taking is governed by medical staff regulations. These notes describe how the patient is progressing and put forth the plan of care for the patient. In an electronic patient record, these notes may be dictated and transcribed or typed by physicians themselves. Physicians are usually taught to document progress notes according to the SOAP format. SOAP stands for the following:

Subjective—The problem in the patient's own words (**chief complaint**)

Objective—The physician identifies the history, physical examination, and diagnostic test results

Assessment—Where the subjective and objective combine for a conclusion

Plan—Approach the physician is taking to solve the patient's problem

See Figure 2-6, *B* for an example of a progress note written in SOAP format.

Nursing Notes

If nursing notes are not integrated, they are often found in their own section of the record on forms that lend themselves to the type of information nurses are required to document. Nursing notes usually consist of an admission note, graphic charts, medication/treatment records, and temperature, pulse, and respiration (TPR) sheets. See Figure 2-7 for an example of an electronic medication administration record (MAR) and Figure 2-8 for an example of laboratory results.

Anesthesia Forms

The anesthesiologist is required to write preanesthesia and postanesthesia notes. The anesthetic agent, amount given, administration technique used, duration of the procedure, amount of blood loss, fluids given, and any complications or additional procedures performed by the anesthesiologist must be documented. See Figure 2-9 for an example of anesthesia documentation.

Operative Report

An operative report must be included in the health record for patients who undergo surgical procedures. The operative report should include a preoperative diagnosis, a postoperative diagnosis, dates, names of surgeons, descriptions of findings, procedures performed, and the condition of the patient at completion of the procedure. The operative report should be dictated and should be in the record within 24 hours of completion of surgery. See Figure 2-10 for a sample of a dictated operative report.

Consultations

Consultations are requested by the attending physician who wishes to gain an expert opinion on treatment of a particular aspect of the patient's condition that is outside the expertise of the attending. A preoperative consultation may be requested as part of the determination of the surgical risk of the patient. Information acquired during consults may be integrated within progress notes or recorded on a separate consult form.

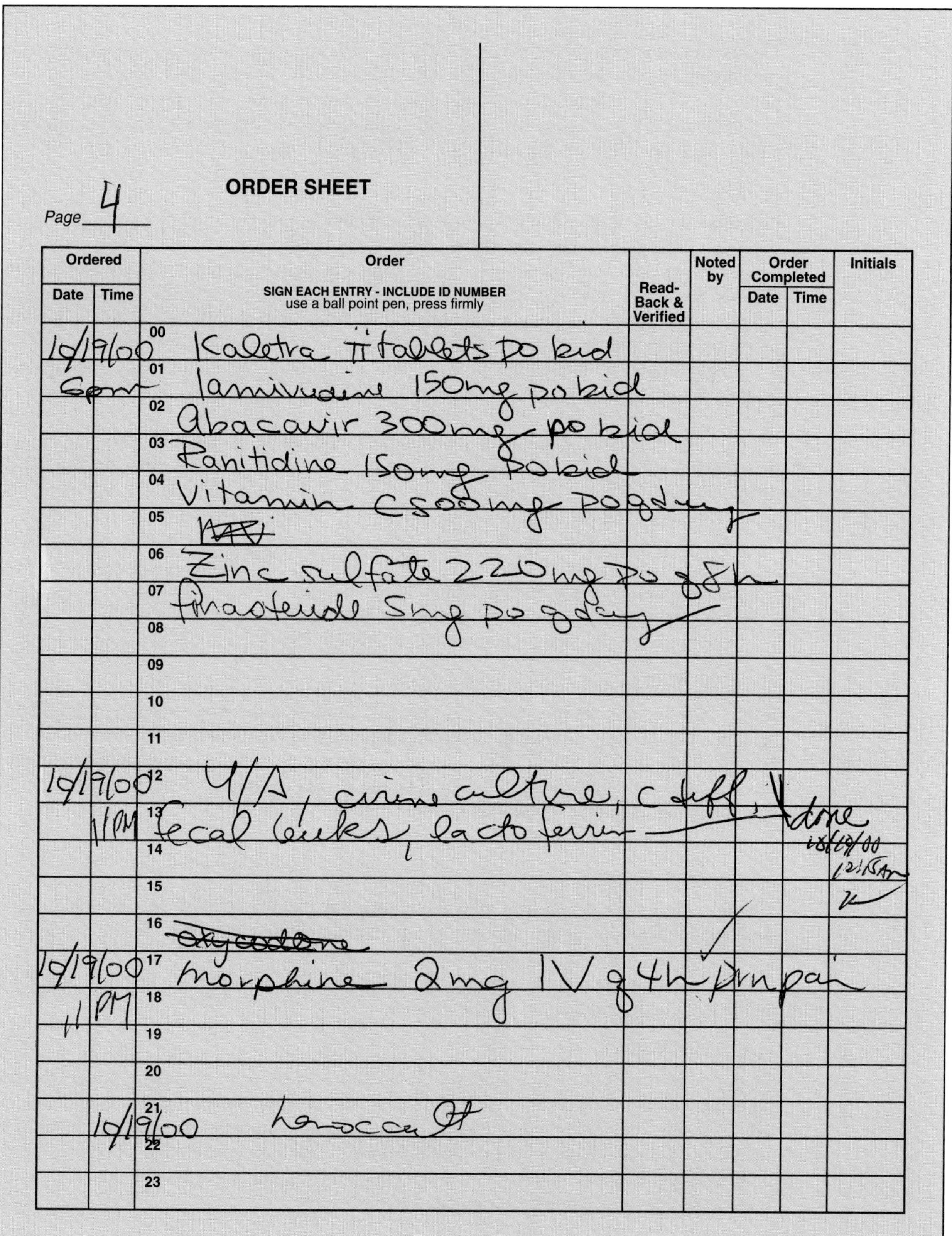

Page 4

ORDER SHEET

Ordered Date	Ordered Time	Order (SIGN EACH ENTRY - INCLUDE ID NUMBER; use a ball point pen, press firmly)	Read-Back & Verified	Noted by	Order Completed Date	Order Completed Time	Initials
10/19/00	6pm	Kaletra II tablets po bid					
		lamivudine 150mg po bid					
		Abacavir 300mg po bid					
		Ranitidine 150mg po bid					
		Vitamin C 500mg po qday					
		Zinc sulfate 220mg po q8h					
		finasteride 5mg po qday					
10/19/00	1PM	U/A, urine culture, c diff, fecal leuks, lactoferrin		done	10/19/00	12:15Am	
10/19/00	1PM	~~oxycodone~~ morphine 2mg IV q4h prn pain		✓			
10/19/00		lorocca					

Figure 2-4. Handwritten physician orders.

Cumulative Order Summary

Orders: ____________

Med Rec No: ____________

Location: ____________ Birth date: ________ Age: ____

Atn: ____________ Sex: ____

ALLERGIES: Swelling-dexamethasone

Ord #	Order name/description	Start date	Ord status	Stop date
001BXMXJH	**Immunofixation-Electro, Serum LAB** Entered DT/TM: ____________ Auth prescriber: ____________ Auth prescriber number: ________	________	1 or more final results received	
001BXMXJJ	**Immunoglobulins, Serum LAB** Entered DT/TM: ____________ Auth prescriber: ____________ Auth prescriber number: ________	________	1 or more final results received	
001BXNBHF	**Transfuse Red Blood Cells** Start date: ________, urgency: when available, transfuse 2 consent obtained units. Transfuse each unit over 2 hours, in dialysis. When the patient is ready and the product is available, call or fax blood bank for delivery. with dialysis ________ Entered DT/TM: ____________ Auth prescriber: ____________ Auth prescriber number: ________	________	Completed	________

Figure 2-5. Electronic physician order.

Laboratory, Radiology, and Pathology Reports

Laboratory data are often captured electronically and may or may not appear in the paper health record. Laboratory data would include such items as complete blood count (CBC), urinalysis, and metabolic levels. Radiology reports are increasingly captured electronically, and the physician may often find the actual image available electronically. Pathology reports, which are also increasingly found in transcribed reports online, consist of a gross description of the tissue removed and microscopic evaluation that includes the diagnosis. See Figures 2-8 and 2-11 for examples of these types of reports.

Discharge Summary

The discharge summary (Figure 2-12) is a summary of the patient's stay in the hospital. It should include the following:

- History of the present illness
- Past medical history
- Significant findings
- Pertinent laboratory data
- Procedures performed or treatment rendered
- Final diagnosis
- Discharge instructions; medications and the condition of the patient on discharge

Text continued on p. 31

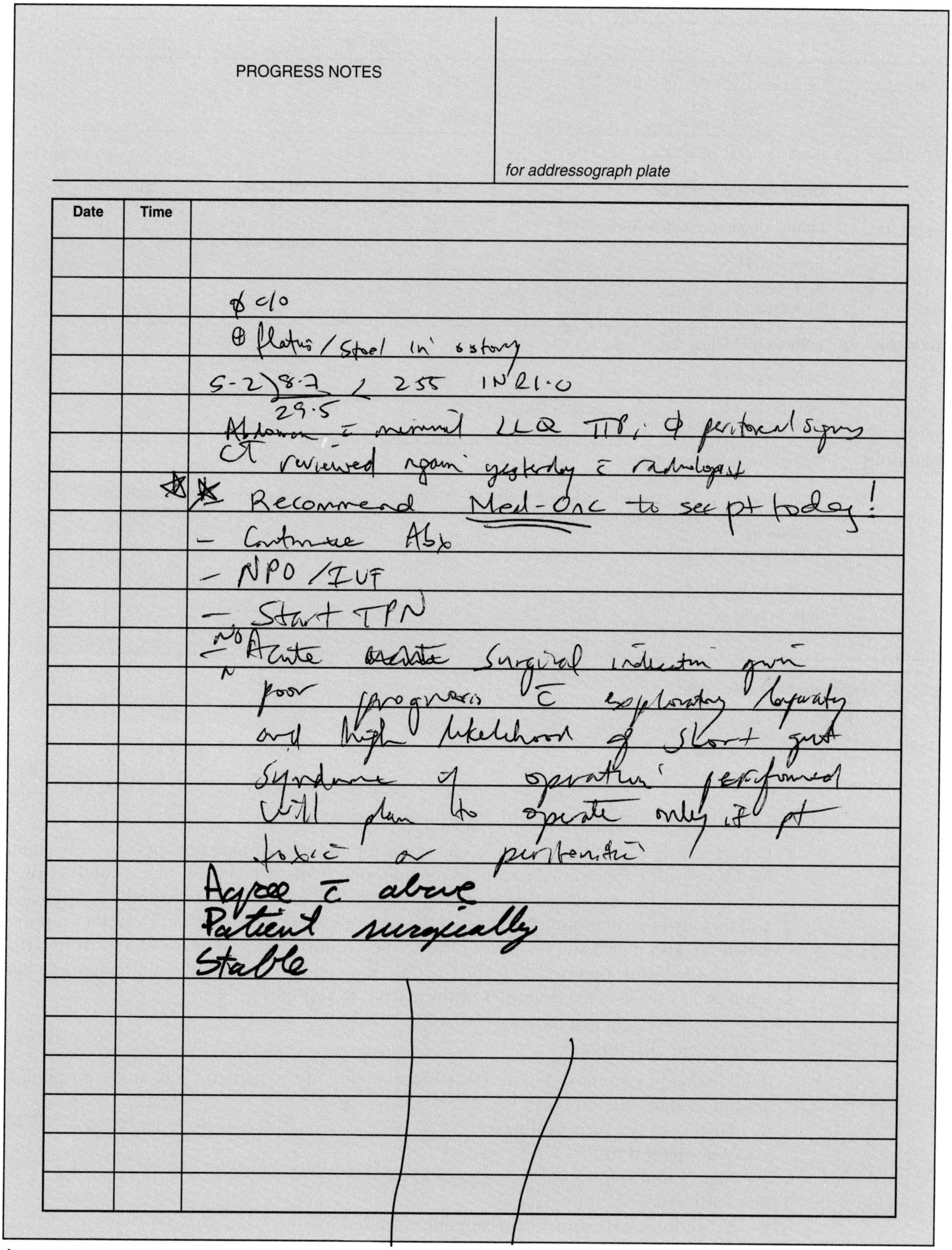

PROGRESS NOTES

for addressograph plate

Date	Time	
		ø c/o
		⊕ flatus / stool in ostomy
		5-2) 8.7 / 29.5 (255 INR 1.0
		Abdomen c̄ minimal LLQ TTP; ø peritoneal signs
		CT reviewed again yesterday c̄ radiologist
		✱ Recommend Med-Onc to see pt today!
		– Continue Abx
		– NPO / IVF
		– Start TPN
		– No acute surgical indication given poor prognosis c̄ exploratory laparoty and high likelihood of short gut syndrome if operation performed. Will plan to operate only if pt toxic or peritonitic
		Agree c̄ above
		Patient surgically
		Stable

A

Figure 2-6. A, progress notes.

Page 1

Patient information

[can use hospital plate]

Inpatient Progress Note

Evaluation type: ☒ Followup care ☐ Discharge note

Meds
Lepirudin
protonix
Odansetron
Dilaudid PCA
Aspart insulin sliding scale

Clinical information

S| Tearful; c/o pain in abd.

O| VS: 37.1 18 95 108/71 97%

⊖icterus

ABD: distended (mod).
well appearing incision
c/d/i c̄ steristrips

EXT: ⊕edema

Assessment & plan:

HD# 10 c̄ Budd Chiari 2° PCV s/p surgical shunt (mesocaval) c̄ bx.

- cont. current management bridging anticoag c̄ Lepirudin given h/o HIT. until ~~ok to start~~ change coumadin c̄ therapeutic INR

Assistant: ______ (Signature) ______ (Print) MD #: ______ Date: ______
(If involved) ☐ Fellow ☐ Resident ☐ NP ☐ PA

Attending: ______ (Signature) ______ (Print) MD #: ______ Date/time ______

(7/03)

B

Figure 2-6, cont'd B, SOAP progress note.

Medication Administration Record

Med Rec No: ____________________
Visit ID No: ____________________

Location: ______________ Age: ______ Sex: ______

Atn DR: __________________ Birthday: __________

ALLERGIES: Swelling-dexamethasone

Scheduled

Medications	Doses	Comments
Routine **Hydroxychloroquine enteral** 200 mg PO bid routine. Administer with food or milk. **Start:** ________ **Stop:** ________	**Ord #: 001BXCBQV** **(Continued...)** Performed __________ 13:00 ________ (RN) Performed __________ 22:00 ________ (RN)	
Routine **Labetalol enteral** 400 mg PO bid, routine **Start:** ________ **Stop:** ________	**Ord #: 001BXTZQD** Not performed– __________ 13:00 ________ (RN) Physician request... Canceled	
Routine **Levothyroxine enteral** 100 mcg PO daily routine **Start:** ________ **Stop:** ________	**Ord #: 001BXBJST** Performed __________ 13:00 ________ (RN)	
Routine **Lisinopril enteral** 40 mg PO daily routine **Start:** ________ **Stop:** ________	**Ord #: 001BXTKKD** Performed __________ 13:00 ________ (RN)	

Figure 2-7. Medication Administration Record.

Laboratory Results

Component	Low range	High range	Range units	16:00:00
Sodium	135	148	mEq/L	140
Potassium, serum	3.5	5.0	mEq/L	4.3
Chloride	99	111	mEq/L	104
Urea-nitrogen	7	22	mg/dL	11
Glucose	60	99	mg/dL	91*
Creatinine, serum	0.5	1.2	mg/dL	0.5
Calcium	8.4	10.5	mg/dL	9.6
Total protein	6.0	8.2	g/dL	7.4
Albumin	3.5	5.3	g/dL	4.6
Total bilirubin	0.1	1.2	mg/dL	0.3
Alanine amino trans	0	31	U/L	5
Aspartate amino tran	0	31	U/L	16
Alkaline phosphatase	100	320	U/L	92
CO_2	21	31	mEq/L	27
Anion gap	11	20	mEq/L	13
Sun/creat ratio				22
Ast/alt ratio				3.2
Est Gfr (Afr Amer)			mL/min/A	Text*
Est Gfr (non-Afr-Am)			mL/min/A	Text*

Figure 2-8. Laboratory results.

Anesthesia Preoperative Assessment

PLEASE WRITE LEGIBLY

PROCEDURE Femoral intramedullar rod

DIAGNOSIS (Rt) Leg shortening

MEDICATIONS

None

for addressograph plate

ALLERGIES (drug/environmental/food) NKDA

PAIN HISTORY ☒ Negative
Intensity (0-10)
Location
Affect quality of life? ☐ Y ☐ N
Pain meds effective? ☐ Y ☐ N
Alleviating / Aggravating factors
Quality: Sharp / dull / other
Onset / duration

Anesthesia Issues ☐ Negative
☐ Difficult Airway
☐ By exam ☐ By history
☐ TMJ problems
☐ Snoring (circled) ☐ OSA mild
☐ Hoarseness
☐ Nasal obstruction
☐ Stridor/croup
☐ Fam Hx Anesth Problems
☐ Malignant Hyperthermia
☐ Obesity
☐ Post-op nausea/vomiting
☐ Organ transplant

Cardiovascular ☒ Negative
☐ Myocard infarct: Date
☐ Hypertension
☐ Arrhythmia: type
☐ Pacemaker ☐ AICD
☐ Angina: ☐ stable ☐ unstable
☐ CHF: Date___ EF___%
☐ Valve disease:
☐ Mod ☐ Severe
☐ Peripheral vascular disease
☐ Past cardiac surgery
☐ Angioplasty
☐ Deep vein thrombus
☐ Pulmonary embolus
☐ Heart murmur
☐ Stress test/cardiac cath
Detail results below

Denies cyanosis or diaphoresis c̄ Activity

Pulmonary ☒ Negative
☐ Smoking hx ☐ current___ppd
☐ Asthma
☐ Hospitalized ☐ Steroid use
☐ Recent wheezing
☐ COPD/BPD
☐ Cough: active / chronic
☐ Other

Renal ☒ Negative
☐ Renal insufficiency
☐ Dialysis
☐ Other

Hepatic ☒ Negative
☐ Hepatitis
☐ Cirrhosis
☐ Other

Endocrine ☒ Negative
☐ Diabetes
☐ Thyroid
☐ Steroid usage
☐ Other

Infections ☐ Negative
☐ SBE prophylaxis
☐ HIV ☐ Sepsis ☐ URI
☐ VRE
☐ MRSA: contact / resp.

Immunized to date

Neurologic ☒ Negative
☐ Seizure
☐ Elevated ICP ☐ Shunt
☐ Spinal cord injury
☐ CVA/TIA
☐ Cerebral palsy
☐ Mental retardation
☐ Chronic pain
☐ Neuropathy/paresthesia
☐ Myopathy/muscular dystrophy
☐ Syncope
☐ Hearing loss
☐ Blind: right / left
☐ Other

Gastrointestinal ☒ Negative
☐ GE reflux / hiatal hernia
☐ Bowel obstruction ☐ Ascites
☐ Ulcers
☐ GI bleed
☐ Dysphagia
☐ Other

Hematol/Onc ☒ Negative
☐ Sickle cell disease ☐ Trait
☐ Coagulopathy
☐ Anemia
☐ Past transfusion
☐ Refuses transfusion
☐ Tumor
☐ Chemo/Rad therapy

Obstetrics ☐ Negative
☐ Preeclampsia/eclampsia
☐ Placenta previa/abruptio
☐ LMP 7/9/06 ☐ HCG
☐ Other

Drug Use ☒ Negative
☐ ETOH ☐ Daily
☐ Never ☐ Occasional
☐ IVDA ☐ Cocaine
☐ Other

Activity Level
☐ Bedridden
☐ Assistance with self-care
☐ <1 flight of stairs
☐ 1–3 flights of stairs
☒ >3 flights of stairs
☒ Able to lie flat one hour

Pediatrics ☐ Negative
☐ Prematurity
☐ Congenital abnl.
☐ Apnea
☐ Passive smoking
☐ Other

FTVD in China

Day of Surgery:
NPO since 10 p.m.

DETAILS OF PRESENT ILLNESS AND PAST MEDICAL HISTORY
16 y.o. ♀ for leg length shortening, ∅ PMH.

PREVIOUS SURGERY AND ANESTHESIA ☒ NONE

140 | 104 | 11 / 4.3 | 27 | 0.5 < 91   4.7 > 12.4 / 37.4 < 232   hcg ⊖

LABS / ECG

BP Range (R) 104/60 (L) 103/54 P 86 R ___ T 36.9 WT 46.4 (lbs/kg) HT 5'0" (in/cm) Room Air Sat 100% Age 16 M/(F)

HISTORY PERFORMED BY: ___ ID Number ___ DATE ___ TIME ___

CHART COPY page 1 of 2

Figure 2-9. Anesthesia record.

Continued

PRE-ANESTHESIA / PRE-OPERATIVE ASSESSMENT
PAGE 2

PLEASE WRITE LEGIBLY

Physical Examination

for addressograph plate

HEENT Normocephaly, NO oral lesions MP=I
Neck: supple c FROM midline trachea
Cardiovascular RRR $S_1 S_2$ NO murmurs or clicks.
Lungs Bil CTA
Pain sites / Pertinent other A OX3 accompanied by Father NAD.
NPO p 12mn Instructions and directions to ccoz were given to pt's Father instructions to avoid NSAIDS preop were given as well to Father

Physical exam performed by: ______ ID Number ______ Date ______ Time ______

ANESTHESIA ATTENDING PRE-ANESTHESIA ASSESSMENT AND CONSENT

Medical record and laboratory data reviewed ☑ Patient examined ☑

Patient is appropriate for the planned anesthesia:
General ☑ Spinal ☐
Regional block ☐ Epidural/caudal ☑
Monitored anesthesia care ☐ Other ☐ ______
Special monitoring ☐ ______

Planned post-operative care: PACU ☑ ICU ☐ Other ☐

ASA STATUS | 1 | 2 | 3 | 4 | 5 | 6 | E | (1 marked)
Airway Assessment:
Oral excursion: FB 1☐ 2☐ 3☐ 4☐
T-M distance: FB 1☐ 2☐ 3☐ 4☐
Dentition: Upper nl☐ dentures☐ caps☐ decayed☐ loose☐
Lower nl☐ dentures☐ caps☐ decayed☐ loose☐
Mallampati: I☐ II☐ III☐ IV☐
Neck Extension: nl☐ 7☐ 77☐
Flexion: nl☐ 7☐ 77☐

Class I /hw

16 y o ♀ for Ⓡ leg shortening
Ⓡ leg length discrepancy
otherwise healthy ⊖ heart/lungs
ASA I for GOTA / epidural for postop analgesia
NO All
NO meds

☐ Informed consent not obtained due to the emergent condition of the patient.

The plan for anesthesia and postoperative pain management, their alternatives, and the risks and benefits of these plans and alternatives have been explained to me and my questions have been answered to my satisfaction. I give my consent.

Signature of Patient / Parent / Guardian, Health Care Agent ______ Telephone consent witness ______ Signature of health care provider securing consent ______

Anesthesiologist Signature ______ **ID Number** ______ **Date** ______ **Time** ______

SURGICAL ATTENDING PRE-OPERATIVE ASSESSMENT–to be completed by surgeon if used as a surgical history and physical

CHIEF COMPLAINT ______

FAMILY HISTORY ______ SOCIAL HISTORY ______

Pre-operative history, physical exam, and pertinent laboratory data reviewed by me with amendments as follows: ☐ NONE

Preoperative diagnosis: ______

Planned procedure: ______

Surgeon Signature ______ **ID Number** ______ **Date** ______ **Time** ______

CHART COPY

page 2 of 2

Figure 2-9, cont'd Anesthesia record.

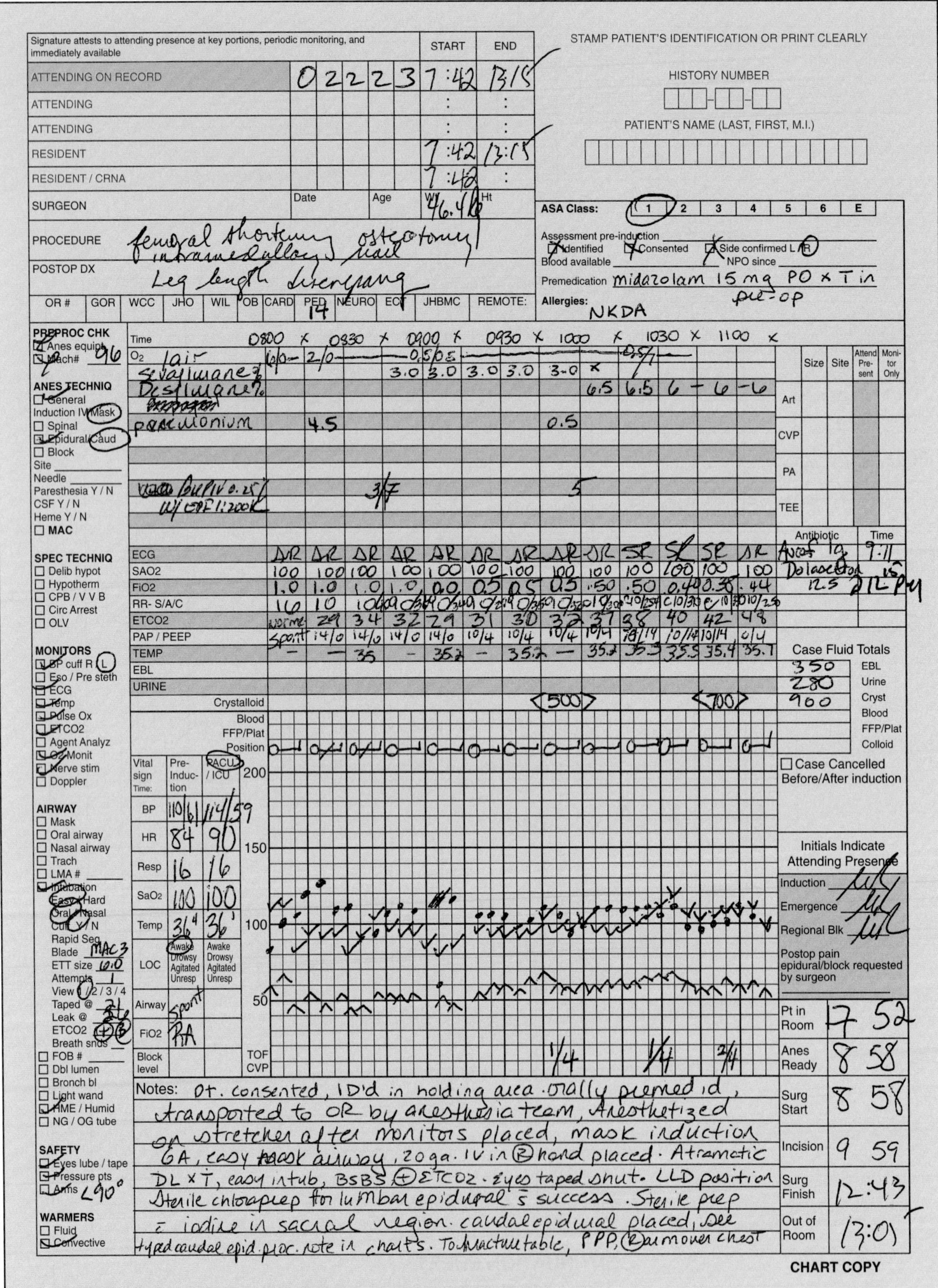

Signature attests to attending presence at key portions, periodic monitoring, and immediately available		START	END
ATTENDING ON RECORD	02223	7:42	13:15
ATTENDING		:	:
ATTENDING		:	:
RESIDENT		7:42	13:15
RESIDENT / CRNA		7:42	:
SURGEON	Date	Age	Wt 46.4 kg Ht
PROCEDURE	femoral shortening osteotomy intramedullary nail		
POSTOP DX	Leg length discrepancy		

OR # | GOR | WCC | JHO | WIL | OB | CARD | PED 14 | NEURO | ECT | JHBMC | REMOTE:

STAMP PATIENT'S IDENTIFICATION OR PRINT CLEARLY

HISTORY NUMBER

PATIENT'S NAME (LAST, FIRST, M.I.)

ASA Class: (1) 2 3 4 5 6 E

Assessment pre-induction
☒ Identified ☒ Consented ☒ Side confirmed L / (R)
Blood available ___ NPO since ___
Premedication midazolam 15 mg PO x 1 in pre-op
Allergies: NKDA

PREPROC CHK: ☒ Anes equip ☒ Mach# 96

ANES TECHNIQ: ☒ General; Induction IV/(Mask); ☐ Spinal; ☒ Epidural/(Caud); ☐ Block; Site; Needle; Paresthesia Y / N; CSF Y / N; Heme Y / N; ☐ MAC

SPEC TECHNIQ: ☐ Delib hypot; ☐ Hypotherm; ☐ CPB / V V B; ☐ Circ Arrest; ☐ OLV

MONITORS: ☒ BP cuff R (L); ☐ Eso / Pre steth; ☒ ECG; ☒ Temp; ☒ Pulse Ox; ☒ ETCO2; ☐ Agent Analyz; ☒ O2 Monit; ☒ Nerve stim; ☐ Doppler

AIRWAY: ☐ Mask; ☐ Oral airway; ☐ Nasal airway; ☐ Trach; ☐ LMA #; ☒ Intubation; (Easy)/Hard; (Oral)/Nasal; Cuff Y/N; Rapid Seq; Blade MAC 3; ETT size 6.0; Attempts 1; View (1)/2/3/4; Taped @ 21; Leak @ ; ETCO2 (+); Breath snds; ☐ FOB #; ☐ Dbl lumen; ☐ Bronch bl; ☐ Light wand; ☒ HME / Humid; ☐ NG / OG tube

SAFETY: ☒ Eyes lube / tape; ☒ Pressure pts; ☒ Arms <90°

WARMERS: ☐ Fluid; ☒ Convective

Time	0800	0830	0900	0930	1000	1030	1100
O2	1 air	10/0 – 2/0	0.5/0.5			0.5/1	
sevoflurane %			3.0 3.0	3.0 3.0	3.0 ×		
Desflurane %					6.5 6.5	6 – 6 – 6	
pancuronium		4.5			0.5		
bupiv 0.25% w/ epi 1:200k			3/7		5		

ECG	AR	AR	AR	AR	AR	AR	AR	AR	AR	SR	SR	SR	AR
SAO2	100	100	100	100	100	100	100	100	100	100	100	100	100
FiO2	1.0	1.0	1.0	1.0	0.0	0.5	0.5	0.5	.50	.50	0.40	0.38	.44
RR- S/A/C	16	10	[illegible]	[illegible]	[illegible]	[illegible]	[illegible]	[illegible]	[illegible]	10/254	c10/30	c10/30	10/25
ETCO2	normal	29	34	32	29	31	30	32	37	38	40	42	48
PAP / PEEP	spont	14/0	14/0	14/0	14/0	10/4	10/4	10/4	10/4	18/14	10/14	10/14	0/4
TEMP	–	–	35	–	35.2	–	35.2	–	35.2	35.3	35.5	35.4	35.7
EBL													
URINE													
Crystalloid						500					700		
Blood													
FFP/Plat													
Position													

	Size	Site	Attend Present	Monitor Only
Art				
CVP				
PA				
TEE				

Antibiotic	Time
Ancef 1g	9:11
Dolasetron 12.5	15

Case Fluid Totals: 350 EBL; 280 Urine; 900 Cryst; Blood; FFP/Plat; Colloid

☐ Case Cancelled Before/After induction

Vital sign	Pre-Induction	(PACU) / ICU
BP	110/61	114/59
HR	84	90
Resp	16	16
SaO2	100	100
Temp	36.4	36.1
LOC	(Awake) Drowsy Agitated Unresp	Awake Drowsy Agitated Unresp
Airway	spont	
FiO2	RA	
Block level		

TOF / CVP: 1/4, 1/4, 2/4

Initials Indicate Attending Presence: Induction; Emergence; Regional Blk; Postop pain epidural/block requested by surgeon

Pt in Room	7 52
Anes Ready	8 58
Surg Start	8 58
Incision	9 59
Surg Finish	12:43
Out of Room	13:01

Notes: Pt. consented, ID'd in holding area. Orally premed'd, transported to OR by anesthesia team, Anesthetized on stretcher after monitors placed, mask induction GA, easy mask airway, 20 ga. IV in (R) hand placed. Atraumatic DL x 1, easy intub, BSBS (+) ETCO2. Eyes taped shut. LLD position Sterile chloraprep for lumbar epidural s̄ success. Sterile prep c̄ iodine in sacral region. caudal epidural placed, see typed caudal epid. proc. note in charts. To fracture table, PPP, (R) arm over chest

CHART COPY

Figure 2-9, cont'd Anesthesia record.

Continued

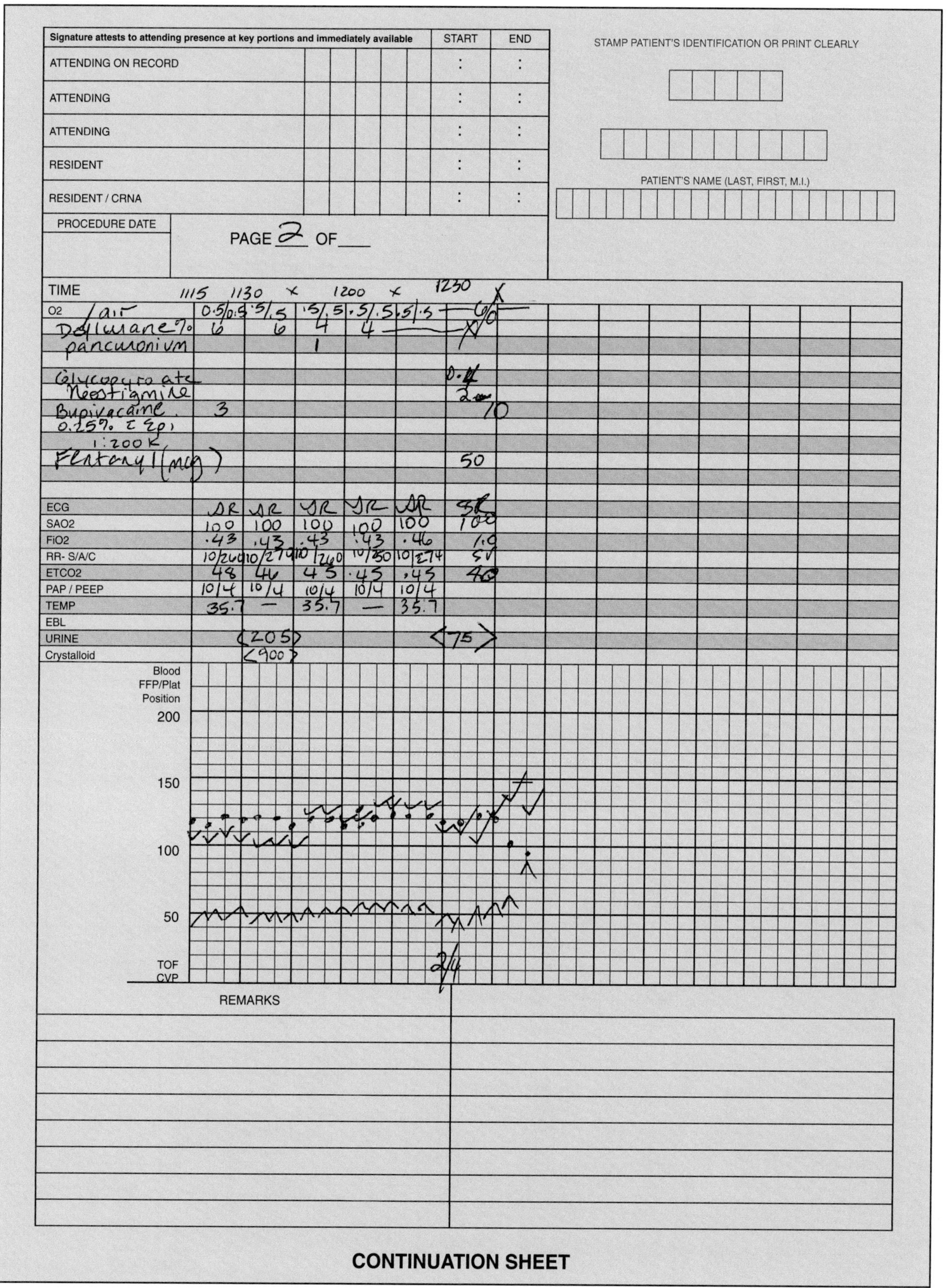

Signature attests to attending presence at key portions and immediately available	START	END
ATTENDING ON RECORD	:	:
ATTENDING	:	:
ATTENDING	:	:
RESIDENT	:	:
RESIDENT / CRNA	:	:

STAMP PATIENT'S IDENTIFICATION OR PRINT CLEARLY

PATIENT'S NAME (LAST, FIRST, M.I.)

PROCEDURE DATE

PAGE 2 OF ___

TIME	1115	1130	×	1200	×	1230
O2 / air	0.5/0.5	.5/.5	.5/.5	.5/.5	.5/.5	0/0
Desflurane %	6	6	4	4		
pancuronium			1			
Glycopyrolate						0.4
Neostigmine						2
Bupivacaine 0.25% c Epi 1:200K	3					10
Fentanyl (mcg)						50
ECG	SR	SR	SR	SR	SR	SR
SAO2	100	100	100	100	100	100
FiO2	.43	.43	.43	.43	.46	1.0
RR- S/A/C	10/260	10/270	10/260	10/250	10/274	SV
ETCO2	48	46	45	45	45	40
PAP / PEEP	10/4	10/4	10/4	10/4	10/4	
TEMP	35.7	—	35.7	—	35.7	
EBL						
URINE		<205>				<75>
Crystalloid		<900>				

Blood
FFP/Plat
Position
200
150
100
50
TOF
CVP

2/4

REMARKS

CONTINUATION SHEET

Figure 2-9, cont'd Anesthesia record.

Patient name ______________________ History # ______________

TIME	pH	pCO2	pO2	HCO3	Na	K	Ca	Glu	HGB				

AS A Physical Status Classification

1: A normal, healthy patient
2: A patient with mild systemic disease
3. A patient with severe systemic disease
4: A patient with severe systemic disease that is a threat to life
5. A moribund patient, not expected to survive without the operation
6: A declared dead patient for organ donation
E: An emergency operation

SYMBOLS		POSITION	TABLE FLAT	OTHER POS.
NIBP	X	Supine	o—┘	Sitting
PULSE	•—•	Prone	o—┐	Lithotomy
ART BP	╪	Lateral L down	o⁄	Jackknife
MAP	✕	Lateral R down	o✕	

CRITERIA FOR DISCHARGE DIRECTLY TO NURSING UNIT	CRITERIA MET	RETURN TO BASELINE
Level of consciousness–awake, alert appropriately conversant or baseline		
Return to usual pattern of mobility or as appropriate per procedure		
BP within normal range. There is no evidence of severe hyper- or hypotension		
Pulse rate (60–100 adults / 80–150 pediatrics) and rhythm regular or baseline		
Respiratory rate: 12–20 (>3 years); 20–40 (<3 years) and pattern normal		
Oxygen saturation >93% or comparable to baseline		
Ability to swallow secretions or baseline		
Dressings, tubes and drains intact with amount of drainage appropriate for procedure		

DISCHARGE TO: Signature Dr. # Date Time

Intraop and Post Anesthesia Notes:

Stable during procedure
Extubated/ventilated in OR
after reversal of paralysis —
Given c 2/4 twitches on TOF
⊕ sust. tetanus, following commands, strong
hand grip.
Alert/awake to PACU O2 FM. Spont vent
MTB pain ⊕ leg. Epidural had just been
redosed + is now connected to infusion.
Report given. No complication

☒ Responsibility for patient management and monitoring after transport and report transferred to: PACU / ICU / Other ________

________ ________ Date ______ Time ______
Signature Provider No.

☐ Transfer of care accepted in ICU:

________ ________ Date ______ Time ______
Signature Provider No.

Figure 2-9, cont'd Anesthesia record.

Operative Report

PATIENT NAME: Sonia Sample
ROOM NUMBER: 222 West
MR NUMBER: 12-34-56

DATE OF PROCEDURE: 04/22/00
PREOPERATIVE DIAGNOSIS: Acute cholecystitis
POSTOPERATIVE DIAGNOSIS: Acute cholecystitis
NAME OF PROCEDURE: 1. Laparoscopic cholecystectomy
2. Intraoperative cystic duct cholangiogram
SURGEON: Claude St. John, M.D.
ASSISTANT: Mark Weiss, D.O.
ANESTHESIOLOGIST: Angela Adams, M.D.
ANESTHESIA: General
DESCRIPTION OF THE OPERATION:

The patient was placed in the supine position under general anesthesia. The oral gastric tube was placed. The Foley catheter was placed. The patient received appropriate antibiotics. The abdomen was prepped with iodine and draped in the usual fashion. Using a midline subumbilical incision, we entered the subcutaneous fat to find the aponeurosis of the rectus abdominis. Two stay sutures were placed 0.5 cm from the midline bilaterally and we left on these sutures, creating an opening in the linea alba.

Under direct vision, the catheter was placed. The Hasson cannula was placed in the abdominal cavity and all was normal except an acute necrotizing and probably gangrenous gallbladder. There were multiple omental adhesions. Three other trocars were placed in the right subcostal plane in the midline, midclavicular line, and midaxillary line using a #10, #5, and #5 mm trocar, respectively. The gallbladder was punctured and emptied of clear white bile indicating a hydrops of the gallbladder. It was grasped at its fundus and at Hartmann's pouch retracted cephalad and to the right, respectively. We found the cystic duct and the cystic artery after circumferential dissection and isolated the cystic duct completely.

When we were sure that this structure was a deep cystic duct, the clip was placed at this most distal aspect to make an opening immediately proximally and we placed a Reddick cholangiocatheter into it via #14 gauge percutaneous catheter. The cholangiogram showed normal arborization of the liver radicals. Normal bifurcation of the common hepatic duct. Normal common hepatic duct. Long large cystic duct. The common bile duct had numerous stones within it. They could not be emptied from the common bile duct. There was good flow into the duodenum.

The impression was choledocholithiasis. This was corroborated by the radiologist. The decision was made to prepare the patient most probably for endoscopic retrograde cholangiopancreatography postoperatively, and no further intervention of the common bile duct was done in this setting.

The cholangiocatheter was removed. An attempt was made to milk the bile out but no stones came out. Three clips were placed on the proximal aspect of the cystic duct and the duct was then cut distally. The artery was isolated and double clipped proximally and single clipped distally and cut in the intervening section. We then peeled the gallbladder off the gallbladder bed with some difficulty because of the intense edema and inflammation. It was then removed from the liver bed completely. Cautery, suctioning and irrigation were used copiously to create a bloodless field. A last check was made and there was no bleeding and no bile leaking. A #15 Jackson-Pratt type drain was placed into Morrison's pouch and brought out through the lateral most port. We then removed, with great difficulty, the gallbladder from the umbilicus. Because of its enormous size and a 3 cm stone within it that was very difficult to macerate, the opening of the umbilicus had to be enlarged.

As this was done, we removed the gallbladder completely and sent it for pathologic section. Two separate figure-of-eight 0 PDS were used to close the abdominal fascia. The Jackson-Pratt drain was then sutured in place with 2.0 nylon. The skin was closed throughout with subcuticular 3-0 PDS after copious irrigation of the subcutaneous plane. Mastisol and Steri-Strips were placed on the wound. The patient remained stable although she did have bigeminy during surgery and was on a Lidocaine drip. She will be going to the intensive care unit but as she left, she was extubated in the recovery room and was fully alert. She is moving all limbs.

I will discuss with the gastroenterologist postoperative endoscopic retrograde cholangiopancreatography.

SPECIMEN: Gallbladder.

Claude St. John, M.D.
CSJ/ld:
D: 04/22/00
T: 04/25/00 9:21 am
CC: Maria Acosta, M.D.

Figure 2-10. Operative report.

EXERCISE 2-1

1. Does every patient encounter have a health record?
   A. Yes
   B. No
2. Is the discharge summary always found in the same place in a health record?
   A. Yes
   B. No
3. List five purposes of a health record.
   1. ______________________________
   2. ______________________________
   3. ______________________________
   4. ______________________________
   5. ______________________________
4. Name one advantage of an electronic patient record.

   ____
5. Name the nonfederal organization that requires reporting of data collected from the health record.

   ____
6. List five elements required by the UHDDS.
   1. ______________________________
   2. ______________________________
   3. ______________________________
   4. ______________________________
   5. ______________________________
7. Where in the record would you find the chief complaint?

   ____
8. If a physician was treating a patient with an antibiotic, where in the record would you look to see that treatment had been discontinued?

   ____
9. Where in the record would you expect to see how the patient was progressing on a daily basis?

   ____
10. Where in the record might you look to find how much blood was lost during surgery?

    ____

UHDDS REPORTING STANDARDS FOR DIAGNOSES AND PROCEDURES

It is the responsibility of a coder to extract from the health record the diagnoses for which a patient is being treated and the procedures that have been performed. To complete this task, a coder must rely on definitions of principal diagnosis, secondary diagnoses, principal procedure, and secondary procedures.

Principal Diagnosis

The **principal diagnosis** is defined as the condition established after study to be chiefly responsible for occasioning the admission of the patient to the hospital for care. This defi-

Radiology Report

EXAM DATE:
HISTORY NUMBER:
AGE: **SEX:** **RACE:**
REQUESTER:

EXAM: MHM 1006-MRI, brain w/wo cont w/diff
RESULT:
SYMPTOMS: Acute change in mental status.
MEDICAL/SURGICAL HISTORY: Pancreatic cancer, bacteremia.
SUSPECTED DIAGNOSIS: Mets.

TECHNIQUE: Sagittal T1, axial T2, axial FLAIR, and post-contrast axial and coronal T1 through brain. Magnevist (0.1 mmol/kg) injected intravenously without complication. Diffusion images obtained.

FINDINGS:
Minimal cerebral atrophy with expected ventricular dilatation appropriate for age.

Minimal scattered foci of increased T2 signal are noted in the periventricular and subcortical white matter and brainstem, cerebellar peduncles which are nonspecific but likely reflective of small vessel ischemia. Old lacunar infarcts noted in the posterior limb of the right internal capsule/right thalamus.

No evidence of mass, hemorrhage, midline shift, or abnormal enhancement. Ventricles and sulci are normal in size, shape, and position. No abnormal intra or extra axial fluid collection. Normal flow voids in carotid and basilar arteries. Normal scalp, calvarium, orbits. Trace ethmoid and maxillary sinus disease. Minimal left mastoiditis.

IMPRESSION:
Minimal cerebral atrophy with expected ventricular dilatation appropriate for age.

Chronic ischemic disease.
Old lacunar infarcts.

Minimal left mastoiditis.

Figure 2-11. Radiology report.

nition is one, if not the most important, concept that a coder must understand and apply. The principal diagnosis, along with the principal procedure, determines the assignment of the Medicare Severity diagnosis-related groups (MS-DRGs), which, in turn, affects reimbursement. Physicians are often not aware of this definition or how it is applied; therefore, the coder must take care to select the correct principal diagnosis after record review.

EXAMPLE

A patient presents to the emergency room with a cough and fever. After the chest x-ray is reviewed, it is determined that the patient has pneumonia.
The principal diagnosis is pneumonia.

EXAMPLE

A patient presents to the emergency room with acute abdominal pain. After the patient is evaluated, he is taken to the OR for an appendectomy. The pathology report reveals an acute appendicitis, which is confirmed by the physician in the discharge summary.
The principal diagnosis is acute appendicitis.

Discharge Summary

PATIENT NAME: Sonia Sample
MR NUMBER: 12-34-56

ADMISSION DATE: 04/19/00
DISCHARGE DATE: 04/27/00
ADMITTING IMPRESSION: Acute abdominal pain, rule out diverticulitis.
HISTORY OF PRESENT ILLNESS:

The patient is a 57-year-old white female who has history of hypertension, valvular heart disease, and cardiomyopathy, who was seen in the emergency room with complaints of acute abdominal pain. On evaluation, she was found to be very tender in the abdomen. She had white blood cell count of 19,000 and was admitted with a diagnosis of rule out diverticulitis.

HOSPITAL COURSE:

CT scan of the abdomen was consistent with cholecystitis and ultrasound of the gallbladder was consistent with cholelithiasis. She was cleared for surgery by cardiologist Dr. Chen and was treated preoperatively with intravenous antibiotics, intravenous fluids, and pain medication. On 4/22/00, the patient underwent laparoscopic cholecystectomy. On 4/26/00, she underwent an endoscopic retrograde cholangiopancreatography. The postoperative course was remarkable for some shortness of breath, otherwise the patient was doing well. She remained very stable, afebrile, and was discharged home.

DISCHARGE DIAGNOSES

1. Cholelithiasis with acute cholecystitis; status post laparoscopic cholecystectomy
2. Mitral valve disorder
3. Hypertensive heart disease with history of angiopathic cardiomyopathy

MEDICATIONS

1. Cozaar
2. Hytrin
3. Lasix
4. Potassium
5. Lanoxin

DIET: The patient is to be on a low-fat diet.
ACTIVITIES: The patient is to be ambulating at home p.r.n.
FOLLOW-UP: Follow-up in two weeks with Dr. St. John and Dr. Glasser.
Medications, diet, activities, and follow-up have all been discussed with the patient and she showed a good understanding

____
Maria Acosta, M.D.
MA/jw: 11931
D: 05/05/00
T: 05/13/00 1:36 pm

Figure 2-12. Discharge summary.

Sometimes, the principal diagnosis is not as easily identifiable as it is in the above two cases. There may be a secondary diagnosis that utilizes more resources during a patient stay but is not the principal diagnosis.

EXAMPLE

A patient is admitted for coronary artery bypass surgery with a diagnosis of coronary artery disease. The surgery is successful, and on the fourth postoperative day, pneumonia develops. The pneumonia is severe, and the patient goes into respiratory failure and must be intubated and treated in the intensive care unit (ICU). The patient remains in the ICU for 10 days because he cannot be weaned from the ventilator. The patient undergoes a tracheostomy procedure and is discharged to a rehab facility.

The principal diagnosis is coronary artery disease, even though most of the treatment was focused on postoperative pneumonia.

Principal Procedure

A **principal procedure** is defined as one that is performed for definitive treatment rather than for diagnostic or exploratory purposes, or a procedure that is necessary to take care of a complication. The principal procedure is sequenced first. If two procedures meet the definition of principal procedure, then the one that is most closely related to the principal diagnosis is the one designated as the principal procedure.

Other Diagnoses

UHDDS requires reporting of other diagnoses that have significance for the specific hospital encounter. Reportable diagnoses are "conditions that coexist at the time of admission, or develop subsequently or affect the treatment received and/or the length of stay. Diagnoses which relate to an earlier episode which have no bearing on the current hospital stay are to be excluded."

This is further clarified in *Coding Clinic* (2000: 2Q:p20-21)[4] where "other diagnoses" are defined as additional conditions that affect patient care because they require one or more of the following:

- Clinical evaluation, or
- Therapeutic treatment, or
- Diagnostic procedures, or
- Extended length of hospital stay, or
- Increased nursing care/or monitoring

Second only to an understanding and application of the definition of "principal diagnosis" is the definition of when to code "other diagnoses." Once again, the importance of these secondary diagnoses comes into play in the MS-DRG reimbursement system. Other diagnoses may be identified as complications and/or **comorbidities** under the MS-DRG system, which may affect payment.

Clinical Evaluation

If the condition of a patient is being clinically evaluated, the coder would expect to see some testing and clinical observations, or perhaps a consultation.

EXAMPLE

During the course of a hospital stay, a patient develops low sodium levels. The physician makes note of this condition and documents that continued laboratory values will be watched. This would constitute clinical evaluation.

Therapeutic Treatment

Medications, physical therapy, and surgery are forms of therapeutic treatment.

EXAMPLE

The physician documents in the patient's past medical history that the patient has a history of a seizure disorder. The medication list contains the drug Dilantin. The fact that the patient is currently being treated for a seizure disorder with this medication constitutes a reportable secondary diagnosis. Physicians often list conditions in the patient's past medical history for which he or she is currently being treated. The coder should be familiar with medications and the conditions they treat.

Diagnostic Procedures

Often in the course of an inpatient hospital stay, physicians are trying to determine the cause of a sign, symptom, or patient complaint; in these cases, tests are often done to deter-

mine the underlying cause. A few examples of types of diagnostic procedures are provided here:

- EKG or ECG (electrocardiogram)
- EEG (electroencephalogram)
- EGD (esophagogastroduodenoscopy)
- Colonoscopy
- Echocardiogram
- MRI (magnetic resonance imaging)
- MRA (magnetic resonance angiography)
- X-rays

EXAMPLE

A patient presents to the emergency room with pain in the leg after a fall down the stairs. An x-ray is performed that reveals a fracture of the tibia.

Extended Length of Hospital Stay

In some cases, a patient is ready to be discharged from the hospital, but develops a condition that requires more intensive investigation, monitoring, or watchful waiting; this may require an additional night's stay.

Increased Nursing Care and/or Other Monitoring

An example of a situation in which increased nursing care or monitoring might be needed is an electrolyte imbalance that is not significant enough to require treatment, although a physician may order additional laboratory draws for monitoring of this condition. In other cases, a patient may have a decubitus ulcer that requires no physician treatment but does require more intensive nursing care. It is important to remember that if the physician does not document the diagnosis for which care is being rendered, the coder must query the physician before adding the code.

Previous Conditions

Often, in a discharge summary or a history and physical, a physician will list diagnoses and/or procedures from previous admissions that are not applicable to the current hospital stay. These conditions are generally not reported. V codes may be used if this historical condition has an impact on current care or influences treatment.

EXAMPLE

A patient is admitted with acute bronchitis. The patient was admitted two years ago for an appendectomy and has a history of shingles. In the discharge summary, the physician documents acute bronchitis, status post appendectomy, and a history of shingles. In this case, the only diagnosis to be coded is acute bronchitis. V codes may be assigned for any history of or status post conditions.

Reporting of Coexisting Chronic Conditions

Clarification of this guideline is reported in *Coding Clinic* (2000:2Q:p20-21)[4]. Often, patients may have multiple chronic conditions when they are admitted to a hospital. *Coding Clinic* says, "Chronic conditions such as, but not limited to, hypertension, congestive heart failure, asthma, emphysema, COPD, Parkinson's disease, and diabetes mellitus are reportable." These chronic conditions may not be specifically treated with medications or procedures; however, they are reported because they may be evaluated and/or monitored.

EXAMPLE

A patient is admitted with benign prostatic hypertrophy (BPH) for a transurethral prostatectomy. The anesthesiologist in the preoperative note documents that the patient has mitral valve prolapse and requires antibiotics prior to undergoing dental procedures. The fact that the patient has mitral valve prolapse and requires antibiotics is a signifi cant factor for the anesthesiologist. This condition is under clinical evaluation by the anesthesiologist and is being treated simultaneously. Therefore, both BPH and mitral valve prolapse (MVP) are reported.

EXAMPLE

A patient is admitted with acute appendicitis. The anesthesiologist and the preoperative consultation indicate that the patient has a history of chronic obstructive pulmonary disease (COPD). The acute appendicitis and the COPD are coded. Refer to *Coding Clinic* (1992:2Q:p16-17)[5]; COPD is a chronic condition that affects patients for the rest of their lives. This, in turn, affects the monitoring and evaluation of this patient.

EXAMPLE

A patient is admitted with a diagnosis of pneumonia. The patient has a history of deep vein thrombosis (DVT) and is on maintenance Coumadin to prevent a recurrence. (For further information, refer to *Coding Clinic* [2002:1Q:p15-16].[6] Pneumonia, a history of deep vein thrombosis, and long-term use of an anticoagulant are the reportable diagnoses. In this case, the fact that the patient no longer has DVT is the reason it is coded as a history of that condition.

Integral versus Nonintegral Conditions

Conditions that are an **integral** part of the disease process are not coded.

EXAMPLE

A patient is admitted to the hospital with a cough. After performing a diagnostic evaluation, the physician determines that the patient has pneumonia. Coughing is a symptom of pneumonia and is not coded.

EXAMPLE

A patient is admitted to the hospital with hypotension, fever, and an elevated white blood count. A blood culture comes back positive, and the physician determines that the patient has sepsis. In this case, only the sepsis and the SIRS are coded; hypotension, fever, and an elevated white blood count are all symptoms of sepsis and are therefore not coded.

Likewise, conditions that are NOT an integral part of the disease process may be coded. Per *Coding Clinic* (1990:2Q:p15)[7]: "Additional conditions that may **not** be associated routinely with a disease process should be coded when present."

EXAMPLE

A patient is admitted to the hospital with a metastatic brain cancer for surgical removal. The patient's history reveals that he has had lung cancer that was surgically removed and now is presenting with seizures, metastatic brain cancer, and headache. Brain cancer is the principal diagnosis, and seizures and history of lung cancer are coded as a secondary diagnoses; headache is not reported because it is a symptom of metastatic brain cancer.

Abnormal Findings (Codes 790-796)

Per *Coding Clinic* (2002:2Q:p17-18),[8] "Abnormal findings (laboratory, x-ray, pathologic, and other diagnostic results) are not coded and reported unless the physician indicates their clinical significance. If the findings are outside the normal range and the physician has

ordered other tests to evaluate the condition or prescribed treatment, it is appropriate to ask the physician whether the abnormal finding should be added."

EXERCISE 2-2

1. What is the most important definition a coder should know?

   ____

2. What determines an MS-DRG?

   ____

3. What is the principal diagnosis in the following scenario?

   A patient is admitted to the hospital with extreme indigestion. A workup ensues, and the patient is found to have GERD (gastroesophageal reflux disease). Three days later, on the day of discharge, the patient is unable to speak. After undergoing MRI, the patient is found to have had a stroke.

   ____

4. A patient is admitted to the hospital with an asthma attack. On his last admission 3 years ago, the diagnosis was community-acquired pneumonia. Is the pneumonia coded, and why or why not?

   ____

5. List five reasons why a secondary diagnosis might be reported.

   1. ____________________
   2. ____________________
   3. ____________________
   4. ____________________
   5. ____________________

6. The physician documents seizure disorder in the patient's past medical history. The patient is receiving Tegretol, according to the list of medications. Should the seizure disorder be coded, and why?

   ____

7. A patient has low urine output after undergoing surgery. The attending writes an order for the nursing staff to record urine output. Should the low urine output be coded, and why?

   ____

8. If a patient is not on any drugs for Parkinson's, should this diagnosis be coded?

   ____

9. If a patient has nausea and vomiting that the attending determines to be gastroenteritis, what diagnosis should be coded?

   ____

CODING FROM DOCUMENTATION FOUND IN THE HEALTH RECORD

The usual advice given to a new coder is to begin to code a record by reading the discharge summary. This, in theory, is the summation of what took place during this patient's hospital admission. The discharge summary is similar to a synopsis of a book. By reading this document, the coder should be able to determine the principal diagnosis. However, the caveat is that the documenting physician may not be aware of the definition of a principal diagnosis and may list a diagnosis that does not meet the requirements of this definition.

Following a review of the discharge summary, the coder should move to the ER record (if applicable), which is the beginning of the patient's story. This will reveal the patient's

chief complaint. The chief complaint is expressed in the words of the patient and gives the reason why he or she is presenting to the ER. The ER record generally provides to the coder the **admission diagnosis**. The admitting diagnosis may be a symptom, and after examination, a working diagnosis may become apparent. By the time the patient leaves the ER to go to the floor, the emergency room physician will have a working diagnosis or will be aware of a symptom that needs additional workup. If this diagnosis is not clear from the ER record, the admission orders should be reviewed for a diagnosis that is listed as the reason for admission.

If no ER record is available, or after the coder has read the ER record, he or she should move on to the admission history and physical (H&P). Generally, the progress notes are reviewed, followed by the OR reports, laboratory results, radiology reports, consults, and orders. Some documents such as the discharge summary, operative report, or pathology report may not be available at the time of coding. Hospitals may have a policy on whether an inpatient record should be coded without these reports or put on hold until the reports are completed. The following examples show documentation inconsistencies.

EXAMPLE

The ER form has a listing of common medical conditions. The ER physician will circle any pertinent diagnoses. The physician has circled ESRD (end-stage renal disease) on the ER form. Throughout the body of the health record, no documentation of ESRD is found, nor does any documentation state that the patient is on dialysis or that the patient is awaiting a transplant. The only documentation in the chart is for chronic renal insufficiency (CRI).

- Differences in coding: with 585.6 or with 585.9

EXAMPLE

Throughout a patient's inpatient chart, it is documented that the patient has a history of pneumonia. This is also documented in the past medical history.

No chest x-ray was performed. Physical exam showed that the lungs were clear. On the discharge summary, pneumonia is documented instead of history of pneumonia.

- Differences in coding: 486 versus V12.61

EXAMPLE

Throughout a patient's chart, documentation of ESLD (end-stage liver disease) is found, along with the fact that the patient is awaiting a liver transplant. The patient has a history of cirrhosis and hepatitis C.

One progress note reads:

Cirrhosis/hep C/ESKD (end-stage kidney disease)

No documentation in the chart describes any abnormal kidney function. It appears that the physician may have meant to write ESLD instead of ESKD.

It is acceptable to code from any documentation provided by a physician. **Physicians** (individuals qualified by education and legally authorized to practice medicine) may be referred to as attendings, consulting physicians, interns, and residents. Physicians may include surgeons, anesthesiologists, oncologists, internists, hospitalists, intensivists, family practitioners, and interventionalists. Medical students have not completed their education and are not included in the category of physician. Some medical staff bylaws may accept documentation by other healthcare providers such as nurse practitioners or physician assistants.

Some confusion has arisen as to what exactly may be coded from radiology and pathology reports. *Coding Clinic* (2002:2Q:p18)[9] attempted to clarify this advice. The coder cannot take information from these reports without obtaining confirmation from the attending. *Coding Clinic* stated that "if the attending physician documents breast mass and the pathologist documents carcinoma of the breast, this would be conflicting documentation and the attending must clarify." Additional details (e.g., area of fracture, location of mass) related

to confirmed diagnoses may be taken from the x-ray report. The example from *Coding Clinic* (2004:1Q:p20-21)[10] says that if the physician has already documented a femur fracture, the coder may pick up additional details on the site of the fracture from this report.

THE USE OF PHYSICIAN QUERIES IN THE CODING PROCESS

Per AHIMA's Practice Brief, *Developing a Physician Query Process,*[11] "the goal of the query process should be to improve physician documentation and coding professionals' understanding of the unique clinical situation, not to improve reimbursement."

Each facility should prepare its own policies and procedures regarding the query process. Some of the best practices for query forms have been recommended by the American Health Quality Association (AHQA).

- Coding queries should be an approved part of the official medical record.
- Query forms should only seek clarification of information that is already present in the record.
- Questions should not be phrased in a way that leads the physician to provide the coder with a particular answer.
- Many facilities have developed standardized query forms for repeated documentation issues. Query forms should contain the following data elements:
    - Date of query
    - Patient name
    - Medical record number
    - Admission date
    - Specific question needing clarification
    - Identification of the coder asking the question
    - Response area
    - Place for physician to sign and date response
    - Instruction for documentation of any correction or addendum in the body of the record

Reasons to Query

- Unclear or questionable diagnoses

EXAMPLE

The use of the term "urosepsis" is often problematic. "Urosepsis" is a term that is frequently used by physicians. It could mean "generalized sepsis," or it could just mean "bacteria in the urine."

EXAMPLE

Conflicting documentation in the record. One physician may document that the patient has type 1 diabetes mellitus, whereas elsewhere in the record, the condition may be documented as type 2 diabetes mellitus.

- Evidence of treatment but no diagnosis.

EXAMPLE

The MAR shows administration of Synthroid, but no documentation is provided by the physician of a diagnosis of hypothyroid. A coder may note that a medication is given, but no diagnosis is documented to correspond with this treatment.

- To determine whether a documented condition is a postoperative complication

EXAMPLE

A patient is admitted 1 week status post radical prostatectomy with a UTI (urinary tract infection). The physician would need to be queried as to whether this is a postoperative infection.

- To determine whether an organism is the cause of a diagnosis

EXAMPLE The physician documents that a patient has a UTI, and the laboratory report shows the causative organism to be *Escherichia coli.*

- To determine a more specific diagnosis

EXAMPLE A physician documents that a patient has an electrolyte disorder but does not specify what type of disorder. The labs show low sodium.

One of the most important aspects of an effective query form is the way the form is worded. Physicians have so little time as it is that a query must get to the point as quickly as possible. It is also important that coders ask only those questions that have significant impact. Asking too many questions may lead to ignoring of questions. AHIMA, in its practice brief,[11] suggests that the query should be presented in the following manner:

- Be clearly and concisely written
- Contain precise language
- Present the facts from the medical record and identify why clarification is needed
- Present the scenario and state a question that asks the physician to make a clinical interpretation of a given diagnosis or condition based on treatment, evaluation, monitoring, and services provided
- Be phrased such that the physician is allowed to specify the correct diagnosis

The AHIMA Practice Brief[11] goes on to say that query forms should NOT

- "Lead" the physician
- Sound presumptive, directing, prodding, probing, or as though the physician is being led to make an assumption
- Ask questions that can be responded to in a "yes" or "no" fashion
- Indicate the financial impact of the response to the query
- Be designed so that all that is required is a physician signature

EXAMPLE In the discharge summary, the attending physician lists hypernatremia as a discharge diagnosis. Lab results indicate hyponatremia. Because of the conflicting information, the coder queries the physician.

> Dr. Smith:
> The discharge diagnosis lists hypernatremia. Lab results list Na values of 128 and 125. Please verify correct diagnosis.
> Thank you.
> Coder

CHAPTER REVIEW EXERCISE

Write the correct answer(s) in the space(s) provided or choose the correct answer option.

1. When coding a record, where is the best place to begin?

____

2. If the discharge summary includes a list of diagnoses, should the coder choose the first in the list as the principal diagnosis?
   A. Yes
   B. No

3. What does TJC stand for?

____

4. What does UHDDS stand for?

____

5. Which report in the record must be on the record within 24 hours?

____

6. What does the term "integral" mean?

____

7. Where in the record would a coder find the admitting diagnosis?

____

8. Name one reason why a coder would query a physician.

____

9. The best place in the record to find the patient's history is in the__________.

____

10. The beginning of the patient's story is usually the discharge summary.
    A. True
    B. False

11. It is permissible for a coder to use documentation provided by an interventionalist.
    A. True
    B. False

12. Once a physician answers a coding question, it should be thrown in the trash.
    A. True
    B. False

13. Physician queries should have only enough room for a physician to sign and date.
    A. True
    B. False

14. When a coding question is asked, it is very important that the financial impact of the response is included.
    A. True
    B. False

15. It is important that the date and the identity of the physician be included for every note.
    A. True
    B. False

16. Is it important for the record to include documentation that supports a code used in billing?
    A. Yes
    B. No

17. Documentation from a consultant cannot be used to assign codes.
    A. True
    B. False

18. A principal diagnosis is one of the elements that determine an MS-DRG.
    A. True
    B. False

19. An example of a diagnostic procedure is an MRI.
    A. True
    B. False

20. Surgery is a form of therapeutic treatment.
    A. True
    B. False

CHAPTER GLOSSARY

Admission Diagnosis: diagnosis that brings the patient to the hospital. This will often be a symptom.

Chief Complaint: reason for presenting to the hospital as stated in the patient's own words.

Comorbidities: preexisting diagnoses or conditions that are present on admission.

Consultant: healthcare provider who is asked to see the patient to provide expert opinion outside the expertise of the requestor.

Disposition: place to which a patient goes when leaving the hospital (e.g., home, nursing home, assisted living).

Documentation: written or typed information supplied by healthcare providers to record and communicate patient data and activity.

Healthcare Provider: person who provides care to a patient.

Hybrid: a combination of formats producing similar results (i.e., paper and electronic records).

Integral: essential part of a disease process.

Physician: licensed medical doctor.

Principal Diagnosis: the condition after study to be chiefly responsible for occasioning the admission of the patient to the hospital for care.

Principal Procedure: procedure performed for definitive treatment rather than for diagnostic or exploratory purposes, or one that was necessary to take care of a complication.

Progress Notes: daily recordings by healthcare providers of patient progress.

Review of Systems: question-and-answer period that occurs between a patient and a healthcare provider during which any healthcare issues are reviewed.

CHAPTER 3

ICD-9-CM Format and Conventions

CHAPTER OUTLINE

LEARNING OBJECTIVES

- Identify the format of the ICD-9-CM code book
- Explain and apply the conventions and guidelines
- Identify the appendices

ABBREVIATIONS

AHFS American Hospital Formulary Service

CPT *Current Procedural Terminology*

DSM-IV *Diagnostic and Statistical Manual of Mental Disorders, Fourth Edition*

ICD-9-CM *International Classification of Diseases, 9th Revision, Clinical Modification*

ICD-O *International Classification of Diseases for Oncology*

MS-DRG Medicare Severity diagnosis-related groups

NEC not elsewhere classifiable

NOS not otherwise specified

WHO World Health Organization

ICD-9-CM Official Guidelines for Coding and Reporting

Please refer to the companion Evolve website for the most current guidelines.

A. Conventions for the ICD-9-CM

The conventions for the ICD-9-CM are the general rules for use of the classification independent of the guidelines. These conventions are incorporated within the index and tabular of the ICD-9-CM as instructional notes. These conventions are as follows:

1. Format

The ICD-9-CM uses an indented format for ease in reference

2. Abbreviations

a. Index abbreviations

NEC "Not elsewhere classifiable"

This abbreviation in the index represents "other specified"; when a specific code is not available for a condition, the index directs the coder to the "other specified" code in the tabular.

b. Tabular abbreviations

NEC "Not elsewhere classifiable"

This abbreviation in the tabular represents "other specified". When a specific code is not available for a condition, the tabular includes an NEC entry under a code to identify the code as the "other specified" code.

(See Section I.A.5.a. "Other" codes).

NOS "Not otherwise specified"

This abbreviation is the equivalent of unspecified.

(See Section I.A.5.b., "Unspecified" codes)

3. Punctuation

[ ] Brackets are used in the tabular list to enclose synonyms, alternative wording or explanatory phrases. Brackets are used in the index to identify manifestation codes. *(See Section I.A.6. "Etiology/manifestations")*

( ) Parentheses are used in both the index and the tabular to enclose supplementary words that may be present or absent in the statement of a disease or procedure without affecting the code number to which it is assigned. The terms within the parentheses are referred to as nonessential modifiers.

: Colons are used in the Tabular list after an incomplete term which needs one or more of the modifiers following the colon to make it assignable to a given category.

4. Includes and Excludes Notes and Inclusion terms

Includes: This note appears immediately under a three-digit code title to further define, or give an example of, the content of the category.

Excludes: An excludes note under a code indicates that the terms excluded from the code are to be coded elsewhere. In some cases the codes for the excluded terms should not be used in conjunction with the code from which it is excluded. An example of this is a congenital condition excluded from an acquired form of the same condition. The congenital and acquired codes should not be used together. In other cases, the excluded terms may be used together with an excluded code. An example of this is when fractures of different bones are coded to different codes. Both codes may be used together if both types of fractures are present.

Inclusion terms: List of terms is included under certain four and five digit codes. These terms are the conditions for which that code number is to be used. The terms may be synonyms of the code title, or, in the case of "other specified" codes, the terms are a list of the various conditions assigned to that code. The inclusion terms are not necessarily exhaustive. Additional terms found only in the index may also be assigned a code.

5. Other and Unspecified codes

a. "Other" codes

Codes titled "other" or "other specified" (usually a code with a 4th digit 8 or a fifth-digit 9 for diagnosis codes) are for use when the information in the medical record provides detail for which a specific code does not exist. Index entries with NEC in the line designate "other" codes in the tabular. These index entries represent specific disease entities for which no specific code exists so the term is included within an "other" code.

b. "Unspecified" codes

Codes (usually a code with a 4th digit 9 or a 5th digit 0 for diagnosis codes) titled "unspecified" are used when the information in the medical record is insufficient to assign a more specific code.

6. Etiology/manifestation convention ("code first," "use additional code," and "in diseases classified elsewhere" notes)

Certain conditions have both an underlying etiology and multiple body system manifestations due to the underlying etiology. For such conditions, the ICD-9-CM has a coding convention that requires the underlying condition be sequenced first followed by the manifestation. Wherever such a combination exists, there is a "use additional code"

note at the etiology code, and a "code first" note at the manifestation code. These instructional notes indicate the proper sequencing order of the codes, etiology followed by manifestation.

In most cases the manifestation codes will have in the code title, "in diseases classified elsewhere." Codes with this title are a component of the etiology/manifestation convention. The code title indicates that it is a manifestation code. "In diseases classified elsewhere" codes are never permitted to be used as first listed or principal diagnosis codes. They must be used in conjunction with an underlying condition code and they must be listed following the underlying condition.

There are manifestation codes that do not have "in diseases classified elsewhere" in the title. For such codes, a "use additional code" note will still be present and the rules for sequencing apply.

In addition to the notes in the tabular, these conditions also have a specific index entry structure. In the index both conditions are listed together with the etiology code first followed by the manifestation codes in brackets. The code in brackets is always to be sequenced second.

The most commonly used etiology/manifestation combinations are the codes for Diabetes mellitus, category 250. For each code under category 250 there is a use additional code note for the manifestation that is specific for that particular diabetic manifestation. Should a patient have more than one manifestation of diabetes, more than one code from category 250 may be used with as many manifestation codes as are needed to fully describe the patient's complete diabetic condition. The category 250 diabetes codes should be sequenced first, followed by the manifestation codes.

"Code first" and "Use additional code" notes are also used as sequencing rules in the classification for certain codes that are not part of an etiology/manifestation combination.

See - Section I.B.9. "Multiple coding for single condition".

7. **"And"**
The word "and" should be interpreted to mean either "and" or "or" when it appears in a title.
8. **"With"**
The word "with" in the alphabetic index is sequenced immediately following the main term, not in alphabetical order.
9. **"See" and "See Also"**
The "see" instruction following a main term in the index indicates that another term should be referenced. It is necessary to go to the main term referenced with the "see" note to locate the correct code.
A "see also" instruction following a main term in the index instructs that there is another main term that may also be referenced that may provide additional index entries that may be useful. It is not necessary to follow the "see also" note when the original main term provides the necessary code.

FORMAT OF ICD-9-CM CODE BOOK

The ICD-9-CM code book contains three volumes:

Volume 1 Tabular List of Diseases and Injuries
Volume 2 Alphabetic Index of Diseases and Injuries
Volume 3 Tabular List and Alphabetic Index of Procedures

Volume 2 (Alphabetic Index) is usually found at the front of the code book and is followed by Volume 1 (Tabular List) and then Volume 3 (Index and Tabular for Procedures).

Several publishers have a variety of ICD-9-CM code books available. Code books are available for use in physician offices that include only Volumes 1 and 2 because ICD-9-CM procedure codes (Volume 3) are not used by physicians. (Physicians use CPT codes to bill for services and procedures.) Expert versions may contain reimbursement edits, color-coded information, Medicare code edits, age and sex edits. Some books are updated with replacement pages quarterly and may include references to *Coding Clinic* articles. At the

Table 3-1. Table of Contents for Tabular List

Diseases: Tabular List, Volume 1

1. Infectious and Parasitic Diseases (001-139)
2. Neoplasms (140-239)
3. Endocrine, Nutritional and Metabolic Diseases, and Immunity Disorders (240-279)
4. Diseases of the Blood and Blood-Forming Organs (280-289)
5. Mental Disorders (290-319)
6. Diseases of the Nervous System and Sense Organs (320-389)
7. Diseases of the Circulatory System (390-459)
8. Diseases of the Respiratory System (460-519)
9. Diseases of the Digestive System (520-579)
10. Diseases of the Genitourinary System (580-629)
11. Complications of Pregnancy, Childbirth, and the Puerperium (630-677)
12. Diseases of the Skin and Subcutaneous Tissue (680-709)
13. Diseases of the Musculoskeletal System and Connective Tissue (710-739)
14. Congenital Anomalies (740-759)
15. Certain Conditions Originating in the Perinatal Period (760-779)
16. Symptoms, Signs, and Ill-Defined Conditions (780-799)
17. Injury and Poisoning (800-999)

V Codes—Supplementary Classification of Factors Influencing Health Status and Contact With Health Services (V01-V89)

E Codes—Supplementary Classification of External Causes of Injury and Poisoning (E800-E999)

beginning of a code book, information is usually provided that explains the conventions used in that version.

Format of Tabular List of Diseases and Injuries

Volume 1, Tabular List of Disease and Injuries (Table 3-1), consists of 17 chapters. Most of these chapters are classified by body system or **etiology** (cause of disease).

Within each chapter, the codes are divided as follows:

- Sections
- Categories
- Subcategories
- Subclassifications

Section

A **section** consists of a group of three-digit categories that represent diseases or conditions that are similar (Figure 3-1).

Categories

Categories are represented by single three-digit codes that describe a disease or a similarly related group of conditions (see Figure 3-1). A category may be an assignable code; however, if it is subcategorized, then the three-digit code is not assignable.

Subcategories

Subcategories consist of fourth-digit codes that provide additional information or specificity. The specificity may provide insight to the etiology of the disease, as well as to the location of the disease or to the manifestation. A **manifestation** is a symptom or condition that is the result of a disease. A fourth digit of .8 usually is used for other specified conditions for that category (see Figure 3-1). A fourth digit of .9 is usually used for unspecified conditions of that category (see Figure 3-1).

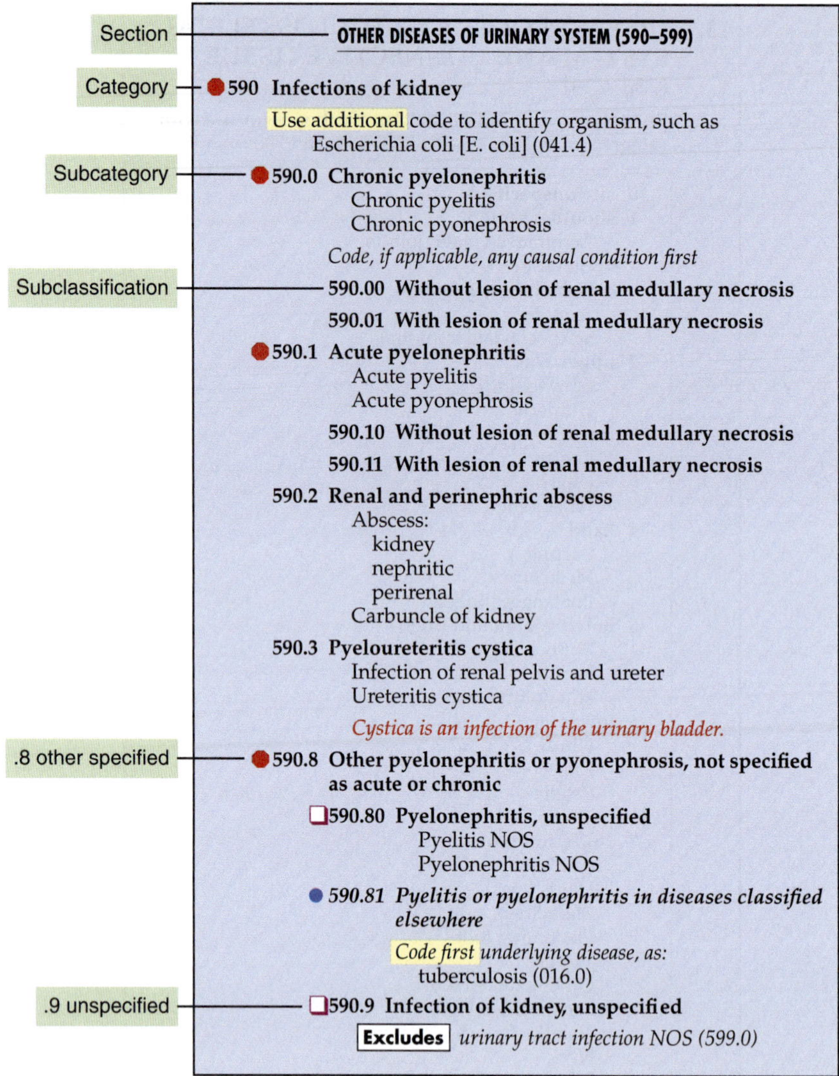

Figure 3-1. Divisions within the Tabular List.

EXERCISE 3-1

Identify the following as a chapter, section, category, or subcategory.

1. Diseases of Veins and Lymphatics, and Other Disease of Circulatory System (451-459) ____________
2. Diseases of the Circulatory System (390-459) ____________
3. 452 Portal vein thrombosis ____________
4. 453 Other venous embolism and thrombosis ____________
5. 453.0 Budd-Chiari syndrome ____________

Subclassification

Fifth-digit **subclassifications** provide even greater specificity. Instructions on the use of fifth digits may appear at the beginning of a chapter, a section, or third- and fourth-digit categories (Figure 3-2).

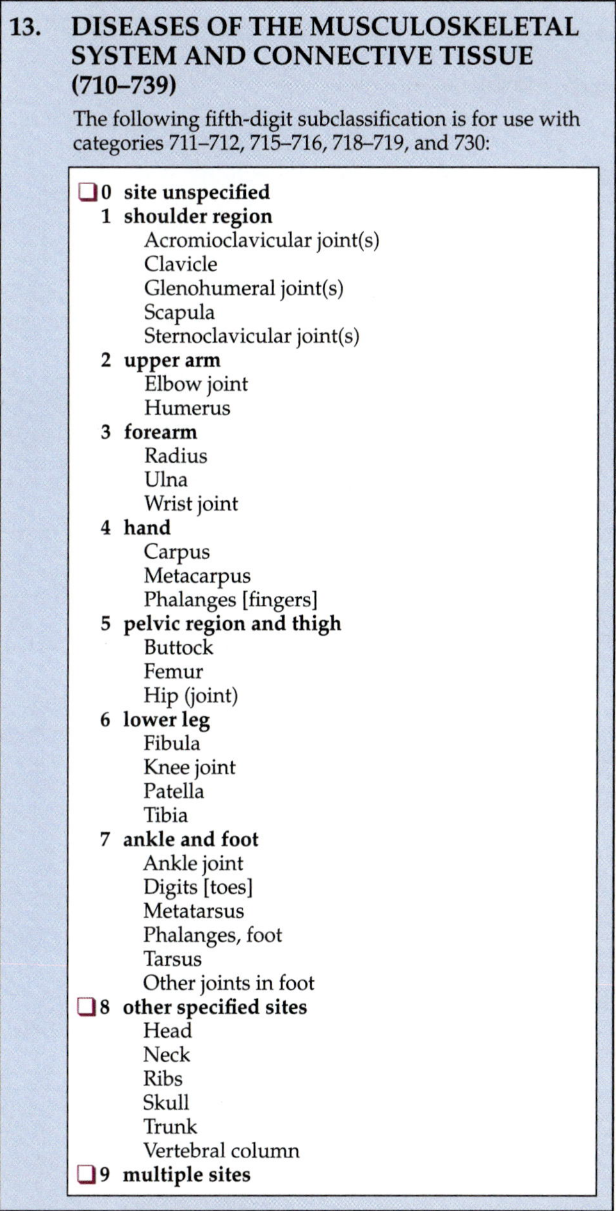

13. DISEASES OF THE MUSCULOSKELETAL SYSTEM AND CONNECTIVE TISSUE (710–739)

The following fifth-digit subclassification is for use with categories 711–712, 715–716, 718–719, and 730:

❑ **0 site unspecified**
1 shoulder region
Acromioclavicular joint(s)
Clavicle
Glenohumeral joint(s)
Scapula
Sternoclavicular joint(s)
2 upper arm
Elbow joint
Humerus
3 forearm
Radius
Ulna
Wrist joint
4 hand
Carpus
Metacarpus
Phalanges [fingers]
5 pelvic region and thigh
Buttock
Femur
Hip (joint)
6 lower leg
Fibula
Knee joint
Patella
Tibia
7 ankle and foot
Ankle joint
Digits [toes]
Metatarsus
Phalanges, foot
Tarsus
Other joints in foot
❑ **8 other specified sites**
Head
Neck
Ribs
Skull
Trunk
Vertebral column
❑ **9 multiple sites**

Figure 3-2. Fifth-digit subclassifications.

EXERCISE 3-2

Using Figure 3-2, assign the appropriate fifth-digit subclassifications.

1. Pyogenic arthritis left knee 711.0 ____
2. Localized osteoarthritis right wrist 715.3 ____
3. Traumatic arthropathy, right ankle 716.1 ____
4. Pain shoulder joint 719.4 ____
5. Swelling elbow joint 719.0 ____

Supplementary Classifications

- Supplementary Classification of Factors Influencing Health Status and Contact With Health Services (V01-V89)
- Supplementary Classification of External Causes of Injury and Poisoning (E800-E999)

Two supplementary classifications contain alphanumeric codes. One of the classifications is found following the Tabular List for Diseases and Injuries and is entitled Supplementary Classification of Factors Influencing Health Status and Contact With Health Services (V01-V89), or V codes. V codes are available to code encounters for circumstances other than disease or injury.

The second supplement is the Supplementary Classification of External Causes of Injury and Poisoning (E800-E999), or E codes. These codes are located after the V codes. The E codes are used as a supplement to ICD-9-CM diagnosis codes to provide data on cause, intent, and place of an injury or poisoning.

Format of Alphabetic Index to Diseases and Injuries

The Alphabetic Index contains three sections:

- Index to Diseases and Injuries
- Table of Drugs and Chemicals
- Alphabetic Index to External Causes of Injury and Poisoning (E codes)

Two tables are located within the Alphabetic Index. These tables are used for further clarification of subterms under the main term entries of Hypertension and Neoplasm. These tables are discussed in their respective chapters.

Index to Diseases and Injuries

Three levels of indentation are used in the Alphabetic Index. These include the following:

- Main terms
- Subterms
- Carryover lines

The **main terms** are identified by bold print and are set flush with the left margin of each column (Figure 3-3). Alphabetization rules apply in locating main terms and subterms in the Alphabetic Index. Numerical entries appear first under the main term or subterm (Figure 3-4). Main terms usually are identified by disease conditions and nouns. The main term is not a body part or site.

EXAMPLE

The patient has been admitted with deep vein thrombosis. The main term is "thrombosis." "Deep" is a location and "vein" refers to a body part.

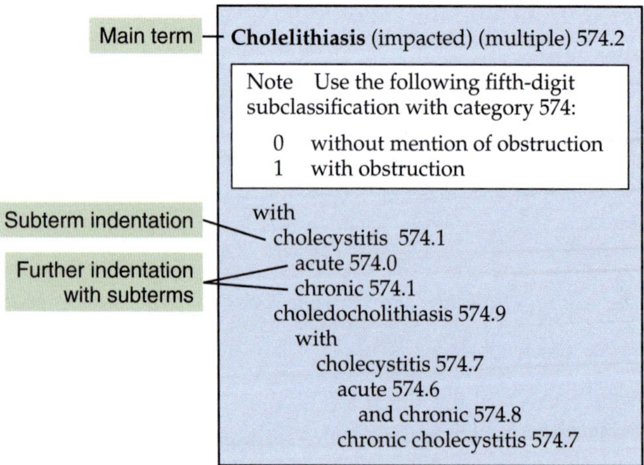

Figure 3-3. Various levels of indentation in the Index. The bold term is the main term, and the various subterms are listed below.

Deficiency, deficient
3-beta-hydroxysteroid dehydrogenase 255.2
6-phosphogluconic dehydrogenase (anemia) 282.2
11-beta-hydroxylase 255.2
17-alpha-hydroxylase 255.2
18-hydroxysteroid dehydrogenase 255.2
20-alpha-hydroxylase 255.2
21-hydroxylase 255.2
AAT (alpha-1 antitrypsin) 273.4
abdominal muscle syndrome 756.79

Figure 3-4. Numerical entries in the Alphabetic Index.

EXAMPLE

The patient is being treated for adhesive bursitis of the shoulder.

The main term is "bursitis." "Adhesive" describes the type of bursitis and "shoulder" is a body part.

EXERCISE 3-3

Underline the main terms to be located in the Alphabetic Index in the following diagnosis statements.

1. Decubitus ulcer of the heel
2. Acute anterior wall myocardial infarction
3. Respiratory anthrax
4. Endometriosis of the ovary
5. Gouty arthritis

The subterms are indented to the right under the main term. They are not bolded and begin with a lowercase letter. **Subterms** modify the main term and sometimes are called essential modifiers. These terms provide greater specificity to the disease or injury. It is possible for a subterm to be followed by additional subterm(s). These additional subterms are indented even farther to the right than are subterms (refer to Figure 3-3).

Some subterms are called **connecting words**. This means that there is a relationship between a main term or a subterm and an associated condition or etiology. Connecting words "with" and "without" are located before any other subterms (Figure 3-5). Additional connecting words include the following:

- Associated with
- Due to
- In
- With
- With mention of

EXERCISE 3-4

Using the Alphabetic Index only, assign codes to the following conditions.

1. Asthma due to detergent ______________
2. Cholelithiasis with acute cholecystitis ______________
3. Parkinsonism associated with orthostatic hypotension ______________
4. Cystocele in pregnancy ______________
5. List the subterms for coryza. ______________

Fever 780.6
  with chills 780.6
    in malarial regions (*see also* Malaria)
      084.6
  abortus NEC 023.9
  aden 061
  African tick-borne 087.1
  American
    mountain tick 066.1
    spotted 082.0
  and ague (*see also* Malaria) 084.6
  aphthous 078.4
  arbovirus hemorrhagic 065.9
  Assam 085.0
  Australian A or Q 083.0
  Bangkok hemorrhagic 065.4

Figure 3-5. Connecting term "with" follows the main term.

Fenestration, fenestrated - *see also* Imper-
  fect, closure
  aorta-pulmonary 745.0
  aorticopulmonary 745.0
  aortopulmonary 745.0
  cusps, heart valve NEC 746.89
    pulmonary 746.09
  hymen 752.49
  pulmonic cusps 746.09

Figure 3-6. Carryover line.

Carryover lines are used when an entry will not fit on a single line. These are indented to the right even farther than a subterm to avoid confusion (Figure 3-6).

CODING CONVENTIONS

Coding **conventions** are addressed by the ICD-9-CM Official Guidelines for Coding and Reporting. It is important for coders to understand these conventions so that accurate assignment of codes can be ensured.

Conventions include the following:

- Abbreviations
- Punctuation/Symbols
- Instructional notes
- Linking terms
- Cross-references

Abbreviations

The two main abbreviations are

- NEC—not elsewhere classifiable
- NOS—not otherwise specified

NEC is used differently in the Alphabetic Index than in the Tabular List. In the Alphabetic Index, NEC represents "other specified." When a specific disease or condition is documented and no specific code is available, the Index will direct the coder with the abbreviation "NEC" to an "other specified" code (Figure 3-7).

The **NEC** abbreviation in the Tabular List means "other specified" or "not elsewhere classifiable" and often is classified to the final digit of 8. The code title may not fully describe the documented disease process or condition (Figure 3-8).

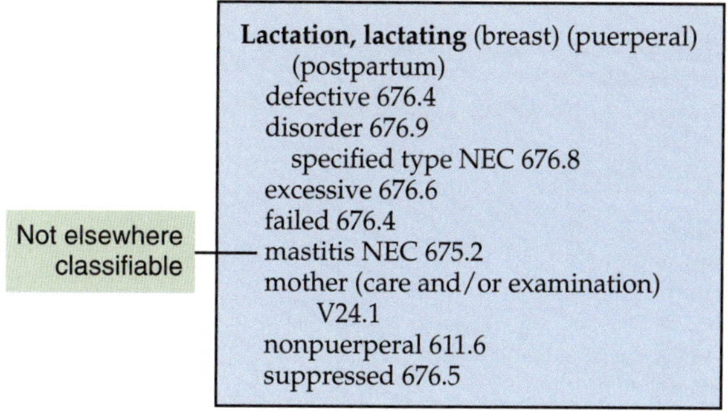

Figure 3-7. The Index entry for lactating mastitis "not elsewhere classifiable" (NEC) is coded to 675.2.

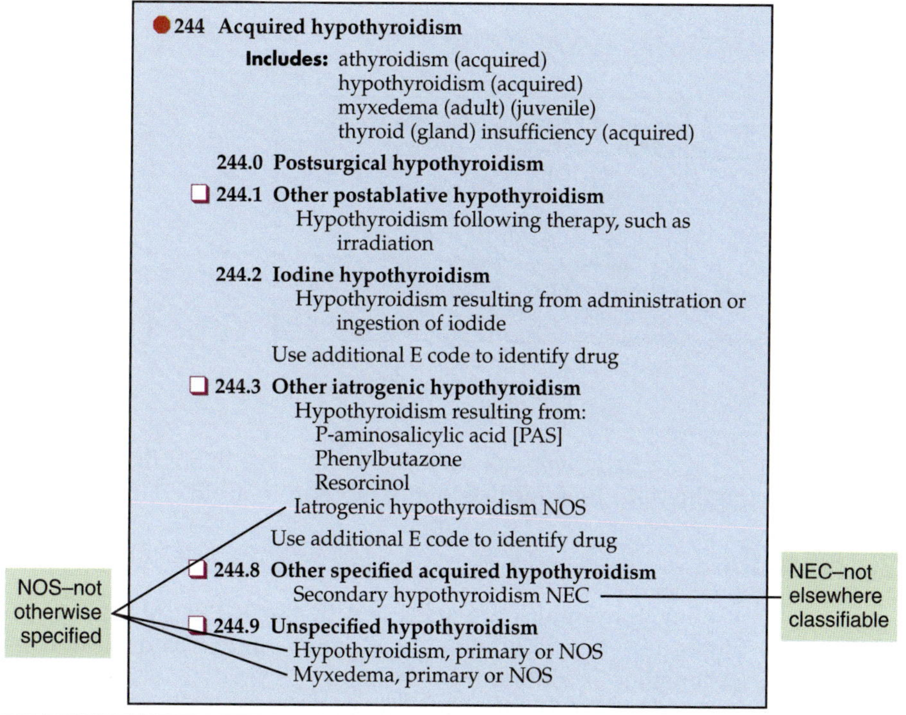

Figure 3-8. Examples of NEC and NOS from the Tabular.

NOS is a Tabular List abbreviation that means "unspecified" (see Figure 3-8). These codes are to be used only when the documentation in the health record does not provide adequate information. The unspecified code often appears as the code following the main term in the Alphabetic Index. The subterms should be reviewed to determine whether a more specific code is available.

Punctuation

Brackets

Square brackets [ ] are used in the Tabular List to enclose synonyms, alternative wording, or explanatory phrases (Figure 3-9).

Slanted brackets *[ ]* are used in the Alphabetic Index to identify manifestation codes (Figure 3-10). The code in brackets is always sequenced second.

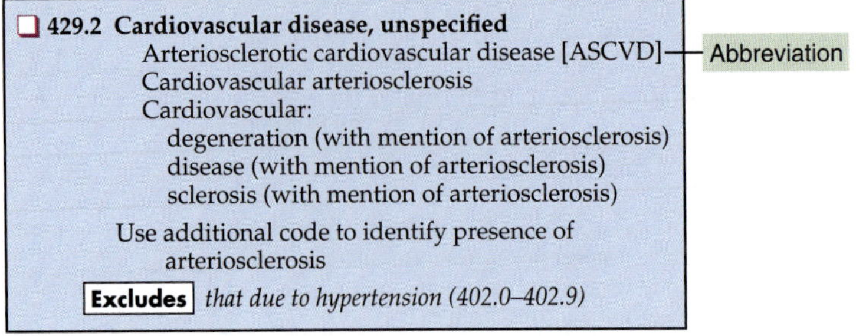

429.2 Cardiovascular disease, unspecified
Arteriosclerotic cardiovascular disease [ASCVD]
Cardiovascular arteriosclerosis
Cardiovascular:
degeneration (with mention of arteriosclerosis)
disease (with mention of arteriosclerosis)
sclerosis (with mention of arteriosclerosis)
Use additional code to identify presence of arteriosclerosis
Excludes *that due to hypertension (402.0–402.9)*

Figure 3-9. Square brackets used to enclose abbreviation.

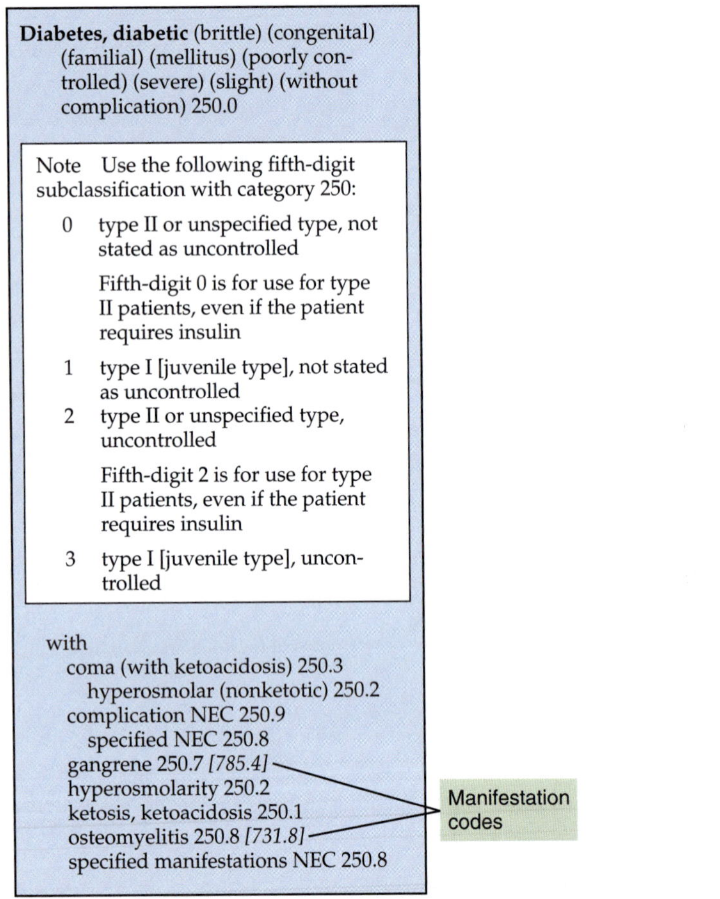

Diabetes, diabetic (brittle) (congenital) (familial) (mellitus) (poorly controlled) (severe) (slight) (without complication) 250.0

Note Use the following fifth-digit subclassification with category 250:

0 type II or unspecified type, not stated as uncontrolled

Fifth-digit 0 is for use for type II patients, even if the patient requires insulin

1 type I [juvenile type], not stated as uncontrolled

2 type II or unspecified type, uncontrolled

Fifth-digit 2 is for use for type II patients, even if the patient requires insulin

3 type I [juvenile type], uncontrolled

with
coma (with ketoacidosis) 250.3
hyperosmolar (nonketotic) 250.2
complication NEC 250.9
specified NEC 250.8
gangrene 250.7 *[785.4]*
hyperosmolarity 250.2
ketosis, ketoacidosis 250.1
osteomyelitis 250.8 *[731.8]*
specified manifestations NEC 250.8

Figure 3-10. Index entry of diabetic manifestation codes enclosed by slanted brackets.

Parentheses

Parentheses are used in both the Alphabetic Index and the Tabular List to enclose supplementary words. The presence or absence of these terms does not affect code assignment, so they are called nonessential modifiers. A **nonessential modifier** is a term that is enclosed in parentheses following a main term or a subterm, whose presence or absence has no effect on code assignment. These are "take it or leave it" terms. Sometimes, the subterm can be found among the nonessential modifiers (Figures 3-11 and 3-12).

If the diagnostic statement is "double pneumonia," (see Figure 3-11), since "double" is a nonessential modifier, it is assigned the same code as "pneumonia" (486). The word "double" makes absolutely no difference in assignment of the code for "double pneumonia."

Also, if the diagnostic statement (see Figure 3-12) is "sliding hiatal hernia with obstruction," the term "sliding" is a nonessential modifier and would not make any difference in assignment of the code.

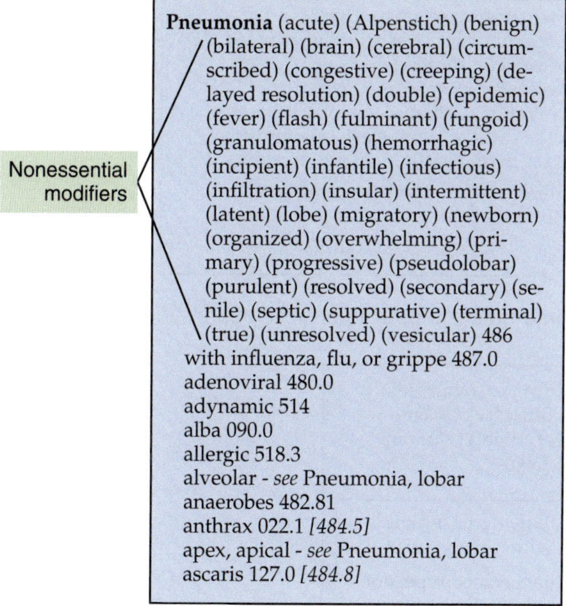

Pneumonia (acute) (Alpenstich) (benign) (bilateral) (brain) (cerebral) (circumscribed) (congestive) (creeping) (delayed resolution) (double) (epidemic) (fever) (flash) (fulminant) (fungoid) (granulomatous) (hemorrhagic) (incipient) (infantile) (infectious) (infiltration) (insular) (intermittent) (latent) (lobe) (migratory) (newborn) (organized) (overwhelming) (primary) (progressive) (pseudolobar) (purulent) (resolved) (secondary) (senile) (septic) (suppurative) (terminal) (true) (unresolved) (vesicular) 486
with influenza, flu, or grippe 487.0
adenoviral 480.0
adynamic 514
alba 090.0
allergic 518.3
alveolar - *see* Pneumonia, lobar
anaerobes 482.81
anthrax 022.1 *[484.5]*
apex, apical - *see* Pneumonia, lobar
ascaris 127.0 *[484.8]*

Figure 3-11. The use of parentheses in the Index for the diagnosis of pneumonia. Multiple nonessential modifiers are used.

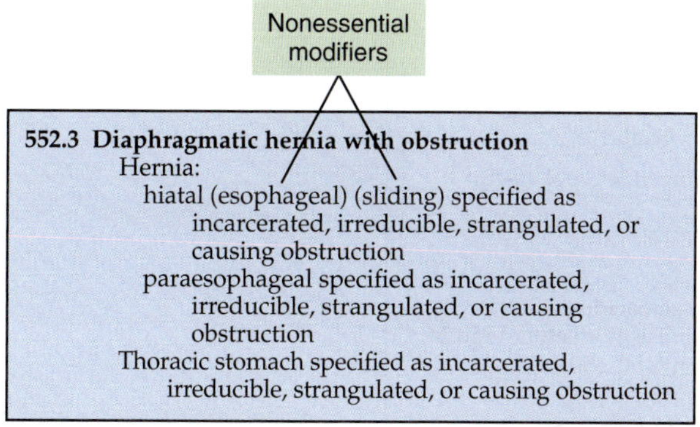

552.3 Diaphragmatic hernia with obstruction
Hernia:
hiatal (esophageal) (sliding) specified as incarcerated, irreducible, strangulated, or causing obstruction
paraesophageal specified as incarcerated, irreducible, strangulated, or causing obstruction
Thoracic stomach specified as incarcerated, irreducible, strangulated, or causing obstruction

Figure 3-12. The nonessential modifier in the Tabular for an incarcerated hiatal or diaphragmatic hernia.

EXERCISE 3-5

Using ICD-9-CM, Volume 2, Alphabetic Index, locate the following main terms, and identify whether the bolded subterm is an essential or a nonessential modifier.

1. **Primary** glaucoma ____________
2. **Narrow-angle** glaucoma ____________
3. **Essential** hypertension ____________
4. **Filarial** infestation ____________
5. **Thyrotoxic** exophthalmos ____________

Colons

Colons are used in the Tabular List after an incomplete term that needs one or more modifiers following the colon to make it assignable to a given category. Colons also are used in

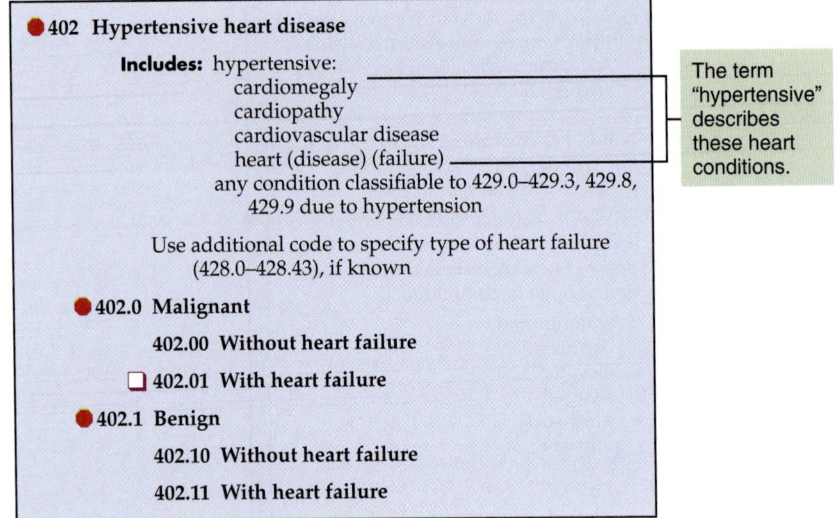

Figure 3-13. Colon used within "Includes" note.

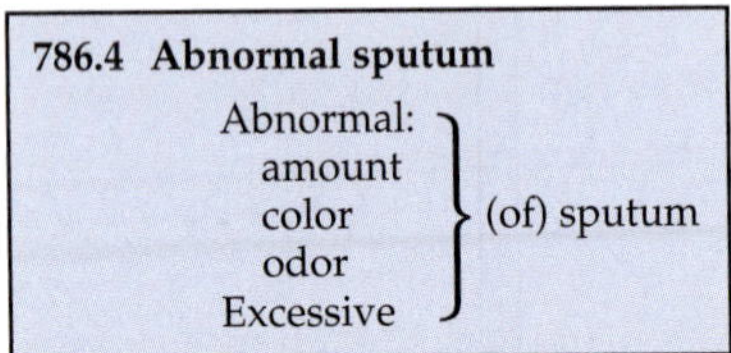

Figure 3-14. Braces.

both Inclusion and Exclusion notes to indicate that one of the words from the indented list must be present for the note to apply (Figure 3-13).

In Figure 3-13, the term "hypertensive" is used to describe various heart conditions. The colon helps to save space and means the same as if it was written in this way:

- Hypertensive cardiomegaly
- Hypertensive cardiopathy
- Hypertensive cardiovascular disease
- Hypertensive heart disease or failure

Braces

The purpose of the brace is to save printing space by reducing the repetition of words. A brace is used to enclose a series of terms, each of which is modified by a statement that appears to the right of the brace (Figure 3-14).

Instructional Notes

Notes with instructions are found in all three volumes. General notes may be found in the Alphabetic Index and the Tabular List. These notes provide additional information (Figure 3-15). Other types of instructional notes are Inclusion; Exclusion; code first; use additional code; and code, if applicable, any causal condition first.

Inclusion Notes

An Includes note is an instructional note that appears immediately under a three-digit code title or category. The purpose of the Includes note is to give examples or further define the content of the category (Figure 3-16).

Inclusion Terms

According to the guidelines, Inclusion terms are a list of terms that are found under some fourth- and fifth-digit codes (Figure 3-17). These terms may be synonyms or various other

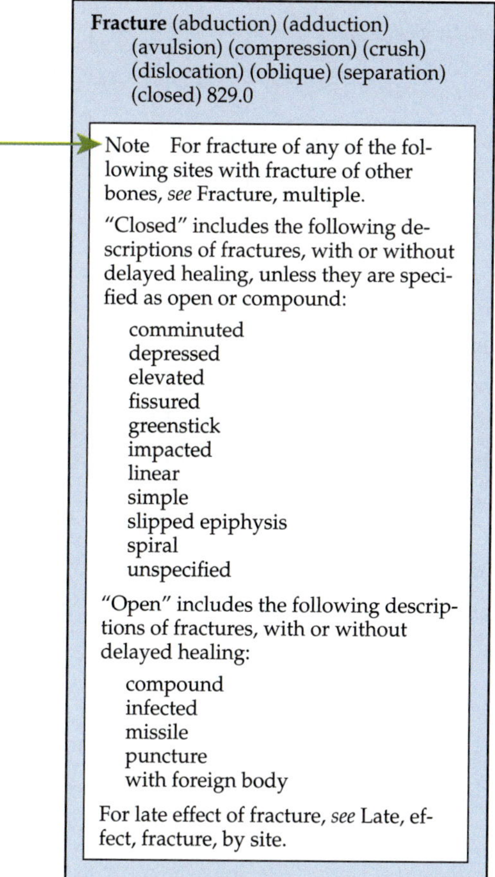

Fracture (abduction) (adduction) (avulsion) (compression) (crush) (dislocation) (oblique) (separation) (closed) 829.0

Note For fracture of any of the following sites with fracture of other bones, *see* Fracture, multiple.

"Closed" includes the following descriptions of fractures, with or without delayed healing, unless they are specified as open or compound:

comminuted
depressed
elevated
fissured
greenstick
impacted
linear
simple
slipped epiphysis
spiral
unspecified

"Open" includes the following descriptions of fractures, with or without delayed healing:

compound
infected
missile
puncture
with foreign body

For late effect of fracture, *see* Late, effect, fracture, by site.

Figure 3-15. General notes found in the Alphabetic Index.

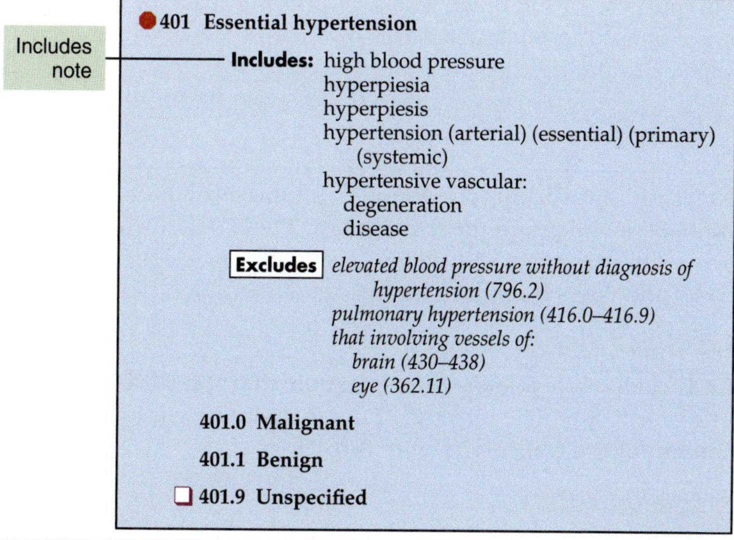

401 Essential hypertension

Includes: high blood pressure
hyperpiesia
hyperpiesis
hypertension (arterial) (essential) (primary) (systemic)
hypertensive vascular:
degeneration
disease

Excludes *elevated blood pressure without diagnosis of hypertension (796.2)*
pulmonary hypertension (416.0–416.9)
that involving vessels of:
brain (430–438)
eye (362.11)

401.0 Malignant

401.1 Benign

401.9 Unspecified

Figure 3-16. This "Includes" note is found under category 401, Essential hypertension.

conditions that are assigned to the code. Inclusion terms do not necessarily constitute a comprehensive list. Additional terms found only in the Alphabetic Index and not in the Tabular List may be assigned a code without mention in the Inclusion terms. In these instances, the Index should be trusted.

Exclusion Notes

An Excludes note is an instructional note that may appear after any code in the Tabular List. One of the purposes of the Excludes note is to direct the coder to another code.

EXAMPLE

The patient has COPD with asthma. Under category 496, an exclusion note indicates that COPD with asthma is coded to 493.2X (Figure 3-18).

Another purpose of an Exclusion note is to instruct the coder that the excluded terms should not be used along with the code that is assigned. The example given in the guidelines is that only one code should be assigned for a condition that has different codes for congenital and acquired (Figure 3-19).

Exclusion notes also are used to instruct the coder that an additional code may be required because this code is excluded from a particular code.

EXAMPLE

A patient has hypertension and pulmonary hypertension. Under the category 401 code for hypertension is an Exclusion note for pulmonary hypertension. In this case, two codes must be assigned: one for hypertension (401.9) and another to identify pulmonary hypertension (416.8) (Figure 3-20).

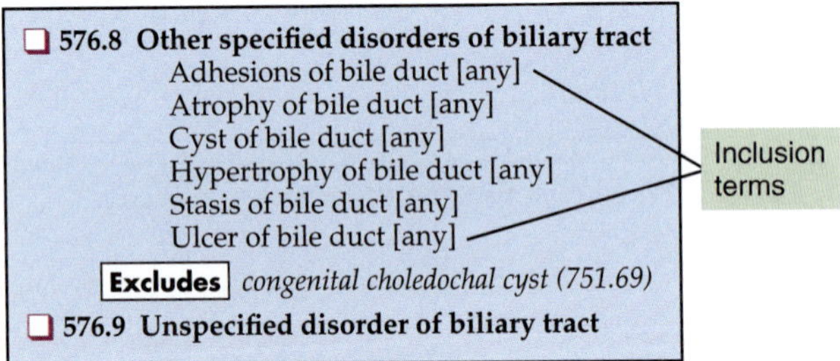

Figure 3-17. Inclusion terms.

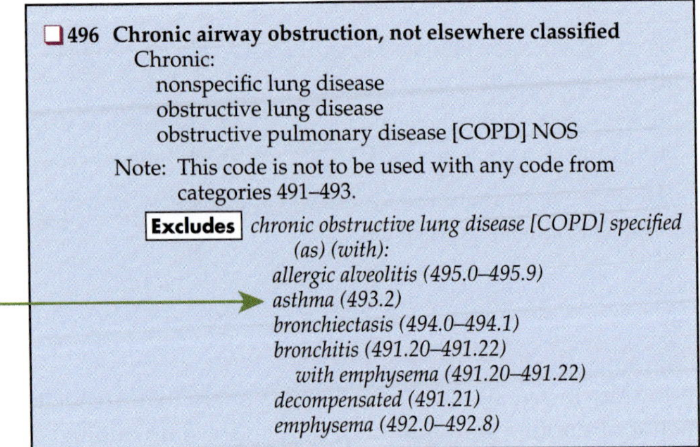

Figure 3-18. Exclusion note.

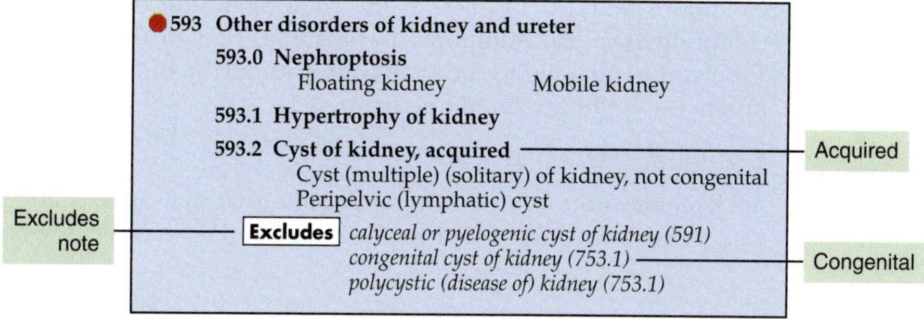

Figure 3-19. Example of a congenital cyst of the kidney that is excluded from the acquired form of a kidney cyst.

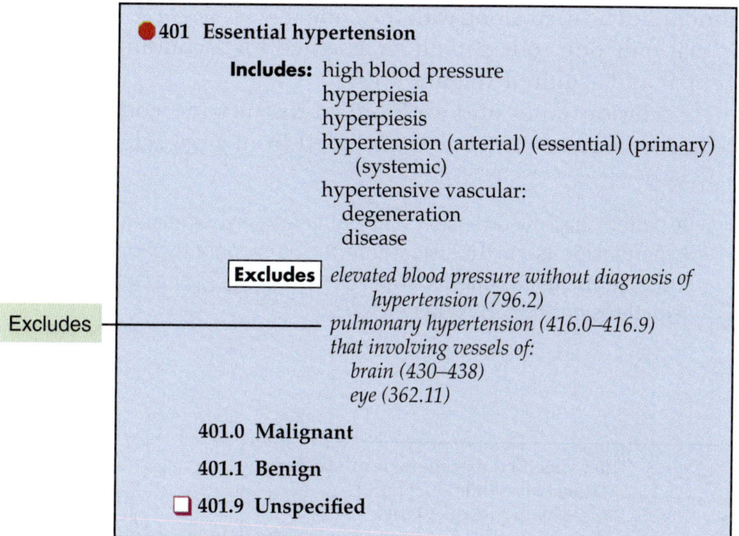

Figure 3-20. Exclusion note directing the coder to another code.

EXERCISE 3-6

Using the Tabular List, answer the following questions.

1. Is bronchitis due to fumes and vapors assigned code 490? ________
   If not, what code is assigned? ________
2. Is chronic sinusitis assigned code category 461? ________
   If not, what code is assigned? ________
3. Is gangrenous tonsillitis assigned to code category 463? ________
   If not, what code is assigned? ________
4. Is hypertensive cardiomegaly included in code category 402? ________
   If not, what code is assigned? ________
5. Are tics due to Tourette's syndrome code category 333.3? ________
   If not, what code is assigned? ________

Etiology and Manifestation Convention

The following instructional notes are designed to instruct the coder regarding proper sequencing of etiology and manifestation codes. The etiology code will include an Instructional note to use an additional code to identify a given manifestation. The manifestation code will have an instructional note to code first the etiology code.

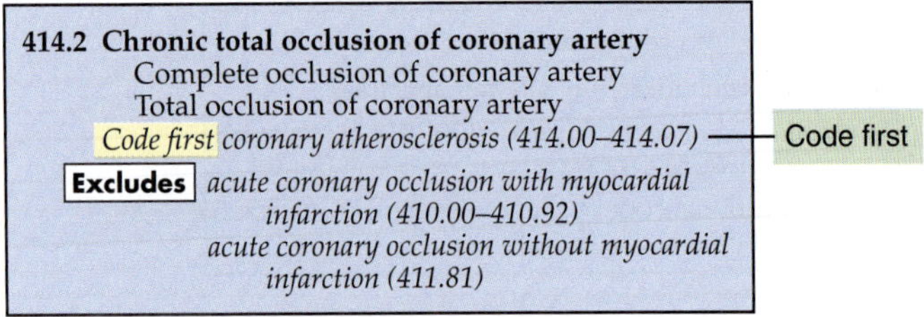

414.2 **Chronic total occlusion of coronary artery**
Complete occlusion of coronary artery
Total occlusion of coronary artery
Code first coronary atherosclerosis (414.00–414.07)
Excludes *acute coronary occlusion with myocardial infarction (410.00–410.92)*
acute coronary occlusion without myocardial infarction (411.81)

Figure 3-21. Instructional note to code first underlying disease.

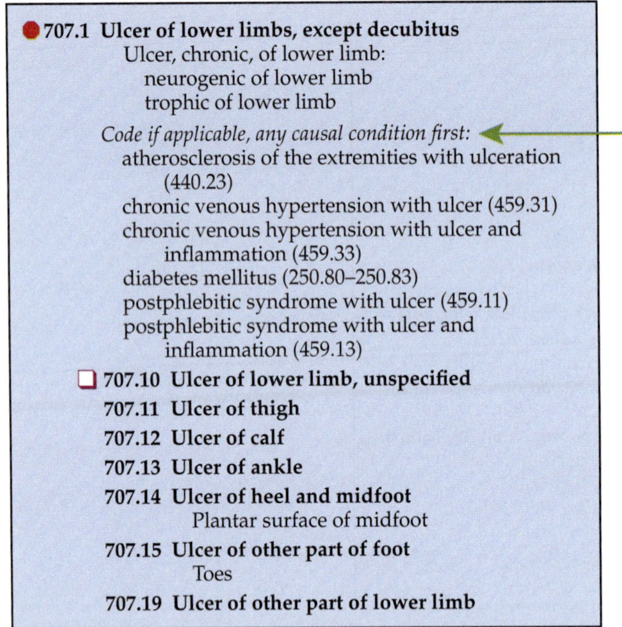

707.1 Ulcer of lower limbs, except decubitus
Ulcer, chronic, of lower limb:
neurogenic of lower limb
trophic of lower limb
Code if applicable, any causal condition first:
atherosclerosis of the extremities with ulceration (440.23)
chronic venous hypertension with ulcer (459.31)
chronic venous hypertension with ulcer and inflammation (459.33)
diabetes mellitus (250.80–250.83)
postphlebitic syndrome with ulcer (459.11)
postphlebitic syndrome with ulcer and inflammation (459.13)
707.10 Ulcer of lower limb, unspecified
707.11 Ulcer of thigh
707.12 Ulcer of calf
707.13 Ulcer of ankle
707.14 Ulcer of heel and midfoot
Plantar surface of midfoot
707.15 Ulcer of other part of foot
Toes
707.19 Ulcer of other part of lower limb

Figure 3-22. Instruction to "Code if applicable any causal condition first."

An instructional note to "code first underlying disease" is used in the Tabular List. The purpose of this is to instruct the coder that there may be a code for the etiology and if so it is to be sequenced first (Figure 3-21).

EXAMPLE

Patient with chronic total occlusion of the coronary artery with coronary atherosclerosis, 414.01, 414.2 (codes must be sequenced in this order).

Code 414.2 includes an instructional note to code the underlying disease first. In this case, the underlying disease is coronary atherosclerosis.

An instructional note to "code, if applicable, any causal condition first" is used in the Tabular List. The purpose of this note is to instruct the coder to sequence the causal condition (etiology) first. Different from the instructional note "code first underlying disease," if no causal condition is present or documented, the code may be sequenced first (Figure 3-22).

EXAMPLE

Patient has ulcer of right ankle due to diabetes, type II, 250.80, 707.13 (codes must be sequenced in this order).

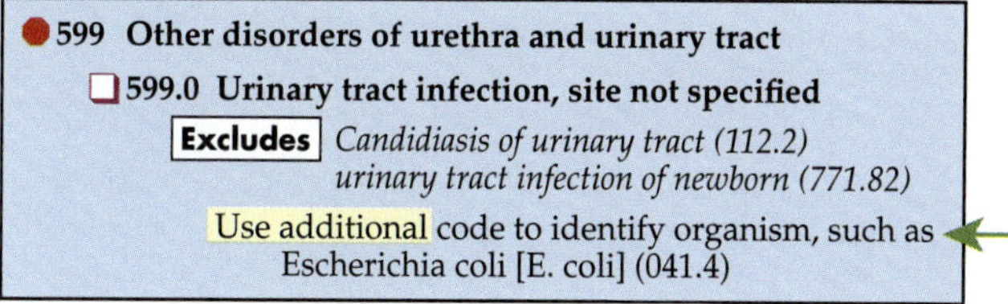

599 Other disorders of urethra and urinary tract

599.0 Urinary tract infection, site not specified

Excludes *Candidiasis of urinary tract (112.2)*
urinary tract infection of newborn (771.82)

Use additional code to identify organism, such as Escherichia coli [E. coli] (041.4)

Figure 3-23. Instructional note to use an additional code.

Diabetes, diabetic *(Continued)*
hypoglycemia 250.8
hypoglycemic shock 250.8
insipidus 253.5
nephrogenic 588.1
pituitary 253.5
vasopressin-resistant 588.1
intercapillary glomerulosclerosis 250.4 *[581.81]*
iritis 250.5 *[364.42]*
ketosis, ketoacidosis 250.1
Kimmelstiel (-Wilson) disease or syndrome (intercapillary glomerulosclerosis) 250.4 *[581.81]*
Lancereaux's (diabetes mellitus with marked emaciation) 250.8 *[261]*
latent (chemical) 790.29
complicating pregnancy, childbirth, or puerperium 648.8
lipoidosis 250.8 *[272.7]*
macular edema 250.5 *[362.07]*
maternal
with manifest disease in the infant 775.1
affecting fetus or newborn 775.0
microaneurysms, retinal 250.5 *[362.01]*
mononeuropathy 250.6 *[355.9]*
neonatal, transient 775.1
nephropathy 250.4 *[583.81]*
nephrosis (syndrome) 250.4 *[581.81]*

Diabetic nephropathy 250.4X *[583.81]*

Figure 3-24. Slanted brackets enclosing manifestation code.

Code 707.1 includes an instructional note to code first any applicable causal condition. In this case, the causal condition is diabetes.

An instructional note to "use additional code" is found in the Tabular List. The purpose of this is to instruct the coder to use an additional code to provide a complete picture of the diagnosis or condition. These codes should be assigned only if they are documented by a physician (Figure 3-23).

EXAMPLE

Patient has a urinary tract infection due to *Escherichia coli*, 599.0, 041.4 (must be sequenced in this order).

The "use additional code" note instructs the coder to assign an additional code for the organism.

In the Alphabetic Index, some manifestation codes are enclosed in slanted brackets. The etiology code is listed first and is sequenced first. The manifestation code is assigned as an additional code. The Index entry for diabetes is a good example of the use of etiology and manifestation codes (Figure 3-24).

EXERCISE 3-7

Using the Tabular List and instructional notes, assign and sequence the following code(s).

1. See category 331 and assign code(s) for a patient who has Alzheimer's disease with behavioral disturbances. ______________
2. See code 484.3 and assign code(s) for a patient with pneumonia due to whooping cough. ______________
3. See code 707.1 and assign code(s) for a patient with atherosclerosis of the lower extremities with a toe ulcer. ______________
4. See code 600.91 and assign code(s) for a patient with hyperplasia of the prostate with urinary retention. ______________
5. See code 456.2 and assign code(s) for a patient with bleeding esophageal varices and cirrhosis of the liver. ______________

Linking Terms

As in the Index, terms such as "and," "with," "due to," and "in" are used to link terms. These terms have special definitions within ICD-9-CM and code assignment.

The term "and" means "and/or" when it appears in a code title in the Tabular List. The code 474.8, Other chronic disease of tonsils and adenoids, could mean any of the following:

- Chronic disease of tonsils
- Chronic disease of adenoids
- Chronic disease of tonsils and adenoids

The term "with" (with "mention of," "associated with," and "in") indicates that both elements in the title must be present and documented for this code to be assigned.

EXAMPLE

Viral pneumonia with influenza is assigned codes 487.0 and 480.9 (Figure 3-25). Both the pneumonia and the influenza must be present for code 487.0 to be assigned.

The term "due to" indicates a causal relationship between two conditions. It is found in both the Alphabetic Index and the Tabular List. If it is documented that a condition is due to another condition and there is an Alphabetic Index entry for the subterm "due to," the coder must follow the Index (Figure 3-26).

Cross-References

Cross-reference terms are used in the Alphabetic Index to instruct a coder to look elsewhere prior to code assignment. These terms include "see," "see also," "see category," and "see condition" (Figure 3-27).

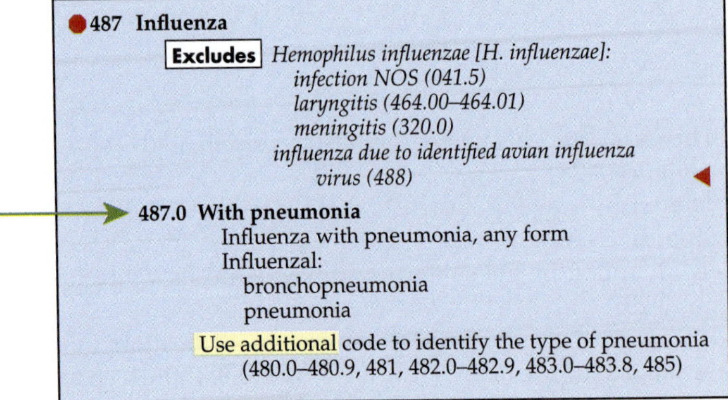

487 Influenza

Excludes *Hemophilus influenzae [H. influenzae]:*
infection NOS (041.5)
laryngitis (464.00–464.01)
meningitis (320.0)
influenza due to identified avian influenza virus (488)

487.0 With pneumonia
Influenza with pneumonia, any form
Influenzal:
bronchopneumonia
pneumonia
Use additional code to identify the type of pneumonia (480.0–480.9, 481, 482.0–482.9, 483.0–483.8, 485)

Figure 3-25. Influenza with pneumonia.

Cataract *(Continued)*
complicated NEC 366.30
congenital 743.30
capsular or subcapsular 743.31
cortical 743.32
nuclear 743.33
specified type NEC 743.39
total or subtotal 743.34
zonular 743.32
coronary (congenital) 743.39
acquired 366.12
cupuliform 366.14
diabetic 250.5 *[366.41]*
drug-induced 366.45
due to
chalcosis 360.24 *[366.34]*
chronic choroiditis (*see also* Choroiditis) 363.20 *[366.32]*
degenerative myopia 360.21 *[366.34]*
glaucoma (*see also* Glaucoma) 365.9 *[366.31]*
infection, intraocular NEC 366.32
inflammatory ocular disorder NEC 366.32
iridocyclitis, chronic 364.10 *[366.33]*
pigmentary retinal dystrophy 362.74 *[366.34]*
radiation 366.46

Figure 3-26. "Due to" indicates a relationship between the cataract and subsequent subterms.

Hereditary - *see* condition
Heredodegeneration 330.9
macular 362.70
Heredopathia atactica polyneuritiformis 356.3

Figure 3-27. Under the main term "Hereditary," mandatory instructions are given to "*see*" condition.

Angioblastoma (M9161/1) - *see* Neoplasm, connective tissue, uncertain behavior

Figure 3-28. Cross-reference to "*see*" another main term.

The term "**see**" is a mandatory instruction that advises the coder to go to another main term (Figure 3-28).

The term "**see also**" instructs the coder about the possibility that a better main term may appear elsewhere in the Alphabetic Index. If the specific diagnosis cannot be completely identified by the subterms, it may be necessary to follow the "see also" instruction (Figure 3-29).

If a patient has hives because of use of a medication, in the Alphabetic Index, the only code available for the main term "hives" is 780.9. If the "see also" instruction is not followed, the wrong code would be assigned. When you go to "urticaria" in the Index, several subterm selections are available, including 708.0 for "urticaria due to a drug" (see Figure 3-29).

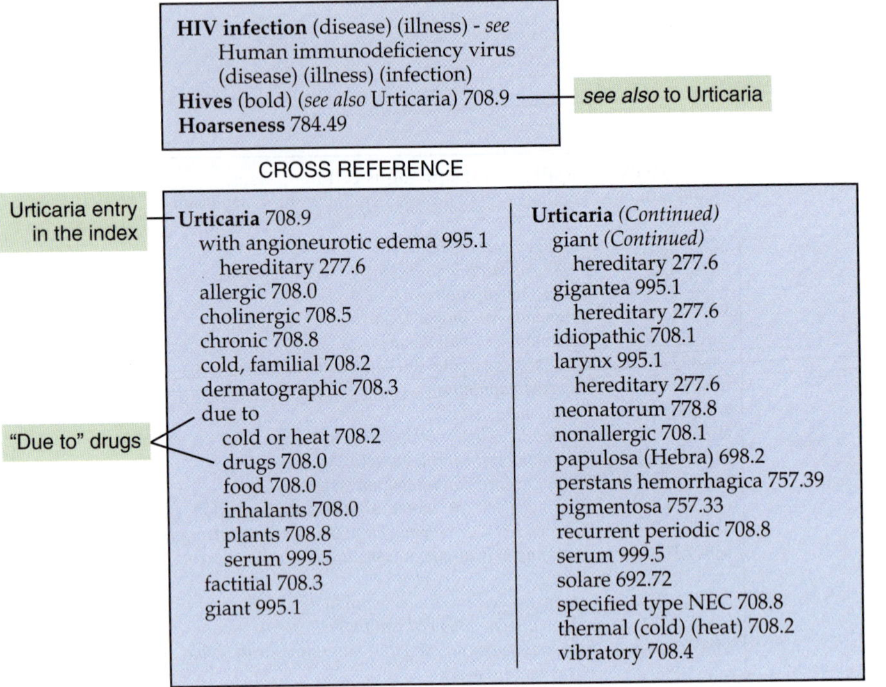

Figure 3-29. "*See also*" instruction to go to the main term "urticaria."

EXERCISE 3-8

Using the Alphabetic Index, answer the following questions.

1. Locate the main term "arthropathy" in the Index. Is there another term for "arthropathy" that may be located in the Index, and if so, what is the term? ____________
2. Locate the main term "climacteric" in the Index. Is there another term for "climacteric" that may be located in the Index, and if so, what is the term? ____________
3. Locate the main term "Endamebiasis" in the Index. Is there another term for "Endamebiasis" that may be located in the Index, and if so, what is the term? ____________
4. Locate the main term "enteric" in the Index. Is there another term for "enteric" that may be located in the Index, and if so, what is the term? ____________
5. Locate the main term "late effect of phlebitis of the intracranial venous sinuses." What cross-reference is given? ____________

APPENDICES

As noted at the beginning of the chapter, book content and format may vary depending on the publisher. The following are the most commonly found appendices.

M805-M808	**Papillary and squamous cell neoplasms**
M8050/0	*Papilloma NOS (except Papilloma of urinary bladder M8120/1)*
M8050/2	*Papillary carcinoma in situ*
M8050/3	*Papillary carcinoma NOS*
M8051/0	*Verrucous papilloma*
M8051/3	*Verrucous carcinoma NOS*
M8052/0	*Squamous cell papilloma*
M8052/3	*Papillary squamous cell carcinoma*
M8053/0	*Inverted papilloma*
M8060/0	*Papillomatosis NOS*
M8070/2	*Squamous cell carcinoma in situ NOS*
M8070/3	*Squamous cell carcinoma NOS*
M8070/6	*Squamous cell carcinoma, metastatic NOS*
M8071/3	*Squamous cell carcinoma, keratinizing type NOS*
M8072/3	*Squamous cell carcinoma, large cell, nonkeratinizing type*
M8073/3	*Squamous cell carcinoma, small cell, nonkeratinizing type*
M8074/3	*Squamous cell carcinoma, spindle cell type*
M8075/3	*Adenoid squamous cell carcinoma*
M8076/2	*Squamous cell carcinoma in situ with questionable stromal invasion*
M8076/3	*Squamous cell carcinoma, microinvasive*
M8080/2	*Queyrat's erythroplasia*
M8081/2	*Bowen's disease*
M8082/3	*Lymphoepithelial carcinoma*

Figure 3-30. Example from Appendix A, Morphology of Neoplasms.

24:00	**CARDIOVASCULAR DRUGS**	
24:04	Cardiac Drugs	972.9
	cardiotonic agents	972.1
	rhythm regulators	972.0
24:06	Antilipemic Agents	972.2
	thyroid derivatives	962.7
24:08	Hypotensive Agents	972.6
	adrenergic blocking agents	971.3
	ganglion-blocking agents	972.3
	vasodilators	972.5
24:12	Vasodilating Agents	972.5
	coronary	972.4
	nicotinic acid derivatives	972.2
24:16	Sclerosing Agents	972.7

Figure 3-31. Example from Appendix C, Classification of Drugs by American Hospital Formulary Service List Number and Their ICD-9-CM Equivalents.

A. Morphology of Neoplasms

The World Health Organization (WHO) has published an adaptation of the International Classification of Diseases for Oncology (ICD-O). The ICD-O contains codes for the **topography** (location) and morphology of tumors. **Morphology** is the study of neo-plasms. Morphology codes consist of five digits; the first four identify the histologic type, and the fifth indicates its behavior (Figure 3-30). Not all facilities use the "M codes." These are discussed in greater detail in Chapter 15 of this textbook, Neoplasms.

B. Glossary of Mental Disorders

The psychiatric terms that appear in ICD-9-CM, Chapter 5, Mental Disorders, used to be listed in alphabetical order along with definitions in Appendix B. This Appendix was deleted in 2004. Most psychiatric conditions are classified according to the *Diagnostic and Statistical Manual of Mental Disorders, Fourth Edition* (DSM-IV).

C. Classification of Drugs by American Hospital Formulary: Service List Number and Their ICD-9-CM Equivalents

Appendix C contains codes from the American Hospital Formulary Services (AHFS) along with corresponding codes from ICD-9-CM (Figure 3-31).

A division of the AFHS regularly published a coded listing of drugs. These AHFS codes have as many as five digits. Each code has a number, then a colon, and can include up to four additional digits to provide specificity. An associated ICD-9-CM poisoning code follows the drug. The American Hospital Formulary list can be useful to the coder in assigning appropriate ICD-9-CM poisoning codes.

D. Classification of Industrial Accidents According to Agency

Appendix D contains three-digit codes for use in identifying occupational hazards. These codes can be very useful in assessment of statistical data and analysis of occupational hazards.

The subsection is divided into the following categories:

- Machines
- Means of Transport and Lifting Equipment
- Other Equipment
- Materials, Substances, and Radiations
- Working Environment
- Other Agencies, Not Elsewhere Classified
- Agencies Not Classified for Lack of Sufficient Data

E. List of Three-Digit Categories

Appendix E is a complete listing of all the three-digit code categories used in the ICD-9-CM.

All fourth- and fifth-digit codes can be condensed back down to the three-digit categories. This allows for comparability of worldwide data with the use of ICD-9.

CHAPTER REVIEW EXERCISE

Match the term, symbol, or punctuation with the appropriate description.

________ **1.** Appendix that contains a listing of all three-digit code categories

________ **2.** Stands for "not otherwise specified"

________ **3.** Appendix that contains the Morphology of Neoplasm codes

________ **4.** Used in both the Index and the Tabular to enclose supplementary words that may be present or absent in the statement of a disease or procedure, without affecting the code number to which it is assigned

________ **5.** Used in the Tabular List after an incomplete term that needs one or more of the modifiers to make it assignable to a given category

________ **6.** This note appears immediately under a three-digit code title to further define, or give examples of, the content of the category

_______ 7. A note under a code indicates that the terms excluded from the code are to be coded elsewhere

_______ 8. A word that should be interpreted to mean either "and" or "or" when it appears in a title

_______ 9. Appendix that was deleted October 1, 2004

_______ 10. List of terms that is included under particular four- and five-digit codes

_______ 11. Stands for "not elsewhere classifiable"

_______ 12. Term that is used to indicate that no code should be assigned

A. Omit code	**G.** See category	**M.** Use additional code
B. ( )	**H.** Inclusion terms	**N.** Appendix A
C. NOS	**I.** See also	**O.** Appendix B
D. Includes	**J.** Etiology	**P.** Appendix C
E. NEC	**K.** Excludes	**Q.** Appendix D
F. :	**L.** And	**R.** Appendix E

Using ICD-9-CM, Volume 1, Tabular List, locate the first pages of Chapter 8, and answer the following questions about the chapter.

13. The name of the chapter: _______
14. The name of the first section: _______
15. The description of the first category: _______
16. The description of the first subcategory: _______
17. The description of the first subclassification: _______
18. What instructional note applies to the entire chapter? _______
19. What Excludes note applies to the first section? _______

Underline the main terms to be located in the Alphabetic Index in the following diagnostic statements.

20. Profound anemia
21. Chronic prostatitis
22. Mild protein-calorie malnutrition
23. Granuloma lung
24. Pain in shoulder

Using ICD-9-CM, Volume 2, Alphabetic Index, locate the following main terms and identify whether the bolded subterm is an essential or a nonessential modifier.

25. **Immature** cataract _______
26. **Senile** cataract _______
27. **Contact** dermatitis _______
28. **Classical** migraine _______
29. **Congential** strabismus _______

Using the Alphabetic Index, answer the following questions.

30. Locate the main term "acquired immune deficiency syndrome" in the Index. Is there another term for "acquired immune deficiency syndrome" that may be located in the Index, and if so, what is the term? _______
31. Locate the main term "malarial" in the Index. Is there another term for "malarial" that may be located in the Index, and if so, what is the term? _______

Using the Tabular List, answer the following questions.

32. Is acute exacerbation of chronic myeloid leukemia assigned code 205.00? __________
If not, what code is assigned? __________

33. Is rupture of the esophagus assigned code 530.4? __________
If not, what code is assigned? __________

Using the Tabular List and instructional notes, assign and sequence the following code(s).

34. See category 331 and assign code(s) for a patient who has Pick's disease with behavioral disturbances. __________

35. See code 484.6 and assign code(s) for a patient with pneumonia due to aspergillosis. __________

36. See code 707.1 and assign code(s) for a patient with atherosclerosis of the lower extremities with an ankle ulcer. __________

CHAPTER GLOSSARY

Carryover line: used when an entry will not fit on a single line.

Category: a single three-digit code that describes a disease or a similarly related group of conditions.

Connecting words: subterms that denote a relationship between a main term or a subterm and an associated condition or etiology.

Conventions: general rules for use in classification that must be followed for accurate coding.

Etiology: cause or origin of a disease or condition.

Main terms: identified in bold print and set flush with the left margin of each column in the Alphabetic Index.

Manifestation: symptom of a condition that is the result of a disease.

Morphology: the study of neoplasms.

NEC: abbreviation for "not elsewhere classifiable" that means "other specified."

Nonessential modifier: term that is enclosed in parentheses; its presence or absence does not affect code assignment.

NOS: abbreviation for "not otherwise specified" that means "unspecified."

Section: consists of a group of three-digit categories that represent diseases or conditions that are similar.

See: a mandatory cross-reference that advises the coder to go to another main term.

See also: cross-reference that instructs the coder about the possibility that there may be a better main term elsewhere in the Alphabetic Index.

Subcategory: a fourth-digit code that provides additional information or specificity.

Subclassification: a fifth-digit code that provides even greater specificity.

Subterms: modifiers that are indented to the right of the main term.

Topography: location.

CHAPTER 4

Basic Steps of Coding

CHAPTER OUTLINE

LEARNING OBJECTIVES

- Assign a diagnosis or procedure from the Alphabetic Index using main terms, subterms, and essential modifiers
- Explain the necessity of referencing the Alphabetic Index and the Tabular List
- Describe basic steps of coding
- Explain how to use both Alphabetic Index and the Tabular List

ABBREVIATIONS

CC chief complaint
DS discharge summary
ER Emergency Room
OR operating room

BASIC STEPS OF CODING

- Review the health record.
- Identify the diagnoses and procedures to be coded.
- Identify the principal diagnosis and the principal procedure.
- Identify main term(s) in the Alphabetic Index.
- Review any subterms under the main term in the Index.
- Follow any cross-reference instructions, such as "*see also.*"
- Verify in the Tabular List the code(s) selected from the Index.
- Refer to any instructional notation in the Tabular.
- Assign codes to the highest level of specificity.
- Assign codes to the diagnoses and procedures, reporting all applicable codes and sequence in accordance with the guidelines.

REVIEW OF THE HEALTH RECORD

As described in Chapter 2 of this textbook, the first step in coding the **principal diagnosis** (condition established after study to be chiefly responsible for occasioning admission of the patient to the hospital for care), other reportable diagnoses, and procedures is review of the health record.

The discharge summary (DS) if available may be the first document to be reviewed for code selection. The coder reads the summary to understand the highlights of this encoun-

ter. The discharge summary is a synopsis of the events included in a patient's hospital stay. Most pertinent information is contained in the discharge summary. A physician should list the diagnoses and the procedures that were performed during this encounter. The coder should not solely rely on the discharge summary to capture all diagnoses and procedures that occurred during this encounter.

For many reasons, the discharge summary is not the only document from which codes are captured.

- Coders may not have a discharge summary at the time of coding.
- If the patient is in the hospital for a long stay, often the attending physician will focus only on those diagnoses that were treated during the latter part of the stay.
- Physicians list conditions that are not currently under treatment and that appear only in the patient's history.
- Likewise, physicians describe diagnoses as "history of" when, in fact, they represent conditions that are being currently treated.

Most coders start the coding process as they begin their document review. A coder is continually trying to determine the principal diagnosis during the record review. Clues to determination of the principal diagnosis can be found in the ER record or in the admitting orders. Physicians, in their admitting orders, give a reason for admitting the patient. When evaluating an ER record, a coder first looks for the chief complaint (CC), which is the reason in the patient's own words for presenting to the hospital.

EXAMPLE

CC: I have a bad cough, fever, and headache, and my throat is so sore I can't even swallow liquids.

As the coder continues the review of the ER document, the ER physician provides a diagnosis for admission to the hospital. This may be a known diagnosis or a probable diagnosis, or it may include a differential diagnosis. In the previous example, the ER physician might document "Admit patient to the hospital for possible pneumonia and dehydration." In this case, the pneumonia has not yet been confirmed, but the dehydration is known.

A differential diagnosis occurs when a patient presents with a symptom that could represent a variety of diagnoses.

EXAMPLE

A patient presents with abdominal pain, and the physician suspects that this might represent appendicitis, gastroenteritis, or cholecystitis. Appendicitis, gastroenteritis, and cholecystitis are differential diagnoses.

A coder continues on through the health record, reviewing all progress notes, operative reports, anesthesiology notes, and consults to arrive at all diagnoses and procedures that need to be captured or reported.

The second most important concept that a coder must remember (after the definition of principal diagnosis and principal procedure) is that once a term has been located in the Alphabetic Index, the code must then be verified in the Tabular Index.

ALPHABETIC INDEX

The Alphabetic Index consists of an Alphabetic Index to Diseases and an Alphabetic Index to Procedures.

Locate the Main Term in the Index to Diseases

Once the coder begins to establish diagnoses and procedures, the first task in selecting a code is to locate the main term, which is always identified by bold type, in the Alphabetic Index.

EXAMPLE

Using pneumonia as the principal diagnosis, locate this term in the Alphabetic Index. The code for pneumonia is 486 (Figure 4-1).

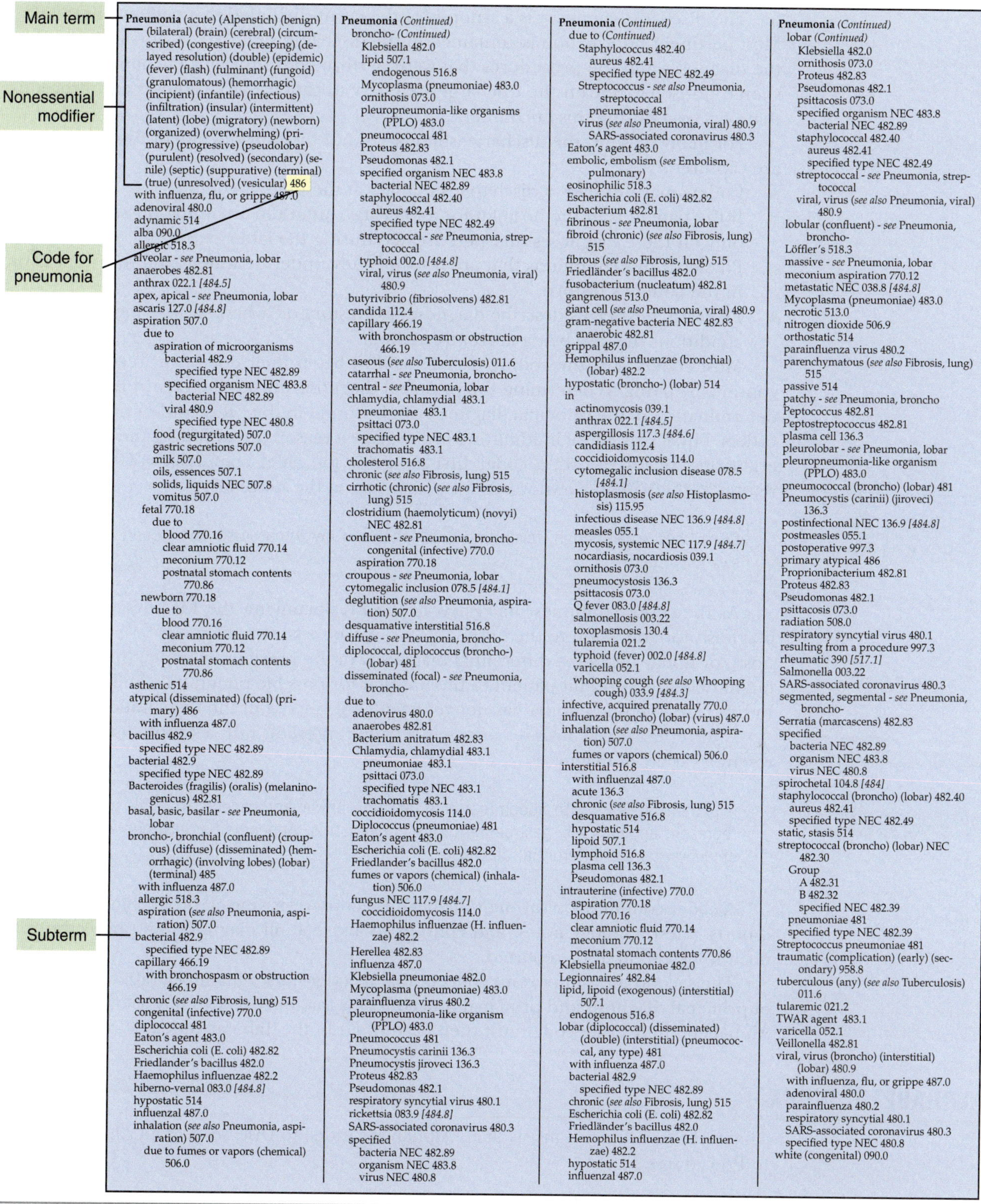

Pneumonia (acute) (Alpenstich) (benign) (bilateral) (brain) (cerebral) (circumscribed) (congestive) (creeping) (delayed resolution) (double) (epidemic) (fever) (flash) (fulminant) (fungoid) (granulomatous) (hemorrhagic) (incipient) (infantile) (infectious) (infiltration) (insular) (intermittent) (latent) (lobe) (migratory) (newborn) (organized) (overwhelming) (primary) (progressive) (pseudolobar) (purulent) (resolved) (secondary) (senile) (septic) (suppurative) (terminal) (true) (unresolved) (vesicular) 486
with influenza, flu, or grippe 487.0
adenoviral 480.0
adynamic 514
alba 090.0
allergic 518.3
alveolar - *see* Pneumonia, lobar
anaerobes 482.81
anthrax 022.1 *[484.5]*
apex, apical - *see* Pneumonia, lobar
ascaris 127.0 *[484.8]*
aspiration 507.0
due to
aspiration of microorganisms
bacterial 482.9
specified type NEC 482.89
specified organism NEC 483.8
bacterial NEC 482.89
viral 480.9
specified type NEC 480.8
food (regurgitated) 507.0
gastric secretions 507.0
milk 507.0
oils, essences 507.1
solids, liquids NEC 507.8
vomitus 507.0
fetal 770.18
due to
blood 770.16
clear amniotic fluid 770.14
meconium 770.12
postnatal stomach contents 770.86
newborn 770.18
due to
blood 770.16
clear amniotic fluid 770.14
meconium 770.12
postnatal stomach contents 770.86
asthenic 514
atypical (disseminated) (focal) (primary) 486
with influenza 487.0
bacillus 482.9
specified type NEC 482.89
bacterial 482.9
specified type NEC 482.89
Bacteroides (fragilis) (oralis) (melaninogenicus) 482.81
basal, basic, basilar - *see* Pneumonia, lobar
broncho-, bronchial (confluent) (croupous) (diffuse) (disseminated) (hemorrhagic) (involving lobes) (lobar) (terminal) 485
with influenza 487.0
allergic 518.3
aspiration (*see also* Pneumonia, aspiration) 507.0
bacterial 482.9
specified type NEC 482.89
capillary 466.19
with bronchospasm or obstruction 466.19
chronic (*see also* Fibrosis, lung) 515
congenital (infective) 770.0
diplococcal 481
Eaton's agent 483.0
Escherichia coli (E. coli) 482.82
Friedlander's bacillus 482.0
Haemophilus influenzae 482.2
hiberno-vernal 083.0 *[484.8]*
hypostatic 514
influenzal 487.0
inhalation (*see also* Pneumonia, aspiration) 507.0
due to fumes or vapors (chemical) 506.0

Pneumonia *(Continued)*
broncho- *(Continued)*
Klebsiella 482.0
lipid 507.1
endogenous 516.8
Mycoplasma (pneumoniae) 483.0
ornithosis 073.0
pleuropneumonia-like organisms (PPLO) 483.0
pneumococcal 481
Proteus 482.83
Pseudomonas 482.1
specified organism NEC 483.8
bacterial NEC 482.89
staphylococcal 482.40
aureus 482.41
specified type NEC 482.49
streptococcal - *see* Pneumonia, streptococcal
typhoid 002.0 *[484.8]*
viral, virus (*see also* Pneumonia, viral) 480.9
butyrivibrio (fibriosolvens) 482.81
candida 112.4
capillary 466.19
with bronchospasm or obstruction 466.19
caseous (*see also* Tuberculosis) 011.6
catarrhal - *see* Pneumonia, broncho-
central - *see* Pneumonia, lobar
chlamydia, chlamydial 483.1
pneumoniae 483.1
psittaci 073.0
specified type NEC 483.1
trachomatis 483.1
cholesterol 516.8
chronic (*see also* Fibrosis, lung) 515
cirrhotic (chronic) (*see also* Fibrosis, lung) 515
clostridium (haemolyticum) (novyi) NEC 482.81
confluent - *see* Pneumonia, broncho-
congenital (infective) 770.0
aspiration 770.18
croupous - *see* Pneumonia, lobar
cytomegalic inclusion 078.5 *[484.1]*
deglutition (*see also* Pneumonia, aspiration) 507.0
desquamative interstitial 516.8
diffuse - *see* Pneumonia, broncho-
diplococcal, diplococcus (broncho-) (lobar) 481
disseminated (focal) - *see* Pneumonia, broncho-
due to
adenovirus 480.0
anaerobes 482.81
Bacterium anitratum 482.83
Chlamydia, chlamydial 483.1
pneumoniae 483.1
psittaci 073.0
specified type NEC 483.1
trachomatis 483.1
coccidioidomycosis 114.0
Diplococcus (pneumoniae) 481
Eaton's agent 483.0
Escherichia coli (E. coli) 482.82
Friedlander's bacillus 482.0
fumes or vapors (chemical) (inhalation) 506.0
fungus NEC 117.9 *[484.7]*
coccidioidomycosis 114.0
Haemophilus influenzae (H. influenzae) 482.2
Herellea 482.83
influenza 487.0
Klebsiella pneumoniae 482.0
Mycoplasma (pneumoniae) 483.0
parainfluenza virus 480.2
pleuropneumonia-like organism (PPLO) 483.0
Pneumococcus 481
Pneumocystis carinii 136.3
Pneumocystis jiroveci 136.3
Proteus 482.83
Pseudomonas 482.1
respiratory syncytial virus 480.1
rickettsia 083.9 *[484.8]*
SARS-associated coronavirus 480.3
specified
bacteria NEC 482.89
organism NEC 483.8
virus NEC 480.8

Pneumonia *(Continued)*
due to *(Continued)*
Staphylococcus 482.40
aureus 482.41
specified type NEC 482.49
Streptococcus - *see also* Pneumonia, streptococcal
pneumoniae 481
virus (*see also* Pneumonia, viral) 480.9
SARS-associated coronavirus 480.3
Eaton's agent 483.0
embolic, embolism (*see* Embolism, pulmonary)
eosinophilic 518.3
Escherichia coli (E. coli) 482.82
eubacterium 482.81
fibrinous - *see* Pneumonia, lobar
fibroid (chronic) (*see also* Fibrosis, lung) 515
fibrous (*see also* Fibrosis, lung) 515
Friedländer's bacillus 482.0
fusobacterium (nucleatum) 482.81
gangrenous 513.0
giant cell (*see also* Pneumonia, viral) 480.9
gram-negative bacteria NEC 482.83
anaerobic 482.81
grippal 487.0
Hemophilus influenzae (bronchial) (lobar) 482.2
hypostatic (broncho-) (lobar) 514
in
actinomycosis 039.1
anthrax 022.1 *[484.5]*
aspergillosis 117.3 *[484.6]*
candidiasis 112.4
coccidioidomycosis 114.0
cytomegalic inclusion disease 078.5 *[484.1]*
histoplasmosis (*see also* Histoplasmosis) 115.95
infectious disease NEC 136.9 *[484.8]*
measles 055.1
mycosis, systemic NEC 117.9 *[484.7]*
nocardiasis, nocardiosis 039.1
ornithosis 073.0
pneumocystosis 136.3
psittacosis 073.0
Q fever 083.0 *[484.8]*
salmonellosis 003.22
toxoplasmosis 130.4
tularemia 021.2
typhoid (fever) 002.0 *[484.8]*
varicella 052.1
whooping cough (*see also* Whooping cough) 033.9 *[484.3]*
infective, acquired prenatally 770.0
influenzal (broncho) (lobar) (virus) 487.0
inhalation (*see also* Pneumonia, aspiration) 507.0
fumes or vapors (chemical) 506.0
interstitial 516.8
with influenzal 487.0
acute 136.3
chronic (*see also* Fibrosis, lung) 515
desquamative 516.8
hypostatic 514
lipoid 507.1
lymphoid 516.8
plasma cell 136.3
Pseudomonas 482.1
intrauterine (infective) 770.0
aspiration 770.18
blood 770.16
clear amniotic fluid 770.14
meconium 770.12
postnatal stomach contents 770.86
Klebsiella pneumoniae 482.0
Legionnaires' 482.84
lipid, lipoid (exogenous) (interstitial) 507.1
endogenous 516.8
lobar (diplococcal) (disseminated) (double) (interstitial) (pneumococcal, any type) 481
with influenza 487.0
bacterial 482.9
specified type NEC 482.89
chronic (*see also* Fibrosis, lung) 515
Escherichia coli (E. coli) 482.82
Friedländer's bacillus 482.0
Hemophilus influenzae (H. influenzae) 482.2
hypostatic 514
influenzal 487.0

Pneumonia *(Continued)*
lobar *(Continued)*
Klebsiella 482.0
ornithosis 073.0
Proteus 482.83
Pseudomonas 482.1
psittacosis 073.0
specified organism NEC 483.8
bacterial NEC 482.89
staphylococcal 482.40
aureus 482.41
specified type NEC 482.49
streptococcal - *see* Pneumonia, streptococcal
viral, virus (*see also* Pneumonia, viral) 480.9
lobular (confluent) - *see* Pneumonia, broncho-
Löffler's 518.3
massive - *see* Pneumonia, lobar
meconium aspiration 770.12
metastatic NEC 038.8 *[484.8]*
Mycoplasma (pneumoniae) 483.0
necrotic 513.0
nitrogen dioxide 506.9
orthostatic 514
parainfluenza virus 480.2
parenchymatous (*see also* Fibrosis, lung) 515
passive 514
patchy - *see* Pneumonia, broncho
Peptococcus 482.81
Peptostreptococcus 482.81
plasma cell 136.3
pleurolobar - *see* Pneumonia, lobar
pleuropneumonia-like organism (PPLO) 483.0
pneumococcal (broncho) (lobar) 481
Pneumocystis (carinii) (jiroveci) 136.3
postinfectional NEC 136.9 *[484.8]*
postmeasles 055.1
postoperative 997.3
primary atypical 486
Proprionibacterium 482.81
Proteus 482.83
Pseudomonas 482.1
psittacosis 073.0
radiation 508.0
respiratory syncytial virus 480.1
resulting from a procedure 997.3
rheumatic 390 *[517.1]*
Salmonella 003.22
SARS-associated coronavirus 480.3
segmented, segmental - *see* Pneumonia, broncho-
Serratia (marcascens) 482.83
specified
bacteria NEC 482.89
organism NEC 483.8
virus NEC 480.8
spirochetal 104.8 *[484]*
staphylococcal (broncho) (lobar) 482.40
aureus 482.41
specified type NEC 482.49
static, stasis 514
streptococcal (broncho) (lobar) NEC 482.30
Group
A 482.31
B 482.32
specified NEC 482.39
pneumoniae 481
specified type NEC 482.39
Streptococcus pneumoniae 481
traumatic (complication) (early) (secondary) 958.8
tuberculous (any) (*see also* Tuberculosis) 011.6
tularemic 021.2
TWAR agent 483.1
varicella 052.1
Veillonella 482.81
viral, virus (broncho) (interstitial) (lobar) 480.9
with influenza, flu, or grippe 487.0
adenoviral 480.0
parainfluenza 480.2
respiratory syncytial 480.1
SARS-associated coronavirus 480.3
specified type NEC 480.8
white (congenital) 090.0

Figure 4-1. Alphabetic Index entry for "pneumonia."

EXERCISE 4-1

Using Figure 4-1, assign ICD-9-CM codes to the following diagnoses:

1. Aspiration pneumonia __________
2. Pneumonia due to *Klebsiella pneumoniae* __________
3. Mycoplasma pneumonia __________
4. Varicella pneumonia __________
5. Viral pneumonia __________

After the main term, "pneumonia," in the Alphabetic Index, is a long list of **nonessential modifiers** (words in parentheses). Remember that nonessential modifiers have no effect on the main term. They are "take it or leave it" terms. Sometimes, the subterm that a coder is searching for can be found among the nonessential modifiers.

EXAMPLE

Granulomatous pneumonia is coded to 486.
Acute pneumonia, 486.
Fulminant pneumonia, 486. (See Figure 4-1)

In locating the main term, the coder must remember that main terms are usually identified by disease conditions and nouns. They are not body parts or sites. If a physician documents *Klebsiella pneumoniae* pneumonia, the noun is the main term and the one to be located in the Alphabetic Index. To find *Klebsiella pneumoniae* in the Alphabetic Index, the coder goes to "pneumonia" and looks for the subterm, "Klebsiella" (Figure 4-2).

Subterms are modifiers of main terms, and in contrast to nonessential modifiers, they do have an effect on the appropriate code assignment. To determine the main term, the coder must decide what condition the patient has (in this case, pneumonia), which is the main term; subterms are modifiers of the main term, which in this case is *Klebsiella pneumoniae.*

EXAMPLE

If a patient has a diagnosis of hiatal hernia, the main term is "hernia," and the subterm is "hiatal."

The main terms usually are nouns and/or disease conditions. The main terms below are underlined.

Gastric <u>upset</u>
Chronic <u>mastoiditis</u>
<u>Herpes</u> simplex

Likewise, in locating procedures, the coder starts by looking in the Alphabetic Index to procedures.

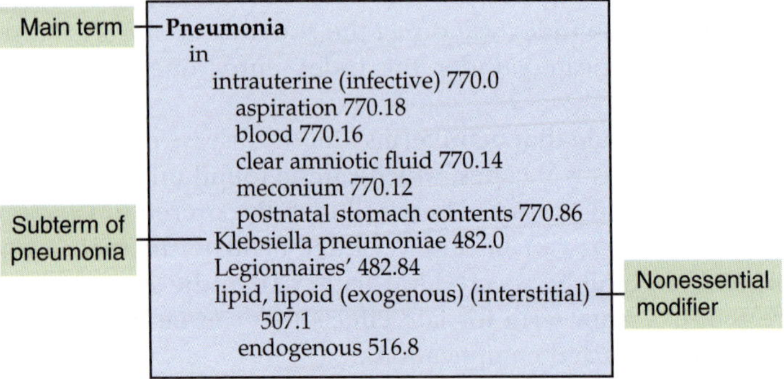

Figure 4-2. Example of subterm "Klebsiella," under "pneumonia."

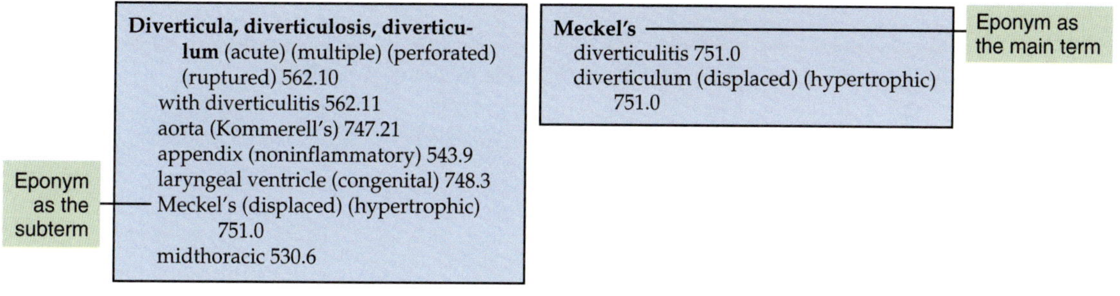

Figure 4-3. Example of multiple Alphabetic Index entries for Meckel's diverticulum.

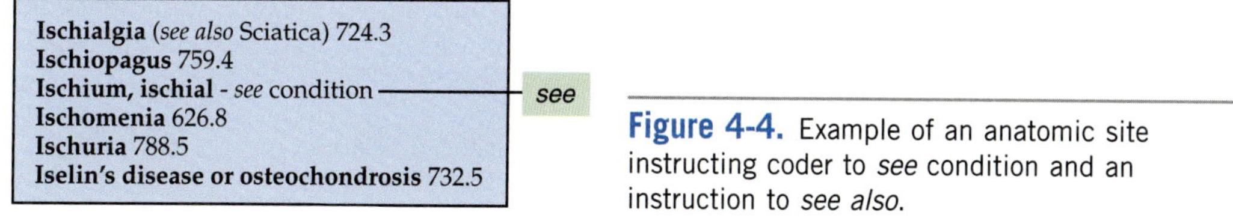

Figure 4-4. Example of an anatomic site instructing coder to *see* condition and an instruction to *see also*.

EXAMPLE

The patient has a diagnosis of appendicitis, and the operative report (OR) describes the procedure as a laparoscopic appendectomy.

Look up "appendectomy" in the Alphabetic Index and the subterm "laparoscopic," 47.01.

Sometimes, a main term may be found under more than one index entry (Figure 4-3). This is most often true of **eponyms** (a disease, syndrome or a procedure, named for a person). Adjectives and anatomic sites do appear as main terms, but they instruct the coder to see the condition (Figure 4-4).

EXAMPLE

Diagnosis of ischial fracture: The Index for "ischial" would direct the coder to go to the condition or, in this case, fracture.

Ischium, ischial—*see* condition

EXAMPLE

Chronic otitis media—look up "chronic" in the Alphabetic Index

Chronic—*see* condition

The term ***see*** is a mandatory direction to look elsewhere in the Alphabetic Index.

Sometimes, the Index will direct the coder to *see also*. This instruction means that if the term cannot be located under the Index entry, one should go to the suggested Index entry.

The general rule that main terms identify disease conditions has some exceptions. One of these exceptions is V codes, which can be found under main terms such as "admission," "examination," and "status." These will be fully covered in Chapter 8 on V codes. Likewise, obstetric conditions can be found under main terms such as "pregnancy," "labor," and "puerperal" and will be covered in Chapter 16 in the section on obstetrics and gynecology. There is also a main term for late effects that can be used to identify residuals of various disease conditions and complications.

Locating a main term may be difficult because of the terminology used by the physician or because an eponym is used. For example, physicians often describe arterial lines used

for monitoring as Swan Ganz (pulmonary capillary wedge monitoring). If the coder were to look under "Swan Ganz" in the procedural Alphabetic Index, no listing would be found. In these cases, the coder should try alternative terminology.

EXAMPLE

Swan Ganz is a type of catheter. Try looking under "Catheterization, Swan Ganz" in the procedure Alphabetic Index, 89.64.

Locate the Main Term in the Index to Procedures

Just as in diagnoses, once a procedure is determined to have been performed, a coder searches for that procedure in the Alphabetic Index to Procedures. The main terms for procedures are identified by the type of procedure performed and not by the anatomic site. When one is having trouble locating a procedure, it is wise to remember that many procedures can be found under the terms, "excision," "incision," or "removal."

EXAMPLE

Removal of a skin lesion, 86.4 (Figure 4-5).
Needle biopsy of the liver, 50.11 (Figure 4-6).

- **Excision** *(Continued)*
  - lesion *(Continued)*
    - odontogenic 24.4
    - omentum 54.4
    - orbit 16.92
    - ovary 65.29
      - by wedge resection 65.22
        - laparoscopic 65.24
      - that by laparoscope 65.25
    - palate (bony) 27.31
      - by wide excision 27.32
      - soft 27.49
    - pancreas (local) 52.22
      - endoscopic 52.21
    - parathyroid 06.89
    - parotid gland or duct NEC 26.29
    - pelvic wall 54.3
    - pelvirectal tissue 48.82
    - penis 64.2
    - pericardium 37.31
    - perineum (female) 71.3
      - male 86.3
    - periprostatic tissue 60.82
    - perirectal tissue 48.82
    - perirenal tissue 59.91
    - peritoneum 54.4
    - perivesical tissue 59.91
    - pharynx 29.3
      - diverticulum 29.32
    - pineal gland 07.53
    - pinna 18.29
      - radical 18.31
    - pituitary (gland) - *see also* Hypophysectomy, partial 07.63
      - by stereotactic radiosurgery 92.30
        - cobalt 60 92.32
        - linear accelerator (LINAC) 92.31
        - multi-source 92.32

- **Excision** *(Continued)*
  - lesion *(Continued)*
        - particle beam 92.33
        - particulate 92.33
        - radiosurgery NEC 92.39
        - single source photon 92.31
    - pleura 34.59
    - pouch of Douglas 70.32
    - preauricular (ear) 18.21
    - presacral 54.4
    - prostate (transurethral) 60.61
    - pulmonary (fibrosis) 32.29
      - endoscopic 32.28
    - rectovaginal septum 48.82
    - rectum 48.35
      - polyp (endoscopic) 48.36
    - retroperitoneum 54.4
    - salivary gland or duct NEC 26.29
      - en bloc 26.32
    - sclera 12.84
    - scrotum 61.3
    - sinus (nasal) - *see* Excision, lesion, nasal sinus
    - Skene's gland 71.3
    - skin 86.3 — Excision lesion skin
      - breast 85.21
      - nose 21.32
      - radical (wide) (involving underlying or adjacent structure) (with flap closure) 86.4
      - scrotum 61.3
    - skull 01.6
    - soft tissue NEC 83.39
      - hand 82.29
    - spermatic cord 63.3
    - sphincter of Oddi 51.62
      - endoscopic 51.64
    - spinal cord (meninges) 03.4
    - spleen (cyst) 41.42
    - stomach NEC 43.42

- **Excision** *(Continued)*
  - lesion *(Continued)*
      - endoscopic 43.41
        - polyp 43.41
      - polyp (endoscopic) 43.41
    - subcutaneous tissue 86.3
      - breast 85.21
    - subgingival 24.31
    - sweat gland 86.3
    - tendon 83.39
      - hand 82.29
      - ocular 15.13
      - sheath 83.31
        - hand 82.21
    - testis 62.2
    - thorax 34.4
    - thymus 07.81
    - thyroid 06.31
      - substernal or transsternal route 06.51
    - tongue 25.1
    - tonsil 28.92
    - trachea 31.5
    - tunica vaginalis 61.92
    - ureter 56.41
    - urethra 58.39
      - endoscopic 58.31
    - uterine ligament 69.19
    - uterosacral ligament 69.19
    - uterus 68.29
    - vagina 70.33
    - vein 38.60
      - abdominal 38.67
      - head and neck NEC 38.62
      - intracranial NEC 38.61
      - lower limb 38.69
      - thoracic NEC 38.65
      - upper limb 38.63
    - ventricle (heart) 37.33
    - vocal cords 30.09
    - vulva 71.3

Figure 4-5. Example from entry for "excision skin lesion" in the Index to Procedures.

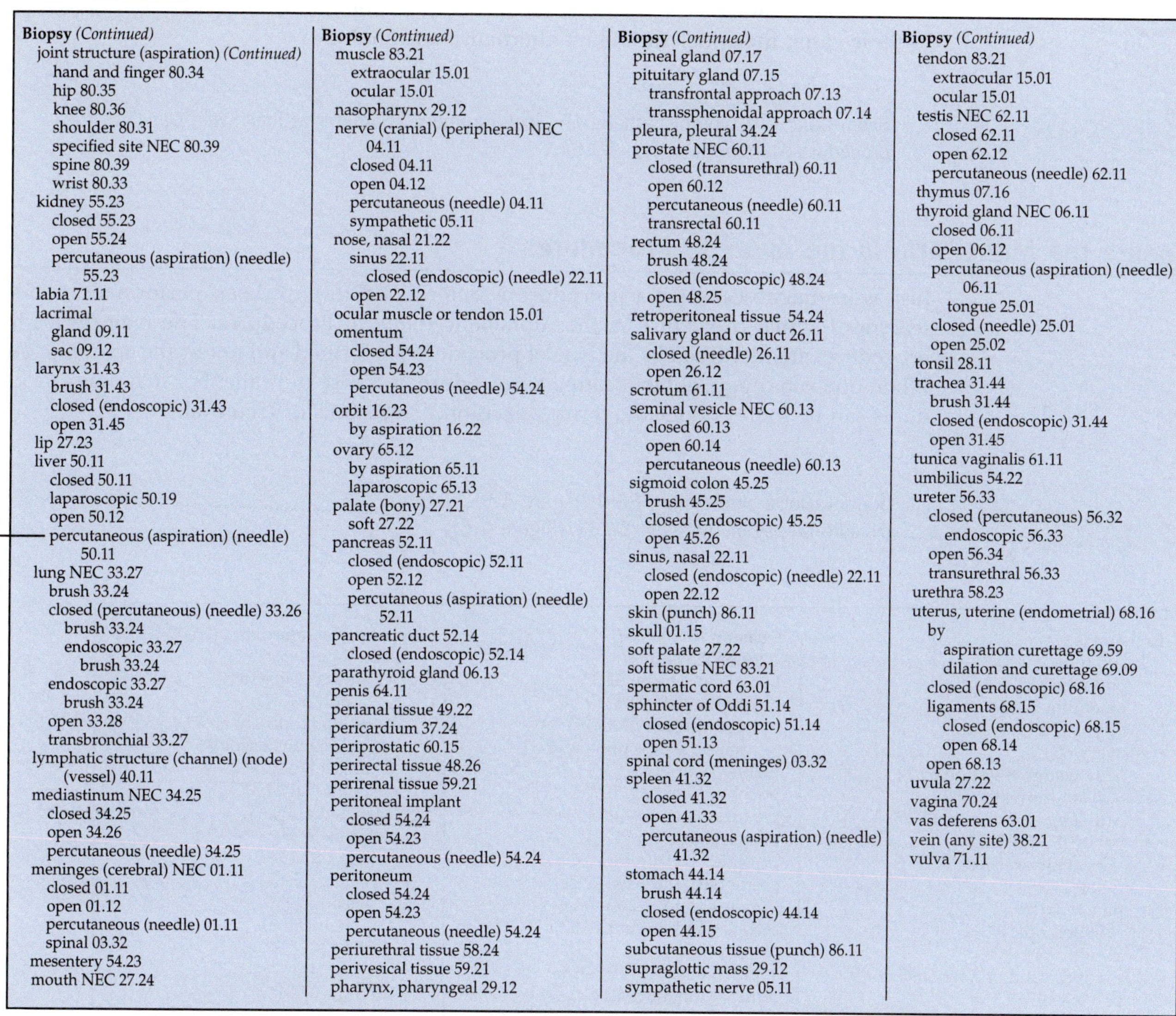

Biopsy *(Continued)*
- joint structure (aspiration) *(Continued)*
  - hand and finger 80.34
  - hip 80.35
  - knee 80.36
  - shoulder 80.31
  - specified site NEC 80.39
  - spine 80.39
  - wrist 80.33
- kidney 55.23
  - closed 55.23
  - open 55.24
  - percutaneous (aspiration) (needle) 55.23
- labia 71.11
- lacrimal
  - gland 09.11
  - sac 09.12
- larynx 31.43
  - brush 31.43
  - closed (endoscopic) 31.43
  - open 31.45
- lip 27.23
- liver 50.11
  - closed 50.11
  - laparoscopic 50.19
  - open 50.12
  - percutaneous (aspiration) (needle) 50.11
- lung NEC 33.27
  - brush 33.24
  - closed (percutaneous) (needle) 33.26
    - brush 33.24
    - endoscopic 33.27
      - brush 33.24
  - endoscopic 33.27
    - brush 33.24
  - open 33.28
  - transbronchial 33.27
- lymphatic structure (channel) (node) (vessel) 40.11
- mediastinum NEC 34.25
  - closed 34.25
  - open 34.26
  - percutaneous (needle) 34.25
- meninges (cerebral) NEC 01.11
  - closed 01.11
  - open 01.12
  - percutaneous (needle) 01.11
  - spinal 03.32
- mesentery 54.23
- mouth NEC 27.24

Biopsy *(Continued)*
- muscle 83.21
  - extraocular 15.01
  - ocular 15.01
- nasopharynx 29.12
- nerve (cranial) (peripheral) NEC 04.11
  - closed 04.11
  - open 04.12
  - percutaneous (needle) 04.11
  - sympathetic 05.11
- nose, nasal 21.22
  - sinus 22.11
    - closed (endoscopic) (needle) 22.11
  - open 22.12
- ocular muscle or tendon 15.01
- omentum
  - closed 54.24
  - open 54.23
  - percutaneous (needle) 54.24
- orbit 16.23
  - by aspiration 16.22
- ovary 65.12
  - by aspiration 65.11
  - laparoscopic 65.13
- palate (bony) 27.21
  - soft 27.22
- pancreas 52.11
  - closed (endoscopic) 52.11
  - open 52.12
  - percutaneous (aspiration) (needle) 52.11
- pancreatic duct 52.14
  - closed (endoscopic) 52.14
- parathyroid gland 06.13
- penis 64.11
- perianal tissue 49.22
- pericardium 37.24
- periprostatic 60.15
- perirectal tissue 48.26
- perirenal tissue 59.21
- peritoneal implant
  - closed 54.24
  - open 54.23
  - percutaneous (needle) 54.24
- peritoneum
  - closed 54.24
  - open 54.23
  - percutaneous (needle) 54.24
- periurethral tissue 58.24
- perivesical tissue 59.21
- pharynx, pharyngeal 29.12

Biopsy *(Continued)*
- pineal gland 07.17
- pituitary gland 07.15
  - transfrontal approach 07.13
  - transsphenoidal approach 07.14
- pleura, pleural 34.24
- prostate NEC 60.11
  - closed (transurethral) 60.11
  - open 60.12
  - percutaneous (needle) 60.11
  - transrectal 60.11
- rectum 48.24
  - brush 48.24
  - closed (endoscopic) 48.24
  - open 48.25
- retroperitoneal tissue 54.24
- salivary gland or duct 26.11
  - closed (needle) 26.11
  - open 26.12
- scrotum 61.11
- seminal vesicle NEC 60.13
  - closed 60.13
  - open 60.14
  - percutaneous (needle) 60.13
- sigmoid colon 45.25
  - brush 45.25
  - closed (endoscopic) 45.25
  - open 45.26
- sinus, nasal 22.11
  - closed (endoscopic) (needle) 22.11
  - open 22.12
- skin (punch) 86.11
- skull 01.15
- soft palate 27.22
- soft tissue NEC 83.21
- spermatic cord 63.01
- sphincter of Oddi 51.14
  - closed (endoscopic) 51.14
  - open 51.13
- spinal cord (meninges) 03.32
- spleen 41.32
  - closed 41.32
  - open 41.33
  - percutaneous (aspiration) (needle) 41.32
- stomach 44.14
  - brush 44.14
  - closed (endoscopic) 44.14
  - open 44.15
- subcutaneous tissue (punch) 86.11
- supraglottic mass 29.12
- sympathetic nerve 05.11

Biopsy *(Continued)*
- tendon 83.21
  - extraocular 15.01
  - ocular 15.01
- testis NEC 62.11
  - closed 62.11
  - open 62.12
  - percutaneous (needle) 62.11
- thymus 07.16
- thyroid gland NEC 06.11
  - closed 06.11
  - open 06.12
  - percutaneous (aspiration) (needle) 06.11
    - tongue 25.01
  - closed (needle) 25.01
  - open 25.02
- tonsil 28.11
- trachea 31.44
  - brush 31.44
  - closed (endoscopic) 31.44
  - open 31.45
- tunica vaginalis 61.11
- umbilicus 54.22
- ureter 56.33
  - closed (percutaneous) 56.32
    - endoscopic 56.33
  - open 56.34
  - transurethral 56.33
- urethra 58.23
- uterus, uterine (endometrial) 68.16
  - by
    - aspiration curettage 69.59
    - dilation and curettage 69.09
  - closed (endoscopic) 68.16
  - ligaments 68.15
    - closed (endoscopic) 68.15
    - open 68.14
  - open 68.13
- uvula 27.22
- vagina 70.24
- vas deferens 63.01
- vein (any site) 38.21
- vulva 71.11

Figure 4-6. Example from the entry for "needle, biopsy liver" in the Index to Procedures.

EXERCISE 4-2

Underline all main terms to be located in the Alphabetic Index.

1. Esophageal reflux
2. Tourette's disease
3. Iatrogenic thyroiditis
4. Infantile eczema
5. Coronary artery disease
6. Congestive heart failure
7. Rheumatoid arthritis
8. Atrial fibrillation
9. Sickle cell anemia
10. Coronary artery bypass, one-vessel

11. Inguinal hernia repair
12. Excision herniated disc
13. Balloon angioplasty
14. Open reduction internal fixation
15. Vaginal hysterectomy
16. Calculus of the ureter

TABULAR LIST

Once the code has been selected from the Alphabetic Index, it must then be verified in the **Tabular List**. Sometimes, a code that is selected from the Alphabetic Index does not seem to match what is described in the Tabular. If this is the case, the coder should review the Alphabetic Index and the Tabular for all exclusion notes and other instructional notes. It may require that the coder browse the category in the Tabular for a more representative code. It also may require that the coder access *Coding Clinic* for any up-to-date information on how to code a specific diagnosis. It is possible that coding advice given in *Coding Clinic* may override the Index (see "arteriovenous malformation" example below).

EXAMPLE

Documentation in the chart describes the patient as having anorexia. She has been admitted to the psychiatric unit of the hospital.

Look up "Anorexia" in the Alphabetic Index, 783.0.

Go to the Tabular List and review the Excludes notes.

Because this is a psychiatric admission, reviewing the codes excluded may assist in assigning the correct code.

EXAMPLE

The diagnosis is stated as arteriovenous malformation of the intestine.

Look under "Malformation, colon" in the Alphabetic Index.

This directs the coder to "*see also* Anomaly."

"Anomaly colon" directs the coder to 751.5.

Look up 751.5 in the Tabular, and decide whether this appears to be the correct code.

Look up "arteriovenous malformation" in *Coding Clinic.*

Coding Clinic (1986:Nov-Dec:p11)[1] directs the coder to use "557.1, Chronic vascular insufficiency of intestine."

The rule of never coding directly from the Alphabetic Index without reviewing the Tabular also applies to never coding from instructional notes within the Tabular without first reviewing the actual Tabular Listing of the code.

EXAMPLE

The instructional notes found in category 601 recommend the use of an additional code to identify the organism Staph (041.1) or Strep (041.0). If these codes were captured without review of the Tabular, an invalid code would be assigned because both require fifth digits.

CHAPTER REVIEW EXERCISE

Using the Alphabetic Index and the Tabular List, code all the following diagnoses and procedures.

1. Acute subendocardial infarction, initial episode of care ____________
2. *Clostridium difficile* enteritis ____________
3. Refractory megaloblastic anemia ____________
4. Acute suppurative appendicitis with laparoscopic appendectomy ____________
5. Decubitus ulcer of the sacrum treated with excisional debridement ____________
6. Abdominal aortic aneurysm treated with aneurysm repair ____________
7. Small-bowel obstruction treated with left hemicolectomy ____________
8. Partial psychomotor epilepsy ____________
9. Paroxysmal supraventricular tachycardia ____________
10. Streptococcal group A pneumonia ____________
11. Deep vein thrombosis of the femoral artery ____________
12. Acute congenital syphilitic laryngotracheitis ____________
13. Dysphagia as a late effect of a stroke ____________
14. Adhesive bursitis of the shoulder ____________
15. History of cardiovascular disease in the family ____________

CHAPTER GLOSSARY

Alphabetic Index: the index found in the ICD-9-CM book for both disease conditions and procedures.

Chief Complaint: the reason in the patient's own words for presenting to the hospital.

Differential Diagnosis: when a symptom may represent a variety of diagnoses.

Discharge Summary: a review of the patient's hospital course. This summary details the reason for admission or tests or procedures performed and how the patient responded.

Eponym: term for a disease, structure, procedure, or syndrome that has been named for a person.

Main term: term that identifies disease conditions or injuries in the Alphabetic Index.

Nonessential Modifier: term that is enclosed in parentheses; its presence or absence does not affect code assignment.

Principal Diagnosis: condition established after study to be chiefly responsible for occasioning admission of the patient to the hospital for care.

See: mandatory term to look elsewhere in the Alphabetic Index.

Specificity: coding to the greatest detail of a code. Coding to the fourth or fifth digit as necessary.

Subterm: gives more specific information about a main term. Subterms identify site, type, or etiology of a disease condition or injury. Also, modifiers that are indented to the right of the main term.

Tabular List: section of the ICD-9-CM book that contains the code listing, along with exclusion or inclusion notes.

CHAPTER 5

General Coding Guidelines for Diagnosis

(Volumes 1 and 2)

CHAPTER OUTLINE

LEARNING OBJECTIVES

- Apply ICD-9-CM Official Guidelines for Coding and Reporting
- Sequence ICD-9-CM diagnosis codes as directed by coding guidelines or ICD-9-CM conventions
- Determine whether signs, symptoms, or manifestations require separate code assignments

ABBREVIATIONS

AHA American Hospital Association
AHIMA American Health Information Management Association
CMS Centers for Medicare and Medicaid Services
DHHS U.S. Department of Health and Human Services
DRA Deficit Reduction Act
GPO Government Printing Office
HIPAA Health Insurance Portability and Accountability Act
ICD-9-CM *International Classification of Diseases, 9th Revision, Clinical Modification*
NCHS National Center for Health Statistics
POA Present on Admission

ICD-9-CM OFFICIAL GUIDELINES FOR CODING AND REPORTING

The ICD-9-CM Official Guidelines for Coding and Reporting were developed by the cooperating parties to provide further guidance regarding coding and sequencing that is not provided in the ICD-9-CM manual. These guidelines do not cover every situation and have been formatted in a manner that will allow for expansion as new guidelines are developed. The guidelines may be changed each year and changes may have greater impact in some years than in others.

In this chapter, the coder will review the general guidelines and coding examples as applicable. The convention guidelines with examples were presented in Chapter 3, "ICD-9-CM, Format and Conventions." Chapter-specific guidelines are provided and explained in the respective disease or body system chapter.

ICD-9-CM Official Guidelines for Coding and Reporting

Please refer to the companion Evolve website for the most current guidelines.

Effective October 1, 2007

Narrative changes appear in bold text

Items underlined have been moved within the guidelines since November 15, 2006

The guidelines include the updated V Code Table

The Centers for Medicare and Medicaid Services (CMS) and the National Center for Health Statistics (NCHS), two departments within the U.S. Federal Government's Department of Health and Human Services (DHHS) provide the following guidelines for coding and reporting using the International Classification of Diseases, 9th Revision, Clinical Modification (ICD-9-CM). These guidelines should be used as a companion document to the official version of the ICD-9-CM as published on CD-ROM by the U.S. Government Printing Office (GPO).

These guidelines have been approved by the four organizations that make up the Cooperating Parties for the ICD-9-CM: the American Hospital Association (AHA), the American Health Information Management Association (AHIMA), CMS, and NCHS. These guidelines are included on the official government version of the ICD-9-CM, and also appear in "*Coding Clinic for ICD-9-CM*" published by the AHA.

These guidelines are a set of rules that have been developed to accompany and complement the official conventions and instructions provided within the ICD-9-CM itself. These guidelines are based on the coding and sequencing instructions in Volumes I, II and III of ICD-9-CM, but provide additional instruction. Adherence to these guidelines when assigning ICD-9-CM diagnosis and procedure codes is required under the Health Insurance Portability and Accountability Act (HIPAA). The diagnosis codes (Volumes 1-2) have been adopted under HIPAA for all healthcare settings. Volume 3 procedure codes have been adopted for inpatient procedures reported by hospitals. A joint effort between the healthcare provider and the coder is essential to achieve complete and accurate documentation, code assignment, and reporting of diagnoses and procedures. These guidelines have been developed to assist both the healthcare provider and the coder in identifying those diagnoses and procedures that are to be reported. The importance of consistent, complete documentation in the medical record cannot be overemphasized. Without such documentation accurate coding cannot be achieved. The entire record should be reviewed to determine the specific reason for the encounter and the conditions treated.

The term encounter is used for all settings, including hospital admissions. In the context of these guidelines, the term provider is used throughout the guidelines to mean physician or any qualified health care practitioner who is legally accountable for establishing the patient's diagnosis. Only this set of guidelines, approved by the Cooperating Parties, is official.

The guidelines are organized into sections. Section I includes the structure and conventions of the classification and general guidelines that apply to the entire classification, and chapter-specific guidelines that correspond to the chapters as they are arranged in the classification. Section II includes guidelines for selection of principal diagnosis for non-outpatient settings. Section III includes guidelines for reporting additional diagnoses in non-outpatient settings. Section IV is for outpatient coding and reporting.

GENERAL CODING GUIDELINES

General coding guidelines apply to all healthcare settings and to the entire ICD-9-CM classification system.

Section I. Conventions, general coding guidelines and chapter specific guidelines

B. General Coding Guidelines

1. Use of Both Alphabetic Index and Tabular List

Use both the Alphabetic Index and the Tabular List when locating and assigning a code. Reliance on only the Alphabetic Index or the Tabular List leads to errors in code assignments and less specificity in code selection.

Threatened
abortion or miscarriage 640.0
with subsequent abortion (*see also* Abortion, spontaneous) 634.9
affecting fetus 762.1
labor 644.1
affecting fetus or newborn 761.8
premature 644.0
miscarriage 640.0
affecting fetus 762.1
premature
delivery 644.2
affecting fetus or newborn 761.8
labor 644.0
before 22 completed weeks of gestation 640.0

Figure 5-1. Alphabetic Index entry for "threatened miscarriage."

EXAMPLE

Patient presents with threatened miscarriage. She is discharged home the next day with viable pregnancy. Threatened miscarriage: Under the main term "threatened" and the subterm "miscarriage" in the Alphabetic Index, code 640.0 is listed. If the coder were to assign this code, it would be an invalid code. Verification in the Tabular List reveals that a fifth digit is required. The correct code assignment for "threatened miscarriage" is 640.03. (see Figures 5-1 and 5-2)

2. **Locate each term in the Alphabetic Index**
Locate each term in the Alphabetic Index and verify the code selected in the Tabular List. Read and be guided by instructional notations that appear in both the Alphabetic Index and the Tabular List. (See Figures 5-3 and 5-4.)

Instructional notes can be found in all three volumes. It is important to review the Tabular code category for notes that may apply to the entire category. These notes can be found at the beginning of a chapter, section, code category, or individual code classification. For additional details on various instructional notes, refer to Chapter 3 in this text.

3. **Level of Detail in Coding**
Diagnosis and procedure codes are to be used at their highest number of digits available.

ICD-9-CM diagnosis codes are composed of codes with either 3, 4, or 5 digits. Codes with three digits are included in ICD-9-CM as the heading of a category of codes that may be further subdivided by the use of fourth and/or fifth digits, which provide greater detail.

A three-digit code is to be used only if it is not further subdivided. Where fourth-digit subcategories and/or fifth-digit subclassifications are provided, they must be assigned. A code is invalid if it has not been coded to the full number of digits required for that code. For example, Acute myocardial infarction, code 410, has fourth digits that describe the location of the infarction (e.g., 410.2, Of inferolateral wall), and fifth digits that identify the episode of care. It would be incorrect to report a code in category 410 without a fourth and fifth digit.

ICD-9-CM Volume 3 procedure codes are composed of codes with either 3 or 4 digits. Codes with two digits are included in ICD-9-CM as the heading of a category of codes that may be further subdivided by the use of third and/or fourth digits, which provide greater detail.

EXAMPLE

Bronchitis, 490 (three-digit code).
Chronic bronchitis, 491.9 (four-digit code).
Emphysematous bronchitis, 491.20 (five-digit code).

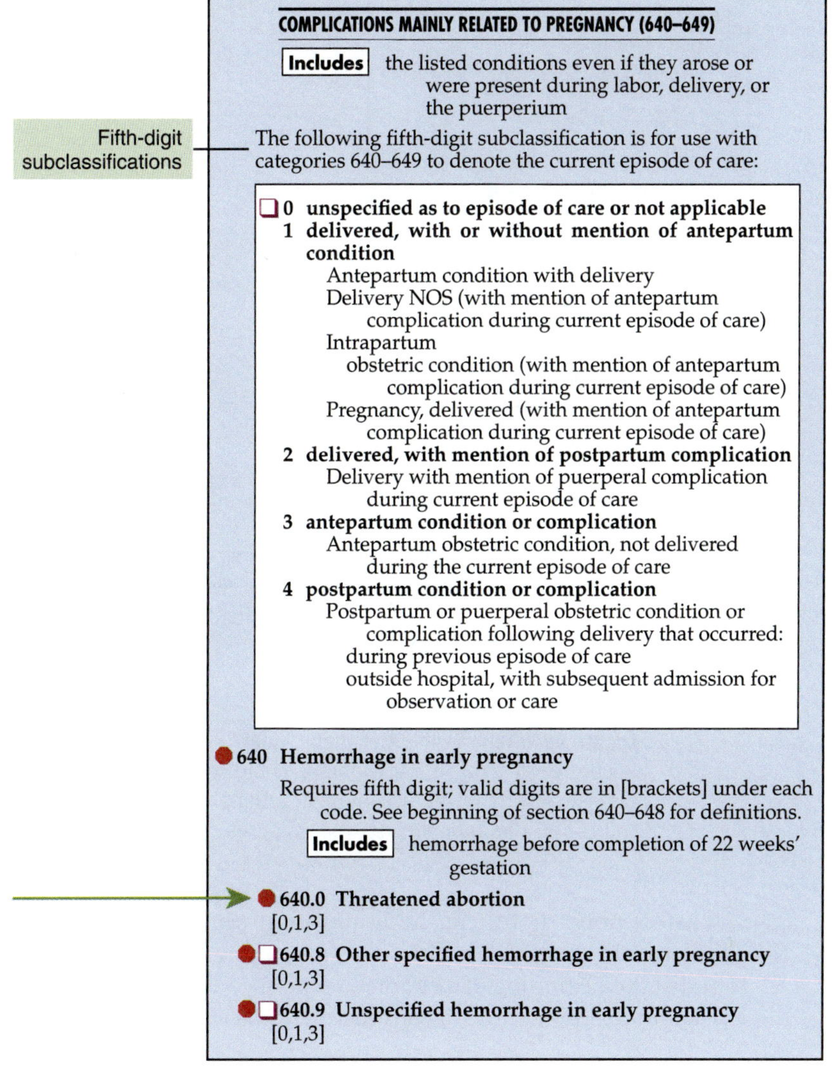

COMPLICATIONS MAINLY RELATED TO PREGNANCY (640–649)

Includes the listed conditions even if they arose or were present during labor, delivery, or the puerperium

The following fifth-digit subclassification is for use with categories 640–649 to denote the current episode of care:

0 unspecified as to episode of care or not applicable
1 delivered, with or without mention of antepartum condition
Antepartum condition with delivery
Delivery NOS (with mention of antepartum complication during current episode of care)
Intrapartum
obstetric condition (with mention of antepartum complication during current episode of care)
Pregnancy, delivered (with mention of antepartum complication during current episode of care)
2 delivered, with mention of postpartum complication
Delivery with mention of puerperal complication during current episode of care
3 antepartum condition or complication
Antepartum obstetric condition, not delivered during the current episode of care
4 postpartum condition or complication
Postpartum or puerperal obstetric condition or complication following delivery that occurred:
during previous episode of care
outside hospital, with subsequent admission for observation or care

640 Hemorrhage in early pregnancy
Requires fifth digit; valid digits are in [brackets] under each code. See beginning of section 640–648 for definitions.
Includes hemorrhage before completion of 22 weeks' gestation

640.0 Threatened abortion
[0,1,3]
640.8 Other specified hemorrhage in early pregnancy
[0,1,3]
640.9 Unspecified hemorrhage in early pregnancy
[0,1,3]

Figure 5-2. Tabular List entry with fifth-digit subclassifications.

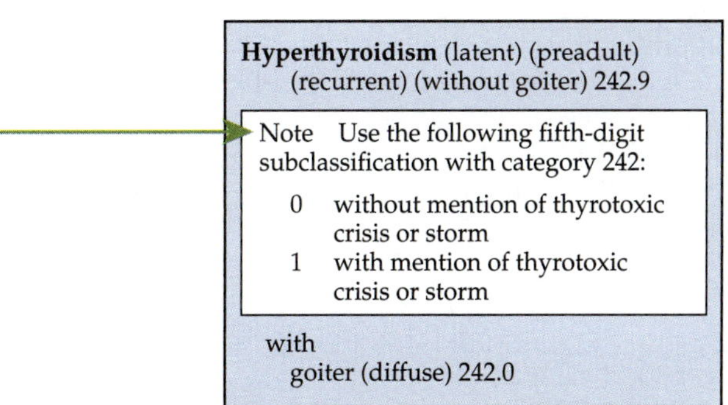

Hyperthyroidism (latent) (preadult) (recurrent) (without goiter) 242.9

Note Use the following fifth-digit subclassification with category 242:
0 without mention of thyrotoxic crisis or storm
1 with mention of thyrotoxic crisis or storm

with
goiter (diffuse) 242.0

Figure 5-3. Instructional note from Alphabetic Index.

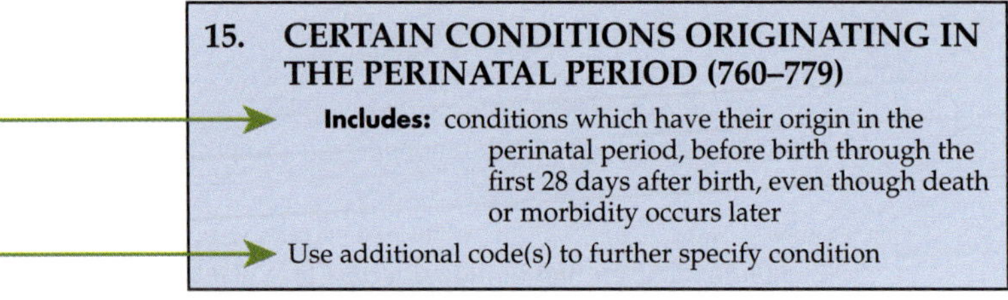
15. CERTAIN CONDITIONS ORIGINATING IN THE PERINATAL PERIOD (760–779)

Includes: conditions which have their origin in the perinatal period, before birth through the first 28 days after birth, even though death or morbidity occurs later

Use additional code(s) to further specify condition

Figure 5-4. Instructional notes from Tabular List.

EXERCISE 5-1

Using the Alphabetic Index and the Tabular List, assign the appropriate code(s).

1. Status asthmaticus
   Code from Alphabetic Index ______________
   Code following verification in Tabular List ______________
2. Hairy cell leukemia in remission
   Code from Alphabetic Index ______________
   Code following verification in Tabular List ______________
3. Closed fracture humerus
   Code from Alphabetic Index ______________
   Code following verification in Tabular List ______________
4. Epilepsy
   Code from Alphabetic Index ______________
   Code following verification in Tabular List ______________
5. Right upper quadrant pain
   Code from Alphabetic Index ______________
   Code following verification in Tabular List ______________

4. **Code or codes from 001.0 through V89**
   The appropriate code or codes from 001.0 through V89 must be used to identify diagnoses, symptoms, conditions, problems, complaints, or other reason(s) for the encounter/visit.
5. **Selection of codes 001.0 through 999.9**
   The selection of codes 001.0 through 999.9 will frequently be used to describe the reason for the admission/encounter. These codes are from the section of ICD-9-CM for the classification of diseases and injuries (e.g., infectious and parasitic diseases; neoplasms; symptoms, signs, and ill-defined conditions, etc.).
6. **Signs and symptoms**
   Codes that describe symptoms and signs, as opposed to diagnoses, are acceptable for reporting purposes when a related definitive diagnosis has not been established (confirmed) by the provider. Chapter 16 of ICD-9-CM, Symptoms, Signs, and Ill-defined conditions (codes 780.0-799.9) contain many, but not all codes for symptoms.

EXAMPLE

Pyrexia of unknown origin, 780.6.

7. **Conditions that are an integral part of a disease process**
   Signs and symptoms that are **associated routinely with** a disease process should not be assigned as additional codes, unless otherwise instructed by the classification.

EXAMPLE

Hematuria due to calculus of kidney, 592.0.
Code 599.70 for "hematuria" would not be assigned because hematuria is integral to a kidney stone. According to *Coding Clinic* (1995:3Q:p8)[1], "hematuria is a usual finding in a patient with renal stones and is considered integral to the condition."

8. **Conditions that are not an integral part of a disease process**
   Additional signs and symptoms that may not be associated routinely with a disease process should be coded when present.

EXAMPLE

Ascites due to cirrhosis of the liver, 571.5, 789.59

Chapter 16 of ICD-9-CM contains most but not all codes used to identify signs and symptoms (780.0 to 799.9).

Signs and symptoms codes are acceptable to code:

- When no definitive diagnosis has been established
- When they are not an integral part of the disease process

It is not acceptable to code signs or symptoms:

- When a definitive diagnosis has been established
- When they are an integral part of the disease process

EXERCISE 5-2

Identify integral and nonintegral conditions by answering the following questions.

1. List two common symptoms of gallstones. _______________
2. List the symptom most commonly associated with costochondritis. _______________
3. List two common symptoms of urinary tract infection. _______________
4. A patient has osteoarthritis and anemia. The anemia is integral to the osteoarthritis.
   A. True
   B. False
5. A patient has dyspnea caused by congestive heart failure. Dyspnea should be assigned as an additional code.
   A. True
   B. False

9. **Multiple coding for a single condition**
   In addition to the etiology/manifestation convention that requires two codes to fully describe a single condition that affects multiple body systems, there are other single conditions that also require more than one code. "Use additional code" notes (Figure 5-5) are found in the tabular at codes that are not part of an etiology/manifestation pair where a secondary code is useful to fully describe a condition. The sequencing rule is the same as the etiology/manifestation pair - , "use additional code" indicates that a secondary code should be added.

   For example, for infections that are not included in chapter 1, a secondary code from category 041, Bacterial infection in conditions classified elsewhere and of unspecified site, may be required to identify the bacterial organism causing the infection. A "use additional code" note will normally be found at the infectious disease code, indicating a need for the organism code to be added as a secondary code.

● 590 **Infections of kidney**
Use additional code to identify organism, such as Escherichia coli [E. coli] (041.4)

Figure 5-5. Instruction to "Use additional code" if applicable.

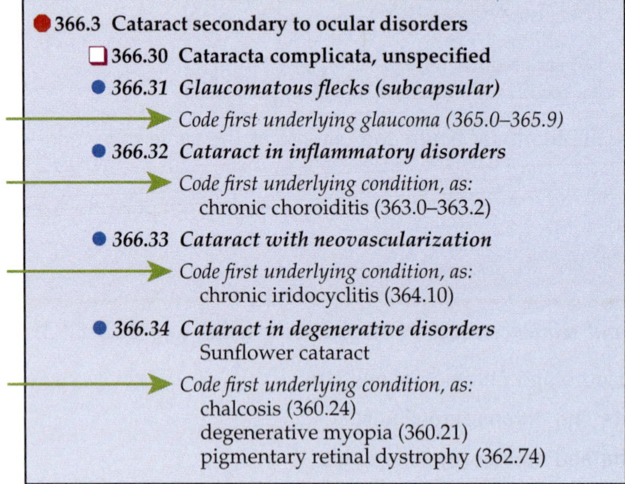
● 366.3 **Cataract secondary to ocular disorders**
❑ 366.30 **Cataracta complicata, unspecified**
● 366.31 ***Glaucomatous flecks (subcapsular)***
Code first underlying glaucoma (365.0–365.9)
● 366.32 ***Cataract in inflammatory disorders***
Code first underlying condition, as:
chronic choroiditis (363.0–363.2)
● 366.33 ***Cataract with neovascularization***
Code first underlying condition, as:
chronic iridocyclitis (364.10)
● 366.34 ***Cataract in degenerative disorders***
Sunflower cataract
Code first underlying condition, as:
chalcosis (360.24)
degenerative myopia (360.21)
pigmentary retinal dystrophy (362.74)

Figure 5-6. Examples of "Code first" instructions.

EXAMPLE Acute pyelonephritis due to *Escherichia coli (E coli)*, 590.10, 041.4.

"Code first" notes (Figure 5-6) are also under certain codes that are not specifically manifestation codes but may be due to an underlying cause. When a "code first" note is present and an underlying condition is present the underlying condition should be sequenced first.

"Code, if applicable, any causal condition first", notes indicate that this code may be assigned as a principal diagnosis when the causal condition is unknown or not applicable. If a causal condition is known, then the code for that condition should be sequenced as the principal or first-listed diagnosis.

EXAMPLE Chronic pyelonephritis due to vesicoureteral reflux, 593.70, 590.00.

Multiple codes may be needed for late effects, complication codes and obstetric codes to more fully describe a condition. See the specific guidelines for these conditions for further instruction.

10. Acute and Chronic Conditions

If the same condition is described as both acute (subacute) and chronic, and separate subentries exist in the Alphabetic Index at the same indentation level (Figure 5-7), code both and sequence the acute (subacute) code first.

EXAMPLE Acute and chronic pancreatitis, 577.0, 577.1.

EXAMPLE Acute and chronic cholecystitis, 575.12.
Separate subterms are included for "acute" and "chronic," but a subterm for "acute and chronic" is also provided.

EXAMPLE Acute and chronic otitis media, 382.9.
Separate subterms are provided for "acute" and "chronic," but they use the same code.

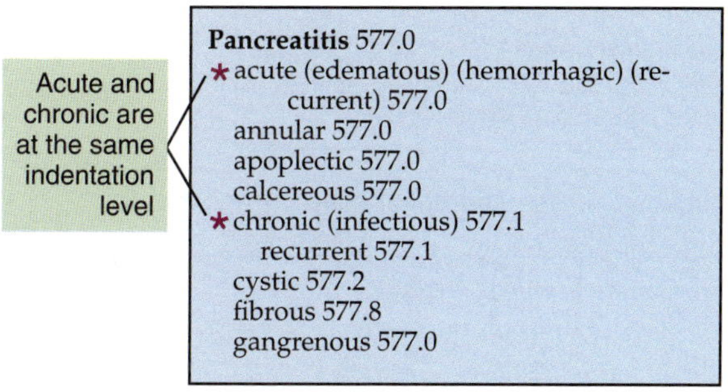
Acute and chronic are at the same indentation level
Pancreatitis 577.0
*acute (edematous) (hemorrhagic) (recurrent) 577.0
annular 577.0
apoplectic 577.0
calcereous 577.0
*chronic (infectious) 577.1
recurrent 577.1
cystic 577.2
fibrous 577.8
gangrenous 577.0

Figure 5-7. Subterms for acute and chronic at the same indention level.

EXERCISE 5-3

Assign and sequence codes to the following using your ICD-9-CM code book.

1. Subacute and chronic appendicitis __________
2. Acute and chronic bronchitis __________
3. Acute and chronic pyelonephritis __________
4. Acute on chronic renal failure __________
5. Acute on chronic respiratory failure __________

11. Combination Code

A combination code is a single code used to classify:
Two diagnoses, or
A diagnosis with an associated secondary process (manifestation)
A diagnosis with an associated complication

Combination codes are identified by referring to subterm entries in the Alphabetic Index and by reading the inclusion and exclusion notes in the Tabular List.

Assign only the combination code when that code fully identifies the diagnostic conditions involved or when the Alphabetic Index so directs. Multiple coding should not be used when the classification provides a combination code that clearly identifies all of the elements documented in the diagnosis. When the combination code lacks necessary specificity in describing the manifestation or complication, an additional code should be used as a secondary code.

EXAMPLE

Pseudomonas pneumonia, 482.1.
The combination code includes the infection and the organism responsible for the infection (Pseudomonas). It would be incorrect to assign separate codes such as 486 for pneumonia and 041.7 to identify the *Pseudomonas* organism.

EXERCISE 5-4

Assign codes to the following using your ICD-9-CM code book.

1. Urinary tract infection due to candidiasis __________
2. Streptococcal group A pneumonia __________
3. Food poisoning due to *Salmonella* __________

12. Late Effects

A late effect is the residual effect (condition produced) after the acute phase of an illness or injury has terminated. There is no time limit on when a late effect code can be used. The residual may be apparent early, such as in cerebrovascular accident cases, or it may occur months or years later, such as that due to a previous injury. Coding of late effects generally requires two codes sequenced in the following order: The condition or nature of the late effect is sequenced first. The late effect code is sequenced second.

EXAMPLE

Paraplegia due to traumatic spinal cord injury suffered in a motor vehicle accident 3 years ago, 344.1 (residual), 907.2 (cause, late effect code), E929.0 (late effect E code).

An exception to the above guidelines are those instances where the code for late effect is followed by a manifestation code identified in the Tabular List and title, or the late effect code has been expanded (at the fourth and fifth-digit levels) to include the manifestation(s). The code for the acute phase of an illness or injury that led to the late effect is never used with a code for the late effect.

EXAMPLE

Aphasia due to cerebrovascular accident 4 months ago 438.11, Includes the residual, aphasia, and describes the cause, cerebrovascular accident.

EXAMPLE

Scoliosis due to past history of poliomyelitis, 138, 737.43.

This is an example of the exception to sequencing the residual first. In the Alphabetic Index, under the main term "scoliosis" and the subterm "due to poliomyelitis," the 138 (cause) is listed first with the scoliosis code 737.43 in brackets. This means that 138 must be sequenced first (Figure 5-8).

13. Impending or Threatened Condition

Code any condition described at the time of discharge as "impending" or "threatened" as follows:

If it did occur, code as confirmed diagnosis.

If it did not occur, reference the Alphabetic Index to determine if the condition has a subentry term for "impending" or "threatened" and also reference main term entries for "Impending" and for "Threatened."

If the subterms are listed, assign the given code.

If the subterms are not listed, code the existing underlying condition(s) and not the condition described as impending or threatened.

Scoliosis (acquired) (postural) 737.30
  congenital 754.2
  due to or associated with
    Charcôt-Marie-Tooth disease 356.1 *[737.43]*
    mucopolysaccharidosis 277.5 *[737.43]*
    neurofibromatosis 237.71 *[737.43]*
    osteitis
      deformans 731.0 *[737.43]*
      fibrosa cystica 252.01 *[737.43]*
    osteoporosis (*see also* Osteoporosis) 733.00 *[737.43]*
    poliomyelitis 138 *[737.43]* ★

Figure 5-8. Alphabetic Index entry for scoliosis due to poliomyelitis.

Occasionally, conditions will be treated and documented as impending conditions. According to the guidelines, if the diagnosis has been confirmed, it should be coded as an active and current condition. If it is impending or threatened rather than active and current, check the Alphabetic Index to see whether a code is available that describes the impending condition. If no code is available, code the existing underlying condition(s).

EXAMPLE Impending cerebrovascular accident (CVA), 435.9

EXAMPLE Impending fracture of the humerus due to multiple myeloma, 203.00

EXERCISE 5-4

Assign codes to the following conditions using your ICD-9-CM code book.

1. Impending delirium tremens ____________
2. Threatened miscarriage ____________
3. Evolving myocardial infarction ____________
4. Impending fracture of femur due to severe osteoporosis ____________
5. Impending stroke ____________

Section II. Selection of Principal Diagnosis

The circumstances of inpatient admission always govern the selection of principal diagnosis. The principal diagnosis is defined in the Uniform Hospital Discharge Data Set (UHDDS) as "that condition established after study to be chiefly responsible for occasioning the admission of the patient to the hospital for care."

The UHDDS definitions are used by hospitals to report inpatient data elements in a standardized manner. These data elements and their definitions can be found in the July 31, 1985, Federal Register (Vol. 50, No, 147), pp. 31038-40.

Since that time the application of the UHDDS definitions has been expanded to include all non-outpatient settings (acute care, short term, long term care and psychiatric hospitals; home health agencies; rehab facilities; nursing homes, etc).

In determining principal diagnosis the coding conventions in the ICD-9-CM, Volumes I and II take precedence over these official coding guidelines.

(See Section I.A., Conventions for the ICD-9-CM)

The importance of consistent, complete documentation in the medical record cannot be overemphasized. Without such documentation the application of all coding guidelines is a difficult, if not impossible, task.

A. Codes for symptoms, signs, and ill-defined conditions

Codes for symptoms, signs, and ill-defined conditions from Chapter 16 are not to be used as principal diagnosis when a related definitive diagnosis has been established.

EXAMPLE Right lower quadrant abdominal pain due to acute appendicitis. The code for the abdominal pain is 789.03 (from Chapter 16), and it is due to acute appendicitis. The only code necessary is 540.9, for acute appendicitis.

B. Two or more interrelated conditions, each potentially meeting the definition for principal diagnosis.

When there are two or more interrelated conditions (such as diseases in the same ICD-9-CM chapter or manifestations characteristically associated with a certain disease) potentially meeting the definition of principal diagnosis, either condition may be sequenced first, unless the circumstances of the admission, the therapy provided, the Tabular List, or the Alphabetic Index indicate otherwise.

EXAMPLE

The patient had severe dehydration and hypokalemia that were treated with IV fluids and IV potassium supplements, 276.51, 276.8 or 276.8, 276.51.

C. Two or more diagnoses that equally meet the definition for principal diagnosis

In the unusual instance when two or more diagnoses equally meet the criteria for principal diagnosis as determined by the circumstances of admission, diagnostic workup and/or therapy provided, and the Alphabetic Index, Tabular List, or another coding guidelines does not provide sequencing direction, any one of the diagnoses may be sequenced first.

EXAMPLE

The patient was admitted with an exacerbation of her chronic obstructive pulmonary disease and decompensation of her congestive heart failure. Either 496 or 428.0 could be selected for the principal diagnosis, and the other code would be a secondary diagnosis code.

D. Two or more comparative or contrasting conditions.

In those rare instances when two or more contrasting or comparative diagnoses are documented as "either/or" (or similar terminology), they are coded as if the diagnoses were confirmed and the diagnoses are sequenced according to the circumstances of the admission. If no further determination can be made as to which diagnosis should be principal, either diagnosis may be sequenced first.

EXAMPLE

Peptic ulcer disease versus cholecystitis, 533.90, 575.10 or 575.10, 533.90.

E. A symptom(s) followed by contrasting/comparative diagnoses

When a symptom(s) is followed by contrasting/comparative diagnoses, the symptom code is sequenced first. All the contrasting/comparative diagnoses should be coded as additional diagnoses.

EXAMPLE

Abdominal pain due to peptic ulcer disease versus cholecystitis, 789.00, 533.90, 575.10.

F. Original treatment plan not carried out

Sequence as the principal diagnosis the condition, which after study occasioned the admission to the hospital, even though treatment may not have been carried out due to unforeseen circumstances.

EXAMPLE

The patient was admitted for cholecystectomy because of cholelithiasis. The patient was noted to be having an exacerbation of congestive heart failure (CHF), so the surgery was canceled and IV Lasix was administered to treat the CHF, 574.20, 428.0, V64.1. No procedure code would be assigned because the procedure was cancelled before it was started.

G. Complications of surgery and other medical care

When the admission is for treatment of a complication resulting from surgery or other medical care, the complication code is sequenced as the principal diagnosis. If the complication is classified to the 996-999 series and the code lacks the necessary specificity in describing the complication, an additional code for the specific complication should be assigned.

EXAMPLE The patient was admitted for dehiscence of an abdominal incision, 998.32, E879.9.

H. Uncertain Diagnosis

If the diagnosis documented at the time of discharge is qualified as "probable", "suspected", "likely", "questionable", "possible", or "still to be ruled out", or other similar terms indicating uncertainty, code the condition as if it existed or was established. The bases for these guidelines are the diagnostic workup, arrangements for further workup or observation, and initial therapeutic approach that correspond most closely with the established diagnosis.

Note: This guideline is applicable only to inpatient admissions to short-term, acute, long-term care and psychiatric hospitals.

EXAMPLE Possible adenovirus meningitis, 049.1.

In the chapter specific guidelines, there are two exceptions to the uncertain diagnosis guideline.

- Code 042 AIDS should only be assigned for confirmed cases
- Code 488 Avian influenza should only be assigned for confirmed cases

I. Admission from Observation Unit

1. Admission Following Medical Observation

When a patient is admitted to an observation unit for a medical condition, which either worsens or does not improve, and is subsequently admitted as an inpatient of the same hospital for this same medical condition, the principal diagnosis would be the medical condition which led to the hospital admission.

EXAMPLE The patient was admitted for medical observation because of chest pain. After further investigation and testing, it was determined that the patient had a NSTEMI, and the patient was admitted for inpatient care, 410.71.

2. Admission Following Post-Operative Observation

When a patient is admitted to an observation unit to monitor a condition (or complication) that develops following outpatient surgery, and then is subsequently admitted as an inpatient of the same hospital, hospitals should apply the Uniform Hospital Discharge Data Set (UHDDS) definition of principal diagnosis as "that condition established after study to be chiefly responsible for occasioning the admission of the patient to the hospital for care."

J. Admission from Outpatient Surgery

When a patient receives surgery in the hospital's outpatient surgery department and is subsequently admitted for continuing inpatient care at the same hospital, the following guidelines should be followed in selecting the principal diagnosis for the inpatient admission:

- If the reason for the inpatient admission is a complication, assign the complication as the principal diagnosis.

EXAMPLE The patient was admitted following an outpatient esophagogastroduodenoscopy for gastroesophageal reflux. The patient went into atrial fibrillation in the recovery room and was admitted. 997.1, 427.31, 530.81, 45.13, E878.8, E849.7.

- If no complication, or other condition, is documented as the reason for the inpatient admission, assign the reason for the outpatient surgery as the principal diagnosis.
- If the reason for the inpatient admission is another condition unrelated to the surgery, assign the unrelated condition as the principal diagnosis.

Section III. Reporting Additional Diagnoses

GENERAL RULES FOR OTHER (ADDITIONAL) DIAGNOSES

For reporting purposes the definition for "other diagnoses" is interpreted as additional conditions that affect patient care in terms of requiring:

clinical evaluation; or
therapeutic treatment; or
diagnostic procedures; or
extended length of hospital stay; or
increased nursing care and/or monitoring.

The UHDDS item #11-b defines Other Diagnoses as "all conditions that coexist at the time of admission, that develop subsequently, or that affect the treatment received and/or the length of stay. Diagnoses that relate to an earlier episode which have no bearing on the current hospital stay are to be excluded." UHDDS definitions apply to inpatients in acute care, short-term, long term care and psychiatric hospital setting. The UHDDS definitions are used by acute care short-term hospitals to report inpatient data elements in a standardized manner. These data elements and their definitions can be found in the July 31, 1985, Federal Register (Vol. 50, No, 147), pp. 31038-40.

Since that time the application of the UHDDS definitions has been expanded to include all non-outpatient settings (acute care, short term, long term care and psychiatric hospitals; home health agencies; rehab facilities; nursing homes, etc).

The following guidelines are to be applied in designating "other diagnoses" when neither the Alphabetic Index nor the Tabular List in ICD-9-CM provide direction. The listing of the diagnoses in the patient record is the responsibility of the attending provider.

A. Previous conditions

If the provider has included a diagnosis in the final diagnostic statement, such as the discharge summary or the face sheet, it should ordinarily be coded. Some providers include in the diagnostic statement resolved conditions or diagnoses and status-post procedures from previous admission that have no bearing on the current stay. Such conditions are not to be reported and are coded only if required by hospital policy.

However, history codes (V10-V19) may be used as secondary codes if the historical condition or family history has an impact on current care or influences treatment.

EXAMPLE

The patient is being treated for congestive heart failure and has a history of allergy to shellfish. A code is available for history of shellfish allergy, V15.04, but it would not be necessary to assign this code unless facility policy directs the coder to do so. Some physicians list allergies and previous surgeries as diagnoses, 428.0.

EXAMPLE

The patient is being treated for prostate cancer. A significant family history of prostate cancer has been reported, 185, V16.42.

B. Abnormal findings

Abnormal findings (laboratory, x-ray, pathologic, and other diagnostic results) are not coded and reported unless the provider indicates their clinical significance. If the findings are outside the normal range and the attending provider has ordered other tests to evaluate the condition or prescribed treatment, it is appropriate to ask the provider whether the abnormal finding should be added.

Please note: This differs from the coding practices in the outpatient setting for coding encounters for diagnostic tests that have been interpreted by a provider.

EXAMPLE

Potassium is noted to be low on laboratory testing. Potassium 20 mEq was ordered. Query the physician regarding the significance of the abnormal lab value and subsequent treatment.

C. Uncertain Diagnosis

If the diagnosis documented at the time of discharge is qualified as "probable", "suspected", "likely", "questionable", "possible", or "still to be ruled out" or other similar terms indicating uncertainty, code the condition as if it existed or was established. The bases for these guidelines are the diagnostic workup, arrangements for further workup or observation, and initial therapeutic approach that correspond most closely with the established diagnosis.

Note: This guideline is applicable only to inpatient admissions to short-term, acute, long-term care and psychiatric hospitals.

EXAMPLE — Suspected aspiration pneumonitis, 507.0.

Section IV. Diagnostic Coding and Reporting Guidelines for Outpatient Services

These coding guidelines for outpatient diagnoses have been approved for use by hospitals/providers in coding and reporting hospital-based outpatient services and provider-based office visits.

These guidelines will not be presented in this chapter because the focus of this text is on Inpatient coding. In the hospital setting, however, many coders must be familiar with both inpatient and outpatient guidelines. The Diagnostic Coding and Reporting Guidelines for Outpatient Services will be presented in detail in Chapter 26 on coding outpatient encounters.

PRESENT ON ADMISSION

The **Deficit Reduction Act** (DRA) mandates that as of October 1, 2007, all acute-care facilities reimbursed under Medicare Severity diagnosis-related groups (MS-DRGs) must identify and report diagnoses that are present at the time of a patient's admission. This policy change was implemented to save lives and dollars by no longer paying the extra costs of treating preventable errors, injuries, and infections that occur in hospitals. Medicare does not want to pay for conditions they consider preventable, such as pressure ulcers, injuries due to falls, infections caused by genitourinary catheters and central venous lines, or complications such as a sponge left in a patient during surgery.

The **present on admission** (POA) indicator (which follows) is to differentiate between conditions that develop during a particular hospital encounter and conditions that were present at the time of admission. Hospitals will have a 1-year grace period before their payment will be affected by conditions that were not present at the time of admission. Most of these conditions will be identified by a particular ICD-9-CM diagnosis code, and the POA indicator on the UB-04. Coding staff will have to assign POA indicators to the ICD-9-CM codes that are assigned. This requirement places even more importance on accurate and complete documentation within the health record. In some instances it may be necessary to query the physician about whether a condition was present at the time of admission.

The Cooperating Parties have developed POA guidelines that are supplemental to the *ICD-9-CM Official Guidelines for Coding and Reporting* to assist with the application of the POA requirement. The indicators that are reported are the following:

- Y = Yes (present at the time of inpatient admission)
- N = No (not present at the time of inpatient admission)
- U = Unknown (documentation is insufficient to determine whether condition is present on admission)
- W = Clinically undetermined (provider is unable to clinically determine whether condition was present on admission)
- Unreported/Not used (Exempt from POA reporting). Electronic claims will have a "1."

The Centers for Medicare and Medicaid Services (CMS) has identified certain hospital-acquired conditions and will no longer reimburse for the extra costs that are incurred as a result of these conditions. These conditions include the following:

- Catheter-associated urinary tract infection (UTI)
- Decubitus ulcers (pressure)
- Object left in surgery
- Air embolism
- Blood incompatibility (transfusion)
- Vascular catheter–associated infections (central line)
- Surgical site infections
- Falls

After October 1, 2008, these diagnoses will not count as an MCC/CC (major complication/comorbidity and complication/comorbidity) if they developed after the patient's admission to the hospital.

Appendix I
Present on Admission Reporting Guidelines
[Added to the Official Coding Guidelines October 1, 2006]

Introduction

These guidelines are to be used as a supplement to the *ICD-9-CM Official Guidelines for Coding and Reporting* to facilitate the assignment of the Present on Admission (POA) indicator for each diagnosis and external cause of injury code reported on claim forms (UB-04 and 837 Institutional).

These guidelines are not intended to replace any guidelines in the main body of the *ICD-9-CM Official Guidelines for Coding and Reporting*. The POA guidelines are not intended to provide guidance on when a condition should be coded, but rather, how to apply the POA indicator to the final set of diagnosis codes that have been assigned in accordance with Sections I, II, and III of the official coding guidelines. Subsequent to the assignment of the ICD-9-CM codes, the POA indicator should then be assigned to those conditions that have been coded.

As stated in the Introduction to the ICD-9-CM Official Guidelines for Coding and Reporting, a joint effort between the healthcare provider and the coder is essential to achieve complete and accurate documentation, code assignment, and reporting of diagnoses and procedures. The importance of consistent, complete documentation in the medical record cannot be overemphasized. Medical record documentation from any provider involved in the care and treatment of the patient may be used to support the determination of whether a condition was present on admission or not. In the context of the official coding guidelines, the term "provider" means a physician or any qualified healthcare practitioner who is legally accountable for establishing the patient's diagnosis.

General Reporting Requirements

All claims involving inpatient admissions to general acute care hospitals or other facilities that are subject to a law or regulation mandating collection of present on admission information.

Present on admission is defined as present at the time the order for inpatient admission occurs—conditions that develop during an outpatient encounter, including emergency department, observation, or outpatient surgery, are considered as present on admission.

POA indicator is assigned to principal and secondary diagnoses (as defined in Section II of the Official Guidelines for Coding and Reporting) and the external cause of injury codes.

Issues related to inconsistent, missing, conflicting or unclear documentation must still be resolved by the provider.

If a condition would not be coded and reported based on UHDDS definitions and current official coding guidelines, then the POA indicator would not be reported.

Reporting Options

Y - Yes
N - No
U - Unknown
W – Clinically undetermined
Unreported/Not used – (Exempt from POA reporting)

Continued

Reporting Definitions

Y = present at the time of inpatient admission
N = not present at the time of inpatient admission
U = documentation is insufficient to determine if condition is present on admission
W = provider is unable to clinically determine whether condition was present on admission or not

Assigning the POA Indicator

Condition is on the "Exempt from Reporting" list

Leave the "present on admission" field blank if the condition is on the list of ICD-9-CM codes for which this field is not applicable. This is the only circumstance in which the field may be left blank.

POA Explicitly Documented

Assign Y for any condition the provider explicitly documents as being present on admission.

Assign N for any condition the provider explicitly documents as not present at the time of admission.

Conditions diagnosed prior to inpatient admission

Assign "Y" for conditions that were diagnosed prior to admission (example: hypertension, diabetes mellitus, asthma)

Conditions diagnosed during the admission but clearly present before admission

Assign "Y" for conditions diagnosed during the admission that were clearly present but not diagnosed until after admission occurred.

Diagnoses subsequently confirmed after admission are considered present on admission if at the time of admission they are documented as suspected, possible, rule out, differential diagnosis, or constitute an underlying cause of a symptom that is present at the time of admission.

Condition develops during outpatient encounter prior to inpatient admission

Assign Y for any condition that develops during an outpatient encounter prior to a written order for inpatient admission.

Documentation does not indicate whether condition was present on admission

Assign "U" when the medical record documentation is unclear as to whether the condition was present on admission. "U" should not be routinely assigned and used only in very limited circumstances. Coders are encouraged to query the providers when the documentation is unclear.

Documentation states that it cannot be determined whether the condition was or was not present on admission

Assign "W" when the medical record documentation indicates that it cannot be clinically determined whether or not the condition was present on admission.

Chronic condition with acute exacerbation during the admission

If the code is a combination code that identifies both the chronic condition and the acute exacerbation, see POA guidelines pertaining to combination codes.

If the combination code only identifies the chronic condition and not the acute exacerbation (e.g., acute exacerbation of CHF), assign "Y."

Conditions documented as possible, probable, suspected, or rule out at the time of discharge

If the final diagnosis contains a possible, probable, suspected, or rule out diagnosis, and this diagnosis was suspected at the time of inpatient admission, assign "Y."

If the final diagnosis contains a possible, probable, suspected, or rule out diagnosis, and this diagnosis was based on symptoms or clinical findings that were not present on admission, assign "N".

Conditions documented as impending or threatened at the time of discharge

If the final diagnosis contains an impending or threatened diagnosis, and this diagnosis is based on symptoms or clinical findings that were present on admission, assign "Y".

If the final diagnosis contains an impending or threatened diagnosis, and this diagnosis is based on symptoms or clinical findings that were **not** present on admission, assign "N".

Acute and Chronic Conditions

Assign "Y" for acute conditions that are present at time of admission and N for acute conditions that are not present at time of admission.

Assign "Y" for chronic conditions, even though the condition may not be diagnosed until after admission.

If a single code identifies both an acute and chronic condition, see the POA guidelines for combination codes.

Combination Codes

Assign "N" if any part of the combination code was not present on admission (e.g., obstructive chronic bronchitis with acute exacerbation and the exacerbation was not present on admission; gastric ulcer that does not start bleeding until after admission; asthma patient develops status asthmaticus after admission)

Assign "Y" if all parts of the combination code were present on admission (e.g., patient with diabetic nephropathy is admitted with uncontrolled diabetes)

If the final diagnosis includes comparative or contrasting diagnoses, and both were present, or suspected, at the time of admission, assign "Y".

For infection codes that include the causal organism, assign "Y" if the infection (or signs of the infection) was present on admission, even though the culture results may not be known until after admission (e.g., patient is admitted with pneumonia and the provider documents pseudomonas as the causal organism a few days later).

Obstetrical conditions

Whether or not the patient delivers during the current hospitalization does not affect assignment of the POA indicator. The determining factor for POA assignment is whether the pregnancy complication or obstetrical condition described by the code was present at the time of admission or not.

If the pregnancy complication or obstetrical condition was present on admission (e.g., patient admitted in preterm labor), assign "Y".

If the pregnancy complication or obstetrical condition was not present on admission (e.g., 2nd degree laceration during delivery, postpartum hemorrhage that occurred during current hospitalization, fetal distress develops after admission), assign "N".

If the obstetrical code includes more than one diagnosis and any of the diagnoses identified by the code were not present on admission assign "N".

(e.g., Code 642.7, Pre-eclampsia or eclampsia superimposed on pre-existing hypertension).

If the obstetrical code includes information that is not a diagnosis, do not consider that information in the POA determination.

(e.g., Code 652.1x, Breech or other malpresentation successfully converted to cephalic presentation should be reported as present on admission if the fetus was breech on admission but was converted to cephalic presentation after admission since the conversion to cephalic presentation does not represent a diagnosis, the fact that the conversion occurred after admission has no bearing on the POA determination).

Perinatal conditions

Newborns are not considered to be admitted until after birth. Therefore, any condition present at birth or that developed in utero is considered present at admission and should be assigned "Y". This includes conditions that occur during delivery (e.g., injury during delivery, meconium aspiration, exposure to streptococcus B in the vaginal canal).

Congenital conditions and anomalies

Assign "Y" for congenital conditions and anomalies. Congenital conditions are always considered present on admission.

External cause of injury codes

Assign "Y" for any E code representing an external cause of injury or poisoning that occurred prior to inpatient admission (e.g., patient fell out of bed at home, patient fell out of bed in emergency room prior to admission)

Assign "N" for any E code representing an external cause of injury or poisoning that occurred during inpatient hospitalization (e.g., patient fell out of hospital bed during hospital stay, patient experienced an adverse reaction to a medication administered after inpatient admission)

Categories and Codes
Exempt from
Diagnosis Present on Admission Requirement (Table 5-1)

Note: "Diagnosis present on admission" for these code categories are exempt because they represent circumstances regarding the healthcare encounter or factors influencing health status that do not represent a current disease or injury or are always present on admission

Table 5-1. Categories and Codes Exempt From Diagnosis Present on Admission Requirement*

Code/Code Range	Description
137-139	Late effects of infectious and parasitic diseases
268.1	Rickets, late effect
326	Late effects of intracranial abscess or pyogenic infection
412	**Old myocardial infarction**
438	Late effects of cerebrovascular disease
650	Normal delivery
660.7	Failed forceps or vacuum extractor, unspecified
677	Late effect of complication of pregnancy, childbirth, and the puerperium
905-909	Late effect of injuries, poisonings, toxic effects, and other external causes
V02	Carrier or suspected carrier of infectious diseases
V03	Need for prophylactic vaccination and inoculation against bacterial diseases
V04	Need for prophylactic vaccination and inoculation against certain viral diseases
V05	Need for other prophylactic vaccination and inoculation against single diseases
V06	Need for prophylactic vaccination and inoculation against combinations of diseases
V07	Need for isolation and other prophylactic measure
V10	Personal history of malignant neoplasm
V11	Personal history of mental disorder
V12	Personal history of certain other diseases
V13	Personal history of other diseases
V14	Personal history of allergy to medicinal agents
V15	Other personal history presenting hazards to health
V16	Family history of malignant neoplasm
V17	Family history of certain chronic disabling diseases
V18	Family history of certain other specific conditions
V19	Family history of other conditions
V20	Health supervision of infant or child
V21	Constitutional states in development
V22	Normal pregnancy
V23	Supervision of high-risk pregnancy
V24	Postpartum care and examination
V25	Encounter for contraceptive management
V26	Procreative management
V27	Outcome of delivery
V28	Antenatal screening
V29	Observation and evaluation of newborn for suspected condition not found
V30-V39	Liveborn infant according to type of birth
V42	Organ or tissue replaced by transplant
V43	Organ or tissue replaced by other means
V44	Artificial opening status
V45	Other postprocedural states
V46	Other dependence on machines
V49.60-V49.77	Upper and lower limb amputation
V49.81-V49.84	Other specified conditions influencing health status
V50	Elective surgery for purposes other than remedying health states
V51	Aftercare involving the use of plastic surgery
V52	Fitting and adjustment of prosthetic device and implant
V53	Fitting and adjustment of other device
V54	Other orthopedic aftercare
V55	Attention to artificial openings
V56	Encounter for dialysis and dialysis catheter care
V57	Care involving use of rehabilitation procedures

*Note: "Diagnosis present on admission" for those code categories are exempt because they represent circumstances regarding the healthcare encounter or factors influencing health status that do not represent a current disease or injury or are always present on admission.

Table 5-1. Categories and Codes Exempt From Diagnosis Present on Admission Requirement*—cont'd

Code/Code Range	Description
V58	Encounter for other unspecified procedures and aftercare
V59	Donors
V60	Housing, household, and economic circumstances
V61	Other family circumstances
V62	Other psychosocial circumstances
V64	Persons encountering health services for specific procedures, not carried out
V65	Other persons seeking consultation
V66	Convalescence and palliative care
V67	Follow-up examination
V68	Encounter for administrative purposes
V69	Problems related to lifestyle
V70	General medical examination
V71	Observation and evaluation for suspected condition not found
V72	Special investigations and examinations
V73	Special screening examination for viral and chlamydial diseases
V74	Special screening examination for bacterial and spirochetal diseases
V75	Special screening examination for other infectious diseases
V76	Special screening for malignant neoplasms
V77	Special screening for endocrine, nutritional, metabolic, and immunity disorders
V78	Special screening for disorders of blood and blood-forming organs
V79	Special screening for mental disorders and developmental handicaps
V80	Special screening for neurologic, eye, and ear diseases
V81	Special screening for cardiovascular, respiratory, and genitourinary diseases
V82	Special screening for other conditions
V83	Genetic carrier status
V84	Genetic susceptibility to disease
V85	Body mass index
V86	Estrogen receptor status
E800-E807	Railway accidents
E810-E819	Motor vehicle traffic accidents
E820-E825	Motor vehicle nontraffic accidents
E826-E829	Other road vehicle accidents
E830-E838	Water transport accidents
E840-E845	Air and space transport accidents
E846-E848	Vehicle accidents not elsewhere classifiable
E849.0-E849.6	Place of occurrence
E849.8-E849.9	Place of occurrence
E883.1	Accidental fall into well
E883.2	Accidental fall into storm drain or manhole
E884.0	Fall from playground equipment
E884.1	Fall from cliff
E885.0	Fall from (nonmotorized) scooter
E885.1	Fall from roller skates
E885.2	Fall from skateboard
E885.3	Fall from skis
F885.4	Fall from snowboard
E886.0	Fall on same level from collision, pushing, or shoving, by or with another person, in sports
E890.0-E890.9	Conflagration in private dwelling
E893.0	Accident caused by ignition of clothing, from controlled fire in private dwelling
E893.2	Accident caused by ignition of clothing, from controlled fire not in a building or structure
E894	Ignition of highly inflammable material
E895	Accident caused by controlled fire in private dwelling

Continued

Table 5-1. Categories and Codes Exempt From Diagnosis Present on Admission Requirement*—cont'd

Code/Code Range	Description
E897	Accident caused by controlled fire not in building or structure
E898.0-E898.1	Accident caused by other specified fire and flames
E917.0	Striking against or struck accidentally by objects or persons, in sports without subsequent fall
E917.1	Striking against or struck accidentally by objects or persons, caused by a crowd, by collective fear or panic without subsequent fall
E917.2	Striking against or struck accidentally by objects or persons, in running water without subsequent fall
E917.5	Striking against or struck accidentally by objects or persons, object in sports with subsequent fall
E917.6	Striking against or struck accidentally by objects or persons, caused by a crowd, by collective fear or panic with subsequent fall
E919.0-E919.1	**Accidents caused by machinery**
E919.3-E919.9	**Accidents caused by machinery**
E921.-E921.9	Accident caused by explosion of pressure valves
E922.0-E922.9	Accident caused by firearm and air gun missile
E924.1	Caustic and corrosive substances
E926.2	Visible and ultraviolet light sources
E927	Overexertion and strenuous movements
E928.0-E928.8	Other and unspecified environmental and accidental causes
E929.0-E929.9	Late effects of accidental injury
E959	Late effects of self-inflicted injury
E970-E978	Legal intervention
E979	Terrorism
E981.0-E980	**Poisoning by gases in domestic use, undetermined whether accidentally or purposely inflicted**
E982.0-E982.9	Poisoning by other gases, undetermined whether accidentally or purposely inflicted
E985.0-E985.7	Injury by firearms, air guns, and explosives; undetermined whether accidentally or purposely inflicted
E987.0	Falling from high place; undetermined whether accidentally or purposely inflicted
E987.2	Falling from a high place, undetermined whether accidentally or purposely inflicted; natural sites
E989	Late effects of injury, undetermined whether accidentally or purposely inflicted
E990-E999	Injury resulting from operations of war

*Note: "Diagnosis present on admission" for those code categories are exempt because they represent circumstances regarding the healthcare encounter or factors influencing health status that do not represent a current disease or injury or are always present on admission.

POA Examples

General Medical Surgical

1. Patient is admitted for diagnostic work-up for cachexia. The final diagnosis is malignant neoplasm of lung with metastasis.
   Assign "Y" on the POA field for the malignant neoplasm. The malignant neoplasm was clearly present on admission, although it was not diagnosed until after the admission occurred.
2. A patient undergoes outpatient surgery. During the recovery period, the patient develops atrial fibrillation and the patient is subsequently admitted to the hospital as an inpatient.
   Assign "Y" on the POA field for the atrial fibrillation since it developed prior to a written order for inpatient admission.
3. A patient is treated in observation and while in Observation, the patient falls out of bed and breaks a hip. The patient is subsequently admitted as an inpatient to treat the hip fracture.

Assign "Y" on the POA field for the hip fracture since it developed prior to a written order for inpatient admission.

4. A patient with known congestive heart failure is admitted to the hospital after he develops decompensated congestive heart failure.
   Assign "Y" on the POA field for the congestive heart failure. The ICD-9-CM code identifies the chronic condition and does not specify the acute exacerbation.
5. A patient undergoes inpatient surgery. After surgery, the patient develops fever and is treated aggressively. The physician's final diagnosis documents "possible postoperative infection following surgery."
   Assign "N" on the POA field for the postoperative infection since final diagnoses that contain the terms "possible", "probable", "suspected" or "rule out" and that are based on symptoms or clinical findings that were not present on admission should be reported as "N".
6. A patient with severe cough and difficulty breathing was diagnosed during his hospitalization to have lung cancer.
   Assign "Y" on the POA field for the lung cancer. Even though the cancer was not diagnosed until after admission, it is a chronic condition that was clearly present before the patient's admission.
7. A patient is admitted to the hospital for a coronary artery bypass surgery. Postoperatively he developed a pulmonary embolism.
   Assign "N" on the POA field for the pulmonary embolism. This is an acute condition that was not present on admission.
8. A patient is admitted with a known history of coronary atherosclerosis, status post myocardial infarction five years ago is now admitted for treatment of impending myocardial infarction. The final diagnosis is documented as "impending myocardial infarction."
   Assign "Y" to the impending myocardial infarction because the condition is present on admission.
9. A patient with diabetes mellitus developed uncontrolled diabetes on day 3 of the hospitalization.
   Assign "N" to the diabetes code because the "uncontrolled" component of the code was not present on admission.
10. A patient is admitted with high fever and pneumonia. The patient rapidly deteriorates and becomes septic. The discharge diagnosis lists sepsis and pneumonia. The documentation is unclear as to whether the sepsis was present on admission or developed shortly after admission.
    Query the physician as to whether the sepsis was present on admission, developed shortly after admission, or it cannot be clinically determined as to whether it was present on admission or not.
11. A patient is admitted for repair of an abdominal aneurysm. However, the aneurysm ruptures after hospital admission.
    Assign "N" for the ruptured abdominal aneurysm. Although the aneurysm was present on admission, the "ruptured" component of the code description did not occur until after admission.
12. A patient with viral hepatitis B progresses to hepatic coma after admission.
    Assign "N" for the viral hepatitis B with hepatic coma because part of the code description did not develop until after admission.
13. A patient with a history of varicose veins and ulceration of the left lower extremity strikes the area against the side of his hospital bed during an inpatient hospitalization. It bleeds profusely. The final diagnosis lists varicose veins with ulcer and hemorrhage.
    Assign "Y" for the varicose veins with ulcer. Although the hemorrhage occurred after admission, the code description for varicose veins with ulcer does not mention hemorrhage.
14. **The initial nursing assessment upon admission documents the presence of a decubitus ulcer. No mention of the decubitus ulcer is provided in the physician documentation until several days after admission.**
    Query the physician as to whether the decubitus ulcer was present on admission, or whether it developed after admission. Both diagnosis code assignment and determination of whether a condition was present on admission must be based on provider documentation in the medical record (per the definition of "provider" found at the beginning of these POA

guidelines and in the introductory section of the ICD-9-CM Official Guidelines for Coding and Reporting). If it cannot be determined from the provider documentation whether or not a condition was present on admission, the provider should be queried.

Obstetrics

1. A female patient was admitted to the hospital and underwent a normal delivery.
   Leave the "present on admission" (POA) field blank. Code 650, Normal delivery, is on the "exempt from reporting" list.
2. Patient admitted in late pregnancy due to excessive vomiting and dehydration. During admission patient goes into premature labor.
   Assign "Y" for the excessive vomiting and the dehydration.
   Assign "N" for the premature labor.
3. Patient admitted in active labor. During the stay, a breast abscess is noted when mother attempted to breast feed. Provider is unable to determine whether the abscess was present on admission.
   Assign "W" for the breast abscess.
4. Patient admitted in active labor. After 12 hours of labor it is noted that the infant is in fetal distress and a Cesarean section is performed.
   Assign "N" for the fetal distress.

Newborn

1. A single liveborn infant was delivered in the hospital via Cesarean section. The physician documented fetal bradycardia during labor in the final diagnosis in the newborn record.
   Assign "Y" because the bradycardia developed prior to the newborn admission (birth).
2. A newborn developed diarrhea which was believed to be due to the hospital baby formula.
   Assign "N" because the diarrhea developed after admission.

CHAPTER REVIEW EXERCISE

Select the correct answer for each of the following:

1. Conditions that are integral to a disease or condition should be coded as additional diagnoses.
   A. True
   B. False

2. When separate codes are used to identify acute and chronic conditions, the chronic code is sequenced first.
   A. True
   B. False

3. Reliance on only the Alphabetic Index or only the Tabular List can lead to errors in code assignments and less specificity in code selection.
   A. True
   B. False

4. A patient has anemia due to chronic renal failure. The anemia is integral to the chronic renal failure.
   A. True
   B. False

5. A patient has right lower quadrant abdominal pain due to acute appendicitis. The abdominal pain should be assigned an additional code.
   A. True
   B. False

6. In the inpatient setting, it is acceptable to code diagnoses that have not yet been confirmed but that are questionable or suspected.
   A. True
   B. False

7. If the principal diagnosis was abdominal pain due to acute appendicitis, abdominal pain would be coded as the principal diagnosis.
   A. True
   B. False

Assign codes to the following conditions using your ICD-9-CM code book.

8. Acute exacerbation of asthma
Code from Alphabetic Index ____________
Code following verification in Tabular List ____________

9. Non-ST elevation myocardial infarction
Code from Alphabetic Index ____________
Code following verification in Tabular List ____________

10. Spastic hemiplegia affecting dominant side
Code from Alphabetic Index ____________
Code following verification in Tabular List ____________

Identify integral and nonintegral conditions by answering the following questions.

11. List two common symptoms of kidney stones. ____________

12. List two common symptoms associated with rheumatoid arthritis. ____________

13. List two common symptoms of acute renal failure. ____________

Assign and sequence codes to the following conditions using your ICD-9-CM code book.

14. Acute and chronic cystitis ____________

15. Acute on chronic oophoritis ____________

16. Acute and chronic prostatitis ____________

17. Viral gastroenteritis ____________

18. Viral meningitis ____________

CHAPTER GLOSSARY

This chapter is unique in that the glossary definitions are not provided within the chapter. These terms are used within the guidelines without definition. All of these terms will be better defined in other areas of this text. The glossary definitions are provided in this section for quick reference.

Acute: a short and relatively severe course.

Asymptomatic: without any symptoms.

Chronic: persistent over a long period.

Combination code: a single code used to classify two diagnoses; or a diagnosis with an associated secondary process (manifestation); or a diagnosis with an associated complication.

Conventions: general rules for use in classification that must be followed for accurate coding.

Deficit Reduction Act: mandates all acute-care facilities reimbursed under MS-DRGs to identify and report diagnoses that are present at the time of a patient's admission.

Etiology: cause or origin of a disease or condition.

Late effect code: used when the acute phase of an illness or injury has passed, but a residual condition or health problem remains.

Manifestation: symptom or condition that is the result of a disease.

Present on admission: an indicator to differentiate between conditions that develop during a particular hospital encounter or if a condition was present at the time of admission.

Residual condition or effect: when the acute phase of an illness or injury has passed, but a residual condition or health problem remains.

Sequelae: residual conditions or effects; time when the acute phase of an illness or injury has passed, but residual conditions or health problems remain.

Sign: objective evidence of a disease or of a patient's condition as perceived by the patient's examining physician.

Subacute: somewhat acute; between chronic and acute.

Symptom: subjective evidence of a disease or of a patient's condition as perceived by the patient.

CHAPTER 6

General Coding Guidelines for Procedures

(Volume 3)

CHAPTER OUTLINE

Format of Volume 3, Tabular List and Alphabetic Index of Procedures
- Alphabetic Index

UHDDS Definitions
- Principal Procedure
- Significant Procedure

ICD-9-CM Official Guidelines for Coding and Reporting

Procedure Codes That Should Be Reported
- Valid OR Procedure
- Non-OR Procedure Affecting MS-DRG Assignment
- Noncovered OR Procedure
- Limited Coverage

Surgical Hierarchy

Bilateral Procedures

Operative Approaches and Closures

Closed Surgical Procedures and Conversion to Open Procedures

Endoscopic Approaches

Planned and Canceled Procedures

Biopsies

Facility Policy

Chapter Review Exercise

Chapter Glossary

LEARNING OBJECTIVES

- Identify the format of Volume 3, Tabular List and Alphabetic Index of Procedures
- Apply the conventions and ICD-9-CM Official Guidelines for Coding and Reporting
- Define principal procedure
- Define significant procedures
- Explain the surgical hierarchy
- Explain when to code operative approaches and closures
- Assign codes for canceled or converted to open procedures
- Compare and contrast endoscopic versus open procedures
- Discuss the importance of having a hospital policy regarding procedure code assignment

ABBREVIATIONS

BMI body mass index
CMS Centers for Medicare and Medicaid Services
COPD chronic obstructive pulmonary disease
ECMO extracorporeal membrane oxygenation
ER Emergency Room
ICD-9-CM *International Classification of Diseases, 9th Revision, Clinical Modification*
ICU intensive care unit
MCE Medicare code editor
MS-DRG Medicare Severity diagnosis-related group
NPI National Provider Identifier
OB obstetrics
OR Operating Room
UHDDS Uniform Hospital Discharge Data Set
VAD vascular access device

There are only a few references made to procedural coding within the ICD-9-CM Official Guidelines for Coding and Reporting. These will be reviewed briefly in this chapter.

FORMAT OF VOLUME 3, TABULAR LIST AND ALPHABETIC INDEX OF PROCEDURES

The format of Volume 3, Alphabetic Index and Tabular List, follows the same format and conventions that are used in Volume 1, Tabular List of Diseases and Injuries, and Volume 2, Alphabetic Index of Disease and Injuries. These procedural codes are used to code hospital inpatient procedures. ICD-9-CM procedures codes are not used by hospital outpatient departments or by physician practices. Physicians and hospital outpatient services are coded using *Current Procedural Terminology* (CPT) for procedural coding. According to Coding Clinic (2008:1Q:p15),[1] "The use of ICD-9-CM procedure codes is restricted to the reporting of inpatient procedures by hospitals." This is in accordance with HIPAA regulations. A hospital may still collect ICD-9-CM procedural data but only for internal or non–claim-related purposes.

Volume 3 consists of 17 chapters (Table 6-1). Most of these chapters are classified by body system. It should be noted that Chapter 0 contains procedures and interventions that represent new technology.

Table 6-1. Table of Contents for Volume 3, Procedures

Procedures: Volume 3
Index to Procedures
Tabular List of Procedures
0. Procedures and Interventions, Not Elsewhere Classifiable (00)
1. Operations on the Nervous System (01-05)
2. Operations on the Endocrine System (06-07)
3. Operations on the Eye (08-16)
4. Operations on the Ear (18-20)
5. Operations on the Nose, Mouth, and Pharynx (21-29)
6. Operations on the Respiratory System (30-34)
7. Operations on the Cardiovascular System (35-39)
8. Operations on the Hemic and Lymphatic System (40-41)
9. Operations on the Digestive System (42-54)
10. Operations on the Urinary System (55-59)
11. Operations on the Male Genital Organs (60-64)
12. Operations on the Female Genital Organs (65-71)
13. Obstetrical Procedures (72-75)
14. Operations on the Musculoskeletal System (76-84)
15. Operations on the Integumentary System (85-86)
16. Miscellaneous Diagnostic and Therapeutic Procedures (87-99)

Alphabetic Index

The location of procedures in the Alphabetic Index can be found under the common name of a procedure (e.g., appendectomy, hysterectomy). However, procedures may be listed under the general type of procedure with terminology such as the following:

- Insertion
- Incision
- Excision
- Clipping
- Repair
- Implantation
- Examination
- Removal

EXERCISE 6-1

Underline the main terms for the following procedures using the Alphabetic Index.

1. Cataract removal
2. Incision and drainage abscess right arm
3. Excisional debridement ulcer ankle
4. Inguinal hernia repair
5. Laparoscopic cholecystectomy

Omit Code

Omit code is an instructional note that is found only in the Alphabetic Index and Tabular List of Volume 3. This instruction denotes that no code is to be assigned. The omit code instruction is generally found under codes that are used for approaches and closures and therefore may be integral to the operative procedure (Figure 6-1). This convention is explained in further detail in this chapter under Operative Approaches and Closures.

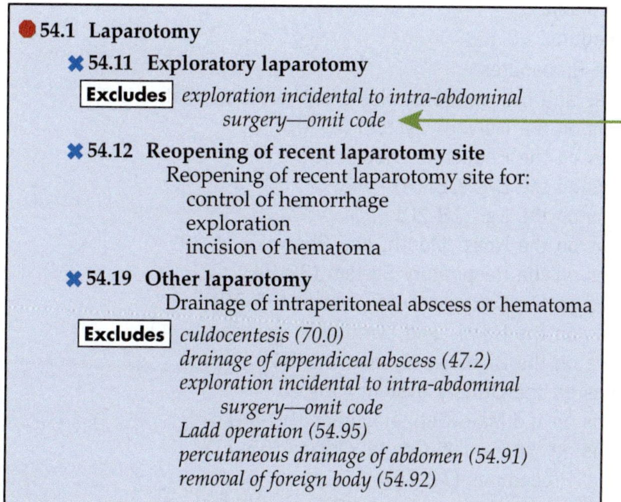

54.1 Laparotomy

54.11 Exploratory laparotomy

Excludes *exploration incidental to intra-abdominal surgery—omit code*

54.12 Reopening of recent laparotomy site

Reopening of recent laparotomy site for:
control of hemorrhage
exploration
incision of hematoma

54.19 Other laparotomy

Drainage of intraperitoneal abscess or hematoma

Excludes *culdocentesis (70.0)*
drainage of appendiceal abscess (47.2)
exploration incidental to intra-abdominal surgery—omit code
Ladd operation (54.95)
percutaneous drainage of abdomen (54.91)
removal of foreign body (54.92)

Figure 6-1. Instruction to "Omit code" if the laparotomy approach to intra-abdominal surgery is used.

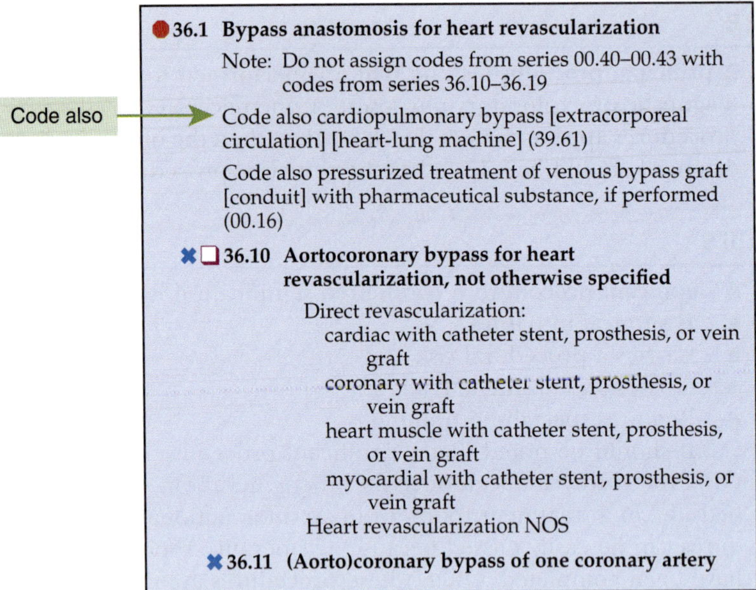

Code also

36.1 Bypass anastomosis for heart revascularization

Note: Do not assign codes from series 00.40–00.43 with codes from series 36.10–36.19

Code also cardiopulmonary bypass [extracorporeal circulation] [heart-lung machine] (39.61)

Code also pressurized treatment of venous bypass graft [conduit] with pharmaceutical substance, if performed (00.16)

36.10 Aortocoronary bypass for heart revascularization, not otherwise specified

Direct revascularization:
- cardiac with catheter stent, prosthesis, or vein graft
- coronary with catheter stent, prosthesis, or vein graft
- heart muscle with catheter stent, prosthesis, or vein graft
- myocardial with catheter stent, prosthesis, or vein graft

Heart revascularization NOS

36.11 (Aorto)coronary bypass of one coronary artery

Figure 6-2. "Code also" instructional note.

Code Also

"Code also" is an instructional note found in Volume 3 that directs the coder to code an additional procedure if it was performed.

EXAMPLE

Aortocoronary bypass, one coronary vessel with cardiopulmonary bypass, 36.11, 39.61 (Figure 6-2)

Adjunct Codes

Adjunct codes are assigned as add-on codes to a primary procedure to provide additional information about the primary procedure performed. These codes cannot be used alone and are assigned as a secondary procedure code.

EXAMPLE

Percutaneous transluminal coronary angioplasty is performed with drug-eluting stent placement into the LAD from coronary atherosclerosis, 414.01, 00.66, 36.07, 00.45, 00.40.

Codes 00.45 and 00.40 are adjunct vascular system procedure codes. These codes cannot be used alone and are used only to provide more information about the procedure that was performed.

EXERCISE 6-2

Assign and sequence the following procedures using your ICD-9-CM code book.

1. Partial ventriculectomy with synchronous open mitral valve repair __________
2. Total abdominal hysterectomy with bilateral salpingo-oophorectomy __________
3. Pelvic evisceration with application of adhesion barrier __________

UHDDS DEFINITIONS

Uniform Hospital Discharge Data Set (UHDDS) definitions are used by acute care, short-term hospitals to report inpatient data elements in a standardized manner. Definitions that pertain to the assignment of procedure codes are presented in the following sections.

Principal Procedure

A **principal procedure** is one that was performed for definitive treatment rather than for diagnostic or exploratory purposes, or one necessary to take care of a complication. If two procedures appear to meet this definition, then the one most closely related to the principal diagnosis should be selected as the principal procedure.

Significant Procedure

A **significant** procedure is considered significant if it

- Is surgical in nature
- Carries a procedural risk
- Carries an anesthetic risk
- Requires specialized training

It should be noted that a significant procedure does not have to be performed in an OR. Procedures can be done in the emergency room (ER) before admission, at the patient's bedside, in a treatment room, or in an interventional radiology department. These procedures can be easily missed because an operative report describing the procedure may not have been completed. Often, these procedures are documented with a brief, handwritten note on the ER record or in a progress note. Consent for treatment may assist the coder in attempting to verify a procedure, but not all procedures require consent forms. Also, a signed consent form does not confirm that the procedure was actually performed. A complete review of the entire health record is necessary to ensure that all completed procedures have been coded.

Other UHDDS data elements that must be coded include the date of the procedure and the NPI (National Provider Identifier) of the person who performed the procedure. It may be the coder's responsibility to abstract these data elements.

ICD-9-CM Official Guidelines for Coding and Reporting

Please refer to the companion Evolve site for the most current guidelines.

Under the specific chapter guidelines, there are only a few references to procedure codes.

The first is in the OB chapter and references the assignment of the principal diagnosis when a certain procedure was performed. It guides the selection of the principal diagnosis when a vaginal or a cesarean delivery occurs.

Chapter 11: Complications of Pregnancy, Childbirth, and the Puerperium (630-677)
b. Selection of OB Principal or First-listed Diagnosis
3) Episodes when no delivery occurs
In episodes when no delivery occurs, the principal diagnosis should correspond to the principal complication of the pregnancy, which necessitated the encounter. Should more than one complication exist, all of which are treated or monitored, any of the complications codes may be sequenced first.

EXAMPLE

Vomiting due to mild hyperemesis gravidarum. Patient is 10 weeks' pregnant, 643.03 (No procedure performed).

4) When a delivery occurs

When a delivery occurs, the principal diagnosis should correspond to the main circumstances or complication of the delivery. In cases of cesarean delivery, the selection of the principal diagnosis should correspond to the reason the cesarean delivery was performed unless the reason for admission/encounter was unrelated to the condition resulting in the cesarean delivery.

EXAMPLE

Obstructed labor due to breech position. Lower segment cesarean section was performed with delivery of a single liveborn infant, 660.01, 652.21, V27.0, 74.1.

The next reference to procedures involves debridements, which are frequently documented within the physician's progress notes or physical therapy notes.

Chapter 17. Injury and Poisoning (800-999)

d. Coding of Debridement of Wound, Infection, or Burn

Excisional debridement involves surgical removal or cutting away, as opposed to mechanical (brushing, scrubbing, washing) debridement.

For coding purposes, excisional debridement is assigned to code 86.22.

Nonexcisional debridement is assigned to code 86.28.

Excisional debridement, as defined by *Coding Clinic* (1988:4Q:p5),[2] is "the surgical removal or cutting away of devitalized tissue, necrosis, or slough." Excisional debridement may be performed in a variety of settings (operating room, emergency room, or bedside) and by a variety of healthcare providers (physicians, nurse practitioners, physician assistants, and physical therapists). For a debridement to qualify as excisional, documentation provided by the healthcare provider who performed this service must indicate that the procedure involved definite cutting away of the skin (i.e., sharp)—not just minor scissoring of loose fragments. When a laser is used to perform debridement, it qualifies as excisional.

According to *Coding Clinic* (1999:1Q:p8-9),[3] when an extensive debridement goes beyond the skin and subcutaneous tissue into the muscle, tendon, and/or bone, it is appropriate to "assign only a code for the deepest layer of debridement when multiple layers of the same site are debrided." If a patient underwent debridement of skin, subcutaneous tissue, muscle, and bone, the bone is the deepest layer, and debridement of the bone, 77.67, is the only procedure code assigned.

Any debridement that does not meet the criteria described for an excisional debridement would be coded as nonexcisional. A **nonexcisional debridement** may be performed by brushing, irrigating, scrubbing, or washing to remove devitalized tissue. Once again, this procedure may be performed in a variety of settings by a variety of healthcare providers.

It is important to remember that if debridement of the skin is performed in preparation for further surgery, the debridement should not be coded separately. For example, prior to reduction of an open fracture, a debridement may be performed.

EXAMPLE

Excisional debridement of right heel ulcer performed by physical therapist, 707.14, 86.22.

EXAMPLE

Excisional debridement of gangrenous sacral decubitus ulcer by physician, 707.03, 785.4, 86.22.

EXAMPLE

Debridement by scrubbing of the left foot ulcer by physical therapist, 707.15, 86.28.

The last reference to procedures is in the V code section, Classification of Factors Influencing Health Status and Contact with Health Service. The guideline emphasizes the fact that V codes are not procedure codes.

18. Classification of Factors Influencing Health Status and Contact with Health Service (Supplemental V01-V84)

c. V Codes indicate a reason for an encounter

They are not procedure codes. A corresponding procedure code must accompany a V code to describe the procedure performed.

Although V codes can be a reason for an encounter when a procedure is performed, a procedure code is still required.

EXAMPLE

A female patient is admitted for elective sterilization. Endoscopic ligation is performed with a Falope ring, V25.2, 66.29. The V code is the reason for the encounter and the 66.29 identifies the specific procedure that was performed.

PROCEDURE CODES THAT SHOULD BE REPORTED

Any procedures that affect payment or reimbursement must be reported. Other procedures may be reported at a hospital's discretion or in accordance with hospital policy. Encoders (ICD-9-CM coding software) may also have special popup notices that alert the coder about noncovered or limited coverage OR procedures.

After assigning procedure codes, the coder should review the diagnosis codes to ensure the assignment of diagnosis codes that support the performance of a procedure.

EXAMPLE

If it was determined that lysis of peritoneal adhesions was sufficient to warrant a procedure code in this male patient, it would make sense that a diagnosis code should be assigned to identify the peritoneal adhesions.

Procedure: Lysis of peritoneal adhesions, 54.59.
Diagnosis: Peritoneal adhesions, 568.0.

The Centers for Medicare and Medicaid Services (CMS) has categorized procedures into different classifications through the Medicare Code Editor (MCE). In some code books, these procedures may be highlighted to facilitate assignment of procedure codes. The **Medicare Code Editor** is software that detects errors in coding on Medicare claims. For example, it would identify a male-only procedure performed on a female patient.

During a patient's hospitalization, it may be necessary for a procedure to be performed at an outside facility. This could be for reasons such as the service may not be offered at the admitting hospital or equipment may malfunction. The patient may be transported by ambulance to this outside facility and after the procedure, returns for continued care at the admitting hospital. In these cases, the admitting hospital may assign procedure codes for services performed at the outside facility. The admitting hospital also would include these charges on the hospital bill, and the admitting hospital would reimburse the outside facility for the procedure.

Valid OR Procedure

A **valid OR procedure** is a procedure that may affect MS-DRG assignment.

EXAMPLE

Radical vaginal hysterectomy is designated as a valid OR procedure, 68.79.

Designation of a procedure as a valid OR procedure does not mean that it must be performed in the inpatient setting. Many surgical procedures can be safely performed on an outpatient basis, and many third party payers and/or insurance companies require that certain surgical procedures be performed in an outpatient setting. Repair of direct inguinal hernia is designated as a valid OR procedure, but this procedure is usually performed and billed as an outpatient procedure.

Non-OR Procedure Affecting MS-DRG Assignment

A procedure designated as a **"non-OR procedure affecting MS-DRG assignment"** is a procedure that may affect MS-DRG assignment, even though the procedure is not routinely performed in the OR.

EXAMPLE Insertion of a totally implantable vascular access device (VAD), 86.07. VADs may be used in patients who require long-term vascular access for chemotherapy, drug administration, or hemodialysis.

In some cases, the procedure code 86.07 will make a difference in MS-DRG assignment; in other cases, it will not.

EXAMPLE The patient was admitted with progressive chronic renal failure, stage V. A VAD was implanted for future hemodialysis, 585.5, 86.07.

In this case, the codes group to a surgical MS-DRG: MS-DRG 675, Other Kidney & Urinary Tract Procedures without CC/MCC.

EXAMPLE The patient was admitted with primary liver cancer. It was decided to implant a VAD for future chemotherapy, 155.0, 86.07.

In this case, the codes group to a medical MS-DRG: MS-DRG 437, Malignancy of Hepatobiliary System or Pancreas without CC/MCC.

Noncovered OR Procedure

Noncovered OR procedure codes are identified by the Medicare Code Editor as procedures for which Medicare does not provide reimbursement.

EXAMPLE Vasectomy is identified as a noncovered OR procedure, V25.2, 63.73.

Sterilization procedures are usually not covered by Medicare. It is possible to assign an MS-DRG but that does not guarantee payment.

Limited Coverage

Limited coverage procedures are identified by the Medicare Code Editor as procedures covered under limited circumstances.

EXAMPLE Patient with cystic fibrosis had a bilateral lung transplantation, 277.02, 33.52.

For a transplant facility to obtain Medicare coverage for organ transplantation, it must meet preapproved guidelines. Criteria are set forth and updated in *Federal Register* notices.

SURGICAL HIERARCHY

The **MS-DRG grouper** software (computer program that assigns an MS-DRG), using diagnosis and procedure codes, identifies whether a particular patient falls into a medical MS-DRG or a surgical MS-DRG. The MS-DRG grouper is able to determine which procedure is the most resource intensive and assigns the procedure to that particular surgical MS-DRG.

EXAMPLE

A patient has a breast biopsy during the same operative episode as a modified radical mastectomy. The patient also has congestive heart failure. The pathology report confirms that the patient has cancer of the right upper outer quadrant.

CODE ASSIGNMENTS: 174.4, 428.0, 85.43, 85.12
(The codes were put into the MS-DRG grouper in this order.)
MS-DRG: 583, MASTECTOMY FOR MALIGNANCY W/O CC/MCC

In this case, the patient was admitted and after study was determined to have breast cancer of the right upper outer quadrant (174.4). She also has a comorbidity of congestive heart failure (428.0). The principal procedure is one that is performed for definitive treatment; in this case, that would be the modified radical mastectomy (85.43). The mastectomy is more resource intensive than a breast biopsy. It is appropriate to code the diagnostic breast biopsy (85.12) as an additional procedure code.

EXAMPLE

CODE ASSIGNMENTS: 174.4, 428.0, 85.12, 85.43
MS-DRG: 583, MASTECTOMY FOR MALIGNANCY W/O CC/MCC

In this case, all the codes are the same, but the breast biopsy is incorrectly sequenced as the principal procedure instead of the mastectomy. Because of the surgical hierarchy within the grouper, it groups to the mastectomy MS-DRG, so the reimbursement and MS-DRG assignment would be correct. Even if the grouper will automatically arrange the codes to fit the surgical hierarchy, the code should be sequenced as the principal procedure on the basis of the UHDDS definition.

EXAMPLE

CODE ASSIGNMENTS: 428.0, 174.4, 85.43, 85.12
MS-DRG: 983, EXTENSIVE OR PROCEDURE UNRELATED TO PRINCIPAL DIAGNOSIS W/O CC/MCC

In this case, a data entry error was made and congestive heart failure was incorrectly sequenced as the principal diagnosis, resulting in a 983 MS-DRG assignment. Although MS-DRG 983 may be the correct assignment in some cases, it is not appropriate in this case, and the coder should review the entered codes.

In this case, the principal diagnosis combined with the procedure codes resulted in the MS-DRG assignment. If the data entry error had not been corrected before billing, the facility would have been incorrectly reimbursed.

BILATERAL PROCEDURES

A **bilateral procedure** occurs when the same procedure is performed on paired anatomic organs or tissues (i.e., eyes, ears, joints such as shoulder or knee). According to *Coding Clinic* (1988:1Q:p9)[4] "when the same procedures are performed bilaterally and ICD-9-CM provides a single code that identifies the procedure as bilateral, assign that code. When the same procedure is performed bilaterally and ICD-9-CM does not provide a code to identify that procedure as being performed bilaterally, record the procedure code twice. When there is a difference in the procedure performed on one side as opposed to the other side involving different code assignments, report both codes."

The coding of bilateral procedures should be addressed by facility policy. For major procedures such as joint replacements, the coder must assign two codes. As procedures become less invasive, more bilateral procedures may be performed during the same operative episode.

EXAMPLE

Repair of bilateral direct and indirect inguinal hernia with prosthesis, 550.92, 53.16.

EXAMPLE Osteoarthritis knees for bilateral total knee replacement, 715.36, 81.54, 81.54.

OPERATIVE APPROACHES AND CLOSURES

An important convention in Volume 3 is the "Omit code." Main terms in the Alphabetic Index may be used to identify incisions. If an incision is made only for the purpose of performing further surgery, the instruction "Omit code" is given.

EXAMPLE Laminectomy (decompression) (for exploration), 03.09 as operative approach—Omit code.

Other examples of incisions include laparotomy, thoracotomy, arthrotomy, and craniotomy. Often, the surgeon will indicate the approach in the operative procedure statement. Documentation of laparotomy by the physician does not necessarily mean that it should be coded. It is necessary to review the entire operative report to determine the extent of the procedure and to decide what should be coded. Sometimes, a physician will document that an exploratory laparotomy was performed along with an appendectomy for acute appendicitis. It is not necessary to code the exploratory laparotomy. Usually, some component of exploration occurs during a surgical procedure.

EXAMPLE Exploratory laparotomy with appendectomy for acute appendicitis, 540.9, 47.09.

The exploratory laparotomy was incidental to the intra-abdominal surgery.

Closure of the operative wound is a routine part of most surgical procedures, so it is not necessary to code this separately. In some instances, a surgical wound is not closed at the time of a surgical operation but is allowed to heal and will be closed at a later date. In this case, a closure would be coded.

EXAMPLE A patient is admitted for delayed closure of the laparotomy site, V58.41, 54.62.

CLOSED SURGICAL PROCEDURES AND CONVERSION TO OPEN PROCEDURES

As technology has advanced, procedures are increasingly being performed through scopes which are less invasive than open procedures. This has resulted in quicker recoveries, shorter hospital stays, and fewer complications.

Common closed surgical approaches include laparoscopic, thoracoscopic, and arthroscopic procedures. The **laparoscopic approach** involves use of a laparoscope to examine and perform closed procedures within the abdomen. With a **thorascopic approach**, a thoracoscope is used to examine and perform closed procedures within the thorax. The **arthroscopic approach** requires the use of an arthroscope to examine and perform closed procedures within a joint. Closed procedures may be diagnostic and/or therapeutic in nature.

A surgical procedure may start with a closed approach that may need to be converted to an open procedure. V codes describe the conversion from a closed surgical procedure to an open procedure. These codes are found in the index under the main term, Conversion.

V64.41 Laparoscopic surgical procedure converted to open procedure
V64.42 Thoracoscopic surgical procedure converted to open procedure
V64.43 Arthroscopic surgical procedure converted to open procedure

In the case of conversion from closed to open, only assign the open procedure code. Some reasons for conversion to an open procedure include adhesions, bleeding, technical difficulties due to anatomic body structure and/or inflammatory changes, and injury to an organ.

EXAMPLE

A patient was admitted for a laparoscopic cholecystectomy for chronic cholecystitis with cholelithiasis. Because of excessive bleeding from the liver bed, the procedure was converted to an open cholecystectomy and the bleeding was controlled, 574.10, 998.11, V64.41, 51.22.

Because the variety of procedures that can be performed via a scope is constantly changing, a code that describes the approach accurately may not be available. In these instances, the open code is used.

EXAMPLE

A patient is admitted for laparoscopic nephrectomy as a donor, V59.4, 55.51.

Coding Clinic (1992:3Q:p12)[5] states "until specific codes for laparoscopic and thorascopic approaches can be created, the codes for open approaches must be applied. Do not assign a separate code for the laparoscopy or thorascopy."

It may be the policy of some facilities to assign an additional procedure code for the laparoscopy (54.21) so that data can be collected on the number of laparoscopic procedures performed.

ENDOSCOPIC APPROACHES

Endoscopic examinations and procedures are performed with an instrument that allows examination of any cavity of the body through a rigid or flexible scope. The scope is usually inserted into the body through an orifice or stoma. When a colonoscopy is performed, the anus is the body orifice that allows entry of the scope.

As the scope is inserted and various parts of the body are examined, the coder would not code every body part that is viewed. The coder would code the farthest site that was reached. If a procedure such as a biopsy is performed, only the biopsy code is assigned.

EXAMPLE

A flexible colonoscopy is performed for gastrointestinal bleeding. During the procedure, the physician examines the ascending, transverse, descending, and sigmoid colon, 578.9, 45.23.

Only the colonoscopy code is assigned because examination of all these areas is included within that code.

PLANNED AND CANCELED PROCEDURES

When patients are admitted to the hospital for a scheduled procedure(s), under some circumstances, the procedure(s) may be canceled or not completed. If a patient's procedure is canceled prior to the time that he or she presents to the hospital, no code will be required because no services were provided, no bill was generated, and there is no health record. On some occasions, a patient presents to have a procedure performed, but for whatever reason the procedure has to be canceled. The principal diagnosis in this case is the reason why the patient was going to have the procedure performed. If a complication arose that resulted in the cancellation, a diagnosis code for that condition would be assigned as a secondary diagnosis. Also, V codes describe the reason for the cancellation. They can be located in the index under the main term, procedure (surgical) not done.

V64.1 Surgical or other procedure not carried out because of contraindication (medical reason to delay the procedure)
V64.2 Surgical or other procedure not carried out because of patient's decision
V64.3 Procedure not carried out for other reasons (staffing, equipment problems, unavailability of OR due to emergency)

EXAMPLE

A patient was admitted for hysterectomy because of uterine fibroids. Shortly after admission, the patient told the nurse that she was having second thoughts and had decided not to go through with the procedure; the patient was discharged, 218.9, V64.2. No procedure code is assigned because the procedure was never started.

EXAMPLE

A patient was admitted for coronary artery bypass grafting because of coronary atherosclerosis of the native arteries. The cardiac surgeon became ill, and the surgery was rescheduled. The patient was discharged, 414.01, V64.3.

EXAMPLE

A patient was admitted for laparoscopic cholecystectomy for cholelithiasis. It was noted that the patient was having an acute exacerbation of his COPD. The patient was treated with steroids and nebulizer treatments and was discharged. The cholecystectomy was rescheduled for next week, 574.20, 491.21, V64.1.

Occasionally, a surgical procedure will be started that for whatever reason cannot be completed. The surgical procedure should be coded to the extent that it was performed. These circumstances are different from those surrounding a procedure that is canceled, in that the patient received anesthesia and surgery was begun. No V codes are available for these situations.

EXAMPLE

A patient was admitted for colon resection because of cancer of the descending colon. A laparotomy incision was made, and the patient became unstable with atrial fibrillation. It was decided that the procedure should be terminated and the patient transferred to the ICU for further management. The incision was closed before any definitive surgery could be performed, 153.2, 997.1, 427.31, 54.19.

EXAMPLE

The patient was admitted for colonoscopy, but because of the obstructing lesion, the scope could not be inserted beyond the sigmoid colon. A biopsy specimen of the lesion was taken, and cancer of the sigmoid colon was confirmed, 153.3, 45.25 (sigmoidoscopy with biopsy).

BIOPSIES

Biopsy is a very common diagnostic procedure that is often performed before more definitive treatment is provided. **Biopsy** is defined as "the removal of tissue followed by pathologic examination to establish a precise diagnosis." The entire abnormality is not removed during a biopsy.

If the entire specimen is removed, it is no longer a biopsy but an excision of tissue. The physician may document in the OR report that the lesion was totally removed. Biopsies may be performed in a number of different ways, such as by aspiration, brush, core, endoscopic, excisional, incisional, percutaneous, punch, shave, stereotactic, and washing methods. Different codes may be assigned, depending on the biopsy method used. According to *Coding Clinic* (1984:J-A:p3-4),[6] biopsies that are performed by endoscopy or percutaneous aspiration are coded as "closed" biopsies. An incisional approach for removal of tissue is coded as an "open biopsy." A patient may be undergoing an open abdominal procedure while a percutaneous biopsy of the liver is also performed. Biopsy of the liver would be coded to percutaneous and not to open biopsy, even though the abdominal cavity was open at the time per *Coding Clinic* (1988:4Q:p12).[7]

Facility Policy

DEPARTMENT: HEALTH INFORMATION SERVICES
POLICY: Coding of ICD-9-CM Procedure Codes **POLICY NUMBER:** HIM 03.005
DEVELOPED BY: Karla Lovaasen, RHIA, CCS, CCS-P
ORIGINATED: October 2001
REVISED: 10/02 **REVIEWED:** 10/03
SCOPE: All personnel responsible for performing, supervising or monitoring coding services.
PURPOSE: To facilitate the coding of ICD-9-CM procedure codes from Volume 3.
POLICY: To assign procedure codes consistently to optimize reimbursement and capture facility data for quality and statistical monitoring.

PROCEDURE:

Assign ICD-9-CM diagnosis and procedure codes according to UHDDS guidelines and definitions and The Official Guidelines for Coding and Reporting.

ICD-9-CM procedure codes will be assigned to any procedures that are identified as a valid OR procedure or as a non-OR procedure affecting MS-DRG assignment.

Code all procedures that fall within 00.01 and 86.99 EXCEPT insertion of Foley catheter (57.94).

Bilateral procedures will be coded separately. Example: Bilateral knee replacement 81.54, 81.54.

It is not necessary to code minor procedures such as a blood transfusion that is given on multiple days.

Do NOT code procedures that fall within the code range 87.01 to 99.99 EXCEPT:

Some procedures that fall in this range, but may need to be performed under sedation/anesthesia on certain patients should be coded. Example: A gynecologic exam (89.26) performed under anesthesia due to patient's severe mental retardation.

87.53	Intraoperative cholangiogram
88.40 to 88.58	Arteriography and angiography
88.96	Intraoperative MRI
89.41	Cardiovascular stress test
89.50	Holter monitor
89.62	CVP monitoring
89.64	Swan-Ganz catheterization
92.21 to 92.29	Radiation therapy
92.30 to 92.39	Sterotactic radiosurgery
93.51 to 93.59	Immobilization, pressure and attention to wound
94.24 to 94.27	Psychiatric therapy
94.61 to 94.69	Alcohol/drug detoxification and rehabilitation
95.04	Eye examination under anesthesia
96.01 to 96.09	Nonoperative intubation and irrigation
96.21 to 96.29	Nonoperative dilation and manipulation
96.31 to 96.39	Nonoperative alimentary tract irrigation, cleaning and local instillation
96.49	Prostaglandin instillation
96.51 to 96.52	Irrigation of eye and ear
96.6	Enteral infusion
96.70 to 96.72	Mechanical ventilation
97.01 to 97.05	Nonoperative replacement of gastrointestinal appliances
97.11 to 97.16	Nonoperative replacement of musculoskeletal and integumentary system appliance
97.29	Other nonoperative replacements
98.01 to 98.29	Nonoperative removal of foreign body or calculus
98.51 to 98.59	ESWL
99.00 to 99.09	Transfusion of blood products
99.10 to 99.11	Injections of thrombolytic agent and Rh immune globulin
99.15	TPN
99.20 to 99.29	Injection or infusion of other therapeutic or prophylactic substance (coded primarily in outpatient setting)
99.31 to 99.59	Vaccinations and Inoculations
99.61 to 99.69	Conversions of cardiac rhythm

Any interventional procedures charged by radiology will be assigned a corresponding ICD-9-CM procedure code.

Procedures done at another facility can be coded if they are billed to the patient and/or third party payer by facility.

This policy will be reviewed at least annually to incorporate any procedure code changes that may be effective April and October 1.

Figure 6-3. This policy is a sample policy, and any policies should be designed to fit the needs of a facility.

EXAMPLE

The patient was admitted for elective open cholecystectomy for gallstones. An abnormality of the liver (pathology is consistent with patient's chronic hepatitis C) was noted during exploration, and percutaneous biopsy was performed, 574.20, 070.54, 51.22, 50.11.

Cholecystectomy is the principal procedure because it was performed for definitive treatment.

The documentation should be reviewed closely when excisional biopsies are performed. In some instances, the surgeon will document that he/she performed an "excisional biopsy" of a breast mass or lump. Upon reading the OR report and confirming findings through review of the pathology report, the coder may discover that the entire lump or mass was removed. This changes the coding from a biopsy code (85.12) to a lumpectomy code (85.21).

FACILITY POLICY

Each facility should have its own written policy (Figure 6-3) regarding the assignment of ICD-9-CM procedure codes. This policy should consider reimbursement, but it should also take into account other uses of a procedure database and how that information can be extracted. It may be necessary to determine what types of procedures are being performed for physician profiles and credentialing. Research is an important aspect of data collection.

As has been stated previously, because not all procedures are performed in the operating room, it may be difficult to locate documentation of all procedures performed. Procedures that are easy to overlook include mechanical ventilation, debridement, lumbar puncture, suturing, ECMO (extracorporeal membrane oxygenation), and procedures performed by interventional radiology.

CHAPTER REVIEW EXERCISE

Complete the following review exercises.

1. If a surgical procedure was canceled because of a medical condition or complication, which V code would be assigned?
   - **A.** V64.1 Surgical or other procedure not carried out because of contraindication
   - **B.** V64.2 Surgical or other procedure not carried our because of patient's decision
   - **C.** V64.3 Procedure not carried out for other reasons
   - **D.** None of the above
2. The principal diagnosis that is assigned when a surgical procedure is canceled is
   - **A.** V64.1 Surgical or other procedure not carried out because of contraindication
   - **B.** V64.2 Surgical or other procedure not carried our because of patient's decision
   - **C.** V64.3 Procedure not carried out for other reasons
   - **D.** None of the above
3. The approach of the surgical procedure should always be coded.
   - **A.** True
   - **B.** False
4. It is not necessary to code closure of a routine surgical incision.
   - **A.** True
   - **B.** False
5. If a procedure has been designated as a valid OR procedure, the procedure should be performed as an inpatient hospital stay.
   - **A.** True
   - **B.** False
6. It is a good idea for facilities to have a policy regarding which procedures are coded and which procedures are not coded.
   - **A.** True
   - **B.** False

7. A biopsy is the removal of tissue and pathologic examination to establish a precise diagnosis.
   A. True
   B. False
8. The surgical hierarchy within an MS-DRG grouper assists with sequencing the most resource-intensive procedure performed.
   A. True
   B. False
9. With the laparoscopic approach, a thoracoscope is used to examine and perform closed procedures within the thorax.
   A. True
   B. False
10. When a procedure is canceled because of a medical contraindication, the principal diagnosis is the medical contraindication and not the reason for which the patient was to undergo the procedure.
   A. True
   B. False

Underline the main terms.

11. Laparoscopic appendectomy
12. Creation of arteriovenous fistula for dialysis
13. Clipping aneurysm of brain
14. Insertion central venous catheter
15. Excision lesion of eyelid

Assign procedure codes to the following using your ICD-9-CM code book.

16. Low cervical cesarean section with bilateral tubal ligation, Pomeroy technique ____________
17. Partial esophagectomy with end-to-end anastomosis ____________
18. Excisional debridement performed by physical therapist ____________

Using the sample facility procedure policy, answer the following questions.

19. Would a code be assigned for TPN? ____________
20. Would the code 87.41 be assigned for CT of thorax? ____________
21. Absolutely no procedure codes can be assigned unless the procedure is performed at the facility, true or false? ____________
22. Would the code 87.53 be assigned for an intraoperative cholangiogram? ____________

CHAPTER GLOSSARY

Adjunct codes: add-on codes to a primary procedure to provide additional information about the primary procedure that was performed.

Arthroscopic approach: an arthroscope is used to examine and perform closed procedures within a joint.

Bilateral procedure: operative procedure performed on paired anatomic organs or tissues during the same operative session.

Biopsy: removal of tissue and pathologic examination to establish a precise diagnosis.

Endoscopic: examinations and procedures performed with an instrument that examines any cavity of the body with a rigid or flexible scope.

Excisional debridement: surgical removal or cutting away of devitalized tissue, necrosis, or slough.

Laparoscopic approach: uses a laparoscope is used to examine and perform closed procedures within the abdomen.

Limited coverage: procedures that are identified by the Medicare Code Editor as procedures covered under limited circumstances.

Medicare Code Editor: software that detects errors in coding on Medicare claims.

MS-DRG grouper: software that assigns MS-DRG using diagnosis and procedure codes.

Noncovered OR procedure: procedure code categorized by the Medicare Code Editor as a noncovered operating room procedure for which Medicare does not provide reimbursement.

Nonexcisional debridement: removal of devitalized tissue by brushing, irrigating, scrubbing, or washing.

Non-OR procedure affecting MS-DRG assignment: procedure code recognized by the MS-DRG Grouper as a non–operating room procedure that may affect MS-DRG assignment.

Omit code: an instructional note found in Volume 3 that denotes that no code is to be assigned; it generally is used for coding approaches and closures that are integral to an operative procedure.

Principal procedure: procedure that is performed for definitive treatment rather than for diagnostic or exploratory purposes, or one performed that was necessary to take care of a complication.

Significant procedure: a procedure is considered significant if it is surgical in nature, carries a procedural risk, carries an anesthetic risk, and/or requires specialized training.

Thoracoscopic approach: a thoracoscope is used to examine and perform closed procedures within the thorax.

Valid OR procedure: a procedure that may affect MS-DRG assignment.

CHAPTER 7

Reimbursement Methodologies

CHAPTER OUTLINE

LEARNING OBJECTIVES

- Describe the complexities of MS-DRGs and hospital reimbursement
- Explain the difference between optimization and maximization
- Calculate case-mix index (CMI)
- Explain the role of Quality Improvement Organizations (QIOs)
- Explain the purpose of PEPPER
- Describe the purpose of a clinical documentation improvement program
- Identify key elements of a UB-04

ABBREVIATIONS

AHIMA American Health Information Management Association

ALOS average length of stay

CC complication/comorbidity

CDIP Clinical Documentation Improvement Program

CHF congestive heart failure

CMI case-mix index

CMS Centers for Medicare and Medicaid Services

COPD chronic obstructive pulmonary disease

CPT *Current Procedural Terminology*

DHHS U.S. Department of Health and Human Services

GMLOS geometric length of stay

HH Home Health

HMO Health Maintenance Organization

HPR hospital payment rate

ICD-9-CM *International Classification of Diseases, 9th Revision, Clinical Modification*

IPPS Inpatient Prospective Payment System

LOS Length of stay

LTC long-term care

MDC major diagnostic category

MI myocardial infarction

MS-DRG Medicare Severity diagnosis-related group

NPI National Provider Identifier

PEPPER Program for Evaluating Payment Patterns Electronic Report

PPO Preferred Provider Organization

PPS Prospective Payment System

ABBREVIATIONS—*cont'd*

QIO Quality Improvement Organization
RPS retrospective payment system
RW relative weight
SNF skilled nursing facility
SOW scope of work
TEFRA Tax Equity and Fiscal Responsibility Act
UB-04 Uniform Bill-04

INTRODUCTION TO REIMBURSEMENT

Reimbursement or payment for healthcare services has evolved over time into a complicated system with many rules and guidelines that must be followed if proper payment is to be received from third party payers. Rules and guidelines vary, depending on which healthcare setting or third party payer is involved. A **third party payer** payments on behalf of the patient for health services. Third party payers may include government programs, insurance companies, and managed care plans.

Private Plans

A variety of private plans (commercial payer) are provided by companies such as Blue Cross/Blue Shield, Aetna, Cigna, and Travelers. These plans are available in different formats, including the following:

- **Self-insured plans**—self-insurance fund set up by an employer to provide health claim benefits for employees.
- **Health Maintenance Organization (HMO)**—type of managed care in which hospitals, physicians, and other providers contract to provide health care for patients, usually at a discounted rate.
- **Preferred Provider Organizations (PPO)**—type of managed care in which hospitals, physicians, and other providers have an arrangement with a third party payer to provide health care at discounted rates to third party payer clients.

Because Medicare is the predominant payer for healthcare services, this text focuses on Medicare's reimbursement system. Of note, many private and commercial payers have adopted the Medicare reimbursement system.

Government Plans

Medicare is a federal entitlement program administered by the Centers for Medicare and Medicaid Services (CMS) for patients over 65 years of age, certain disabled individuals, and those with end-stage renal disease.

Medicaid is a federal and state insurance plan, administered by the states and managed by the Social Security Administration of the federal government for patients whose income and resources are insufficient to pay for health care.

TRICARE, previously known as CHAMPUS (Civilian Health and Medical Program for the Uniformed Services), is a medical program for active duty military members, qualified family members, non–Medicare eligible retirees and their family members.

Workers' Compensation is a requirement of the federal government for employers to cover employees who are injured or become sick on the job. It is managed by various plans chosen by the employer or by state governments.

Medicare

After many years of debate in Congress, in July 1965, the House and Senate passed the bill that established Medicare, an insurance program designed to provide all older adults with comprehensive health care coverage at an affordable cost. In 1972, Medicare eligibility was extended to people with disabilities and those with end-stage renal disease.

The Social Security Act was responsible for the establishment of the Medicare program. As a result of this, the government became more involved in the delivery of health care. The government wanted to ensure that Medicare participants received both quality health care and medically necessary services.

Medicare is a federal health insurance program that is divided into parts according to the type of coverage.

Part A: Hospital Insurance. To be eligible for Part A hospital insurance, one must have worked or must have had a spouse who worked a minimum of 40 quarters of Medicare-covered employment. Part A of Medicare pays for inpatient hospital, skilled nursing facility, and some home health care. Medicare pays all costs for each benefit period (60 days), except for the deductible (which changes each year).

Part B: Medical Insurance. To be eligible for Part B insurance, one must meet the same requirements as for Part A. A premium (changes each year) is deducted from a person's social security check for Part B coverage. Part B Medicare covers Medicare-eligible physician services, outpatient hospital services, certain home health services, and durable medical equipment. A yearly deductible (that changes each year) and a 20% co-payment amount are applied to these services.

Part C: Medicare Advantage Plans. Medicare Advantage Plans are run by private companies and are similar to HMOs and PPOs. They provide more choices and sometimes additional benefits. They offer all the benefits provided by Part A and Part B, but some also may provide prescription drug coverage (Part D). Patients may be required to use certain hospitals and physicians in the service area.

Part D: Prescription Drug Coverage. This is an optional program for prescription drug coverage. Medicare prescription drug coverage is available to anyone who is covered by Medicare.

DIAGNOSIS-RELATED GROUPS/MEDICARE SEVERITY DIAGNOSIS-RELATED GROUPS

DRGs were developed at Yale University in the late 1960s to monitor quality of care and utilization of services. DRGs were not intended to be a means of determining hospital reimbursement. In 1982, the Tax Equity and Fiscal Responsibility Act (TEFRA) mandated limits on Medicare payments to hospitals. The government decided to use the DRG classification system, a prospective payment system (PPS), to pay for services rendered to Medicare inpatients. A **prospective payment system** is a method of reimbursement in which payment is made according to a predetermined, fixed amount rather than on the basis of billed charges.

The government implemented a prospective payment system in an effort to control the costs of inpatient hospital stays. The DRG system had some inequities in that a patient with multiple complication(s) or comorbid condition(s) is assigned that same DRG and receives the same payment as the patient who has just one complication or comorbid condition. Larger hospitals and tertiary care centers may present greater financial risks because they routinely care for patients who are severely ill. As a result, CMS implemented the Medicare Severity diagnosis-related groups (MS-DRGs), which became effective on October 1, 2007.

ICD-9-CM codes are used to determine the Medicare Severity diagnosis-related group (MS-DRG). First, a patient is assigned to an MDC (Figure 7-1) on the basis of the principal diagnosis code; next, it is determined whether the case is a "medical" or a "surgical" case. If no procedures are identified, a medical MS-DRG is assigned. Patients who undergo a valid operating room procedure or another non–operating room procedure that affects MS-DRG assignment are assigned a surgical MS-DRG. It is logical that a patient who has undergone a surgical procedure would use more resources because of costs associated with anesthesia, operating and recovery rooms, and additional nursing care.

The MS-DRG classification system is divided into 25 major diagnostic categories (MDCs), which are based on all possible principal diagnoses that often correspond with an organ system.

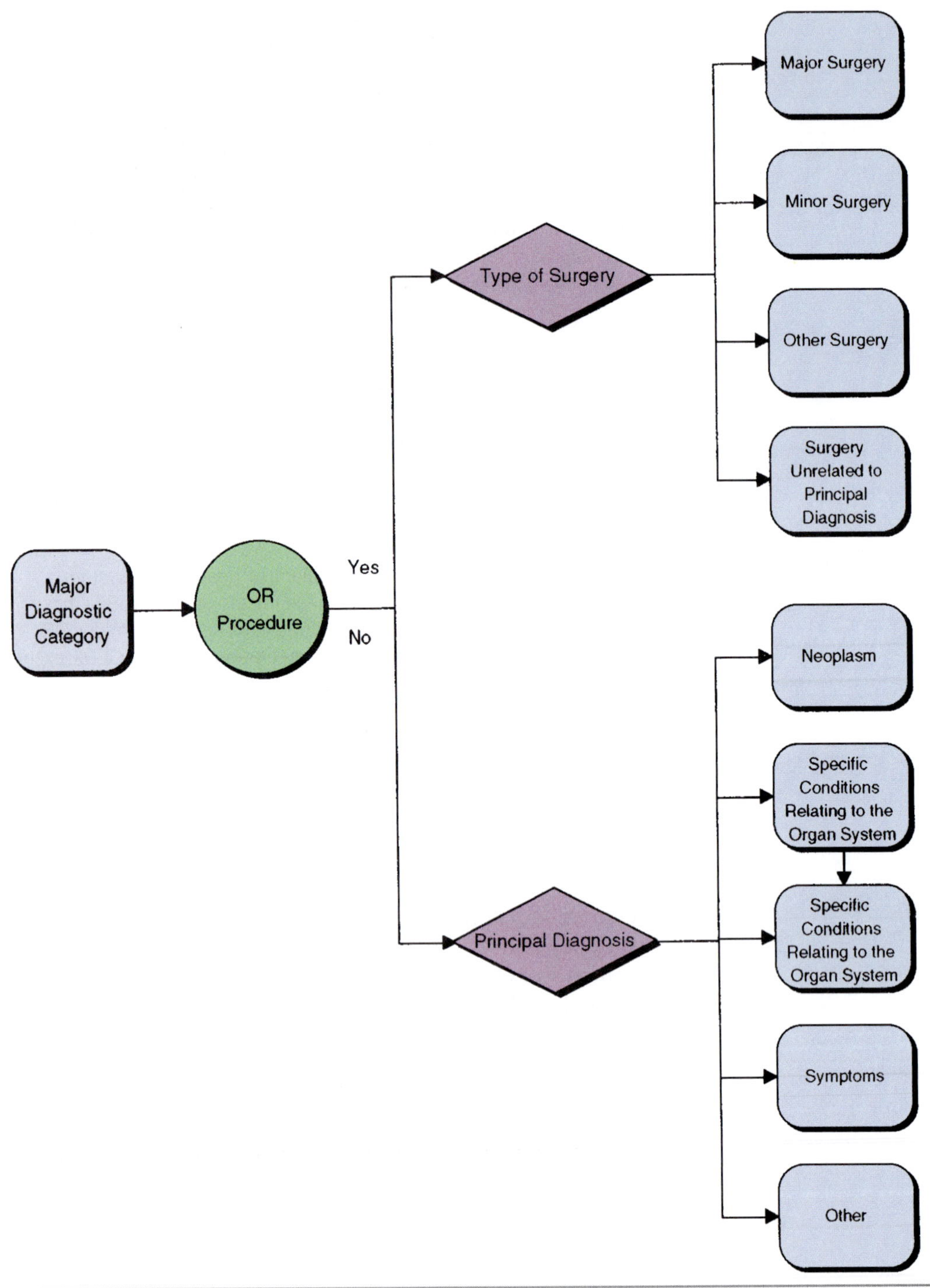

Figure 7-1. MS-DRG structure for a major diagnostic category (MDC).

MDC 1	Diseases and Disorders of the Nervous System
MDC 2	Diseases and Disorders of the Eye
MDC 3	Diseases and Disorders of the Ear, Nose, Mouth, and Throat
MDC 4	Diseases and Disorders of the Respiratory System
MDC 5	Diseases and Disorders of the Circulatory System
MDC 6	Diseases and Disorders of the Digestive System

MDC 7	Diseases and Disorders of the Hepatobiliary System and Pancreas	
MDC 8	Diseases and Disorders of the Musculoskeletal System and Connective Tissue	
MDC 9	Diseases and Disorders of the Skin, Subcutaneous Tissue, and Breast	
MDC 10	Endocrine, Nutritional, and Metabolic Diseases and Disorders	
MDC 11	Diseases and Disorders of the Kidney and Urinary Tract	
MDC 12	Diseases and Disorders of the Male Reproductive System	
MDC 13	Diseases and Disorders of the Female Reproductive System	
MDC 14	Pregnancy, Childbirth, and the Puerperium	
MDC 15	Newborns and Other Neonates with Conditions Originating in the Perinatal Period	
MDC 16	Diseases and Disorders of the Blood and Blood-Forming Organs and Immunologic Disorders	
MDC 17	Myeloproliferative Diseases and Disorders, and Poorly Differentiated Neoplasms	
MDC 18	Infectious and Parasitic Diseases (Systemic or unspecified sites).	
MDC 19	Mental Diseases and Disorders	
MDC 20	Alcohol/Drug Use and Alcohol/Drug-Induced Organic Mental Disorders	
MDC 21	Injuries, Poisonings, and Toxic Effects of Drugs	
MDC 22	Burns	
MDC 23	Factors Influencing Health Status and Other Contacts with Health Services	
MDC 24	Multiple Significant Trauma	
MDC 25	Human Immunodeficiency Virus Infections	
PreMDC	Heart transplant or implant of heart assist system	MS-DRG 001/002
	ECMO or trach with mechanical ventilation 96+ hr or PDX except face, mouth, and neck with major OR	MS-DRG 003
	Trach with mechanical ventilation 96+ hr or PDX except Face, mouth, and neck without major OR	MS-DRG 004
	Liver transplant	MS-DRG 005/006
	Lung transplant	MS-DRG 007
	Simultaneous pancreas/kidney transplant	MS-DRG 008
	Bone marrow transplant	MS-DRG 009
	Pancreas transplant	MS-DRG 010
	Tracheostomy for face, mouth, and neck diagnoses	MS-DRG 011/012/013

Other factors influencing MS-DRG assignment include:

- Patient's sex
- Patient's discharge disposition or status
- Secondary diagnoses and the presence or absence of complications or comorbidities (CC) or major complication or comorbidities (MCC)
- Birth weight for neonates
- Procedures used as proxy for CC/MCC

There are 745 MS-DRGs which group patients who have similar diagnoses, lengths of stay, and need for resources into a particular MS-DRG with a set payment rate. Specialized software called a **grouper** is used to assign the appropriate MS-DRG. Groupers are often included in the **encoder** or coding software that is used to assign diagnosis and procedure codes.

After completing a thorough review of the health record, the coder must determine the principal diagnosis on the basis of the UHDDS definition. The **principal diagnosis** is "the condition established after study to be chiefly responsible for occasioning the admission of the patient to the hospital for care." Then, codes for all secondary diagnoses and procedures can be assigned. Grouper software is used to determine the appropriate MS-DRG.

Changes may be made to ICD-9-CM codes on April 1 and/or October 1 each year. The government also makes changes to the MS-DRG system annually on October 1. These changes are published in the *Federal Register*, which is the official daily publication for rules, proposed rules, and notices of U.S. federal agencies and organizations, as well as for Executive Orders and other Presidential documents. MS-DRG changes are first published as a proposed rule, and a comment period is generally provided for the public prior to publishing of the final rule.

MS-DRG OPTIMIZATION

Optimization is the process of striving to obtain optimal reimbursement or the highest possible payment to which the facility is legally entitled on the basis of coded data supported by documentation in the health record. It is often said that "If it is not documented, it was not done." If services were performed and not documented, payment for these services may be denied. On the other hand, **maximization** is the manipulation of codes to receive maximum reimbursement without supporting documentation in the health record or with disregard for coding conventions, guidelines, and UHDDS definitions. Maximization is unethical and is addressed in the American Health Information Management Association (AHIMA) Standards of Ethical Coding, which can be found in Chapter 1.

Not all MS-DRGs are affected by the presence of a secondary diagnosis. It can be determined by the MS-DRG title whether the MS-DRG is affected by the absence or presence of a CC or MCC. A **complication** is a condition that arises during a patient's hospitalization which may lead to increased resource use. A **comorbidity** is a preexisting condition (is present on admission) which may lead to increased resource use. The fact that a physician documents that a diagnosis is a complication during a patient's stay does not necessarily mean that diagnosis will fit the definition of a complication in the MS-DRG assignment. A physician may also document that the patient had no complications during hospital stay, and an assigned secondary diagnosis may qualify as a CC or MCC for that particular MS-DRG.

EXAMPLE

MS-DRG 193, Simple pneumonia and pleurisy with MCC, 1.2505
MS-DRG 192, Simple pneumonia and pleurisy with CC, 1.0235
MS-DRG 191, Simple pneumonia and pleurisy without MCC/CC, 0.8398

In the above example, one way to optimize MS-DRG 191 would be to review the record further for documentation of a secondary diagnosis that would qualify as CC or MCC.

Ways to optimize in the above case would be to review the record for the following:

- An organism that is responsible for the pneumonia
- Respiratory neoplasm
- Septicemia
- Mechanical ventilation
- Opportunistic lung infection in a patient with HIV
- Tracheostomy with mechanical ventilation over 96 hours

Remember to optimize, supporting documentation must be included in the health record, and the definition for principal diagnosis must be met.

Some of the most commonly missed CCs or MCCs include the following:

- Atrial flutter
- Atelectasis
- Cachexia
- Cardiogenic shock
- Cardiomyopathy
- Cellulitis
- Chronic kidney disease, stages IV-VI
- Chronic obstructive pulmonary disease (COPD)—exacerbation
- Diabetes mellitus with complications
- Hematemesis
- Hyponatremia
- Malnutrition
- Melena
- Pleural effusion

- Pneumothorax
- Respiratory failure
- Urinary tract infection

MS-DRG REIMBURSEMENT

Each MS-DRG payment is determined by two basic factors:

1. Relative weight of assigned MS-DRG
2. Individual hospital payment rate or base rate

Each of the more than 745 MS-DRGs is assigned a relative weight (see Appendix B). The average relative weight factor is 1.0000. If a particular MS-DRG used twice as many resources as the average, it would be assigned a relative weight of 2.0000. If a particular MS-DRG used half as many resources as the average, it would be assigned a relative weight of 0.5000. Each year, MS-DRG relative weights are updated to reflect the following:

- Changes in treatment patterns
- Technology
- Any other factors that may change the use of hospital resources

Each hospital is assigned a base dollar amount as the hospital payment rate for a relative weight of 1.0000. Larger facilities that have more complicated cases and provide additional services may have higher hospital payment rates than smaller rural facilities. The individual hospital payment rate or base dollar amount is determined by the following:

- A regional or national adjusted standardized amount that considers the type of hospital
- Designation of large urban, urban, or rural hospital
- Wage index for the geographic area where the hospital is located

A hospital payment rate can change from time to time. It usually changes once a year, effective on October 1.

Relative weight (RW) is multiplied by the hospital's payment rate (HPR), to equal that hospital's MS-DRG reimbursement.

RW × HPR = MS-DRG payment

EXAMPLE

A patient who is admitted with pneumonia (486) and is being treated for a urinary tract infection (599.0) which is a CC, and assigned to MS-DRG 194

Simple pneumonia and pleurisy with CC is assigned. If this hospital's payment rate is $4000.00, the MS-DRG payment would be calculated as follows. MS-DRG 194 has a relative weight of 1.0235.

RW × HPR = MS-DRG payment
1.0235 × $4000.00 = $4094.00

The MS-DRG payment is not based on actual charges for that patient during the hospital stay. If the patient had actual charges that totaled more than $10,000.00, the hospital would be paid only the above amounts. The hospital would not be able to bill the patient for any additional charges other than deductible and/or coinsurance amounts. If the patient had a hospital bill that totaled $3500.00, the hospital would still be paid the above amount. The hospital would lose reimbursement in the first scenario but would gain reimbursement in the second case scenario.

The intent with a PPS system is that hospitals would know what they are going to be reimbursed for a particular type of patient before they render any services. The old payment method, or a retrospective payment system (RPS), was based on actual charges or a percentage of charges; this did not promote best practices and quality care because the hospital was paid on the basis of charges, and the higher the charges, the higher the payment. The amount of the payment is determined after the patient has been cared for and the charges assessed. If a patient experienced complications and the hospital bill went higher,

the hospital was still paid. PPS provides incentive to decrease patient complications. Hospitals must provide quality care in an efficient manner to maintain a healthy bottom line.

Each hospital stay will fit into one and only one MS-DRG category. For example, if a patient was admitted because of osteoarthritis for a hip replacement and had a myocardial infarction (MI) 2 days after the procedure, the hip replacement MS-DRG is the one that will be assigned. No additional MS-DRG is assigned to pay for the costs associated with the MI. However, the MI is an MCC, and increased reimbursement would be received because of the assignment of an MS-DRG with MCC.

If more than one procedure is performed, the procedure in the highest surgical group will determine the MS-DRG assignment. For example, if the patient had a breast biopsy and a mastectomy during the same hospital stay, the mastectomy would determine the surgical MS-DRG.

UB-04

Uniform Bill-04, or UB-04, is the claim form (Figure 7-2) that is used to submit bills to Medicare and other third party payers. For the most part, hospital billing is done electronically. The first uniform bill was introduced in 1982 and was called the UB-82. Prior to that time, each and every insurance or third party payer had its own forms. The uniform bill made it much easier for patients and hospital billing offices to submit claims to all insurance companies in a timely manner. Some different completion requirements may apply for an individual payer.

The UB-04 consists of fields for 12 diagnosis codes (9 diagnosis codes and 3 E codes) and 6 procedure codes. Codes affecting reimbursement need to be sequenced in the top nine codes in order for codes to be submitted on the UB-04. The same applies to the top six procedure codes. A code for the admitting diagnosis is also required. The admitting diagnosis does not have to be the same as the principal diagnosis.

When errors in coding occur, the hospital may resubmit the billing data with revised codes on the claim or UB-04. For Medicare patients, the hospital has 60 days from the date of the MS-DRG payment to request a review of the original MS-DRG assignment. After 60 days, no resubmissions for higher payment can be made. If an error was found that meant a lower payment for the hospital, the adjustment should be made as soon as possible.

POST–ACUTE CARE TRANSFER POLICY

The U.S. Congress, through the Balanced Budget Act of 1997, required CMS to begin applying a slightly different payment methodology when transferring from acute care to a post–acute care setting. This payment methodology was already in place for transfers from an acute facility to another short-term acute care facility. Complicated formulas are used to determine the transfer-adjusted payment.

It was found that shortly after admission, many patients were transferred to other post–acute care settings, so CMS figured it was overpaying the hospitals for these patients. CMS created special rules for certain MS-DRGs when patients were discharged immediately after their hospitalization to a rehabilitation hospital, a skilled nursing facility (SNF), a long-term care (LTC) hospital, or home health care. These MS-DRGs are called “transfer MS-DRGs” (see Appendix B). This started in 1999 with 10 transfer MS-DRGs. It had expanded to 273 transfer MS-DRGs. Although a patient may be grouped in a transfer MS-DRG, a payment reduction occurs only if all of the following conditions are met:

- The patient is in a transfer MS-DRG.
- The patient was a “short-stay” or early discharge (LOS+1 < GMLOS).
- The patient was transferred to a SNF, home health care, a rehab hospital, or a long-term care hospital.

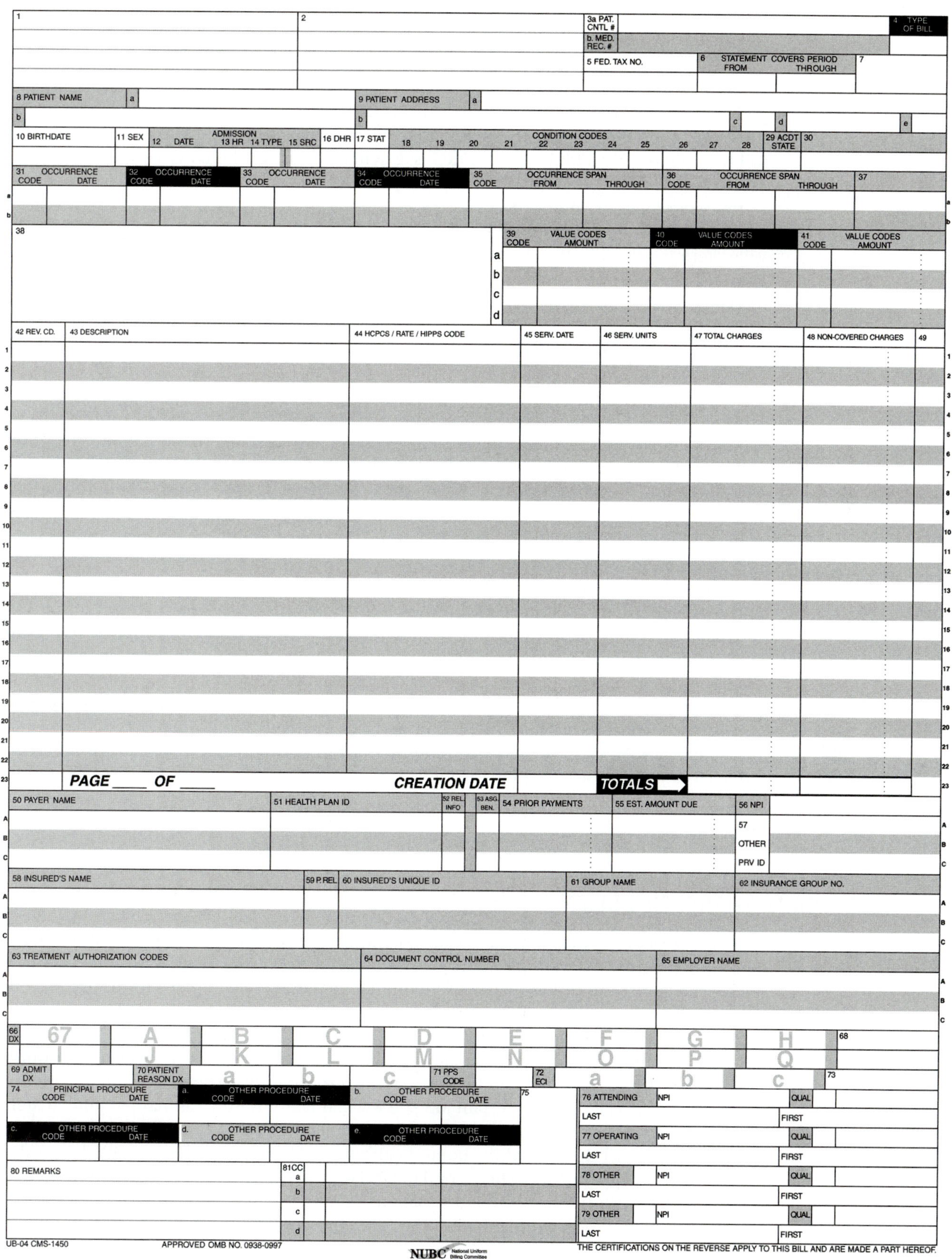

1
2
3a PAT. CNTL #
b. MED. REC. #
4 TYPE OF BILL
5 FED. TAX NO.
6 STATEMENT COVERS PERIOD FROM THROUGH
7
8 PATIENT NAME a b
9 PATIENT ADDRESS a b c d e
10 BIRTHDATE | 11 SEX | ADMISSION 12 DATE 13 HR 14 TYPE 15 SRC | 16 DHR | 17 STAT | CONDITION CODES 18 19 20 21 22 23 24 25 26 27 28 | 29 ACDT STATE | 30
31 OCCURRENCE CODE DATE | 32 OCCURRENCE CODE DATE | 33 OCCURRENCE CODE DATE | 34 OCCURRENCE CODE DATE | 35 CODE OCCURRENCE SPAN FROM THROUGH | 36 CODE OCCURRENCE SPAN FROM THROUGH | 37
a
b
38
39 CODE VALUE CODES AMOUNT | 40 CODE VALUE CODES AMOUNT | 41 CODE VALUE CODES AMOUNT
a
b
c
d
42 REV. CD. | 43 DESCRIPTION | 44 HCPCS / RATE / HIPPS CODE | 45 SERV. DATE | 46 SERV. UNITS | 47 TOTAL CHARGES | 48 NON-COVERED CHARGES | 49
1
2
3
4
5
6
7
8
9
10
11
12
13
14
15
16
17
18
19
20
21
22
23 PAGE ____ OF ____ CREATION DATE TOTALS
50 PAYER NAME | 51 HEALTH PLAN ID | 52 REL. INFO | 53 ASG. BEN. | 54 PRIOR PAYMENTS | 55 EST. AMOUNT DUE | 56 NPI
A | 57
B | OTHER
C | PRV ID
58 INSURED'S NAME | 59 P. REL | 60 INSURED'S UNIQUE ID | 61 GROUP NAME | 62 INSURANCE GROUP NO.
A
B
C
63 TREATMENT AUTHORIZATION CODES | 64 DOCUMENT CONTROL NUMBER | 65 EMPLOYER NAME
A
B
C
66 DX | 67 A B C D E F G H | 68
I J K L M N O P Q
69 ADMIT DX | 70 PATIENT REASON DX a b c | 71 PPS CODE | 72 ECI a b c | 73
74 PRINCIPAL PROCEDURE CODE DATE | a. OTHER PROCEDURE CODE DATE | b. OTHER PROCEDURE CODE DATE | 75
c. OTHER PROCEDURE CODE DATE | d. OTHER PROCEDURE CODE DATE | e. OTHER PROCEDURE CODE DATE
76 ATTENDING NPI QUAL LAST FIRST
77 OPERATING NPI QUAL LAST FIRST
80 REMARKS | 81CC a b c d
78 OTHER NPI QUAL LAST FIRST
79 OTHER NPI QUAL LAST FIRST
UB-04 CMS-1450 APPROVED OMB NO. 0938-0997 NUBC National Uniform Billing Committee THE CERTIFICATIONS ON THE REVERSE APPLY TO THIS BILL AND ARE MADE A PART HEREOF.

Figure 7-2. UB-04—form used to submit inpatient claims.

CASE-MIX INDEX

MS-DRGs provide a means of defining and measuring a hospital's **case-mix index** (CMI), in other words, how sick its patients are. Following are interrelated parts of case-mix:

- Severity of illness
- Prognosis
- Treatment difficulty
- Need for intervention
- Resource intensity

To calculate case-mix, add the relative weight of the MS-DRG assigned to each patient discharged during a specific time period. Then divide the total relative weight by the number of patients in that time period. The resultant value represents the case-mix index. Some facilities may calculate their Medicare case-mix, along with overall case-mix, which includes all patients. This value may be calculated each month, quarterly, and/or at the end of each fiscal year. If great variations in the case-mix are seen from month to month, hospital administration may want an explanation. For example, if the hospital was undergoing renovations in the surgery department and the number of surgeries for the month was significantly lower than usual, this change may cause a facility's case-mix to drop.

EXAMPLE

During the month of June, the following Medicare patients were discharged from Hospital A:

2 patients	MS-DRG 194	RW 1.0235
2 patients	MS-DRG 292	RW 1.0134
1 patient	MS-DRG 192	RW 0.8145
3 patients	MS-DRG 302	RW 0.8236
2 patients	MS-DRG 065	RW 1.1901

A total of 10 patients are included. To perform a manual calculation, add the following:

1.0235
1.0235
1.0134
1.0134
0.8145
0.8236
0.8236
0.8236
1.1901
1.1901
TOTAL 9.7393 is the total of the relative weights of the 10 patients listed above.

The next step is to divide the total relative weight by the number of patients. 9.7393 divided by 10 = 0.9739. This is the CMI for this group of patients.

Usually, these figures are calculated with the use of software programs and can be calculated using certain parameters such as specific third party payer, by date, by physician, or by clinical service. If significant coding errors and/or errors in MS-DRG assignment occur, the CMI may not be accurate.

QUALITY IMPROVEMENT ORGANIZATION

Quality improvement organizations (QIOs) work for consumers. Healthcare providers and hospitals to make sure that patients are getting the "right care at the right time in the appropriate setting." A total of 53 QIOs have been created, one for each state and territory and the District of Columbia. This network acts under the direction of CMS and is contracted to monitor the quality of health care, and to make sure that Medicare pays only for

services that are reasonable and necessary. QIO functions under 3-year contract cycles called *scopes of work* (SOWs).

PEPPER

The Program for Evaluating Payment Patterns Electronic Report (PEPPER) is an electronic report that is sent to a hospital that contains hospital-specific information for 13 target areas. These target areas are specific MS-DRGs that have been identified as being at risk for payment errors. PEPPER was developed to assist QIOs with their Hospital Payment Monitoring Programs (HPMPs) to identify and prevent payment errors due to billing, MS-DRG assignment, coding, and/or admission necessity issues.

DATA QUALITY

In Chapter 1, it was mentioned that coded data have many purposes.[1] In November 2007, AHIMA published a position statement on the "Consistency of Healthcare Diagnostic and Procedural Coding." It states that accurate and complete coded data are critical for:

- Healthcare delivery
- Research
- Public reporting
- Reimbursement
- Policy making

All users must consistently apply the same official coding rules, conventions, guidelines, and definitions. AHIMA promotes the idea that coding professionals are educated and certified to assign and validate codes and to assist with policy development related to coding accuracy.

As reimbursement and coding systems evolve, it is important to remember that the codes that are assigned today will have a role in the reimbursement system(s) of tomorrow, so it is imperative that each health record be coded accurately and completely.

CLINICAL DOCUMENTATION IMPROVEMENT PROGRAM

Incomplete, inaccurate, and illegible documentation has been a problem in health care for years. With the evolution of reimbursement systems that are based on documentation and coded data, it is imperative that hospitals make improvements in their clinical documentation. A clinical documentation improvement program (CDIP) will depend on the facility's needs and must work within the culture and framework of the organization. The success of any improvement type of program is dependent on the participation of the "right" team players. It is extremely important to get physician support and buy-in because physicians are responsible for much of the documentation within the health record.

One of the goals of a CDIP is to improve the facility's case-mix index (CMI). Case-mix data can be used for comparison with other facilities and for monitoring trends within the facility. Better documentation, along with accurate and complete coding of the health record, should lead to better reimbursement and increased CMI.

The manner in which documentation is collected should be analyzed, so improvements can be made to capture complete and accurate clinical documentation. As hospitals convert from paper to electronic records, the time is ideal for assessing all forms of documentation.

Many facilities are employing Clinical Documentation Specialists who concurrently review patient records and query the attending physician about documentation that may be missing or incomplete within the patient's record. Most documentation issues can be resolved before the patient is discharged, and the record will have more complete and accurate documentation for assigning codes. This should reduce the number of physician queries asked by the coder.

CHAPTER REVIEW EXERCISE

Choose the best answer to the followings questions.

1. A preexisting condition that is present on admission and may lead to increased resource use
   A. Complication
   B. Comorbidity
   C. Morbidity
   D. Other diagnosis
2. The condition that, after study, is established as chiefly responsible for occasioning the admission of the patient to the hospital is called the
   A. Primary diagnosis
   B. Provisional diagnosis
   C. Principal diagnosis
   D. Major diagnosis
3. DRG stands for
   A. drug-related gastritis
   B. diagnostic related groups
   C. diagnosis related group
   D. diagnostic regulation by government
4. The billing form that is currently in use in hospitals is
   A. UB-87
   B. UB-04
   C. UB-82
   D. UB-92
5. Calculate the case-mix for the following patients using the weights from Appendix B:
   2 patients MS-DRG 690
   3 patients MS-DRG 292
   1 patient MS-DRG 069
   2 patients MS-DRG 378

Complete the following questions.

6. Identify four MS-DRGs that appear on the post-transfer policy listing.
   ______________ ______________
   ______________ ______________
7. List four commonly missed CCs or MCCs.
   ______________ ______________
   ______________ ______________
8. What organization is the QIO in your state?
   ____

CHAPTER GLOSSARY

Case-mix index: a measurement used by hospitals to define how sick their patients are.

Comorbidity: a preexisting condition (it is present on admission) which may lead to increased resource use.

Complication: a condition that arises during a patient's hospitalization which may lead to increased resource use.

Encoder: coding software that is used to assign diagnosis and procedure codes.

Federal Register: the official daily publication for rules, proposed rules, and notices of U.S. federal agencies and organizations, as well as for Executive Orders and other Presidential documents.

Grouper: specialized software used to assign the appropriate MS-DRG.

Health Maintenance Organizations (HMOs): type of managed care in which hospitals, physicians, and other providers contract to provide health care for patients, usually at a discounted rate.

Maximization: the manipulation of codes to result in maximum reimbursement without supporting documentation in the health record or with disregard for coding conventions, guidelines, and UHDDS definitions.

Optimization: the process of striving to obtain optimal reimbursement or the highest possible payment to which a facility is legally entitled on the basis of documentation in the health record.

Preferred Provider Organizations (PPOs): type of managed care in which hospitals, physicians, and other providers have an arrangement with a third party payer to provide health care at discounted rates to third party payer clients.

Principal Diagnosis: "the condition established after study to be chiefly responsible for occasioning the admission of the patient to the hospital for care."

Prospective payment system: method of reimbursement in which payment is made on the basis of a predetermined, fixed amount rather than for billed charges.

Reimbursement: payment for healthcare services.

Self-insured plans: self-insurance fund is set up by an employer to provide health claim benefits for employees.

Third Party Payer: makes payments for health services on behalf of the patients; may be a government program, insurance company, or managed care plan.

CHAPTER 8

Symptoms, Signs, and Ill-defined Conditions, V Codes, E Codes, and Late Effects

(V Codes, E Codes, and ICD-9-CM Chapter 16, Codes 780-799)

CHAPTER OUTLINE

LEARNING OBJECTIVES

- Apply and assign the correct ICD-9-CM codes in accordance with Official Guidelines for Coding and Reporting
- Determine when to assign signs and symptoms codes
- Assign the correct V codes
- Explain the importance of documentation in relation to MS-DRGs for reimbursement

ABBREVIATIONS

ASCUS atypical squamous cells of undetermined significance
BMI body mass index
COPD chronic obstructive pulmonary disease
CT computerized tomography
CVA cerebrovascular accident
MS-DRG Medicare Severity diagnosis-related group
FUO fever of unknown origin
HGSIL high-grade squamous intraepithelial lesion
HIV human immunodeficiency virus
ICD-9-CM *International Classification of Diseases, 9th Revision, Clinical Modification*
OR Operating Room

ABBREVIATIONS—*cont'd*

PSA prostate-specific antigen
RW relative weight
SIDS sudden infant death syndrome
UTI urinary tract infection

ANATOMY AND PHYSIOLOGY

Signs, symptoms, ill-defined conditions, V codes, E codes, and late effects can affect any of the body systems. The anatomy and physiology of these body systems are outlined in their respective chapters.

DISEASE CONDITIONS

Symptoms, Signs, and Ill-Defined Conditions (780-799), Chapter 16 in the ICD-9-CM code book, is divided into the following categories:

CATEGORY	SECTION TITLES
780-789	Symptoms
790-796	Nonspecific Abnormal Findings
797-799	Ill-Defined and Unknown Causes of Morbidity and Mortality

See Figure 8-1 for details on an instructional note that appears at the very beginning of Chapter 16 of the Tabular List and applies to the entire chapter. This note provides information on to the appropriate use of signs and symptoms codes.

V codes and E codes are found in the supplemental sections of the code book, and codes are assigned in the same manner as other codes, that is, by looking up the main term in the Alphabetic Index or E code index and verifying the code in the Tabular.

A few V code guidelines are explained with the various chapter guidelines; these will be addressed in those chapters. Some of them are repeated in the guidelines for V codes

16. SYMPTOMS, SIGNS, AND ILL-DEFINED CONDITIONS (780–799)

This section includes symptoms, signs, abnormal results of laboratory or other investigative procedures, and ill-defined conditions regarding which no diagnosis classifiable elsewhere is recorded.

Signs and symptoms that point rather definitely to a given diagnosis are assigned to some category in the preceding part of the classification. In general, categories 780–796 include the more ill-defined conditions and symptoms that point with perhaps equal suspicion to two or more diseases or to two or more systems of the body, and without the necessary study of the case to make a final diagnosis. Practically all categories in this group could be designated as "not otherwise specified," or as "unknown etiology," or as "transient." The Alphabetic Index should be consulted to determine which symptoms and signs are to be allocated here and which to more specific sections of the classification; the residual subcategories numbered .9 are provided for other relevant symptoms which cannot be allocated elsewhere in the classification.

The conditions and signs or symptoms included in categories 780–796 consist of: (a) cases for which no more specific diagnosis can be made even after all facts bearing on the case have been investigated; (b) signs or symptoms existing at the time of initial encounter that proved to be transient and whose causes could not be determined; (c) provisional diagnoses in a patient who failed to return for further investigation or care; (d) cases referred elsewhere for investigation or treatment before the diagnosis was made; (e) cases in which a more precise diagnosis was not available for any other reason; (f) certain symptoms which represent important problems in medical care and which it might be desired to classify in addition to a known cause.

Figure 8-1. Instructional note that appears at the beginning of Chapter 16.

and are reviewed in this chapter. These codes are addressed at the beginning of the book because they apply to all body systems. V codes, E codes, late effects, and signs and symptoms are common throughout the book.

ICD-9-CM Official Guidelines for Coding and Reporting

Please refer to the companion Evolve site for the most current guidelines.

16. Chapter 16: Signs, Symptoms and Ill-Defined Conditions (780-799)
Reserved for future guideline expansion

Although there are no guidelines in the Chapter 16 section, there are very specific guidelines in the general coding guideline section that address the coding of signs and symptoms, late effects and impending conditions. Only guidelines applicable to this chapter are included; therefore the numbering is not sequential.

B. General Coding Guidelines

6. Signs and symptoms
Codes that describe symptoms and signs, as opposed to diagnoses, are acceptable for reporting purposes when a related definitive diagnosis has not been established (confirmed) by the provider. Chapter 16 of ICD-9-CM, Symptoms, Signs, and Ill-Defined conditions (codes 780.0 - 799.9) contain many, but not all codes for symptoms.

7. Conditions that are an integral part of a disease process
Signs and symptoms that are **associated routinely with a** disease process should not be assigned as additional codes, unless otherwise instructed by the classification.

8. Conditions that are not an integral part of a disease process
Additional signs and symptoms that may not be associated routinely with a disease process should be coded when present.

Symptoms (780-789)

A **symptom** is subjective evidence of a disease or of a patient's condition as perceived by the patient.

EXAMPLE

The patient presents to the ER complaining of a severe headache. The headache is an example of a symptom because it is a description of the patient's condition as perceived by the patient, 784.0.

A **sign** is objective evidence of a disease or of a patient's condition as perceived by the patient's examining physician.

EXAMPLE

The patient has a fever. This can be discerned by noting the patient's elevated temperature, 780.6.

It can be difficult to determine whether a sign or a symptom from Chapter 16 is integral to the disease. It may be necessary to access resource books or the Internet to find the most common symptoms of a disease or condition. As was previously stated in Chapter 5 of this text, signs and symptoms codes are acceptable to code:

- When no definitive diagnosis has been established
- When they are not an integral part of the disease process

It is not acceptable to code signs or symptoms:

- When a definitive diagnosis has not been established
- When they are an integral part of the disease process

EXAMPLE

Fever due to pneumonia, 486.

Fever is one of the symptoms of pneumonia that is integral to the disease process. Only the pneumonia should be coded.

EXAMPLE

Dehydration due to pneumonia, 486, 276.51.

Although many patients who are admitted to the hospital may be dehydrated, not all patients who have pneumonia become dehydrated.

EXAMPLE

Patient was admitted with right lower quadrant abdominal pain with nausea and vomiting. Patient has a low-grade fever. A diagnosis of acute appendicitis was confirmed upon removal of the patient's appendix in the operating room (OR), 540.9, 47.09. The fever, abdominal pain, and nausea/vomiting are all symptoms of appendicitis and are not coded.

EXERCISE 8-1

Assign codes to the following conditions using your ICD-9-CM code book.

1. Alteration in mental status ____________
2. Fever of unknown origin (FUO) ____________
3. Right upper quadrant abdominal pain due to cholecystitis versus peptic ulcer disease ____________
4. Ascites due to cirrhosis of liver ____________
5. Oliguria ____________
6. Renal colic ____________
7. Change in bowel habits ____________
8. Substernal chest pain ____________
9. Loss of appetite ____________
10. Ataxia ____________
11. Generalized pain ____________
12. Delirium ____________

Nonspecific Abnormal Findings (790-796)

Many times, an abnormality or elevation in a test result will lead to further investigation or repeat performance of certain tests. The patient may be without any signs or symptoms, and no definitive diagnosis may explain the abnormality. Some of the main terms that may be used to assist with location of these codes include "abnormal," "abnormality," "abnormalities," "elevation," and "findings, abnormal, without diagnosis." These abnormal findings must be documented by the physician to be coded. A coder should not code an abnormal finding on the basis of a review of laboratory results or reports of other diagnostic procedures (Coding Clinic 1990:2Q:pp 15-16).[1]

EXAMPLE

Elevated blood pressure. Patient does not have a history of hypertension, 796.2.

EXAMPLE

Abnormal lung x-ray. Patient will be scheduled for a computerized tomography (CT) of the chest, 793.1.

EXERCISE 8-2

Assign codes to the following conditions using your ICD-9-CM code book.

1. Significant drop in hematocrit __________
2. Abnormal coagulation profile __________
3. Proteinuria __________
4. Abnormal Pap smear with atypical squamous cells of undetermined signifi cance (ASCUS) __________
5. Abnormal mammogram __________
6. Bacteremia __________
7. Abnormal lead levels in blood __________
8. Positive Mantoux test __________
9. Elevated CA-125 __________
10. Transaminasemia __________

Ill-Defined and Unknown Causes of Morbidity and Mortality (797-799)

The title of this section is fitting because the codes included in this section are ill-defined and of unknown causes, ranging from sudden infant death syndrome (SIDS) to decreased libido.

EXAMPLE Elderly patient is receiving physical therapy for debility, 799.3.

EXERCISE 8-3

Assign codes to the following conditions using your ICD-9-CM code book.

1. Respiratory arrest __________
2. Sudden infant death syndrome (SIDS) __________
3. Decreased libido __________
4. Hypoxia __________
5. Nervousness __________

B. General Coding Guidelines

12. Late Effects

A late effect is the residual effect (condition produced) after the acute phase of an illness or injury has terminated. There is no time limit on when a late effect code can be used. The residual may be apparent early, such as in cerebrovascular accident cases, or it may occur months or years later, such as that due to a previous injury. Coding of late effects generally requires two codes sequenced in the following order: The condition or nature of the late effect is sequenced first. The late effect code is sequenced second.

An exception to the above guidelines are those instances where the code for late effect is followed by a manifestation code identified in the Tabular List and title, or the late effect code has been expanded (at the fourth and fifth-digit levels) to include the manifestation(s). The code for the acute phase of an illness or injury that led to the late effect is never used with a code for the late effect.

LATE EFFECTS

Late effect codes are not assigned to a separate chapter in the Tabular. A **late effect** code is used when the acute phase of an illness or injury has passed but a residual condition or health problem remains. The residual is coded first, and the appropriate late effects code is assigned to indicate the cause of the residual. In most instances, two codes are assigned—one for the residual that is being treated and the other to indicate the cause. As the guidelines state, no time limit applies, and it is possible that a residual may not be immediately apparent. It is also possible for a patient to have more than one residual condition.

EXAMPLE Sensorineural deafness due to meningitis, 389.10, 326.

EXAMPLE Facial droop as a result of previous stroke (CVA). The CVA late effect codes include the residual and its cause in a combination code, so only one code is necessary, 438.83.

Sometimes, it may be difficult to determine what is the residual and what is the late effect. The following exercise will help with that differentiation.

EXERCISE 8-4

Write the term(s) that represent the residual and its cause in the following cases on the lines provided, and assign the appropriate codes.

1. Keloid scar left forearm, resulting from second-degree burns. Injury occurred 1 year ago

Residual: ______________________ Code: __________

Cause: ______________________ Code: __________

2. Foreign body (bullet) in soft tissue of thigh due to gunshot injury years ago

Residual: ______________________ Code: __________

Cause: ______________________ Code: __________

3. Traumatic arthritis in the ankle due to previous ankle fracture

Residual: ______________________ Code: __________

Cause: ______________________ Code: __________

4. Dysphagia due to CVA 3 months ago

Residual: ______________________ Code: __________

Cause: ______________________ Code: __________

V CODES

The V codes are located after Chapter 17 in the Tabular List. According to the guidelines, ICD-9-CM provides codes that should be assigned to encounters for circumstances other than a disease or injury. The Supplementary Classification of Factors Influencing Health Status and Contact with Health Services (V01.0-V89) is provided to deal with occasions when circumstances other than a disease or injury (codes 001-999) are recorded as a diagnosis or problem.

18. Classification of Factors Influencing Health Status and Contact with Health Service (Supplemental V01-V89)

Note: The chapter specific guidelines provide additional information about the use of V codes for specified encounters.

a. Introduction

ICD-9-CM provides codes to deal with encounters for circumstances other than a disease or injury. The Supplementary Classification of Factors Influencing Health Status and Contact with Health Services (V01.0-V89) is provided to deal with occasions when circumstances other than a disease or injury (codes 001-999) are recorded as a diagnosis or problem.

There are four primary circumstances for the use of V codes:

1) A person who is not currently sick encounters the health services for some specific reason, such as to act as an organ donor, to receive prophylactic care, such as inoculations or health screenings, or to receive counseling on health related issues.

EXAMPLE

The patient was admitted to donate a kidney for a brother's kidney transplant. A nephrectomy was performed without complication, V59.4, 55.51.

2) A person with a resolving disease or injury, or a chronic, long-term condition requiring continuous care, encounters the health care system for specific aftercare of that disease or injury (e.g., dialysis for renal disease; chemotherapy for malignancy; cast change). A diagnosis/symptom code should be used whenever a current, acute, diagnosis is being treated or a sign or symptom is being studied.

EXAMPLE

A patient was admitted for hemodialysis for ESRD, V56.0, 585.6, 39.95.

EXAMPLE

Patient with hydrocephalus was admitted for removal of ventricular shunt, V53.01, 331.4, 02.43.

3) Circumstances or problems influence a person's health status but are not in themselves a current illness or injury.

EXAMPLE

A patient was admitted with congestive heart failure and coronary artery disease. The patient has a history of coronary artery bypass graft and a family history of coronary artery disease, 428.0, 414.00, V45.81, V17.3.

4) Newborns, to indicate birth status

EXAMPLE

A newborn is delivered by vaginal delivery and receives prophylactic vaccination for hepatitis B before discharge, V30.00, V05.3, 99.55.

EXAMPLE

Healthy liveborn twins born via cesarean section: Twin A, V30.01; Twin B, V30.01

b. V codes use in any healthcare setting

V codes are for use in any healthcare setting. V codes may be used as either a first listed (principal diagnosis code in the inpatient setting) or secondary code, depending on the circumstances of the encounter. Certain V codes may only be used as first listed, others only as secondary codes.

See Section I.C.18.e, V Code Table.

c. V Codes indicate a reason for an encounter

They are not procedure codes. A corresponding procedure code must accompany a V code to describe the procedure performed.

EXAMPLE A female patient was admitted for elective sterilization and endoscopic ligation with Falope ring was performed, V25.2, 66.29.

d. Categories of V Codes

1) Contact/Exposure

Category V01 indicates contact with or exposure to communicable diseases. These codes are for patients who do not show any sign or symptom of a disease but have been exposed to it by close personal contact with an infected individual or are in an area where a disease is epidemic. These codes may be used as a first listed code to explain an encounter for testing, or, more commonly, as a secondary code to identify a potential risk.

EXAMPLE Exposure to anthrax, V01.81.

2) Inoculations and vaccinations

Categories V03-V06 are for encounters for inoculations and vaccinations. They indicate that a patient is being seen to receive a prophylactic inoculation against a disease. The injection itself must be represented by the appropriate procedure code. A code from V03-V06 may be used as a secondary code if the inoculation is given as a routine part of preventive health care, such as a well-baby visit.

EXAMPLE Vaccination for influenza, V04.81, 99.52.

3) Status

Status codes indicate that a patient is either a carrier of a disease or has the sequelae or residual of a past disease or condition. This includes such things as the presence of prosthetic or mechanical devices resulting from past treatment. A status code is informative, because the status may affect the course of treatment and its outcome. A status code is distinct from a history code. The history code indicates that the patient no longer has the condition.

A status code should not be used with a diagnosis code from one of the body system chapters, if the diagnosis code includes the information provided by the status code. For example, code V42.1, Heart transplant status, should not be used with code 996.83, Complications of transplanted heart. The status code does not provide additional information. The complication code indicates that the patient is a heart transplant patient.

Assignment of V codes can be problematic because some can be used only as the principal diagnosis, others can be used as both principal and secondary diagnoses, and some can be used only as secondary diagnoses. It can be difficult to locate V codes in the Alphabetic Index. Coders will often say, "I did not know there was a V code for that." It is very important to be familiar with the different types and uses of V codes. Because appropriate main terms are difficult to find in the Alphabetic Index, some common main terms are as follows:

Admission
Aftercare
Attention to
Boarder
Care (of)
Carrier
Checking
Contraception
Counseling
Dialysis
Donor
Examination
Fitting of
Follow-up
Health, Healthy
History
Maintenance
Maladjustment
Observation
Problem
Procedure (surgical)
Prophylactic
Replacement
Screening
Status
Supervision (of)
Test
Transplant
Unavailability of medical facilities
Vaccination

Guidelines for V codes provide a lot of detail and descriptions of the various sections of V codes. It may be necessary to review these guidelines frequently; V codes will also be addressed in most of the following chapters because some V codes are specific to certain body systems.

Screening V codes should be assigned only when the service fits the definition of a screening. A **screening examination** is one that occurs in the absence of any signs or symptoms. It consists of examination of an asymptomatic individual to detect a given disease, typically by means of an inexpensive diagnostic test. There are V codes for prophylactic organ removal. A **prophylactic** measure is the use of medication or treatment to prevent a disease from occurring.

EXAMPLE Screening mammogram for 45-year-old patient, V76.12.

EXAMPLE Screening mammogram in a 45-year-old patient with nipple discharge, 611.79.

In this case, even though it was documented as a screening mammogram, it does not fit the definition because the nipple discharge is a symptom and a reason for the test. It would be inappropriate to assign the screening V code.

Several V codes identify the history of certain conditions. Documentation of a patient's medical and surgical history may be found within the History and Physical or the Admit Note.

Sometimes, documentation in the health record may indicate a history of a particular disease or condition, and the disease or condition is actually a current or active problem. If any question arises as to whether a condition is currently an active problem, a physician query may be necessary.

Relevant family history is often documented. It may be important to code a family history of malignant neoplasm of the breast when a patient has been admitted with breast cancer and is having a mastectomy. In the Index under "History," "Family history" is a subterm, and it may be difficult to locate where the family history subterms start and stop (Figure 8-2).

EXAMPLE Patient has a past history of chronic obstructive pulmonary disease (COPD). You would not assign a V code to indicate a previous history of a respiratory condition but the code for the active disease. COPD is a chronic condition that cannot be cured, 496.

EXAMPLE The patient has a history of urinary tract infections (UTIs). In this case, no documentation, such as antibiotic therapy, indicates that the patient currently has a UTI, so a history of UTI V code is appropriate, V13.02.

EXAMPLE Patient has a history of thrombocytopenia. The physician documents that the patient still has a low platelet count, (thrombocytopenia and low platelets are assigned the same code). A V code is not necessary as the patient continues to be thrombocytopenic, 287.5.

The status V codes/categories are:

V02	Carrier or suspected carrier of infectious diseases Carrier status indicates that a person harbors the specific organisms of a disease without manifest symptoms and is capable of transmitting the infection.
V08	Asymptomatic HIV infection status This code indicates that a patient has tested positive for HIV but has manifested no signs or symptoms of the disease.
V09	Infection with drug-resistant microorganisms This category indicates that a patient has an infection that is resistant to drug treatment. Sequence the infection code first.
V21	Constitutional states in development
V22.2	Pregnant state, incidental This code is a secondary code only for use when the pregnancy is in no way complicating the reason for visit. Otherwise, a code from the obstetric chapter is required.

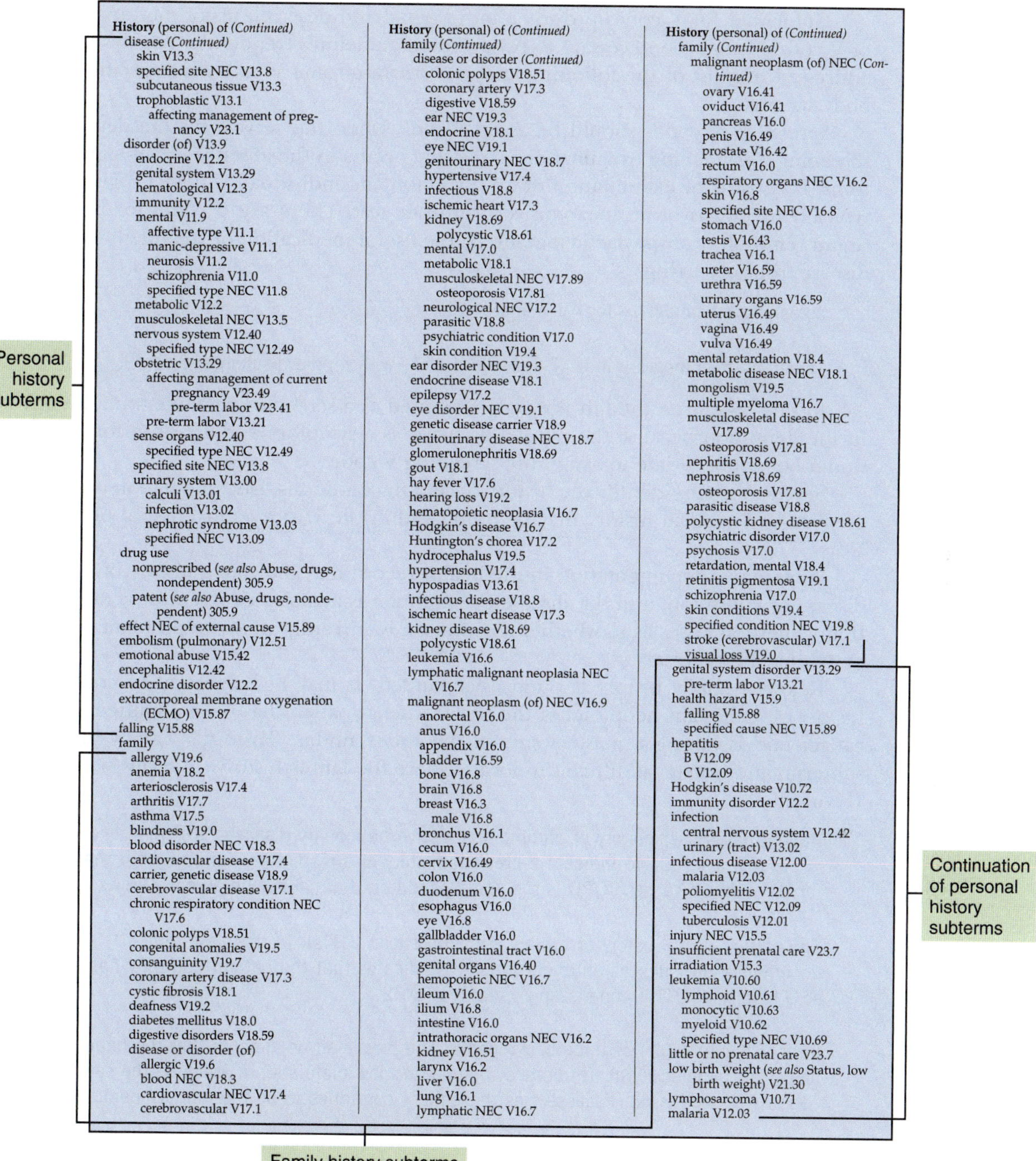

History (personal) of *(Continued)*
disease *(Continued)*
skin V13.3
specified site NEC V13.8
subcutaneous tissue V13.3
trophoblastic V13.1
affecting management of pregnancy V23.1
disorder (of) V13.9
endocrine V12.2
genital system V13.29
hematological V12.3
immunity V12.2
mental V11.9
affective type V11.1
manic-depressive V11.1
neurosis V11.2
schizophrenia V11.0
specified type NEC V11.8
metabolic V12.2
musculoskeletal NEC V13.5
nervous system V12.40
specified type NEC V12.49
obstetric V13.29
affecting management of current pregnancy V23.49
pre-term labor V23.41
pre-term labor V13.21
sense organs V12.40
specified type NEC V12.49
specified site NEC V13.8
urinary system V13.00
calculi V13.01
infection V13.02
nephrotic syndrome V13.03
specified NEC V13.09
drug use
nonprescribed (*see also* Abuse, drugs, nondependent) 305.9
patent (*see also* Abuse, drugs, nondependent) 305.9
effect NEC of external cause V15.89
embolism (pulmonary) V12.51
emotional abuse V15.42
encephalitis V12.42
endocrine disorder V12.2
extracorporeal membrane oxygenation (ECMO) V15.87
falling V15.88
family
allergy V19.6
anemia V18.2
arteriosclerosis V17.4
arthritis V17.7
asthma V17.5
blindness V19.0
blood disorder NEC V18.3
cardiovascular disease V17.4
carrier, genetic disease V18.9
cerebrovascular disease V17.1
chronic respiratory condition NEC V17.6
colonic polyps V18.51
congenital anomalies V19.5
consanguinity V19.7
coronary artery disease V17.3
cystic fibrosis V18.1
deafness V19.2
diabetes mellitus V18.0
digestive disorders V18.59
disease or disorder (of)
allergic V19.6
blood NEC V18.3
cardiovascular NEC V17.4
cerebrovascular V17.1

History (personal) of *(Continued)*
family *(Continued)*
disease or disorder *(Continued)*
colonic polyps V18.51
coronary artery V17.3
digestive V18.59
ear NEC V19.3
endocrine V18.1
eye NEC V19.1
genitourinary NEC V18.7
hypertensive V17.4
infectious V18.8
ischemic heart V17.3
kidney V18.69
polycystic V18.61
mental V17.0
metabolic V18.1
musculoskeletal NEC V17.89
osteoporosis V17.81
neurological NEC V17.2
parasitic V18.8
psychiatric condition V17.0
skin condition V19.4
ear disorder NEC V19.3
endocrine disease V18.1
epilepsy V17.2
eye disorder NEC V19.1
genetic disease carrier V18.9
genitourinary disease NEC V18.7
glomerulonephritis V18.69
gout V18.1
hay fever V17.6
hearing loss V19.2
hematopoietic neoplasia V16.7
Hodgkin's disease V16.7
Huntington's chorea V17.2
hydrocephalus V19.5
hypertension V17.4
hypospadias V13.61
infectious disease V18.8
ischemic heart disease V17.3
kidney disease V18.69
polycystic V18.61
leukemia V16.6
lymphatic malignant neoplasia NEC V16.7
malignant neoplasm (of) NEC V16.9
anorectal V16.0
anus V16.0
appendix V16.0
bladder V16.59
bone V16.8
brain V16.8
breast V16.3
male V16.8
bronchus V16.1
cecum V16.0
cervix V16.49
colon V16.0
duodenum V16.0
esophagus V16.0
eye V16.8
gallbladder V16.0
gastrointestinal tract V16.0
genital organs V16.40
hemopoietic NEC V16.7
ileum V16.0
ilium V16.8
intestine V16.0
intrathoracic organs NEC V16.2
kidney V16.51
larynx V16.2
liver V16.0
lung V16.1
lymphatic NEC V16.7

History (personal) of *(Continued)*
family *(Continued)*
malignant neoplasm (of) NEC *(Continued)*
ovary V16.41
oviduct V16.41
pancreas V16.0
penis V16.49
prostate V16.42
rectum V16.0
respiratory organs NEC V16.2
skin V16.8
specified site NEC V16.8
stomach V16.0
testis V16.43
trachea V16.1
ureter V16.59
urethra V16.59
urinary organs V16.59
uterus V16.49
vagina V16.49
vulva V16.49
mental retardation V18.4
metabolic disease NEC V18.1
mongolism V19.5
multiple myeloma V16.7
musculoskeletal disease NEC V17.89
osteoporosis V17.81
nephritis V18.69
nephrosis V18.69
osteoporosis V17.81
parasitic disease V18.8
polycystic kidney disease V18.61
psychiatric disorder V17.0
psychosis V17.0
retardation, mental V18.4
retinitis pigmentosa V19.1
schizophrenia V17.0
skin conditions V19.4
specified condition NEC V19.8
stroke (cerebrovascular) V17.1
visual loss V19.0
genital system disorder V13.29
pre-term labor V13.21
health hazard V15.9
falling V15.88
specified cause NEC V15.89
hepatitis
B V12.09
C V12.09
Hodgkin's disease V10.72
immunity disorder V12.2
infection
central nervous system V12.42
urinary (tract) V13.02
infectious disease V12.00
malaria V12.03
poliomyelitis V12.02
specified NEC V12.09
tuberculosis V12.01
injury NEC V15.5
insufficient prenatal care V23.7
irradiation V15.3
leukemia V10.60
lymphoid V10.61
monocytic V10.63
myeloid V10.62
specified type NEC V10.69
little or no prenatal care V23.7
low birth weight (*see also* Status, low birth weight) V21.30
lymphosarcoma V10.71
malaria V12.03

Figure 8-2. Family history subterms.

V26.5x	Sterilization status
V42	Organ or tissue replaced by transplant
V43	Organ or tissue replaced by other means
V44	Artificial opening status
V45	Other postsurgical states
V46	Other dependence on machines
V49.6	Upper limb amputation status
V49.7	Lower limb amputation status

Note: Categories V42-V46, and subcategories V49.6, V49.7 are for use only if there are no complications or malfunctions of the organ or tissue replaced, the amputation site or the equipment on which the patient is dependent.

V49.81 Postmenopausal status

V49.82 Dental sealant status

V49.83 Awaiting organ transplant status

V58.6**x** Long-term (current) drug use

Codes from this subcategory indicate a patient's continuous use of a prescribed drug (including such things as aspirin therapy) for the long-term treatment of a condition or for prophylactic use. It is not for use for patients who have addictions to drugs. Assign a code from subcategory V58.6, Long-term (current) drug use, if the patient is receiving a medication for an extended period as a prophylactic measure (such as for the prevention of deep vein thrombosis) or as treatment of a chronic condition (such as arthritis) or a disease requiring a lengthy course of treatment (such as cancer). Do not assign a code from subcategory V58.6 for medication being administered for a brief period of time to treat an acute illness or injury (such as a course of antibiotics to treat acute bronchitis).

V83 Genetic carrier status

Genetic carrier status indicates that a person carries a gene, associated with a particular disease, which may be passed to offspring who may develop that disease. The person does not have the disease and is not at risk of developing the disease.

V84 Genetic susceptibility status

Genetic susceptibility indicates that a person has a gene that increases the risk of that person developing the disease.

Codes from category V84, Genetic susceptibility to disease, should not be used as principal or first-listed codes. If the patient has the condition to which he/she is susceptible, and that condition is the reason for the encounter, the code for the current condition should be sequenced first. If the patient is being seen for follow-up after completed treatment for this condition, and the condition no longer exists, a follow-up code should be sequenced first, followed by the appropriate personal history and genetic susceptibility codes. If the purpose of the encounter is genetic counseling associated with procreative management, a code from subcategory V26.3, Genetic counseling and testing, should be assigned as the first-listed code, followed by a code from category V84. Additional codes should be assigned for any applicable family or personal history.

See Section I.C. 18.d.14 for information on prophylactic organ removal due to a genetic susceptibility.

V86 Estrogen receptor status

EXAMPLE

A patient was admitted for myocardial infarction. The patient is status post mitral valve replacement with porcine valve, 410.91, V42.2.

4) History (of)

There are two types of history V codes, personal and family. Personal history codes explain a patient's past medical condition that no longer exists and is not receiving any treatment, but that has the potential for recurrence, and therefore may require continued monitoring. The exceptions to this general rule are category V14, Personal history of allergy to medicinal agents, and subcategory V15.0, Allergy, other than to medicinal agents. A person who has had an allergic episode to a substance or food in the past should always be considered allergic to the substance.

Family history codes are for use when a patient has a family member(s) who has had a particular disease that causes the patient to be at higher risk of also contracting the disease.

Personal history codes may be used in conjunction with follow-up codes and family history codes may be used in conjunction with screening codes to explain the need for a test or procedure. History codes are also acceptable on any medical record regardless of the reason for visit. A history of an illness, even if

no longer present, is important information that may alter the type of treatment ordered.

The history V code categories are:

V10 Personal history of malignant neoplasm
V12 Personal history of certain other diseases
V13 Personal history of other diseases
Except: V13.4, Personal history of arthritis, and V13.6, Personal history of congenital malformations. These conditions are life-long so are not true history codes.
V14 Personal history of allergy to medicinal agents
V15 Other personal history presenting hazards to health
Except: V15.7, Personal history of contraception.
V16 Family history of malignant neoplasm
V17 Family history of certain chronic disabling diseases
V18 Family history of certain other specific diseases
V19 Family history of other conditions

EXAMPLE Family history of polycystic kidney disease, V18.61.

EXAMPLE Personal history of exposure to asbestos, V15.84.

5) Screening

Screening is the testing for disease or disease precursors in seemingly well individuals so that early detection and treatment can be provided for those who test positive for the disease. Screenings that are recommended for many subgroups in a population include: routine mammograms for women over 40, a fecal occult blood test for everyone over 50, an amniocentesis to rule out a fetal anomaly for pregnant women over 35, because the incidence of breast cancer and colon cancer in these subgroups is higher than in the general population, as is the incidence of Down's syndrome in older mothers.

The testing of a person to rule out or confirm a suspected diagnosis because the patient has some sign or symptom is a diagnostic examination, not a screening. In these cases, the sign or symptom is used to explain the reason for the test.

A screening code may be a first listed code if the reason for the visit is specifically the screening exam. It may also be used as an additional code if the screening is done during an office visit for other health problems. A screening code is not necessary if the screening is inherent to a routine examination, such as a pap smear done during a routine pelvic examination.

Should a condition be discovered during the screening then the code for the condition may be assigned as an additional diagnosis.

The V code indicates that a screening exam is planned. A procedure code is required to confirm that the screening was performed.

The screening V code categories:

V28 Antenatal screening
V73-V82 Special screening examinations

EXAMPLE Screening for prostate cancer, V76.44.

6) Observation

There are two observation V code categories. They are for use in very limited circumstances when a person is being observed for a suspected condition that is ruled out. The observation codes are not for use if an injury or illness or any signs or symptoms related to the suspected condition are present. In such cases the diagnosis/symptom code is used with the corresponding E code to identify any external cause.

The observation codes are to be used as principal diagnosis only. The only exception to this is when the principal diagnosis is required to be a code from the V30, Live born infant, category. Then the V29 observation code is sequenced after the V30 code. Additional codes may be used in addition to the observation code but only if they are unrelated to the suspected condition being observed.

The observation V code categories:

V29	Observation and evaluation of newborns for suspected condition not found. For the birth encounter, a code from category V30 should be sequenced before the V29 code.
V71	Observation and evaluation for suspected condition not found

EXAMPLE

The driver of a motor vehicle was admitted for observation after a rollover, V71.4, E816.0, E849.5.

7) Aftercare

Aftercare visit codes cover situations when the initial treatment of a disease or injury has been performed and the patient requires continued care during the healing or recovery phase, or for the long-term consequences of the disease. The aftercare V code should not be used if treatment is directed at a current, acute disease or injury. The diagnosis code is to be used in these cases. Exceptions to this rule are codes V58.0, Radiotherapy, and codes from subcategory V58.1, Encounter for chemotherapy and immunotherapy for neoplastic conditions. These codes are to be first listed, followed by the diagnosis code when a patient's encounter is solely to receive radiation therapy or chemotherapy for the treatment of a neoplasm. Should a patient receive both chemotherapy and radiation therapy during the same encounter code V58.0 and V58.1 may be used together on a record with either one being sequenced first.

The aftercare codes are generally first listed to explain the specific reason for the encounter. An aftercare code may be used as an additional code when some type of aftercare is provided in addition to the reason for admission and no diagnosis code is applicable. An example of this would be the closure of a colostomy during an encounter for treatment of another condition.

Certain aftercare V code categories need a secondary diagnosis code to describe the resolving condition or sequelae, for others, the condition is inherent in the code title.

Additional V code aftercare category terms include, fitting and adjustment, and attention to artificial openings.

Status V codes may be used with aftercare V codes to indicate the nature of the aftercare. For example code V45.81, Aortocoronary bypass status, may be used with code V58.73, Aftercare following surgery of the circulatory system, NEC, to indicate the surgery for which the aftercare is being performed. Also, a transplant status code may be used following code V58.44, Aftercare following organ transplant, to identify the organ transplanted. A status code should not be used when the aftercare code indicates the type of status, such as using V55.0, Attention to tracheostomy with V44.0, Tracheostomy status.

The aftercare V category/codes:

V52	Fitting and adjustment of prosthetic device and implant
V53	Fitting and adjustment of other device
V54	Other orthopedic aftercare
V55	Attention to artificial openings
V56	Encounter for dialysis and dialysis catheter care
V57	Care involving the use of rehabilitation procedures
V58.0	Radiotherapy
V58.11	Encounter for antineoplastic chemotherapy
V58.12	Encounter for antineoplastic immunotherapy
V58.3x	Attention to dressings and sutures
V58.41	Encounter for planned postoperative wound closure

V58.42	Aftercare, surgery, neoplasm
V58.43	Aftercare, surgery, trauma
V58.44	Aftercare involving organ transplant
V58.49	Other specifi ed aftercare following surgery
V58.7x	Aftercare following surgery
V58.81	Fitting and adjustment of vascular catheter
V58.82	Fitting and adjustment of nonvascular catheter
V58.83	Monitoring therapeutic drug
V58.89	Other specifi ed aftercare

EXAMPLE

A patient was admitted for takedown of a colostomy placed 3 months ago for diverticular disease, Patient still has diverticulosis, V55.3, 562.10, 46.52.

8) Follow-up

The follow-up codes are used to explain continuing surveillance following completed treatment of a disease, condition, or injury. They imply that the condition has been fully treated and no longer exists. They should not be confused with aftercare codes that explain current treatment for a healing condition or its sequelae. Follow-up codes may be used in conjunction with history codes to provide the full picture of the healed condition and its treatment. The follow-up code is sequenced first, followed by the history code.

A follow-up code may be used to explain repeated visits. Should a condition be found to have recurred on the follow-up visit, then the diagnosis code should be used in place of the follow-up code.

The follow-up V code categories:

V24	Postpartum care and evaluation
V67	Follow-up examination

EXAMPLE

Routine postpartum follow-up at 6 weeks. No problems or medical issues, V24.2.

9) Donor

Category V59 is the donor codes. They are used for living individuals who are donating blood or other body tissue. These codes are only for individuals donating for others, not for self donations. They are not for use to identify cadaveric donations.

EXAMPLE

Bone marrow donor, V59.3, 41.91.

10) Counseling

Counseling V codes are used when a patient or family member receives assistance in the aftermath of an illness or injury, or when support is required in coping with family or social problems. They are not necessary for use in conjunction with a diagnosis code when the counseling component of care is considered integral to standard treatment.

The counseling V categories/codes:

V25.0	General counseling and advice for contraceptive management
V26.3	Genetic counseling
V26.4	General counseling and advice for procreative management
V61	Other family circumstances
V65.1	Person consulted on behalf of another person
V65.3	Dietary surveillance and counseling
V65.4	Other counseling, not elsewhere classified

EXAMPLE

Dietary counseling for diabetic diet, V65.3, 250.00.

11) Obstetrics and related conditions

See Section I.C.11., the Obstetrics guidelines for further instruction on the use of these codes.

V codes for pregnancy are for use in those circumstances when none of the problems or complications included in the codes from the Obstetrics chapter exist (a routine prenatal visit or postpartum care). Codes V22.0, Supervision of normal first pregnancy, and V22.1, Supervision of other normal pregnancy, are always first listed and are not to be used with any other code from the OB chapter.

The outcome of delivery, category V27, should be included on all maternal delivery records. It is always a secondary code.

V codes for family planning (contraceptive) or procreative management and counseling should be included on an obstetric record either during the pregnancy or the postpartum stage, if applicable.

Obstetrics and related conditions V code categories:

V22	Normal pregnancy
V23	Supervision of high-risk pregnancy Except: V23.2, Pregnancy with history of abortion, Code 646.3, Habitual aborter, from the OB chapter is required to indicate a history of abortion during a pregnancy.
V24	Postpartum care and evaluation
V25	Encounter for contraceptive management Except V25.0x *(See Section I.C.18.d.11, Counseling)*
V26	Procreative management Except V26.5x, Sterilization status, V26.3 and V26.4 *(See Section I.C.18.d.11., Counseling)*
V27	Outcome of delivery
V28	Antenatal screening *(See Section I.C.18.d.6., Screening)*

EXAMPLE Vaginal delivery of a single female infant with no complications, 650, V27.0.

12) Newborn, infant and child

See Section I.C.15, the Newborn guidelines for further instruction on the use of these codes.

Newborn V code categories:

V20	Health supervision of infant or child
V29	Observation and evaluation of newborns for suspected condition not found *(See Section I.C.18.d.7, Observation)*
V30-V39	Liveborn infant according to type of birth

EXAMPLE Single liveborn female infant born via vaginal delivery, V30.00.

13) Routine and administrative examinations

The V codes allow for the description of encounters for routine examinations, such as, a general check-up, or, examinations for administrative purposes, such as, a preemployment physical. The codes are not to be used if the examination is for diagnosis of a suspected condition or for treatment purposes. In such cases the diagnosis code is used. During a routine exam, should a diagnosis or condition be discovered, it should be coded as an additional code. Preexisting and chronic conditions and history codes may also be included as additional codes as long as the examination is for administrative purposes and not focused on any particular condition.

Pre-operative examination V codes are for use only in those situations when a patient is being cleared for surgery and no treatment is given.

The V codes categories/code for routine and administrative examinations:

V20.2 Routine infant or child health check
Any injections given should have a corresponding procedure code.

V70 General medical examination

V72 Special investigations and examinations

Codes V72.5 and V72.6 may be used if the reason for the patient encounter is for routine laboratory/radiology testing in the absence of any signs, symptoms, or associated diagnosis. If routine testing is performed during the same encounter as a test to evaluate a sign, symptom, or diagnosis, it is appropriate to assign both the V code and the code describing the reason for the non-routine test.

EXAMPLE Preoperative examination for respiratory clearance for surgery. The patient has emphysema and is scheduled for cholecystectomy for cholelithiasis, V72.82, 492.8, 574.20.

14) Miscellaneous V codes

The miscellaneous V codes capture a number of other healthcare encounters that do not fall into one of the other categories. Certain of these codes identify the reason for the encounter, others are for use as additional codes that provide useful information on circumstances that may affect a patient's care and treatment.

Prophylactic Organ Removal

For encounters specifically for prophylactic removal of breasts, ovaries, or another organ due to a genetic susceptibility to cancer or a family history of cancer, the principal or first listed code should be a code from subcategory V50.4, Prophylactic organ removal, followed by the appropriate genetic susceptibility code and the appropriate family history code.

If the patient has a malignancy of one site and is having prophylactic removal at another site to prevent either a new primary malignancy or metastatic disease, a code for the malignancy should also be assigned in addition to a code from subcategory V50.4. A V50.4 code should not be assigned if the patient is having organ removal for treatment of a malignancy, such as the removal of the testes for the treatment of prostate cancer.

Miscellaneous V code categories/codes:

V07 Need for isolation and other prophylactic measures
V50 Elective surgery for purposes other than remedying health states
V58.5 Orthodontics
V60 Housing, household, and economic circumstances
V62 Other psychosocial circumstances
V63 Unavailability of other medical facilities for care
V64 Persons encountering health services for specific procedures, not carried out
V66 Convalescence and Palliative Care
V68 Encounters for administrative purposes
V69 Problems related to lifestyle
V85 Body Mass Index

EXAMPLE A patient was admitted for cosmetic surgery (bilateral breast implants), V50.1, 85.54.

15) Nonspecific V codes

Certain V codes are so non-specific, or potentially redundant with other codes in the classification, that there can be little justification for their use in the inpatient setting. Their use in the outpatient setting should be limited to those instances when there is no further documentation to permit more precise coding. Otherwise, any sign or symptom or any other reason for visit that is captured in another code should be used.

Nonspecific V code categories/codes:

V11	Personal history of mental disorder A code from the mental disorders chapter, with an in remission fifth-digit, should be used.
V13.4	Personal history of arthritis
V13.6	Personal history of congenital malformations
V15.7	Personal history of contraception
V23.2	Pregnancy with history of abortion
V40	Mental and behavioral problems
V41	Problems with special senses and other special functions
V47	Other problems with internal organs
V48	Problems with head, neck, and trunk
V49	Problems with limbs and other problems

Exceptions:

V49.6	Upper limb amputation status
V49.7	Lower limb amputation status
V49.81	Postmenopausal status
V49.82	Dental sealant status
V49.83	Awaiting organ transplant status

V51	Aftercare involving the use of plastic surgery
V58.2	Blood transfusion, without reported diagnosis
V58.9	Unspecified aftercare

See Section IV.K. and Section IV.L. of the Outpatient guidelines.

V CODE TABLE

Please refer to Appendix A to locate this table. This table lists all V codes and identifies which V codes may be used as a first diagnosis only, as a first or additional diagnosis, as an additional diagnosis only, or as a nonspecific diagnosis.

EXERCISE 8-5

Assign codes to the following conditions using your ICD-9-CM code book.

1. Patient receives long-term oxygen therapy for emphysema; patient has a history of tobacco abuse ____________
2. Dietary counseling for morbid obesity; body mass index (BMI) is 41 ____________
3. Screening for prostate cancer; patient has no signs or symptoms ____________
4. Family history of ischemic heart disease ____________
5. Personal history of malaria ____________
6. History of urinary calculi ____________
7. Personal history of diabetes mellitus, type II; patient currently takes insulin for diabetes ____________
8. Awaiting liver transplant for end-stage liver disease ____________
9. Patient on Coumadin (anticoagulant) because of mechanical heart valve ____________
10. Patient is noncompliant with diet and medications ____________

Using the V code table found in Appendix A, select the correct answer.

11. V52.1 Fitting and adjustment of artificial leg
    - **A.** First diagnosis only
    - **B.** First or additional diagnosis
    - **C.** Additional diagnosis only
    - **D.** Nonspecific diagnosis

12. V46.11 Dependence on respiratory status
- **A.** First diagnosis only
- **B.** First or additional diagnosis
- **C.** Additional diagnosis only
- **D.** Nonspecific diagnosis

13. V42.0 Kidney replaced by transplant
- **A.** First diagnosis only
- **B.** First or additional diagnosis
- **C.** Additional diagnosis only
- **D.** Nonspecific diagnosis

14. V27.0 Outcome of delivery—single liveborn
- **A.** First diagnosis only
- **B.** First or additional diagnosis
- **C.** Additional diagnosis only
- **D.** Nonspecific diagnosis

15. V22.0 Supervision of normal first pregnancy
- **A.** First diagnosis only
- **B.** First or additional diagnosis
- **C.** Additional diagnosis only
- **D.** Nonspecific diagnosis

EXTERNAL CAUSES

As with V codes, detailed guidelines have been put forth for the use of E codes. The Index for E codes is located after the Alphabetic Index for diseases. Codes are located by using the Index and then verifying the appropriate E code in the Tabular. The assignment of E codes may depend on facility policy and particular state requirements. For example, the assignment of E codes could be helpful in determining the number of head injuries that occur as the result of bicycle accidents. These data may be used to support bicycle helmet programs in a particular city or state. Codes for external causes are never used as a principal diagnosis; E codes are always assigned as an additional code. E codes identify the cause of an injury, adverse effects or poisoning, and the intent and place of occurrence. E codes for an adverse effect or poisoning can be found in the Table of Drugs and Chemicals. It may be necessary to assign more than one E code to fully describe the event. The use of E codes is addressed in greater detail later in Chapters 19, 20, and 21.

According to the guidelines, E codes only need to be assigned for the initial visit (except when acute fracture codes are still applicable). Insufficient documentation can make it difficult to assign E codes and especially place of occurrence E codes. Although a place of occurrence code, E849.9 is in the code book to designate an unspecified place, the guidelines state not to use an E code if the place of occurrence is not stated. It takes practice to figure out which main terms to look up in the Alphabetic Index.

EXAMPLE Concussion due to accidental fall down steps at home, 850.9, E880.9, E849.0.

19. Supplemental Classification External Causes Injury and Poisoning (E-codes, E800-E999)

Introduction: These guidelines are provided for those who are currently collecting E codes in order that there will be standardization in the process. If your institution plans to begin collecting E codes, these guidelines are to be applied. The use of E codes is supplemental to the application of ICD-9-CM diagnosis codes. E codes are never to be recorded as principal diagnoses (first-listed in non-inpatient setting) and are not required for reporting to CMS.

External causes of injury and poisoning codes (E codes) are intended to provide data for injury research and evaluation of injury prevention strategies. E codes capture how the injury or poisoning happened (cause), the intent (unintentional or accidental; or intentional, such as suicide or assault), and the place where the event occurred.

Some major categories of E codes include:

- transport accidents
- poisoning and adverse effects of drugs, medicinal substances and biologicals
- accidental falls
- accidents caused by fire and flames
- accidents due to natural and environmental factors
- late effects of accidents, assaults or self injury
- assaults or purposely inflicted injury
- suicide or self inflicted injury

These guidelines apply for the coding and collection of E codes from records in hospitals, outpatient clinics, emergency departments, other ambulatory care settings and provider offices, and nonacute care settings, except when other specific guidelines apply.

The Supplementary Classification of E codes is divided into the following categories:

CATEGORY	SECTION TITLES
E800-E807	Railway accidents
E810-E819	Motor vehicle traffic accidents
E820-E825	Motor vehicle nontraffic accidents
E826-E829	Other road vehicle accidents
E830-E838	Water transport accidents
E840-E845	Air and space transport accidents
E846-E848	Vehicle accidents, not elsewhere classifiable
E849	Place of occurrence
E850-E858	Accidental poisoning by drugs, medicinal substances, and biologicals
E860-E869	Accidental poisoning by other solid and liquid substances, gases, and vapors
E870-E876	Misadventures of patients during surgical and medical care
E878-E879	Surgical and medical procedure as the cause of abnormal reaction of patient or later complication, without mention of misadventure at the time of procedure
E880-E888	Accidental falls
E890-E899	Accidents caused by fire and flames
E900-E909	Accidents due to natural and environmental factors
E910-E915	Accidents caused by submersion, suffocation, and foreign bodies
E916-E928	Other accidents
E929	Late effects of accidental injury
E930-E949	Drugs, medicinal and biological substances causing adverse effects in therapeutic use
E950-E959	Suicide and self-inflicted injury
E960-E969	Homicide and injury purposely inflicted by other persons
E970-E978	Legal intervention
E980-E989	Injury undetermined whether accidentally or purposely inflicted
E990-E999	Injury resulting from operations of war

a. General E Code Coding Guidelines

1) Used with any code in the range of 001-V89

An E code may be used with any code in the range of 001-V89, which indicates an injury, poisoning, or adverse effect due to an external cause.

2) Assign the appropriate E code for all initial treatments

Assign the appropriate E code for the initial encounter of an injury, poisoning, or adverse effect of drugs, not for subsequent treatment.

External cause of injury codes (E-codes) may be assigned while the acute fracture codes are still applicable.

See Section 1.C.17.b.1 for coding of acute fractures.

EXAMPLE

Injury left knee due to twisting movement while playing basketball at the gym, 959.7, E927, E849.4.

3) Use the full range of E codes

Use the full range of E codes to completely describe the cause, the intent and the place of occurrence, if applicable, for all injuries, poisonings, and adverse effects of drugs.

EXAMPLE

Injury left wrist and dislocation right elbow from fall on escalator in public building. Dislocation was reduced, 832.00, 959.3, 79.72, E880.0, E849.6.

4) Assign as many E codes as necessary

Assign as many E codes as necessary to fully explain each cause. If only one E code can be recorded, assign the E code most related to the principal diagnosis.

5) The selection of the appropriate E code

The selection of the appropriate E code is guided by the Index to External Causes, which is located after the alphabetical index to diseases and by Inclusion and Exclusion notes in the Tabular List.

6) E code can never be a principal diagnosis

An E code can never be a principal (first listed) diagnosis.

Usually, E codes are reported in a specific designated area within a computer system or on an abstracting form. A limited number of fields may be available for reporting of E codes. When this occurs, the coder will need to refer to these guidelines to aid in the selection of the most important E codes. Facility policy may also provide instruction.

7) External cause code(s) with systemic inflammatory response syndrome (SIRS)

An external cause code is not appropriate with a code from subcategory 995.9, unless the patient also has an injury, poisoning, or adverse effect of drugs.

b. Place of Occurrence Guideline

Use an additional code from category E849 to indicate the Place of Occurrence for injuries and poisonings. The Place of Occurrence describes the place where the event occurred and not the patient's activity at the time of the event.

Do not use E849.9 if the place of occurrence is not stated.

EXAMPLE

Injury to the wrist occurred on the playground. Patient fell off slide, 959.3, E884.0, E849.4.

c. Adverse Effects of Drugs, Medicinal and Biological Substances Guidelines

1) Do not code directly from the Table of Drugs

Do not code directly from the Table of Drugs and Chemicals. Always refer back to the Tabular List.

2) Use as many codes as necessary to describe

Use as many codes as necessary to describe completely all drugs, medicinal or biological substances.

EXAMPLE

Patient was treated for epistaxis which is likely due to the patient's long term use of Coumadin for atrial fibrillation. Patient was taking the Coumadin as prescribed. 784.7, 427.31, V58.61, E934.2.

3) **If the same E code would describe the causative agent**
   If the same E code would describe the causative agent for more than one adverse reaction, assign the code only once.
4) **If two or more drugs, medicinal or biological substances**
   If two or more drugs, medicinal or biological substances are reported, code each individually unless the combination code is listed in the Table of Drugs and Chemicals. In that case, assign the E code for the combination.
5) **When a reaction results from the interaction of a drug(s)**
   When a reaction results from the interaction of a drug(s) and alcohol, use poisoning codes and E codes for both.

EXAMPLE

A patient combined Percodan with beer and was stuporous and drowsy, 965.09, 980.0, 780.09, E980.0, E980.9.

6) **If the reporting format limits the number of E codes**
   If the reporting format limits the number of E codes that can be used in reporting clinical data, code the one most related to the principal diagnosis. Include at least one from each category (cause, intent, place) if possible.

   If there are different fourth digit codes in the same three digit category, use the code for "Other specified" of that category. If there is no "Other specified" code in that category, use the appropriate "Unspecified" code in that category.

   If the codes are in different three digit categories, assign the appropriate E code for other multiple drugs and medicinal substances.
7) **Codes from the E930-E949 series**
   Codes from the E930-E949 series must be used to identify the causative substance for an adverse effect of drug, medicinal and biological substances, correctly prescribed and properly administered. The effect, such as tachycardia, delirium, gastrointestinal hemorrhaging, vomiting, hypokalemia, hepatitis, renal failure, or respiratory failure, is coded and followed by the appropriate code from the E930-E949 series.

EXAMPLE

Hypokalemia due to Lasix therapy for congestive heart failure, 276.8, 428.0, E944.4.

d. Multiple Cause E Code Coding Guidelines

If two or more events cause separate injuries, an E code should be assigned for each cause. The first listed E code will be selected in the following order:

E codes for child and adult abuse take priority over all other E codes.
See Section I.C.19.e., Child and Adult abuse guidelines.

E codes for terrorism events take priority over all other E codes except child and adult abuse.

E codes for cataclysmic events take priority over all other E codes except child and adult abuse and terrorism.

E codes for transport accidents take priority over all other E codes except cataclysmic events and child and adult abuse and terrorism.

The first-listed E code should correspond to the cause of the most serious diagnosis due to an assault, accident, or self-harm, following the order of hierarchy listed above.

e. Child and Adult Abuse Guideline

1) **Intentional injury**
   When the cause of an injury or neglect is intentional child or adult abuse, the first listed E code should be assigned from categories E960-E968, Homicide and injury purposely inflicted by other persons, (except category E967). An E code from category E967, Child and adult battering and other maltreatment, should be added as an additional code to identify the perpetrator, if known.

EXAMPLE A wife was seen with head and face injuries due to spousal beatings and abuse, 995.81, 959.01, 959.09, E968.9, E967.3.

2) Accidental intent

In cases of neglect when the intent is determined to be accidental E code E904.0, Abandonment or neglect of infant and helpless person, should be the first listed E code.

f. Unknown or Suspected Intent Guideline

1) If the intent (accident, self-harm, assault) of the cause of an injury or poisoning is unknown

If the intent (accident, self-harm, assault) of the cause of an injury or poisoning is unknown or unspecified, code the intent as undetermined E980-E989.

EXAMPLE Poisoning due to phenobarbital and Seconal, 967.0, E980.1.

2) If the intent (accident, self-harm, assault) of the cause of an injury or poisoning is questionable

If the intent (accident, self-harm, assault) of the cause of an injury or poisoning is questionable, probable or suspected, code the intent as undetermined E980-E989.

EXAMPLE Suspected intentional poisoning due to phenobarbital and Seconal, 967.0, E980.1.

g. Undetermined Cause

When the intent of an injury or poisoning is known, but the cause is unknown, use codes: E928.9, Unspecified accident, E958.9, Suicide and self-inflicted injury by unspecified means, and E968.9, Assault by unspecified means.

These E codes should rarely be used, as the documentation in the medical record, in both the inpatient outpatient and other settings, should normally provide sufficient detail to determine the cause of the injury.

h. Late Effects of External Cause Guidelines

1) Late effect E codes

Late effect E codes exist for injuries and poisonings but not for adverse effects of drugs, misadventures and surgical complications.

2) Late effect E codes (E929, E959, E969, E977, E989, or E999.1)

A late effect E code (E929, E959, E969, E977, E989, or E999.1) should be used with any report of a late effect or sequela resulting from a previous injury or poisoning (905-909).

EXAMPLE Keloid scar due to previous burns from fire (accidental), 701.4, 906.9, E929.4.

3) Late effect E code with a related current injury

A late effect E code should never be used with a related current nature of injury code.

4) Use of late effect E codes for subsequent visits

Use a late effect E code for subsequent visits when a late effect of the initial injury or poisoning is being treated. There is no late effect E code for adverse effects of drugs. Do not use a late effect E code for subsequent visits for follow-up care (e.g., to assess healing, to receive rehabilitative therapy) of the injury or poisoning when no late effect of the injury has been documented.

EXAMPLE Malunion fracture of right tibia from motor vehicle accident, 733.81, 905.4, E929.0, E849.5.

i. Misadventures and Complications of Care Guidelines

1) Code range E870-E876

Assign a code in the range of E870-E876 if misadventures are stated by the provider.

EXAMPLE The colon was accidentally perforated during routine screening colonoscopy. The colon was sutured, V76.51, 998.2, 46.75, 45.23, E870.8, E849.7.

2) Code range E878-E879

Assign a code in the range of E878-E879 if the provider attributes an abnormal reaction or later complication to a surgical or medical procedure, but does not mention misadventure at the time of the procedure as the cause of the reaction.

EXAMPLE Rejection of liver transplant, 996.82, E878.0.

j. Terrorism Guidelines

1) Cause of injury identified by the Federal Government (FBI) as terrorism

When the cause of an injury is identified by the Federal Government (FBI) as terrorism, the first-listed E-code should be a code from category E979, Terrorism. The definition of terrorism employed by the FBI is found at the inclusion note at E979. The terrorism E-code is the only E-code that should be assigned. Additional E codes from the assault categories should not be assigned.

EXAMPLE The patient had a head injury due to a terrorist explosion, 959.01, E979.2.

2) Cause of an injury is suspected to be the result of terrorism

When the cause of an injury is suspected to be the result of terrorism a code from category E979 should not be assigned. Assign a code in the range of E codes based circumstances on the documentation of intent and mechanism.

EXAMPLE The patient was observed for injury after a terrorist attack involving an explosion, V71.6, E979.2.

3) Code E979.9, Terrorism, secondary effects

Assign code E979.9, Terrorism, secondary effects, for conditions occurring subsequent to the terrorist event. This code should not be assigned for conditions that are due to the initial terrorist act.

EXAMPLE The patient had posttraumatic stress syndrome after a terrorist attack, 309.81, E979.9.

4) Statistical tabulation of terrorism codes

For statistical purposes these codes will be tabulated within the category for assault, expanding the current category from E960-E969 to include E979 and E999.1.

EXERCISE 8-6

For the purposes of this exercise, assign only the appropriate E codes. Opportunities will be provided throughout the text to assign all necessary codes.

1. Fall from a ladder in the backyard ____________
2. Injury due to lightning ____________
3. Patient was bitten by a dog at a public park ____________
4. Farmer was injured by a hay mower while making hay in the field ____________
5. Child was accidentally burned by hot water ____________
6. Patient was assaulted with a baseball bat in the alley ____________
7. Patient was physically abused by a babysitter ____________
8. Suicide attempt by jumping from the balcony of an apartment ____________
9. Accidental poisoning by carbon monoxide due to a faulty furnace in the house ____________
10. Motor vehicle accident occurring on highway; patient was a passenger in vehicle ____________

PROCEDURES

Procedures can be taken from any of the chapters in Volume 3. When a V code is used as a diagnosis for a given procedure or a reason for the encounter, a procedure code is still necessary to identify that the procedure was performed. It can be confusing when a V code seems to describe a procedure.

EXAMPLE Patient was admitted for sterilization. A laparoscopic division of the fallopian tubes was performed, V25.2, 66.22.

EXAMPLE Patient is donating a kidney. A left laparoscopic nephrectomy was performed, V59.4, 55.51.

EXERCISE 8-7

Assign codes for all diagnoses and procedures using your ICD-9-CM code book.

1. Encounter for dialysis due to end-stage renal disease ____________
2. Admission for chemotherapy for ovarian cancer ____________
3. Admission for replacement of tracheostomy tube ____________
4. Admission following delivery in ambulance ____________
5. Encounter for removal of internal fixation device, right femur ____________

DOCUMENTATION/REIMBURSEMENT/MS-DRGs

Often, coding difficulties are due to lack of documentation. Lack of documentation may be defined as scanty information concerning the intent and place of occurrence for injuries, poisonings, and adverse effects. Signs and symptoms are often not correlated with a definitive diagnosis in the health record. Sometimes, pathology and other test results are not available at the time of discharge, or when the physician is dictating the discharge summary or reporting the final diagnoses. As a general rule, MS-DRGs that are assigned and have a principal diagnosis from Chapter 16 may have lower reimbursement than an MS-DRG that has a principal diagnosis of a definitive condition or disease.

Symptoms That Are Integral to a Disease Process

EXAMPLE

Patient was admitted with chest pain due to costochondritis. 733.6.

DIAGNOSES	CODES	MS-DRG	RW
Costochondritis	733.6	206	0.7848
Chest pain due to costochondritis	786.50, 733.6	313	0.5489

In this case, the symptom (chest pain) is due to a specific cause, and the chest pain is an integral part of costochondritis, so to assign a code for the chest pain would be incorrect, and would not be in accordance with the coding guidelines. The hospital would receive less reimbursement.

MS-DRG With and Without MCC/CC

EXAMPLE

Patient was admitted with abdominal pain. The patient has end-stage renal disease on dialysis. No cause was determined for the abdominal pain.

DIAGNOSES	CODES	MS-DRG	RW
Abd pain	789.00	392	0.7121
Abd pain	789.00	391	0.9565
ESRD	585.6, V45.1		

In this case, the patient has a chronic condition of ESRD so it should be reported as a secondary diagnosis. No cause was determined for the patient's abdominal pain, so assignment of 789.00 symptom code is correct for the principal diagnosis. The hospital receives less reimbursement than it deserves if the 585.6 code for the comorbidity is not assigned.

CHAPTER REVIEW EXERCISE

Assign codes for all diagnoses and procedures, including all applicable V and E codes and procedures.

1. Paresthesia __________
2. Abnormal Pap smear with high-grade squamous intraepithelial lesion (HGSIL) __________
3. History of cardiac arrest __________
4. Anasarca __________
5. Chest pain due to unstable angina __________
6. Adult failure to thrive __________
7. Insulin pump training for Type I diabetic __________
8. Complex febrile seizure __________
9. Cachexia __________
10. Sleep apnea __________
11. Debility __________
12. Patient has a gastrostomy tube and receives tube feedings __________
13. Headache due to migraine __________
14. Absence of kidney due to surgical removal __________

15. Constrictive pericarditis due to old tuberculosis infection ______________
16. Fussy baby ______________
17. Elevated blood pressure ______________
18. Screening mammogram in a high-risk patient with family history of breast cancer ______________
19. Mild mental retardation due to previous poliomyelitis ______________
20. Elevated prostate-specific antigen (PSA) ______________
21. Admission for elective circumcision ______________
22. Occult blood in stool ______________
23. Aphasia due to CVA 2 months ago ______________
24. Renal colic due to kidney stone ______________
25. Abnormal liver function tests ______________
26. Changing of gastrostomy tube in patient with dysphagia ______________
27. Diarrhea due to gastroenteritis ______________
28. Vaccination for influenza ______________
29. Patient has type I diabetes mellitus and has an insulin pump ______________
30. Prophylactic removal of both ovaries due to strong family history of ovarian cancer and genetic susceptibility. A bilateral salpingo-oophorectomy was performed ______________

Assign only the appropriate E codes to the following statements.

31. Motor vehicle accident involving collision with pedestrian. The patient was the pedestrian ______________
32. Patient in a nursing home fell out of wheelchair ______________
33. Frostbite injury due to exposure ______________
34. Injury during hurricane ______________
35. Injury due to human bite, intentional ______________

CHAPTER GLOSSARY

Late effect code: used when the acute phase of an illness or injury has passed, but a residual condition or health problem remains.

Prophylactic: medication or treatment used to prevent a disease from occurring.

Screening examination: one that occurs in the absence of any signs or symptoms. It involves examination of an asymptomatic individual to detect a given disease, typically by means of an inexpensive diagnostic test.

Sign: objective evidence of a disease or of a patient's condition as perceived by the patient's examining physician.

Symptom: subjective evidence of a disease or of a patient's condition as perceived by the patient.

CHAPTER 9

Infectious and Parasitic Diseases

(ICD-9-CM Chapter 1, Codes 001-139)

CHAPTER OUTLINE

LEARNING OBJECTIVES

- Apply and assign the correct ICD-9-CM codes in accordance with Official Guidelines for Coding and Reporting
- Recognize infectious and parasitic diseases
- Assign the correct V codes and procedure codes related to infectious and parasitic diseases
- Identify common treatments, medications, laboratory values, and diagnostic tests
- Explain the importance of documentation as it relates to MS-DRGs for reimbursement

ABBREVIATIONS

AIDS acquired immunodeficiency syndrome
C. DIFF *Clostridium difficile*
CD4 Cluster of differentiation 4
CDC Centers for Disease Control and Prevention
DMAC disseminated *Mycobacterium avium-intracellulare* complex

ABBREVIATIONS—*cont'd*

EGD esophogastroduodenoscopy
HAART highly active antiretroviral therapy
HIV human immunodeficiency virus
HIVAN HIV-associated nephropathy
HPV Human papilloma virus
HSV herpes simplex virus
IVDU intravenous drug use
MAC *Mycobacterium avium-intracellulare* complex
MAI *Mycobacterium avium-intracellulare*
MRSA methicillin-resistant *Staphylococcus aureus*
MSSA methicillin-sensitive *Staphylococcus aureus*
RPR rapid plasma reagin
SARS severe acute respiratory syndrome
SIRS systemic inflammatory response syndrome
STD sexually transmitted disease
TB tuberculosis
UTI urinary tract infection
VDRL Venereal Disease Research Laboratory
VRE Vancomycin resistant enterococcus

ICD-9-CM Official Guidelines for Coding and Reporting

Please refer to the companion Evolve website for the most current guidelines.

1. **Chapter 1: Infectious and Parasitic Diseases (001-139)**
   a. **Human Immunodeficiency Virus (HIV) Infections**
      1) **Code only confirmed cases**
      Code only confirmed cases of HIV infection/illness. This is an exception of the hospital inpatient guideline Section II, H.
      In this context, "confirmation" does not require documentation of positive serology or culture for HIV; the provider's diagnostic statement that the patient is HIV positive, or has an HIV-related illness is sufficient.

EXAMPLE

Patient with possible human immunodeficiency virus (HIV). Even though in the inpatient setting, it is acceptable to code diagnoses that are possible or suspected, in the case of possible HIV, you would not assign 042. You would have to query the physician regarding the patient's exact HIV status. This is one of the only exceptions to coding a diagnosis as if it exists when it is documented as possible or probable.

2) **Selection and sequencing of HIV codes**
(a) **Patient admitted for HIV-related condition**
If a patient is admitted for an HIV-related condition, the principal diagnosis should be 042, followed by additional diagnosis codes for all reported HIV-related conditions.

EXAMPLE

The patient was admitted for treatment of Kaposi's sarcoma of the skin. The patient's HIV has been symptomatic for the past year, 042, 176.0.

(b) **Patient with HIV disease admitted for unrelated condition**
If a patient with HIV disease is admitted for an unrelated condition (such as a traumatic injury), the code for the unrelated condition (e.g., the nature of injury code) should be the principal diagnosis. Other diagnoses would be 042 followed by additional diagnosis codes for all reported HIV-related conditions.

EXAMPLE

Fracture of the left femur in a patient who has acquired immunodeficiency syndrome (AIDS), 821.00, 042.

(c) Whether the patient is newly diagnosed
Whether the patient is newly diagnosed or has had previous admissions/encounters for HIV conditions is irrelevant to the sequencing decision.

(d) Asymptomatic human immunodeficiency virus
V08 Asymptomatic human immunodeficiency virus [HIV] infection, is to be applied when the patient without any documentation of symptoms is listed as being "HIV positive," "known HIV," "HIV test positive," or similar terminology. Do not use this code if the term "AIDS" is used or if the patient is treated for any HIV-related illness or is described as having any condition(s) resulting from his/her HIV positive status; use 042 in these cases.

EXAMPLE

The patient's HIV test last week was positive; the patient is asymptomatic, V08.

(e) Patients with inconclusive HIV serology
Patients with inconclusive HIV serology, but no definitive diagnosis or manifestations of the illness, may be assigned code 795.71, Inconclusive serologic test for Human Immunodeficiency Virus [HIV].

(f) Previously diagnosed HIV-related illness
Patients with any known prior diagnosis of an HIV-related illness should be coded to 042. Once a patient had developed an HIV-related illness, the patient should always be assigned code 042 on every subsequent admission/encounter. Patients previously diagnosed with any HIV illness (042) should never be assigned to 795.71 or V08.

EXAMPLE

HIV patient with prior history of *Pneumocystis carinii* pneumonia (PCP), 042. PCP is an opportunistic lung infection that has been identified as an AIDS-defining illness.

(g) HIV Infection in Pregnancy, Childbirth and the Puerperium
During pregnancy, childbirth or the puerperium, a patient admitted (or presenting for a health care encounter) because of an HIV-related illness should receive a principal diagnosis of 647.6X, Other specified infectious and parasitic diseases in the mother classifiable elsewhere, but complicating the pregnancy, childbirth or the puerperium, followed by 042 and the code(s) for the HIV-related illness(es). Codes from Chapter 15 always take sequencing priority.

EXAMPLE

The patient is 20 weeks pregnant and is admitted for treatment of esophageal candidiasis due to AIDS, 647.63, 042, 112.84.

Patients with asymptomatic HIV infection status admitted (or presenting for a health care encounter) during pregnancy, childbirth, or the puerperium should receive codes of 647.6X and V08.

EXAMPLE

A mother delivered liveborn twins vaginally during her hospital stay. The mother's HIV has remained asymptomatic, 651.01, 647.61, V08, V27.2.

(h) Encounters for testing for HIV
If a patient is being seen to determine his/her HIV status, use code V73.89, Screening for other specified viral disease. Use code V69.8, Other problems related to lifestyle, as a secondary code if an asymptomatic patient is in a known high risk group for HIV. Should a patient with signs or symptoms or illness, or a confirmed HIV related diagnosis be tested for HIV, code the signs and symptoms or the diagnosis. An additional counseling code V65.44 may be used if counseling is provided during the encounter for the test.

When a patient returns to be informed of his/her HIV test results use code V65.44, HIV counseling, if the results of the test are negative.

If the results are positive but the patient is asymptomatic use code V08, Asymptomatic HIV infection. If the results are positive and the patient is symptomatic use code 042, HIV infection, with codes for the HIV related symptoms or diagnosis. The HIV counseling code may also be used if counseling is provided for patients with positive test results.

EXAMPLE

Because of high-risk sexual behaviors, the patient is seen in the clinic for HIV screening, V73.89, V69.2.

EXAMPLE

The patient returns for test results that are negative and is counseled regarding HIV prevention, V65.44.

EXAMPLE

The patient returns for test results that are positive and is asymptomatic. She is instructed regarding symptoms to watch for and means of prevention, V08, V65.44.

b. Septicemia, Systemic Inflammatory Response Syndrome (SIRS), Sepsis, Severe Sepsis, and Septic Shock

1) SIRS, Septicemia, and Sepsis

(a) The terms *septicemia* and *sepsis* are often used interchangeably by providers, however they are not considered synonymous terms. The following descriptions are provided for reference but do not preclude querying the provider for clarification about terms used in the documentation:

(i) Septicemia generally refers to a systemic disease associated with the presence of pathological microorganisms or toxins in the blood, which can include bacteria, viruses, fungi or other organisms.

(ii) Systemic inflammatory response syndrome (SIRS) generally refers to the systemic response to infection, trauma/burns, or other insult (such as cancer) with symptoms including fever, tachycardia, tachypnea, and leukocytosis.

(iii) Sepsis generally refers to SIRS due to infection.

(iv) Severe sepsis generally refers to sepsis with associated acute organ dysfunction.

(b) The Coding of SIRS, Sepsis and Severe Sepsis
The coding of SIRS, sepsis and severe sepsis requires a minimum of 2 codes: a code for the underlying cause (such as infection or trauma) and a code from subcategory 995.9 Systemic inflammatory response syndrome (SIRS).

(i) The code for the underlying cause (such as infection or trauma) must be sequenced before the code from subcategory 995.9 Systemic inflammatory response syndrome (SIRS).

(ii) Sepsis and severe sepsis require a code for the systemic infection (038.xx, 112.5, etc.) and either code 995.91, Sepsis, or 995.92, Severe sepsis. If the causal organism is not documented, assign code 038.9, Unspecified septicemia.

(iii) Severe sepsis requires additional code(s) for the associated acute organ dysfunction(s).

(iv) If a patient has sepsis with multiple organ dysfunctions, follow the instructions for coding severe sepsis.

(v) Either the term sepsis or SIRS must be documented to assign a code from subcategory 995.9.

(vi) *See Section I.C.17.g.), Injury and poisoning, for information regarding systemic inflammatory response syndrome (SIRS) due to trauma/burns and other non-infectious processes.*

(c) Due to the complex nature of sepsis and severe sepsis, some cases may require querying the provider prior to assignment of the codes.

2) Sequencing sepsis and severe sepsis

(a) Sepsis and severe sepsis as principal diagnosis

If sepsis or severe sepsis is present on admission, and meets the definition of principal diagnosis, the systemic infection code (e.g., 038.xx, 112.5, etc) should be assigned as the principal diagnosis, followed by code 995.91, Sepsis, or 995.92, Severe sepsis, as required by the sequencing rules in the Tabular List. Codes from subcategory 995.9 can never be assigned as a principal diagnosis. A code should also be assigned for any localized infection, if present.

If the sepsis or severe sepsis is due to a postprocedural infection, see Section I.C.10 for guidelines related to sepsis due to postprocedural infection.

EXAMPLE

The patient was admitted and treated for SIRS with sepsis due to streptococcus, group D; the patient has cellulitis of the leg, 038.0, 995.91, 682.6.

(b) Sepsis and severe sepsis as secondary diagnoses

When sepsis or severe sepsis develops during the encounter (it was not present on admission), the systemic infection code and code 995.91 or 995.92 should be assigned as secondary diagnoses.

EXAMPLE

The patient was admitted with pneumonia due to *Staphylococcus aureus.* Two days after admission, the patient developed signs of SIRS due to the staph infection, 482.41, 038.11, 995.91.

(c) Documentation unclear as to whether sepsis or severe sepsis is present on admission

Sepsis or severe sepsis may be present on admission but the diagnosis may not be confirmed until sometime after admission. If the documentation is not clear whether the sepsis **or severe sepsis** was present on admission, the provider should be queried.

3) Sepsis/SIRS with Localized Infection

If the reason for admission is both sepsis, severe sepsis, or SIRS and a localized infection, such as pneumonia or cellulitis, a code for the systemic infection (038.xx, 112.5, etc) should be assigned first, then code 995.91 or 995.92, followed by the code for the localized infection. If the patient is admitted with a localized infection, such as pneumonia, and sepsis/SIRS doesn't develop until after admission, see guideline **I.C.1.b.**2.b).

If the localized infection is postprocedural, *see Section I.C.10 for guidelines related to sepsis due to postprocedural infection.*

EXAMPLE

The patient was admitted with pneumonia due to *Staphylococcus aureus* and SIRS due to staph infection, 038.11, 482.41, 995.91.

Note: The term urosepsis is a nonspecific term. If that is the only term documented then only code 599.0 should be assigned based on the default for the term in the ICD-9-CM index, in addition to the code for the causal organism if known.

EXAMPLE The patient was treated for urosepsis due to *E coli*, 599.0, 041.4.

4) **Bacterial Sepsis and Septicemia**
In most cases, it will be a code from category 038, Septicemia, that will be used in conjunction with a code from subcategory 995.9 such as the following:
   (a) **Streptococcal sepsis**
   If the documentation in the record states streptococcal sepsis, codes 038.0, Streptococcal septicemia, and code 995.91 should be used, in that sequence.
   (b) **Streptococcal septicemia**
   If the documentation states streptococcal septicemia, only code 038.0 should be assigned, however, the provider should be queried whether the patient has sepsis, an infection with SIRS.

5) **Acute organ dysfunction that is not clearly associated with the sepsis**
If a patient has sepsis and an acute organ dysfunction, but the medical record documentation indicates that the acute organ dysfunction is related to a medical condition other than the sepsis, do not assign code 995.92, Severe sepsis. An acute organ dysfunction must be associated with the sepsis in order to assign the severe sepsis code. If the documentation is not clear as to whether an acute organ dysfunction is related to the sepsis or another medical condition, query the provider.

EXAMPLE The patient was admitted in acute respiratory failure due to *Staphylococcus aureus* pneumonia. The patient also presented with SIRS due to staph infection associated with respiratory failure, 038.11, 482.41, 995.92, 518.81.

6) **Septic shock**
   (a) **Sequencing of septic shock**
   Septic shock generally refers to circulatory failure associated with severe sepsis, and, therefore, it represents a type of acute organ dysfunction.
   For all cases of septic shock, the code for the systemic infection should be sequenced first, followed by codes 995.92 and 785.52. Any additional codes for other acute organ dysfunctions should also be assigned. As noted in the sequencing instructions in the Tabular List, the code for septic shock cannot be assigned as a principal diagnosis.

EXAMPLE The patient was admitted with pneumonia due to *Staphylococcus aureus*. Two days after admission, the patient developed septic shock due to *Staphylococcus* sepsis, 482.41, 038.11, 995.92, 785.52.

   (b) **Septic Shock without documentation of severe sepsis**
   Septic shock indicates the presence of severe sepsis.
   Code 995.92, Severe sepsis, must be assigned with code 785.52, Septic shock, even if the term severe sepsis is not documented in the record. The "use additional code" note and the "code first" note in the tabular support this guideline. (Figure 9-1)

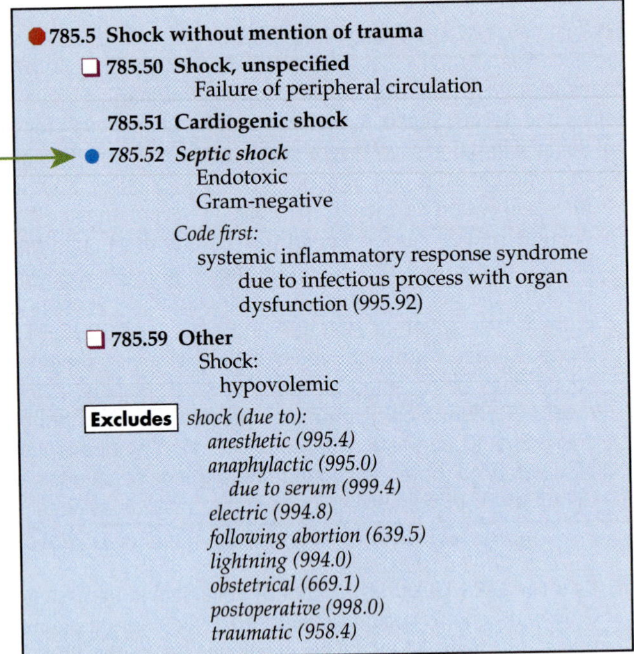

785.5 Shock without mention of trauma

785.50 Shock, unspecified
Failure of peripheral circulation

785.51 Cardiogenic shock

785.52 Septic shock
Endotoxic
Gram-negative

Code first:
systemic inflammatory response syndrome due to infectious process with organ dysfunction (995.92)

785.59 Other
Shock:
hypovolemic

Excludes *shock (due to):*
anesthetic (995.4)
anaphylactic (995.0)
due to serum (999.4)
electric (994.8)
following abortion (639.5)
lightning (994.0)
obstetrical (669.1)
postoperative (998.0)
traumatic (958.4)

Figure 9-1. Tabular entry for septic shock.

EXAMPLE

The patient was admitted with septic shock and acute renal failure and was treated for urosepsis due to *E coli*, 038.42, 995.92, 584.9, 785.52, 599.0.

7) Sepsis and septic shock complicating abortion and pregnancy
Sepsis and septic shock complicating abortion, ectopic pregnancy, and molar pregnancy are classified to category codes in Chapter 11 (630-639).
See section I.C.11.

8) Negative or inconclusive blood cultures
Negative or inconclusive blood cultures do not preclude a diagnosis of septicemia or sepsis in patients with clinical evidence of the condition, however, the provider should be queried.

9) Newborn sepsis
See Section I.C.15.j. for information on the coding of newborn sepsis.

10) Sepsis due to a Postprocedural Infection

(a) Documentation of causal relationship
As with all postprocedural complications, code assignment is based on the provider's documentation of the relationship between the infection and the procedure.

(b) Sepsis due to postprocedural infection
In cases of postprocedural sepsis, the complication code, such as code 998.59, Other postoperative infection, or 674.3x, Other complication of obstetrical surgical wounds should be coded first followed by the appropriate sepsis codes (systemic infection code and either code 995.91 or 995.92). An additional code(s) for any acute organ dysfunction should also be assigned for cases of severe sepsis.

EXAMPLE

The patient was readmitted after undergoing surgery last week; the patient is being treated for postoperative septicemia, 998.59, 038.9, E879.9.

11) **External cause of injury codes with SIRS**
Refer to Section I.C.19.a.7 for instruction on the use of external cause of injury codes with codes for SIRS resulting from trauma.

12) **Sepsis and Severe Sepsis Associated with Non-infectious Process**

(a) **Sequencing of sepsis/severe sepsis associated with non-infectious process**
In some cases, a non-infectious process, such as trauma, may lead to an infection which can result in sepsis or severe sepsis. If sepsis or severe sepsis is documented as associated with a noninfectious condition, such as a burn or serious injury, and this condition meets the definition for principal diagnosis, the code for the noninfectious condition should be sequenced first, followed by the code for the systemic infection and either code 995.91, Sepsis, or 995.92, Severe sepsis. Additional codes for any associated acute organ dysfunction(s) should also be assigned for cases of severe sepsis. If the sepsis or severe sepsis meets the definition of principal diagnosis, the systemic infection and sepsis codes should be sequenced before the noninfectious condition. When both the associated non-infectious condition and the sepsis or severe sepsis meet the definition of principal diagnosis, either may be assigned as principal diagnosis.
See Section I.C.1.b.2) (a) for guidelines pertaining to sepsis or severe sepsis as the principal diagnosis.

(b) **Only one SIRS (subcategory 995.9) code should be assigned**
Only one code **from subcategory 995.9 should be assigned for SIRS associated with trauma or other non-infectious condition. Assign the SIRS code (subcategory 995.9) that corresponds to the principal diagnosis. That is, if trauma or a non-infectious condition is the underlying cause, assign code 995.93 or 995.94. If an infection is the underlying cause, assign code 995.91 or 995.92.**
See Section I.C.17.g for information on the coding of SIRS due to trauma/burns or other noninfectious disease processes.

EXAMPLE

Acute *Staphylococcus* vaginitis, 616.10 and 041.10.

To locate the code for *Staphylococcus,* the coder must look under the main term, "Infection," and then under the subterm "*Staphylococcus.*" Sometimes, the organism and the disease condition have a combination code; this is the case for many of the pneumonia codes.

Klebsiella pneumonia, 482.0.

Apply the General Coding Guidelines as found in Chapter 5.

ANATOMY AND PHYSIOLOGY

This chapter focuses on diseases that are **communicable** (easily spread from one to another) and **parasitic** (organism taking nourishment from another organism) and the organisms that are responsible for the disease conditions. Many times, two codes are required. If a condition is not considered communicable, it will be found in a body system chapter; in this case, an additional code from category 041 or 079 may be assigned to identify causative organisms.

There is no one body system that causes or is affected by infectious disease. These organisms can be found in any or all of the body systems.

DISEASE CONDITIONS

Infectious and Parasitic Diseases (001-139), Chapter 1 in the ICD-9-CM code book, is divided into the following categories:

CATEGORY	SECTION TITLES
001-009	Intestinal Infectious Diseases
010-018	Tuberculosis
020-027	Zoonotic Bacterial Diseases
030-041	Other Bacterial Diseases
042	Human Immunodeficiency Virus (HIV) Infections
045-049	Poliomyelitis and Other Non–Arthropod-Borne Viral Diseases of Central Nervous System
050-058	Viral Diseases Accompanied by Exanthem
060-066	Arthropod-Borne Viral Diseases
070-079	Other Diseases Due to Viruses and Chlamydiae
080-088	Rickettsioses and Other Arthropod-Borne Diseases
090-099	Syphilis and Other Venereal Diseases
100-104	Other Spirochetal Diseases
110-118	Mycoses
120-129	Helminthiases
130-136	Other Infectious and Parasitic Diseases
137-139	Late Effects of Infectious and Parasitic Diseases

Intestinal Infectious Diseases (001-009)

Clostridium difficile

Clostridium difficile, which is also known as *C. diff*, is a leading cause of pseudomembranous colitis. It can be found in the Index under "Enteritis, clostridium."

C. diff is one of the most common **nosocomial** infections (hospital acquired). In the hospital setting, it may be spread from healthcare worker to patient. Spores associated with this disease can survive up to 70 days. It can also be caused by antibiotic use. This disease is characterized by watery diarrhea and abdominal cramping. The intestinal tract has usually been altered in some way to allow *C. diff* bacteria to flourish.

If a physician suspects *C. diff* (often seen in elderly hospitalized patients), a stool specimen is tested for *C. diff* toxins (cytotoxicity assay). The test results can take between 24 and 48 hours to complete. Treatment depends on the severity of infection. Often, antibiotics are changed or discontinued; however, in severe cases, a patient is treated with metronidazole (Flagyl). Patients with *C. diff* are placed on isolation protocol.

EXAMPLE *Clostridium difficile*, 008.45.

Tuberculosis (010-018)

Tuberculosis (TB) is an infection caused by *Mycobacterium tuberculosis* (Figure 9-2). These bacteria can attack any part of the body but most often attack the lungs. TB was the leading cause of death in the United States prior to the discovery of medicines to treat the disease. TB was almost eradicated but made a resurgence in the late 1980s.

TB is spread through the air via coughing or sneezing. TB of the lung is the only infectious form of TB. If TB occurs in the bones or kidney, it is not likely to be contagious. TB can be infectious only if it is an active disease. It may be necessary to isolate a patient who is suspected of having this condition pending confirmation. A form of TB called "latent TB" occurs when a person breathes the bacteria but the immune system fights them off, and they remain alive in the body but are inactive. Latent TB can become active TB. Persons with latent TB usually have a positive TB test result.

Active TB usually occurs in the population whose immune systems are too weak to fight off this disease. This group would include individuals with human immunodeficiency virus (HIV), leukemia, substance abusers, young children, and organ transplant recipients.

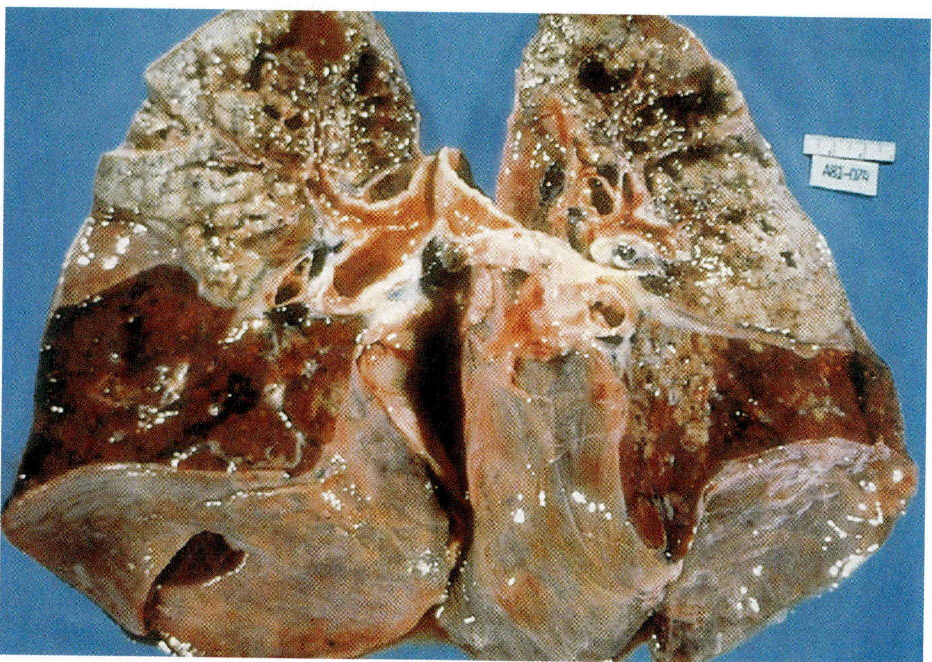

Figure 9-2. Tuberculosis.

Coding TB (010-018) requires the use of a fifth digit. The fifth digits are as follows:

- 0 unspecified
- 1 bacteriological or histological examination not done
- 2 bacteriological or histological examination unknown (at present)
- 3 tubercle bacilli found (in sputum) by microscopy
- 4 tubercle bacilli not found (in sputum) by microscopy, but found by bacterial culture
- 5 tubercle bacilli not found by bacteriological examination, but tuberculosis confirmed histologically
- 6 tubercle bacilli not found by bacteriological or histological examination, but tuberculosis confirmed by other methods [inoculation of animals]

More often than not, a fifth digit of 0, unspecified is assigned because further detail is not documented.

EXAMPLE

Patient admitted for pneumonia due to tuberculosis, which was confirmed by bacterial culture, 001.64.

EXERCISE 9-1

Assign codes to the following conditions using your ICD-9-CM code book.

1. Pyelonephritis caused by tuberculosis ____________
2. Acute miliary tuberculosis ____________
3. Interstitial keratitis caused by tuberculosis; bacterial culture performed, results unknown. ____________
4. Cavitation of the lung caused by tuberculosis ____________
5. *Salmonella* septicemia ____________
6. Food poisoning caused by *Salmonella* ____________
7. Enteritis caused by the rotavirus ____________
8. Norwalk virus ____________
9. Diarrhea caused by dysentery ____________
10. Giardiasis ____________

Zoonotic Bacterial Diseases (020-027)

Anthrax

Anthrax is a bacterial infection that is usually found in wild or domestic animals. It is most common in agricultural regions of Central America, Africa, Asia, and the Caribbean. Anthrax occurs in three forms: cutaneous, inhalation, and gastrointestinal. The most serious form is the inhalation type, which causes severe breathing problems that are most often fatal. Since the 9/11 attack on the United States and threats of anthrax attacks, a code was developed for contact or exposure to anthrax.

EXAMPLE

Contact with or exposure to anthrax, V01.81.

This code can be used for anyone who has been exposed to anthrax, or who is closely linked to persons with known exposure. See *Coding Clinic* (2002:4Q:p78).[1]

Other Bacterial Diseases (030-040)

Mycobacterium Avium Complex

Mycobacterium avium complex (MAC) or ***Mycobacterium avium-intercellulare*** (MAI) is a bacterium which attacks immunocompromised individuals. This bacterium is found in soil and water; an individual who is not immunocompromised does not succumb to the disease. This has been classified as an acquired immunodeficiency syndrome (AIDS)–defining illness. Tests that show high blood levels of the liver enzyme alkaline phosphatase may indicate MAC. Symptoms of this disease include night sweats, weight loss, and diarrhea. Prior to the advent of highly active antiretroviral therapy (HAART), which is a group of drugs given to patients with AIDS for prophylaxis, a high incidence of this condition was reported. It generally affects individuals whose T4 cell count is under 50. A variety of antibiotics are used to treat patients with this disease. Individuals with advanced AIDS often develop disseminated *Mycobacterium avium-intracellulare* complex (DMAC). Per *Coding Clinic* (1997:4Q:p3),[2] the single unique presentation of patients with DMAC is severe anemia.

EXAMPLE

Infection from *Mycobacterium avium*, 031.0.

Meningococcal Infection

Meningococcal infections are caused by the bacterium, meningococcus (Figure 9-3). These bacteria may be found in around 10% of the population (in the nose or throat) and cause no ill effects. These people are known as asymptomatic carriers. This bacterium can cause **meningitis**, which is an infection in the fluid of a person's spinal cord and brain. It also can cause septicemia (blood infection), which is known as meningococcal septicemia.

EXAMPLE

Meningococcal meningitis, 036.0.

EXAMPLE

Meningococcemia, 036.2.

Septicemia

Septicemia is the presence in the blood of pathologic microorganisms that causes systemic illness. It is also known as blood poisoning. Per *Coding Clinic* (2000:2Q:p5-6),[3] "bacteremia is bacteria in the blood, as confirmed by culture." Bacteremia is a laboratory finding, whereas septicemia is an illness. *Coding Clinic* (2003:4Q:p79-81)[4] gives a detailed explanation of the differences between the terms.

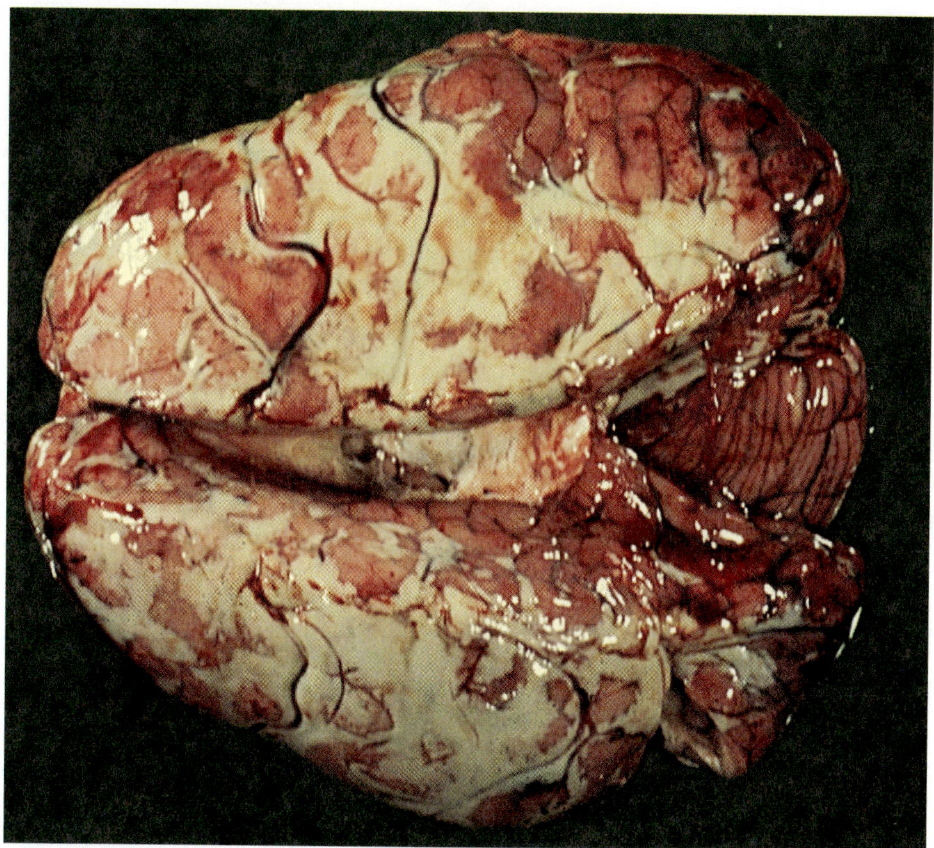

Figure 9-3. Bacterial meningitis. The surface of the brain is covered with pus.

Bacteremia—bacteria in blood, 790.7

Septicemia—systemic disease characterized by the presence of microorganisms or toxins in the blood. These organisms may include bacteria, virus, fungi, and others, 038.XX.

SIRS—systemic inflammatory response syndrome to infection or trauma. Includes symptoms such as fever, tachycardia, tachypnea, and leukocytosis

Sepsis—SIRS due to infection. Code first 038.X or trauma plus 995.91. If underlying cause of infection is something other than 038, code as follows: 038.XX, 995.91, or 995.93. Code for causative infection (i.e., pneumonia, cellulitis).

Sepsis with organ failure or severe sepsis—SIRS due to infection with organ failure. Code first 038.XX or causative trauma, 995.92 or 995.94. Then code any organ failure codes.

Septic shock, also known as endotoxic shock and/or Gram-negative shock. It is caused by a failure of the cardiovascular system and therefore meets the definition of severe sepsis. Code first 038.XX or causative trauma, 995.92 or 995.94; then code 785.2, septic shock and then code any specified organ failures.

Urosepsis is an infection of urinary site only. Code 599.0.

Sepsis due to urosepsis is an infection of the urinary site that has spread to the blood and has initiated a systemic response, 038.9, 995.91, 599.0.

If a physician documents septicemia alone and does not document sepsis, then only a code from 038.XX would be used. It would be appropriate to query the physician for the presence of sepsis.

Sepsis that occurs in the newborn or pregnant patient is governed by coding guidelines found in their respective chapters.

Negative blood cultures do not preclude a diagnosis of sepsis or septicemia in patients who exhibit clinical evidence of these conditions.

When a patient develops sepsis due to an infection following a procedure, this is coded as a complication of care. Code first 998.59, 038.XX, 995.91.

An external cause code is not required when the codes 995.91 and 995.92 are used.

EXAMPLE Patient admitted with pneumonia, fever, and tachycardia. Physician suspects sepsis and orders blood cultures. Two days after admittance, cultures are positive for pneumococcal bacteria and physician confirms pneumococcal sepsis, 038.2, 995.91, 486.

EXERCISE 9-2

Assign codes to the following conditions using your ICD-9-CM code book.

1. Respiratory anthrax ____________
2. Cutaneous anthrax ____________
3. *Mycobacterium kansasii* ____________
4. MAI ____________
5. MAC ____________
6. Whooping cough ____________
7. Patient has MAC and is on HAART. What other disease could you query for? ____________
8. Meningococcal infection in the heart muscle ____________
9. Septicemia due to meningococcal bacteria ____________
10. Urosepsis ____________
11. Gonococcal septicemia ____________
12. Severe sepsis with acute respiratory failure ____________
13. Sepsis of the newborn ____________
14. Patient presents with fever, chills, and hypotension. The physician orders blood cultures for suspected sepsis. Results are negative. The discharge summary lists sepsis due to *Escherichi coli.* ____________
15. Patient with SIRS secondary to pneumonia ____________

Bacterial Infection in Conditions Classified Elsewhere and of Unspecified Site (041)

Often, infectious diseases are characterized by a condition and a bacterial organism. When this occurs, it is appropriate to use two codes to fully describe the infection and the causative organism. Practitioners sometimes define organisms as resistant to certain antibiotics. MRSA is methicillin-resistant *Staphyloccus aureus.* If a patient has pneumonia caused by *Staphylococcus aureus* and the organism is resistant to methicillin it would be coded as 482.41 and V09.0. Likewise, practitioners may identify organisms that are sensitive to antibiotics, such as MSSA, which is methicillin-sensitive *Staphylococcus aureus.* If a patient has pneumonia caused by *Staphylococcus aureus*, which is sensitive to methicillin, it would be coded to 482.41.

EXAMPLE Urinary tract infection (UTI) caused by *E. coli*, 599.0, 041.4.

EXAMPLE UTI due to strep group D resistant to vancomycin, 599.0, 0.41.04, V09.88.

Human Immunodeficiency Virus (HIV) Infection (042)

It is important to note that codes within this section are used only when the diagnosis has been confirmed. This is an exception to the hospital inpatient guideline that allows the coding of possible, probable, or suspected diagnoses.

AIDS is an incurable disease of the immune system caused by the human immunodeficiency (HIV) virus and it is the final stage of HIV disease. This virus was believed to have originated in Africa, with the source of this infection coming from the chimpanzee. It first appeared in the United States in 1981. In the beginning this virus was seen in the homosexual and intravenous drug user (IVDU) population and later spread to the heterosexual population. The virus is found in and is transmitted by blood, semen, vaginal secretions, and breast milk. Transmission occurs through sexual contact, blood transfusions, needle sharing, or breastfeeding.

People who are infected with the HIV virus may not have any symptoms for up to 10 years. Once the immune system becomes weakened they become susceptible to opportunistic infections. Once a CD4 count goes below 350 cells/ml a patient may be at risk to develop herpes, TB, thrush, Kaposi's sarcoma, or non-Hodgkins lymphoma. When the count goes below 50 a patient may develop *Mycobacterium avium* or cytomegalovirus (CMV).

AIDS may be treated with HAART (highly active antiretroviral therapy). Sometimes drugs are given on a prophylactic basis to prevent opportunistic infections. With the use of today's drugs a patient's CD4 count can rebound above 200. However, this does not change the fact that they have AIDS and should be coded as 042. For example, it may be documented that a patient's CD4 nadir is 150. **Nadir** means the lowest level this patient's CD4 count has ever been. A patient with a nadir of 150 would be coded to 042.

Once a patient develops AIDS, from then on he or she is always assigned code 042. When a patient is admitted for treatment of an HIV-related condition, the principal diagnosis should always be 042.

EXAMPLE Patient admitted with Kaposi's sarcoma of subcutaneous tissue. Code first 042 AIDS; then, code 176.1, Kaposi's sarcoma.

If a patient is admitted with an AIDS-defining illness (Box 9-1), the principal diagnosis is 042. Likewise, if a patient is admitted with an HIV-related condition, the principal diagnosis is 042.

EXAMPLE A patient presents with severely elevated blood pressure and known hypertension and HIVAN (HIV-associated nephropathy). The patient has ESRD and is currently on dialysis. The principal diagnosis in this case is 042.

When a patient is admitted with a condition unrelated to AIDS, then the code for the unrelated condition is the principal diagnosis.

EXAMPLE A patient with a history of AIDS is admitted in alcohol withdrawal, 291.81 303.90 042.

Sometimes, patients test HIV positive but have no symptoms. V08 is the code that should be used for these patients. Tests may have inconclusive results; then, the code 795.71 should be assigned, nonspecific serologic evidence of HIV. This code can be found in the Alphabetic Index under Finding, abnormal, serological, HIV, inconclusive.

BOX 9-1 LIST OF AIDS-DEFINING CONDITIONS[5]

The Centers for Disease Control and Prevention (CDC) considers a patient to have acquired immunodeficiency syndrome (AIDS) if a CD4+ T-cell count is below 200 cells/μl (or a CD4+ T-cell percentage of total lymphocytes is less than 14%), or if the patient has one of the following defining illnesses:

- Conditions included in the 1993 AIDS surveillance case definition
- Candidiasis of bronchi, trachea, or lungs
- Candidiasis, esophageal
- Cervical cancer, invasive
- Coccidioidomycosis, disseminated or extrapulmonary
- Cryptococcosis, extrapulmonary
- Cryptosporidiosis, chronic intestinal (longer than 1 month duration)
- Cytomegalovirus disease (other than liver, spleen, or nodes)
- Cytomegalovirus retinitis (with loss of vision)
- Encephalopathy, human immunodefi ciency virus (HIV)-related
- Herpes simplex: chronic ulcer(s) (longer than 1 month duration); or bronchitis, pneumonitis, or esophagitis
- Histoplasmosis, disseminated or extrapulmonary
- Isosporiasis, chronic intestinal (longer than 1 month duration)
- Kaposi's sarcoma
- Lymphoma, Burkitt's (or equivalent term)
- Lymphoma, immunoblastic (or equivalent term)
- Lymphoma, primary, of brain
- *Mycobacterium avium* complex or *Mycobacterium kansasii*, disseminated or extrapulmonary
- *Mycobacterium tuberculosis,* any site (pulmonary or extrapulmonary)
- *Mycobacterium,* other species or unidentifi ed species, disseminated or extrapulmonary
- *Pneumocystis carinii* pneumonia
- Pneumonia, recurrent
- Progressive multifocal leukoencephalopathy
- *Salmonella* septicemia, recurrent
- Toxoplasmosis of brain
- Wasting syndrome due to HIV

EXAMPLE

Patient is being treated for thrush and is HIV positive. 112.0, V08 (thrush is not an AIDS-defining illness).

AIDS and Pregnancy

If a woman has AIDS and is pregnant, code 647.6X should be used, along with 042. Codes from Chapter 15 in the code book always take precedence.

Encounters for Testing for HIV

- Encounter for determining HIV status, V73.89, Screening for other specified viral disease
- Encounter for counseling for an HIV-negative patient, V65.44
- Encounter for an HIV-positive patient who is asymptomatic, V08; counseling code may also be used
- Encounter for HIV-positive patient who is symptomatic, 042; counseling code may also be used.

Poliomyelitis and Other Non–Arthropod-Borne Viral Diseases of the Central Nervous System (045-049)

Poliomyelitis (polio) is a viral disease that affects the nerves and is caused by the poliovirus. It is also known as infantile paralysis. This disease has been nearly eradicated in the United States as the result of mandatory vaccination. Polio is rarely seen except in four countries: Nigeria, India, Pakistan, and Afghanistan.

If people are unvaccinated, this disease may be contracted through direct contact with infected persons. The virus usually enters the body through the mouth or nose. Symptoms can resemble the flu, and a person may or may not become paralyzed. Treatment consists of alleviating the symptoms and letting the virus run its course. Essentially three types of polio infection may occur: subclinical infection, nonparalytic, and paralytic. If the spinal cord or the brain is not affected (which is the case 90% of the time), then complete recovery can occur.

EXAMPLE

A patient presents to the hospital with headache, muscle weakness, fever, and muscle spasms of the neck. After a battery of testing, it is determined that the patient has type I acute poliomyelitis, 045.91.

Viral meningitis, also known as aseptic meningitis, is an infection of the fluid in the spinal cord and the fluid around the brain. Viral meningitis is far less serious than bacterial meningitis and is rarely fatal. No treatment is available for viral meningitis other than relieving the symptoms, which usually consist of headache, stiff neck, and photophobia. Many different viruses may cause meningitis, but most cases are caused by the enteroviruses, and these viruses may be associated with other diseases. Meningitis also may be transmitted via mosquito bites.

EXAMPLE

A patient presents to the hospital with severe headache and stiff neck. A lumbar puncture is performed, and it is determined that the patient has meningitis due to Echo virus, 047.1, 03.31.

EXERCISE 9-3

Assign codes to the following conditions using your ICD-9-CM code book.

1. Patient with HIV and CD4 nadir of 100. ____________
2. Patient has HIV and a history of invasive cervical cancer. ____________
3. Patient is admitted with *Pneumocystis* pneumonia (PCP) and has a history of AIDS. ____________
4. Patient is admitted with dehydration and has AIDS. ____________
5. Patient is tested for AIDS in the physician's office, and the results are inconclusive. ____________
6. Patient is pregnant and is positive for AIDS. ____________
7. Patient is admitted with bacteremia and is an AIDS patient. ____________
8. Patient is admitted with tuberculosis and has AIDS. ____________
9. Patient is admitted with *E coli* sepsis and a CD4 count of 32, with known HIV. ____________
10. Patient is admitted with difficulty swallowing; after an esophagogastroduodenoscopy (EGD) was performed, it was discovered that the patient had candidal esophagitis and a history of being HIV positive. ____________

Viral Diseases Accompanied by Exanthem (050-058)

Herpes Zoster

Herpes zoster, or shingles, is a disease that is caused by the same virus that causes chickenpox. Once a person has contracted chickenpox, the virus remains dormant in the body in certain nerves. Shingles usually occurs in people over 50 years of age but sometimes is reported in younger people. It is caused by conditions that weaken the body's immune system such as cancer, aging, and stress.

Shingles starts as a rash that turns into fluid-filled blisters that may become very painful. Sometimes, a case of shingles results in long-term pain, known as "postherpetic neuralgia."

EXAMPLE Shingles with eye complication, 053.29.

EXAMPLE Trigeminal neuralgia as a result of shingles, 053.12.

Herpes Simplex I and II

Herpes simplex virus is another name for a cold sore or fever blister, also known as HSV type I. The disease manifests as small fluid-filled blisters (Figure 9-4). It usually occurs on the face but occasionally is noted in the genital area. People usually acquire HSV I during infancy or childhood from people who kiss them or share towels or eating utensils. In type II or genital herpes, sores appear on the vagina, penis, or buttocks. Type II is transmitted via sexual intercourse. Antiviral medications are being used to suppress recurrences of herpes.

EXAMPLE Fever blister, 054.9.

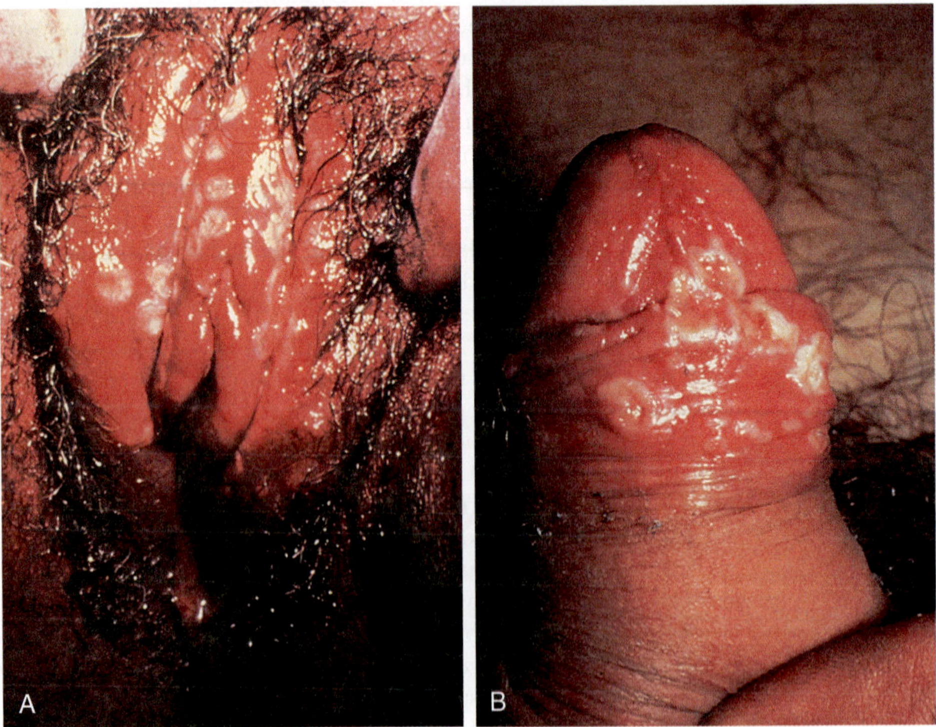

Figure 9-4. Genital herpes in the female patient **(A)** and the male patient **(B)**.

EXAMPLE Septicemia due to herpes simplex, 054.5.

EXAMPLE Otitis externa caused by herpes simplex, 054.73.

Arthropod-Borne Viral Diseases (060-066)

West Nile

West Nile virus is a disease that is spread to individuals by a mosquito bite. People with healthy immune systems may be infected with this disease and have only mild symptoms such as fever or headache. Those people with weakened immune systems and the elderly may experience complications.

EXAMPLE West Nile virus, 066.40.

EXAMPLE West Nile encephalitis, 066.41.

Other Diseases Due to Viruses and Chlamydiae (070-079)

Hepatitis

Hepatitis is inflammation of the liver and can be caused by among other things several different viruses, namely, A, B, C, D, and E. All of theses strains of hepatitis cause acute viral hepatitis. Only B, C, and D viruses cause chronic hepatitis. In chronic hepatitis, the infection may last a lifetime. Symptoms of hepatitis include fatigue, jaundice, nausea and vomiting, headache, diarrhea, and fever.

Hepatitis A is most commonly spread via food or water that has been contaminated by feces from an infected person. International travelers are at risk for this disease. A vaccine is available. If contracted, this disease usually resolves on its own.

Hepatitis B is spread through contact with infected blood, via sex with an infected person, or during childbirth. A hepatitis B vaccine is available. In the past, this disease may have been acquired during a blood transfusion, but in 1992, testing was instituted to control infection transmitted through the blood supply. Acute hepatitis B usually resolves on its own, but chronic cases require drug treatment. Hepatitis B may cause cirrhosis of the liver, liver failure, and liver cancer. About 10% of those infected with the B virus may become carriers. A carrier will have B virus in his or her blood for 6 months or longer after the original infection subsides.

Hepatitis C is spread through infected blood, sexual contact and childbirth. No vaccine is available for this disease; the only way to prevent it is through avoidance of risky behaviors such as needle sharing. Patients with chronic hepatitis C are treated with medications.

Hepatitis D is spread through infected blood. To acquire hepatitis D, a patient must already have hepatitis B infection. Those with chronic hepatitis D are treated with medications. This form was formerly known as delta.

Hepatitis E is spread through food or water that has been contaminated by feces from an infected person; it is unusual in the United Sates. No vaccine is available, and an outbreak usually resolves on its own.

The 070 category for Viral hepatitis can be used with the following fifth digits:

- 0 Acute and unspecified, without mention of hepatitis delta
- 1 Acute or unspecified, with hepatitis delta
- 2 Chronic, without mention of hepatitis delta
- 3 Chronic, with hepatitis delta

EXAMPLE Patient admitted is jaundiced and has chronic hepatitis B, 070.32.

EXAMPLE Patient has elevated liver function tests and was diagnosed with alcoholic hepatitis. Patient drinks alcohol on a daily basis, 571.1, 303.91.

Codes are also available for carriers of viral hepatitis B, C, or D. These people have no symptoms, but the condition is identified by laboratory testing.

EXAMPLE Hepatitis B carrier, V02.61.

Rickettsioses and Other Arthropod-Borne Diseases (080-088)

Lyme disease, also known as borreliosis, is an inflammatory disease caused by bacteria carried by ticks. Ticks acquire this bacterium through biting deer that are infected. It was first reported in the Northeast United States but now has spread throughout the Midwest, as well as the Pacific Coast. The symptoms of this disease resemble the flu and include headache, fever, and muscle aches. Sometimes, a bull's-eye rash appears at the site of the tick bite.

A blood test can be performed to look for antibodies to the bacteria that cause Lyme disease. Treatment for Lyme disease consists of antibiotics and anti-inflammatory medicines. If this disease is left untreated, complications such as Lyme arthritis, heart problems, or neurologic disorders can occur.

EXAMPLE A patient presents with severe joint pain. Blood work reveals Lyme disease. The physician documents that the patient has Lyme arthritis, 088.81, 711.8.

EXERCISE 9-4

Assign codes to the following conditions using your ICD-9-CM code book.

1. Shingles __________
2. Stomatitis due to herpes zoster __________
3. Genital herpes __________
4. Mumps __________
5. Hepatitis B __________
6. Acute hepatitis C with hepatitis delta __________
7. Patient is a carrier of hepatitis C. __________

Syphilis and Other Venereal Diseases (090-099)

Syphilis

Syphilis is a sexually transmitted disease (STD) that is caused by bacteria. Syphilis is passed through direct contact with syphilis sores. Sores occur in the vagina, penis, anus, or rectum. They can also occur on the lips and in the mouth. Syphilis can be passed on to babies through pregnant women. Syphilis occurs in three stages: primary, secondary, and late.

Primary syphilis is revealed by sores called **"chancres"** (Figure 9-5). These sores can last for 3 to 6 weeks. Treatment with a single injection of penicillin can cure the patient at this stage of the disease.

Secondary syphilis, which usually presents as a rash on the palms of the hands and feet, may be accompanied by fever, sore throat, headache, and fatigue. Lesions also may appear

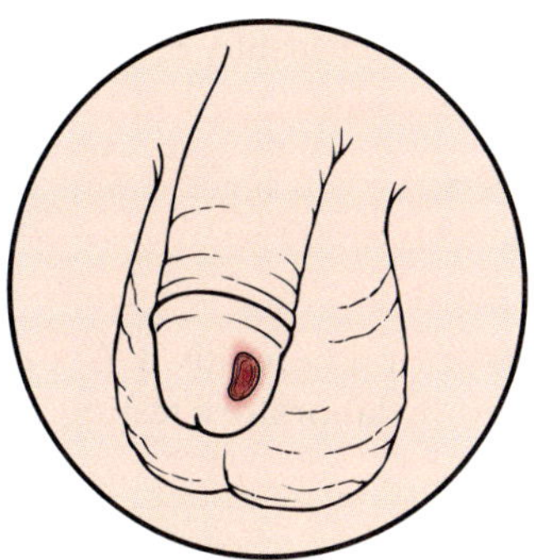

Figure 9-5. Chancre of primary syphilis.

in the mouth, vagina, or penis. Sometimes, warty patches called "**condylomata** lata" may appear on the genitalia. These secondary signs eventually disappear even without treatment, but the infection then progresses to late stages.

Late syphilis is the hidden stage of the disease. No signs or symptoms are noted until it begins to damage internal organs, which may occur years later.

A blood test is performed to test for syphilis. This test is called VDRL (Venereal Disease Research Laboratory), or RPR (rapid plasma reagin).

EXAMPLE Late neurosyphilis with ataxia, 094.0.

EXAMPLE Two-year-old presents with syphilitic pemphigus, 090.0.

EXAMPLE Genital chancre, 091.0.

Gonorrhea

Gonorrhea is caused by a bacterium and transmitted by sexual contact. Women may have no symptoms, but men usually report burning while urinating and discharge from the penis. Gonorrhea is treated with an antibiotic. If gonorrhea is not treated, complications usually occur.

EXAMPLE Female patient presents with acute gonococcal cervicitis, 098.15.

EXAMPLE Male patient presents with chronic prostatitis due to gonorrhea, 098.7, 601.1.

Mycoses (110-118)

Candidiasis

Candidiasis is caused by *Candida* fungi. These fungi often live harmlessly within the body until a patient's immune system becomes weak, or until he or she is taking medications that reduce the native bacteria that control this fungus. Usual spots in which *Candida* infections are found include the following:

Mouth—Thrush is found as white plaques on lips, cheeks, or tongue. It can be seen in babies, people with cancer, and diabetics.

Esophagus—often found in patients with AIDS and those on chemotherapy

Cutaneous—found in warm, moist areas that receive little ventilation, such as diaper areas, buttocks, and skin folds of the abdomen or breasts

Vaginal yeast infections are often caused by birth control pills, pregnancy, or frequent douching. Candidal infections are treated according to the area infected. Patients with

thrush are generally treated with nystatin swish and swallow while those with candidal esophagitis are treated with fluconazole. Patients with vaginal yeast infection are treated with antifungals such as Monistat, nystatin, or Vagistat.

EXAMPLE Patient is being treated for candidal intertrigo under breast, 112.3.

Late Effects of Infectious and Parasitic Diseases (137-139)

Some infections result in **sequelae** or late effects of an acute disease or that may be due to an inactive condition. Hemoptysis can be a late effect of tuberculosis caused by residual cavitation of the lung. When late effects are coded, two codes are required. Residual conditions/sequelae are coded first, and the cause of the late effect is coded next. If sequelae are unknown or unspecified, the late effect code may be used alone.

EXAMPLE Patient with hemiplegia following acute poliomyelitis, 342.90; hemiplegia, 138.

EXERCISE 9-5

Assign codes to the following conditions using your ICD-9-CM code book.

1. Patient has a chancre on the penis. ____________
2. Patient presents with condyloma latum. ____________
3. Latent syphilis with unknown date of infection ____________
4. Dementia due to syphilis ____________
5. Early congenital syphilis ____________
6. Exposure to gonorrhea ____________
7. Suspected carrier of gonorrhea ____________
8. Yeast infection of the vagina ____________
9. Late effect of tuberculosis ____________
10. Myalgia as a late effect of Lyme disease ____________

V CODES

In the past, V codes were primarily considered for use in the outpatient setting. This has changed with the addition of more V codes each year. As was discussed in Chapter 8, it may be difficult to locate V codes in the Index. Coders often say, "I did not know there was a V code for that." Refer to Chapter 8 for a listing of common main terms to locate V codes.

A review of the Tabular reveals that some V codes pertain to infectious and parasitic diseases:

V01.0	Contact or exposure to cholera
V01.1	Contact or exposure to tuberculosis
V01.2	Contact or exposure to poliomyelitis
V01.3	Contact or exposure to smallpox
V01.4	Contact or exposure to rubella
V01.5	Contact or exposure to rabies
V01.6	Contact or exposure to venereal diseases
V01.71	Contact or exposure to varicella
V01.79	Contact or exposure to other viral diseases

V01.81	Contact or exposure to anthrax
V01.82	Exposure to severe acute respiratory syndrome (SARS)-associated coronavirus
V01.83	Contact or exposure to *Escherichia coli*
V01.81	Contact or exposure to *meningococcus*
V01.89	Contact or exposure to other communicable diseases
V02.0	Carrier or suspected carrier of cholera
V02.1	Carrier or suspected carrier of typhoid
V02.2	Carrier or suspected carrier of amebiasis
V02.3	Carrier or suspected carrier of other gastrointestinal pathogens
V02.4	Carrier or suspected carrier of diphtheria
V02.51	Carrier or suspected carrier of group B streptococcus
V02.52	Carrier or suspected carrier of other streptococcus
V02.59	Carrier or suspected carrier of other specified bacterial disease
V02.60	Carrier or suspected carrier of viral hepatitis, unspecified
V02.61	Carrier or suspected carrier of hepatitis B
V02.62	Carrier or suspected carrier of hepatitis C
V02.69	Carrier or suspected carrier of other viral hepatitis
V02.7	Carrier or suspected carrier of gonorrhea
V02.8	Carrier or suspected carrier of other venereal diseases
V02.9	Carrier or suspected carrier of another specified infectious organism
V03.81	Haemophilus influenzae, type B [Hib]
V03.82	*Streptococcus pneumoniae* [pneumococcus]
V03.89	Other specified vaccination
V04.0	Need for prophylactic vaccination and inoculation against poliomyelitis
V04.1	Need for prophylactic vaccination and inoculation against Smallpox
V04.2	Need for prophylactic vaccination and inoculation against Measles alone
V04.3	Need for prophylactic vaccination and inoculation against Rubella alone
V04.4	Need for prophylactic vaccination and inoculation against Yellow fever
V04.5	Need for prophylactic vaccination and inoculation against Rabies
V04.6	Need for prophylactic vaccination and inoculation against Mumps alone
V04.7	Need for prophylactic vaccination and inoculation against Common cold
V04.81	Need for prophylactic vaccination and inoculation against Influenza
V04.82	Need for prophylactic vaccination and inoculation against Respiratory syncytial virus (RSV)
V04.89	Need for prophylactic vaccination and inoculation against other viral disease
V05.0	Need for prophylactic vaccination and inoculation against arthropod-borne viral encephalitis
V05.1	Need for prophylactic vaccination and inoculation against other arthropod-borne viral diseases
V05.2	Need for prophylactic vaccination and inoculation against Leishmaniasis
V05.3	Need for prophylactic vaccination and inoculation against viral hepatitis
V05.4	Need for prophylactic vaccination and inoculation against Varicella
V05.8	Need for prophylactic vaccination and inoculation against other specified disease
V05.9	Need for prophylactic vaccination and inoculation against unspecified single disease
V06.0	Need for prophylactic vaccination and inoculation against cholera with typhoid-paratyphoid [cholera TAB]
V06.1	Need for prophylactic vaccination and inoculation against diphtheria-tetanus-pertussis, combined [DTP[DtaP]]
V06.2	Need for prophylactic vaccination and inoculation against Diphtheria-tetanus-pertussis with typhoid-paratyphoid [DTP-TAB]
V06.3	Need for prophylactic vaccination and inoculation against Diphtheria-tetanus-pertussis with poliomyelitis [DTP + polio]

V06.4	Need for prophylactic vaccination and inoculation against Measles-mumps-rubella [MMR]
V06.5	Need for prophylactic vaccination and inoculation against Tetanus-diphtheria [Td][DT]
V06.6	Need for prophylactic vaccination and inoculation against Streptococcus pneumoniae [pneumococcus] and influenza
V06.8	Need for prophylactic vaccination and inoculation against other combinations
V06.9	Need for prophylactic vaccination and inoculation against unspecified combined vaccine
V07.0	Need for isolation
V07.1	Need for desensitization to allergens
V07.2	Need for prophylactic immunotherapy
V07.31	Need for prophylactic fluoride administration
V07.39	Need for other prophylactic chemotherapy
V07.4	Need for hormone replacement therapy (post menopausal)
V07.8	Need for other specified prophylactic measure
V07.9	Need for unspecified prophylactic measure
V09.0	Infection with microorganisms resistant to penicillins
V09.1	Infection with microorganisms resistant to cephalosporins and other beta-lactam antibiotics
V09.2	Infection with microorganisms resistant to macrolides
V09.3	Infection with microorganisms resistant to tetracyclines
V09.4	Infection with microorganisms resistant to aminoglycosides
V09.50	Infection with microorganisms resistant to quinolones and fluoroquinolones without mention of resistance to multiple quinolones and fluoroquinolones
V09.51	Infection with microorganisms resistant to quinolones and fluoroquinolones with resistance to multiple quinolones and fluoroquinolones
V09.6	Infection with microorganisms resistant to sulfonamides
V09.70	Infection with microorganisms resistant to other specified antimycobacterial agents without mention of resistance to multiple antimycobacterial agents
V09.71	Infection with microorganisms resistant to other specified antimycobacterial agents with resistance to multiple antimycobacterial agents
V09.80	Infection with microorganisms resistant to other specified drugs without mention of multiple drug resistance
V09.81	Infection with microorganisms resistant to other specified drugs without resistance to multiple drugs
V09.90	Infection with drug-resistant microorganism without mention of multiple drug resistance
V09.91	Infection with drug-resistant microorganism with multiple drug resistance
V12.00	Personal history of unspecified infectious and parasitic disease
V12.01	Personal history of tuberculosis
V12.02	Personal history of poliomyelitis
V12.03	Personal history of malaria
V12.09	Personal history of other infectious and parasitic diseases
V64.00	Vaccination not carried out, unspecified reason
V64.01	Vaccination not carried out because of acute illness
V64.02	Vaccination not carried out because of chronic illness or condition
V64.03	Vaccination not carried out because of immune compromised state
V64.04	Vaccination not carried out because of allergy to vaccine or component
V64.05	Vaccination not carried out because of caregiver refusal
V64.06	Vaccination not carried out because of patient refusal
V64.07	Vaccination not carried out for religious reasons
V64.08	Vaccination not carried out because patient had disease being vaccinated against

V64.09	Vaccination not carried out for other reason
V65.45	Counseling on other sexually transmitted diseases
V69.2	Problems related to high-risk sexual behavior
V71.2	Observation for suspected tuberculosis
V71.82	Observation and evaluation for suspected exposure to anthrax
V73.0	Special screening examination for poliomyelitis
V73.1	Special screening examination for smallpox
V73.2	Special screening examination for measles
V73.3	Special screening examination for rubella
V73.4	Special screening examination for yellow fever
V73.5	Special screening examination for other arthropod-borne viral diseases
V73.6	Special screening examination for trachoma
V73.81	Special screening examination, Human papilloma virus (HPV)
V73.88	Special screening examination for other specified chlamydial diseases
V73.89	Special screening examination for unspecified viral disease
V74.0	Special screening examination for cholera
V74.1	Special screening examination for pulmonary tuberculosis
V74.2	Special screening examination for leprosy [Hansen's disease]
V74.3	Special screening examination for diphtheria
V74.4	Special screening examination for bacterial conjunctivitis
V74.5	Special screening examination for venereal disease
V74.6	Special screening examination for yaws
V74.8	Special screening examination for other specified bacterial and spirochetal diseases
V74.9	Special screening examination for unspecified bacterial and spirochetal disease
V75.0	Special screening examination for rickettsial diseases
V75.1	Special screening examination for malaria
V75.2	Special screening examination for leishmaniasis
V75.3	Special screening examination for Trypanosomiasis
V75.4	Special screening examination for Mycotic infections
V75.5	Special screening examination for Schistosomiasis
V75.6	Special screening examination for Filariasis
V75.7	Special screening examination for Intestinal helminthiasis
V75.8	Special screening examination for Other specified parasitic infections
V75.9	Special screening examination for unspecified infectious disease

EXAMPLE Student presents to health clinic after exposure to meningitis, V01.81.

EXAMPLE Patient with cough, fever, and recent incarceration. Admitted for observation for TB, V71.2.

EXERCISE 9-6

Assign codes to the following condition using your ICD-9-CD code book.

1. History of malaria __________
2. Exposure to chickenpox at daycare __________
3. Patient returning from China; was exposed to SARS __________
4. Patient needs vaccination for cholera __________
5. Influenza vaccination not administered because patient is hospitalized with pneumonia __________

Table 9-1. Drugs for Infectious Diseases[6]

Drug Category	Drug Action	Examples	Side Effects	Comments
Antibiotics	Destroy or inhibit the growth of bacterial strains or microorganisms but have not been found to be effective for viral infections	Penicillin v Potassium (Pen-V-K) Tetracycline (Sumycin) Amoxicillin (Amoxil) Cephalosporins (Kefl ex, Ceclor) Ciprofloxacin (Cipro)	Common side effects of any are nausea, GI upset, urticaria	Caution must be used when administering penicillin IM regarding observation after infection for potential of anaphylaxis Cipro: acute infections and prophylactic postanthrax exposure
Antifungals	Inhibit and kill fungal growth	Griseofulvin (Grisactin) Ketoconazole (Nizoral) Clotrimazole (Lotrimin)	Nausea, vomiting, abdominal, pain, itching, urticaria	Some are available in oral for systemic treatment, others are available in topical form
Antivirals	Inhibit viral growth	Acyclovir (Zovirax) Zidovudine (Retrovir) Amantadine (Symmetrel)	GI disturbances, headache, malaise, insomnia, dizziness	Should be taken at first sign of onset of viral attack for best relief of symptoms
Antiprotozoals	Inhibit protozoal infections	Chloroquine HCl (Aralen HCl)	Headache, pruritus, GI disturbances, tinnitus	Also known as antimalarials
Antipyretics	Reduce fever	Acetaminophen (Tylenol) Acetylsalicylic acid (aspirin) Ibuprofen (Motrin)	Toxic doses of acetaminophen may cause irreversible and fatal liver damage	Caution must be exercised when administering Tylenol drops and syrup to infants and children; check dosage for either before administering
Antitubercular	Suppress mycobacterium causing tuberculosis	Isoniazid (INH) Ethambutol (Myambutol)	GI disturbances and hepatic disturbances	These drugs usually are given in combination

COMMON TREATMENTS

See Table 9-1 for drugs commonly used to treat infectious diseases.

PROCEDURES

There are multiple therapeutic and diagnostic procedures that can be performed for infectious and parasitic diseases. There is no specific procedure chapter for infectious and parasitic diseases.

DOCUMENTATION/REIMBURSEMENT/MS-DRGs

Often, coding difficulties are due to lack of documentation. Sometimes pathology and other test results are not available at the time of discharge, or when the physician is dictating the discharge summary or is reporting the final diagnoses.

Causative Organism

When coding meningitis, the record should be reviewed for the causative organism.

EXAMPLE

DIAGNOSES	CODE	MS-DRG	RW
Viral meningitis	047.9	076	1.1439
Salmonella meningitis	003.21	096	2.3482

AIDS and AIDS Manifestations

Coding AIDS, HIV, and any manifestations correctly is very important to MS-DRG assignment.

EXAMPLE

DIAGNOSES	CODE	MS-DRG	RW
AIDS	042	977	1.0387
AIDS with candidal esophagitis	042, 112.84	976	1.3357
AIDS with candidal esophagitis and acute renal failure	042, 112.84, 584.9	974	2.1382

For reimbursement purposes, the coder must be aware of possible sepsis on admission. This condition may be suspected at the time of admission, and blood cultures may be taken. Results of the blood cultures may not become positive until several days into the patient's hospital stay. This does not mean that the patient did not have this condition on admission.

CHAPTER REVIEW EXERCISE

Where applicable, assign codes for diagnoses, procedures, and V codes and E codes.

1. Gastroenteritis due to *Salmonella* ____________
2. Food poisoning ____________
3. UTI due to candidiasis ____________
4. Diarrhea due to *Clostridium difficile* ____________
5. Rotavirus ____________
6. Infectious colitis ____________
7. Primary TB. Patient in isolation. ____________
8. TB of the hip bone. ____________
9. Tuberculosis lichenoides ____________
10. Bubonic plague ____________
11. Gastrointestinal anthrax ____________
12. Whooping cough with pneumonia ____________
13. DMAC ____________

14. Meningococcal endocarditis ______
15. MSSA sepsis ______
16. *Haemophilus influenzae* septicemia ______
17. Acute prostatitis due to *E coli* ______
18. HIV positive ______
19. AIDS with Burkitt's lymphoma ______
20. Postherpetic syndrome ______

CHAPTER GLOSSARY

AIDS: an incurable disease of the immune system caused by a virus.

Anthrax: a bacterial infection usually found in wild or domestic animals.

Bacteremia: bacteria in blood.

Candidiasis: a fungal infection and is also known as a yeast infection.

Chancre: an ulcer that forms during the first stage of syphilis.

Clostridium difficile: microorganisms that are a leading cause of pseudomembranous cells; also known as *C. diff.*

Communicable: easily spread from one person to another.

Condyloma: wart-type growth found usually in the genital or anal area.

Gonorrhea: caused by a bacterium and transmitted by sexual contact.

Hepatitis: an inflammation of the liver that has a variety of causes.

Herpes simplex: a virus also known as a *cold sore* or *fever blister.*

Herpes zoster: a disease caused by the same virus that causes chickenpox.

Lyme disease: an inflammatory disease caused by bacteria carried by ticks.

Meningitis: an infection in the fluid of a person's spinal cord and brain.

Mycobacterium avium intercellulare: a mycobacteria found in soil and water.

Mycosis: fungal infection.

Nadir: the lowest level.

Nosocomial: hospital-acquired infection.

Parasite: organism that lives on or takes nourishment from another organism.

Poliomyelitis: a viral disease that affects the nerves.

Sepsis: SIRS due to infection

Septic shock: a condition caused by *infection* and *sepsis.* It can cause *multiple organ failure* and *death.*

Septicemia: the presence in the blood of pathologic microorganisms that causes systemic illness.

Sequelae: late affect or residual of an acute disease.

SIRS: systemic inflammatory response syndrome, which can be caused by infection or trauma.

Syphilis: a sexually transmitted disease (STD) that is caused by bacteria.

Tuberculosis (TB): an infection caused by *Mycobacterium tuberculosis.*

Viral meningitis: a viral infection of the fluid in the spinal cord and around the brain.

West Nile: a viral disease that is spread to individuals by a mosquito bite.

CHAPTER 10

Diseases of the Blood and Blood-Forming Organs

(ICD-9-CM Chapter 4, Codes 280-289)

CHAPTER OUTLINE

LEARNING OBJECTIVES

- Apply and assign the correct ICD-9-CM codes in accordance with Official Guidelines for Coding and Reporting
- Identify pertinent anatomy and physiology of the blood and blood-forming organs
- Identify diseases of the blood and blood-forming organs
- Assign the correct V codes and procedure codes related to the blood-forming organs
- Identify laboratory values and diagnostic tests
- Explain the importance of documentation in relation to MS-DRGs for reimbursement

ABBREVIATIONS

ASA aspirin
CBC complete blood count
DIC disseminated intravascular coagulation
ESRD end-stage renal disease
Hct hematocrit
Hgb hemoglobin
HIV human immunodeficiency virus
ICD-9-CM *International Classification of Diseases, 9th Revision, Clinical Modification*
ITP idiopathic thrombocytopenic purpura
MS-DRG Medicare Severity diagnosis-related group
PT prothrombin time
PTT partial thromboplastin time
WBC white blood cell

ICD-9-CM Official Guidelines for Coding and Reporting

Please refer to the companion Evolve website for the most current guidelines.

Chapter 4: Diseases of Blood and Blood Forming Organs (280-289)

a. Anemia of chronic disease

Subcategory 285.2, Anemia in chronic illness, has codes for anemia in chronic kidney disease, code. 285.21; anemia in neoplastic disease, code 285.22; and anemia in other chronic illness, code 285.29. These codes can be used as the principal/first listed code if the reason for the encounter is to treat the anemia. They may also be used as secondary codes if treatment of the anemia is a component of an encounter, but not the primary reason for the encounter. When using a code from subcategory 285 it is also necessary to use the code for the chronic condition causing the anemia.

1) Anemia in chronic kidney disease

When assigning code 285.21, Anemia in chronic kidney disease, it is also necessary to assign a code from category 585, Chronic kidney disease, to indicate the stage of chronic kidney disease.

See I.C.10.a. Chronic kidney disease (CKD).

EXAMPLE

Anemia due to end-stage renal disease (ESRD), 285.21, 585.6

2) Anemia in neoplastic disease

When assigning code 285.22, Anemia in neoplastic disease, it is also necessary to assign the neoplasm code that is responsible for the anemia. Code 285.22 is for use for anemia that is due to the malignancy, not for anemia due to antineoplastic chemotherapy drugs, which is an adverse effect.

See I.C.2.c.1 Anemia associated with malignancy.

See I.C.2.c.2 Anemia associated with chemotherapy, immunotherapy and radiation therapy.

See I.C.17.e.1. Adverse effects.

EXAMPLE

Anemia due to metastatic bone cancer. The patient has a history of primary breast cancer that was treated with mastectomy 4 years ago, 285.22, 198.5, V10.3, V45.71.

Apply the General Coding Guidelines as found in Chapter 5.

ANATOMY AND PHYSIOLOGY

Blood is a viscous fluid that circulates through the vessels of the circulatory system as a result of the pumping action of the heart. Blood has three major functions. First, it transports oxygen, nutrients, hormones, enzymes, waste products, and carbon dioxide to and from cells. Second, blood promotes hemostasis and regulates body temperature. **Homeostasis** means balance or equilibrium. It is the ability of an organism or cell to maintain internal equilibrium by adjusting its physiologic processes. Third, blood provides a protective mechanism that combats foreign materials and assists in the body's defense against disease. Blood loss is prevented by clotting mechanisms within the body.

Blood is composed of plasma and formed elements or corpuscles. Corpuscles include erythrocytes (red blood cells), leukocytes (white blood cells), and platelets or thrombocytes. All of these components differ in terms of appearance, structure and type, functions, life span, numbers, and means of production. **Erythrocytes**, or red blood cells, are made within the marrow of the bones; their main responsibility is to carry oxygen throughout the body and remove carbon dioxide. These are the cells that give blood its red color. **Leukocytes**, or white blood cells, increase in number to battle infection, inflammation, and other diseases. Five different types of white blood cells have been identified, and each has a role in

fighting infection. White cells are comprised of neutrophils, monocytes, lymphocytes, eosinophils, and basophils. **Platelets** or **thrombocytes** circulate in the blood and assist in the clotting process.

Complete blood count (CBC) is a blood test that is commonly used to evaluate a patient's overall health; it detects a variety of disorders such as anemia, infection, and leukemia. This test measures the following:

- Hemoglobin (Hgb), a protein in red blood cells that carries oxygen to body tissues
- Hematocrit (Hct), the percentage of blood volume made up of red blood cells
- White blood cells (WBCs), which fight infection
- Platelets, which are essential to blood clotting

See Table 10-1 for normal values.

DISEASE CONDITIONS

Chapter 4 in the ICD-9-CM code book focuses on Diseases of the Blood and Blood-Forming Organs (280-289). This relatively small chapter is the only chapter that is not divided into sections. Of interest is an Excludes note that appears at the very beginning of the chapter. This signifies that the instructions given in the note pertain to the entire chapter. The Excludes note shown in Figure 10-1 instructs the coder to refer to code 648.2 for anemia complicating pregnancy or the puerperium. Because anemia is a condition that is commonly associated with pregnancy and the puerperium, this topic will be covered in Chapter 16, Complications of Pregnancy, Childbirth, and the Puerperium.

Neoplastic diseases of the blood such as leukemia are discussed in Chapter 15, Neoplasms; hematologic disorders involving newborns are addressed in Chapter 17, Congenital Anomalies and Perinatal Conditions. The Excludes note under code 282.0, hereditary spherocytosis, excludes hemolytic anemia of the newborn (773.0-773.5), as is illustrated in Figure 10-2.

Deficiency Anemias (280-281)

The first two code categories, 280 and 281, identify the deficiency anemias. **Anemia** occurs when hemoglobin drops, which interrupts the transport of oxygen throughout the body. The most common type of anemia is iron deficiency anemia. In women, this condition is often due to heavy blood loss during menstrual periods. In older men and women, it may be an indication of gastrointestinal blood loss. Pregnant women and children need more iron, so a deficiency is likely due to insufficient iron in the diet. Testing may be necessary to determine a cause.

Table 10-1. Normal Laboratory Values[1]

WBC 5000-10,000/mm³ or µL	
Differential:	
Segs (polyps)	54%-62%
Lymphs	20%-40%
Eos	1%-3%
Baso	0%-1%
Mono	3%-7%
RBC	(M) 4.5-6.0 million per mm³ or µL
	(F) 4.0-5.5 million per mm³ or µL
Hct	(M) 40%-50%
	(F) 37%-47%
HGB	(M) 14-16 g/dL
	(F) 12-14 g/dL
Platelets	150,000-350,000/mm³ or µL

Baso, Basophils; *Eos*, eosinophils; *Hct*, hematocrit; *HGB*, hemoglobin; *Lymphs*, lymphocytes; *Mono*, monocytes; *RBC*, red blood cell; *Segs*, segments; *WBC*, white blood cell.

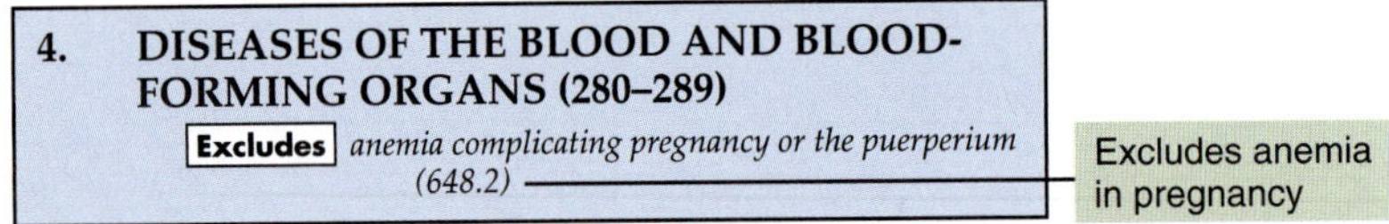

Figure 10-1. Excludes note that affects the entire chapter.

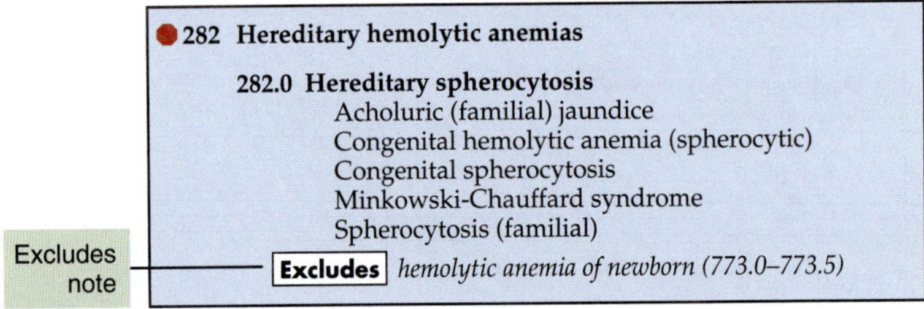

Figure 10-2. The Excludes note under code 282.0, hereditary spherocytosis, excludes hemolytic anemia of newborn (773.0-773.5).

If a particular cause were determined, it would be appropriate to code the underlying condition. The sequencing of diagnoses would be determined by the general coding guidelines. Some of the reasons for iron deficiency include the following:

- Inadequate intake of iron in the diet
- Chronic blood loss
- Impaired absorption during digestion
- Liver disease
- Infection
- Cancers (neoplasms)

Numerous symptoms can indicate anemia; these include pallor, fatigue, lethargy, cold intolerance, irritability, stomatitis, headache, loss of appetite, numbness and tingling sensations, brittle hair, spoon-shaped and brittle nails, and edema, especially of the ankles. Severe anemia can result in tachycardia, palpitations, dyspnea (difficulty breathing), and syncope (fainting). Treatment depends on the cause, but the approach may be as simple as eating iron-rich foods or taking an iron supplement such as ferrous sulfate or ferrous gluconate. Blood transfusions may be necessary.

Look up the main term "Anemia" in the Index, and see the many subterms for the various types of anemia. "Deficiency" is also a subterm with many subterms, as is shown in Figure 10-3. At the subterm "in," entries are found for anemia in chronic illness, anemia in end-stage renal disease/chronic kidney disease, and anemia in neoplastic disease. The term *chronic anemia* is not equated to "chronic simple anemia" or "anemia in chronic disease" (Figure 10-4). Chronic anemia is coded to 285.9 because no specific subterm is available for chronic, so the default code for anemia (285.9) code is assigned.

EXAMPLE Patient has anemia due to inadequate dietary iron intake, 280.1.

EXAMPLE Patient is being treated for folate deficiency anemia, 281.2.

EXERCISE 10-1

Assign codes to the following conditions using your ICD-9-CM code book.

1. Iron deficiency anemia due to chronic blood loss __________
2. Vitamin B_{12} deficiency anemia __________
3. Megaloblastic anemia __________

Anemia *(Continued)*
congenital *(Continued)*
pernicious 281.0
spherocytic (*see also* Spherocytosis) 282.0
Cooley's (erythroblastic) 282.49
crescent - *see* Disease, sickle-cell
cytogenic 281.0
Dacie's (nonspherocytic)
type I 282.2
type II 282.3
Davidson's (refractory) 284.9
deficiency 281.9
2,3 diphosphoglycurate mutase 282.3
2,3 PG 282.3
6-PGD 282.2
6-phosphogluronic dehydrogenase 282.2
amino acid 281.4
combined B_{12} and folate 281.3
enzyme, drug-induced (hemolytic) 282.2
erythrocytic glutathione 282.2
folate 281.2
dietary 281.2
drug-induced 281.2
folic acid 281.2
dietary 281.2
drug-induced 281.2

Subterm "deficiency"

Figure 10-3. Alphabetic Index entry for "anemia" and the subterm "deficiency."

Anemia *(Continued)*
in
chronic illness NEC 285.29
chronic kidney disease 285.21
end-stage renal disease 285.21
neoplastic disease 285.22

Figure 10-4. Anemia due to chronic diseases.

Hemolytic Anemias (282-283)

The hemolytic anemias are assigned to 282 (hereditary) and 283 (acquired) code categories (Figure 10-5). **Hemolytic anemia** results from abnormal or excessive destruction of red blood cells. **Sickle cell anemia** is one of the more common types of hereditary hemolytic anemia; it is found often in the African American population and among people living in Africa, the Mediterranean, Arabia, and South Asia. Red blood cells change from a disc shape to a crescent or "sickle" shape. This causes obstruction of the small blood vessels and eventual damage from thrombus formation, repeated organ infarctions, and tissue necrosis throughout the body. Varying degrees of disease severity and symptoms have been reported. Reported symptoms include severe anemia, hyperbilirubinemia or jaundice, splenomegaly, delayed and impaired growth and development, vascular occlusion, and infarctions, which can result in permanent damage, pain, frequent infection, and congestive heart failure. Most treatment is supportive in nature. A drug called Hydrea (hydroxyurea) has reduced the number of crises.

Look up "Sickle cell" in the Index; both subterms of anemia and disease instruct the coder to *see also* Disease, sickle cell. When looking up "Anemia," under the subterm "Sickle cell," the coder is instructed to *see also* Disease, sickle cell (Figure 10-6). Under the main term "Disease" and the subterm "Sickle cell," code selections are more detailed (Figure 10-7). Remember to follow these cross-references for identification of the code

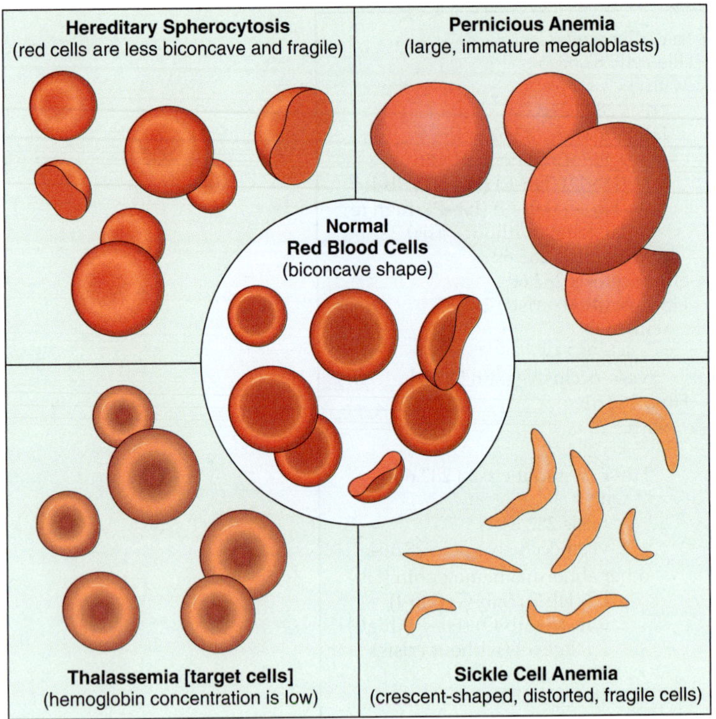

Figure 10-5. Normal red blood cells and red blood cells in several types of anemia.

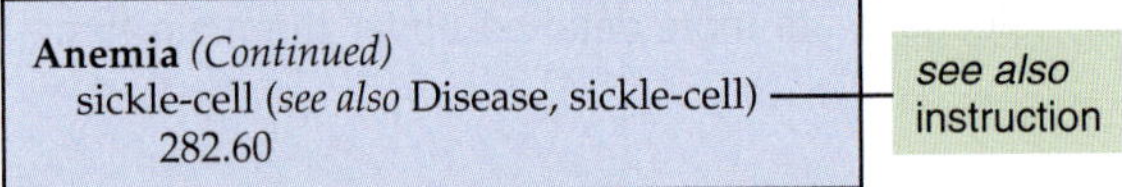

Figure 10-6. *See also* Disease, sickle cell.

that best describes the patient's condition. Code 282.5 for sickle cell trait is assigned when a patient is a carrier and the disease has remained asymptomatic. When both sickle cell trait and sickle cell anemia are present, only sickle cell anemia is coded (282.6X). Codes under the subcategory 282.6X have an additional fifth digit that relates to the absence or presence of a "crisis." The crisis may include additional conditions such as an infarct, acute chest syndrome, and splenic sequestration. These conditions would be coded additionally, and the sequencing of the codes depends on the reason for admission and the coding guidelines.

EXAMPLE

Patient was admitted with sickle cell crisis with acute chest syndrome. Patient has Hb-SS disease, 282.62, 517.3.

Another hereditary disease that is prevalent among people from Greece and Italy (Mediterranean countries), the Middle East, South Asia, and Africa is **thalassemia**. Similar to sickle cell anemia, the disease manifests in varying degrees. Cooley's anemia is another name that is used to describe the beta thalassemias. Frequent blood transfusions are administered, along with treatment with an iron chelation drug, which helps the body get rid of excess iron resulting from repeated transfusions. Occasionally, bone marrow transplant is performed, but this is a risky procedure, and a suitable donor is required.

EXAMPLE

Patient admitted with sickle cell thalassemia with vaso-occlusive pain crisis, 282.42.

Disease, diseased *(Continued)*
sickle-cell 282.60
with
crisis 282.62
Hb-S disease 282.61
other abnormal hemoglobin (Hb-D) (Hb-E) (Hb-G) (Hb-J) (Hb-K) (Hb-O) (Hb-P) (high fetal gene) (without crisis) 282.68
with crisis 282.69
elliptocytosis 282.60
Hb-C (without crisis) 282.63
with
crisis 282.64
vaso-occlusive pain 282.64
Hb-S 282.61
with
crisis 282.62
Hb-C (without crisis) 282.63
with
crisis 282.64
vaso-occlusive pain 282.64
other abnormal hemoglobin (Hb-D) (Hb-E) (Hb-G) (Hb-J) (Hb-K) (Hb-O) (Hb-P) (high fetal gene) (without crisis) 282.68
with crisis 282.69
spherocytosis 282.60
thalassemia (without crisis) 282.41
with
crisis 282.42
vaso-occlusive pain 282.42

Figure 10-7. Code selections are more detailed under the main terms "Disease" and subterm "sickle cell."

EXERCISE 10-2

Assign codes to the following conditions using your ICD-9-CM code book.

1. Cooley's anemia ____________
2. Sickle cell trait with sickle cell anemia ____________
3. Acholuric jaundice ____________
4. Sickle cell Hb-C with vaso-occlusive crisis ____________
5. Sickle cell thalassemia ____________

Aplastic Anemias (284)

Aplastic anemias are identified by the code category 284. **Aplastic anemia** is characterized by a reduction in red blood cells due to impairment or failure of bone marrow function. Decreased production of erythrocytes (red blood cells), leukocytes (white blood cells), and thrombocytes (platelets), also defined as pancytopenia, can lead to many complications. In 50% of cases, the cause of pancytopenia is unknown or **idiopathic** in nature. Some drugs, industrial agents, chemicals, or radiation can affect the bone marrow. If these are the cause an additional E code is required. If the causative factor can be identified and eliminated, the bone marrow possibly can recover. Viruses such as hepatitis C may also cause aplastic anemia.

If a patient has the following three conditions—neutropenia, thrombocytopenia, and anemia, also known as **pancytopenia**—the code 284.1 would be assigned. According to *Coding Clinic* (2005:3Q:p11-12),[2] an exception occurs when a patient is admitted with neutropenic fever and is also pancytopenic; in this case, it is acceptable to assign the neutropenia code (288.00) as the principal diagnosis, with an additional code 284.1 used to describe the pancytopenia and 780.6 for the fever.

EXAMPLE Patient has pancytopenia due to oral methotrexate which is taken for treatment of rheumatoid arthritis. 284.89, 714.0, E933.1.

EXAMPLE Infant with congenital aplastic anemia 284.01.

EXERCISE 10-3

Assign codes to the following conditions using your ICD-9-CM code book.

1. Aplastic anemia due to hepatitis C __________
2. Idiopathic aplastic anemia __________
3. Fanconi's anemia __________

Other and Unspecified Anemias (285)

Other and unspecified anemias are identified by code category 285. This category includes 285.1, acute posthemorrhagic anemia or anemia due to acute blood loss. Confusion arises regarding anemia related to blood loss and whether blood loss is acute or chronic and/or both. Sometimes, blood loss is well documented, but the resultant anemia may not be documented by the physician. Whenever doubt occurs, the coder should query the physician. If acute and chronic blood loss anemias are present, both are coded, and acute blood loss anemia is sequenced first.

EXAMPLE Patient has anemia due to gastric cancer, 285.22, 151.9.

EXAMPLE Patient treated for anemia due to acute blood loss 285.1.

EXERCISE 10-4

Assign codes to the following conditions using your ICD-9-CM code book.

1. Anemia due to end-stage renal disease (ESRD) __________
2. Normocytic anemia __________
3. Congenital sideroblastic anemia __________
4. Anemia due to chronic disease __________

Coagulation Disorders (286)

Coagulation defects are classified as code category 286. Excessive bleeding that occurs after a minor injury may be a sign of a **coagulation defect**, which is a breakdown in the blood clotting process. Multiple reasons may account for excessive bleeding:

- Acute viral infection in children
- Autoimmune reactions in adults

- End-stage renal failure
- Ingestion of aspirin (acetylsalicylic acid [ASA])
- Vitamin K deficiency
- Liver disease
- Inherited disorders
- Hemorrhagic fever viruses

Multiple warning signs may indicate a coagulation defect; these include bleeding from gums or repeated nosebleeds, petechiae (Figure 10-8), ecchymoses (bruises), hemarthroses (bleeding into a joint), hemoptysis (coughing up blood), hematemesis (vomiting blood), melena (blood in feces), anemia, feeling faint and anxious, low blood pressure, and increased pulse. Blood tests that involve bleeding time, prothrombin time (PT), or partial thromboplastin time (PTT) can measure the coagulation of blood. Occasionally, patients who take anticoagulants such as warfarin (Coumadin) will have complications. Some common complications include gastrointestinal bleeding, epistaxis, hematuria, or hemorrhage from any tissue. Their coagulation laboratory test results may be abnormal, but this does not mean that they have a coagulopathy, and the condition should not be coded as such. It should be coded to abnormal coagulation profile, 790.92, which can be located in the Alphabetic Index under the main term "Findings, abnormal, without diagnosis." It is a common mistake to assign code 286.5 (coagulopathy) when a patient is taking an anticoagulant. Per *Coding Clinic* (2006:2Q:p17),[3] a code from category 286, coagulation defects, is not appropriate for patients on anticoagulant therapy. The V code V58.61 is assigned to identify the long-term use of anticoagulant medication such as Coumadin, which is located in the Alphabetic Index under the main term "Long-term drug use." A code would also be assigned for the diagnosis for which the patient is on anticoagulation therapy.

EXAMPLE Patient is taking Coumadin for previous history of pulmonary embolism, V12.51, V58.61.

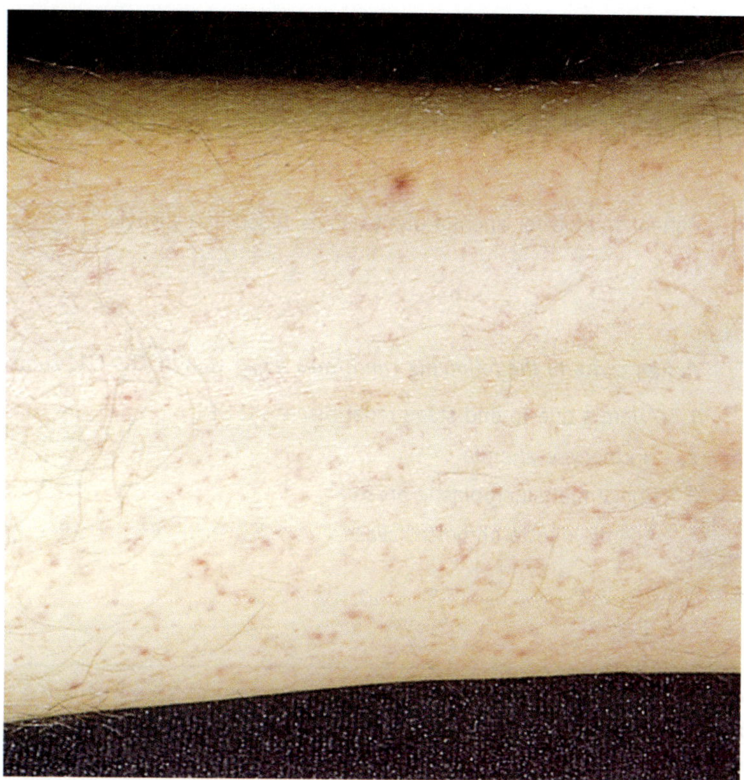

Figure 10-8. Petechiae.

patient will donate his or her own blood to be used in the event a transfusion is needed. This is known as an **autologous transfusion**.

Apheresis is a procedure that separates the different components of the blood and removes a certain part of the blood, such as occurs in leukapheresis, plateletpheresis, and plasmapheresis. A therapeutic plasmapheresis or plasma exchange occurs when the plasma is removed and is replaced with fresh plasma.

Bone marrow biopsy and/or aspiration is a diagnostic procedure that can be used to identify types of blood disorders. It may also be performed to evaluate the patient's response to treatment.

Peripheral stem cell and bone marrow transplants (Figure 10-9) are used to treat patients with certain leukemias and cancers, bone marrow failure syndromes, and genetic disease. Prior to transplant, the patient is prepared with radiation and/or chemotherapy to get rid of the defective or malignant cells and reduce the body's immunity, so it will not reject the transplanted cells.

EXERCISE 10-9

Assign codes for all diagnoses and procedures using your ICD-9-CM code book.

1. Patient with profound pancytopenia had a bone marrow biopsy __________
2. Thrombocytopenia was treated with transfusion of platelets __________
3. Therapeutic plasmapheresis performed on patient with thrombotic thrombocytopenic purpura __________
4. DIC with transfusion of fresh frozen plasma __________
5. Post operative blood loss anemia with autologous transfusion of red blood cells __________

DOCUMENTATION/REIMBURSEMENT/MS-DRGs

Often, coding difficulties are due to lack of documentation. Sometimes pathology and other test results are not available at the time of discharge or when the physician is dictating the discharge summary or is reporting the final diagnoses.

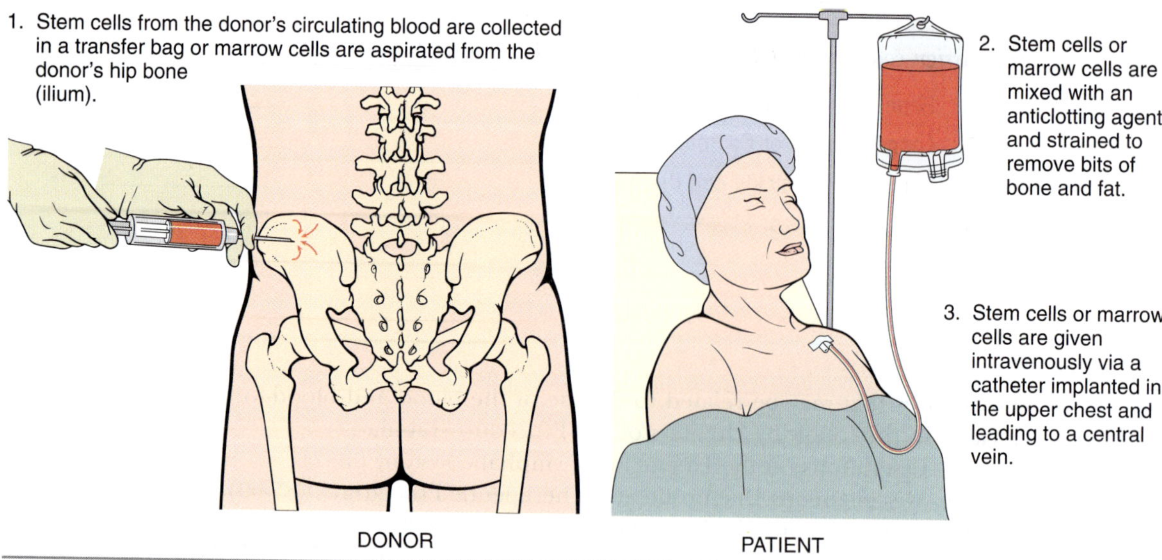

Figure 10-9. Peripheral stem cell and bone marrow transplants.

V42.81	Organ or tissue replaced by transplant—bone marrow
V42.82	Organ or tissue replaced by transplant—peripheral stem cells
V58.2	Blood transfusion without reported diagnosis
V58.61	Long-term (current) use of anticoagulants
V58.63	Long-term (current) use of antiplatelets/antithrombotics
V58.66	Long-term (current) use of aspirin
V59.01	Donor whole blood
V59.02	Donor stem cells
V59.09	Donor, other
V59.3	Donor bone marrow
V78.0	Special screening for iron deficiency anemia
V78.1	Special screening for other and unspecified deficiency anemia
V78.2	Special screening sickle cell disease or trait
V78.3	Special screening, other hemoglobinopathies
V78.8	Special screening, other disorders of blood and blood-forming organs
V78.9	Special screening, unspecified disorder of blood and blood-forming organs
V83.01	Asymptomatic hemophilia A carrier
V83.02	Symptomatic hemophilia A carrier

Some V codes describe the long-term use of a particular type of medication such as anticoagulants or antiplatelets/antithrombotics. **Anticoagulants** are medications that are used to prevent venous thrombi. They can be administered parenterally with heparin, or warfarin (Coumadin) can be taken orally. **Parenteral** drug administration is when medications are administered other than through the digestive tract, such as by intravenous or intramuscular injection. **Antiplatelet** drugs are used to prevent clumping of platelets or formation of an arterial thrombus. Medications that are used as antiplatelet therapy include clopidgrogrel (Plavix), ticlopidine (Ticlid), dipyridamole (Persantin), and aspirin (ASA).

EXAMPLE Screening for iron deficiency anemia, V78.0.

EXAMPLE Long-term use of ASA due to family history of stroke, V58.66, V17.1.

EXERCISE 10-8

Assign codes to the following conditions using your ICD-9-CM code book.

1. Bone marrow donor ____________
2. Long-term use of Coumadin ____________
3. Screening for sickle cell disease ____________
4. Long-term use of Plavix ____________

PROCEDURES

Procedures that may be related to disease of the blood and blood-forming organs can be located in the following chapters of the Procedure Tabular:

8. Operations on the Hemic and Lymphatic System (40-21)
16. Miscellaneous Diagnostic and Therapeutic Procedures (87-99)

Blood transfusion, which can be performed for many reasons, is the administration of donor blood cells into a patient. The most common types of transfusions consist of red blood cells, plasma, and platelets. Sometimes, before undergoing an elective surgery, a

Diseases of the White Blood Cells (288)

Diseases of the white blood cells (leukocytes) are classified to code category 288. **Leukocytosis** (neutrophilia or granulocytosis) is characterized by an increase in the number of white cells in the blood. Usually, no treatment is required. If leukocytosis persists, investigation to rule out a neoplastic process or infection may become necessary. Leukocytosis may also be related to certain drugs or may occur in response to stress. The most common white blood cell condition is agranulocytosis, or **neutropenia**, which is an abnormal decrease in granular leukocytes in the blood. Radiation therapy, drugs used for chemotherapy, and other chemicals may cause neutropenia. With severe neutropenia, a patient may become immunocompromised; his or her ability to fight infection may be hampered, and treatment often consists of antibiotics. Testing may be necessary to determine cause and select appropriate treatment.

EXAMPLE Infant is being treated for congenital agranulocytosis, 288.01.

Other Diseases of Blood and Blood-Forming Organs (289)

Other diseases of the blood and blood-forming organs are classified to category 289. This includes conditions of the spleen, lymphatic system, and bone marrow. The spleen serves as a blood reservoir, filters the blood and removes old or defective blood cells, and serves as part of the immune system by helping to fight infection. The spleen can become enlarged **(splenomegaly)** due to infections or other diseases. A swollen spleen is at risk for rupturing, which could result in significant blood loss. **Lymphadenitis** is the inflammation of a lymph node that is typically caused by a bacterial infection and can easily be treated with antibiotics.

EXAMPLE Ultrasound exam showed that the patient has a splenic infarction, 289.59.

EXERCISE 10-7

Assign codes to the following conditions using your ICD-9-CM code book.

1. Neutropenic fever ____________
2. Leukocytosis ____________
3. Eosinophilia ____________
4. Leukopenia ____________
5. Factor V Leiden mutation ____________
6. Mesenteric lymphadenitis ____________

V CODES

In the past, V codes were primarily considered for use in the outpatient setting. This has changed with the addition of more V codes each year. As was discussed in Chapter 8, it may be difficult to locate V codes in the Index. Coders often say, "I did not know there was a V code for that." Refer to Chapter 8 for a listing of common main terms used to locate V codes.

A review of the Tabular reveals that some V codes pertain to diseases of the blood and blood-forming organs:

V12.3	Personal history of diseases of blood and blood-forming organs
V18.2	Family history of anemia
V18.3	Family history of other blood disorders

Hemophilia is an inherited clotting disorder. **Hemophilia A**, the most common form, is a deficiency or abnormality of clotting factor VIII. **Hemophilia B** (Christmas disease) is the result of a deficiency of factor IX, and **Hemophilia C** is a mild form characterized by a decrease in factor XI. As with some of the other diseases of the blood, varying degrees of severity are reported. A common treatment consists of replacement therapy for factor VIII with cryoprecipitate. Unfortunately, transmission of viruses such as hepatitis and human immunodeficiency virus (HIV) has resulted from this treatment. Currently, blood products are treated in an effort to destroy known viruses, but risk of unknown infection or immune reaction is still present.

Disseminated intravascular coagulation (DIC) is a disorder that causes depletion of clotting factors in the blood. Risk factors include recent sepsis, severe injury or trauma, recent surgery and anesthesia, complications of labor and delivery, cancer, transfusion reaction, and liver disease. Treatment may include transfusion of coagulation factors with fresh frozen plasma; the underlying cause must be determined so the appropriate treatment can be provided.

EXAMPLE Patient was treated for coagulopathy due to chronic liver disease, 286.7, 571.9.

EXERCISE 10-5

Assign codes to the following conditions using your ICD-9-CM code book.

1. Rosenthal's hemophilia ____________
2. Classic hemophilia ____________
3. Christmas disease ____________
4. DIC ____________
5. von Willebrand's disease ____________

Purpura and Other Hemorrhagic Conditions (287)

Purpura and other hemorrhagic conditions are identified by code category 287. **Purpura** is characterized by ecchymoses or small hemorrhages in the skin, mucous membranes, or serosal surfaces that are due to blood disorders, vascular abnormalities, or trauma. A patient with idiopathic thrombocytopenic purpura (ITP) experiences a decrease in the number of platelets with no identifiable cause. Following laboratory testing, a bone marrow biopsy may be necessary. Treatments may include corticosteroids, immunosuppressive therapy, and possibly splenectomy.

Secondary thrombocytopenia is characterized by a decrease in the number of platelets; it is due to specific diseases such as congestive splenomegaly, Felty's syndrome, tuberculosis, sarcoidosis, lupus erythematosus, and chronic alcoholism. Some external causes include drugs, blood transfusions, and overhydration.

EXAMPLE Thrombocytopenia due to chronic alcoholism, 287.4, 303.90.

EXAMPLE Patient admitted with idiopathic thrombocytopenic purpura, 287.31.

EXERCISE 10-6

Assign codes to the following conditions using your ICD-9-CM code book.

1. Idiopathic nonthrombocytopenic purpura ____________
2. Thrombocytopenia due to lupus erythematosus ____________
3. Schönlein-Henoch purpura ____________
4. Low platelets ____________

V42.81	Organ or tissue replaced by transplant—bone marrow
V42.82	Organ or tissue replaced by transplant—peripheral stem cells
V58.2	Blood transfusion without reported diagnosis
V58.61	Long-term (current) use of anticoagulants
V58.63	Long-term (current) use of antiplatelets/antithrombotics
V58.66	Long-term (current) use of aspirin
V59.01	Donor whole blood
V59.02	Donor stem cells
V59.09	Donor, other
V59.3	Donor bone marrow
V78.0	Special screening for iron deficiency anemia
V78.1	Special screening for other and unspecified deficiency anemia
V78.2	Special screening sickle cell disease or trait
V78.3	Special screening, other hemoglobinopathies
V78.8	Special screening, other disorders of blood and blood-forming organs
V78.9	Special screening, unspecified disorder of blood and blood-forming organs
V83.01	Asymptomatic hemophilia A carrier
V83.02	Symptomatic hemophilia A carrier

Some V codes describe the long-term use of a particular type of medication such as anticoagulants or antiplatelets/antithrombotics. **Anticoagulants** are medications that are used to prevent venous thrombi. They can be administered parenterally with heparin, or warfarin (Coumadin) can be taken orally. **Parenteral** drug administration is when medications are administered other than through the digestive tract, such as by intravenous or intramuscular injection. **Antiplatelet** drugs are used to prevent clumping of platelets or formation of an arterial thrombus. Medications that are used as antiplatelet therapy include clopidgrogrel (Plavix), ticlopidine (Ticlid), dipyridamole (Persantin), and aspirin (ASA).

EXAMPLE Screening for iron deficiency anemia, V78.0.

EXAMPLE Long-term use of ASA due to family history of stroke, V58.66, V17.1.

EXERCISE 10-8

Assign codes to the following conditions using your ICD-9-CM code book.

1. Bone marrow donor __________
2. Long-term use of Coumadin __________
3. Screening for sickle cell disease __________
4. Long-term use of Plavix __________

PROCEDURES

Procedures that may be related to disease of the blood and blood-forming organs can be located in the following chapters of the Procedure Tabular:

8. Operations on the Hemic and Lymphatic System (40-21)
16. Miscellaneous Diagnostic and Therapeutic Procedures (87-99)

Blood transfusion, which can be performed for many reasons, is the administration of donor blood cells into a patient. The most common types of transfusions consist of red blood cells, plasma, and platelets. Sometimes, before undergoing an elective surgery, a

patient will donate his or her own blood to be used in the event a transfusion is needed. This is known as an **autologous transfusion**.

Apheresis is a procedure that separates the different components of the blood and removes a certain part of the blood, such as occurs in leukapheresis, plateletpheresis, and plasmapheresis. A therapeutic plasmapheresis or plasma exchange occurs when the plasma is removed and is replaced with fresh plasma.

Bone marrow biopsy and/or aspiration is a diagnostic procedure that can be used to identify types of blood disorders. It may also be performed to evaluate the patient's response to treatment.

Peripheral stem cell and bone marrow transplants (Figure 10-9) are used to treat patients with certain leukemias and cancers, bone marrow failure syndromes, and genetic disease. Prior to transplant, the patient is prepared with radiation and/or chemotherapy to get rid of the defective or malignant cells and reduce the body's immunity, so it will not reject the transplanted cells.

EXERCISE 10-9

Assign codes for all diagnoses and procedures using your ICD-9-CM code book.

1. Patient with profound pancytopenia had a bone marrow biopsy ____________
2. Thrombocytopenia was treated with transfusion of platelets ____________
3. Therapeutic plasmapheresis performed on patient with thrombotic thrombocytopenic purpura ____________
4. DIC with transfusion of fresh frozen plasma ____________
5. Post operative blood loss anemia with autologous transfusion of red blood cells ____________

DOCUMENTATION/REIMBURSEMENT/MS-DRGs

Often, coding difficulties are due to lack of documentation. Sometimes pathology and other test results are not available at the time of discharge or when the physician is dictating the discharge summary or is reporting the final diagnoses.

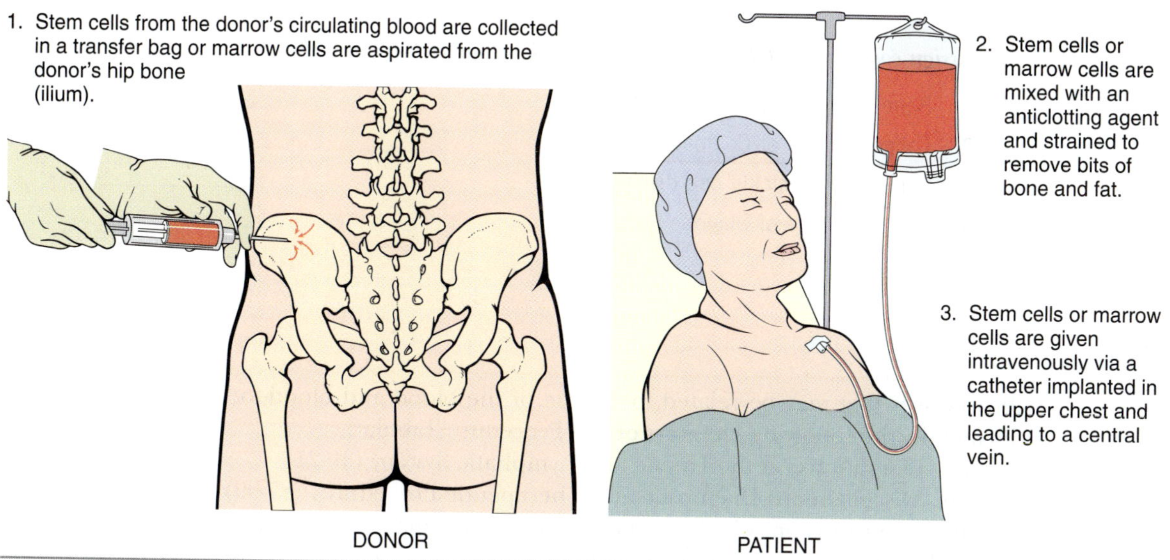

Figure 10-9. Peripheral stem cell and bone marrow transplants.

Documentation difficulties include lack of documentation regarding various types of anemia and the relationship of anemia to other chronic illnesses and diseases such as ESRD and neoplastic disease. Sometimes, acute and/or chronic blood loss is documented, but in the record, no mention of associated anemia is made by the physician.

MS-DRG With and Without MCC/CC

EXAMPLE

A patient had a total abdominal hysterectomy for fibroid uterus. The patient was symptomatic with menorrhagia. Patient has von Willebrand's disease.

DIAGNOSES	CODES	MS-DRG	RW
Fibroid uterus with menorrhagia and von Willebrand's disease Total abdominal hysterectomy	218.9, 626.2, 286.4, 68.49	742	1.2422
Fibroid uterus with menorrhagia Total abdominal hysterectomy	218.9, 626.2 68.49	743	0.8672

In this case, von Willebrand's disease is a CC, and this affects reimbursement.

CHAPTER REVIEW EXERCISE

Assign codes for all diagnoses and procedures, including all applicable V and E codes.

1. Vitamin K deficiency __________
2. Pernicious anemia __________
3. Coagulopathy due to Coumadin taken for atrial fibrillation. Patient has been on Coumadin for 1 year. __________
4. Hemophilia A carrier __________
5. Pseudocholinesterase deficiency __________
6. Polycythemia, benign __________
7. Severe congenital aplastic anemia treated with bone marrow transplant, allogeneic from related donor __________
8. Sickle cell Hb-SS disease with crisis treated with plasma exchange __________
9. Anemia due to AIDS __________
10. Anemia due to acute and chronic blood loss treated with transfusion of 2 units of packed red blood cells __________
11. Idiopathic thrombocytopenic purpura treated with a splenectomy __________
12. History of bone marrow transplant __________
13. Chronic agranulocytosis __________
14. Chronic lymphadenitis __________
15. Hypersplenism __________
16. Congestive splenomegaly __________
17. Hemochromatosis __________
18. Lymphocytic leukemoid reaction __________

19. Lupus anticoagulant ____________

20. Neutropenia due to infection ____________

Write the correct answer(s) in the space(s) provided.

21. Which blood component is essential for clotting?

____

22. Describe apheresis.

____

23. List two warning signs of a coagulation disorder.

____

24. Which cells fight infection, inflammation and other diseases?

____

25. Define idiopathic.

____

CHAPTER GLOSSARY

Anemia: occurs when hemoglobin drops, which interrupts the transport of oxygen throughout the body.

Anticoagulant medications: medications that are used to prevent venous thrombi.

Antiplatelet medications: medications that are used to prevent clumping of platelets or formation of an arterial thrombus.

Apheresis: procedure that separates different components of blood and removes a certain part of the blood, such as occurs in leukapheresis, plateletpheresis, and plasmapheresis.

Aplastic anemia: reduction in red blood cells due to impairment or failure of bone marrow function.

Autologous transfusion: transfusion of a patient's own blood. Blood may have been donated prior to an elective procedure.

Blood: viscous fluid that circulates through the vessels of the circulatory system as a result of the pumping action of the heart.

Bone marrow biopsy: diagnostic procedure that is used to identify types of anemia and cell deficiencies, and to detect leukemia.

Coagulation defect: breakdown in the clotting process of the blood.

Disseminated intravascular coagulation: disorder that results in depletion of clotting factors in the blood.

Erythrocytes: another name for red blood cells that are made in the marrow of bones; their main responsibility is to carry oxygen around the body and remove carbon dioxide. These are the cells that give blood its red color.

Hemolytic anemias: result from abnormal or excessive destruction of red blood cells.

Hemophilia A: most common type of hemophilia; deficiency or abnormality in clotting factor VIII.

Hemophilia B: another name for Christmas disease, which is results from a deficiency of factor IX.

Hemophilia C: mild form of hemophilia with decreased factor XI.

Homeostasis: the ability of an organism or cell to maintain internal equilibrium by adjusting its physiologic processes.

Idiopathic: causative factor is unknown.

Leukocytes: white blood cells increase in number to battle infection, inflammation, and other diseases.

Leukocytosis: increase in the number of white cells in the blood; it may be a sign of infection or may indicate stress on the body.

Lymphadenitis: inflammation of a lymph node that is usually caused by a bacterial infection.

Neutropenia: abnormal decrease in granular leukocytes in the blood.

Pancytopenia: decrease in production of erythrocytes (red blood cells), leukocytes (white blood cells), and thrombocytes (platelets).

Parenteral: when medications are administered other than through the digestive tract, such as by intravenous or intramuscular injection.

Platelets: another name for thrombocytes. Platelets circulate in the blood and assist in the clotting process.

Purpura: ecchymoses or small hemorrhages in the skin, mucous membranes, or serosal surfaces due to blood disorders, vascular abnormalities, or trauma.

Secondary thrombocytopenia: decrease in the number of platelets due to specific diseases or external causes, such as drugs, blood transfusions, and overhydration.

Sickle cell anemia: one of the most common hemolytic anemias, in which the shape of the red blood cell changes from a disc to a crescent or "sickle," causing obstruction of small blood vessels and eventual damage throughout the body.

Splenomegaly: enlarged spleen.

Thalassemia: hereditary disease that is similar to sickle cell anemia and occurs in varying degrees.

Thrombocytes: another name for platelets. Thrombocytes circulate in the blood and assist in the clotting process.

CHAPTER 11

Diseases of the Genitourinary System

(ICD-9-CM Chapter 10, Codes 580-629)

CHAPTER OUTLINE

LEARNING OBJECTIVES

- Apply and assign the correct ICD-9-CM codes in accordance with Official Guidelines for Coding and Reporting
- Identify pertinent anatomy and physiology of diseases of the genitourinary system
- Identify diseases of the genitourinary system
- Assign the correct V codes and procedure codes related to the genitourinary system
- Identify common treatments, medications, laboratory values, and diagnostic tests
- Explain the importance of documentation in relation to MS-DRGs for reimbursement

ABBREVIATIONS

ARF acute renal failure
ARI acute renal insufficiency
AV arteriovenous
BUN blood urea nitrogen
CAPD continuous ambulatory peritoneal dialysis
CC chief complaint
CCPD continuous cycling peritoneal dialysis
CKD chronic kidney disease
CRF chronic renal failure
CRI chronic renal insufficiency
D&C dilatation and curettage
ESRD end-stage renal disease
ESWL extracorporeal shock wave lithotripsy
FSG focal segmental glomerulosclerosis
GFR glomerular filtration rate
GN glomerulonephritis
ICD-9-CM *International Classification of Diseases, 9th Revision, Clinical Modification*
Ig immunoglobulin
LAVH laparoscopically assisted vaginal hysterectomy
LDMF latissimus dorsi musculocutaneous flap
LUTS lower urinary tract symptoms
MRSA methicillin-resistant Staphylococcus aureus
MS-DRG Medicare Severity diagnosis-related group
NEC not elsewhere classifiable
NKF National Kidney Foundation
NOS not otherwise specified
OIG Office of the Inspector General
PID pelvic inflammatory disease
RPGN rapidly progressive glomerulonephritis
TRAM transverse rectus abdominis musculocutaneous
TULIP transurethral ultrasound-guided laser-induced prostatectomy
TUMT transurethral microwave thermotherapy
TUNA transurethral needle ablation of prostate
TURP transurethral resection of the prostate
UHDDS Uniform Hospital Discharge Data Set
UTI urinary tract infection
VLAP visual laser ablation of the prostate

ICD-9-CM Official Guidelines for Coding and Reporting

Please refer to the companion Evolve website for the most current guidelines.

10. Chapter 10: Diseases of Genitourinary System (580-629)

a. Chronic kidney disease

1) Stages of chronic kidney disease (CKD)

The ICD-9-CM classifies CKD based on severity. The severity of CKD is designated by stages I-V. Stage II, code 585.2, equates to mild CKD; stage III, code 585.3, equates to moderate CKD; and stage IV, code 585.4, equates to severe CKD. Code 585.6, End stage renal disease (ESRD), is assigned when the provider has documented end-stage-renal disease (ESRD).

If both a stage of CKD and ESRD are documented, assign code 585.6 only.

2) Chronic kidney disease and kidney transplant status

Patients who have undergone kidney transplant may still have some form of CKD, because the kidney transplant may not fully restore kidney function. Therefore, the presence of CKD alone does not constitute a transplant complication. Assign the appropriate 585 code for the patient's stage of CKD and code V42.0. If a transplant complication such as failure or rejection is documented, see section I.C.17.f.1.b for information on coding complications of a kidney transplant. If the documentation is unclear as to whether the patient has a complication of the transplant, query the provider.

3) Chronic kidney disease with other conditions

Patients with CKD may also suffer from other serious conditions, most commonly diabetes mellitus and hypertension. The sequencing of the CKD code in relationship to codes for other contributing conditions is based on the conventions in the tabular list.

See I.C.3.a.4 for sequencing instructions for diabetes.
See I.C.4.a.1 for anemia in CKD.
See I.C.7.a.3 for hypertensive chronic kidney disease.
See I.C.17.f.1.b, Kidney transplant complications, for instructions on coding of documented rejection or failure.

EXAMPLE Patient was admitted to the hospital for fluid overload due to noncompliance with attending renal dialysis sessions. Patient has stage V CKD. Hemodialysis was performed, 276.6, 585.6, V45.12, 39.95.

Apply the General Coding Guidelines as found in Chapter 5.

ANATOMY AND PHYSIOLOGY

Urinary Tract

The kidneys, ureters, urinary bladder, and urethra form the urinary tract (Figure 11-1). Its main function involves producing, storing, and excreting urine. The kidneys and ureters make up the upper urinary tract, and the bladder and urethra constitute the lower urinary tract. The kidneys are two bean-shaped organs that are located on either side of the spine or retroperitoneally. The kidneys form a complex filtration system that cleanses the blood of waste products that become urine. Each kidney has a ureter that allows the urine to travel to the bladder for storage. The bladder is expandable, and openings into the ureters close so that urine cannot flow backward or reflux into the kidneys. The urine is excreted out of the body through a tube called the urethra. It is easy to confuse the terminology for urethra and ureter. Less than half of a single kidney is needed to do all the work that can be accomplished by two kidneys. The main difference between the male and female urinary tracts is the length of the urethra. The male urethra is 20 cm long; the female urethra measures only 3 cm.

Male Genital Tract

The main parts of the male genital or reproductive tract are the testes, epididymis, vas deferens, seminal vesicles, prostate, and penis (Figure 11-2). Its primary function is the production of sperm. The main diseases related to the male genital tract are infertility, infection, and tumor.

Female Genital Tract

The main parts of the female genital or reproductive tract are the vulva, vagina, uterus, fallopian tubes, and ovaries (Figure 11-3). Reproduction is its primary function. The main diseases and conditions of the female genital tract are related to infection, tumor, hormonal disorders, and pregnancy.

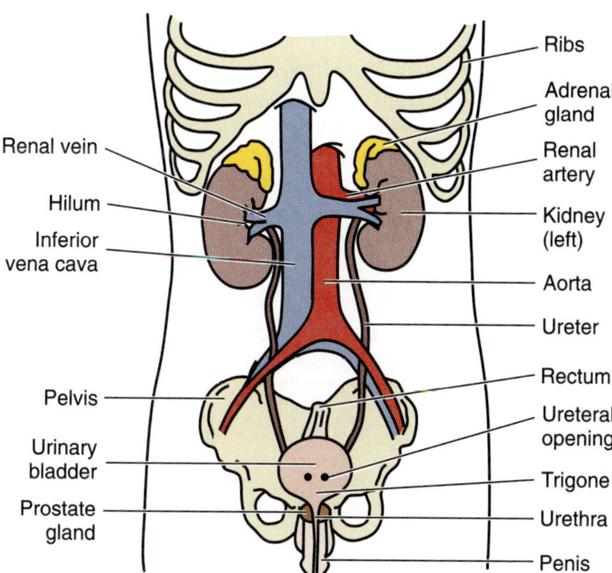

Figure 11-1. Gross anatomy of the urinary system (male).

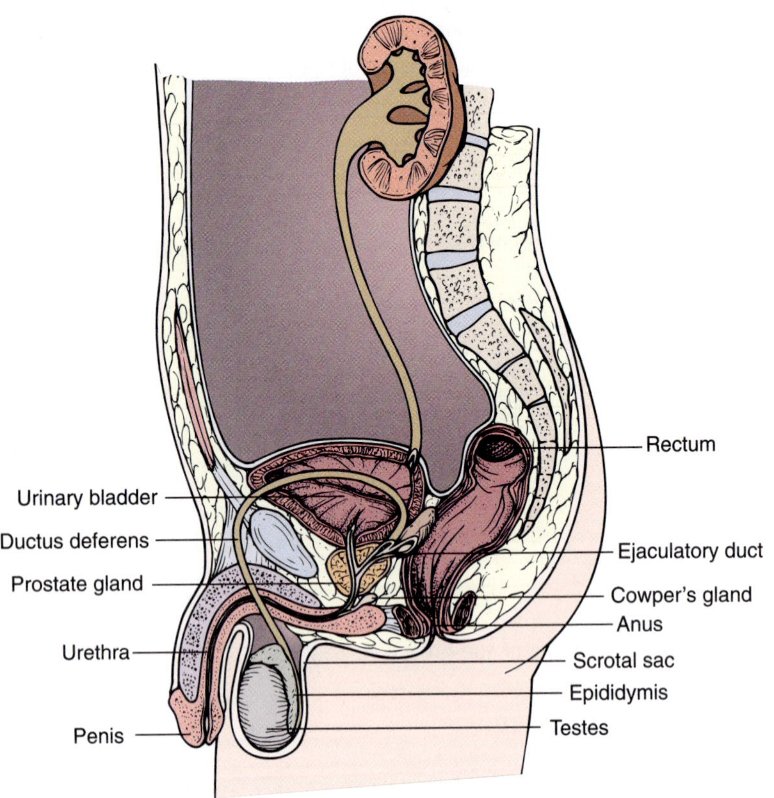

Figure 11-2. Normal male reproductive system.

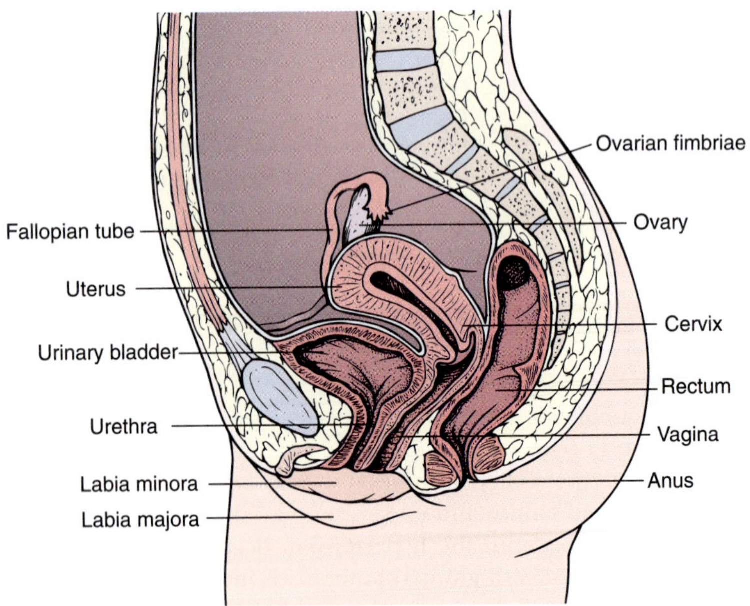

Figure 11-3. Normal female reproductive system.

Breast

Male and female breasts are similar in that they are formed embryologically from the same tissues. It is possible for males to have breast disorders also. The female breast (Figure 11-4) will start to develop during puberty due to the hormone estrogen. Female breasts are considered an accessory organ of reproduction and are composed of fat and fibrous tissue with mammary glands for the production of milk **(lactation)**.

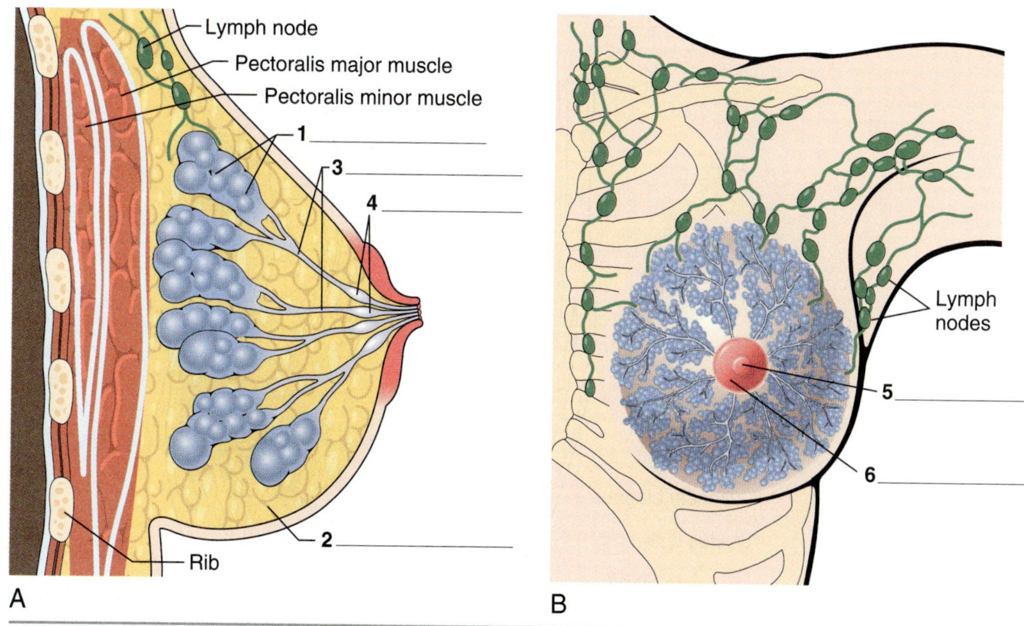

Figure 11-4. Views of the breast. **A,** Sagittal. **B,** Frontal. Notice the numerous lymph nodes.

DISEASE CONDITIONS

Diseases of the genitourinary system (580-629) are located in Chapter 10 of the ICD-9-CM code book and are divided into the following categories:

CATEGORY	SECTION TITLES
580-589	Nephritis, Nephrotic Syndrome, and Nephrosis
590-599	Other Diseases of the Urinary System
600-608	Disease of the Male Genital Organs
610-611	Disorders of Breast
614-616	Inflammatory Disease of Female Pelvic Organs
617-629	Other Disorders of Female Genital Tract

It is important to note that disorders of the breast are classified as Diseases of the Genitourinary System in ICD-9-CM.

Nephritis, Nephrotic Syndrome, and Nephrosis (580-589)

Glomerulonephritis

Glomerulonephritis (GN) (Figure 11-5) is inflammation of the glomeruli of the kidneys. (See Figure 11-6 for illustration of the anatomy of the kidney.) Glomerulonephritis can be a temporary, reversible condition, or it may be a chronic progressive condition that results in chronic renal failure and end-stage renal disease. GN may cause hypertension and may not be discovered until the hypertension becomes difficult to control. Specific disorders that are associated with glomerulonephritis include the following:

- Focal segmental glomerulosclerosis (FSG)
- Goodpasture's syndrome
- Immunoglobulin (Ig)A nephropathy (Berger's disease)
- IgM mesangial proliferative glomerulonephritis
- Lupus nephritis
- Membranoproliferative glomerulonephritis I
- Membranoproliferative glomerulonephritis II
- Poststreptococcal glomerulonephritis
- Rapidly progressive (crescentic) glomerulonephritis
- Rapidly progressive glomerulonephritis (RPGN)

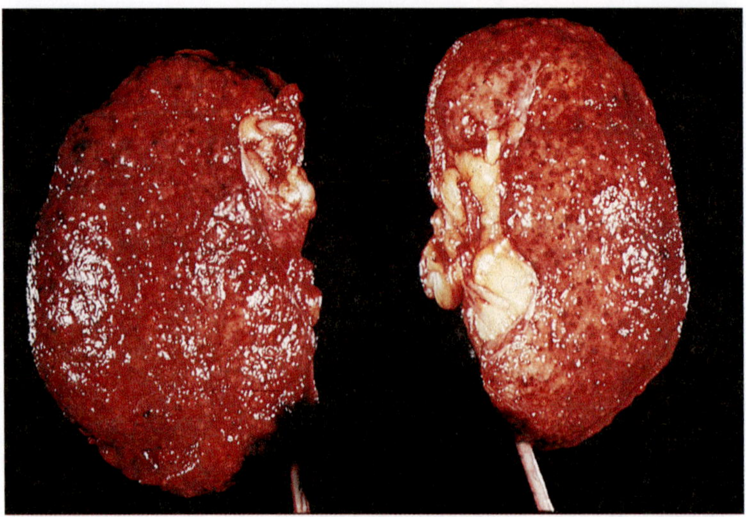

Figure 11-5. End-stage glomerulopathy–chronic glomerulonephritis.

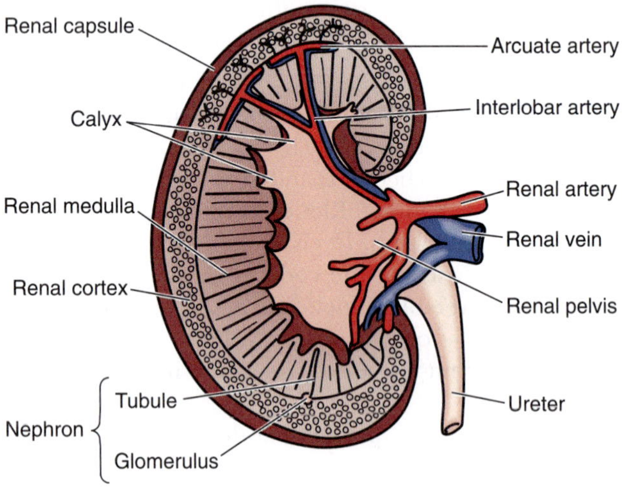

Figure 11-6. Anatomy of the kidney.

EXAMPLE Minimal change glomerulonephritis, 581.3.

EXAMPLE Chronic RPGN, 582.4.

Nephrotic Syndrome/Nephrosis

Nephrotic syndrome is a condition that is marked by **proteinuria** (protein in the urine), low levels of protein in the blood, hypercholesterolemia, and swelling of the eyes, feet, and hands. Damage to the kidneys' glomeruli can result in nephrotic syndrome. Treatment focuses on identifying the underlying cause and reducing cholesterol, blood pressure, and protein in urine through diet and medications.

EXAMPLE Lupus nephritis, 710.0, 583.81.

Acute Renal Failure

Acute renal failure (ARF) is sudden and severe impairment in renal function characterized by oliguria, increased serum urea, and acidosis. With treatment, ARF is usually reversible. ARF often occurs in hospitalized patients with serious systemic illness such as infection, low blood pressure, shock, and as an adverse effect of the use of certain antibiotics and drugs. Obstruction of the urinary tract and dehydration may also cause ARF. It is possible for a patient with chronic renal failure or chronic kidney disease to also develop ARF. In this case, codes are assigned for both the acute and chronic renal failure.

EXAMPLE Acute renal failure due to dehydration, 584.9, 276.51.

When a patient is admitted to the hospital with acute renal failure and dehydration, according to *Coding Clinic* (2002:3Q:p21-22),[1] ARF is the principal diagnosis, and the dehydration is a secondary diagnosis. Patients with both conditions are generally treated with IV fluids, and ARF is more serious than dehydration. A patient who is dehydrated and has no impairment in renal function may be given IV fluids and sent home instead of being admitted to the hospital.

Chronic Renal Failure (CRF)/Chronic Kidney Disease (CKD)

According to *Coding Clinic* (2005:4Q:p77-79),[2] "Changes were made to the ICD-9-CM classification to recognize more current terminology related to chronic kidney disease (CKD) rather than imprecise terms like chronic renal failure [CRF] and chronic renal insufficiency (CRI). The descriptor for code 585, Chronic renal failure, has been changed to chronic kidney disease. Code 585 has been expanded to recognize current staging of chronic kidney disease developed by the National Kidney Foundation (NKF)" (Table 11-1).

Using these NKF guidelines, levels of kidney damage and kidney function must be determined to accurately assign the code for CKD. A patient's glomerular filtration rate (GFR) indicates the level of kidney function and indicates the stage of the disease, which may slowly progress over many years. Early detection through laboratory tests and proper treatment can limit the effects of CKD, if the disease is discovered in the early stages.

If CKD is left untreated, a patient will develop end-stage renal disease (ESRD). This condition is characterized by the near or complete failure of kidney function, which leaves the patient unable to process waste material. Dialysis or transplantation may be needed to treat the condition.

Table 11-1. Five Stages of Chronic Kidney Disease

Stage	Description	Glomerular Filtration Rate (GFR)
At increased risk	Risk factors for kidney disease (e.g., diabetes, high blood pressure, family history, older age, ethnic group)	Higher than 90
1	Kidney damage (protein in the urine) and normal GFR	Higher than 90
2	Kidney damage and mild decrease in GFR	60-89
3	Moderate decrease in GFR	30-59
4	Severe decrease in GFR	15-29
5	Kidney failure (dialysis or kidney transplant needed)	Less than 15

Data from the National Kidney Foundation.

CRF or CKD can develop from ARF if renal function is not restored through dialysis or treatment. This may take several weeks or months. Documentation in the health record that might indicate the presence of renal failure could include the following:

1. Markedly elevated values of serum creatinine or blood urea nitrogen (BUN), or diminished creatinine clearance
2. Other clinical and laboratory manifestations of renal impairment are as follows:
   - Anemia
   - Hyperphosphatemia
   - Hypocalcemia
   - Hyperkalemia
   - Renal osteodystrophy
   - Uremic symptoms: nausea, vomiting, itching, hemorrhagic conditions, hypertension, edema, dyspnea, lethargy, coma, etc.

EXAMPLE Hyperkalemia due to chronic kidney disease (CKD), 276.7, 585.9.

Hypertension and Chronic Kidney Disease/Renal Failure

ICD-9-CM presumes a cause-and-effect relationship with hypertension and renal failure or kidney disease. This is addressed in the coding guidelines and in the "Excludes notes" for codes 586, and 587 (Figure 11-7). Code 585 has instructions to code first hypertensive chronic kidney disease, if applicable. The physician would have to specifically document that CKD or renal failure is NOT due to hypertension to negate the cause-and-effect relationship. Hypertension and hypertensive manifestations are discussed more extensively in Chapter 14, Diseases of the Circulatory System.

EXAMPLE Patient has chronic kidney disease, stage III, and benign hypertension, 403.10, 585.3.

EXAMPLE Patient has chronic renal insufficiency and hypertension, 403.90, 585.9.

Diabetic Nephropathy

Diabetes mellitus can have effects on many organs, including the kidneys. If diabetes is not well controlled, it may cause renal complications such as glomerulosclerosis, pyelonephritis, and papillary necrosis. Diabetic patients with renal manifestations may be prone to infections that can cause further damage to the kidneys.

Unlike the relationship between renal failure/chronic kidney disease and hypertension, diabetes and renal disease must be linked in a manner that denotes a direct relationship. For example, diabetic nephropathy or intercapillary glomerulosclerosis due to diabetes shows a cause-and-effect relationship with diabetes. It is possible for a patient to have nephropathy and diabetes, and no documentation indicates that nephropathy is due to diabetes. In Chapter 12 of this book, diabetes mellitus and manifestations of the disease are discussed in greater depth.

EXAMPLE Patient is admitted for treatment of uncontrolled diabetes mellitus, type II. Patient is on hemodialysis for end-stage renal disease, 250.02, 585.6, V45.1.

EXAMPLE Patient had intercapillary glomerulosclerosis due to diabetes mellitus type I, 250.41, 581.81.

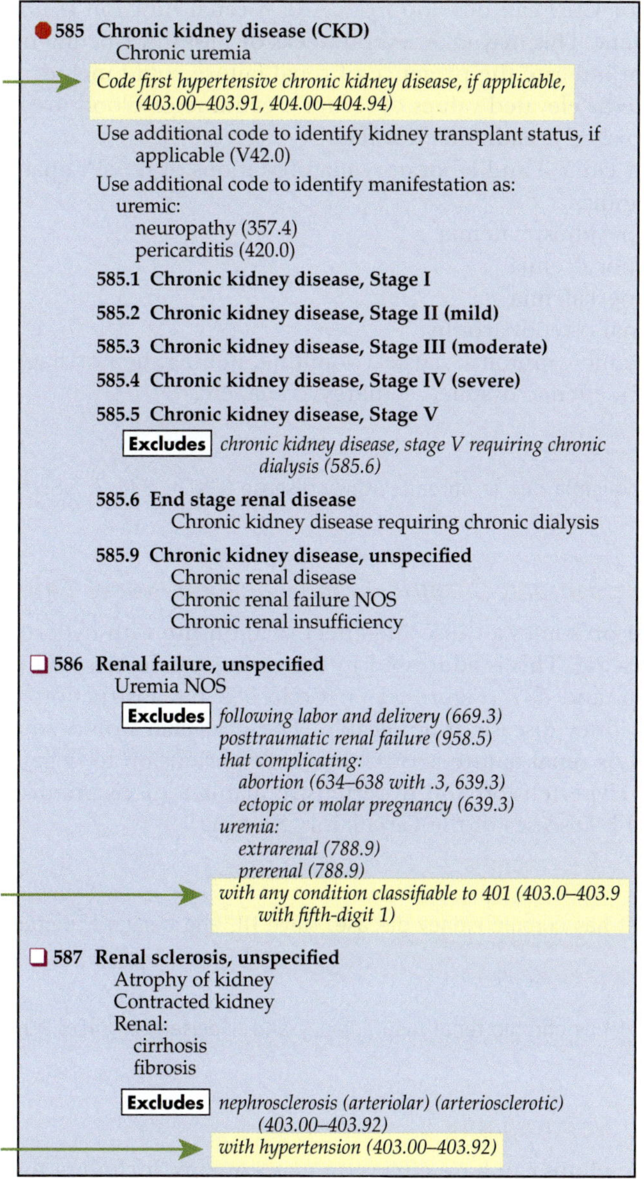

585 Chronic kidney disease (CKD)
Chronic uremia

Code first hypertensive chronic kidney disease, if applicable, (403.00–403.91, 404.00–404.94)

Use additional code to identify kidney transplant status, if applicable (V42.0)

Use additional code to identify manifestation as:
uremic:
neuropathy (357.4)
pericarditis (420.0)

585.1 Chronic kidney disease, Stage I

585.2 Chronic kidney disease, Stage II (mild)

585.3 Chronic kidney disease, Stage III (moderate)

585.4 Chronic kidney disease, Stage IV (severe)

585.5 Chronic kidney disease, Stage V

Excludes *chronic kidney disease, stage V requiring chronic dialysis (585.6)*

585.6 End stage renal disease
Chronic kidney disease requiring chronic dialysis

585.9 Chronic kidney disease, unspecified
Chronic renal disease
Chronic renal failure NOS
Chronic renal insufficiency

586 Renal failure, unspecified
Uremia NOS

Excludes *following labor and delivery (669.3)*
posttraumatic renal failure (958.5)
that complicating:
abortion (634–638 with .3, 639.3)
ectopic or molar pregnancy (639.3)
uremia:
extrarenal (788.9)
prerenal (788.9)
with any condition classifiable to 401 (403.0–403.9 with fifth-digit 1)

587 Renal sclerosis, unspecified
Atrophy of kidney
Contracted kidney
Renal:
cirrhosis
fibrosis

Excludes *nephrosclerosis (arteriolar) (arteriosclerotic) (403.00–403.92)*
with hypertension (403.00–403.92)

Figure 11-7. Instructions for coding 585, 586, and 587 with hypertension.

EXERCISE 11-1

Assign codes to the following conditions using your ICD-9-CM code book.

1. Acute on chronic renal failure ______________
2. Nephrotic syndrome ______________
3. Nephritis due to tuberculosis ______________
4. Focal segmental glomerulosclerosis ______________
5. Essential hypertension; stage IV CKD ______________

Other Diseases of the Urinary System (590-599)

Hematuria

Hematuria is the presence of blood in the urine. Hematuria may be grossly visible, or it may be detected only through microscopic analysis. The causes of hematuria are varied,

and some are more serious than others. The extent of diagnostic investigation required to determine a cause depends on the amount of hematuria, its duration, and risk factors the patient may have that indicate a more serious disease. Causes include inflammation due to drugs or medications, stones, infections, cancers or malignancies, trauma, and blockages or obstructions of flow. A patient with renal stones often has hematuria. Hematuria would not be assigned as an additional code because it is considered integral to the renal stones according to *Coding Clinic* (1995:3Q:p8)[3]. This corresponds with the general coding guideline that signs and symptoms that are integral to the disease process should not be assigned as additional codes.

EXAMPLE

Hematuria due to nephrolithiasis, 592.0.

EXAMPLE

Hematuria due to Coumadin, which is taken for atrial fibrillation, 599.70, E934.2, 427.31, V58.61.

Hematuria in this case is the adverse effect of medication that was properly prescribed and properly taken. An E code for the therapeutic use of Coumadin is also assigned.

Occasionally, hematuria occurs as the result of a traumatic injury due to catheterization or removal of a urinary catheter. According to *Coding Clinic* (1985:Nov-Dec:p15),[4] this is coded as injury of the urethra (867.0), with hematuria (599.70) assigned as an additional code. In some cases, it may be appropriate to assign an E code to indicate the cause and intent of the injury.

EXAMPLE

Hematuria due to patient pulling out indwelling urinary catheter, 867.0, 599.70, E928.9.

EXAMPLE

Hematuria due to catheterization, 867.0, 599.70, E879.6.

Hematuria is expected after many urinary procedures and should not be coded unless it is excessive and has been documented as such by the physician.

Urinary Tract Infections

Urinary tract infection (UTI) is a general term that is used to describe infection of any area of the urinary tract. **Cystitis** is a lower tract infection that affects the bladder (Figure 11-8), and **urethritis** affects the urethra. An upper tract infection that involves the kidneys is called **pyelonephritis** (Figure 11-9).

According to *Coding Clinic* (1999:2Q:p15-16),[5] "physicians commonly use the term "urinary tract infection" when referring to cystitis, urethritis, or pyelonephritis. UTIs are

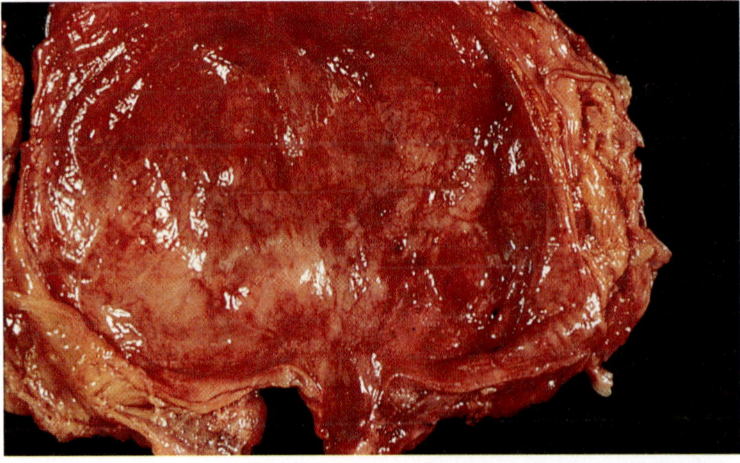

Figure 11-8. Acute cystitis. The mucosa of the bladder is red and swollen.

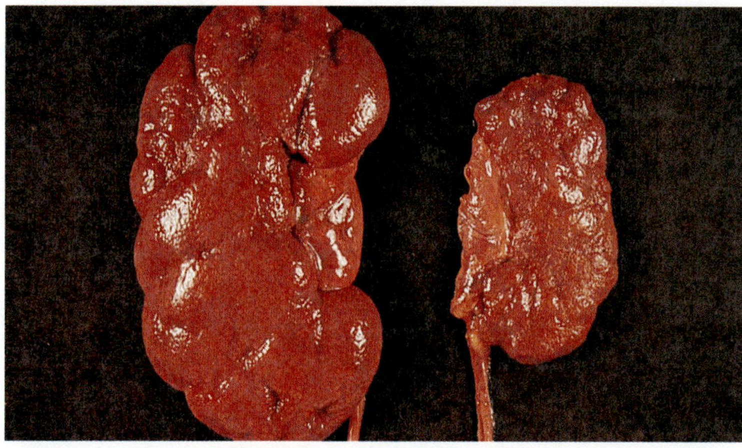

Figure 11-9. Small, shrunken, irregularly scarred kidney of a patient with chronic pyelonephritis. The other kidney is of normal size but has scarring on the upper pole.

assigned codes based on the site of infection, if known, although it is not always possible to distinguish between the three conditions on clinical grounds alone." Based on this reference, only 595.9, cystitis, should be assigned when the physician indicates the bladder as the infection site. Additional sites may be coded if the infection has spread. However, if the documentation includes both UTI and cystitis as diagnoses, only 595.9 should be used. If the site of the UTI is not documented or identified, code 599.0, urinary tract infection, NOS, should be assigned; this code can ONLY be used if the site is not identified and not in combination with any other codes where the site is identified.

EXAMPLE

Urinary tract infection due to acute pyelonephritis, 590.10.

The code 599.0 is not assigned because the site of infection has been identifi ed as the kidneys. No bacteria have been identified, so no organism code is assigned.

Most UTIs are due to bacteria. Urinalysis (Table 11-2) and culture and sensitivity tests may be performed to identify the causative organism and to determine which drugs are more effective in treating the infection. Less common are infections caused by viruses, fungi, or parasites. Infections that are due to sexually transmitted disease such as chlamydia or candidiasis are discussed in the infectious and parasitic disease chapter. An instructional note is provided about the use of an additional code to identify the organism as well as the code for the urinary tract infection (Figure 11-10). The following are the most common organisms responsible for UTIs:

- 041.4 *Escherichia coli* (*E coli*)
- 041.6 *Proteus* (*mirabilis*) (*morganii*)
- 041.11 *Staphylococcus aureus*
- 041.19 *Staphylococcus saprophyticus*
- 041.02 Group B *Streptococcus*
- 041.3 *Klebsiella pneumoniae*

If a causative organism is documented by the physician, this should be coded, in addition to the infection. It would not be appropriate to code an organism on the basis of a urine culture or sensitivity report only. Sometimes the documentation will indicate that the urine grew gram negative bacteria, awaiting sensitivity report. The next progress note will indicate that the urine culture is positive for *Escherichia coli (E. coli)*. The *E. coli* is the gram negative bacteria that was identified and the only code necessary to show the causative organism is 041.4 for the *E. coli*. It would be incorrect to also assign 041.85, other gram negative organisms.

EXAMPLE

Urinary tract infection due to *E coli*, 599.0, 041.4.

Table 11-2. Routine Urinalysis*[6]

	Normal	Abnormal	Pathology
Characteristics			
Color and clarity	Pale to darker yellow, and clear	Very pale Cloudy, milky white blood cells Hematuria, red blood cells, reddish to reddish brown	Excessive water Pus, urinary tract infection Bleeding in infection, calculi, or cancer
Odor	Aromatic	Fishy Fruity Foul	Cystitis Diabetes mellitus Urinary tract infection
Chemical nature	pH is generally slightly acidic, 6.5	Alkaline	Infections cause ammonia to form
Specific gravity	1.003-1.030—reflects quantity of waste, minerals, and solids in urine	Higher—causes precipitation of solutes Lower—polyuria	Kidney stones, diabetes mellitus, diabetes insipidus
Constituent Compounds			
Protein	None, or small amount	Albuminuria	Nephritis, renal failure, infection
Glucose	None	Glycosuria	Faulty carbohydrate metabolism, as in diabetes mellitus
Ketone bodies	None	Ketonuria	Diabetic acidosis
Bile and bilirubin	None	Bilirubinuria	Hepatic or gallbladder disease
Casts	None—or small number of hyaline casts	Urinary casts composed of red or white blood cells, fat, or pus	Nephritis, renal disease, inflammation, metal poisoning
Nitrogenous wastes	Ammonia, creatinine, urea, and uric acid	Azoturia, creatinine, and urea clearance tests disproportionate to normal BUN/creatinine ratio	Hepatic disease, renal disease
Crystals	None to trace	Acidic urine, alkaline urine, hypercalcemia, metabolism error	Not signifi cant unless the crystals are large (stones); certain types are interpreted by physician
Fat droplets	None	Lipoiduria	Nephrosis

BUN, Blood urea nitrogen.
*Routine urinalysis is the physical, chemical, and microscopic examination of urine for abnormal elements; this may help the clinician to estimate renal function and may provide clues of systemic disease. This table includes some important characteristics and elements that are screened for in basic urinalysis. Other normal constituents of urine that are studied routinely for diagnosis include calcium, potassium, sodium, phosphorus, creatinine, and volume in a 24-hour period.

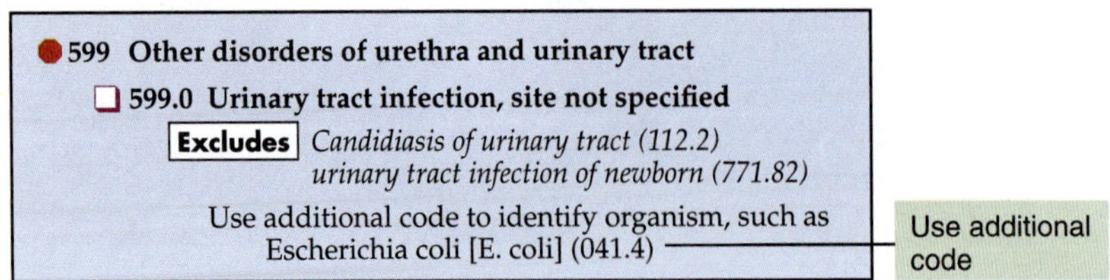

● **599 Other disorders of urethra and urinary tract**

❑ **599.0 Urinary tract infection, site not specified**

Excludes *Candidiasis of urinary tract (112.2)*
urinary tract infection of newborn (771.82)

Use additional code to identify organism, such as Escherichia coli [E. coli] (041.4)

Figure 11-10. Instruction is given to use an additional code to identify the organism.

EXAMPLE Acute cystitis due to Friedlander's bacillus, 595.0, 041.3.

Some patients are plagued by recurrent (chronic) UTIs. For this reason, they are sometimes treated with a daily dose of antibiotic to prevent an infection or for prophylactic measures. According to *Coding Clinic* (1996:2Q:p7),[7] "the patient doesn't have any symptoms of UTI, so it would be inappropriate to assign a code for the condition." This should be coded as V58.62, long-term (current) use of antibiotic, and V13.02 to identify the personal history of urinary tract infection.

The term "urosepsis" can cause confusion. Some physicians use the term "urosepsis" to mean an infection of the urinary tract without systemic infection. Other physicians may document urosepsis and mean that the patient has a UTI that has progressed to sepsis. Thus, a physician query may be required to establish the appropriate code(s). According to the Alphabetic Index, the term "urosepsis" defaults to 599.0, so unless other information is available, the urinary tract infection code should be assigned.

EXAMPLE Urosepsis due to *Proteus mirabilis,* 599.0, 041.6.

EXAMPLE Sepsis due to *Staphylococcus aureus* with urinary tract infection as the source, 038.11, 995.91, 599.0.

Calculus

Calculi or stones (Figure 11-11) may develop anywhere in the urinary tract and can vary in size. "**Urolithiasis**" describes a stone in the urinary tract. The terms "nephrolithiasis" and "**ureterolithiasis**" provide greater specificity with regard to location of the stone. Patients with stones are often asymptomatic unless they result in infection or start to move and obstruct the flow of urine. Obstructions due to stones are very painful and may result in admission to the hospital for pain control, identification, and treatment of the stone. Procedures such as extracorporeal shock wave lithotripsy (ESWL) and laser lithotripsy can be used to break up larger stones. "**Renal colic**" describes the intense pain associated with the body's efforts to try to force the stone through the ureters. According to *Coding Clinic* (1991:1Q:p11),[8] renal colic is not coded separately from a renal or ureteral calculus. Pain or renal colic is integral to the presence of urinary tract calculus.

On the other hand, hydronephrosis (due to urinary obstruction) should be assigned as an additional code. **Hydronephrosis** is abnormal dilatation of the renal pelvis that is caused by pressure from urine that cannot flow past an obstruction in the urinary tract (Figure 11-12). **Hydroureter** is the accumulation of urine in the ureters. These conditions may be documented in x-ray reports, ultrasound, or other diagnostic tests, but they must be documented by a physician before code assignment. Obstruction can result from a stone, tumor, infection, prostatic hypertrophy, or congenital abnormalities.

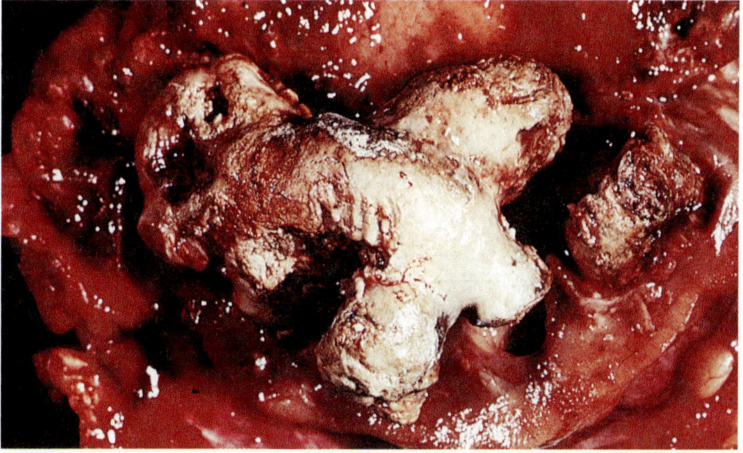

Figure 11-11. Irregularly shaped struvite stone in the renal pelvis.

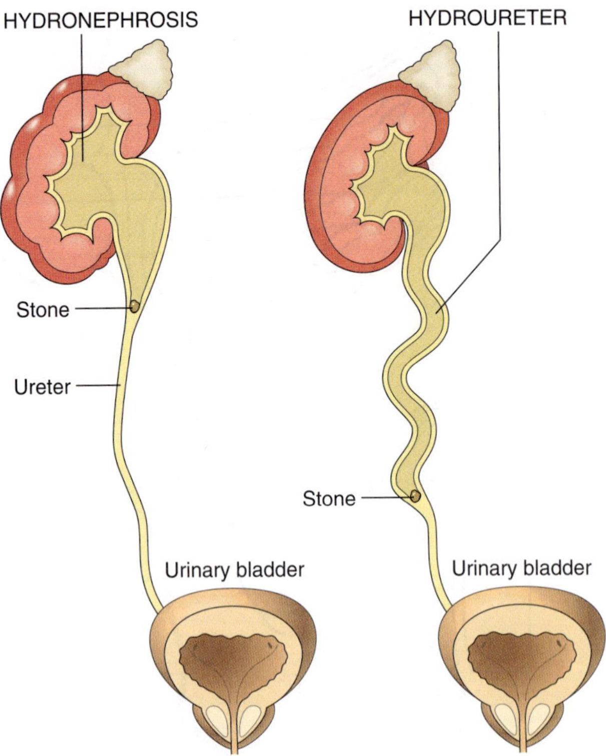

Figure 11-12. Hydronephrosis caused by a stone (obstruction) in the proximal part of the ureter and hydroureter with hydronephrosis caused by a stone in the distal part of the ureter.

EXAMPLE Hydroureter due to ureterolithiasis, 592.1, 593.5.

EXAMPLE Hematuria due to renal stone, 592.0.

EXERCISE 11-2

Assign codes to the following conditions using your ICD-9-CM code book.

1. Acute and chronic pyelonephritis due to *Pseudomonas* __________
2. Neurogenic bladder __________
3. Flank pain due to ureteral stone __________
4. Stricture of the urethra __________
5. Hydronephrosis due to kinking of ureter __________

Diseases of the Male Genital Organs (600-608)

Prostate

The most common diseases of the male genitourinary tract are those that affect the prostate. The prostate gland can become inflamed or enlarged, causing urinary problems. The prostate surrounds the urethra, through which urine flows. The flow of urine can be obstructed by the prostate. **Benign prostatic hyperplasia** and **benign prostatic hypertrophy** are conditions that result in enlargement of the prostate gland; these conditions usually occur in men who are older than 50 years of age (Figure 11-13). Symptoms may include frequency, nocturia, difficulty starting urination, a weak stream of urine, and inability to completely empty the bladder. Some subclassifications within the 600 code category contain special instructions for coding lower urinary tract symptoms (LUTS) (Figure 11-14). This corresponds with the general coding guideline that signs and symptoms that are integral to the disease process should not be assigned as additional codes, *unless otherwise instructed by the classification.*

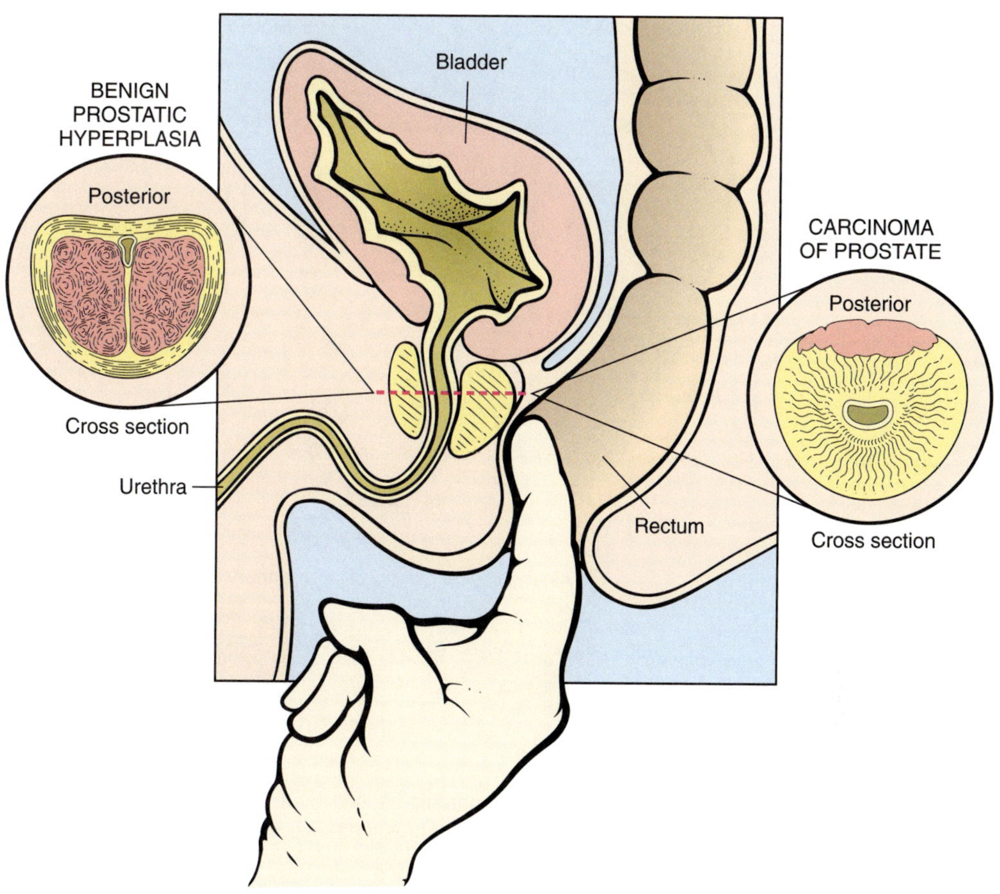

Figure 11-13. Digital prostate examination to identify prostatic abnormalities.

Prostatitis or inflammation of the prostate may be acute and/or chronic in nature and may be due to a bacteria or to inflammation that is not caused by a bacterial infection. Bacterial infections can be easily treated with antibiotics. Nonbacterial prostatitis involves treatment of urinary symptoms, which may be ongoing. There is an instructional note to use an additional code to identify the organism, if known (Figure 11-15). Use the Index and the Tabular to verify the accuracy of organism codes as referenced in the Tabular instructional note. If the code 041.1 is assigned as shown in Figure 11-15 for staphylococcal infection, an invalid code would have been assigned. A fifth digit is required to identify the type of staphylococcal infection.

041.1	*Staphylococcus* (invalid code because a fifth digit is available, see below)
041.10	*Staphylococcus,* unspecified
041.11	*Staphylococcus aureus*
041.19	Other *Staphylococcus*

EXAMPLE Chronic prostatitis due to staphylococcus 601.1, 041.10.

EXERCISE 11-3

Assign codes to the following conditions using your ICD-9-CM code book.

1. Nocturia due to benign prostatic hypertrophy __________
2. Acute prostatitis due to *Escherichia coli* __________
3. Scrotal pain and swelling due to epididymitis __________
4. Hydrocele __________
5. Phimosis __________

● 600 **Hyperplasia of prostate**
Includes: enlarged prostate

● 600.0 **Hypertrophy (benign) of prostate**
Benign prostatic hypertrophy
Enlargement of prostate
Smooth enlarged prostate
Soft enlarged prostate

600.00 **Hypertropy (benign) of prostate without urinary obstruction and other lower urinary tract symptoms (LUTS)**
Hypertrophy (benign) of prostate NOS

600.01 **Hypertrophy (benign) of prostate with urinary obstruction and other lower urinary tract symptoms (LUTS)**
Hypertrophy (benign) of prostate with urinary retention

→ Use additional code to identify symptoms:
incomplete bladder emptying (788.21)
nocturia (788.43)
straining on urination (788.65)
urinary frequency (788.41)
urinary hesitancy (788.64)
urinary incontinence (788.30–788.39)
urinary obstruction (599.69)
urinary retention (788.20)
urinary urgency (788.63)
weak urinary stream (788.62)

● 600.1 **Nodular prostate**
Hard, firm prostate
Multinodular prostate
Excludes *malignant neoplasm of prostate (185)*

600.10 **Nodular prostate without urinary obstruction**
Nodular prostate NOS

600.11 **Nodular prostate with urinary obstruction**
Nodular prostate with urinary retention

● 600.2 **Benign localized hyperplasia of prostate**
Adenofibromatous hypertrophy of prostate
Adenoma of prostate
Fibroadenoma of prostate
Fibroma of prostate
Myoma of prostate
Polyp of prostate
Excludes *benign neoplasms of prostate (222.2)*
hypertrophy of prostate (600.00–600.01)
malignant neoplasm of prostate (185)

600.20 **Benign localized hyperplasia of prostate without urinary obstruction and other lower urinary tract symptoms (LUTS)**
Benign localized hyperplasia of prostate NOS

600.21 **Benign localized hyperplasia of prostate with urinary obstruction and other lower urinary tract symptoms (LUTS)**
Benign localized hyperplasia of prostate with urinary retention

→ Use additional code to identify symptoms:
incomplete bladder emptying (788.21)
nocturia (788.43)
straining on urination (788.65)
urinary frequency (788.41)
urinary hesitancy (788.64)
urinary incontinence (788.30–788.39)
urinary obstruction (599.69)
urinary retention (788.20)
urinary urgency (788.63)
weak urinary stream (788.62)

600.3 **Cyst of prostate**

● 600.9 **Hyperplasia of prostate, unspecified**
Median bar
Prostatic obstruction NOS

❑ 600.90 **Hyperplasia of prostate, unspecified, without urinary obstruction and other lower urinary tract symptoms (LUTS)**
Hyperplasia of prostate NOS

❑ 600.91 **Hyperplasia of prostate, unspecified, with urinary obstruction and other lower urinary tract symptoms (LUTS)**
Hyperplasia of prostate, unspecified, with urinary retention

→ Use additional code to identify symptoms:
incomplete bladder emptying (788.21)
nocturia (788.43)
straining on urination (788.65)
urinary frequency (788.41)
urinary hesitancy (788.64)
urinary incontinence (788.30–788.39)
urinary obstruction (599.69)
urinary retention (788.20)
urinary urgency (788.63)
weak urinary stream (788.62)

Figure 11-14. Instructions to use additional code(s) for lower urinary tract symptoms (LUTS).

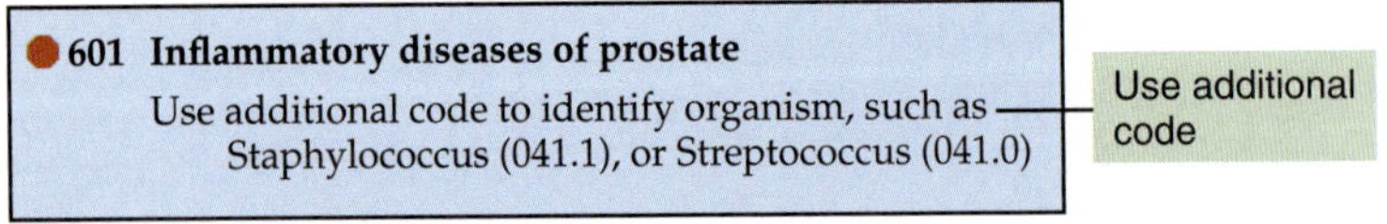
● 601 **Inflammatory diseases of prostate**
Use additional code to identify organism, such as Staphylococcus (041.1), or Streptococcus (041.0)

Figure 11-15. Instruction is given to use an additional code to identify the organism.

Disorders of Breast (610-611)

Breast

Many conditions of the breast described in this chapter are treated in the outpatient setting. Conditions of the breast in a pregnant woman are coded in the obstetrical chapter, or Chapter 11, of the ICD-9-CM code book. Male patients can also have conditions that are classified to the breast. **Mastitis** is inflammation or infection of the breast (Figure 11-16). Swelling, redness, tenderness, and pain may be noted. A breast abscess may form if mastitis is not treated. An abscess may require incision and drainage.

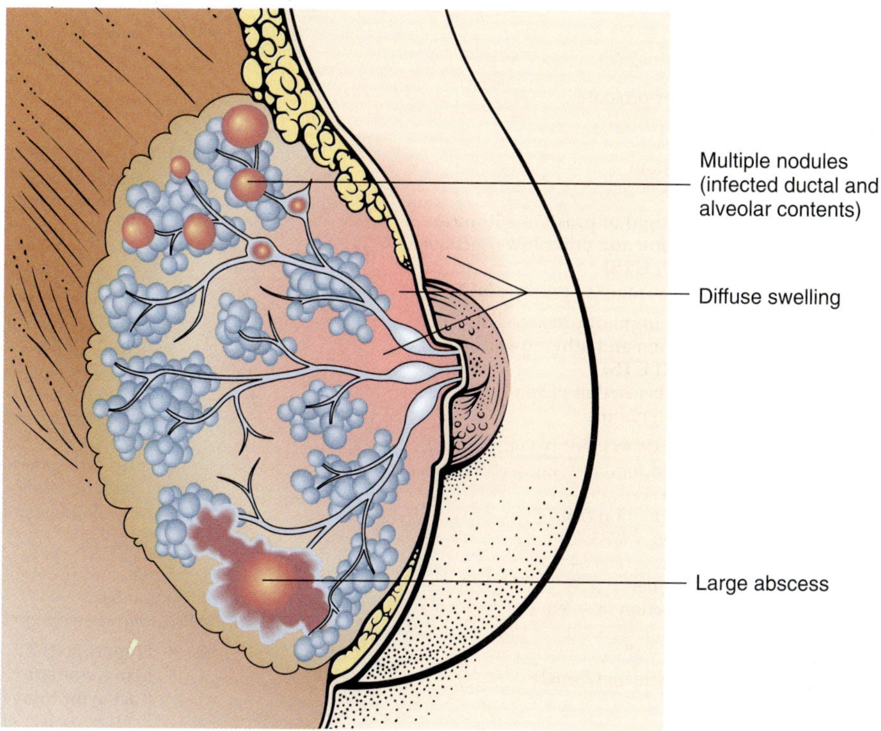

Figure 11-16. Acute mastitis typically occurs during lactation.

Some patients undergo prophylactic breast removal because they have a strong family history of breast cancer and/or genetic susceptibility or a personal history of breast cancer. After breast reconstruction is performed, complications such as infection, pain, and malfunction or failure of the implant or tissue expander, may occur. Complications of breast reconstruction are discussed in Chapter 21 of this text.

EXAMPLE Patient has diffuse fibroadenosis of both breasts, 610.2.

EXERCISE 11-4

Assign codes to the following conditions using your ICD-9-CM code book.

1. Fibrocystic disease of breast ____________
2. Nipple discharge ____________
3. Male patient with gynecomastia ____________
4. Mastodynia ____________

Inflammatory Disease of Female Pelvic Organs (614-616)

Pelvic Inflammatory Disease

Pelvic inflammatory disease (PID) occurs when vaginal or cervical infection spreads and involves the uterus, fallopian tubes, ovaries, and surrounding tissues. **Salpingitis** is inflammation of the fallopian tubes, which are the most common site of pelvic inflammation. **Endometritis** is inflammation of the uterus, and **oophoritis** is inflammation of the ovaries. The most prevalent symptoms of these infections include vaginal discharge, pain, and possibly a fever. Complications that may result include infertility, chronic pain, tubal pregnancy, recurrent inflammation, and abscess.

EXAMPLE Acute and chronic right salpingo-oophoritis, 614.0, 614.1.

EXERCISE 11-5

Assign codes to the following conditions using your ICD-9-CM code book.

1. Tubo-ovarian abscess ____________
2. Cervicitis ____________
3. Bartholin's cyst ____________
4. Pelvic adhesions, female ____________
5. PID ____________

Other Disorders of Female Genital Tract (617-629)

Endometriosis

Endometriosis is a chronic condition in which endometrial material, the tissue that lines the inside of the uterus, grows outside the uterus and attaches to other organs in the pelvic cavity. Code assignment is based on site of implantation (Figure 11-17). The most common sites are the ovaries and fallopian tubes. Although it is uncommon, endometrial tissue can spread to sites throughout the body to areas such as the lungs. Pain and infertility are the two most common symptoms.

EXAMPLE Endometriosis of the uterus, 617.0.

Genital Prolapse

Genital prolapse occurs when pelvic organs such as the uterus, bladder, and rectum shift from their normal anatomic positions and protrude into the vagina or press against the wall of the vagina (Figure 11-18). Weakening or damage to the ligaments, muscles, and

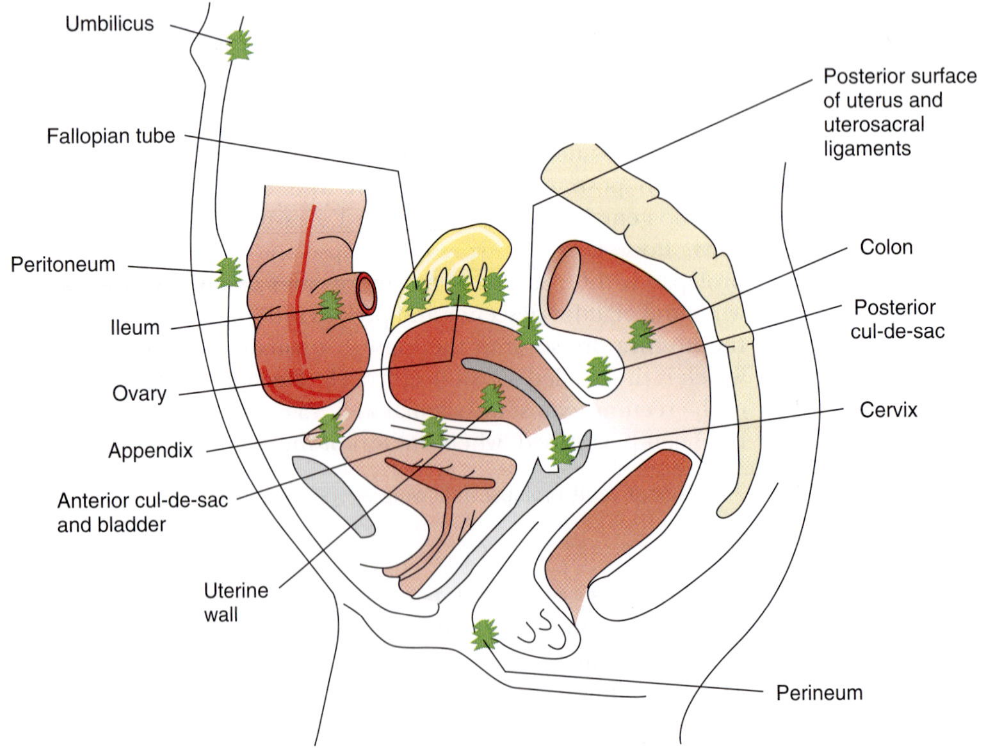

Figure 11-17. Possible sites for endometriosis implantation.

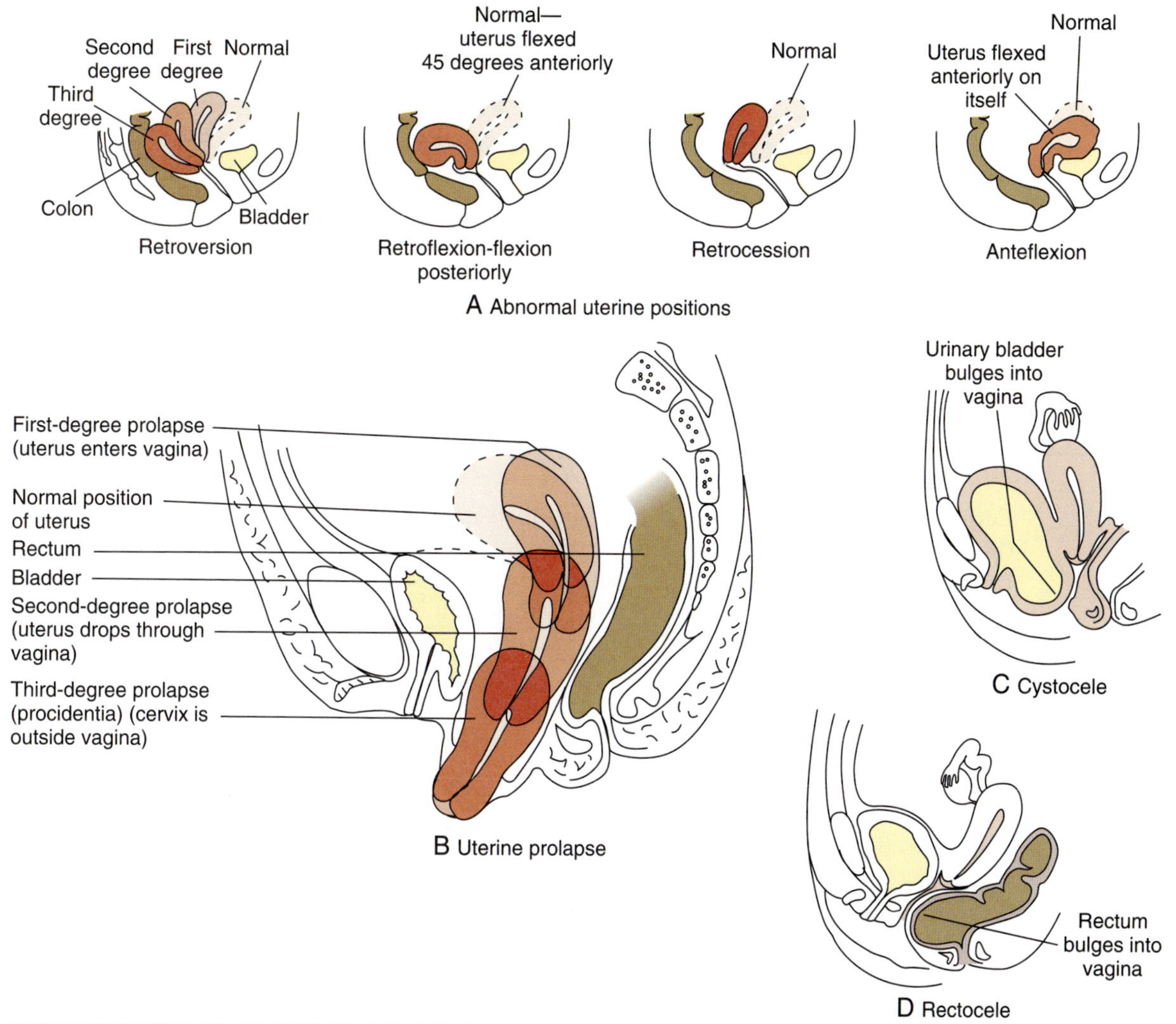

Figure 11-18. Structural abnormalities of the uterus.

connective tissues that support these organs is the cause of genital prolapse. It occurs commonly in postmenopausal women who have had children. Other contributing factors include genetics, pelvic surgery, and pressures within the abdomen that would weaken the pelvic floor. Different types of prolapse are usually graded on the basis of severity. **Uterine prolapse** is the descent of the uterus and cervix into the vaginal canal. **Cystocele** occurs when the bladder descends and presses into the wall of the vagina. **Urethrocele** results when the urethra presses into the vagina; it usually is reported in conjunction with a cystocele, which is then called a cystourethrocele. **Rectocele** is the descent of the rectum and pressing of the rectum against the vaginal wall. **Vaginal vault prolapse** may occur after a hysterectomy has been performed, when the top of the vagina descends into the vault.

EXAMPLE Vaginal vault prolapse following a hysterectomy, 618.5.

Fistulas

A **fistula** is an abnormal passage or communication between two internal organs, or leading from an organ to the surface of the body (Figure 11-19). A **urethrovaginal fistula** is an abnormal passage between the urethra and the vagina. The bladder has the potential to communicate with the uterus, vagina, and rectum, forming a **vesicouterine fistula, vesicovaginal fistula**, and/or **rectovesical fistula**, respectively.

EXAMPLE Rectovesicovaginal fistula, 619.1.

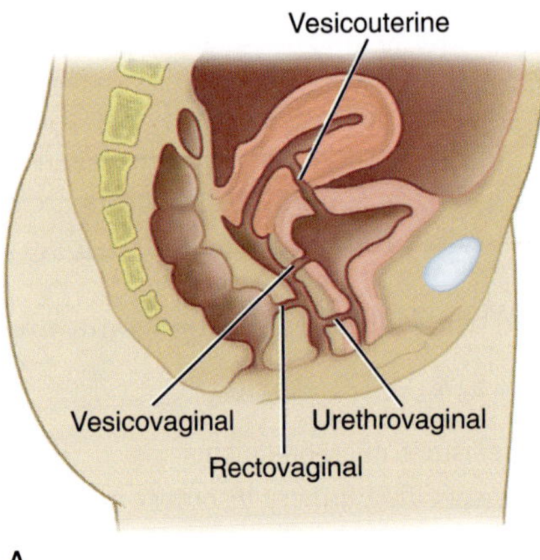

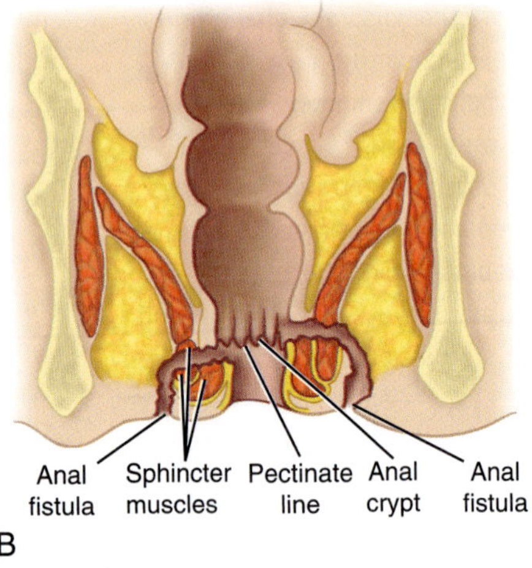

Figure 11-19. Various types of fistulas, designated according to site or to organs with which they communicate. **A,** Genitourinary fistulas. **B,** Anal fistulas.

Urinary Incontinence

Urinary incontinence can be a significant health problem that interferes with a patient's activities of daily living. This problem is more common among women because of specific features of their anatomy and as the result of childbearing. Incontinence often occurs after radical prostatectomy but usually resolves in time.

Types of incontinence include stress, urge, mixed, and overflow incontinence. **Stress incontinence** is the involuntary loss of small amounts of urine due to increased pressure from coughing, sneezing, or laughing. **Urge incontinence** is the sudden and involuntary loss of large amounts of urine. **Mixed incontinence** is a combination of stress and urge incontinence. **Overflow incontinence** is the constant dribbling of urine. Treatments include diet, Kegel exercises, biofeedback, and bladder training.

EXAMPLE Neurogenic bladder with stress incontinence, 596.54, 625.6.

EXERCISE 11-6

Assign codes to the following conditions using your ICD-9-CM code book.

1. Endometriosis of fallopian tube ____________
2. Cystocele with stress incontinence ____________
3. Corpus luteum cyst ____________
4. Chocolate cyst of the ovary ____________
5. Vaginal stenosis ____________

V CODES

In the past, V codes have been considered primarily for use in the outpatient setting. This has changed with the addition of more V codes each year. As was discussed in Chapter 8, it may be difficult to locate V codes in the Index. Coders often say, "I did not know there was a V code for that." Refer to Chapter 8 for a listing of common main terms used to locate V codes.

V codes that may be used with diseases of the genitourinary system include the following:

V09.X	Infection with drug-resistant microorganisms
V13.00	Personal history of unspecified urinary disorder
V13.01	Personal history of urinary calculi
V13.02	Personal history of urinary (tract) infection
V13.03	Personal history of nephrotic syndrome
V13.09	Personal history of other disorder of the urinary system
V13.22	Personal history of cervical dysplasia
V18.61	Family history of polycystic kidney
V18.69	Family history of other kidney disease
V18.7	Family history of other genitourinary diseases
V42.0	Organ or tissue replaced by transplant—kidney
V43.5	Organ or tissue replaced by other means—bladder
V44.50	Artificial opening status—cystostomy, unspecified
V44.51	Artificial opening status—cutaneous vesicostomy
V44.52	Artificial opening status—appendico-vesicostomy
V44.59	Artificial opening status—other cystostomy
V44.6	Artificial opening status—other artificial opening of urinary tract
V44.7	Artificial vagina
V45.11	Renal dialysis status
V45.12	Noncompliance with renal dialysis
V45.71	Acquired absence of organ—breast and nipple
V45.73	Acquired absence of organ—kidney
V45.74	Acquired absence of organ—other parts of urinary tract
V45.77	Acquired absence of organ—genital organs
V45.83	Other postprocedural status—breast implant removal status
V47.4	Other problems of internal organs—other urinary problems
V47.5	Other problems of internal organs—other genital problems
V50.2	Routine or ritual circumcision
V50.41	Prophylactic organ removal—breast
V50.42	Prophylactic organ removal—ovary
V52.4	Fitting and adjustment of breast prosthesis and implant
V53.6	Fitting and adjustment of urinary devices
V55.5	Attention to cystostomy
V55.6	Attention to other artificial opening of urinary tract
V55.7	Attention to artificial vagina
V56.0	Encounter for extracorporeal dialysis
V56.1	Encounter for fitting and adjustment of extracorporeal dialysis catheter
V56.2	Encounter for fitting and adjustment of peritoneal dialysis catheter
V56.31	Encounter for adequacy testing for hemodialysis
V56.32	Encounter for adequacy testing for peritoneal dialysis
V56.8	Encounter for other dialysis
V58.62	Long-term (current) use of antibiotics

V58.76	Aftercare following surgery of the genitourinary system, NEC
V59.4	Donor—kidney
V72.3	Gynecologic examination
V88.01	Acquired absence of both cervix and uterus
V88.02	Acquired absence of uterus with remaining cervical stump
V88.03	Acquired absence of cervix with remaining uterus

EXAMPLE

Adult male is admitted for elective routine circumcision, V50.2, 64.0.

The V code indicates that a procedure is going to be performed, but it is not the procedure code. A diagnosis code is not assigned because no medical condition is present.

EXAMPLE

Urinary tract infection due to methicillin-resistant *Staphylococcus aureus* (MRSA), 599.0, 041.11, V09.0.

The V code that identifies drug resistance can be used only as a secondary diagnosis code.

EXAMPLE

Patient is admitted for kidney donation. A laparoscopic nephrectomy is performed, V59.4, 55.51.

EXERCISE 11-7

Assign codes to the following conditions using your ICD-9-CM code book.

1. Status post kidney transplant ____________
2. Admission for dialysis for ESRD due to diabetic nephropathy. ____________
3. Personal history of kidney stones ____________
4. Family history of polycystic kidney disease ____________
5. Acquired absence of uterus and cervix ____________

COMMON TREATMENTS

CONDITION	MEDICATION/TREATMENT
Glomerulonephritis	If due to infection, antibiotics. Diuretics, antihypertensives, and diet. Serious cases may be treated with corticosteroids and/or Cytoxan.
Acute renal failure	Fluid management and treat the underlying cause. Dialysis, if necessary.
Chronic renal failure	Determine cause. Control blood pressure and diet.
Cystitis	Fluids and possibly antibiotics.
Urethritis	Antibiotics.
Pyelonephritis	Antibiotics.
Calculus of urinary tract	Fluids, pain control, blood pressure control, and antibiotics, if associated infection.
Urinary incontinence	Kegel exercises, biofeedback, and medications such as Detrol.
Prostatitis	Antibiotics.
Benign prostatic hyperplasia	Medications such as tamsulosin hydrochloride (Flomax) and terazosin hydrochloride (Hytrin).
Mastitis	Compresses, massage, fluids, and possibly antibiotics.
PID	Antibiotics.
Endometriosis	Pain medication and/or hormonal therapy.

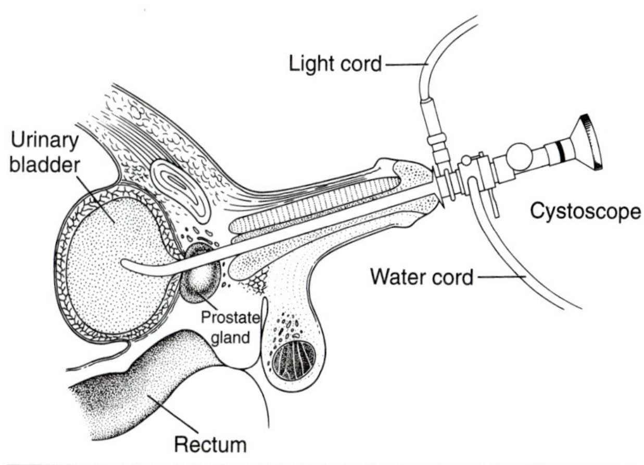

Figure 11-20. Cystoscopy.

PROCEDURES

Procedures that may be related to diseases of the genitourinary system can be located in the following chapters of the Procedure Tabular:

10. Operations of the Urinary System (55-59)
11. Operations on the Male Genital Organs (60-64)
12. Operations on the Female Genital Organs (65-71)
15. Operations on the Integumentary System (85-86)

Cystoscopy may be the approach used for many procedures involving the urinary tract (Figure 11-20). Code 57.32 is assigned for a diagnostic cystoscopy. Often, another diagnostic or therapeutic procedure, such as biopsy, removal of a stone, dilatation of a stricture, or control of hemorrhage, is performed during a cystoscopic examination. When a procedure is performed in addition to cystoscopy, it is not necessary to code the cystoscopy as it is the approach.

EXAMPLE Bladder lesion with transurethral biopsy of the bladder, 596.9, 57.33.

EXAMPLE Cystoscopy with control of hemorrhage of bladder, 596.8, 57.93.

Dialysis

Dialysis is needed when the kidneys can no longer filter the blood and form urine. Two basic types of dialysis are available. **Hemodialysis** uses a machine called a hemodialyzer to remove wastes from the blood (Figure 11-21). Access is obtained through a surgically created internal (arteriovenous [AV]) fistula that allows blood to pass from the body to the machine for cleansing. Sometimes, an AV graft (Figure 11-22) is used for permanent access. If treatment must be begun before permanent access is ready or available, temporary access can be obtained through a catheter. Usually, hemodialysis is conducted at dialysis centers, and it is often scheduled 3 times per week. A dialysis session may take 3 to 5 hours to complete.

If the encounter is for dialysis, a V code is assigned as the principal diagnosis. In cases where the patient is receiving treatment in preparation for dialysis (e.g., creation of an arteriovenous fistula), the principal diagnosis will be the medical condition for which the dialysis is required.

EXAMPLE Patient with ESRD is admitted for hemodialysis, V56.0, 585.6, 39.95.

EXAMPLE Patient with ESRD and hypertension is admitted for creation of an AV fistula. Patient has dialysis on M, W, and F. 403.91, 585.6, V45.1, 39.27.

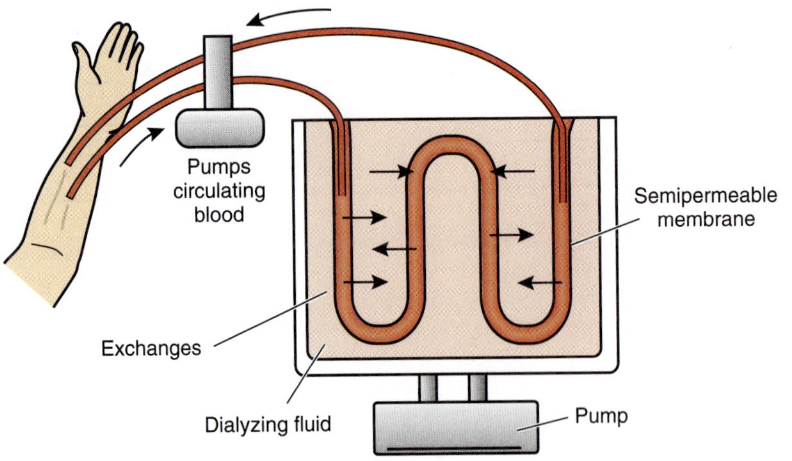

Figure 11-21. Hemodialysis.

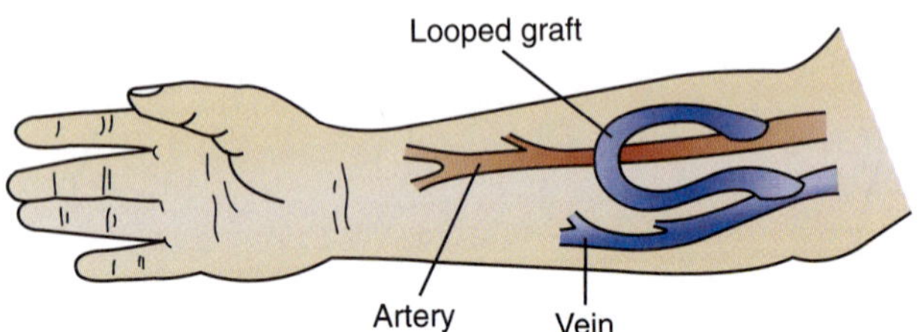

Figure 11-22. Arteriovenous graft for dialysis.

Peritoneal dialysis uses the peritoneal membrane in the patient's own body along with a dialysate solution to filter out wastes and excess fluid (Figure 11-23). Dialyzing fluid passes into the peritoneal cavity through a permanent indwelling peritoneal catheter (Tenckhoff catheter) and is then drained from the peritoneal cavity. **Continuous ambulatory peritoneal dialysis** (CAPD) takes about 15 minutes and is performed 3 to 4 times per day and once at night. **Continuous cycling peritoneal dialysis** (CCPD) uses a cycling machine and is performed while the patient sleeps. In some cases, a combination of the two may be needed to achieve the best results.

EXAMPLE

Patient with end-stage renal failure has peritoneal dialysis while hospitalized for acute prostatitis, 601.0, 585.6, V45.1, 54.98.

Kidney Transplantation

A kidney transplant (Figure 11-24) is one of the most common transplant operations. Prior to performance of a transplant procedure, a thorough pretransplant evaluation is necessary to assess the patient's overall health and identify potential problems to increase the chances of a successful transplant. A couple of different types of kidney transplants may be performed—transplant from a live related donor, transplant from a live nonrelated donor, and transplant from a cadaver. Transplants from a living donor are generally scheduled in advance, and the kidney may be transplanted immediately following removal from the donor.

Patients who are on a waiting list for a kidney are notified when a kidney becomes available that is a good match; they must report to the hospital immediately. The transplanted kidney will usually start making urine as soon as the blood starts to flow through it, and most patients feel much better after their surgery has been completed. In most cases, only one kidney is necessary to take over for two failed kidneys. Most of the time, diseased kidneys are left in place.

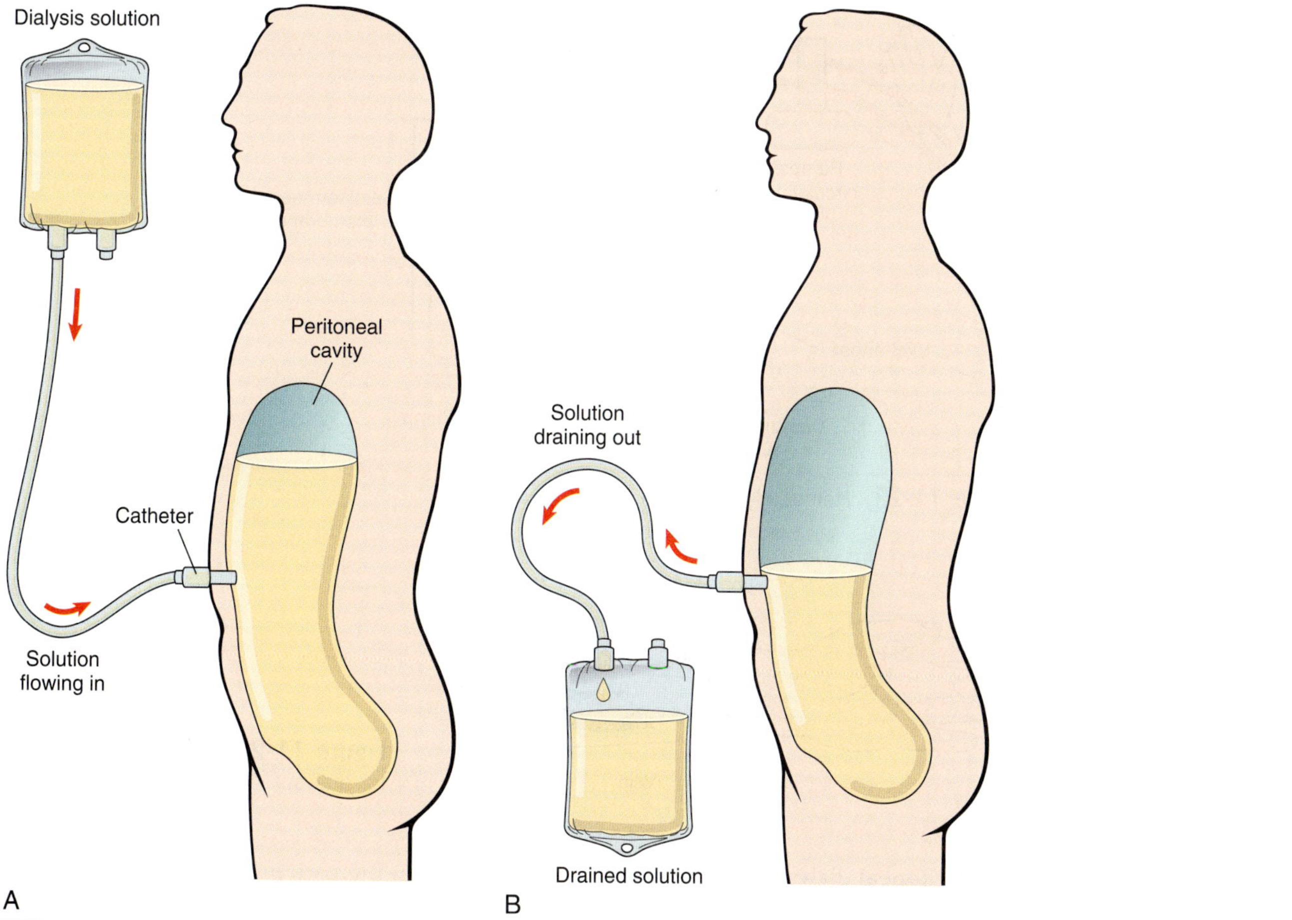

Dialysis solution

Peritoneal cavity

Catheter

Solution flowing in

A

Solution draining out

Drained solution

B

Figure 11-23. Continuous ambulatory peritoneal dialysis. **A,** The dialysis solution (dialysate) flows from a collapsible plastic bag through a Tenckhoff catheter into the patient's peritoneal cavity. The empty bag is folded and inserted into undergarments. **B,** After 4 to 8 hours, the bag is unfolded, and the fluid is allowed to drain into it with the help of gravity. The full bag is discarded, and a new bag of fresh dialysate is attached.

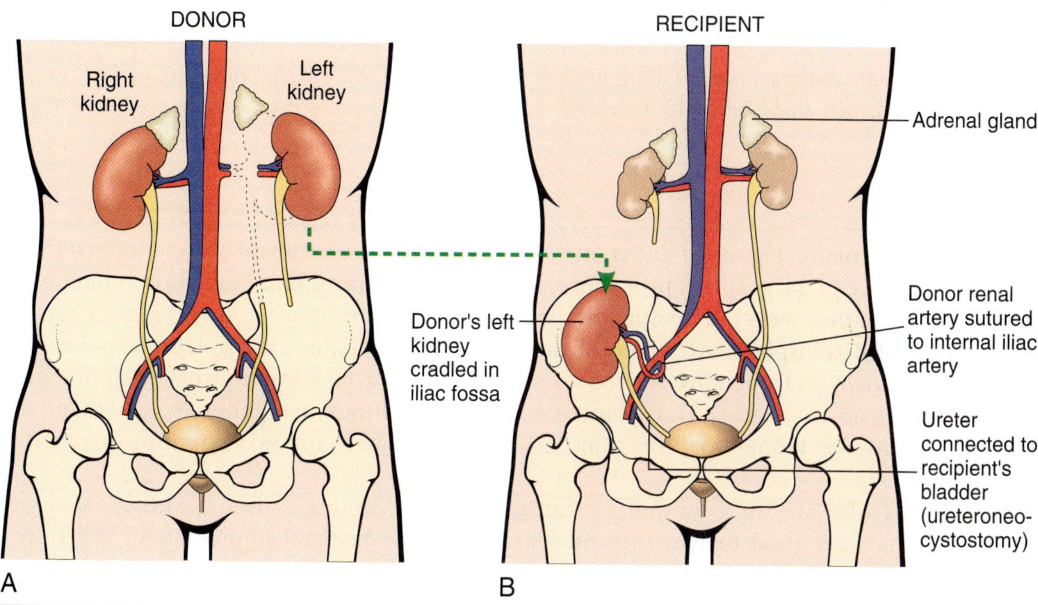

Figure 11-24. Kidney transplantation. **A,** Left kidney of the donor is removed for transplant. **B,** The kidney is transplanted to the right pelvis of the recipient.

Prostate Procedures

Prostate procedures are most often performed for benign prostatic hypertrophy or for prostate cancer. A biopsy is usually performed prior to a prostatectomy. Correct procedural code assignment depends on the method of the procedure performed. When **transurethral resection of the prostate** (TURP) is performed, it is not necessary to code the cystoscopy that is performed in the course of the surgical procedure. Cystoscopy is the approach that is used in transurethral procedures. Transurethral ultrasound-guided laser-induced prostatectomy (TULIP) and visual laser ablation of the prostate (VLAP) are two types of laser treatments used for ablation of prostatic tissue. Transurethral microwave thermotherapy (TUMT) and transurethral needle ablation (TUNA) of the prostate use radiofrequency energy to ablate obstructive prostatic tissue; these procedures can be performed in the physician's office.

EXAMPLE

Cancer of the prostate with radical prostatectomy with bilateral regional lymphadenectomy, 185, 60.5, 40.3.

EXAMPLE

Benign prostatic hypertrophy with urinary obstruction. Transurethral ultrasound-guided laser-induced prostatectomy, 600.01, 599.69, 60.21.

Breast Biopsies and Reconstruction

Breast biopsies are performed for diagnostic purposes to determine the nature of a breast abnormality or mass. A code is used for open biopsy of the breast and for local excision of a lesion of the breast (lumpectomy). In an open biopsy of the breast, a tissue sample is taken for diagnostic examination. In a local excision of the breast, the entire specimen is removed for pathologic examination. It is important to read the operative note and the pathology report to verify how much of the specimen was removed. Physicians may document an excisional biopsy when a lumpectomy is performed.

Sometimes, a needle or **mammographic localization** is necessary to assist the surgeon in identifying the area of breast tissue that must be biopsied or excised. An additional code would be assigned for the localization. This procedure is often perfomed by a radiologist.

At times, breast biopsy is performed during the same operative episode as a therapeutic procedure or more definitive treatment such as lumpectomy or mastectomy. In these cases, the biopsy is coded in addition to the lumpectomy or the mastectomy. Per Uniform Hospital Discharge Data Set (UHDDS) guidelines for selection of a principal procedure, either lumpectomy or mastectomy would fit the definition of a principal procedure.

Breast reconstructions are often performed following a mastectomy. Reconstruction may be done immediately or as a delayed procedure. The type of reconstruction and the timing of when it is done vary according to the patient's need for radiation and the type of mastectomy that is performed. Reconstruction may also be performed in stages. Implants and tissue expanders are sometimes used to create the breast. Tissue expanders are removed after the skin and muscles have been expanded to accommodate the breast implant or further reconstruction.

Tissue flap procedures use tissue from the abdomen, back, thighs, or buttocks to reconstruct the breast. Several flap procedures are currently used (Figure 11-25); these include the following:

- Transverse rectus abdominis musculocutaneous (TRAM)
- Latissimus dorsi musculocutaneous flap (LDMF)
- Gluteal free flap
- Lateral transverse thigh flap
- Nipple—Areola reconstruction
- Flap and microsurgical procedures

A **pedicle flap** involves a flap that remains attached to its original blood supply and tunneling it under the skin to the breast area. A **free flap** involves the cutting of skin, fat,

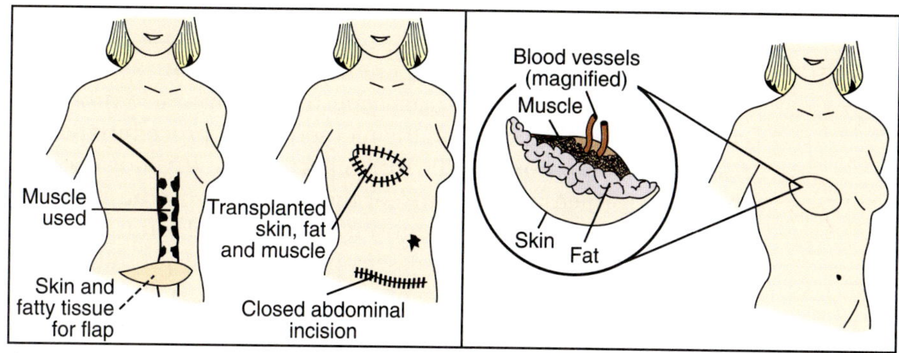

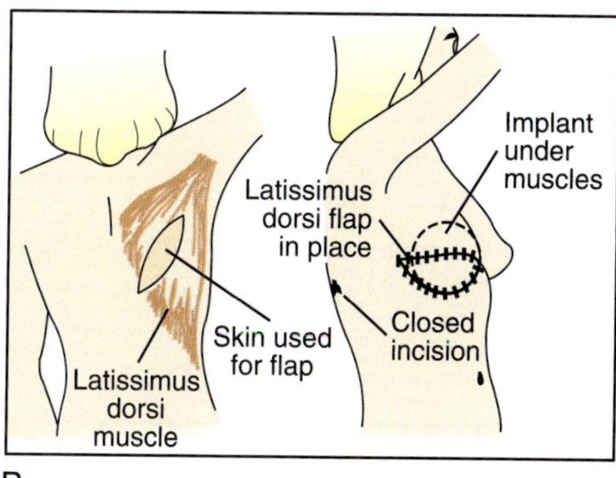

Figure 11-25. Various flaps used for breast reconstruction.

blood vessels, and muscle free from their locations and moving them to the chest area. Blood vessels are connected with the use of a microscope. A free flap takes more time to complete.

EXAMPLE Patient admitted for bilateral breast reduction due to hypertrophy, 611.1, 85.32.

Removal of Stones

Extracorporeal shock wave lithotripsy (ESWL) is used to break up kidney stones into small particles that can then pass through the urinary tract in the urine. Different devices can be used to transmit shock waves, and usually, x-ray or ultrasound is used to reveal the exact location of the stone.

If the stone is quite large, or the location is such that ESWL is not very effective, a **percutaneous nephrolithotomy** is performed. The stone is removed by the surgeon with the use of a nephroscope. At times, an ultrasonic or electrohydraulic probe is used to break up the stone, and the fragments are then removed. A nephrostomy tube may have to remain within the kidney during the postoperative phase.

Ureteroscopic stone removal is necessary when a kidney stone has traveled into one of the ureters. The ureteroscope is inserted through the urethra and bladder and into the ureter until the stone can be removed or is broken into pieces.

EXAMPLE Patient was treated with percutaneous removal of kidney stone with fragmentation, 592.0, 55.04.

EXERCISE 11-8

Assign codes for all diagnosis and procedures using your ICD-9-CM code book.

1. Right solitary renal cyst with right partial laparoscopic nephrectomy ____________
2. Transurethral needle ablation of prostate (TUNA) in patient with benign prostatic hyperplasia ____________
3. Laparoscopically assisted vaginal hysterectomy (LAVH) in patient with endometriosis of the uterus ____________
4. Extracorporeal shock wave lithotripsy bladder stone ____________
5. Bilateral modified radical mastectomy, and breast reconstruction with latissimus dorsi musculocutaneous flap (LDMF) following prophylactic removal due to strong family history of breast cancer ____________
6. Peritoneal dialysis in patient with ESRD and anemia of chronic renal disease ____________
7. Kidney transplant in patient with with hypertensive renal disease and end-stage renal failure The patient's spouse was the donor. ____________
8. Left breast cyst with percutaneous breast aspiration ____________

DOCUMENTATION/REIMBURSEMENT/MS-DRGs

Often, coding difficulties are due to lack of documentation. Sometimes pathology and other test results are not available at the time of discharge, or when the physician is dictating the discharge summary or is reporting the final diagnoses.

Definitions and ways a physician uses terms such as "urosepsis" versus "sepsis," and "acute renal insufficiency" versus "acute renal failure" can be problematic and may require a physician query.

Urosepsis Versus Sepsis

EXAMPLE

Urosepsis compared with sepsis as the principal diagnosis

DIAGNOSES	CODES	MS-DRG	RW
Urosepsis	599.0	690	0.8000
Sepsis	038.9 995.91	872	1.3783

MS-DRG With and Without MCC/CC

The presence of a complication and/or comorbidity (CC) can make a difference in reimbursement, depending on the principal diagnosis and the MS-DRG assigned. The code for acute renal failure (584.9) is an MCC, and the code for acute renal insufficiency (593.9) is not an MCC/CC when it is used as a secondary diagnosis.

EXAMPLE

Patient with pneumonia and acute renal failure (ARF) compared with patient with pneumonia and acute renal insufficiency (ARI)

DIAGNOSES	CODES	MS-DRG	RW
Pneumonia with ARF	486,584.9	193	1.2505
Pneumonia with ARI	486,593.9	195	0.8398

CHAPTER REVIEW EXERCISE

Assign codes for all diagnoses and procedures, including all applicable V and E codes and procedures.

1. Pelvic pain due to interstitial cystitis ______
2. Benign hyperplasia of the prostate with urinary obstruction ______
3. Benign prostatic hypertrophy with urinary obstruction and slight hematuria due to TURP. History of renal calculi ______
4. Complete ureterovaginal prolapse ______
5. Prerenal azotemia ______
6. Vesicoureteral reflux ______
7. Menometrorrhagia with chronic blood loss anemia ______
8. Infertility due to tubal endometriosis ______
9. Hematuria with diagnostic cystoscope performed ______
10. Acute tubular necrosis in patient with labile hypertension ______
11. Berger's disease ______
12. Rectovesical fistula ______
13. Chronic glomerulonephritis due to amyloidosis ______
14. Multinodular prostate ______
15. Infertility due to azoospermia ______
16. Incision and drainage of Bartholin's abscess ______
17. Total abdominal hysterectomy with right salpingo-oophorectomy for symptomatic uterine fibroids and follicular cyst right ovary. Family history of cervical cancer ______
18. Infertility due to dysmucorrhea ______
19. Urethroscrotal fistula ______
20. Nonfunctioning kidney with laparoscopic nephrectomy ______
21. Postmenopausal bleeding. Diagnostic dilatation and curettage of uterus (D&C) ______
22. Hematuria due to traumatic injury from indwelling genitourinary catheterization for urinary retention in the ER ______
23. Descensus of uterus ______
24. Ureteral stent was placed due to obstruction from kidney stone ______
25. Bilateral laparoscopic oophorectomy with salpingectomy due to polycystic ovarian syndrome ______
26. Which MS-DRG is reimbursed at a higher rate: MS-DRG 690 or MS-DRG 872? ______

Write the correct answer(s) in the space(s) provided.

27. Define fistula.

______

28. Pyelonephritis involves what organ?

______

29. Describe the main difference in the female and male genitourinary tract.

______

30. Define ARF.

______

CHAPTER GLOSSARY

Acute renal failure: sudden and severe impairment of renal function characterized by oliguria, increased serum urea, and acidosis.

Benign prostatic hyperplasia: condition resulting in enlargement of the prostate gland; usually occurs in men older than 50 years of age.

Benign prostatic hypertrophy: condition resulting in enlargement of the prostate gland; usually occurs in men older than 50 years of age.

Calculus: a stone. Calculi, which vary in size, can develop anywhere in the urinary tract.

Continuous ambulatory peritoneal dialysis: type of peritoneal dialysis that takes about 15 minutes and is performed 3 to 4 times per day and once at night.

Continuous cycling peritoneal dialysis: type of peritoneal dialysis that uses a cycling machine and is performed while the patient sleeps.

Cystitis: lower tract infection that affects the bladder.

Cystocele: when the bladder descends and presses into the wall of the vagina.

Cystoscopy: approach used for many procedures of the urinary tract.

Cystourethrocele: a urethrocele in conjunction with a cystocele.

Endometriosis: chronic condition in which endometrial material, the tissue that lines the inside of the uterus, grows outside the uterus and attaches to other organs in the pelvic cavity

Endometritis: inflammation of the uterus.

Extracorporeal shock wave lithotripsy: used to break up kidney stones into small particles that can then pass through the urinary tract into the urine.

Fistula: abnormal passage or communication between two internal organs, or leading from an organ to the surface of the body.

Free flap: involves the cutting of skin, fat, blood vessels, and muscle free from its location and moving it to the chest area.

Genital prolapse: when pelvic organs such as the uterus, bladder, and rectum shift from their normal anatomic positions and protrude into the vagina or press against the wall of the vagina.

Glomerulonephritis: inflammation of the glomeruli of the kidneys.

Hematuria: the presence of blood in the urine.

Hemodialysis: process that uses a machine called a hemodialyzer to remove wastes from the blood.

Hydronephrosis: abnormal dilatation of the renal pelvis caused by pressure from urine that cannot flow past an obstruction in the urinary tract.

Hydroureter: accumulation of urine in the ureters.

Lactation: the secretion of milk from mammary glands.

Mammographic localization: procedure that may be necessary to assist the surgeon in identifying the area of breast tissue that must be biopsied or excised.

Mastitis: inflammation or infection of the breast.

Mixed incontinence: combination of stress and urge incontinence.

Nephrolithiasis: kidney stone.

Nephrotic syndrome: condition marked by proteinuria (protein in the urine), low levels of protein in the blood, hypercholesterolemia, and swelling of the eyes, feet, and hands.

Oophoritis: inflammation of the ovaries.

Overflow incontinence: the constant dribbling of urine.

Pedicle flap: involves identifying a flap that remains attached to its original blood supply and tunneling it under the skin to a particular area such as the breast.

Pelvic inflammatory disease: when vaginal or cervical infections spread and involve the uterus, fallopian tubes, ovaries, and surrounding tissues.

Percutaneous nephrolithotomy: procedure in which the surgeon uses a nephroscope to remove a stone. At times, an ultrasonic or electrohydraulic probe is used to break up the stone, and the fragments are then removed.

Peritoneal dialysis: when the peritoneal membrane in the patient's own body is used with a dialysate solution to filter out the wastes and excess fluids.

Prostatitis: inflammation of the prostate that can be acute and/or chronic in nature and is due to a bacterium or inflammation that is not caused by a bacterial infection.

Proteinuria: protein in urine.

Pyelonephritis: upper tract infection that involves the kidneys.

Rectocele: descent of the rectum and pressing of the rectum against the vaginal wall.

Rectovesical fistula: a communication between the bladder and the rectum.

Renal colic: intense pain associated with the body's efforts to try to force the stone through the ureters.

Salpingitis: inflammation of the fallopian tubes, which are the most common site of pelvic inflammation.

Stress incontinence: involuntary loss of small amounts of urine due to increased pressure resulting from coughing, sneezing, or laughing.

Transurethral resection of the prostate: endoscopic removal of prostate tissue.

Ureterolithiasis: ureter stone.

Urethritis: infection of the urethra.

Urethrocele: when the urethra presses into the vagina.

Urethrovaginal fistula: abnormal passage between the urethra and the vagina.

Urge incontinence: sudden and involuntary loss of large amounts of urine.

Urinary tract infection: general term used to describe infection in any area of the urinary tract.

Urolithiasis: a stone in the urinary tract.

Uterine prolapse: descent of the uterus and the cervix into the vaginal canal.

Vaginal vault prolapse: condition that may occur following a hysterectomy when the top of the vagina descends.

Vesicouterine fistula: communication between the bladder and the uterus.

Vesicovaginal fistula: communication between the bladder and the vagina.

CHAPTER 12

Endocrine, Nutritional, and Metabolic Diseases, and Immunity Disorders

(ICD-9-CM Chapter 3, Codes 240-279)

CHAPTER OUTLINE

LEARNING OBJECTIVES

- Apply and assign the correct ICD-9-CM codes in accordance with Official Guidelines for Coding and Reporting
- Identify pertinent anatomy and physiology of the endocrine, nutritional, and metabolic diseases and immunity disorders
- Identify endocrine, nutritional, and metabolic diseases and immunity disorders
- Assign the correct V codes and procedure codes related to the endocrine, nutritional, and metabolic diseases and immunity disorders
- Identify common treatments, medications, laboratory values, and diagnostic tests
- Explain the importance of documentation in relation to MS-DRGs for reimbursement

ABBREVIATIONS

AIDS acquired immunodeficiency syndrome
BMI body mass index
BPD biliopancreatic diversion
CC complication/comorbidity
CDC Centers for Disease Control and Prevention
CF cystic fibrosis
DI diabetes insipidus
DM diabetes mellitus
hGH human growth hormone
IDC-9-CM *International Classification of Diseases, 9th Revision, Clinical Modification*
IDDM insulin-dependent diabetes mellitus
IV intravenous
MEN multiple endocrine neoplasia
MS-DRG Medicare Severity diagnosis-related group
NIDDM non–insulin-dependent diabetes mellitus
OIG Office of the Inspector General
PKU phenylketonuria
SCID severe combined immunodeficiency
SIADH syndrome of inappropriate antidiuretic hormone secretion
TPN total parenteral nutrition
TSH thyroid-stimulating hormone
UTI urinary tract infection
VBG vertical banded gastroplasty

ICD-9-CM Official Guidelines for Coding and Reporting

Please refer to the companion Evolve website for the most current guidelines

3. Chapter 3: Endocrine, Nutritional, and Metabolic Diseases and Immunity Disorders (240-279)

a. Diabetes mellitus

Codes under category 250, Diabetes mellitus, identify complications/manifestations associated with diabetes mellitus. A fifth-digit is required for all category 250 codes to identify the type of diabetes mellitus and whether the diabetes is controlled or uncontrolled.

1) Fifth-digits for category 250:

The following are the fifth-digits for the codes under category 250:
0 type II or unspecified type, not stated as uncontrolled
1 type I, [juvenile type], not stated as uncontrolled
2 type II or unspecified type, uncontrolled
3 type I, [juvenile type], uncontrolled

The age of a patient is not the sole determining factor, though most type I diabetics develop the condition before reaching puberty. For this reason type I diabetes mellitus is also referred to as juvenile diabetes.

EXAMPLE Juvenile diabetes, 250.01.

EXAMPLE The patient is a 16-year-old with obesity and diabetes mellitus, type 2, uncontrolled, 250.02, 278.00.

2) Type of diabetes mellitus not documented

If the type of diabetes mellitus is not documented in the medical record the default is type II.

EXAMPLE The patient takes daily insulin for diabetes, 250.00, V58.67.

3) Diabetes mellitus and the use of insulin

All type I diabetics must use insulin to replace what their bodies do not produce. However, the use of insulin does not mean that a patient is a type I diabetic. Some patients with type II diabetes mellitus are unable to control their blood sugar through diet and oral medication alone and do require insulin. If the documentation in a medical record does not indicate the type of diabetes but does indicate that the patient uses insulin, the appropriate fifth-digit for type II must be used. For type II

patients who routinely use insulin, code V58.67, Long-term (current) use of insulin, should also be assigned to indicate that the patient uses insulin. Code V58.67 should not be assigned if insulin is given temporarily to bring a type II patient's blood sugar under control during an encounter.

EXAMPLE

A patient with type II diabetes has been undergoing changes to daily insulin dosages. The patient's diabetes is uncontrolled, 250.02, V58.67.

4) Assigning and sequencing diabetes codes and associated conditions

When assigning codes for diabetes and its associated conditions, the code(s) from category 250 must be sequenced before the codes for the associated conditions. The diabetes codes and the secondary codes that correspond to them are paired codes that follow the etiology/manifestation convention of the classification. *(See Section I. A.6., Etiology/manifestation convention).* Assign as many codes from category 250 as needed to identify all of the associated conditions that the patient has. The corresponding secondary codes are listed under each of the diabetes codes (Figure 12-1).

● **250.4 Diabetes with renal manifestations**

Use additional code to identify manifestation, as:
chronic kidney disease (585.1–585.9) diabetic:
nephropathy NOS (583.81)
nephrosis (581.81)
intercapillary glomerulosclerosis (581.81)
Kimmelstiel-Wilson syndrome (581.81)

● **250.5 Diabetes with ophthalmic manifestations**

Use additional code to identify manifestation, as:
diabetic:
blindness (369.00–369.9)
cataract (366.41)
glaucoma (365.44)
macular edema (362.07)
retinal edema (362.07)
retinopathy (362.01–362.07)

● **250.6 Diabetes with neurological manifestations**

Use additional code to identify manifestation, as:
diabetic:
amyotrophy (358.1)
gastroparalysis (536.3)
gastroparesis (536.3)
mononeuropathy (354.0–355.9)
neurogenic arthropathy (713.5)
peripheral autonomic neuropathy (337.1)
polyneuropathy (357.2)

● **250.7 Diabetes with peripheral circulatory disorders**

Use additional code to identify manifestation, as:
diabetic:
gangrene (785.4)
peripheral angiopathy (443.81)

● ❑ **250.8 Diabetes with other specified manifestations**

Diabetic hypoglycemia
Hypoglycemic shock

Use additional code to identify manifestation, as:
any associated ulceration (707.10–707.9)
diabetic bone changes (731.8)

Use additional E code to identify cause, if drug-induced

Figure 12-1. Tabular entry for diabetes mellitus.

EXAMPLE

The patient was admitted for care of a diabetic foot ulcer. The patient also had chronic kidney disease due to diabetes, 250.80, 707.15, 250.40, 585.9.

(a) **Diabetic retinopathy/diabetic macular edema**
Diabetic macular edema, code 362.07, is only present with diabetic retinopathy. Another code from subcategory 362.0, Diabetic retinopathy, must be used with code 362.07. Codes under subcategory 362.0 are diabetes manifestation codes, so they must be used following the appropriate diabetes code.

5) **Diabetes mellitus in pregnancy and gestational diabetes**
(a) For diabetes mellitus complicating pregnancy, see Section I.C.11.f., Diabetes mellitus in pregnancy.
(b) For gestational diabetes, see Section I.C.11.g., Gestational diabetes.

6) **Insulin pump malfunction**
(a) **Underdose of insulin due to insulin pump failure**
An underdose of insulin due to an insulin pump failure should be assigned 996.57, Mechanical complication due to insulin pump, as the principal or first listed code, followed by the appropriate diabetes mellitus code based on documentation.
(b) **Overdose of insulin due to insulin pump failure**
The principal or first listed code for an encounter due to an insulin pump malfunction resulting in an overdose of insulin, should also be 996.57, Mechanical complication due to insulin pump, followed by code 962.3, Poisoning by insulins and antidiabetic agents, and the appropriate diabetes mellitus code based on documentation.

Apply the General Coding Guidelines as found in Chapter 5.

ANATOMY AND PHYSIOLOGY

The **endocrine system** (Figure 12-2) works with the nervous system to maintain body functions, homeostasis and to respond to stress. The **endocrine system** is composed of many glands that are located throughout the body. These glands secrete **hormones** that can regulate bodily functions such as urinary output, cellular metabolic rate, growth, and development.

Major endocrine glands include the following:

- Anterior pituitary
- Posterior pituitary
- Thyroid
- Parathyroid
- Adrenal cortex
- Adrenal medulla
- Pancreas
- Ovaries
- Testes
- Thymus
- Pineal gland

See Table 12-1 for a listing of the glands, corresponding hormones, and expected hormonal response.

Endocrine diseases may result from an abnormal decrease or increase in hormone production. Changes in the size of a gland can alter hormone production. If the gland becomes larger, this is called **hyperplasia** and/or **hypertrophy**. If the gland becomes smaller, this is called **hypoplasia** and/or **atrophy**. Infection, inflammation, radiation, trauma, and surgical procedures can produce changes in the gland and hormonal dysfunction.

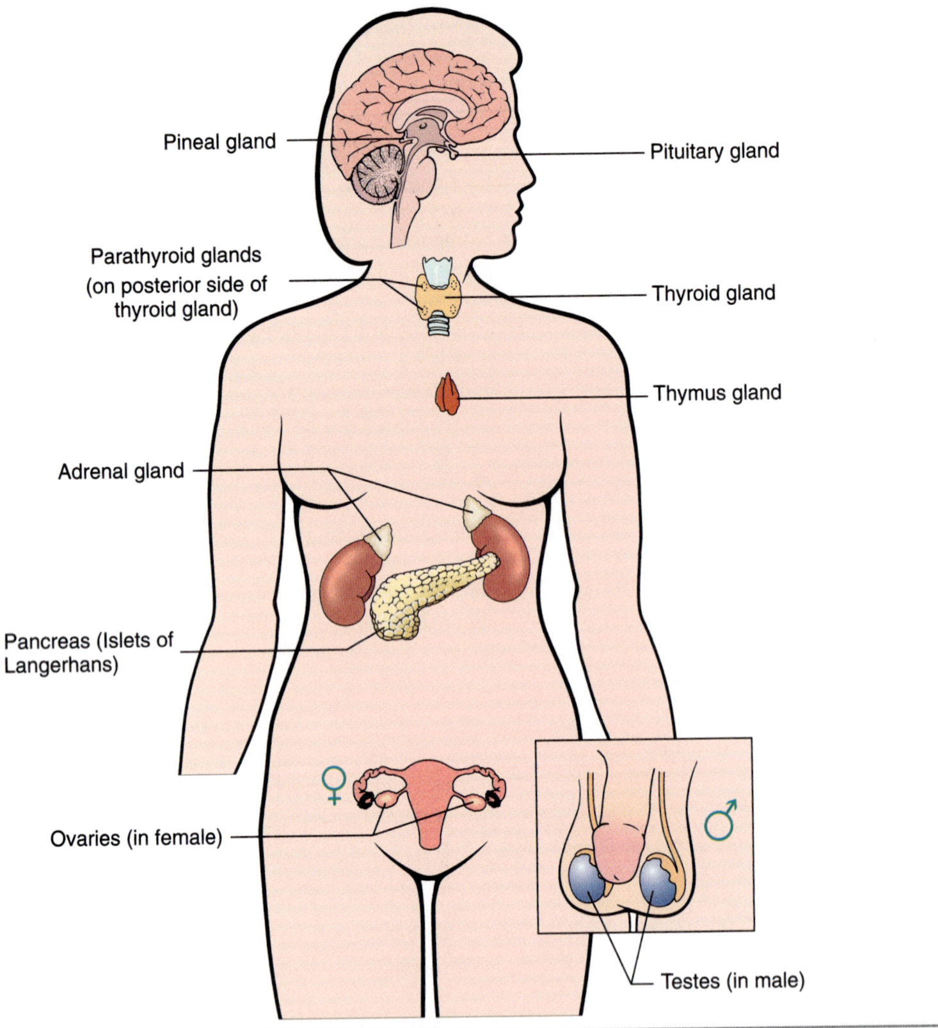

Figure 12-2. The endocrine system.

Some common mental and physical symptoms include the following:

- Growth abnormalities
- Emotional disturbances
- Skin, hair, and nail changes
- Edema
- Hypertension or hypotension
- Cardiac arrhythmias
- Changes in urine output
- Muscle weakness or atrophy
- Menstrual irregularities
- Impotence
- Changes in libido
- Infertility
- Fatigue

Table 12-1. Major Endocrine Gland Secretions and Functions[1]

Endocrine Gland	Hormone	Target Action
Anterior pituitary	Growth hormone (GH)	Promotes bone and tissue growth
	Thyrotropin (thyroid-stimulating hormone [TSH])	Stimulates thyroid gland and production of thyroxine
	Corticotropin (adrenocorticotropic hormone [ACTH])	Stimulates adrenal cortex to produce glucocorticoids
	Gonadotropin	
	Follicle-stimulating hormone (FSH)	Initiates growth of eggs in ovaries; stimulates spermatogenesis in testes
	Luteinizing hormone (LH)	Causes ovulation; stimulates ovaries to produce estrogen and progesterone; stimulates testosterone production
	Prolactin	Stimulates breast development and formation of milk during pregnancy and after delivery
	Melanocyte-stimulating hormone (MSH)	Regulates skin pigmentation
Posterior pituitary	Vasopressin (antidiuretic hormone [ADH])	Stimulates water resorption by renal tubules; has antidiuretic effect
	Oxytocin	Stimulates uterine contractions; stimulates ejection of milk in mammary glands; causes ejection of secretions in male prostate gland
Thyroid	Thyroxine (T_4) and triiodothyronine (T_3)—thyroid hormone (TH)	Regulates rate of cellular metabolism (catabolic phase)
	Calcitonin	Promotes retention of calcium and phosphorus in bone; opposes effect of parathyroid hormone
Parathyroid	Parathyroid hormone (parathormone, PTH)	Regulates metabolism of calcium; elevates serum calcium levels by drawing calcium from bones
Adrenal cortex	Mineralocorticoids (MCs), primarily aldosterone	Promote retention of sodium by kidneys; regulate electrolyte and fluid homeostasis
	Glucocorticoids (GCs): cortisol, corticosterone, cortisone	Regulate metabolism of carbohydrates, proteins, and fats in cells
	Gonadocorticoids: androgens, estrogens, progestins	Govern secondary sex characteristics and masculinization
Adrenal medulla	Catecholamines: epinephrine and norepinephrine	Produce quick-acting "fight or flight" response during stress; increase blood pressure, heart rate, and blood glucose level; dilate bronchioles
Pancreas	Insulin	Regulates metabolism of glucose in body cells; maintains proper blood glucose level
	Glucagon	Increases concentration of glucose in blood by causing conversion of glycogen to glucose
Ovaries	Estrogens	Cause development of female secondary sex characteristics
	Progesterone	Prepares and maintains endometrium for implantation and pregnancy
Testes	Testosterone	Stimulates and promotes growth of male secondary sex characteristics and is essential for erections
Thymus	Thymosin	Promotes development of immune cells (gland atrophies during adulthood)
Pineal gland	Melatonin	Regulates daily patterns of sleep and wakefulness; inhibits hormones that affect ovaries; other functions unknown

DISEASE CONDITIONS

Diseases of the Endocrine, Nutritional and Metabolic Disease, and Immunity Disorders (240-279), Chapter 3 in the ICD-9-CM code book, is divided into the following categories:

CATEGORY	SECTION TITLES
240-246	Disorders of Thyroid Gland
249-259	Diseases of Other Endocrine Glands
260-269	Nutritional Deficiencies
270-279	Other Metabolic and Immunity Disorders

Disorders of Thyroid Gland (240-246)

Goiter

Goiter is an enlargement of the thyroid gland (Figure 12-3). This enlargement may be uniform throughout the gland, or diffuse. Enlargement may also occur in the form of nodules or nodular goiter. A goiter can cause difficulties in swallowing and/or breathing and may or may not be associated with hormonal disturbances. The most common cause is lack of iodine in the diet. Goiters due to iodine deficiency are rare in the United States since the introduction of iodized salt.

EXAMPLE Patient has a multinodular goiter, 241.1.

Hypothyroidism

Hypothyroidism is diminished production of thyroid hormone, manifested by low metabolic rate, tendency toward weight gain, somnolence, and sometimes myxedema. **Myxedema** is a skin and tissue disorder that is usually due to severe prolonged hypothyroidism (Figure 12-4). Symptoms include dull, puffy, yellowed skin; coarse, sparse hair; and periorbital edema and prominent tongue.

EXAMPLE Patient has primary hypothyroidism, 244.9.

Hashimoto's disease is an inflammation of the thyroid gland that often results in hypothyroidism. It is most common in women and individuals who have a family history of

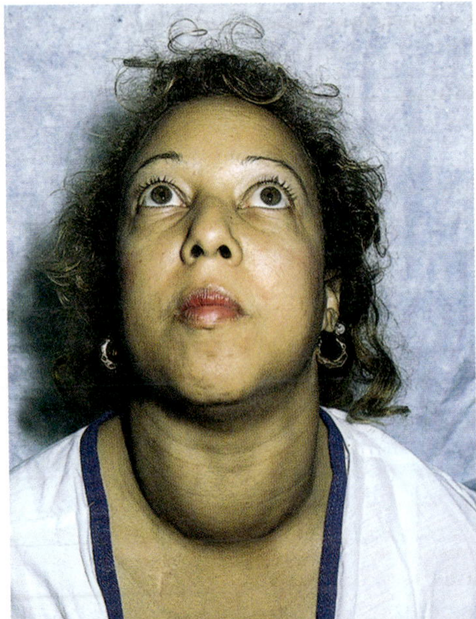

Figure 12-3. Goiter. Note the enlarged neck due to enlargement of the thyroid gland.

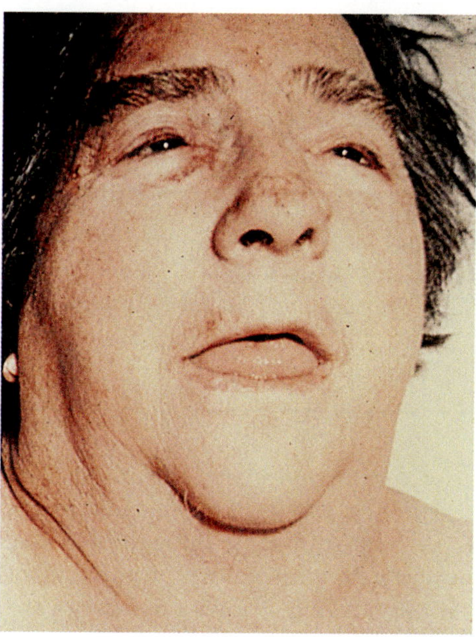

Figure 12-4. Myxedema.

thyroid disease. Onset of Hashimoto's is slow, and it may not be detected for years. The most common signs and symptoms of Hashimoto's disease include the following:

- Intolerance to cold
- Weight gain
- Fatigue
- Constipation
- Goiter
- Dry skin
- Hair loss
- Heavy or irregular menses
- Difficulty with concentration

EXAMPLE

Patient has constipation and fatigue due to autoimmune thyroiditis, 245.2, 564.00 (the fatigue code comes from the symptom chapter).

Hyperthyroidism/Graves' Disease

Hyperthyroidism (Figure 12-5) is an abnormality of the thyroid gland in which secretion of thyroid hormone is usually increased and is no longer under the regulatory control of hypothalamic-pituitary centers.

Graves' disease, the most common form of hyperthyroidism, occurs as the result of an autoimmune response that attacks the thyroid gland, resulting in overproduction of the thyroid hormone thyroxine. Graves' disease is most common among women between 20 and 40 years of age. The most common signs and symptoms include the following:

- Anxiety
- Irritability
- Difficulty sleeping
- Rapid or irregular heartbeat
- Tremor of hands or fingers
- Increased perspiration
- Sensitivity to heat
- Weight loss
- Brittle hair
- Goiter
- Light menstrual periods
- Frequent bowel movements

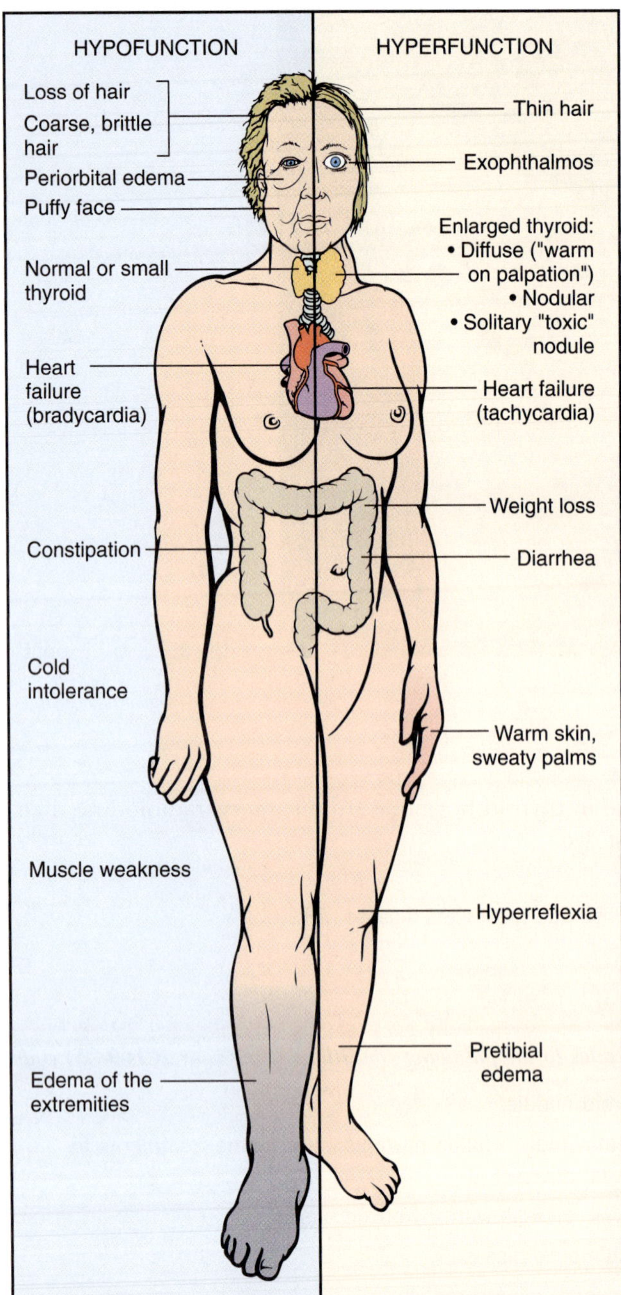

Figure 12-5. Comparison of hyperthyroidism and hypothyroidism.

Graves' ophthalmopathy is also fairly common and may result in **exophthalmos**, or bulging eyes (Figure 12-6). A complication of hyperthyroidism is **thyrotoxic crisis or storm**. This is a sudden intensification of symptoms combined with fever, rapid pulse, and delirium. Medical attention is required when a crisis episode occurs.

Common causes of a thyrotoxic storm or crisis include a medical illness or infection. Other causes include the following:

- Emotional stress
- Diabetic ketoacidosis
- Hypoglycemia
- Cerebrovascular accident
- Pulmonary embolism
- Bowel infarct

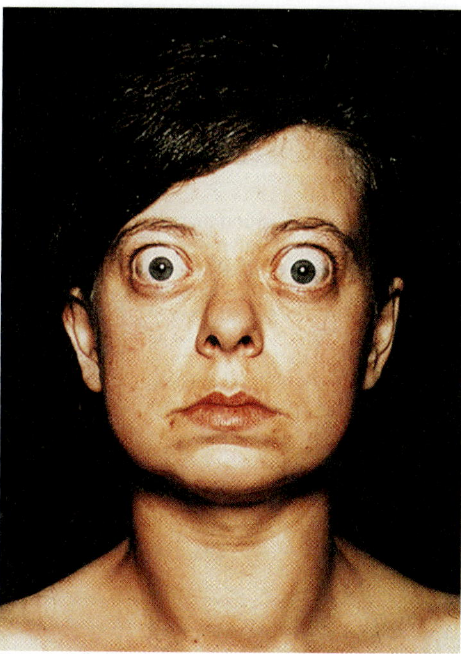

Figure 12-6. Exophthalmos in Graves' disease.

- Trauma
- Increase in thyroid hormone from surgery, radioiodine therapy, or iodinated contrast dye

EXAMPLE Weight loss due to Graves' disease, 242.00.

EXERCISE 12-1

Assign codes to the following conditions using your ICD-9-CM code book.

1. Thyroid nodule ____________
2. Hypothyroidism following radioactive iodine treatments for Graves' disease ____________
3. Graves' disease with thyrotoxic crisis ____________
4. Hashimoto's disease ____________
5. Congenital hypothyroidism ____________

Disorders of Other Endocrine Glands (249-259)

Diabetes Mellitus

Diabetes mellitus is a chronic syndrome of impaired carbohydrate, protein, and fat metabolism caused by insufficient production of insulin by the pancreas or faulty utilization of insulin by the cells. The coding of diabetes mellitus (DM) may be complicated because various manifestations are associated with the disease.

There are two major types of diabetes mellitus: type I and type II. These types vary in origin, pathology, genetics, age of onset, and treatment (Table 12-2). Patients with type I diabetes are insulin dependent; this condition usually develops early in life. The pancreas produces insulin in very small amounts or not at all. Type II diabetes usually is of adult onset. The pancreas continues to produce insulin, but it is not properly metabolized. Occasionally, patients with type II diabetes must be treated with insulin so that acceptable

Table 12-2. Comparison of Type I and Type II Diabetes Mellitus[2]

	Type I	Type II
Features	Usually occurs before age 30	Usually occurs after age 30
Symptoms	Abrupt, rapid onset	Gradual onset; asymptomatic
	Little or no insulin production	Insulin usually present
	Thin or normal body weight at onset	85% are obese
	Ketoacidosis often occurs	Ketoacidosis seldom occurs
	Polyuria (glycosuria promotes loss of water)	Polyuria sometimes seen
	Polydipsia (dehydration causes thirst)	Polydipsia sometimes seen
	Polyphagia (tissue breakdown causes hunger)	Polyphagia sometimes seen
Treatment	Insulin	Diet; oral hypoglycemics or insulin

glucose levels are maintained; the fact that they are taking insulin does not mean that they are dependent on insulin, or that they have type I diabetes. Type II diabetes is much more common than type I; 90% to 95% of diabetic patients have type II diabetes. Type II diabetes in adolescents and children is a relatively new phenomenon, and statistics are still being collected. Sometimes, diabetes is documented as insulin-dependent diabetes mellitus (IDDM) or non–insulin-dependent diabetes mellitus (NIDDM). Documentation of insulin dependence does not determine appropriate fifth digit assignment, because a patient with type II diabetes may be on insulin. If only IDDM is documented, and type I or type II is not specified, according to coding guidelines, the appropriate fifth digit code should be assigned for type II diabetes.

According to *Coding Clinic* (1991:3Q:p6),[3] "Two types of complications may occur with diabetes mellitus. One of these is the acute metabolic complication that is part of diabetes itself and does not require an additional code. The other is the late effect or chronic effect that occurs in another body system due to the diabetes and requires a code from the 250.4X to 250.8X series with an additional code for the manifestation" (Figure 12-7).

EXAMPLE

The patient is treated for diabetic ketoacidosis, 250.13.

Acidosis would not be coded as an additional code in a diabetic patient with ketoacidosis, per the Excludes note under code 276.2.

Category 250.0X, Diabetes mellitus without mention of complication, would have no additional diabetic subcategory codes or manifestation codes (i.e., 205.4X, Diabetes with renal manifestation codes) (Figure 12-8).

There are subcategories for metabolic complications that require no additional manifestation code (Figure 12-9). Subcategories are available for the following diabetic complications and manifestations (Figure 12-10).

Subcategory 250.9X is reserved for diabetes with unspecified complication (Figure 12-11). In the inpatient setting, it may be beneficial to query the physician for specific documentation regarding any diabetic complications and/or manifestations.

The appropriate diabetes and manifestation codes as documented in the health record, as well as the correct fifth digits must be assigned. See Figure 12-12 for fifth digit subclassifications for use with category 250.

According to *Coding Clinic* (2002:2Q:p13),[4] the coder must query the physician if diabetes has been documented as "poorly controlled" or "poor control," to verify whether "uncontrolled" is meant, so that the fifth digit can be assigned. There may be conflicting information regarding which diabetes code should be used for a patient with uncontrolled diabetes, type I or type II. According to *Coding Clinic* (1997:4Q:p33),[5] the correct code for a patient with uncontrolled diabetes mellitus, adult-onset type, requiring insulin is 250.02.

It is possible for a diabetic patient to have more than one complication and/or manifestation of diabetes, so it is necessary for the coder to use as many codes as necessary to

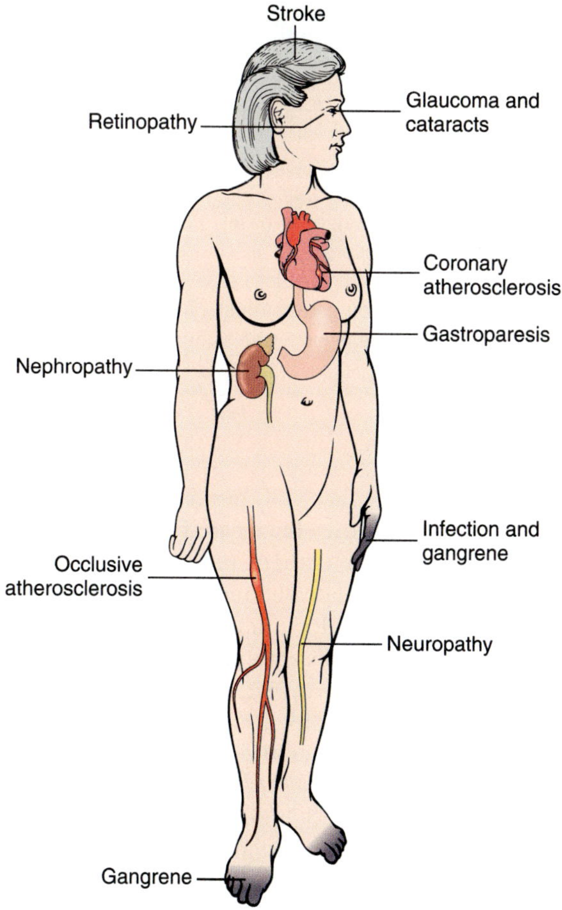

Figure 12-7. Possible manifestations/complication of diabetes mellitus.

● **250.0 Diabetes mellitus without mention of complication**
Diabetes mellitus without mention of complication
or manifestation classifiable to 250.1–250.9
Diabetes (mellitus) NOS

Figure 12-8. Diabetes mellitus without complications.

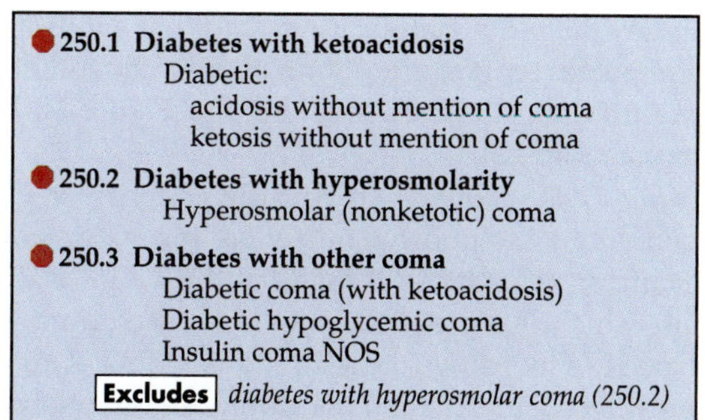

● **250.1 Diabetes with ketoacidosis**
Diabetic:
acidosis without mention of coma
ketosis without mention of coma

● **250.2 Diabetes with hyperosmolarity**
Hyperosmolar (nonketotic) coma

● **250.3 Diabetes with other coma**
Diabetic coma (with ketoacidosis)
Diabetic hypoglycemic coma
Insulin coma NOS
Excludes *diabetes with hyperosmolar coma (250.2)*

Figure 12-9. Diabetes with metabolic complication subcategories.

● 250.4 **Diabetes with renal manifestations**

Use additional code to identify manifestation, as:
chronic kidney disease (585.1–585.9) diabetic:
nephropathy NOS (583.81)
nephrosis (581.81)
intercapillary glomerulosclerosis (581.81)
Kimmelstiel-Wilson syndrome (581.81)

● 250.5 **Diabetes with ophthalmic manifestations**

Use additional code to identify manifestation, as:
diabetic:
blindness (369.00–369.9)
cataract (366.41)
glaucoma (365.44)
macular edema (362.07)
retinal edema (362.07)
retinopathy (362.01–362.07)

● 250.6 **Diabetes with neurological manifestations**

Use additional code to identify manifestation, as:
diabetic:
amyotrophy (358.1)
gastroparalysis (536.3)
gastroparesis (536.3)
mononeuropathy (354.0–355.9)
neurogenic arthropathy (713.5)
peripheral autonomic neuropathy (337.1)
polyneuropathy (357.2)

● 250.7 **Diabetes with peripheral circulatory disorders**

Use additional code to identify manifestation, as:
diabetic:
gangrene (785.4)
peripheral angiopathy (443.81)

●❑ 250.8 **Diabetes with other specified manifestations**

Diabetic hypoglycemia
Hypoglycemic shock

Use additional code to identify manifestation, as:
any associated ulceration (707.10–707.9)
diabetic bone changes (731.8)

Use additional E code to identify cause, if drug-induced

Figure 12-10. Diabetes with complications/manifestations.

●❑ 250.9 **Diabetes with unspecified complication**

Figure 12-11. Diabetes with unspecified complication.

● 250 **Diabetes mellitus**

Excludes *gestational diabetes (648.8)*
hyperglycemia NOS (790.6)
neonatal diabetes mellitus (775.1)
nonclinical diabetes (790.29)

The following fifth-digit subclassification is for use with category 250:

0 **type II or unspecified type, not stated as uncontrolled**
Fifth-digit 0 is for use for type II patients, even if the patient requires insulin
Use additional code, if applicable, for associated long-term (current) insulin use V58.67

1 **type I [juvenile type], not stated as uncontrolled**

2 **type II or unspecified type, uncontrolled**
Fifth-digit 2 is for use for type II patients, even if the patient requires insulin
Use additional code, if applicable, for associated long-term (current) insulin use V58.67

3 **type I [juvenile type], uncontrolled**

Figure 12-12. Fifth digit subclassification for use with category 250.

Diabetes, diabetic (brittle) (congenital) (familial) (mellitus) (poorly controlled) (severe) (slight) (without complication) 250.0

> Note Use the following fifth-digit subclassification with category 250:
>
> 0 type II or unspecified type, not stated as uncontrolled
>
> Fifth-digit 0 is for use for type II patients, even if the patient requires insulin
>
> 1 type I [juvenile type], not stated as uncontrolled
>
> 2 type II or unspecified type, uncontrolled
>
> Fifth-digit 2 is for use for type II patients, even if the patient requires insulin
>
> 3 type I [juvenile type], uncontrolled

→ with
- coma (with ketoacidosis) 250.3
- hyperosmolar (nonketotic) 250.2
- complication NEC 250.9
- specified NEC 250.8
- gangrene 250.7 *[785.4]*
- hyperosmolarity 250.2
- ketosis, ketoacidosis 250.1
- osteomyelitis 250.8 *[731.8]*
- specified manifestations NEC 250.8

Figure 12-13. Alphabetic index of "Diabetes with ...".

completely describe the patient's diabetic conditions. The 250.4X to 250.8X codes should be sequenced before the associated manifestation codes. It is very important to follow the guidelines with regard to coding and sequencing of manifestation codes.

EXAMPLE A patient is admitted with diabetic gangrene of the left little toe. The toe was amputated. The patient has uncontrolled type I diabetes, 250.73, 785.4, 84.11.

EXAMPLE Patient is admitted with diabetic ketoacidosis. Patient also has diabetic gastroparesis, 250.13, 250.63, 536.3.

Before a diagnosis can be coded as a diabetic manifestation, a direct cause-and-effect relationship must be established. The manifestation must be documented as diabetic or due to diabetes. For a patient who has diabetes and a cataract, diabetic cataract may not be assigned without documentation linking the cataract to the diabetes.

EXAMPLE Patient has diabetes and senile cataracts bilaterally, 250.00, 366.10.

EXAMPLE Patient has cataracts due to diabetes, 250.50, 366.41.

A couple of exceptions to this rule should be noted. See Figure 12-13 for index terms under the main term "Diabetes." Note the term "with" and the selections underneath that term. If a patient has diabetes, and if that patient also has osteomyelitis, a cause-and-effect relationship may be assumed, unless it is documented as unrelated. This is supported by *Coding Clinic* (2004:1Q:p14-15):[6] "If the physician indicates diabetic osteomyelitis, or the

patient has both diabetes and acute osteomyelitis and no other cause of the osteomyelitis is documented, it would be appropriate to assign codes 250.80, Diabetes with other specified manifestations, Type II, or unspecified type, not stated as uncontrolled, 731.8, Other bone involvement in diseases classified elsewhere, and 730.0X, Acute osteomyelitis. ICD-9-CM assumes a relationship between diabetes and osteomyelitis when both conditions are present, unless the physician has indicated in the medical record that the acute osteomyelitis is totally unrelated to the diabetes."

EXAMPLE

Acute osteomyelitis right calcaneus in patient with type I diabetes that is poorly controlled, 250.81, 731.8, 730.07. The physician would have to be queried about whether "poorly controlled" meant "uncontrolled" for assignment of code 250.83.

Hypoglycemia

Hypoglycemia occurs when glucose or blood sugar becomes abnormally low. This is a relatively common occurrence in a diabetic patient. Hypoglycemia can also occur in patients who do not have diabetes mellitus. Normal fasting blood glucose levels range from 70 to 99 mg/dL.

EXAMPLE

Patient with hypoglycemia, 251.2.

EXAMPLE

Patient who has type II diabetes with hypoglycemia, 250.80.

Hyperglycemia

Hyperglycemia occurs when glucose or blood sugar becomes abnormally high. This also is a relatively common occurrence in a diabetic patient. In contrast to hypoglycemia, hyperglycemia is not assigned to a different fourth digit subcategory. Patients who do not have diabetes may have episodes of hyperglycemia. Sometimes, medication such as steroids can cause hyperglycemia.

EXAMPLE

Patient with diabetes and hyperglycemia, 250.00.

EXAMPLE

Patient with hyperglycemia due to long-term use of prednisone taken for rheumatoid arthritis, 790.29, 714.0, V58.65, E932.0.

Secondary Diabetes

Secondary diabetes mellitus is a form of the disease that develops as a result of another disease or condition. Secondary diabetes can be caused by any condition that damages or interferes with the function of the pancreas. Common conditions that may cause secondary diabetes include pancreatitis, tumor of the pancreas, cystic fibrosis, hemochromatosis, acromegaly, Cushing's syndrome, pheochromocytoma, and drug usage (e.g., corticosteroids). If the underlying cause can be successfully treated, insulin production may improve or return to normal.

Recently, new codes for secondary diabetes were introduced, and they are similar to the 250.XX diabetes codes. There are fourth-digit subcategory codes for metabolic complications and manifestations. There are also fifth-digit subclassification codes to indicate whether the secondary diabetes is controlled or not. A fifth digit of 0 stands for "not stated as uncontrolled, or unspecified," and a fifth digit of 1 stands for "uncontrolled."

Steroid-induced diabetes is diabetes that results from the use of steroids. Steroids enhance insulin resistance, making insulin less effective. If the pancreas cannot make enough insulin to keep blood glucose within a normal range and the patient is on steroids, this is steroid-induced diabetes. Steroid-induced diabetes may go away when steroids are discontinued. If the patient has a condition that requires long-term treatment with steroids, diabetes may remain. An episode of steroid-induced diabetes may be an indicator that the patient is at risk for developing diabetes later in life.

EXAMPLE Patient with steroid-induced diabetes due to long-term use of prednisone taken for rheumatoid arthritis. 249.00, 714.0, V58.65, E932.0.

EXAMPLE Diabetes due to partial removal of pancreas 251.3.

Gestational Diabetes

Gestational diabetes is discussed in Chapter 16, Complications of Pregnancy, Childbirth, and the Puerperium.

Hyperpituitarism

Hyperpituitarism results from increased production of pituitary hormones, particularly of human growth hormone (hGH). **Gigantism** or **acromegaly** may occur, depending on the time of life when hormonal dysfunction begins (Figure 12-14).

Gigantism occurs when hypersecretion of hGH occurs before puberty, along with proportionate overgrowth of all body tissues, especially of the long bones. Often, a pituitary adenoma results from oversecretion of hGH. Acromegaly results when hypersecretion of hGH occurs after puberty, along with overgrowth of the face, hands, feet, and soft tissues. Pituitary adenoma is often the cause.

EXAMPLE Patient has hypersecretion of growth hormone, 253.0.

Hypopituitarism

Hypopituitarism is a condition that is caused by low levels of pituitary hormones. Hormones secreted by the pituitary gland may affect the function of other glands. Lack of thyroid-

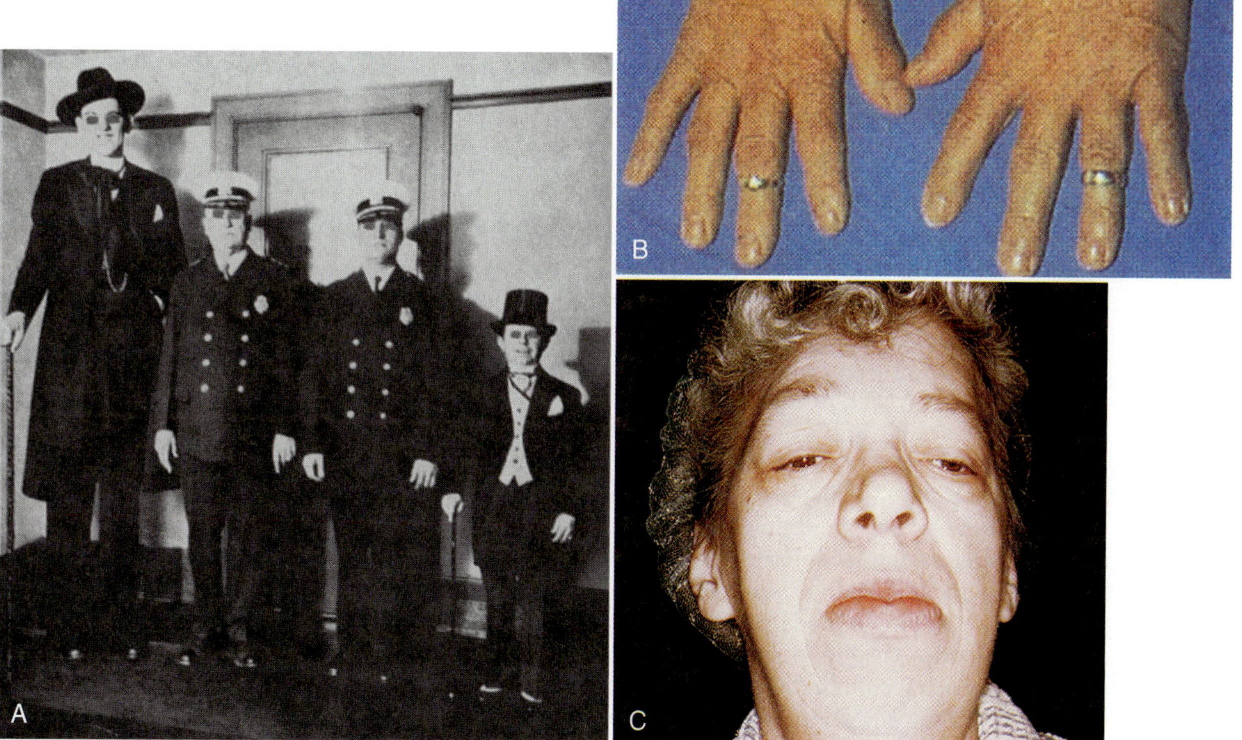

Figure 12-14. Effects of growth hormone. **A,** Comparison of gigantism, normal growth, and dwarfism. **B,** Hands with clinical signs of acromegaly. **C,** Face with clinical signs of acromegaly.

stimulating hormone (TSH) affects the function of the thyroid gland. Hypopituitarism may be caused by a variety of conditions, such as the following:

- Tumor
- Head trauma
- Brain surgery
- Stroke
- Infections of brain

Occasionally, immune system or metabolic disease such as sarcoidosis, histiocytosis X, and hemochromatosis can cause hypopituitarism. The code 253.7 is used to identify hypopituitarism that is hormone induced, hypophysectomy induced, radiotherapy induced, or post ablative in nature.

EXAMPLE The patient has hypopituitarism due to pituitary adenoma, 227.3, 253.2.

EXAMPLE The patient has hypopituitarism due to abscess of the brain, 324.0, 253.2.

Diabetes Insipidus

Diabetes insipidus (DI) or water diabetes is a deficiency in the release of vasopressin by the posterior pituitary gland. The patient excretes volumes of dilute urine and experiences excessive thirst, fatigue, and dehydration. The underlying cause needs to be identified and treated.

Underlying causes of DI include the following:

- Stroke
- Neoplasm
- Polycystic kidney disease
- Neurosurgery

Although DI and DM both include the term *diabetes* in their names, the two conditions are not related.

EXAMPLE The patient suffers from diabetes insipidus, 253.5.

Hyperparathyroidism

Hyperparathyroidism results from an overactive parathyroid gland that secretes excessive parathyroid hormone, causing increased levels of circulating calcium due to loss of calcium in the bone.

Hyperparathyroidism may be primary or secondary. In most cases, primary hyperparathyroidism is caused by a parathyroid adenoma. Secondary hyperparathyroidism is often related to chronic kidney disease.

EXAMPLE The patient was treated for hyperplasia of the parathyroid. The patient was hypercalcemic, 252.01. Note the Excludes note under 725.4, Disorders of calcium metabolism (Figure 12-15). Hypercalcemia or hypocalcemia would not be coded as an additional code with any parathyroid disorder codes (252.00-252.9).

Hypoparathyroidism

Hypoparathyroidism is caused by an underactive parathyroid gland that results in decreased levels of circulating calcium. The primary manifestation is **tetany**, a continuous muscle spasm. Vitamin D and calcium supplements are often used to treat this condition.

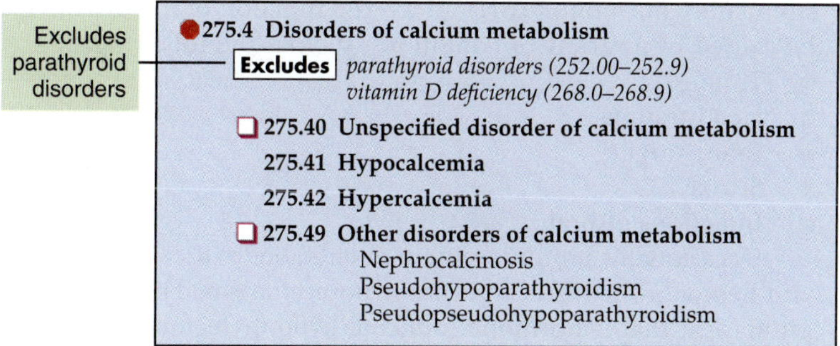

275.4 Disorders of calcium metabolism

Excludes *parathyroid disorders (252.00–252.9)*
vitamin D deficiency (268.0–268.9)

275.40 Unspecified disorder of calcium metabolism

275.41 Hypocalcemia

275.42 Hypercalcemia

275.49 Other disorders of calcium metabolism
Nephrocalcinosis
Pseudohypoparathyroidism
Pseudopseudohypoparathyroidism

Figure 12-15. Disorders of calcium metabolism Excludes note.

EXAMPLE The patient had tetany due to hypoparathyroidism. The patient is hypocalcemic and is treated with calcium supplements, 252.1.

Cushing's Syndrome

Cushing's syndrome is a condition that results in excessive circulating cortisol levels due to chronic hypersecretion of the adrenal cortex. Common signs and symptoms include the following:

- Fatigue
- Muscle weakness
- Changes in body appearance with fat deposits in the scapular and abdominal areas
- Moon face
- Hypertension
- Edema

Other complications include hyperlipidemia, osteoporosis, diabetes, excessive hair growth, amenorrhea, impotence, and psychiatric disturbances (Figure 12-16). The skin becomes thin and bruises easily, and red or purple stretch marks develop.

Administration of glucocorticoids (steroids) to treat other diseases can result in **iatrogenic** (treatment-induced) Cushing's. The patient's appearance may be described as "cushingoid" (Figure 12-16).

EXAMPLE Patient has Cushing's syndrome and hyperlipidemia, 255.0, 272.4.

Addison's Disease

Addison's disease is an adrenocortical insufficiency that may be caused by neoplasms, surgical removal of the adrenal gland, autoimmune processes, tuberculosis, hemorrhage, and/or infection. Addison's is characterized by the following symptoms:

- Hypotension
- Weight loss
- Anorexia
- Weakness
- Bronze skin coloring

Other complications include cardiovascular problems such as irregular pulse, reduced cardiac output, and orthostatic hypotension (Figure 12-17). Emotional disturbances such as depression and anxiety are common. When dehydration and electrolyte imbalances occur, medical attention is required to prevent a life-threatening situation.

EXAMPLE Patient was admitted to the hospital for treatment of dehydration and for prevention of Addison's crisis, 276.51, 255.41.

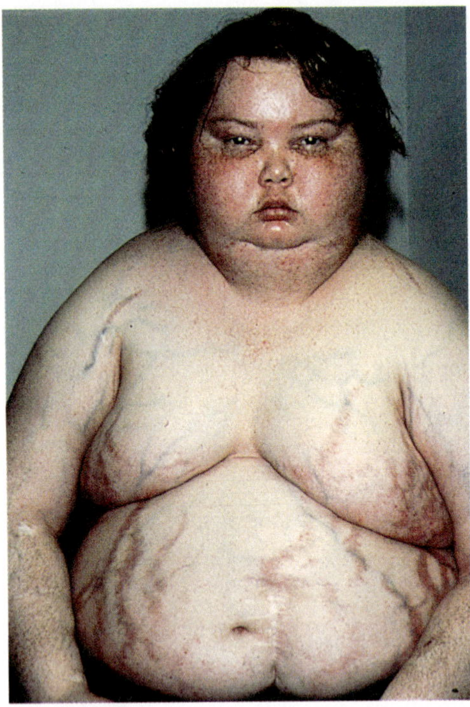

Figure 12-16. Cushingoid features—moon face, obesity, and cutaneous striae.

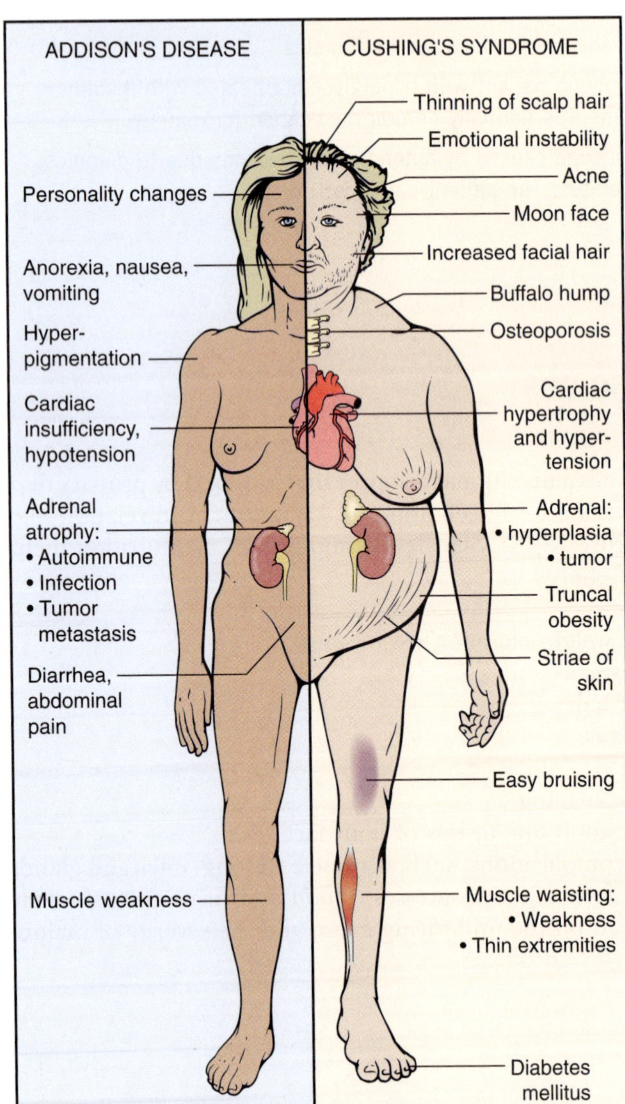

Figure 12-17. Comparison of adrenocortical hyperfunction and hypofunction.

EXERCISE 12-2

Assign codes to the following conditions using your ICD-9-CM code book.

1. Diabetic with episode of hypoglycemia ____________
2. Diabetic retinopathy, DM type II ____________
3. Diabetic hyperosmolar coma ____________
4. Hyperparathyroidism ____________
5. Syndrome of inappropriate antidiuretic hormone secretion (SIADH) ____________
6. Vasopressin deficiency ____________
7. Diabetic gangrene, left big toe ____________
8. Diabetes type II, uncontrolled; Peripheral vascular disease ____________
9. Steroid-induced diabetes; patient has been on long-term steroids for Crohn's disease ____________
10. Multiple endocrine neoplasia, type I ____________
11. Charot's arthropathy right foot due to diabetes, type I uncontrolled ____________
12. Hypoglycemic shock in type I diabetes ____________
13. Overactive bladder due to diabetes ____________
14. Diabetic patient with hyperglycemia treated with insulin. Patient is normally on oral medication for diabetes. ____________
15. Syncope caused by autonomic neuropathy due to diabetes mellitus. The patient has type II diabetes. ____________

Nutritional Deficiencies (260-269)

Malnutrition

Malnutrition is a nutritional disorder that is caused by primary deprivation of protein energy as the result of poverty, self-imposed starvation, or in relation to deficiency diseases such as cancer (Figure 12-18). Signs and symptoms of malnutrition include the following:

- Loss of energy
- Diarrhea
- Drastic weight change (loss or gain)
- Skin lesions
- Loss of hair
- Poor nails
- Edema
- Delayed healing
- Greasy stools due to loss of body fat

Other complications, such as muscle wasting, enlarged glands, and hepatomegaly, may occur as malnutrition progresses. Blood and urine tests show many abnormalities. Treatment is based on the underlying cause and the severity of malnutrition.

EXAMPLE The patient was found to be severely malnourished, 261.

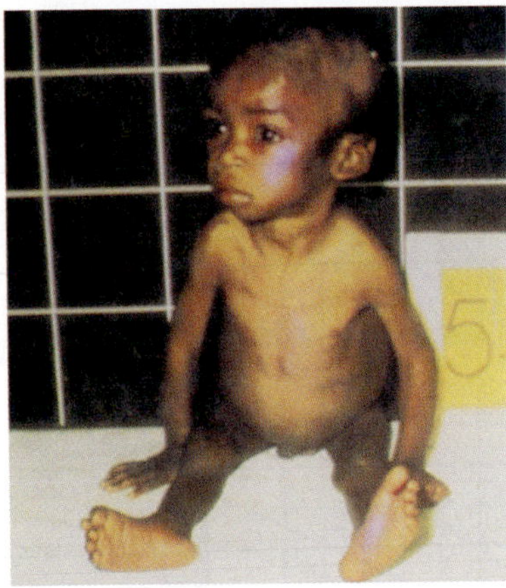

Figure 12-18. Malnourishment.

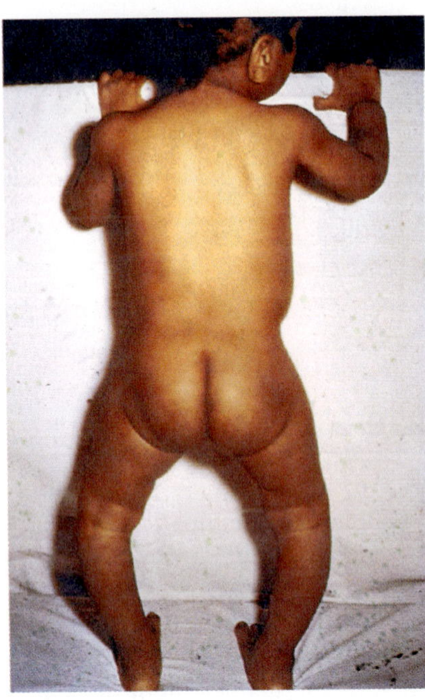

Figure 12-19. Rickets. The bowing of legs in a toddler due to formation of poorly mineralized bones.

Vitamin Deficiencies

Vitamin deficiencies may be caused by many different factors, such as poor nutrient absorption, digestive tract disorders, lifestyle issues (e.g., alcohol, smoking, medications, overexercising), chronic illness, age, and many other factors. Applicable codes are included in the following code categories:

264	Vitamin A deficiency
265	Thiamine and niacin deficiency states
266	Deficiency of B complex components
267	Ascorbic acid deficiency
268	Vitamin D deficiency
269	Other nutritional deficiencies

The deficiency anemias are located in the "Blood and Blood-Forming Organs" chapter. A diagnosis can be stated as a vitamin deficiency, or a specific name may be used for that particular deficiency (Figure 12-19). Another name for vitamin C deficiency is scurvy.

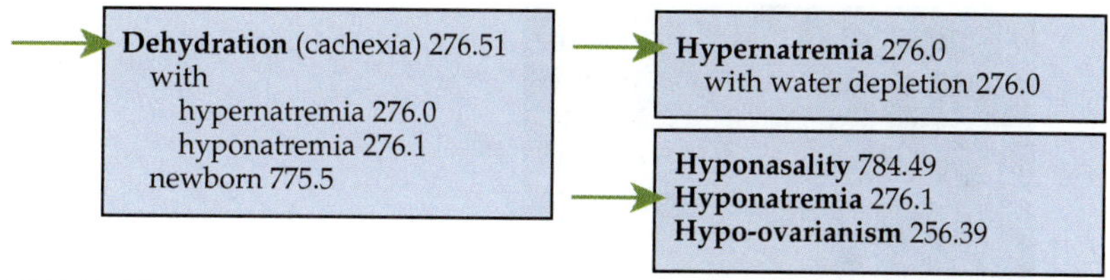

Figure 12-20. Alphabetic Index entries for "dehydration," "hypernatremia," and "hyponatremia."

EXAMPLE Rickets due to vitamin D deficiency, 268.0.

EXERCISE 12-3

Assign codes to the following conditions using your ICD-9-CM code book.

1. Emaciation __________
2. Vitamin B_{12} deficiency __________
3. Night blindness due to vitamin A deficiency __________
4. Severe protein calorie malnutrition __________

Other Metabolic and Immunity Disorders (270-279)

Disorders of Fluid, Electrolyte, and Acid-Base Balance

Category 276 codes are used frequently in the inpatient setting. Occasionally, these codes are assigned for the principal diagnosis, but more often, they are used as secondary diagnoses.

Dehydration occurs frequently as the result of other medical conditions and principal diagnosis selection and sequencing may be confusing. According to the neoplasm guidelines, if an admission occurs for the management of dehydration due to malignancy or therapy for the malignancy, or a combination of both, and only dehydration is being treated, then dehydration is designated as the principal diagnosis, followed by the code(s) for malignancy. According to *Coding Clinic* (2002:3Q:p21-22; 2003:1Q:p22),[7-8] in admissions in which severe dehydration causes acute renal failure, acute renal failure is the principal diagnosis.

Hypernatremia or hyponatremia with dehydration is coded only to the hypernatremia or hyponatremia code; the dehydration code is not assigned. It is clear in the Index under the main term "Dehydration," that hypernatremia/hyponatremia with dehydration requires only one code (Figure 12-20). This is not as clear in the Index under "Hypernatremia" or "Hyponatremia." Hypernatremia includes a subterm "with water depletion." Hyponatremia has no subterm, so if a coder does not look up "Dehydration" the fact that this is a single code assignment could be overlooked.

EXAMPLE Patient was admitted for dehydration and was hypernatremic, with a sodium level of 146, 276.0.

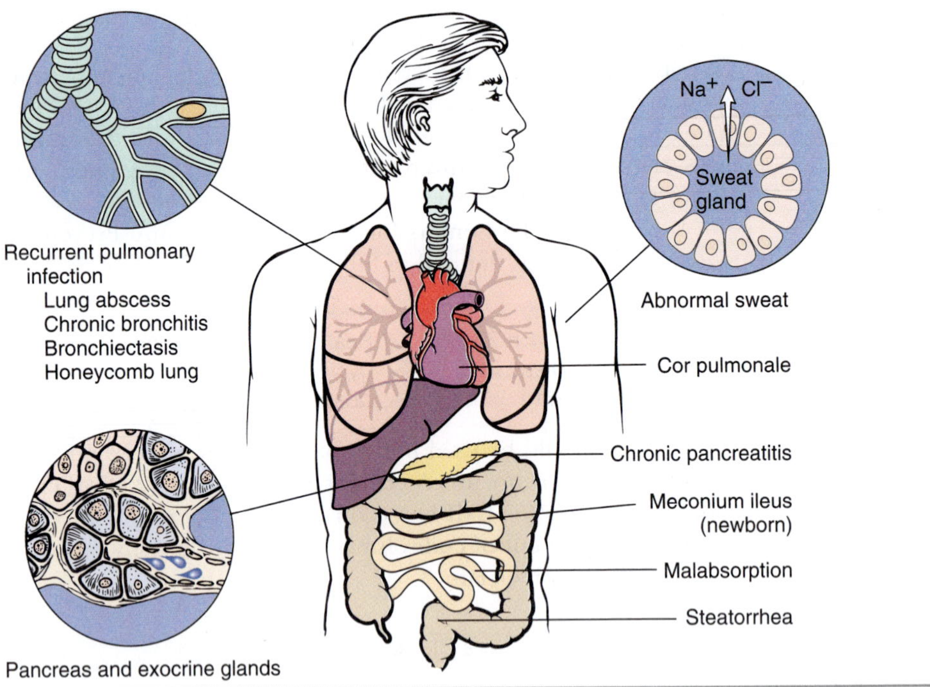

Figure 12-21. Abnormal chloride transport associated with cystic fibrosis affects the secretions of all exocrine glands, especially the pancreas, intestine, and bronchi.

Cystic Fibrosis

Cystic fibrosis (CF) or mucoviscidosis is a **genetic** (inherited) condition that affects the cells that produce mucus, sweat, saliva, and digestive juices (Figure 12-21). Instead of being thin and slippery, these secretions are thick and sticky, plugging up tubes, ducts, and passageways, especially in the pancreas and lungs. No cure is available, and treatment is directed at the complications and manifestations of the disease. The most frequent complications are respiratory infections such as pneumonia, bronchitis, and bronchiectasis. Asthma may also develop. Although the organism *Pseudomonas aeruginosa* does not cause problems in a healthy person, it is a common infective organism in the patient with CF. Presence of *pseudomonas* organism in the patient's sputum does not necessarily indicate that the patient has pneumonia due to *Pseudomonas.*

According to *Coding Clinic* (1990:4Q:p17),[9] when a patient is admitted for a complication of CF, the complication is the principal diagnosis, and CF is a secondary diagnosis. The codes 277.02, cystic fibrosis with pulmonary manifestations, and 277.03, cystic fibrosis with gastrointestinal manifestations, identify the two major systems that are affected by the disease. If the patient has both respiratory and digestive manifestations, both cystic fibrosis codes are used.

EXAMPLE

Patient who suffers from CF is admitted because of acute bronchitis. Patient also has pancreatic insufficiency due to CF, 466.0, 277.02, 277.03.

On occasion, when a patient with CF is admitted primarily for a pulmonary cleanout, in this case, CF is the principal diagnosis.

EXAMPLE

Patient with cystic fibrosis was admitted for pulmonary cleanout, 277.02, 93.99.

Obesity

Obesity is defined as an increase in body weight beyond the limitations of skeletal and physical requirements, as a result of excessive accumulation of fat in the body. In the United States, obesity has reached epidemic proportions, with two thirds of American adults being overweight, and one in three considered obese. **Body mass index** (BMI) uses weight and height to estimate body fat.

According to the Centers for Disease Control and Prevention (CDC), for adults, body mass index (BMI) is defined as follows:

Below 18.5	Underweight
Between 18.5 and 24.9	Healthy weight or normal
Between 25.0 and 29.0	Overweight
30.0 and above	Obese

V codes should be used in combination with overweight and obesity codes to indicate a patient's BMI, if documented. Per *Coding Clinic* (2005:4Q:p96-98),[10] it is acceptable to code the V codes for BMI based on documentation provided in the health record by the dietitian. Assignment of codes for overweight or obesity must be based on documentation provided by the physician.

EXAMPLE Patient is obese with a BMI of 31, 278.00, V85.3.

Morbid obesity is the term that applies to patients who are 100 pounds overweight or over 50% above their ideal body weight. A BMI of 40 or higher defines morbid obesity. Many complications may be related to obesity, including the following:

- Diabetes
- Hypertension
- Heart disease
- Stroke
- Certain cancers such as breast and colon
- Depression
- Osteoarthritis

EXAMPLE Patient is morbidly obese with a BMI of 41 and suffers from DM, 278.01, 250.00, V85.4.

Hypervitaminosis

Hypervitaminosis is toxicity that results from an excess of any vitamin, but especially fat-soluble vitamins such as A, D, and K. If toxicity occurs because of an overdose, a poisoning code would be assigned. Poisonings are discussed in Chapter 20.

EXAMPLE Hypervitaminosis (vitamin D), 278.4.

Immunity Disorders

The **immune system**, the body's major defense mechanism, responds to invasion of the body by foreign substances. The immune system consists of lymphoid tissues such as thymus, bone marrow, tonsils, adenoids, spleen, and appendix. When the immune system malfunctions and homeostasis is interrupted, the response may be classified as one of the following:

- Hyperactive responses (such as allergies)
- Immunodeficiency in which the response is inadequate (such as acquired immunodeficiency syndrome [AIDS])
- Autoimmune disorders in which the immune response is misdirected (such as systemic lupus erythematosus)
- Attacks on beneficial foreign tissues (such as transplants or blood transfusion)

Disorders that are coded in this section include acquired hypogammaglobulinemia, selective immunoglobulin A deficiency, X-linked agammaglobulinemia, severe combined immunodeficiency (SCID), and thymic hypoplasia or DiGeorge's syndrome.

Patients may become immunocompromised by medications; this is seen when patients undergo transplantation and are taking antirejection drugs, or when a patient undergoes chemotherapy treatment for cancer. A patient may also be in an immunocompromised state that is associated with a disease process. According to *Coding Clinic* (1992:3Q:p13-14),[11] an expected side effect for transplant patients or chemotherapy patients is a comprised immune system, and codes should not be assigned for the immunocompromised state. However, if the cause of that state is not identified, code 279.9, Unspecified disorder of immune mechanism, should be assigned.

EXAMPLE Patient has a diagnosis of Wiskott-Aldrich syndrome, 279.12.

EXERCISE 12-4

Assign codes to the following conditions using your ICD-9-CM code book.

1. Hypocalcemia ____________
2. Hypovolemia ____________
3. Alpha 1–antitrypsin deficiency ____________
4. Severe obesity with BMI of 40 ____________
5. Metabolic acidosis ____________

V CODES

In the past, V codes have been considered for use primarily in the outpatient setting. This has changed with the addition of more V codes each year. As was discussed in Chapter 8, it is difficult to locate V codes in the index. Coders will often say, "I did not know there was a V code for that."

Refer to Chapter 8 for a listing of common main terms to locate V codes. V codes that may be used with diseases of the endocrine glands, nutritional and metabolic diseases, and immunity disorders include the following:

V07.4	Hormone replacement therapy (postmenopausal)
V10.87	Personal history of malignant neoplasm—thyroid
V10.88	Personal history of malignant neoplasm—other endocrine glands and related structures
V12.1	Personal history of nutritional deficiency
V12.2	Personal history of endocrine, metabolic, and immunity disorders
V16.8	Family history of other specified malignant neoplasm
V18.0	Family history of diabetes mellitus
V18.11	Family history of multiple endocrine neoplasia [MEN] syndrome
V18.19	Family history of other endocrine and metabolic disease
V42.82	Organ or tissue replaced by transplant—pancreas
V45.86	Bariatric surgery status
V45.79	Acquired absence of organ—other acquired absence of an organ
V45.85	Insulin pump status
V51.0	Encounter for breast reconstruction following mastectomy
V53.91	Fitting and adjustment of insulin pump
V58.67	Long-term (current) use of insulin
V65.3	Dietary surveillance and counseling
V65.46	Encounter for insulin pump training

V76.49	Special screening for malignant neoplasms—other sites
V76.89	Special screening for malignant neoplasms—other neoplasm
V77.0	Special screening for thyroid disorders
V77.1	Special screening for diabetes mellitus
V77.2	Special screening for malnutrition
V77.3	Special screening for phenylketonuria (PKU)
V77.4	Special screening for galactosemia
V77.5	Special screening for gout
V77.6	Special screening for cystic fibrosis
V77.7	Special screening for other inborn errors of metabolism
V77.8	Special screening for obesity
V77.91	Special screening for lipid disorders
V77.99	Special screening for other and unspecified endocrine, nutritional, metabolic, and immunity disorders
V83.81	Cystic fibrosis gene carrier
V84.81	Genetic susceptibility to multiple endocrine neoplasia (MEN)
V85.0	Body mass index (BMI) less than 19, adult
V85.1	Body mass index (BMI) 19-24, adult
V85.21	Body mass index (BMI) 25.0-25.9, adult
V85.22	Body mass index (BMI) 26.0-26.9, adult
V85.23	Body mass index (BMI) 27.0-27.9, adult
V85.24	Body mass index (BMI) 28.0-28.9, adult
V85.25	Body mass index (BMI) 29.0-29.9, adult
V85.30	Body mass index (BMI) 30.0-30.9, adult
V85.31	Body mass index (BMI) 31.0-31.9, adult
V85.32	Body mass index (BMI) 32.0-32.9, adult
V85.33	Body mass index (BMI) 33.0-33.9, adult
V85.34	Body mass index (BMI) 34.0-34.9, adult
V85.35	Body mass index (BMI) 35.0-35.9, adult
V85.36	Body mass index (BMI) 36.0-36.9, adult
V85.37	Body mass index (BMI) 37.0-37.9, adult
V85.38	Body mass index (BMI) 38.0-38.9, adult
V85.39	Body mass index (BMI) 39.0-39.9, adult
V85.4	Body mass index (BMI) 40 and over, adult
V85.51	Body mass index, pediatric, less than 5th percentile for age
V85.52	Body mass index, pediatric, less than 5th percentile to less than 85th percentile for age
V85.53	Body mass index, pediatric, less than 85th percentile to less than 95th percentile for age
V85.54	Body mass index, pediatric, greater than or equal to 95th percentile for age

EXAMPLE Patient has a family history of diabetes, V18.0.

EXAMPLE Patient is a type II diabetic individual who has been treated with insulin, 250.00, V58.67.

EXERCISE 12-5

Assign codes to the following conditions using your ICD-9-CM code book.

1. Status post pancreas transplant __________
2. Dietary counseling for patient with new diagnosis of DM __________

3. Personal history of malignant thyroid neoplasm __________
4. Family history of Graves' disease __________
5. History of rickets as a child __________

COMMON TREATMENTS

CONDITION	MEDICATION/TREATMENT
Goiter	Small doses of iodine if due to iodine deficiency; otherwise, radioactive iodine or surgical treatment if symptomatic
Hypothyroidism/Hashimoto's disease	Levothyroxine or Synthroid is the most common thyroid hormone replacement medication
Hyperthyroidism/Graves' disease	Antithyroid medications such as Tapazole; radioactive iodine or surgery
Diabetes	Diet, monitoring of blood sugars, and insulins such as Regular, Lente, Humalog, NPH; oral medications such as Glyburide, Micronase, Diabeta, Glucophage, etc.
Hyperpituitarism	Decrease the amount of hormone secreted, usually with radiation or surgery
Hypopituitarism	Removal of tumor if that is the cause, or hormone replacement therapy
Diabetes insipidus	Depending on cause, vasopressin medication
Hyperparathyroidism	Treatment depends on the cause
Hypoparathyroidism	Replacement therapy with calcium and vitamin D
Cushing's syndrome	Removal of tumor if that is the cause, or medication to suppress the production of cortisol
Addison's disease	Replacement therapy with corticosteroids
Malnutrition	Treat symptoms and/or underlying cause; nutritional supplements; replace missing nutrients, possibly with TPN (total parenteral nutrition)
Vitamin deficiencies	Treat symptoms and/or underlying cause; replace missing vitamins
Hypokalemia	Replace with potassium supplement, such as K-Dur
Hyperkalemia	Remove potassium from body with Kayexalate, diuretics, sodium bicarbonate, intravenous calcium, glucose, or insulin
Cystic fibrosis	Postural drainage and chest percussion treatments, pancreatic enzymes and vitamins, antibiotics for infection, and possibly lung transplant
Obesity	Diet, exercise, behavior modification, and bariatric surgery
Hypervitaminosis	Stop taking specific vitamin

PROCEDURES

Some of the procedures that may be related to diseases of the endocrine, nutritional and metabolic diseases, and immunity disorders may be located in the following chapters of the procedure tabular:

2. Operations on the Endocrine System (06-07)

Procedures discussed in Chapter 2 include incisional, excisional, and many diagnotic and exploratory procedures such as biopsies on various glands of the endocrine system.

EXAMPLE Goiter with complete thyroidectomy, 240.9, 06.4.

EXAMPLE Adenoma adrenal gland with percutaneous biopsy of adrenal gland, 227.0, 07.12.

Bariatric Procedures

Bariatrics is the branch of medicine that is concerned with the management (prevention or control) of obesity and allied diseases. In some cases, bariatric surgery may be necessary to treat obesity and to control and/or prevent the secondary complications associated with obesity.

Two main types of bariatric surgery are performed: restrictive and malabsorptive gastric procedures that are performed for weight loss. Malabsorptive procedures tend to be more successful for long-term weight loss. Some examples of malabsorptive procedures include the following:

- Roux-en-Y gastric bypass
- Biliopancreatic diversion (BPD)
- "Duodenal switch" procedure
- Some examples of restrictive procedures include the following:
- Gastric banding
- Vertical banded gastroplasty (VBG)

Insulin Pumps

An insulin pump is a small, computerized device that is attached to the body and delivers insulin via a catheter (Figure 12-22). This pump provides a continuous drip of insulin throughout the day. The patient may also administer a bolus of insulin by pushing a button. The code for subcutaneous implantation of the pump is 86.06; 38.91 is used for any associated catheterization, and 99.17 signifies infusion of insulin.

EXERCISE 12-6

Assign codes for all diagnoses and procedures using your ICD-9-CM code book.

1. Multinodular goiter which is symptomatic for dysphagia. Total thyroidectomy was performed __________
2. Biopsy of pituitary gland: pituitary adenoma (transsphenoidal approach) __________
3. Diabetes type I with insertion of insulin pump __________
4. Pheochromocytoma with laparoscopic excision adrenal gland __________
5. Chronic pancreatitis with pseudocyst. Classic Whipple was performed __________
6. Morbid obesity with BMI of 40. Laparoscopic VBG was performed. __________

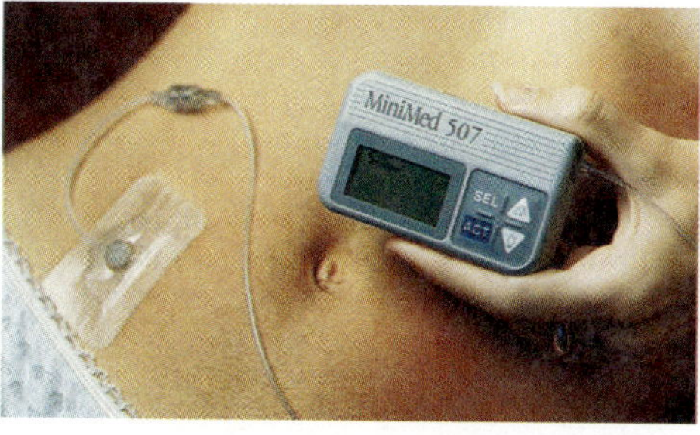

Figure 12-22. Insulin pump.

DOCUMENTATION/REIMBURSEMENT/MS-DRGs

Often, coding difficulties are due to lack of documentation. Sometimes pathology and other test results are not available at the time of discharge, or when the physician is dictating the discharge summary or is reporting the final diagnoses.

Malnutrition may not be well documented by the physician. Nutritional consults or dietitian notes should be reviewed. A physician query would be needed to confirm any diagnoses based on a dietician's assessment.

Many of the conditions and diseases related to nutritional and metabolic disorders are supported by laboratory tests. Coders should not assign a diagnosis code on the basis of abnormal laboratory findings alone. A laboratory value may be higher or lower than the normal range, but this does not necessarily indicate a disorder. If abnormal laboratory value(s) is noted and treatment is given or documentation supports monitoring, it would be appropriate to query the physician regarding the abnormal laboratory value(s). An abnormal finding must be clinically significant to be coded, per *Coding Clinic* (1990:2Q: p15-16).[12]

MS-DRG With and Without MCC/CC

EXAMPLE

Patient was admitted with Addison's crisis, and sodium on admission was 115 (normal, 135-148 mEq/L).

Patient treated with hypertonic saline IVs. The physician documents in the discharge summary that the patient's sodium levels improved dramatically before discharge.

DIAGNOSES	CODES	MS-DRG	RW
Addison's crisis with hyponatremia	255.41, 276.1	644	1.0638
Addison's crisis without hyponatremia	255.41	645	0.8311

The presence of a complication or comorbidity can make a difference in reimbursement, depending on the principal diagnosis and the MS-DRG assigned. The code for hyponatremia (276.1) is a complication/comorbidity. In this case, it would be necessary to query the physician regarding the low sodium levels and treatment with hypertonic saline IV before the hyponatremia code is assigned.

Two Diagnoses That Equally Meet the Definition for Principal Diagnosis

Dehydration may cause confusion when selecting a principal diagnosis because dehydration is often caused by other conditions. If two or more conditions are present on admission and meet the definition for principal diagnosis, either one could be selected as principal.

EXAMPLE

A patient was admitted with urinary tract infection (UTI) and moderate dehydration. The dehydration was treated aggressively with intravenous fluids, and the UTI was treated with intravenous (IV) antibiotics.

DIAGNOSES	CODES	MS-DRG	RW
Dehydration and UTI	276.51, 599.0	641	0.7248
UTI and dehydration	599.0, 276.51	690	0.8000

In this case, both UTI and dehydration were treated by measures that would require inpatient admission, so it would be possible to sequence either diagnosis as the principal diagnosis. If the patient had been treated with IV fluids for dehydration and oral antibiotics

for the UTI, dehydration should be the principal because oral antibiotics would not typically require in-patient hospitalization.

Diabetic Manifestation Versus Not Related to Diabetes

Documentation with regard to diabetes can be conflicting and/or may need clarification. Sometimes documentation is inconsistent, and diabetes has been documented as both type I and type II within the record. A patient is either type I or type II, and it is necessary to query the physician to determine which type is correct. It is also important to make sure that any manifestations are documented as related to diabetes. In addition, when a principal diagnosis is selected, the diabetes codes must be sequenced before any manifestation code. This can make a significant difference in MS-DRG assignment and reimbursement.

EXAMPLE

DIAGNOSES	CODES	MS-DRG	RW
Diabetic ulcer toe	250.80, 707.15	639	0.6742
Ulcer toe, diabetes	707.15, 250.00	594	0.9335

CHAPTER REVIEW EXERCISE

Assign codes for all diagnoses and procedures, including all applicable V and E codes and procedures.

1. Homocystinemia ______
2. Conn's syndrome ______
3. Myxedema ______
4. Idiopathic Cushing's syndrome ______
5. Testicular hypogonadism ______
6. Overproduction of growth hormone ______
7. Hyponatremia due to dehydration ______
8. Gouty arthritis ______
9. Monoclonal gammopathy ______
10. Respiratory acidosis with metabolic alkalosis ______
11. Overweight with BMI of 26.0 ______
12. Volume depletion ______
13. Patient with cystic fibrosis admitted with exacerbation of respiratory symptoms ______
14. Hyperthyroidism with exophthalmos ______
15. Poorly controlled diabetes (type II) with diabetic gastroparesis; patient is on insulin ______
16. Albinism ______
17. Amyloidosis ______
18. Proliferative retinopathy due to DM, type II, out of control ______
19. Diabetes due to prednisone ______
20. Hyperlipidemia due to Cushing's syndrome ______
21. Thiamine deficiency due to chronic alcoholism ______
22. Phenylketonuria (PKU) ______
23. Chronic kidney disease due to diabetic nephropathy; juvenile-onset diabetes ______

24. Severe obesity with BMI 43 and obstructive sleep apnea; patient had Roux-en-Y gastric bypass ____________

25. Erectile dysfunction due to diabetes mellitus, type 2 ____________

26. Inanition ____________

27. Patient is immunocompromised because of medications taken for pancreas transplant ____________

Write the correct answer(s) in the space(s) provided.

28. List a couple of conditions that qualify a person as morbidly obese.

____

____

29. What type of diabetes is the most common?

____

30. What organism may cause complications for a patient with cystic fibrosis?

____

CHAPTER GLOSSARY

Acromegaly: condition that results when hypersecretion of hGH occurs after puberty, along with overgrowth of the face, hands, feet, and soft tissues.

Addison's disease: adrenocortical insufficiency that may be caused by neoplasms, surgical removal of the adrenal gland, autoimmune processes, tuberculosis, hemorrhage, and/or infection.

Atrophy: when a gland becomes smaller.

Bariatrics: branch of medicine that is concerned with the management (prevention or control) of obesity and allied diseases.

Body mass index: uses weight and height to estimate body fat.

Cushing's syndrome: condition that results in excessive circulating cortisol levels caused by chronic hypersecretion of the adrenal cortex.

Cystic fibrosis: genetic (inherited) condition that affects the cells that produce mucus, sweat, saliva, and digestive juices. Instead of being thin and slippery, these secretions are thick and sticky, plugging up tubes, ducts, and passageways, especially in the pancreas and lungs.

Diabetes insipidus: deficiency in the release of vasopressin by the posterior pituitary gland.

Diabetes mellitus: chronic syndrome of impaired carbohydrate, protein, and fat metabolism caused by insufficient production of insulin by the pancreas or faulty utilization of insulin by the cells.

Endocrine system: body system composed of many glands that secrete hormones that regulate bodily functions; it works with the nervous system to maintain body activities and homeostasis and to respond to stress.

Exophthalmos: bulging of the eyes.

Genetic: inherited.

Gigantism: condition that occurs when hypersecretion of hGH occurs before puberty, along with proportionate overgrowth of all bodily tissues, especially the long bones.

Goiter: enlargement of the thyroid gland.

Graves' disease: the most common form of hyperthyroidism; it occurs through an autoimmune response that attacks the thyroid gland, resulting in overproduction of the thyroid hormone thyroxine.

Hashimoto's disease: inflammation of the thyroid gland that often results in hypothyroidism.

Hormones: substances secreted by glands that can regulate bodily functions, such as urinary output, cellular metabolic rate, and growth and development.

Hyperglycemia: condition that results when glucose or blood sugar becomes abnormally high. This is a relatively common event in patients with diabetes.

Hyperparathyroidism: condition that results when an overactive parathyroid gland secretes excessive parathyroid hormone, causing increased levels of circulating calcium associated with loss of calcium in the bone.

Hyperpituitarism: increased production of the pituitary hormones, particularly the human growth hormone (hGH).

Hyperplasia: enlargement of a gland.

Hyperthyroidism: abnormality of the thyroid gland in which secretion of thyroid hormone is usually increased and is no longer under the regulatory control of hypothalamic-pituitary centers.

Hypertrophy: enlargement of a gland.

Hypervitaminosis: toxicity resulting from an excess of any vitamin, especially fat-soluble vitamins such as A, D, and K.

Hypoglycemia: condition that results when glucose or blood sugar becomes abnormally low.

Hypoparathyroidism: underactive parathyroid gland that results in decreased levels of circulating calcium.

Hypopituitarism: condition caused by low levels of pituitary hormones. Hormones secreted by the pituitary gland can affect the functions of other glands.

Hypoplasia: atrophy; condition that results when a gland becomes smaller.

Hypothyroidism: condition caused by low levels of pituitary hormones. Hormones secreted by the pituitary gland can affect the functions of other glands.

Iatrogenic: caused by medical treatment.

Immune system: the body's major defense mechanism that responds to invasion of the body by foreign substances.

Malnutrition: nutrition disorder caused by primary deprivation of protein energy caused by poverty or self-imposed starvation, or associated with deficiency diseases such as cancer.

Morbid obesity: applies to patients who are 50% to 100% or 100 pounds above their ideal body weight. A BMI of 40 or higher defines morbid obesity.

Myxedema: skin and tissue disorder that is usually due to severe prolonged hypothyroidism.

Obesity: condition defined as an increase in body weight beyond the limitation of skeletal and physical requirements, caused by excessive accumulation of fat in the body.

Secondary diabetes mellitus: form of the disease that develops as a result of another disease or condition.

Steroid-induced diabetes: diabetes that is caused by the use of steroids.

Tetany: a continuous muscle spasm.

Thyrotoxic crisis/storm: complication of hyperthyroidism associated with a sudden intensification of symptoms combined with fever, rapid pulse, and delirium.

Vitamin deficiency: condition caused by many different factors, such as lack of absorbance of nutrients taken in, associated with digestive tract disorders, lifestyle issues (e.g., alcohol, smoking, medication, overexercising), chronic illness, age, and many other factors.

CHAPTER 13

Diseases of the Respiratory System

(ICD-9-CM Chapter 8, Codes 460-519)

CHAPTER OUTLINE

LEARNING OBJECTIVES

- Apply and assign the correct ICD-9-CM codes in accordance with Official Guidelines for Coding and Reporting
- Identify pertinent anatomy and physiology of the respiratory system
- Identify diseases of the respiratory system
- Assign the correct V codes and procedure codes related to the respiratory system
- Identify common treatments, medications, laboratory values, and diagnostic tests
- Explain the importance of documentation in relation to MS-DRGs for reimbursement

ABBREVIATIONS

ABG arterial blood gas
AIDS acquired immunodeficiency syndrome
AMI acute myocardial infarction
BAL bronchoalveolar lavage
CAP community-acquired pneumonia
CC complication/comorbidity
CHF congestive heart failure
COPD chronic obstructive pulmonary disease
CVA cerebrovascular accident

ABBREVIATIONS—*cont'd*

E. coli *Escherichia coli*

ER Emergency Room

GERD gastroesophageal reflux disease

H. flu *Haemophilus influenzae*

HIV human immunodeficiency virus

ICD-9-CM *International Classification of Diseases, 9th Revision, Clinical Modification*

IV intravenous

LLL left lower lobe

MS-DRG Medicare Severity diagnosis-related group

NEC not elsewhere classifiable

NOS not otherwise specified

O_2 oxygen

OIG Office of the Inspector General

OR Operating Room

$Paco_2$ partial pressure of carbon dioxide in arterial blood

Pao_2 partial pressure of oxygen in arterial blood

PCP *Pneumocystis carinii* pneumonia

RAD reactive airway disease

RSV respiratory syncytial virus

RUL right upper lobe

RW relative weight

STAPH aureus *Staphylococcus aureus*

VATS video-assisted thoracic surgery

ICD-9-CM Official Guidelines for Coding and Reporting

Please refer to the companion Evolve website for the most current guidelines.

8. Chapter 8: Diseases of Respiratory System (460-519)

a. Chronic Obstructive Pulmonary Disease [COPD] and Asthma

1) Conditions that comprise COPD and Asthma

The conditions that comprise COPD are obstructive chronic bronchitis, subcategory 491.2, and emphysema, category 492. All asthma codes are under category 493, Asthma. Code 496, Chronic airway obstruction, not elsewhere classified, is a nonspecific code that should only be used when the documentation in a medical record does not specify the type of COPD being treated.

2) Acute exacerbation of chronic obstructive bronchitis and asthma

The codes for chronic obstructive bronchitis and asthma distinguish between uncomplicated cases and those in acute exacerbation. An acute exacerbation is a worsening or a decompensation of a chronic condition. An acute exacerbation is not equivalent to an infection superimposed on a chronic condition, though an exacerbation may be triggered by an infection.

3) Overlapping nature of the conditions that comprise COPD and asthma

Due to the overlapping nature of the conditions that make up COPD and asthma, there are many variations in the way these conditions are documented. Code selection must be based on the terms as documented. When selecting the correct code for the documented type of COPD and asthma, it is essential to first review the index, and then verify the code in the tabular list. There are many instructional notes under the different COPD subcategories and codes. It is important that all such notes be reviewed to assure correct code assignment.

4) Acute exacerbation of asthma and status asthmaticus

An acute exacerbation of asthma is an increased severity of the asthma symptoms, such as wheezing and shortness of breath. Status asthmaticus refers to a patient's failure to respond to therapy administered during an asthmatic episode and is a life threatening complication that requires emergency care. If status asthmaticus is documented by the provider with any type of COPD or with acute bronchitis, the status asthmaticus should be sequenced first. It supersedes any type of COPD including that with acute exacerbation or acute bronchitis. It is inappropriate to assign an asthma code with 5th digit 2, with acute exacerbation, together with an asthma code with 5th digit 1, with status asthmatics. Only the 5th digit 1 should be assigned. (See Figure 13-1.)

b. Chronic Obstructive Pulmonary Disease [COPD] and Bronchitis

1) Acute bronchitis with COPD

Acute bronchitis, code 466.0, is due to an infectious organism. When acute bronchitis is documented with COPD, code 491.22, Obstructive chronic bronchitis

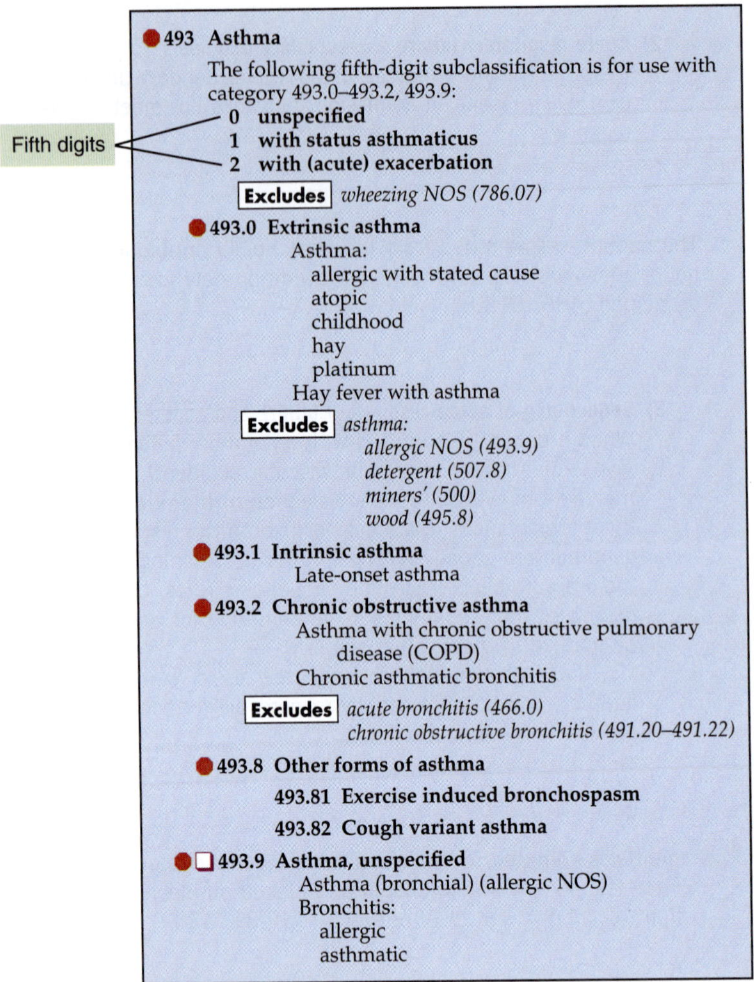

493 Asthma

The following fifth-digit subclassification is for use with category 493.0–493.2, 493.9:

0 unspecified
1 with status asthmaticus
2 with (acute) exacerbation

Excludes *wheezing NOS (786.07)*

493.0 Extrinsic asthma
Asthma:
allergic with stated cause
atopic
childhood
hay
platinum
Hay fever with asthma

Excludes *asthma:*
allergic NOS (493.9)
detergent (507.8)
miners' (500)
wood (495.8)

493.1 Intrinsic asthma
Late-onset asthma

493.2 Chronic obstructive asthma
Asthma with chronic obstructive pulmonary disease (COPD)
Chronic asthmatic bronchitis

Excludes *acute bronchitis (466.0)*
chronic obstructive bronchitis (491.20–491.22)

493.8 Other forms of asthma

493.81 Exercise induced bronchospasm

493.82 Cough variant asthma

493.9 Asthma, unspecified
Asthma (bronchial) (allergic NOS)
Bronchitis:
allergic
asthmatic

Figure 13-1. Fifth digits for asthma.

with acute bronchitis, should be assigned. It is not necessary to also assign code 466.0. If a medical record documents acute bronchitis with COPD with acute exacerbation, only code 491.22 should be assigned. The acute bronchitis included in code 491.22 supersedes the acute exacerbation. If a medical record documents COPD with acute exacerbation without mention of acute bronchitis, only code 491.21 should be assigned.

c. Acute Respiratory Failure

1) Acute respiratory failure as principal diagnosis

Code 518.81, Acute respiratory failure, may be assigned as a principal diagnosis when it is the condition established after study to be chiefly responsible for occasioning the admission to the hospital, and the selection is supported by the Alphabetic Index and Tabular List. However, chapter-specific coding guidelines (such as obstetrics, poisoning, HIV, newborn) that provide sequencing direction take precedence.

EXAMPLE

The patient presented to the ER in acute respiratory failure and was intubated and admitted to ICU. Following admission, the patient was started on antibiotics for pneumonia. The patient was on mechanical ventilation for 24 hours. 518.81, 486, 96.71, 96.04.

(Per guidelines, if respiratory failure and another acute condition are equally responsible for occasioning the admission, the guidelines regarding two or more diagnoses that equally meet the definition for principal diagnoses may be applied.)

2) **Acute respiratory failure as secondary diagnosis**
Respiratory failure may be listed as a secondary diagnosis if it occurs after admission, or if it is present on admission, but does not meet the definition of principal diagnosis.

EXAMPLE

The patient was admitted from the clinic for IV antibiotics for pneumonia. A couple of hours after admission, the patient's condition deteriorated and acute respiratory failure developed, 486, 518.81.

3) **Sequencing of acute respiratory failure and another acute condition**
When a patient is admitted with respiratory failure and another acute condition, (e.g., myocardial infarction, cerebrovascular accident), the principal diagnosis will not be the same in every situation. Selection of the principal diagnosis will be dependent on the circumstances of admission. If both the respiratory failure and the other acute condition are equally responsible for occasioning the admission to the hospital, and there are no chapter-specific sequencing rules, the guideline regarding two or more diagnoses that equally meet the definition for principal diagnosis (*Section II, C.*) may be applied in these situations.

If the documentation is not clear as to whether acute respiratory failure and another condition are equally responsible for occasioning the admission, query the provider for clarification.

EXAMPLE

Patient was admitted to the hospital in acute respiratory failure due to congestive heart failure. The patient was intubated and placed on mechanical ventilation for 2 days. The patient responded well to IV diuretics, 518.81, 428.0, 96.71, 96.04.

d. Influenza due to identified avian influenza virus (avian influenza)
Code only confirmed cases of avian influenza. This is an exception to the hospital inpatient guideline Section II, H. (Uncertain Diagnosis).

In this context, "confirmation" does not require documentation of positive laboratory testing specific for avian influenza. However, coding should be based on the provider's diagnostic statement that the patient has avian influenza.

If the provider records "suspected or possible or probable avian influenza," the appropriate influenza code from category 487 should be assigned. Code 488, Influenza due to identified avian influenza virus, should not be assigned.

EXAMPLE

Patient was admitted with a confirmed case of avian influenza, 488.

EXAMPLE

Patient was admitted with possible avian influenza, 487.1.

Apply the General Coding Guidelines as found in Chapter 5.

ANATOMY AND PHYSIOLOGY

The primary function of the **respiratory system** (Figure 13-2) is to supply the body with oxygen (O_2). Respiration occurs through the nose and mouth, bringing oxygen through the larynx and trachea and into the lungs, where oxygen is delivered and carbon dioxide is exhaled. Dome-shaped muscles at the bottom of the lungs, or the **diaphragm**, assist in

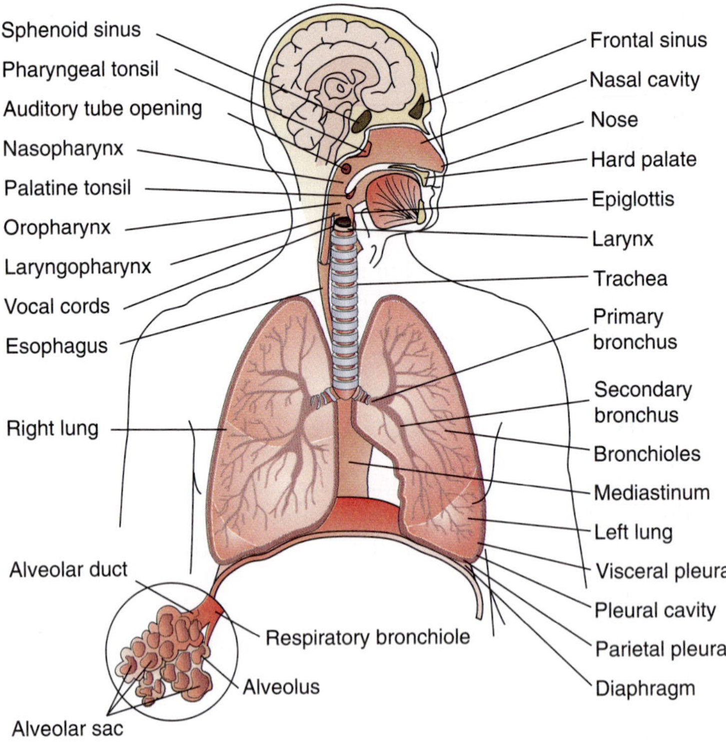

Figure 13-2. Anatomy of the respiratory system.

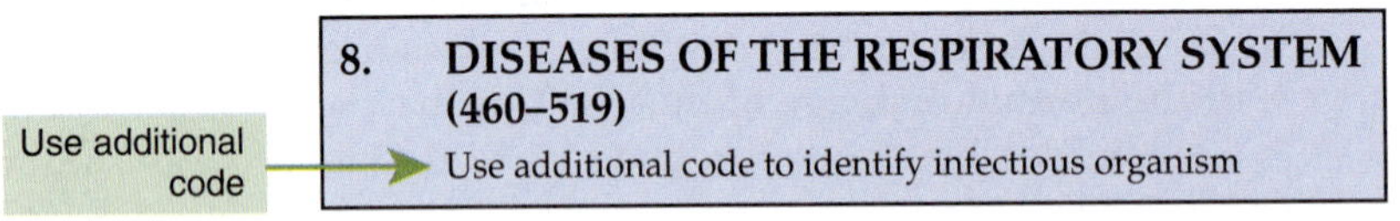

Figure 13-3. Instruction to use additional code to identify infectious organism.

the process of breathing and in the exchange of oxygen/carbon dioxide. The lungs are the major organ of the respiratory system. The right lung is made up of three lobes; the left lung is smaller and contains two lobes. The **bronchi** are the two air tubes that branch off the trachea and deliver air to both lungs. The **trachea**, or windpipe, is responsible for filtering the air that we breathe.

DISEASE CONDITIONS

Diseases of the Respiratory System (460-519), Chapter 8 in the ICD-9-CM code book, is divided into the following categories:

CATEGORY	SECTION TITLES
460-466	Acute Respiratory Infections
470-478	Other Diseases of the Upper Respiratory Tract
480-488	Pneumonia and Influenza
490-496	Chronic Obstructive Pulmonary Disease and Allied Conditions
500-508	Pneumoconioses and Other Lung Disease Due to External Agents
510-519	Other Disease of Respiratory System

At the very beginning of Chapter 8 is an instruction to use an additional code to identify the infectious organism (Figure 13-3). In the respiratory chapter, some codes are provided that do include the organisms. When the organism is included, it is not necessary to assign an additional code.

EXAMPLE Pneumonia due to respiratory syncytial virus, 480.1.

This is a combination code that includes the disease process, pneumonia, and the causative organism, respiratory syncytial virus (RSV). No additional code is necessary to identify the organism.

EXAMPLE Acute laryngitis due to *Haemophilus influenzae,* 464.00, 041.5.

In this case, laryngitis is due to *Haemophilus influenzae* bacteria (H flu). The code for acute laryngitis, 464.0, makes no mention of the causative bacteria; therefore, code 041.5 is assigned as an additional code to identify the bacteria.

Acute Respiratory Infections (460-466) and Other Diseases of the Upper Respiratory Tract (470-478)

Infection is invasion of the body by organisms that have the potential to cause disease. This section deals with infections of the upper respiratory tract and the bronchus. It must be noted that diseases in this section are identified as acute infections. It is possible that an acute infection may be superimposed upon a chronic infection or inflammation. Following general guidelines, "If the same condition is described as both acute (subacute) and chronic, and separate subentries exist in the Alphabetic Index at the same indentation level, code both and sequence the acute (subacute) code first" (Figure 13-4).

EXAMPLE Acute and chronic bronchitis, 466.0, 491.9.

Acute **sinusitis** occurs when the linings of one or more sinuses become infected, usually because of viruses or bacteria. Sinuses may swell, causing an obstruction and interfering with the normal drainage of mucus. This may occur as the result of a cold. Sinusitis can cause considerable discomfort and may lead to more serious infection.

EXAMPLE Acute maxillary sinusitis, 461.0.

EXAMPLE Chronic maxillary sinusitis, 473.0.

Acute **bronchitis** is a lower respiratory tract or bronchial tree infection that may be characterized by cough, sputum production and wheezing. Most cases of acute bronchitis are caused by viruses such as RSV, influenza, and parainfluenza. Bacterial infection with *Mycoplasma pneumoniae, Chlamydia pneumoniae,* and *Bordetella pertussis* (whooping cough), particularly in young adults, can lead to acute bronchitis. Bronchitis may progress to pneumonia or may aggravate respiratory symptoms in those who have chronic respiratory conditions.

EXAMPLE Subacute bronchitis with bronchospasm, 466.0.

EXERCISE 13-1

Assign codes to the following conditions using your ICD-9-CM code book.

1. Headache due to acute pansinusitis ____________
2. Laryngotracheitis ____________
3. Acute streptococcal pharyngitis ____________
4. Acute bronchiolitis due to RSV ____________
5. Upper respiratory infection ____________

Bronchitis (diffuse) (hypostatic) (infectious) (inflammatory) (simple) 490
- with
  - emphysema - *see* Emphysema
  - influenza, flue, or grippe 487.1
  - obstruction airway, chronic 491.20
    - with
      - acute bronchitis 491.22
      - exacerbation (acute) 491.21
  - tracheitis 490
    - acute or subacute 466.0
      - with bronchospasm or obstruction 466.0
    - chronic 491.8
- acute or subacute 466.0 ← Acute
  - with
    - bronchospasm 466.0
    - obstruction 466.0
    - tracheitis 466.0
  - chemical (due to fumes or vapors) 506.0
  - due to
    - fumes or vapors 506.0
    - radiation 508.8
- allergic (acute) (*see also* Asthma) 493.9
- arachidic 934.1
- aspiration 507.0
  - due to fumes or vapors 506.0
- asthmatic (acute) 493.90
  - with
    - acute exacerbation 493.92
    - status asthmaticus 493.91
  - chronic 493.2
- capillary 466.19
  - with bronchospasm or obstruction 466.19
  - chronic 491.8
- caseous (*see also* Tuberculosis) 011.3
- Castellani's 104.8
- catarrhal 490
  - acute - *see* Bronchitis, acute
  - chronic 491.0
- chemical (acute) (subacute) 506.0
  - chronic 506.4
  - due to fumes or vapors (acute) (subacute) 506.0
    - chronic 506.4
- chronic 491.9 ← Chronic
  - with
    - tracheitis (chronic) 491.8
  - asthmatic 493.2
  - catarrhal 491.0

Figure 13-4. Alphabetic Index for acute and chronic bronchitis.

6. Acute and chronic tonsillitis ____________
7. Deviated nasal septum ____________
8. Paralysis, vocal cords ____________
9. Allergic rhinitis ____________
10. Spasm larynx ____________

Pneumonia and Influenza (480-488)

Pneumonia is an infection of the lungs that can be caused by a variety of organisms, including viruses, bacteria, and parasites. Pneumonia frequently follows an upper respiratory infection, and symptoms depend on age and cause of the pneumonia. More than 50

different types of pneumonia have been identified. High-risk individuals include the elderly, the very young, and those with underlying health problems such as chronic obstructive pulmonary disease (COPD), diabetes mellitus, congestive heart failure, asthma, and sickle cell anemia. Those with impaired immune systems as the result of human immunodeficiency virus (HIV)/acquired immunodeficiency syndrome (AIDS), cancer therapy, steroid therapy, or anti-rejection medications are also at risk for developing pneumonia.

Some common symptoms of pneumonia include the following:

- Fever/chills
- Cough
- Chest pain
- Shortness of breath
- Rapid breathing and heart rate

Community-acquired pneumonia (CAP) is a broad term that is used to refer to pneumonias that are contracted outside of the hospital or nursing home setting. The most common cause of CAP is *Streptococcus pneumoniae.* **Nosocomial pneumonia** refers to a pneumonia that is acquired while the patient is hospitalized. Hospital patients are most susceptible to Gram-negative bacteria and staphylococcal pneumonia. **Nursing home–acquired pneumonia** refers to a pneumonia that is acquired in a nursing home or extended care facility. More than one organism may be responsible for pneumonia. In this case, pneumonia codes would be assigned to identify both types of pneumonia. If this was the reason for the hospital stay, either could be sequenced as the principal diagnosis. See Table 13-1 for other pathogens responsible for pneumonia. Complications of pneumonia include the formation of abscesses, respiratory failure, bacteremia, pleural effusion, empyema, and pneumothorax.

According to *Coding Clinic* (1998:2Q:p3),[1] different types of diagnostic tests may be used as part of a "diagnostic workup" to find the "causative organism" that is responsible for the patient's illness. This could include various cultures, x-rays, other minimally invasive tests, such as bronchoscopy, or a lung biopsy, if necessary. A sputum culture from a healthy person would generally have no growth. A mixture of microorganisms, normally found in or on a patient's body, may be identified in a culture. This does not necessarily mean that this organism is responsible for a particular infection. A physician may document that a particular organism is a **contaminant.** This means that the physician does not believe that this organism is responsible for causing the infection. No code would be assigned for an organism that was described as a contaminant. *Coding Clinic* (1998:2Q:p3)[1] goes on to say that it "is inappropriate for coders to assume a causal organism on the basis of laboratory or radiology" findings alone. All code assignments should be based on the physician's documentation. If the documentation is vague or not available, query the physician to confirm whether the culture findings identify the causative organism or identify a contaminant."

Table 13-1. Common Causes of Pneumonia[2]

Causative Agents	Percentage of All Diagnosed Cases
Bacteria	50
Streptococcus pneumoniae	10
Haemophilus influenzae	5
Staphylococcus aureus	5
Mycobacterium tuberculosis	10
Viruses	—
Infl uenza virus	
Fungi*	—
Aspergillus fumigatus	—
Candida albicans	—
Pneumocystis jiroveci	
Bacterium-like organisms	
Mycoplasma pneumoniae	10

*Opportunistic infection: rare except in immunosuppressed, debilitated, or terminally ill patients.

Sometimes, pneumonia may be described as to the lobe that it is located in, for example right upper lobe (RUL) pneumonia or left lower lobe (LLL) pneumonia. Both of these diagnostic statements are coded to 486, pneumonia, unspecified. The location of the pneumonia should not be misinterpreted to mean **lobar pneumonia**, which is a synonym for pneumococcal pneumonia or pneumonia due to *Streptococcus pneumoniae* pneumonia.

Often, **empiric** treatment (initiation of treatment prior to making a definite diagnosis) with antibiotic will be administered before the organism has been identified or the type of pneumonia determined. For example, patients with HIV/AIDS may be treated empirically with antibiotics that treat both *Pneumocystis carinii* pneumonia (PCP) and CAP. Once PCP has been ruled out, the treatment and the type of antibiotic used may be modified. Because *Pneumocystis carinii* pneumonia was ruled out, it cannot be coded, even though the condition was treated as such until test results were complete.

EXAMPLE Pneumonia due to Gram-negative bacteria, 482.83.

EXAMPLE Bronchopneumonia, 485.

Influenza is a contagious viral infection of the respiratory tract that causes coughing, difficulty breathing, headache, muscle aches, and weakness. Possible complications include pneumonia, encephalitis, bronchitis, and sinus and ear infections. Three types of influenza virus have been identified: types A, B, and C. Types A and B cause flu epidemics each winter and are the types that may be prevented with a flu shot. Type A is the most common and the most serious type. Influenza C is a very mild respiratory illness that is not thought to be responsible for epidemics. The type of influenza identified does not affect treatment. Bacterial pneumonia is the most common complication of influenza.

EXAMPLE Influenza with *Klebsiella* pneumonia, 487.0, 482.0

EXAMPLE Influenza, type A, 487.1.

EXERCISE 13-2

Assign codes to the following conditions using your ICD-9-CM code book.

1. Legionnaires' disease __________
2. Pneumonia due to aspergillosis __________
3. Influenza with *Staph aureus* pneumonia __________
4. Viral pneumonia __________
5. *Mycoplasma* pneumonia __________
6. Avian influenza __________
7. Pneumonia due to *E. coli* __________
8. Cough and fever due to pneumonitis __________
9. Community-acquired pneumonia; empiric treatment was started for *Pneumocystis carinii* pneumonia. PCP was ruled out. Patient has AIDS. __________
10. Headache and weakness due to influenza A __________

Chronic Obstructive Pulmonary Disease and Allied Conditions (490-496)

COPD, or **chronic obstructive pulmonary disease**, is a general term that is used to describe a lung disease in which the airways become obstructed, making it difficult for air to get into and out of the lungs. Although cigarette smoking is the most common culprit, other irritants

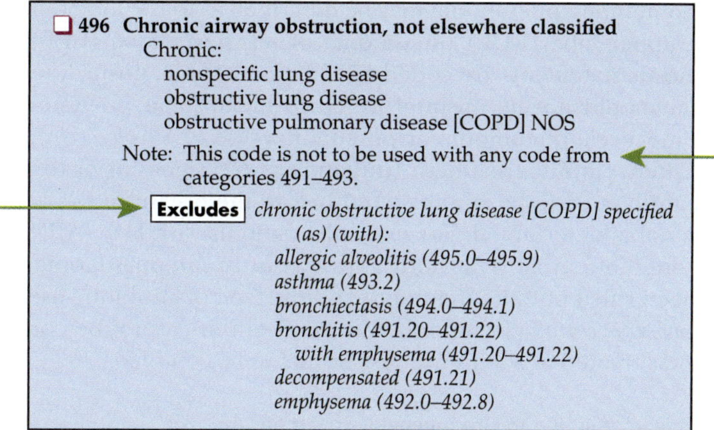

496 Chronic airway obstruction, not elsewhere classified
Chronic:
nonspecific lung disease
obstructive lung disease
obstructive pulmonary disease [COPD] NOS
Note: This code is not to be used with any code from categories 491–493.
Excludes *chronic obstructive lung disease [COPD] specified (as) (with):*
allergic alveolitis (495.0–495.9)
asthma (493.2)
bronchiectasis (494.0–494.1)
bronchitis (491.20–491.22)
with emphysema (491.20–491.22)
decompensated (491.21)
emphysema (492.0–492.8)

Figure 13-5. Note and Excludes notation for category 496.

such as pollution, chemicals, or dust can also play a role. Various diseases can be classified as COPD; these include asthmatic bronchitis, chronic bronchitis, and emphysema. All three affect the bronchial tree and result in wheezing, cough, and shortness of breath. It may be clinically difficult to distinguish among these disorders.

A specific note under category 496, Chronic airway obstruction, not elsewhere classified, instructs as follows: "This code is not to be used with any code from categories 491-493." An Excludes note also assists with proper code assignment (Figure 13-5).

Chronic bronchitis is characterized by a mucus-producing cough most days of the month, 3 months out of a year, for 2 successive years, with no other underlying disease that explains the cough. Smoking cigarettes is the most common cause of chronic bronchitis. Chronic bronchitis often remains untreated because it is thought to be just a "smoker's cough."

Emphysema is a chronic lung disease of gradual onset that can be attributed to chronic infection and inflammation or irritation from cigarette smoke (Figure 13-6).

EXAMPLE Patient was admitted with exacerbation of chronic obstructive bronchitis, 491.21.

Asthma is a disease that affects the airways that carry air into and out of the lungs. Asthma can be controlled to minimize serious symptoms or attacks. Physicians use the terms "asthma" and "reactive airway disease" (RAD) interchangeably.

Asthma is category 493 and the following fifth-digit classifications must be assigned with codes 493.0-493.2, and 493.9:

0 unspecified
1 with status asthmaticus
2 with acute exacerbation

Per *Coding Clinic* (1988:3Q:p9-10),[3] "status asthmaticus can be described with the following terms:

- Intractable asthmatic attack
- Refractory asthma
- Severe, prolonged asthmatic attack
- Airway obstruction (mucous plug) not relieved by bronchodilators
- Severe, intractable wheezing"

If respiratory failure occurs, it should also be coded, and sequencing would depend on whether respiratory failure was present on admission and meets the criteria for principal diagnosis.

Asthmatic bronchitis refers to an underlying asthmatic problem in patients in whom asthma has become so persistent that clinically significant chronic airflow obstruction is

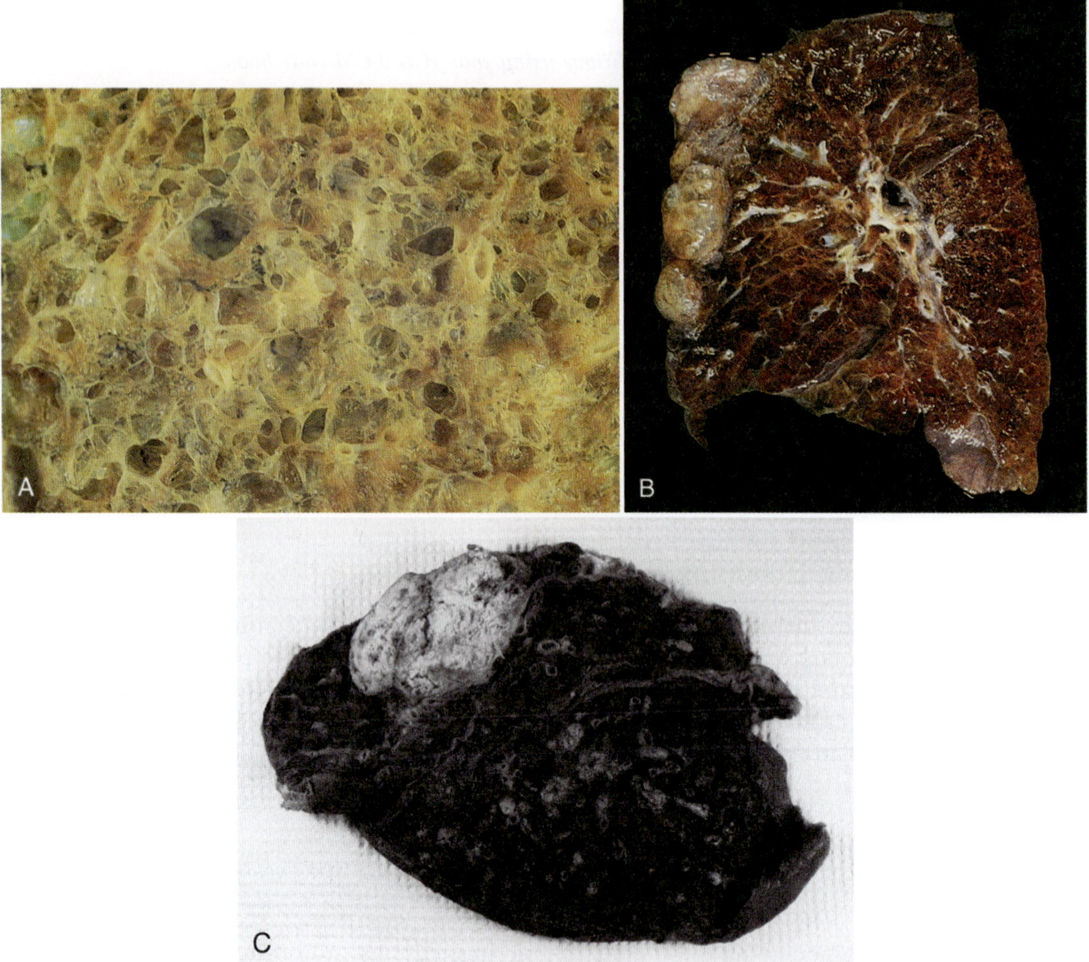

Figure 13-6. **A,** Emphysema. **B,** Bullous emphysema with large subpleural bullae. **C,** Emphysematous lung with tumor.

present, despite antiasthmatic therapy. Symptoms of chronic bronchitis are generally also present.

EXAMPLE

Patient was admitted in respiratory failure caused by an intractable asthmatic attack, 518.81, 493.91.

(Per guidelines, if both the respiratory failure and another acute condition are equally responsible for occasioning the admission, the guidelines regarding two or more diagnoses that equally meet the definition for principal diagnosis may be applied).

EXAMPLE

Patient was admitted with acute exacerbation of asthmatic bronchitis. The patient went into acute respiratory failure 6 hours after admission, 493.92, 518.81.

Category 495, Extrinsic allergic alveolitis, includes conditions that are due to inhalation of organic materials such as grain dust, cotton dust, or animal dander.

EXAMPLE

Patient was diagnosed with farmers' lung, 495.0.

EXERCISE 13-3

Assign codes to the following conditions using your ICD-9-CM code book.

1. Exercise-induced asthma ____________
2. Bronchiectasis ____________
3. Asthma exacerbation with pneumonia ____________
4. Emphysema with chronic bronchitis ____________
5. Ventilation pneumonitis ____________
6. Acute bronchitis with COPD ____________
7. Decompensated COPD ____________
8. Asthma with exacerbation of COPD ____________
9. End-stage COPD with emphysema ____________
10. Mushroom worker's lung ____________

Pneumoconioses and Other Lung Diseases Due to External Agents (500-508)

Pneumoconioses are lung diseases that are caused by chronic inhalation of inorganic (mineral) dust and are often due to occupational exposure. Examples include **siderosis**, which results from inhalation of iron oxide; **baritosis**, caused by inhalation of barium; **stannosis**, resulting from inhalation of tin particles; **black lung or coal workers' pneumoconiosis** (Figure 13-7), caused by inhalation of coal dust; and **asbestosis**, which is caused by inhalation of asbestos.

EXAMPLE Patient has silicosis, caused by working as a sandblaster for many years, 502.

Aspiration pneumonia is an inflammation of the lungs and bronchial tubes that is due to the aspiration of foreign material (e.g., food, saliva, vomit) into the lung. Disorders that affect normal swallowing include: disorders of the esophagus, decreased or absent gag reflex, old age, dental problems, use of sedative drugs, anesthesia, coma, and excessive alcohol consumption. These disorders may cause aspiration.

Per *Coding Clinic* (1991:3Q:p16-17),[4] if both aspiration pneumonia and bacterial pneumonia are present, it is acceptable to assign codes for both.

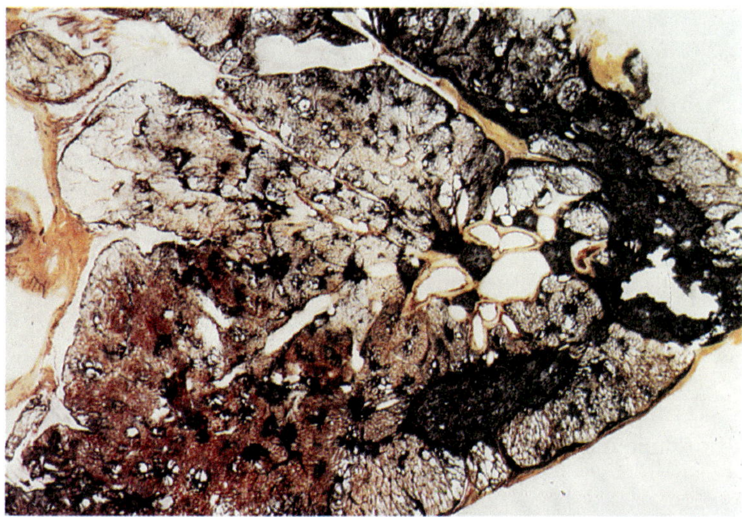

Figure 13-7. Coal workers' lung shows deposits of carbon particles (*black areas*).

EXAMPLE

Aspiration pneumonia with superimposed pneumonia due to *Staphylococcus aureus,* 507.0, 482.41.

If both were present on admission, either could be sequenced as the principal diagnosis.

Several respiratory conditions can be induced by chemical fumes and vapors. These range from acute conditions such as bronchitis and pneumonitis to chronic respiratory conditions such as emphysema and pulmonary fibrosis. The appropriate E code should also be assigned to identify the cause.

EXAMPLE

Acute pulmonary edema due to smoke inhalation from grass fire, 506.1, E892.

EXERCISE 13-4

Assign codes to the following conditions using your ICD-9-CM code book.

1. Aspiration pneumonia; patient has dysphagia due to old CVA ____________
2. Fibrosis due to radiation treatments ____________
3. Black lung disease ____________
4. Pulmonary edema due to anhydrous ammonia; accidental poisoning while working on farm ____________
5. Pleural effusion due to asbestosis ____________

Other Diseases of the Respiratory System (510-519)

Pleural Effusion

Pleural effusion is accumulation of fluid in the pleural space caused by trauma or disease. If blood is present in the accumulating fluid, the condition is called **hemothorax**; if pus is present, it is called **empyema**; if chyle (milky fluid consisting of lymph and fat) is present, it is called **chylothorax**. The most common causes of pleural effusion include the following:

Cardiac: congestive heart failure
Liver: liver failure
Kidney: nephrotic syndrome, peritoneal dialysis, uremia
Lung: infection, pulmonary embolism, pulmonary infarction, cancer (primary lung and metastatic), asbestosis
Vascular: collagen vascular disease (systemic lupus erythematosus, rheumatoid arthritis)
Trauma: hemothorax, chylothorax, rupture of the esophagus
Miscellaneous: pancreatitis, post abdominal or coronary artery bypass graft surgery, and drug reactions

According to *Coding Clinic* (1991:3Q:p19-20),[5] pleural effusion is not usually reported if it appears in conjunction with congestive heart failure because the condition is not separately treated. When the only documentation is a diagnostic x-ray, the coder should not report the condition. However, in certain cases, "special x-rays such as decubitus views are required to confirm the presence of pleural effusion or diagnostic thoracentesis may be performed to identify its etiology. In other cases, it may be necessary to address the effusion by therapeutic thoracentesis or chest tube drainage. In any of these situations, it is acceptable to report pleural effusion as an additional diagnosis since the condition was specifically evaluated or treated, but reporting is not required."

EXAMPLE

Hemothorax due to pulmonary embolism, 415.19, 511.89.

Pneumothorax

When air enters the pleural space, this is called **pneumothorax**. A pneumothorax may be classified as spontaneous (not caused by trauma), traumatic, or iatrogenic. **Spontaneous pneumothorax** may occur in individuals who have no history of lung disease and often is the result of a ruptured subpleural bleb. **Iatrogenic** pneumothorax is the result of a complication of a diagnostic or therapeutic intervention or procedure. Traumatic pneumothorax occurs as the result of an injury and is assigned an injury code.

EXAMPLE Spontaneous pneumothorax, no specific cause found, 512.8.

Pulmonary Edema

Pulmonary edema is a condition whereby fluid accumulates in the lungs. In most cases, heart problems are the cause. According to *Coding Clinic* (1988:3Q:p3),[6] the following codes for heart failure (428.0-428.1) include pulmonary edema that is cardiac in origin:

- Left ventricular failure, 428.1
- Congestive heart failure, 428.0
- Right heart failure secondary to left heart failure, 428.0
- Hypertensive heart disease—see 402.0, 402.1, and 402.9 with fifth digit 1
- Rheumatic heart disease, acute, 391.8
- Rheumatic active chorea, 392.0
- Rheumatic heart disease or chorea, inactive, chronic or quiescent, 398.91
- Rheumatic disease of heart valves (394-396), code also 398.91

EXAMPLE Patient admitted with exacerbation of congestive heart failure (CHF) with pulmonary edema confirmed by chest x-ray, 428.0.

Acute Pulmonary Edema of Noncardiac Origin

According to *Coding Clinic* (1988:3Q:p3-4),[7] pulmonary edema is not always related to a cardiac condition. The "noncardiogenic" type of acute pulmonary edema may also be caused by lung disease or related to patient trauma, and occurs in a variety of conditions. Some of these conditions include the following:

- Postoperative pulmonary edema, [not otherwise specified] (without adult respiratory distress syndrome), is reported with 518.4 (acute edema of the lung, unspecified), which is not used if the edema is actually caused by left ventricular failure (428.1) or CHF (428.0), both of which are cardiac in nature.
- Postoperative pulmonary edema specifically caused by fluid overload is reported with 518.4 and 276.6 (Fluid overload).
- Acute pulmonary edema caused by bacterial pneumonia, 482.0-482.9, or viral pneumonia, 480.0-480.9, is reported with 518.4, unless caused by left ventricular failure (428.1) or congestive heart failure (428.0), because the latter conditions are cardiac in nature.
- Acute pulmonary edema is reported with an additional code of 518.4 when in conjunction with either Endotoxic shock, 785.59, Uremia, 586, or Septicemia, 038.9.

Respiratory Failure

Respiratory failure is a general term that describes ineffective gas exchange across the lungs by the respiratory system. An arterial blood gas (ABG) measurement may be used to detect the presence of respiratory failure. A partial pressure of oxygen in arterial blood (PaO_2) of less than 60 torr and a partial pressure of carbon dioxide in arterial blood ($PaCO_2$) greater than 50 torr indicate respiratory failure.

Some of the most common causes of respiratory failure include the following:

- Obstruction of the airways (chronic bronchitis, emphysema, cystic fibrosis, etc.)
- Weak breathing due to drugs and alcohol, extreme obesity, or sleep apnea

- Muscle weakness from muscular dystrophy, polio, stroke, spinal cord injury, or Lou Gehrig's disease
- Abnormality of lung tissue such as pneumonia, fluid in lungs, lung cancer, pulmonary fibrosis, sarcoidosis, and radiation
- Abnormal chest wall from scoliosis or severe injury to chest wall

Respiratory failure is classified on the basis of acuity. Acute respiratory failure is the result of a sudden, catastrophic event. Chronic respiratory failure is the result of a gradual worsening of respiratory function. Acute on chronic respiratory failure occurs when a patient has chronic respiratory failure that has decompensated or deteriorated.

EXAMPLE

Patient presents to the emergency room (ER) in acute respiratory failure and is admitted. Following admission, the patient was started on antibiotics for pneumonia, 518.81, 486.

(Per guidelines, if both the respiratory failure and another acute condition are equally responsible for occasioning the admission, the guidelines regarding two or more diagnoses that equally meet the definition for principal diagnosis may be applied in these situations).

EXAMPLE

Patient is admitted from the clinic for intravenous (IV) antibiotics for pneumonia. A couple of hours after admission, the patient deteriorated and developed acute respiratory failure, 486, 518.81.

EXAMPLE

Patient is admitted to the hospital in acute respiratory failure and is found to have suffered a myocardial infarction, 410.91, 518.81, or 518.81, 410.91.

(Per guidelines, if both the respiratory failure and another acute condition are equally responsible for occasioning the admission, the guidelines regarding two or more diagnoses that equally meet the definition for principal diagnosis may be applied in these situations).

Lung Involvement in Conditions Classified Elsewhere

Code 516.1 and code category 517 identify conditions that affect the lung that are caused by other diseases. These codes are identified by *italics,* with instructions to "code first underlying disease." Examples of these codes are shown in Figures 13-8 and 13-9.

EXAMPLE

Systemic lupus erythematosus that has affected the patient's lungs, 710.0, 517.8.

EXERCISE 13-5

Assign codes to the following conditions using your ICD-9-CM code book.

1. Empyema ______________
2. Sickle cell disease with vaso-occlusive crisis with acute chest syndrome ______________
3. Tracheal stenosis due to tracheostomy ______________
4. Acute respiratory failure due to pneumonia; patient was intubated and was placed on mechanical ventilation for 48 hours; the respiratory failure developed after admission ______________
5. Asthma with allergic rhinitis ______________
6. Acute respiratory failure due to Lou Gehrig's disease ______________
7. Acute respiratory distress following surgery ______________
8. Acute on chronic respiratory failure in patient with severe emphysema; patient is oxygen dependent ______________
9. Acute pulmonary edema following surgery ______________
10. Respiratory failure due to exacerbation of COPD ______________

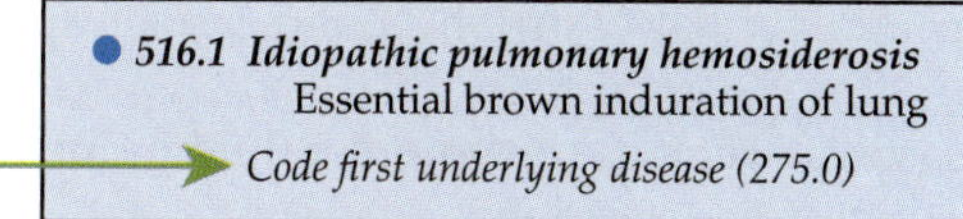

● *516.1 Idiopathic pulmonary hemosiderosis*
Essential brown induration of lung
Code first underlying disease (275.0)

Figure 13-8. Manifestation code for hemosiderosis.

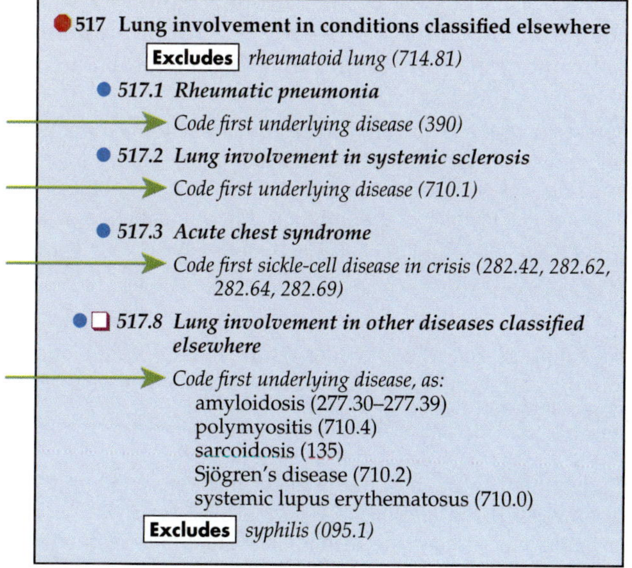

● **517 Lung involvement in conditions classified elsewhere**
Excludes *rheumatoid lung (714.81)*
● ***517.1 Rheumatic pneumonia***
Code first underlying disease (390)
● ***517.2 Lung involvement in systemic sclerosis***
Code first underlying disease (710.1)
● ***517.3 Acute chest syndrome***
Code first sickle-cell disease in crisis (282.42, 282.62, 282.64, 282.69)
● ❑ ***517.8 Lung involvement in other diseases classified elsewhere***
Code first underlying disease, as:
amyloidosis (277.30–277.39)
polymyositis (710.4)
sarcoidosis (135)
Sjögren's disease (710.2)
systemic lupus erythematosus (710.0)
Excludes *syphilis (095.1)*

Figure 13-9. Manifestation lung involvement codes for conditions classified elsewhere.

V CODES

In the past, V codes have been considered for use primarily in the outpatient setting. This has changed with the addition of more V codes each year. As was discussed in Chapter 8, it is difficult to locate V codes in the Index. Coders will often say, "I did not know there was a V code for that." Refer to Chapter 8 for a listing of common main terms to locate V codes.

V codes that may be used with diseases of the respiratory system include the following:

V10.11	Personal history of malignant neoplasm—bronchus and lung
V10.12	Personal history of malignant neoplasm—trachea
V10.20	Personal history of malignant neoplasm—respiratory organ, unspecified
V10.21	Personal history of malignant neoplasm—larynx
V10.22	Personal history of malignant neoplasm—nasal cavities, middle ear, and accessory sinuses
V10.29	Personal history of malignant neoplasm—other
V12.6	Personal history of disease of respiratory system
V15.82	History of tobacco use
V15.84	History of exposure to asbestos
V16.1	Family history of malignant neoplasm—trachea, bronchus, and lung
V16.2	Family history of malignant neoplasm—other respiratory and intrathoracic organs
V17.5	Family history of asthma
V17.6	Family history of other chronic respiratory conditions
V42.5	Organ or tissue replaced by transplant—lung
V43.81	Organ or tissue replaced by other means—larynx

V44.0	Artificial opening status—tracheostomy
V45.76	Acquired absence of organ—lung
V46.0	Other dependence on machines—aspirator
V46.11	Other dependence on machines—respirator, status
V46.12	Encounter for respiratory dependence during power failure
V46.2	Other dependence on machines—supplemental oxygen
V47.2	Other cardiorespiratory problems
V55.0	Attention to artificial openings—tracheostomy
V57.0	Care involving use of rehabilitation procedures—breathing exercises
V58.44	Aftercare following organ transplant
V58.74	Aftercare following surgery of the respiratory system, not elsewhere classified (NEC)
V64.42	Thoracoscopic surgical procedure converted to open procedure
V72.82	Preoperative respiratory examination
V76.0	Special screening for malignant neoplasms—respiratory organs
V81.3	Special screening for chronic bronchitis and emphysema
V81.4	Special screening for other and unspecified respiratory conditions

EXAMPLE Exposure to asbestos, V15.84

EXERCISE 13-6

Assign codes to the following conditions using your ICD-9-CM code book.

1. Status post lung transplant ____________
2. Preoperative examination to assess COPD status prior to elective surgery for cholelithiasis ____________
3. Patient has a tracheostomy and is dependent on a respirator ____________
4. Personal history of lung cancer with previous surgery to remove lung; no recurrence ____________
5. Family history of asthma ____________

COMMON TREATMENTS

Smoking cessation may be beneficial in the prevention of exacerbations and progression of many respiratory conditions. Annual vaccinations against influenza and a once-only vaccination against bacterial pneumococcal pneumonia may help prevent the pulmonary complications of infection.

CONDITION	MEDICATION/TREATMENT
Sinusitis	Decongestant to help sinuses drain; antibiotics
Bronchitis	If viral—rest, fluids, cough medicine If bacterial—an antibiotic may be prescribed
Asthmatic bronchitis	Bronchodilators, steroids, and antibiotics for acute infection
Chronic bronchitis	Bronchodilators, steroids, and antibiotics for acute infection
Emphysema	Bronchodilators, steroids, oxygen therapy, and antibiotics for acute infection
Asthma	Inhalers, nebulizers, and steroids
Pneumonia	Sputum culture and antibiotics, if suspected to be bacterial
Influenza	Influenza vaccination, nasal swab, amantadine, zanamivir, and treatment of symptoms
Respiratory failure	Oxygen, mechanical ventilation, treatment of underlying cause
Pleural effusion	Treatment of underlying cause
Pulmonary edema	Treatment of underlying cause

PROCEDURES

Some of the procedures that may be related to diseases of the respiratory system may be located in the following chapters of the Procedure Tabular:

5. Operations on the Respiratory System (30-34)

Mechanical Ventilation

Mechanical ventilation is the use of a machine to induce alternating inflation and deflation of the lungs for the purpose of regulating the exchange rate of gases in the blood. The most common type of ventilator (or respirator) delivers inspiratory gases directly into the person's airway. Mechanical ventilation codes are time based as follows:

- Continuous mechanical ventilation of unspecified duration 96.70
- Continuous mechanical ventilation for less than 96 consecutive hours 96.71
- Continuous mechanical ventilation for 96 consecutive hours or longer 96.72

Instructions are provided for coding of any associated endotracheal tube insertions or tracheostomy. Specific instructions also explain the calculation of mechanical ventilator hours. To calculate the number of hours (duration) of continuous mechanical ventilation during a hospitalization, begin the count from the start of the (endotracheal) intubation. The duration ends with (endotracheal) extubation. If a patient is intubated prior to admission, begin counting the duration from time of admission. If a patient is transferred (discharged) while intubated, the duration would end at the time of transfer (discharge).

For patients who have been (endotracheal) intubated and subsequently undergo a tracheostomy, duration begins with the (endotracheal) intubation and ends when the mechanical ventilation is turned off (after the weaning period).

In a patient with a tracheostomy, to calculate the number of hours of continuous mechanical ventilation during hospitalization, begin counting the duration when mechanical ventilation is started. Duration ends when the mechanical ventilator is turned off (after the weaning period). If a patient has received a tracheostomy prior to admission and is on mechanical ventilation at the time of admission, begin counting the duration from the time of admission. If a patient is transferred (discharged) while still on mechanical ventilation via tracheostomy, duration would end at the time of transfer (discharge).

For certain procedures or for particular patients, mechanical ventilation may be used during surgery and in the immediate postoperative period. Per *Coding Clinic* (1992:2Q:p14),[8] mechanical ventilation during surgery does not require a code assignment, unless the ventilation is required for "an extended period (several days)" during the post surgical period. *Coding Clinic* (2004:3Q:p11)[9] states "the term 'several' is defined as more than two. Therefore, unless the physician has clearly documented an unexpected extended period of mechanical ventilation (several days), do not assign a code for the mechanical ventilation."

If ventilation is required for a longer period than normal, a medical reason for continuing on ventilation should be documented. If this is not well documented, the coder may have to query the physician. To calculate the hours, begin counting from the time of intubation.

If a patient has been extubated and is no longer on mechanical ventilation, but his or her condition deteriorates, requiring reintubation and mechanical ventilation, this would begin a new ventilation period, and a second code based on hours of ventilation would be assigned, per *Coding Clinic* (1991:4Q:p16-21).[10]

EXAMPLE

Patient was intubated and placed on mechanical ventilation for respiratory failure due to myasthenia gravis. Patient was ventilated for 3 days, 518.81, 358.00, 96.71, 96.04.

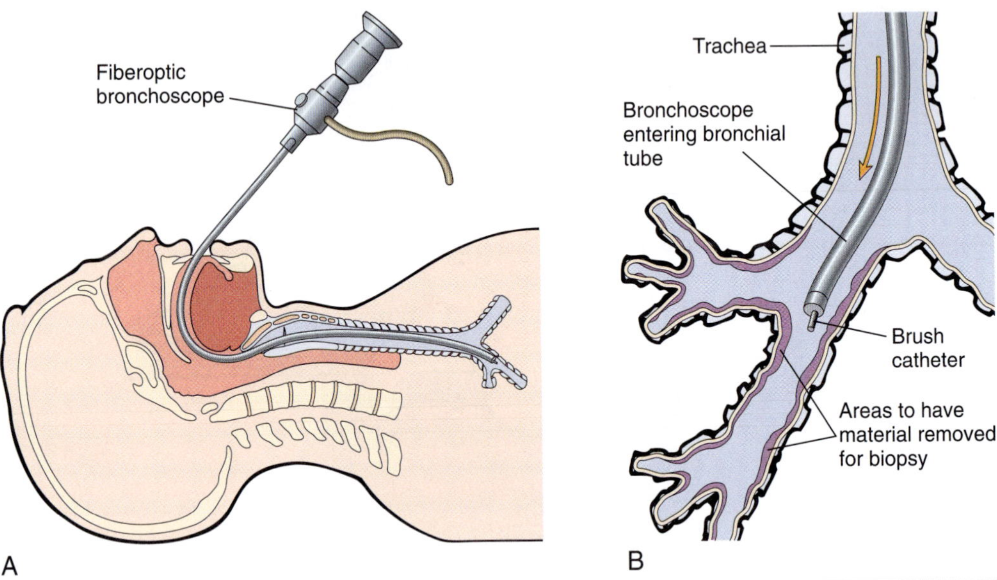

Figure 13-10. **A,** Fiberoptic bronchoscopy—a bronchoscope is passed through the nose, throat, larynx, and trachea into the bronchus. **B,** A bronchoscope with a brush catheter, ready for biopsy of bronchial tissue.

Bronchoscopy

Bronchoscopy is a diagnostic endoscopic procedure in which a tube with a tiny camera on the end is inserted through the nose or mouth into the lungs (Figure 13-10). Different procedure codes are available for a bronchoscopy done through a tracheostomy. This procedure provides a view of the airways of the lung and allows doctors to collect lung secretions or tissue specimens (biopsy). Bronchoalveolar lavage (BAL) is done via bronchoscope. Fluid is squirted into a small part of the lung and is recollected for cytologic examination, microscopy, and culture. Bronchoalveolar lavage is very useful for diagnosing infections such as *P. carinii* pneumonia (PCP) in a patient with HIV/AIDS.

EXAMPLE Bronchoalveolar lavage confirmed the diagnosis of PCP in a patient with AIDS, 042, 136.3, 33.24.

EXAMPLE Transbronchial biopsy of the lung, which confirmed carcinoma of the lung, 162.9, 33.27.

Thoracentesis

Thoracentesis is puncture of the chest wall to remove fluid (pleural effusion) from the space between the lining of the outside of the lungs (pleura) and the wall of the chest (Figure 13-11). Physicians may perform a diagnostic thoracentesis or a therapeutic thoracentesis. The fluid collected is sent to the laboratory for analysis. This may also relieve any shortness of breath caused by compression on the lung by the fluid.

EXAMPLE Patient with pneumonia and large right pleural effusion requiring thoracentesis, 486, 511.9, 34.91.

Thoracostomy

Tube thoracostomy is the term used for insertion of chest tube(s) to drain blood, fluid, or air, and to allow full expansion of the lungs. A tube is placed between the ribs and into the space between the inner lining and the outer lining of the lung (pleural space); fluid is

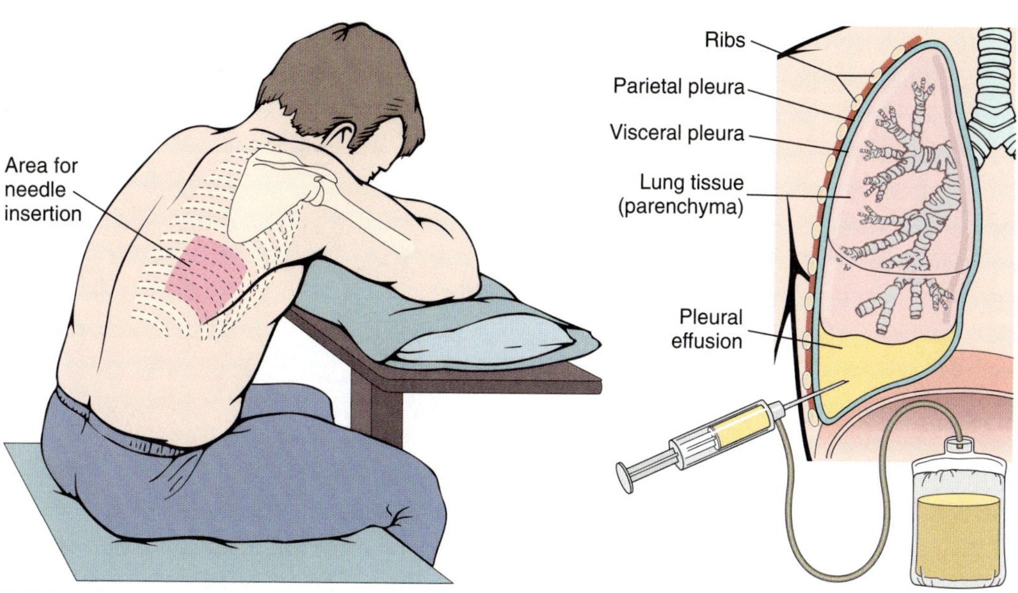

Figure 13-11. Thoracentesis. The needle is inserted close to the base of the effusion so that gravity will help with drainage.

allowed to drain. A suction machine may be used to facilitate drainage. Reasons why chest tubes may be used include pneumothorax, hemothorax, abscess, empyema, and cancer; they also may be used after surgery.

EXAMPLE Insertion of chest tube for continuous drainage of empyema, 510.9, 34.04.

Tracheostomy

Tracheostomy is a procedure in which an artificial opening is made in the front of the windpipe (trachea) through the skin of the neck (Figure 13-12). A tube is inserted, through which breathing may continue until the normal airway can be restored. A tracheostomy may be performed during an emergency at the patient's bedside. In some cases, a tracheostomy is planned and is performed in the operating room (OR). If it is not documented as a permanent tracheostomy, the code for temporary or unspecified tracheostomy should be assigned. If any question arises about the type of tracheostomy, a physician query may be necessary.

EXAMPLE Temporary tracheostomy was performed in the OR because of the patient's recurrent aspiration pneumonitis, 507.0, 31.1.

Pulmonary Resection

The type of pulmonary resection undertaken may depend on the condition that is being diagnosed and/or treated. Wedge resection (Figure 13-13, *A*) is the removal of a small, localized area of diseased tissue near the surface of the lung. Segmental resection (Figure 13-13, *B*) involves the removal of a bronchiole and its alveoli in one or more lung segments. Removal of an entire lobe of the lung is a lobectomy (Figure 13-13, *C*), and the removal of an entire lung is known as pneumonectomy (Figure 13-13, *D*).

A surgical technique known as video-assisted thoracic surgery (VATS) has allowed surgeons to perform thoracic surgery in a minimally invasive manner. Depending on the type of procedure performed, a hospital stay may last only 1 to 3 days, intensive care may not be needed, and recovery may be quicker. Patients may return to their normal activities much sooner than when an "open" procedure is performed.

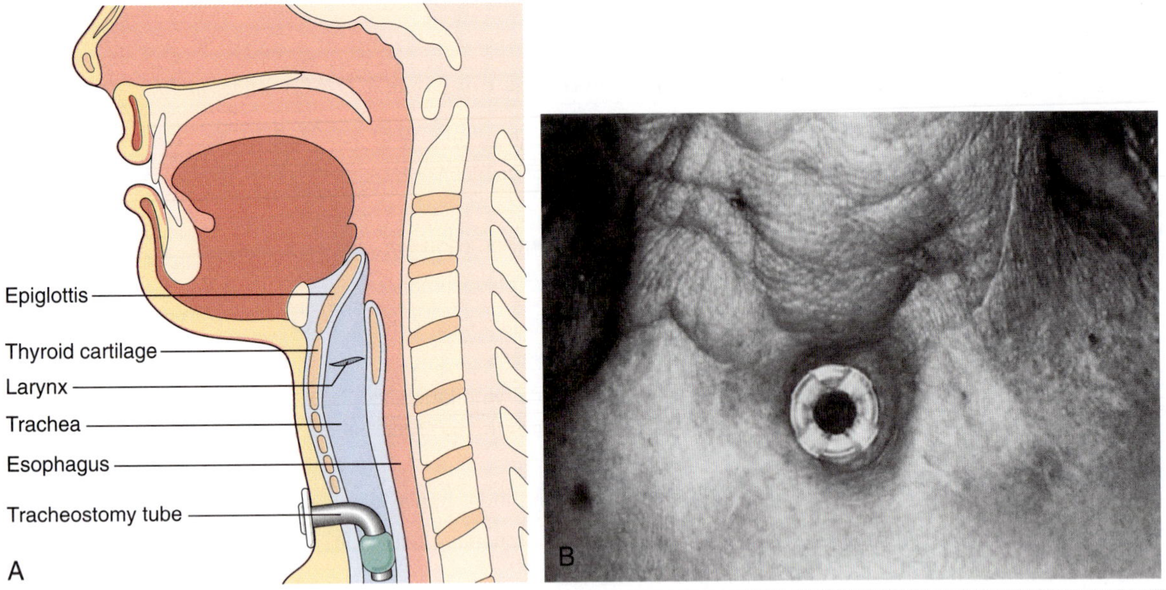

Figure 13-12. **A,** Tracheostomy with tube in place. **B,** Healed tracheostomy incision.

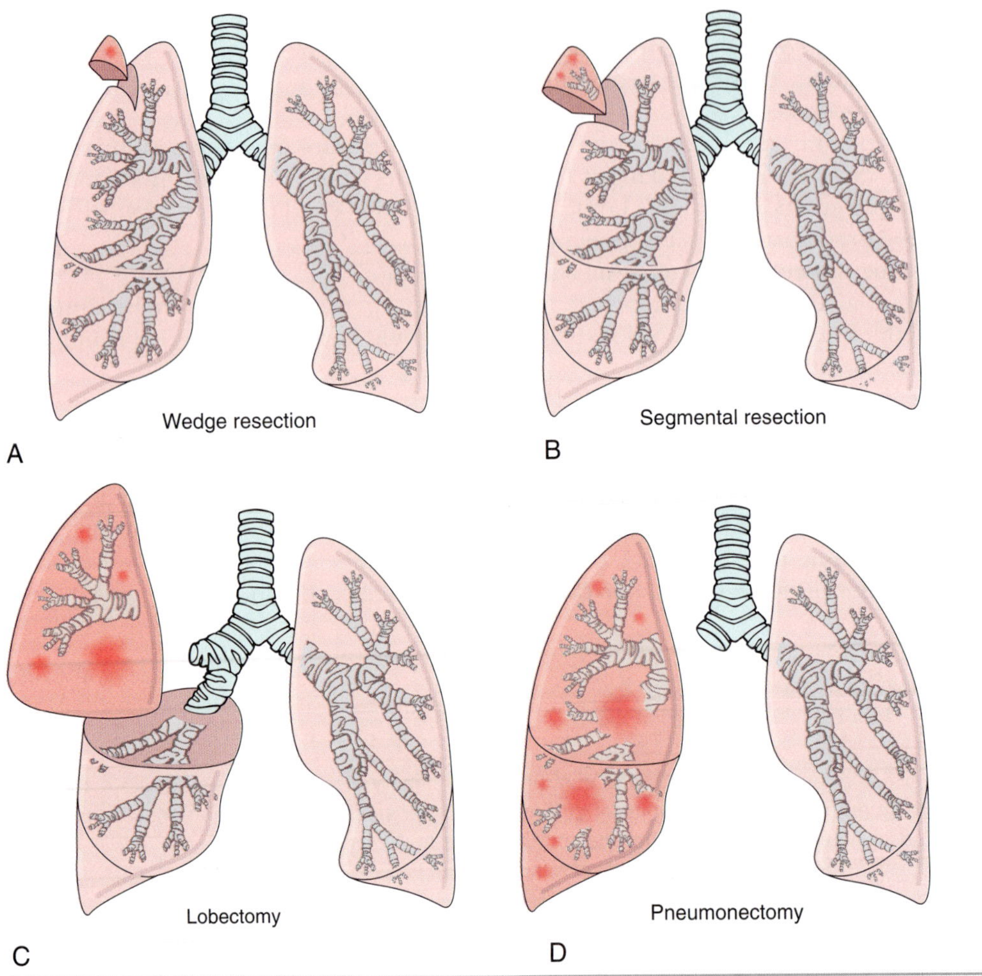

Figure 13-13. Pulmonary resections. **A,** Wedge resection. **B,** Segmental resection. **C,** Lobectomy. **D,** Pneumonectomy.

EXERCISE 13-7

Assign codes for all diagnosis and procedures using your ICD-9-CM code book.

1. Thoracoscopy with removal of lung cancer (lower lobe) ____________
2. Pleurodesis with administration of talc for recurrent spontaneous pneumothorax ____________
3. Diagnostic thoracentesis for large pleural effusion ____________
4. Bronchial alveolar lavage to assess type of pneumonia ____________
5. Temporary tracheostomy in patient with laryngeal cancer who will be having surgery in a couple of weeks ____________
6. Endotracheal intubation with mechanical ventilation for 3 days because of acute respiratory failure due to exacerbation of congestive heart failure ____________
7. Lobectomy for squamous cell carcinoma lung, upper lobe ____________
8. Transbronchial biopsy of the lung and bronchus; histologic exam confirms pulmonary tuberculosis ____________

DOCUMENTATION/REIMBURSEMENT/MS-DRGs

Often, coding difficulties are due to lack of documentation. Sometimes pathology and other test results are not available at the time of discharge, or when the physician is dictating the discharge summary or is reporting the final diagnoses.

Assigning the correct code to identify the COPD can be difficult because of conflicting documentation. Physicians frequently use the general term COPD rather than more specific terminology.

Documentation of pneumonia and the causative organism or sputum culture results may not be directly linked, making it necessary to query the physician. Physicians often document exacerbation of COPD but fail to document any condition that may be responsible for the exacerbation such as pneumonia.

It may be difficult to calculate mechanical ventilation time with the use of physician documentation, and it may be necessary to use respiratory therapy notes to determine the exact length of time. It is also possible that a patient could have more than one continuous episode of ventilation.

Procedures that can be performed at bedside such as tracheostomy, thoracentesis, and insertion of a chest tube may not be well documented by the physician or may be documented only within a progress note and therefore are easy to miss.

An abnormal laboratory test may not necessarily be clinically significant. If abnormal laboratory tests are noted and treatment is given, it would be appropriate to query the physician regarding the abnormal laboratory test(s). An abnormal laboratory test must be clinically significant to be coded, per *Coding Clinic* (1990:2Q:p15-16).[11]

Pneumonia and Causative Organism

EXAMPLE

Patient has a long history of chronic obstructive pulmonary disease and was admitted for the treatment of pneumonia. Sputum cultures grew *Klebsiella.* The physician should be queried to determine whether the pneumonia is due to *Klebsiella.* The patient's COPD was treated due to flare up.

DIAGNOSES	CODES	MS-DRG	RW
Pneumonia in patient with COPD	486, 491.21	194	1.0235
Klebsiella pneumonia with COPD	482.0, 491.21	178	1.5636

The causative organism of pneumonia can make a significant difference in the MS-DRG assignment. Also, the presence of a complication/comorbidity such as an exacerbation of COPD can make a difference in reimbursement, depending on the principal diagnosis and the MS-DRG assigned.

Two Diagnoses That Equally Meet the Definition for Principal Diagnosis

EXAMPLE

Patient was admitted with aspiration pneumonia and *pneumococcal* pneumonia. Patient had severe gastroesophageal reflux disease (GERD). The patient was admitted with both types of pneumonia, and both diagnoses fit the definition of principal diagnosis.

DIAGNOSES	CODES	MS-DRG	RW
Aspiration pneumonia with *pneumococcal* pneumonia	507.0, 481, 530.81	179	1.2754
Pneumococcal pneumonia with aspiration pneumonia	481, 507.0, 530.81	195	0.8398

Note that the aspiration pneumonia groups to an MS-DRG with a higher weight. If both pneumonias meet the definition of a principal diagnosis, it is perfectly acceptable to sequence aspiration pneumonia as the principal. If a patient was admitted with *pneumococcal* pneumonia, and a couple of days after admission aspirated and developed aspiration pneumonia, *pneumococcal* pneumonia is the principal diagnosis and aspiration pneumonia is a secondary diagnosis.

MS-DRG With and Without MCC/CC

In other MS-DRGs, either of the pneumonia diagnoses would qualify as complications/comorbidities, but with pneumonia as the principal and pneumonia as a secondary diagnosis, these case scenarios are grouped into MS-DRGs without complications/comorbidities. Further optimization could be accomplished by reviewing the chart for additional diagnoses, as in the following example:

EXAMPLE

Patient was admitted with aspiration pneumonia and *pneumococcal* pneumonia. Patient has severe GERD. The patient was admitted with both types of pneumonia, and both diagnoses fit the definition of principal diagnosis. It is noted on the history and physical that the patient has a chronic kidney disease, stage IV.

DIAGNOSES	CODES	MS-DRG	RW
Aspiration pneumonia with *pneumococcal* pneumonia	507.0, 481, 530.81, 585.4	178	1.5636
Pneumococcal pneumonia with aspiration pneumonia	481, 507.0, 530.81, 585.4	194	1.0235

Both MS-DRGs are optimized by the addition of 585.4 (CKD), which is a complication/comorbidity in these cases. The difference in relative weight when aspiration pneumonia is sequenced as the principal diagnosis should also be noted.

Frequently missed complications/comorbidities from the respiratory chapter include the following:

- Atelectasis
- Bronchiectasis with acute exacerbation
- Bronchitis, chronic, with exacerbation
- COPD exacerbation
- Effusion, pleural
- Failure, respiratory
- Pneumonia
- Pneumothorax

Respiratory Failure Versus Another Acute Condition

EXAMPLE

Patient was admitted with acute respiratory failure due to pneumonia.

(Per guidelines, if both the respiratory failure and another acute condition are equally responsible for occasioning the admission, the guidelines regarding two or more diagnoses that equally meet the definition for principal diagnosis may be applied in these situations).

DIAGNOSES	CODES	MS-DRG	RW
Respiratory failure due to pneumonia	518.81, 486	189	1.3660
Pneumonia with respiratory failure	486, 518.81	193	1.2505

In this case, either the respiratory failure or the pneumonia could be selected as the principal diagnosis; the reimbursement is higher if the respiratory failure is the principal diagnosis. In MS-DRG 193, the respiratory failure is an MCC.

CHAPTER REVIEW EXERCISE

Assign codes for all diagnoses and procedures, including all applicable V and E codes and procedures.

1. Cough due to *Streptococcus pneumoniae* pneumonia ____________
2. Patient with severe emphysema who is dependent on oxygen; quit smoking 5 years ago ____________
3. Patient is high risk for lung disease due to on-the-job exposure to asbestos, patient has a 20–pack-year history of smoking, currently active ____________
4. Croup ____________
5. Tonsillar abscess. Abscess was drained. ____________
6. Patient with whooping cough has pneumonia ____________
7. *Haemophilus influenzae* pneumonia in a patient who is being treated for influenza ____________
8. Edema larynx ____________
9. Status asthmaticus ____________
10. Bronchospasm with acute exacerbation of COPD ____________
11. Acute on chronic respiratory failure due to sarcoidosis involving the lungs; mechanical ventilation for 3 days; patient was intubated at transferring facility and transferred for evaluation of sarcoidosis ____________
12. Restrictive airway disease ____________
13. Inhalation anthrax with pneumonia ____________
14. Bronchiolitis obliterans organizing pneumonia ____________
15. Acute and chronic sinusitis ____________
16. Chronic tonsillitis and adenitis; tonsillectomy with adenoidectomy performed ____________
17. Nasal cavity polyps with polypectomy ____________
18. Lung nodule ____________
19. Empyema with insertion of chest tubes; empyema was due to *Staphylococcus aureus* ____________
20. Double lung transplant for diffuse idiopathic pulmonary fibrosis; cardiopulmonary bypass was performed in this transplant from a cadaver ____________

21. Congestive heart failure with left pleural effusion that was treated with thoracentesis at bedside ____________

22. Granuloma lung ____________

23. Iatrogenic pneumothorax ____________

24. Acute bronchitis with chronic obstructive bronchitis ____________

25. Postoperative pulmonary edema ____________

Write the correct answer(s) in the space(s) provided.

26. Define contamination of a culture.

____

27. Define empiric treatment.

____

28. Define iatrogenic.

____

29. List two problems/conditions that could cause a patient to aspirate.

____

____

30. List two terms that describe status asthmaticus.

____

____

CHAPTER GLOSSARY

Asbestosis: lung disease due to inhalation of asbestos.

Aspiration pneumonia: inflammation of the lungs and bronchial tubes due to aspiration of foreign material into the lung.

Asthma: chronic disease that affects the airways that carry air into and out of the lungs.

Asthmatic bronchitis: underlying asthmatic problem in patients in whom asthma has become so persistent that clinically significant chronic airflow obstruction is present despite antiasthmatic therapy.

Baritosis: lung disease due to inhalation of barium.

Black lung: lung disease due to inhalation of coal dust.

Bronchi: the two air tubes that branch off the trachea and deliver air to both lungs.

Bronchitis: lower respiratory tract or bronchial tree infection characterized by cough, sputum production, and wheezing.

Bronchoscopy: diagnostic endoscopic procedure in which a tube with a tiny camera on the end is inserted through the nose or mouth into the lungs.

Chronic bronchitis: condition defined by a mucus-producing cough most days of the month, 3 months out of a year for 2 successive years, with no other underlying disease to explain the cough.

Chronic obstructive pulmonary disease: general term used to describe a lung disease in which the airways become obstructed, making it difficult for air to get into and out of the lungs.

Chylothorax: milky fluid consisting of lymph and fat (chyle) that accumulates in the pleural space.

Coal workers' pneumoconiosis: lung disease due to inhalation of coal dust.

Community-acquired pneumonia: broad term used to define pneumonias that are contracted outside of the hospital or nursing home setting.

Contaminant: a cultured organism that a physician does not believe is responsible for causing a particular infection.

Diaphragm: dome-shaped muscles at the bottom of the lungs that assist in the process of breathing and in the exchange of oxygen/carbon dioxide.

Emphysema: chronic lung disease of gradual onset that can be attributed to chronic infection and inflammation or irritation from cigarette smoke.

Empiric: initiation of treatment prior to making a definite diagnosis.

Empyema: pus that accumulates in the pleural space.

Hemothorax: blood that accumulates in the pleural space.

Iatrogenic: caused by medical treatment.

Infection: invasion of the body by organisms that have the potential to cause disease.

Influenza: contagious viral infection of the respiratory tract that causes coughing, difficulty breathing, headache, muscle aches, and weakness.

Lobar pneumonia: synonym for pneumococcal pneumonia or pneumonia due to *Streptococcus pneumoniae.*

Mechanical ventilation: use of a machine to induce alternating inflation and deflation of the lungs, to regulate the exchange rate of gases in the blood.

Nosocomial pneumonia: pneumonia that is acquired while the patient is residing in a hospital-type setting.

Nursing home–acquired pneumonia: pneumonia that is acquired in a nursing home or extended care facility.

Pleural effusion: fluid that accumulates in the pleural space because of trauma or disease.

Pneumoconioses: lung diseases due to chronic inhalation of inorganic (mineral) dust that are often due to occupational exposure.

Pneumonia: infection of the lungs that may be caused by a variety of organisms, including viruses, bacteria, and parasites.

Pneumothorax: air in space around the lung.

Pulmonary edema: condition in which fluid accumulates in the lungs.

Respiratory failure: general term that describes ineffective gas exchange across the lungs by the respiratory system.

Respiratory system: system that supplies the body with oxygen (O_2).

Siderosis: lung disease due to inhalation of iron oxide.

Sinusitis: a condition in which the linings of one or more sinuses become infected, usually because of viruses or bacteria.

Spontaneous pneumothorax: pneumothorax that is not caused by trauma.

Stannosis: lung disease due to inhalation of tin particles.

Thoracentesis: puncture of the chest wall to remove fluid (pleural effusion) from the space between the lining of the outside of the lungs (pleura) and the wall of the chest.

Trachea (windpipe): body part that is responsible for filtering the air that we breathe.

Tracheostomy: procedure in which an artificial opening is made in the front of the windpipe (trachea) through the skin of the neck.

Tube thoracostomy: insertion of chest tube(s) to drain blood, fluid, or air and allow full expansion of the lungs.

CHAPTER 14

Diseases of the Circulatory System

(ICD-9-CM Chapter 7, Codes 390-459)

CHAPTER OUTLINE

LEARNING OBJECTIVES

- Apply and assign the correct ICD-9-CM codes in accordance with Official Guidelines for Coding and Reporting
- Identify pertinent anatomy and physiology of the circulatory system
- Identify diseases of the circulatory system
- Assign the correct V codes and procedure codes related to the circulatory system
- Identify common treatments, medications, laboratory values, and diagnostic tests
- Explain the importance of documentation in relation to MS-DRGs for reimbursement

ABBREVIATIONS

ACS acute coronary syndrome
AF atrial fibrillation
AICD automatic implantable cardioverter-defibrillator
AIDS acquired immunodeficiency syndrome
AMI acute myocardial infarction
AV atrioventricular
AVM arteriovenous malformation
AVR aortic valve replacement
BNP brain natriuretic peptide
BP blood pressure
CAB coronary artery bypass
CABG coronary artery bypass graft
CAD coronary artery disease
CAT computerized axial tomography
CCU coronary care unit
CHF congestive heart failure
CKD chronic kidney disease
COPD chronic obstructive pulmonary disease
CPK creatine phosphokinase
CPK-MB creatine phosphokinase, isoenzyme MB
CRT cardiac resynchronization therapy
CRT-D cardiac resynchronization treatment defibrillator
CRT-P cardiac resynchronization treatment pacemaker
CT computerized tomography
CVA cerebrovascular accident
CVL central venous line
CXR chest x-ray
DES drug-eluting stent
DOE dyspnea on exertion
DM diabetes mellitus
DVT deep vein thrombosis
EKG/ECG electrocardiogram
EP electrophysiologic
ER Emergency Room
HCVD hypertensive cardiovascular disease
HTN hypertension
ICD internal cardiac defibrillator
ICV implantable cardioverter
IV intravenous
IVDU intravenous drug user
LAD left anterior descending
LCA left coronary artery
MI myocardial infarction
MRI magnetic resonance imaging
MS-DRG Medicare Severity diagnosis-related group
MUGA multiple-gated acquisition
MVR mitral valve replacement
NQMI non–Q wave myocardial infarction
NSTEMI non–ST elevation myocardial infarction
OM obtuse marginal
OSA obstructive sleep apnea
PCI percutaneous coronary intervention
PDA posterior descending artery
PHT pulmonary hypertension
PICC peripherally inserted central catheter
PPH primary pulmonary hypertension
PTCA percutaneous transluminal coronary angioplasty
RA right atrium
RBBB right bundle branch block
RCA right coronary artery
RFA radiofrequency ablation
RHD rheumatic heart disease
RW relative weight
SOB shortness of breath
SSS sick sinus syndrome
STEMI ST elevation myocardial infarction
SVT supraventricular tachycardia
TIA transient ischemic attack
TPA tissue plasminogen activator
TPN total parenteral nutrition
USA unstable angina

ICD-9-CM Official Guidelines for Coding and Reporting

Please refer to the companion Evolve website for the most current guidelines.

7. **Chapter 7: Diseases of Circulatory System (390-459)**
   a. **Hypertension**
      Hypertension Table
      The Hypertension Table (Figure 14-1), found under the main term, "Hypertension", in the Alphabetic Index, contains a complete listing of all conditions due to or associated with hypertension and classifies them according to malignant, benign, and unspecified.
      1) **Hypertension, Essential, or NOS**
         Assign hypertension (arterial) (essential) (primary) (systemic) (NOS) to category code 401 with the appropriate fourth digit to indicate malignant (.0), benign (.1), or unspecified (.9). Do not use either .0 malignant or .1 benign unless medical record documentation supports such a designation.

EXAMPLE Hypertension, 401.9.

EXAMPLE Malignant hypertension, 401.0.

EXAMPLE Benign hypertension, 401.1.

SECTION I INDEX TO DISEASES / Hypertension, hypertensive

	Malignant	Benign	Unspecified
Hypertension, hypertensive (arterial) (arteriolar) (crisis) (degeneration) (disease) (essential) (fluctuating) (idiopathic) (intermittent) (labile) (low renin) (orthostatic) (paroxysmal) (primary) (systemic) (uncontrolled) (vascular)	401.0	401.1	401.9
with			
chronic kidney disease	-	-	-
stage I through stage IV, or unspecified	403.00	403.10	403.90
stage V or end stage renal disease	403.01	403.11	403.91
heart involvement (conditions classifiable to 429.0–429.3, 429.8, 429.9 due to hypertension) (*see also* Hypertension, heart)	402.00	402.10	402.90
with kidney involvement - *see* Hypertension, cardiorenal			
renal involvement (only conditions classifiable to 585, 586, 587) (excludes conditions classifiable to 584) (*see also* Hypertension, kidney)	403.00	403.10	403.90
with heart involvement - *see* Hypertension, cardiorenal			
failure (and sclerosis) (*see also* Hypertension, kidney)	403.01	403.11	403.91
sclerosis without failure (*see also* Hypertension, kidney)	403.00	403.10	403.90
accelerated (*see also* Hypertension, by type, malignant)	401.0	-	-
antepartum - *see* Hypertension, complicating pregnancy, childbirth, or the puerperium			
cardiorenal (disease)	404.00	404.10	404.90
with			
chronic kidney disease	-	-	-
stage I through stage IV, or unspecified	404.00	404.10	404.90
and heart failure	404.01	404.11	404.91
stage V or end stage renal disease	404.02	404.12	404.92
and heart failure	404.03	404.13	404.93
heart failure	404.01	404.11	404.91
and chronic kidney disease	404.02	404.12	404.92
stage I through stage IV or unspecified	404.02	404.12	404.92
stage V or end stage renal disease	404.03	404.13	404.93
cardiovascular disease (arteriosclerotic) (sclerotic)	402.00	402.10	402.90
with			
heart failure	402.01	402.11	402.91
renal involvement (conditions classifiable to 403) (*see also* Hypertension, cardiorenal)	404.00	404.10	404.90
cardiovascular renal (disease) (sclerosis) (*see also* Hypertension, cardiorenal)	404.00	404.10	404.90
cerebrovascular disease NEC	437.2	437.2	437.2
complicating pregnancy, childbirth, or the puerperium	642.2	642.0	642.9
with			
albuminuria (and edema) (mild)	-	-	642.4
severe	-	-	642.5
chronic kidney disease	642.2	642.2	642.2
and heart disease	642.2	642.2	642.2
edema (mild)	-	-	642.4
severe	-	-	642.5
heart disease	642.2	642.2	642.2
and chronic kidney disease	642.2	642.2	642.2
renal disease	642.2	642.2	642.2
and heart disease	642.2	642.2	642.2
chronic	642.2	642.0	642.0
with pre-eclampsia or eclampsia	642.7	642.7	642.7
fetus or newborn	760.0	760.0	760.0
essential	-	642.0	642.0
with pre-eclampsia or eclampsia	-	642.7	642.7
fetus or newborn	760.0	760.0	760.0
fetus or newborn	760.0	760.0	760.0
gestational	-	-	642.3
pre-existing	642.2	642.0	642.0
with pre-eclampsia or eclampsia	642.7	642.7	642.7
fetus or newborn	760.0	760.0	760.0
secondary to renal disease	642.1	642.1	642.1
with pre-eclampsia or eclampsia	642.7	642.7	642.7
fetus or newborn	760.0	760.0	760.0
transient	-	-	642.3
due to			
aldosteronism, primary	405.09	405.19	405.99
brain tumor	405.09	405.19	405.99
bulbar poliomyelitis	405.09	405.19	405.99
calculus			
kidney	405.09	405.19	405.99
ureter	405.09	405.19	405.99
coarctation, aorta	405.09	405.19	405.99
Cushing's disease	405.09	405.19	405.99
glomerulosclerosis (*see also* Hypertension, kidney)	403.00	403.10	403.90
periarteritis nodosa	405.09	405.19	405.99
pheochromocytoma	405.09	405.19	405.99
polycystic kidney(s)	405.09	405.19	405.99
polycythemia	405.09	405.19	405.99
porphyria	405.09	405.19	405.99
pyelonephritis	405.09	405.19	405.99
renal (artery)			
aneurysm	405.01	405.11	405.91
anomaly	405.01	405.11	405.91
embolism	405.01	405.11	405.91

Figure 14-1. Hypertension table in Alphabetic Index.

2) Hypertension with Heart Disease

Heart conditions (425.8, 429.0-429.3, 429.8, 429.9) are assigned to a code from category 402 when a causal relationship is stated (due to hypertension) or implied (hypertensive). Use an additional code from category 428 to identify the type of heart failure in those patients with heart failure. More than one code from category 428 may be assigned if the patient has systolic or diastolic failure and congestive heart failure.

The same heart conditions (425.8, 429.0-429.3, 429.8, 429.9) with hypertension, but without a stated causal relationship, are coded separately. Sequence according to the circumstances of the admission/encounter.

EXAMPLE Congestive heart failure due to hypertensive heart disease, 402.91, 428.0.

EXAMPLE Congestive heart failure in a patient with hypertension, 428.0, 401.9.

3) Hypertensive Chronic Kidney Disease

Assign codes from category 403, Hypertensive chronic kidney disease, when conditions classified to categories 585-587 are present. Unlike hypertension with heart disease, ICD-9-CM presumes a cause-and-effect relationship and classifies chronic kidney disease (CKD) with hypertension as hypertensive chronic kidney disease.

Fifth digits for category 403 should be assigned as follows:

- 0 with CKD stage I through stage IV, or unspecified.
- 1 with CKD stage V or end stage renal disease.

The appropriate code from category 585, Chronic kidney disease, should be used as a secondary code with a code from category 403 to identify the stage of chronic kidney disease.

See Section I.C.10.a for information on the coding of chronic kidney disease.

EXAMPLE The patient was admitted with acute renal failure. The patient was given secondary diagnoses of benign hypertension and chronic kidney disease, stage III, 584.9, 403.10, 585.3.

4) Hypertensive Heart and Chronic Kidney Disease

Assign codes from combination category 404, Hypertensive heart and chronic kidney disease, when both hypertensive kidney disease and hypertensive heart disease are stated in the diagnosis. Assume a relationship between the hypertension and the chronic kidney disease, whether or not the condition is so designated. Assign an additional code from category 428, to identify the type of heart failure. More than one code from category 428 may be assigned if the patient has systolic or diastolic failure and congestive heart failure.

Fifth digits for category 404 should be assigned as follows:

- 0 without heart failure and with chronic kidney disease (CKD) stage I through stage IV, or unspecified
- 1 with heart failure and with CKD stage I through stage IV, or unspecified
- 2 without heart failure and with CKD stage V or end stage renal disease
- 3 with heart failure and with CKD stage V or end stage renal disease

The appropriate code from category 585, Chronic kidney disease, should be used as a secondary code with a code from category 404 to identify the stage of kidney disease.

See Section I.C.10.a for information on the coding of chronic kidney disease.

5) Hypertensive Cerebrovascular Disease

First assign codes from 430-438, Cerebrovascular disease, then the appropriate hypertension code from categories 401-405.

EXAMPLE Cerebrovascular accident in a patient with malignant hypertension, 434.91, 401.0.

6) **Hypertensive Retinopathy**
Two codes are necessary to identify the condition. First assign the code from subcategory 362.11, Hypertensive retinopathy, then the appropriate code from categories 401-405 to indicate the type of hypertension.

EXAMPLE The patient is being treated for retinopathy due to labile hypertension, 362.11, 401.9.

7) **Hypertension, Secondary**
Two codes are required: one to identify the underlying etiology and one from category 405 to identify the hypertension. Sequencing of codes is determined by the reason for admission/encounter.

EXAMPLE Hypertension due to periarteritis nodosa, 446.0, 405.99.

8) **Hypertension, Transient**
Assign code 796.2, Elevated blood pressure reading without diagnosis of hypertension, unless patient has an established diagnosis of hypertension.
Assign code 642.3x for transient hypertension of pregnancy.

EXAMPLE The patient has an elevated blood pressure caused by the stress of being in an MVA, 796.2.

9) **Hypertension, Controlled**
Assign appropriate code from categories 401-405. This diagnostic statement usually refers to an existing state of hypertension under control by therapy.

EXAMPLE The patient's benign hypertension has been well controlled since the patient lost 20 pounds and started a regular exercise program, 401.1.

10) **Hypertension, Uncontrolled**
Uncontrolled hypertension may refer to untreated hypertension or hypertension not responding to current therapeutic regimen. In either case, assign the appropriate code from categories 401-405 to designate the stage and type of hypertension. Code to the type of hypertension.

EXAMPLE The patient's hypertension has been uncontrolled for the past 2 months in spite of changes in medication, 401.9.

11) Elevated Blood Pressure

For a statement of elevated blood pressure without further specificity, assign code 796.2, Elevated blood pressure reading without diagnosis of hypertension, rather than a code from category 401.

EXAMPLE The patient has high blood pressure; will recheck at next clinic visit. No medications were given, 796.2.

b. Cerebral infarction/stroke/cerebrovascular accident (CVA)

The terms stroke and CVA are often used interchangeably to refer to a cerebral infarction. The terms stroke, CVA, and cerebral infarction NOS are all indexed to the default code 434.91, Cerebral artery occlusion, unspecified, with infarction. Code 436, Acute, but ill-defined, cerebrovascular disease, should not be used when the documentation states stroke or CVA.

c. Postoperative cerebrovascular accident

A cerebrovascular hemorrhage or infarction that occurs as a result of medical intervention is coded to 997.02, Iatrogenic cerebrovascular infarction or hemorrhage. Medical record documentation should clearly specify the cause-and-effect relationship between the medical intervention and the cerebrovascular accident in order to assign this code. A secondary code from the code range 430-432 or from a code from subcategories 433 or 434 with a fifth digit of "1" should also be used to identify the type of hemorrhage or infarct.

This guideline conforms to the use additional code note instruction at category 997. Code 436, Acute, but ill-defined, cerebrovascular disease, should not be used as a secondary code with code 997.02.

EXAMPLE The patient had a postoperative cerebrovascular accident, which was embolic in nature. The patient had initially been admitted for treatment of coronary artery arteriosclerosis with CABG (left internal mammary artery and two saphenous vein grafts were used). Cardiopulmonary bypass was used during the surgery. 414.01, 997.02, 434.11, 36.12, 36.15, 39.61.

d. Late Effects of Cerebrovascular Disease

1) Category 438, Late Effects of Cerebrovascular Disease

Category 438 is used to indicate conditions classifiable to categories 430-437 as the causes of late effects (neurologic deficits), themselves classified elsewhere. These "late effects" include neurologic deficits that persist after initial onset of conditions classifiable to 430-437. The neurologic deficits caused by cerebrovascular disease may be present from the onset or may arise at any time after the onset of the condition classifiable to 430-437.

EXAMPLE Aphasia due to cerebrovascular accident 3 months ago, 438.11.

EXAMPLE The patient was admitted with left-sided hemiparesis due to a cerebrovascular accident. The patient has a history of previous CVA with residual facial droop, 434.91, 342.90, 438.83.

2) Codes from category 438 with codes from 430-437

Codes from category 438 may be assigned on a healthcare record with codes from 430-437, if the patient has a current cerebrovascular accident (CVA) and deficits from an old CVA.

3) **Code V12.54**

Assign code V12.**54, Transient ischemic attack (TIA), and cerebral infarction without residual deficits** (and not a code from category 438) as an additional code for history of cerebrovascular disease when no neurologic deficits are present.

EXAMPLE The patient had a CVA in 2002 with no residuals, V12.54.

e. Acute myocardial infarction (AMI)

1) ST elevation myocardial infarction (STEMI) and non ST elevation myocardial infarction (NSTEMI)

The ICD-9-CM codes for acute myocardial infarction (AMI) identify the site, such as anterolateral wall or true posterior wall. Subcategories 410.0-410.6 and 410.8 are used for ST elevation myocardial infarction (STEMI). Subcategory 410.7, Subendocardial infarction, is used for non ST elevation myocardial infarction (NSTEMI) and nontransmural MIs (Figure 14-2).

●**410 Acute myocardial infarction**
Includes: cardiac infarction
coronary (artery):
embolism
occlusion
rupture
thrombosis
infarction of heart, myocardium, or ventricle
rupture of heart, myocardium, or ventricle
ST elevation (STEMI) and non-ST elevation (NSTEMI) myocardial infarction
any condition classifiable to 414.1-414.9 specified as acute or with a stated duration of 8 weeks or less

The following fifth-digit subclassification is for use with category 410:

❑ **0 episode of care unspecified**
Use when the source document does not contain sufficient information for the assignment of fifth-digit 1 or 2.

1 initial episode of care
Use fifth-digit 1 to designate the first episode of care (regardless of facility site) for a newly diagnosed myocardial infarction. The fifth-digit 1 is assigned regardless of the number of times a patient may be transferred during the initial episode of care.

2 subsequent episode of care
Use fifth-digit 2 to designate an episode of care following the initial episode when the patient is admitted for further observation, evaluation, or treatment for a myocardial infarction that has received initial treatment, but is still less than 8 weeks old.

●**410.0 Of anterolateral wall**
ST elevation myocardial infarction (STEMI) of anterolateral wall

●❑**410.1 Of other anterior wall**
Infarction:
anterior (wall) NOS (with contiguous portion of intraventricular septum)
anteroapical (with contiguous portion of intraventricular septum)
anteroseptal (with contiguous portion of intraventricular septum)
ST elevation myocardial infarction (STEMI) of other anterior wall

●**410.2 Of inferolateral wall**
ST elevation myocardial infarction (STEMI) of inferolateral wall

●**410.3 Of inferoposterior wall**
ST elevation myocardial infarction (STEMI) of inferoposterior wall

●❑**410.4 Of other inferior wall**
Infarction:
diaphragmatic wall NOS (with contiguous portion of intraventricular septum)
inferior (wall) NOS (with contiguous portion of intraventricular septum)
ST elevation myocardial infarction (STEMI) of other inferior wall

●❑**410.5 Of other lateral wall**
Infarction:
apical-lateral
basal-lateral
high lateral
posterolateral
ST elevation myocardial infarction (STEMI) of other lateral wall

●**410.6 True posterior wall infarction**
Infarction:
posterobasal
strictly posterior
ST elevation myocardial infarction (STEMI) of true posterior wall

●**410.7 Subendocardial infarction**
Nontransmural infarction
Non-ST elevation myocardial infarction (NSTEMI)

●❑**410.8 Of other specified sites**
Infarction of:
atrium
papillary muscle
septum alone
ST elevation myocardial infarction (STEMI) of other specified sites

●❑**410.9 Unspecified site**
Acute myocardial infarction NOS
Coronary occlusion NOS
Myocardial infarction NOS

Figure 14-2. Tabular entry for 410, Acute myocardial infarction.

EXAMPLE The patient was admitted with NSTEMI, 410.71.

EXAMPLE The patient was admitted with anterolateral wall STEMI, 410.01.

2) **Acute myocardial infarction, unspecified**
Subcategory 410.9 is the default for the unspecified term acute myocardial infarction. If only STEMI or transmural MI without the site is documented, query the provider as to the site, or assign a code from subcategory 410.9.
3) **AMI documented as nontransmural or subendocardial but site provided**
If an AMI is documented as nontransmural or subendocardial, but the site is provided, it is still coded as a subendocardial AMI. If NSTEMI evolves to STEMI, assign the STEMI code. If STEMI converts to NSTEMI due to thrombolytic therapy, it is still coded as STEMI.

Apply the General Coding Guidelines as found in Chapter 5.

ANATOMY AND PHYSIOLOGY

The circulatory system is composed of the heart and blood vessels (Figure 14-3). Its function is to supply tissue in the body with oxygen and nutrients. This function is accomplished when the arteries carry blood (oxygen) to the cells. The largest artery, the aorta, branches off the heart and divides into many smaller arteries. The veins carry deoxygenated blood to the lungs to acquire oxygen and then to the heart, whose job it is to pump oxygenated blood back to the arteries.

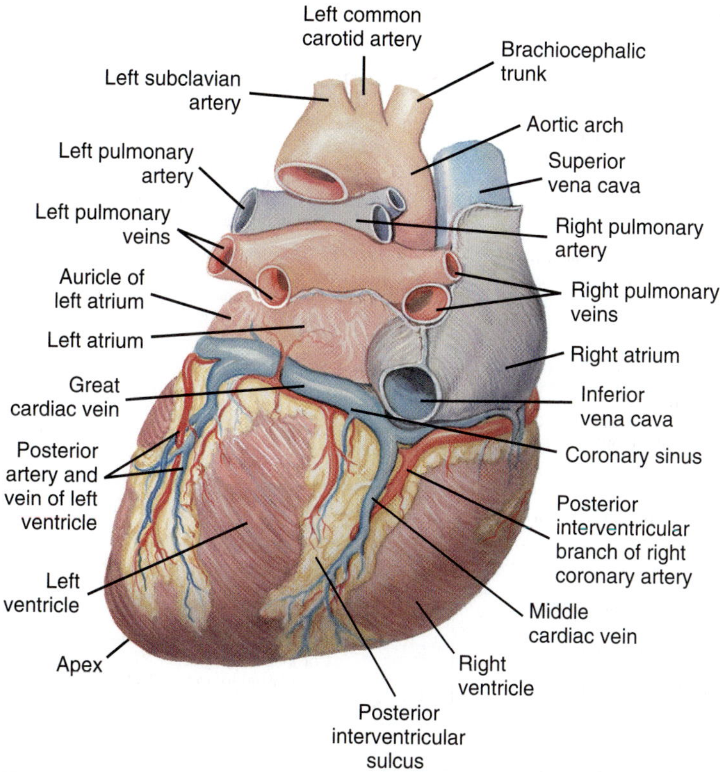

Figure 14-3. The heart and great vessels, posterior view.

The Heart

The function of the heart is to pump oxygen-rich blood to the cells of the body. The heart itself receives oxygenated blood from the coronary arteries; the two major coronary arteries branch off the aorta.

The heart is enclosed laterally by the lungs, posteriorly by the backbone, and anteriorly by the sternum. The wall of the heart is composed of three layers: epicardium, myocardium, and endocardium (Figure 14-4). The epicardium is the outer protective layer, the myocardium is the middle layer and is composed of cardiac muscle, and the endocardium is the inner layer that lines all the heart chambers and covers the heart valves.

The heart consists of four chambers: right atrium, left atrium, right ventricle, and left ventricle. The atrium and the ventricle on the right side are separated from the left by a septum. The top two chambers, the atria, receive blood via the veins from the body or the lungs. The right ventricle pumps blood to the lungs to pick up oxygen, and the left ventricle pumps blood to the rest of the body. Within the heart are four valves (Figure 14-5), and their job is to direct blood flow. The tricuspid valve is located between the right atrium and the right ventricle. The valve between the left atrium and the left ventricle is the mitral or bicuspid valve. The aortic valve is located in the aorta at the point at which the left ventricle empties into the aorta. The pulmonary valve is located in the pulmonary artery at the point of exit from the right ventricle.

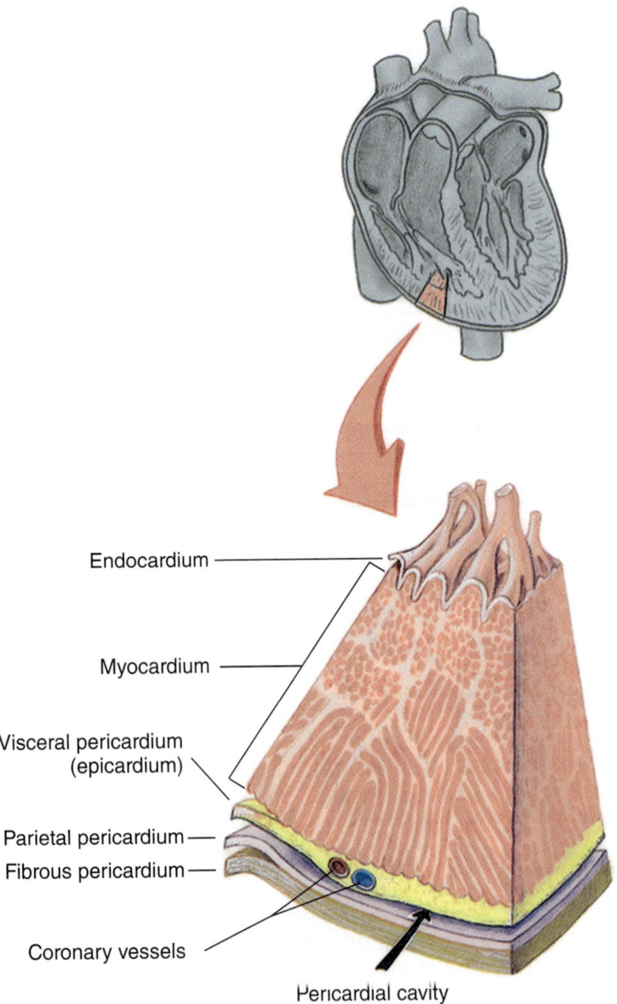

Figure 14-4. Layers of the heart wall.

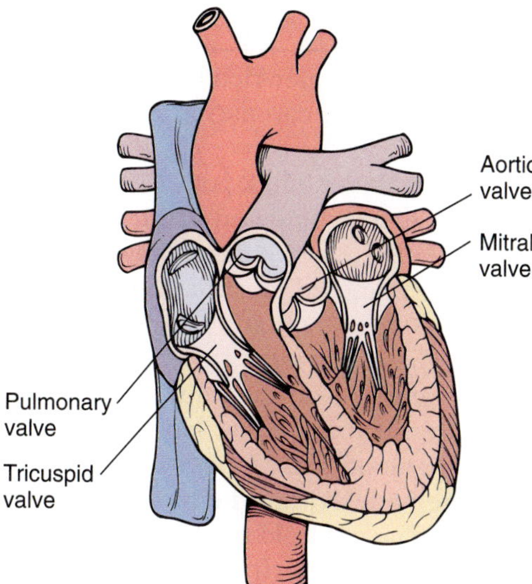

Figure 14-5. Cardiac valves.

Blood Vessels

Blood vessels are the tubes that transport blood from the heart to the cells and back to the heart. Most arteries carry oxygenated blood away from the heart. They continue to get smaller the farther away they are from the heart (arterioles). At this point, arterioles lead to **capillaries**, and exchange is made between blood and body cells; venules and veins return blood back to the heart. The circulation of blood that moves throughout the body is referred to as systemic circulation. Blood pressure measured at the arm indicates systemic pressures.

Lymphatic System

The lymphatic system is closely related to the circulatory system. The lymphatic drainage system returns back to the bloodstream products that have leaked out from the capillaries. The lymph system is also made up of lymph nodes, as well as spleen, thymus, tonsils, and adenoids. The lymph system fights infection by filtering out viruses and bacteria by attacking them with lymphocytes.

DISEASE CONDITIONS

Diseases of the Circulatory System (390-450), Chapter 7 in the ICD-9-CM code book, is divided into the following categories:

CATEGORY	SECTION TITLES
390-392	Acute Rheumatic Fever
393-398	Chronic Rheumatic Heart Disease
401-405	Hypertensive Disease
410-414	Ischemic Heart Disease
415-417	Diseases of Pulmonary Circulation
420-429	Other Forms of Heart Disease
430-438	Cerebrovascular Disease
440-449	Diseases of the Arteries, Arterioles, and Capillaries
451-459	Diseases of the Veins and Lymphatics and Other Diseases of the Circulatory System

Acute Rheumatic Fever (390-392) and Chronic Rheumatic Heart Disease (393-398)

Acute rheumatic fever is an inflammatory disease usually found in children that may affect the heart, joints, skin, or brain following an infection with streptococcal bacteria such as strep throat or scarlet fever.

EXAMPLE Patient was admitted with acute rheumatic fever with endocarditis, 391.1.

EXAMPLE Patient has rheumatic chorea without heart involvement, 392.9.

Chronic rheumatic heart disease is a chronic condition that is usually a late effect of attacks of acute rheumatic fever and most often involves the heart valves. When mitral and aortic valves are both involved ICD-9-CM assumes a causal relationship to rheumatic heart disease.

Index:
- Insufficiency
  - Mitral (valve), 424.0
    - With
      - Aortic (valve) disease, 396.3.

EXAMPLE Aortic stenosis, 424.1.

EXAMPLE Aortic stenosis with mitral stenosis, 396.0.

Mitral stenosis, mitral valve disease unspecified, and mitral valve failure are presumed by ICD-9-CM to be rheumatic in origin.

EXAMPLE Stenosis, mitral, 394.0.

If one mitral valve condition is presumed rheumatic and more than one mitral valve condition exists, ICD-9-CM assumes that both conditions are rheumatic.

Index:
- Stenosis
  - Mitral
    - With
      - Insufficiency, 394.2.

Unless otherwise specified, diseases of the tricuspid valve are presumed to be rheumatic in nature.

Hypertensive Disease (401-405)

The codes for hypertension are located in a table (see figure 14-1) found in the Alphabetic Index of diseases in ICD-9-CM. The three columns within this table identify the course of the disease; malignant, benign, or unspecified.

EXAMPLE Patient has chronic benign hypertension due to renal artery stenosis, 440.1, 405.91.

Hypertension is classified by ICD-9-CM as primary (essential) or secondary. Primary hypertension, or high **blood pressure** (BP), is a condition that is defined as abnormally high blood pressure in the arterial system. The American Heart Association defines hyper-

tension as pressures exceeding 140/90. A diagnosis of hypertension can be made only by a physician and should not be assigned on the basis of BP readings alone. Essential hypertension has no known origin, and its symptoms are insidious. ICD-9-CM uses fourth digits that describe the course of the disease. These fourth digits are as follows:

- 0 for malignant
- 1 for benign
- 9 for unspecified

Secondary hypertension is a consequence of other diseases such as kidney diseases, brain tumor, or polycythermia, and coding requires these same fourth digits. When secondary hypertension is documented, the sequencing of the codes is determined by the reason for admission/encounter.

EXAMPLE Patient has hypertension due to Cushing's disease, 255.0, 405.99.

Benign, Malignant, and Uncontrolled Hypertension

Malignant hypertension is a very severe form of hypertension and may be a life-threatening condition. The coding of malignant hypertension must be documented by a physician. In cases of malignant hypertension, systolic pressure may be greater than 200, and diastolic may be greater than 120. Malignant hypertension is also known as accelerating or necrotizing hypertension. Patients are at greater risk for malignant hypertension if they experience renal failure.

Coding Clinic (1984:July-Aug:p12)[1] describes malignant hypertension as "rapidly rising blood pressure, usually in excess of 140 mm Hg diastolic with findings of visual impairment and symptoms or signs of progressive cardiac failure." The fact that hypertension is uncontrolled does not make it malignant, and a separate code is not used to describe uncontrolled. Benign hypertension is rarely documented by physicians; therefore, coders often must assign the unspecified code. Hypertension that is not specifically documented as malignant or benign must be assigned to the unspecified fourth digit. Often, physicians document a history of hypertension when referring to ongoing hypertension that is under control. The current medication list should be reviewed to determine whether the hypertension is currently under treatment.

EXAMPLE Uncontrolled hypertension, 401.9.

EXAMPLE Hypertension, accelerated, 401.0.

Medications often used for treating hypertension include Accupril, Aldomet, captopril, Cardizem, diltiazem, Cozaar, losartan, Coreg, dyazide, Hytrin, Inderal, Lopressor, Norvasc, Procardia, Tenormin, atenolol, Vasotec, Toprol, Calan, verapamil, Zestril, and lisinopril.

EXAMPLE Patient has a past history of hypertension, currently taking verapamil, 401.9.

For a variety of reasons, patients may have elevated blood pressure readings. Per *Coding Clinic* (1990:3Q:p4),[2] unless a patient has an established diagnosis of hypertension, the code 796.2, elevated blood pressure, should be assigned.

Hypertensive Heart, Renal, and Heart and Renal Disease

Per *Coding Clinic* (2003:1Q:p20-21),[3] "ICD-9-CM assumes a cause-and-effect relationship and classifies chronic real failure with hypertension as hypertensive renal disease." This indicates to the coder that anytime hypertension and renal failure (codes from categories 585, 586, and 587) occur in a patient, category 403 should be assigned. The only time the 403.XX code would not be selected is when the physician documents, "CRF not due to hyperten-

sion." On occasion, a patient will have CKD due to diabetes and also have hypertension, diabetic kidney disease (250.40) and hypertensive kidney disease (403.XX) would be assigned.

Hypertensive heart disease, in contrast to hypertensive renal disease, does not assume a cause-and-effect relationship. A causal relationship must be stated by the physician. For a code from this category to be assigned, the physician must document hypertensive heart disease or must say that heart disease is due to hypertension. This category includes heart failure as the fifth digit. It is important to note that if a patient has hypertensive congestive heart failure, at least two codes—402.X1 and 428.0—are required; if known, the codes for systolic (428.20-428.23), diastolic (428.30-428.33), or a combination systolic and diastolic (428.40-428.43) should also be assigned.

EXAMPLE

Patient is admitted with both diastolic and systolic congestive heart failure due to long history of hypertension, 402.91, 428.40, 428.0.

Hypertensive heart and renal disease requires that the condition be classified to 404. XX. It is important for the coder to become familiar with the Includes as well as Excludes notes in all of the above categories.

EXAMPLE

Patient is admitted with hypertensive renal disease. The patient also has hypertensive cardiomyopathy, 404.90, 585.9, 425.8

EXERCISE 14-1

Assign codes to the following conditions using your ICD-9-CM code book.

1. Patient has hypertension __________
2. Aortic stenosis with mitral insufficiency __________
3. Malignant hypertension __________
4. Labile hypertension __________
5. Portal hypertension __________
6. Heart failure due to hypertensive heart disease __________
7. Cardiomegaly with hypertension __________
8. Hypertension secondary to coarctation of aorta __________
9. Ocular hypertension __________
10. Essential hypertension __________
11. HCVD (hypertensive cardiovascular disease) with chronic renal failure __________
12. High blood pressure reading __________

Ischemic Heart Disease (410-414)

Acute Myocardial Infarction

Acute **myocardial infarction** (AMI, or MI) in layman's terms is known as a heart attack. An MI occurs when complete blockage of blood flow occurs in a coronary artery. When this occurs, blood is prevented from reaching the heart muscle (Figure 14-6). Blockage may be caused by fatty deposits (also known as plaque or atherosclerosis) or blood clots. When the blood cannot reach the heart, the heart muscle may become damaged. Signs of a heart attack include chest pain, shortness of breath, nausea, and pain in the arms and chest.

To determine whether a patient is having a heart attack, several tests, including various types of blood tests, may be performed. One of these tests is called CPK (creatine phospho-

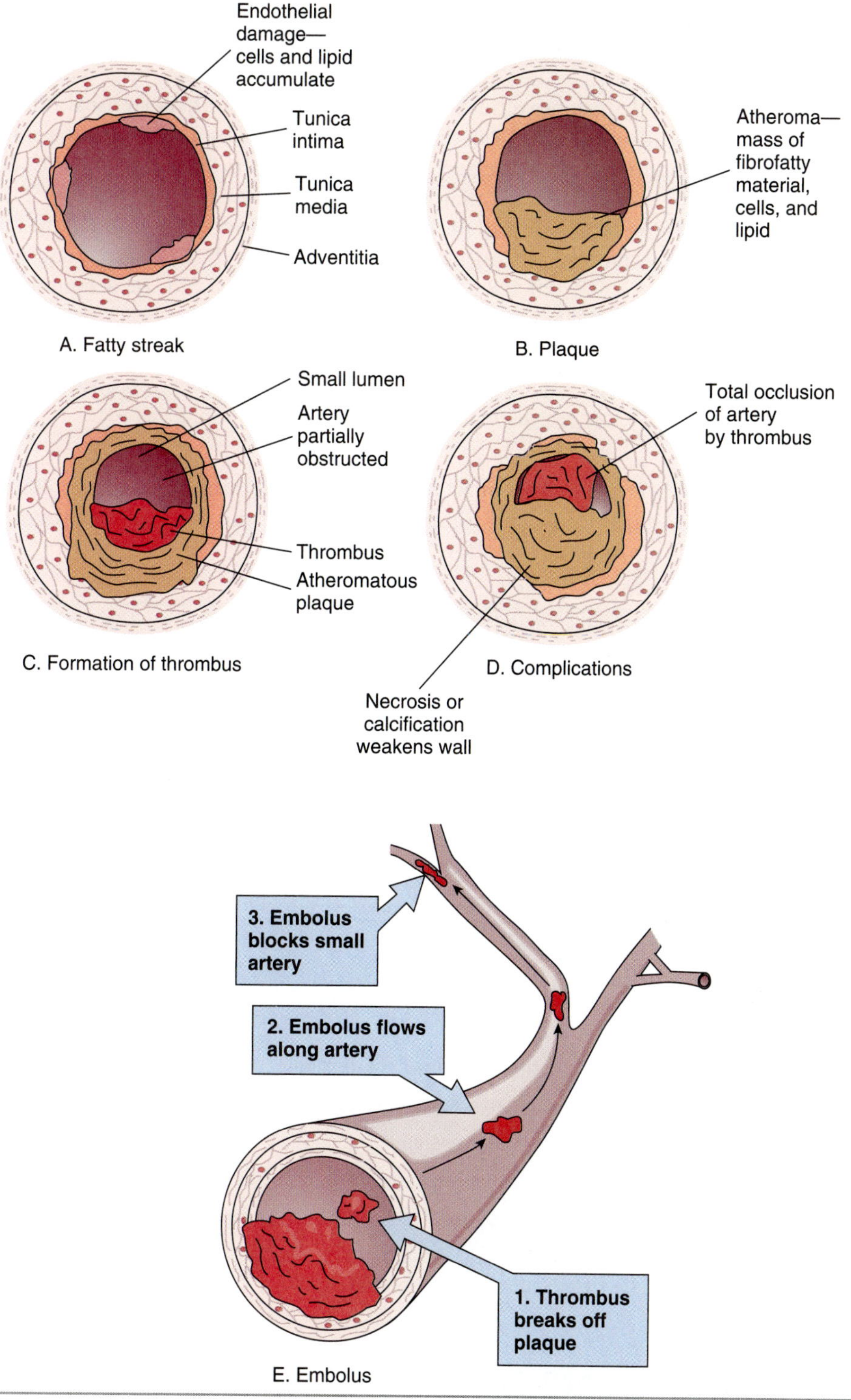

Figure 14-6. Development of an atheroma, leading to arterial occlusion.

kinase, or creatine kinase). CPK is an isoenzyme that occurs in high concentration in the heart and skeletal muscle. The level of CPK-MB (creatine phosphokinase, MB isoenzyme) in the blood rises 3 to 6 hours after an MI and returns to normal 12 to 48 hours after the infarct. Usually, CPK is measured every 8 to 12 hours, and patterns are determined. The normal value for males is 25 to 90; for females, it is 10 to 70. Another type of blood test that is often performed is the measurement of cardiac muscle proteins called troponins. Testing for troponin levels and CPK levels is performed serially. Troponin levels are usually

very low, and elevated levels can indicate damage to the heart. Healthcare providers also perform electrocardiograms (EKGs) to determine whether an MI has occurred. The EKG shows ST segment elevations during episodes of chest pain.

Types of MI may be classified as to the area of heart that suffers damage or the extent of damage, as evidenced by an EKG. The most common areas are the following:

- Anterior
- Inferior
- Lateral
- Posterior
- Right ventricular

STEMI (ST elevation MI) occurs when complete obstruction of the coronary artery causes damage involving the full thickness of the heart muscle. This type of MI is also known as an ST elevation MI or a Q wave MI. **NSTEMI** (non–ST elevation) occurs when a coronary artery is partially obstructed and damage does not involve the full thickness of the heart muscle. This type of MI is often referred to as non–Q wave MI. Old terminology for transmural or nontransmural MI has been replaced by Q or non–Q MI.

Patients suspected of having a MI are usually treated with a combination of medications and/or procedures. Procedures performed to treat the causes of MI include coronary angioplasty (percutaneous transluminal coronary angioplasty [PTCA]), stenting (percutaneous coronary intervention [PCI), and possibly coronary artery bypass surgery (CABG or CAB). Often, upon presentation of the patient to the emergency room (ER), thrombolytic therapy is initiated. Thrombolytics (tissue plasminogen activator [TPA], streptokinase) are used to dissolve blood clots that may be blocking a coronary artery. Thrombolytics must be administered within 6 hours of the onset of chest pain to avoid heart damage. A potential adverse effect of the use of these drugs is severe bleeding; for this reason, they are contraindicated in many patients. All of these procedures are discussed in greater detail in the procedure section of this chapter.

ICD-9-CM provides a fourth digit for the location of the heart attack within the heart and a fifth digit for the episode of care. The record should be reviewed to determine whether the site of the MI is documented. If location of a STEMI or transmural MI is not documented, it may be necessary to query the physician.

Fifth Digits

0 Episode of Care Unspecified This fifth digit would rarely be used in the inpatient setting. The date the infarct occurred is usually documented.

1 Initial Episode of Care This fifth digit is used for a newly diagnosed infarct, regardless of the facility site. In other words, if a patient presents to one facility with an acute MI and then is transferred to another, the fifth digit of one is used in both cases. An MI is coded to this digit if a patient has never been sent home from the hospital after presentation for this diagnosis.

2 Subsequent Episode of Care This fifth digit is used to describe a patient who has had an MI during a previous episode of care but is now being readmitted, This fifth digit is used up to 8 weeks following the original infarct. This digit is used if the patient went home after initial presentation to the hospital for the MI.

Once an MI is greater than 8 weeks old, code 412 is assigned to describe a patient who has had an MI in the past.

EXAMPLE Patient was admitted with NSTEMI. 410.71.

Prior to having an MI, a patient may have had symptoms such as unstable angina (USA), which is often described in today's vernacular as acute coronary syndrome, or ACS. A patient with this condition requires immediate medical treatment, but a patient with chronic angina may be treated with medications on a long-term basis as necessary. Patients with angina may be prescribed sublingual nitroglycerin to relieve pain symptoms. Often, the underlying condition of chest pain, or angina, is coronary artery disease. Coronary artery disease (CAD), 414.0X may be coded with a fifth digit, which describes what type of coronary artery is involved:

- 414.01 is the native coronary artery. (This is the artery the patient was born with.)
- 414.02 is autologous vein bypass graft. (This is a vein that is taken from the patient, usually the saphenous vein, and is placed during a CABG.)
- 414.03 is a nonautologous biological bypass graft. (This is a vessel taken from another patient that is placed during a CABG.)
- 414.04 is an artery bypass graft. (This artery, most often the internal mammary, is used for a bypass.)

Sometimes a patient will present to the ER with acute chest pain. The attending decides to administer TPA and documents that once TPA was administered symptoms were relieved and the patient is admitted for observation with a diagnosis of "aborted MI". Per *Coding Clinic* (2001:2Q:p7-8)[4] an aborted MI is coded to 411.1, Intermediate Coronary Syndrome.

When CAD is present in a patient with a previous CABG, but it is not known whether the CAD is of a graft or a native artery, the code 414.00 for unspecified should be used per *Coding Clinic* (1997:3Q:p15).[5] Also assign code V45.81 to show that the patient had coronary artery bypass surgery. When there is no documentation that the patient had a CABG procedure in the past, then the code for CAD should be assigned to native arteries (414.01).

EXERCISE 14-2

Assign codes to the following conditions using your ICD-9-CM code book.

1. Patient had an MI 1 year prior to this admission ____________
2. Patient had a nontransmural MI 6 weeks ago and now presents with chest pain ____________
3. Patient has CAD and a history of CABG ____________
   Recent coronary catheterization shows coronary artery disease of the native arteries ____________
4. Patient has CAD and a previous MI and coronary artery bypass ____________
5. Patient with an anterolateral MI is transferred to this hospital for further evaluation and treatment ____________

Diseases of Pulmonary Circulation (415-417)

Pulmonary Embolism

A **pulmonary embolism** is a blood clot(s) in the pulmonary artery that causes blockage in the artery. Most often, clots originate in the legs and then travel to the lung. A blood clot that forms and remains in a vein is a **thrombus**. A clot that travels to another part of the body is an **embolus**. Common symptoms of pulmonary embolism include shortness of breath, chest pain, and cough.

A pulmonary embolism may be diagnosed via lung scan or computed tomography (CT) scan. A pulmonary embolism can be life threatening, and once you have had one, the risk for recurrence is increased.

Pulmonary Hypertension

Pulmonary hypertension (PHT) is high blood pressure in the arteries that supply blood to the lungs. Normal pulmonary systolic pressure is 18 to 25 mm Hg. Two types of pulmonary hypertension—primary and secondary—have been identified. Primary pulmonary hypertension (PPH) is a rare condition of unknown origin that is both progressive and ultimately fatal. In recent years, this condition has been linked with the use of anti-obesity drugs such as Fen/Phen. Secondary pulmonary hypertension is caused by other conditions such as chronic obstructive pulmonary disease (COPD), emphysema, pulmonary embolism, or obstructive sleep apnea (OSA). Patients who have prolonged untreated pulmonary hyper-

tension often develop right ventricular failure. Doppler echocardiography is the most useful test for determining the diagnosis of pulmonary hypertension.

Symptoms of pulmonary hypertension may include dyspnea on exertion (DOE), syncope, fatigue, and chest pain. Treatment for this disease may involve correcting the underlying cause, if possible. Medical treatments may include vasodilators, diuretics, anticoagulants, oxygen, and digoxin. In some cases, lung transplantation may be considered.

EXAMPLE Patient has pulmonary hypertension due to COPD, 416.8, 496.

Other Forms of Heart Disease (420-429)

Pericarditis

Pericarditis is inflammation of the covering of the heart. It is often a complication of viral infection and systemic disease such as acquired immunodeficiency syndrome (AIDS). Sometimes, pericarditis follows an MI; it may also arise from bacterial infection. The disease presents with symptoms such as chest pain, breathing difficulties, fever, and cough. The heart sound heard through the stethoscope by the physician in cases of pericarditis is called a pericardial rub. Pericarditis is diagnosed through the use of chest x-ray (CXR), echocardiography, and magnetic resonance imaging (MRI). Usually, these patients also have abnormal EKG results.

EXAMPLE Acute pericardial effusion, 420.90.

EXAMPLE Uremic pericarditis, 585.9, 420.0.

EXAMPLE Acute viral pericarditis, 420.91.

Endocarditis

Endocarditis is inflammation of the lining of the heart chambers and valves. Most often, bacterial infection is the cause of endocarditis. Patients with intravenous drug use (IVDU), central venous lines, and valve replacements (aortic valve replacement [AVR], mitral valve replacement [MVR]) are at greater risk for developing endocarditis. Patients with endocarditis might present with fever, shortness of breath (SOB), fatigue, night sweats, and muscle aches. In determining this diagnosis, physicians order blood cultures and perform echocardiograms. Treatment always consists of intravenous (IV) antibiotics; therefore, the patient must be hospitalized. IV antibiotic treatment may take up to 6 weeks.

EXAMPLE Patient admitted for antibiotics for subacute endocarditis, 421.9.

EXAMPLE Patient admitted for endocarditis caused by typhoid, 002.0, 421.1.

Valve Disorders

Valve disorders of **incompetence, insufficiency**, and **regurgitation** may be classified to the category of 424. A leaking valve is another name for regurgitation, incompetence, or insufficiency. When this occurs, blood flows backward within the valve. If a valve's opening is blocked, or flow of blood is diminished, this is called stenosis. Stenosis, for some valves, is assigned the 424 category. However, tricuspid stenosis is always found under category 397. When diseases of both the mitral valve and the aortic valve are identified, ICD-9-CM assigns them to category 396, whether or not they are specified as rheumatic. Coding of valve disorders requires following the Alphabetic Index closely and pay attention to all instructional notes to assign the appropriate code.

EXAMPLE Tricuspid stenosis, 397.0.

EXAMPLE Mitral insufficiency, 424.0.

EXAMPLE Mitral valve prolapse, 424.0.

Cardiomyopathy

Cardiomyopathy is a disorder of the muscle of the heart chambers that impedes the functioning of the heart. Another term for congestive cardiomyopathy is dilated cardiomyopathy. Cardiomyopathy can be caused by disorders such as CAD, infection, diabetes, or alcohol abuse. Two codes may be required to code cardiomyopathy—one for the underlying condition and one for cardiomyopathy. In subcategories 425.7 and 425.8, the underlying condition would be sequenced first. Cardiomyopathy is diagnosed by echocardiography and is treated with antibiotics if due to an infection or treatment may be targeted to the underlying cause. Congestive cardiomyopathy may be associated with congestive heart failure. When they occur together, congestive heart failure would be the principal diagnosis, because it is often the focus of treatment. The cardiomyopathy would be assigned as an additional code, according to *Coding Clinic* (1990:2Q:p19).[6]

EXAMPLE Cardiomyopathy due to progressive muscular dystrophy, 359.1, 425.8.

EXAMPLE Obstructive hypertrophic cardiomyopathy, 425.1.

EXAMPLE Alcoholic cardiomyopathy, 425.5, 303.90.

Conduction Disorders

A **conduction disorder** is a problem that occurs in the electrical impulses that regulate heartbeat. A heartbeat begins when an electrical impulse is sent through the upper chambers of the heart. A human heart usually beats from 60 to 100 times per minute. **Tachycardia** (fast heart rate) means the heartbeat is greater than 100 beats per minute; **bradycardia** (slow heart rate) is a heartbeat of fewer than 60 beats per minute.

Heart blocks occur when impulses originating in the upper chambers are unable to pass to the lower chambers at the correct rate. Three types of blocks have been observed:

- First degree: Conduction of beats from upper to lower is slower than normal.
- Second degree: Not all beats pass from upper to lower.
- Third degree: Impulses cannot pass from upper to lower.

EXAMPLE ECG shows left bundle branch block, anterior fascicular block with posterior fascicular block, 426.3.

EXAMPLE The patient has a bifascicular block, 426.53.

Cardiac arrhythmias (Table 14-1) occur when the normal sequence of electrical impulses changes, or the rhythm of the heartbeat is disturbed. (Normal sequence = RA [right atrium] through atrioventricular [AV] node through His bundle to ventricles.)

EXAMPLE Atrial fibrillation (AF), 427.31.

EXAMPLE Sick sinus syndrome (SSS), 427.81.

EXAMPLE Supraventricular tachycardia (SVT), 427.8.

Table 14-1. Arrythmias[8]

Types	Symptoms and Signs	Etiology	Diagnosis	Treatment
Normal sinus rhythm	Rate of 60-100 bpm, regular, P wave uniform	Impulse originates in SA node, conduction normal	Normal	None indicated
Sinus tachycardia	Rate >100 bpm, regular, P wave uniform	Rapid impulse originates in SA node, conduction normal	Rapid rate	Beta blockers, calcium channel blockers
Sinus brachycardia	Rate <60 bpm, regular, P wave uniform	Slow impulse originates in SA node, conduction normal	Slow rate	Atropine
Premature atrial contraction	Rate depends on underlying rhythm, usually normal P wave, morphology different from other P waves	Irritable atrium, single ectopic beat that arises prematurely, conduction through ventricle normal	Irregular heartbeat, diagnosis by ECG	Treatment usually unnecessary; if needed, antiarrhythmic drugs
Atrial tachycardia	Rate of 150-250 bpm, rhythm normal, sudden onset	Irritable atrium, firing at rapid rates, normal conduction	Rapid rate with atrial and ventricular rates identical, diagnosis by ECG	Reflex vagal stimulation, calcium channel–blocking drugs (verapamil), cardioversion
Atrial fibrillation	Atrial rate >350 bpm, ventricular rate <100 bpm (controlled) or ≥100 bpm (rapid ventricular response)	Atrial ectopic foci discharging at too rapid and chaotic a rate for muscles to respond and contract, resulting in quivering of atrium; AV node blocks some impulses, and ventricle responds irregularly	ECG show no P waves, grossly irregular ventricular rate	IV verapamil; if unsuccessful, procainamide; if unsuccessful, cardioversion
First-degree heart block	Rate depends on rate of underlying rhythm, PR interval >0.20 second	Delay at AV node, impulse eventually conducted	ECG shows PR interval >0.20 second	Atropine; if unsuccessful, artificial pacemaker insertion
Second-degree heart block, Wenckebach block	Intermittent block with progressively longer delay in conduction until one beat is blocked; atrial rate normal, ventricular rate slower than normal, rhythm irregular	SA node initiates impulse, conduction through AV node is blocked intermittently	ECG shows normal P waves, some P waves not followed by QRS complex; PR interval progressively longer, followed by block of impulse	Mild forms, no treatment; severe, insertion of artificial pacemaker
Classic second-degree heart block	Ventricular rate slow (½, ⅓, or ¼ of atrial rate); rhythm, regular; P waves normal, QRS complex dropped every 2nd, 3rd, or 4th beat	SA node initiates impulse, conduction through AV node is blocked	ECG shows P waves present, QRS complex blocked every 2nd, 3rd, or 4th impulse	Artificial pacemaker is inserted

AV, Atrioventricular; bpm, beats per minute; *ECG*, electrocardiogram; *IV*, intravenous; *PR*, pulse rate; *PVC*, premature ventricular contraction; *SA*, sinoatrial.

Continued

Table 14-1. Arrythmias[8]—cont'd

Types	Symptoms and Signs	Etiology	Diagnosis	Treatment
Third-degree heart block	Atrial rate normal, ventricular rate 20-40 or 40-60 bpm; no relationship between P wave and QRS complex	SA node initiates impulse, which is completely blocked from conduction, causing atria and ventricles to beat independently	ECG shows P waves and QRS complexes with no relationship to each other; rhythms are regular but independent of each other	Insertion of artificial pacemaker is needed
Premature ventricular contraction (single focus)	Single ectopic beat, arising from ventricle, followed by compensatory pause	Ectopic beat originates in irritable ventricle	ECG shows a wide, bizarre QRS complex >0.12 second, usually followed by a compensatory pause	Usually, no treatment if <6 per minute and single focus
Multifocal arrhythmia Coupling, 2 in a row Bigeminy, every other beat Trigeminy, every 3rd beat Quadrigeminy, every 4th beat	Rate dependent on underlying rhythm; rhythm regular or irregular; P wave absent before ectopic beat	Same as single focus	Same as single focus	Same as single focus
Ventricular tachycardia	Rate of 150-250 bpm, rhythm usually regular; focus of pacemaker normally single; patient experiences palpitations, dyspnea, and anxiety followed by chest pain	Four or more consecutive PVCs at a rapid rate due to advanced irritability of myocardium, indicating ventricular command of heart rate	ECG show runs of four or more PVCs; P was buried in QRS complex	Often forerunner of ventricular fibrillation; immediate intervention necessary; IV lidocaine; if unsuccessful, follow by cardioversion; procainamide or bretylium may be used
Ventricular fibrillation (lethal arrhythmia)	Patient loses consciousness immediately after onset; no peripheral pulses palpable, no heart sounds, no blood pressure	Ventricular fibers twitch rather than contract; reason unknown	Pulseless, unconscious patient; ECG shows rapid, repetitive, chaotic waves originating in ventricle	Recognize and terminate rhythm; precordial shock (defibrillation)

AV, Atrioventricular; bpm, beats per minute; *ECG*, electrocardiogram; *IV*, intravenous; *PR*, pulse rate; *PVC*, premature ventricular contraction; *SA*, sinoatrial.

Cardiac arrest, the sudden loss of heart function, is assigned code 427.5. Per *Coding Clinic* (1988:2Q:p8),[7] this may be coded as the principal diagnosis in only two instances:

1. When the patient presents to the ER in cardiac arrest and dies before the underlying cause of the arrest has been established
2. When the patient presents to the hospital in cardiac arrest, is resuscitated, admitted as an inpatient, and subsequently dies before the underlying cause of the arrest has been established

Cardiac arrest may be coded as a secondary diagnosis when a patient has a cardiac arrest and is resuscitated on arrival or during the inpatient stay. The arrest is not coded when a physician documents cardiac arrest as the cause of death.

Heart failure is impaired function of the heart's pumping ability. The heart is unable to pump with enough force or to fill with enough blood. This damage to the heart muscle may be caused by a variety of heart conditions such as CAD, MI, cardiomyopathy, hypertension (HTN), valve disease, diabetes mellitus (DM), and chronic kidney disease (CKD). This impaired pumping function in turn results in insufficient blood reaching the kidneys, which causes the body to retain fluid (Figure 14-7). Symptoms of heart failure include congested lungs, edema, fatigue, and irregular heartbeat.

Two types of heart failure may occur: systolic and diastolic. Systolic heart dysfunction, also known as systolic heart failure, occurs when the heart muscles are not contracting with

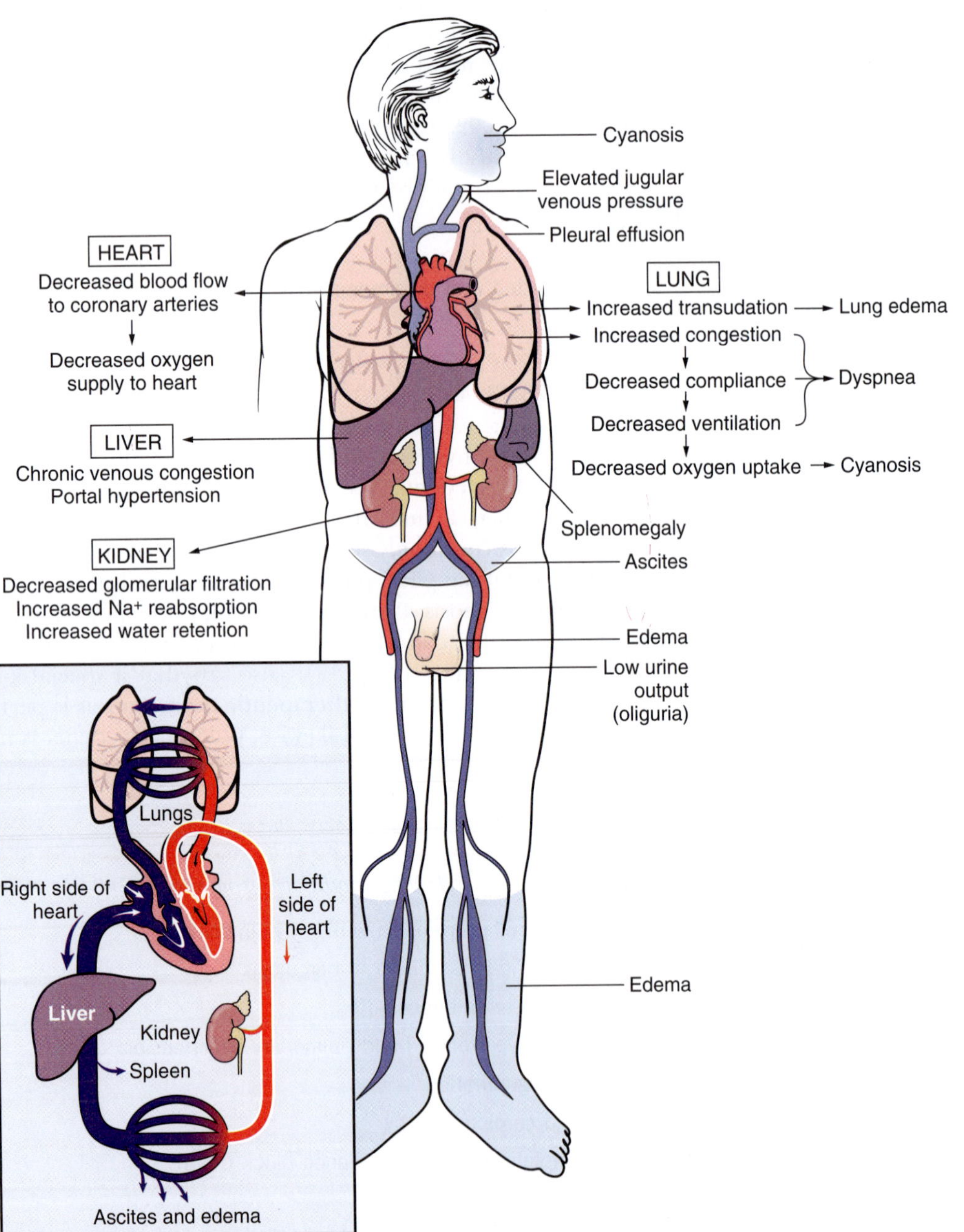

Figure 14-7. Chronic passive congestion. Left-sided heart failure leads to pulmonary edema. Right ventricular failure causes peripheral edema that is most prominent in the lower extremities.

enough force, and therefore, not enough blood is being pumped to the body. Diastolic cardiac dysfunction, also known as diastolic heart failure, occurs when the contraction is normal but the ventricle does not allow enough blood to enter the heart. Physicians can measure the percentage of blood that is pumped out of a filled ventricle with each heartbeat (known as ejection fraction) to determine how the heart is functioning. A normal ejection fraction measures 55% to 70%. Ejection fraction can be determined in several ways: echocardiography, MRI, multiple-gated acquisition (MUGA), or computerized tomography (CT) scan. Another test used to determine whether a patient is in heart failure is the brain natriuretic peptide (BNP) test. **BNP** is a hormone that is produced by the heart; a BNP test measures the amount of BNP that is found in the blood. Normally, levels of BNP are low, but in heart failure, these levels become elevated. A normal value of BNP would be 0 to 99 pg/mL. If this level is greater than 100, heart failure is indicated.

When coding heart failure, it is appropriate to pick up codes for heart failure, as well as codes for systolic, diastolic, or combination systolic/diastolic and codes for the underlying cause, if known. It is also important to look for documentation of acute, chronic, or acute on chronic. Patients may be treated for CHF as a chronic condition and may never be hospitalized. However, should the patient have an exacerbation, he or she may be hospitalized per *Coding Clinic* (2002:4Q:p52-55)[9]. To assign a code for rheumatic congestive heart failure, the heart failure must be classified as rheumatic by ICD-9-CM, or the physician must document that the heart failure is rheumatic in nature, per *Coding Clinic* (2000:2Q:p16-17; 1995:1Q:p6).[10-11]

EXAMPLE Patient admitted with decompensated diastolic congestive heart failure, 428.30, 428.0.

EXAMPLE Patient admitted with congestive heart failure, acute on chronic combined systolic and diastolic, 428.43, 428.0.

In many cases, physicians will refer to heart failure as pulmonary edema or volume overload. Pulmonary edema has other causes, but one of its main causes is heart failure. Also, patients with CHF may have pleural effusions. *Coding Clinic* (1991:3Q:p19)[12] says, "Pleural effusion is commonly seen with CHF with or without pulmonary edema." In cases in which the patient has CHF, pulmonary edema, and pleural effusions, CHF would always be the principal diagnosis. Pleural effusion may be reported as an additional diagnosis if it were specifically evaluated or treated. Pulmonary edema would rarely be coded in addition to CHF. *Coding Clinic* (1991:3Q:p19)[12] also says that if special x-rays are taken to confirm the presence, or if diagnostic or therapeutic thoracentesis is performed, then pleural effusion may be additionally coded. Likewise, pulmonary edema is not assigned an additional code.

EXERCISE 14-3

Assign codes to the following conditions using your ICD-9-CM code book.

1. Pulmonary hypertension with cor pulmonale ____________
2. Acute pericarditis due to tuberculosis ____________
3. Acute bacterial endocarditis ____________
4. Chronic hypertension and pulmonary hypertension ____________
5. Aortic regurgitation ____________
6. Dilated cardiomyopathy ____________
7. Incomplete right bundle branch block (RBBB) ____________
8. Wenckebach heart block ____________
9. Atrial flutter ____________
10. Persistent sinus bradycardia ____________

11. Thyrotoxic cardiomyopathy ____________
12. Hypertensive cardiomyopathy ____________
13. Another name for inflammation of the lining of the heart chambers
____

Cerebrovascular Disease (430-438)

A patient who is admitted with a diagnosis of **stroke** (brain infarction or cerebrovascular accident [CVA]) is similar to a patient who is admitted with a diagnosis of heart attack or MI. The blood supply to a part of the brain is blocked by a broken blood vessel, ischemia, or blood clots (Figure 14-8). When the blood supply is cut off, brain cells die. Several types of stroke or brain infarcts may occur (Figure 14-9). Ischemic stroke, which accounts for 80% of all strokes, happens when blockage to the brain, usually by a blood clot, occurs. A clot that develops in another part of the body and then becomes wedged in a brain artery is a free-roaming clot or an embolus (Figure 14-10).

The most common type of stroke is ischemic (thrombotic/embolic). An ischemic stroke occurs when a blood clot or a piece of plaque breaks loose from an artery and lodges in a

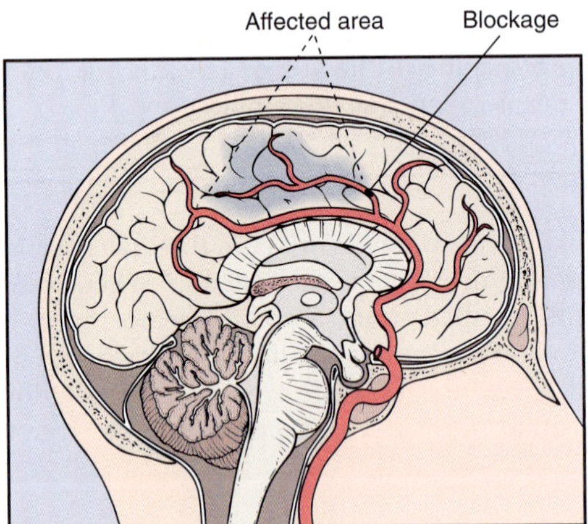

Figure 14-8. Cerebrovascular accident (CVA).

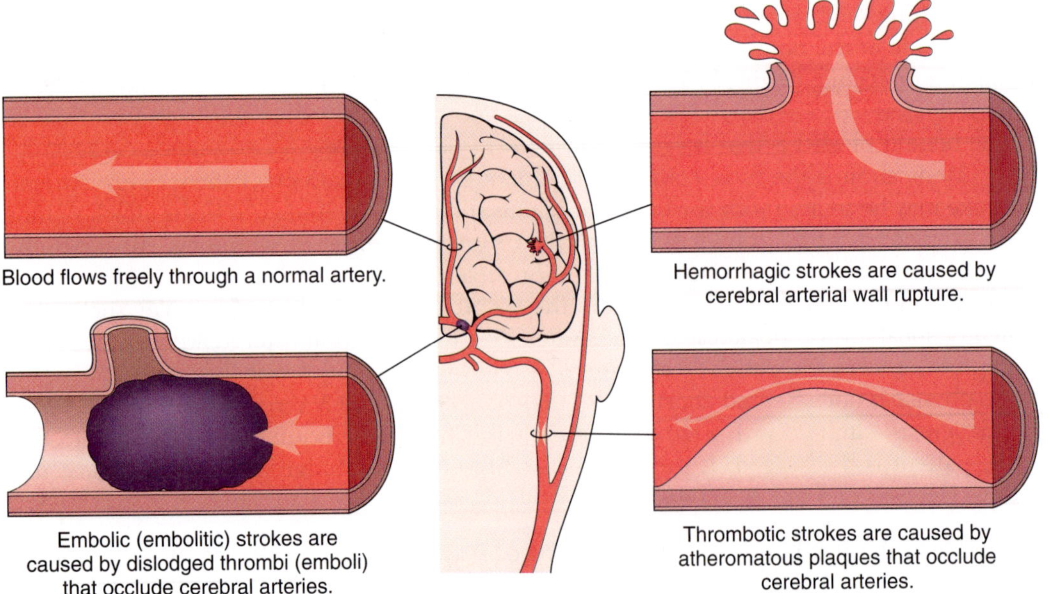

Figure 14-9. Types of stroke: ischemic (thrombotic and embolic) and hemorrhagic.

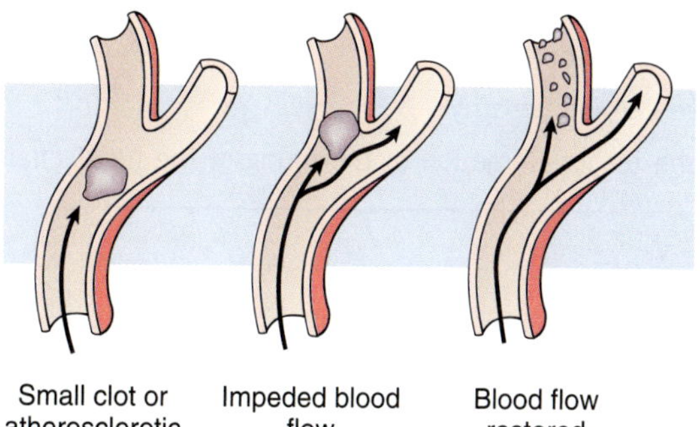

Figure 14-10. Embolus causing transient ischemic attack.

blood vessel of the brain, which then cuts off the blood supply to that area of the brain. A blood clot that forms and remains in a vein is called a **thrombus**, whereas a clot that travels to another part of the body is an **embolus**. Sometimes plaque is dislodged and becomes an embolus. The other type of stroke is hemorrhagic.

EXAMPLE Embolic stroke, 434.11.

Ischemic stroke may be caused by narrowing of the arteries, or **stenosis**. Stenosis is often caused by the buildup of plaque in the artery. This may be referred to as small- or large-vessel disease. Often, this is called a lacunar infarction.

EXAMPLE Ischemic stroke, 434.91.

Hemorrhagic stroke occurs when an artery in the brain bursts and blood seeps into the surrounding tissue, causing the tissue to malfunction. When bleeding from the artery goes into the brain itself, this is called an intracerebral hemorrhage. When bleeding seeps into the meninges or outer membranes, this is called a subarachnoid hemorrhage. Hemorrhagic stroke may be caused by aneurysms, arteriovenous malformations (AVMs), and, possibly, plaque-encrusted walls that rupture. Hypertension can increase the risk of rupture of the artery wall.

EXAMPLE Subarachnoid hemorrhage, 430.

Symptoms of a stroke often appear suddenly. These may occur as weakness or numbness of one side of the body, arm, leg, or face; confusion; difficulty talking or speaking; trouble walking or seeing; dizziness; and headache. A CT scan is often used to determine whether a patient has had a hemorrhagic stroke; MRI is another useful tool in the diagnosis of stroke. The benefit of MRI is that it can rapidly detect small infarcts.

Medication is the most common treatment for stroke patients. Patients with ischemic stroke may be treated with thrombolytic agents such as TPA. Similar to heart attack victims, stroke patients need to be treated with TPA soon after onset of symptoms. Most patients are treated with anticoagulants or with antiplatelet agents.

Sometimes a patient will present to the hospital with symptoms of a stroke, such as difficulty speaking or weakness on one side. TPA may be administered with considerable improvement in the patient's symptoms. According to *Coding Clinic* (2007:1Q:p23-24)[13] if the physician documented aborted CVA the code 434.91 for CVA would be assigned. Often, a patient is admitted with a stroke with deficits. These deficits are often gone by the time the patient is discharged. If the deficits are present at discharge, they are coded; if they have cleared, they are not coded.

EXAMPLE Subdural hemorrhage, with dysphagia at time of discharge, 432.1, 787.20.

EXAMPLE Stenosis of the carotid artery with cerebral infarction, 433.11.

Patient has a history of bilateral carotid stenosis. Upon presentation to the hospital it is determined that the patient has had a CVA due to thrombosis. (*Coding Clinic* 1995:2Q: p14).[14] In this case both the codes for the carotid stenosis without infarct, 433.10 and 433.30, and the code for the CVA, 434.01, would be assigned.

When coding bilateral carotid artery stenosis it is necessary to assign two codes; one for the site, code 433.1X, as well as one for laterality code, 433.3X. (*Coding Clinic* 2006:1Q: p17).[15]

Transient Ischemic Attack

A **transient ischemic attack** (TIA) is a stroke that lasts for only a few minutes. Patients who present with a TIA usually have the same symptoms as occur with a stroke. Most symptoms of a TIA are gone within an hour, but they may last up to 24 hours.

It is important for the coder to be aware of the Excludes notes in this chapter, excluding codes found in this category that occur during pregnancy or the puerperium and strokes that occur as a result of treatment.

Late Effects of Cerebrovascular Disease

Stroke is one of the leading causes of disability in the United States. Types of disability that may result from stroke consist of paralysis, particularly on one side of the body (hemiplegia), or weakness on one side (hemiparesis). Other disabilities include **cognitive deficits**, **aphasia** (impairment of language comprehension and production), emotional problems, and pain. When an inpatient has had a stroke, has current deficits, and also has late effects from a previous stroke, all codes should be assigned. Late effect codes may be listed as principal diagnoses when the purpose of the admission is to treat the late effect. The code for a history of CVA with no residuals is V12.54.

EXAMPLE

Patient presents with carotid artery stenosis with infarct and current hemiparesis. Patient has residual aphasia from a previous stroke, 433.11, 342.90, 438.11.

EXERCISE 14-4

Assign codes to the following conditions using your ICD-9-CM code book.

1. Transient ischemic attack with right sided weakness, which cleared shortly following admission ____________
2. Cerebral hemorrhage ____________
3. Patient was admitted with CVA and aphasia; the aphasia cleared before discharge ____________
4. Cerebral thrombosis without infarction ____________
5. Ruptured berry aneurysm ____________
6. Patient with a history of cerebrovascular accident, no residuals ____________ ____________
7. Quadriplegia resulting from a stroke last year
8. Patient is being treated for cognitive deficits following a stroke ____________

Diseases of the Arteries, Arterioles, and Capillaries (440-449)

Atherosclerosis or arteriosclerosis is a stricture or hardening of the artery that is caused by deposits of plaque. These deposits restrict blood flow through the artery; plaques can rupture and travel to other parts of the body or can form blood clots that block a blood vessel. If a blood vessel to the heart is blocked, this causes a heart attack; if a vessel to the brain is blocked, this causes a stroke; and if vessels to the extremities are blocked, this can cause claudication, ulcers, and eventually, gangrene. Codes found in subcategory 440.2 are hierarchical. Per *Coding Clinic* (1993:4Q:p27-28),[16] "Thus all patients in this subcategory who

have gangrene (regardless of whether ulceration, rest pain, and/or intermittent claudication [is] present) are coded to 440.24." For example, if a patient presents with atherosclerosis of the extremities with ulceration and gangrene, only the code for gangrene, 440.24, is assigned. The ulcer code 707.1X is assigned in addition to the 440.23.

EXAMPLE Arteriosclerotic renal artery, 440.1.

EXAMPLE Atherosclerosis of extremity autologous bypass graft, 440.31.

An **aneurysm** is a bulging or ballooning out of a vessel. Aneurysms are often caused by atherosclerosis and tend to have no symptoms, unless dissection occurs. Dissection is typically accompanied by severe pain in the area of dissection. Aneurysms tend to form in areas where vessels branch out. Aortic aneurysms (Figure 14-11) can occur anywhere along the aorta, which is the largest artery in the body; it runs from the heart through the chest into the abdominal area and then divides into vessels that supply blood to the legs. The most common aneurysms occur in the abdominal area. Rupture of an aneurysm is a life-threatening event. The risk of rupture increases as the aneurysm becomes larger. Sometimes, an aneurysm becomes **dissecting**, which means a tear begins in the wall of the vessel that causes layers to separate. Physicians use the terms type I, type II, and type III to describe dissecting aneurysms.

EXAMPLE Patient presents to hospital with Type I thoracoabdominal aneurysm, 441.03.

Aneurysms are usually not treated until they reach a certain size or begin to enlarge quickly. Treatment for an aneurysm consists of open or endovascular surgery, which is discussed in the Procedure section of this chapter.

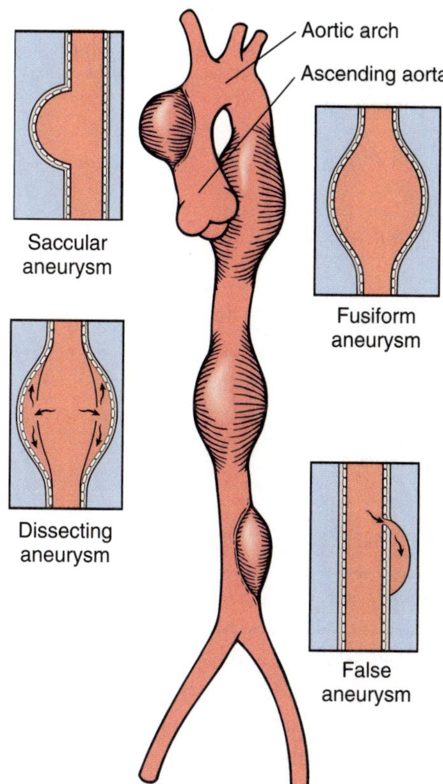

Figure 14-11. Types of aortic aneurysm.

EXAMPLE Abdominal aortic aneurysm, 441.4.

EXAMPLE Ruptured thoracic aneurysm, 441.1.

EXAMPLE Femoral aneurysm, 442.3.

An arteriovenous **fistula** is an abnormal passage between an artery and a vein. Blood typically flows from arteries into capillaries and then to veins; however, when blood bypasses the capillaries and goes directly to the vein, an arteriovenous fistula results.

EXAMPLE Patient has an arteriovenous fistula, acquired, 447.0.

Diseases of Veins and Lymphatics, and Other Diseases of Circulatory System (451-459)

Phlebitis, Thrombophlebitis, and Deep Vein Thrombosis

Phlebitis is inflammation of a vein; thrombophlebitis occurs when a clot forms in the vein and then causes inflammation or phlebitis. **Deep vein thrombosis** (DVT) is a blood clot that forms in a deep vein, usually in the leg or hip (Figures 14-12 and 14-13). *Coding Clinic*

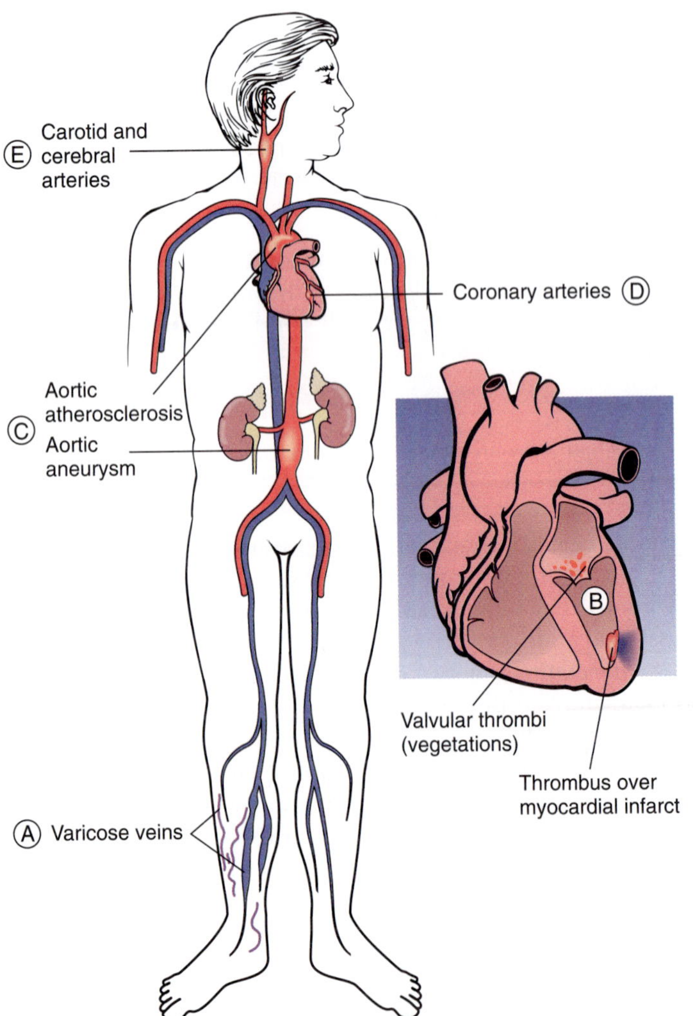

Figure 14-12. Common sites of thrombus formation.

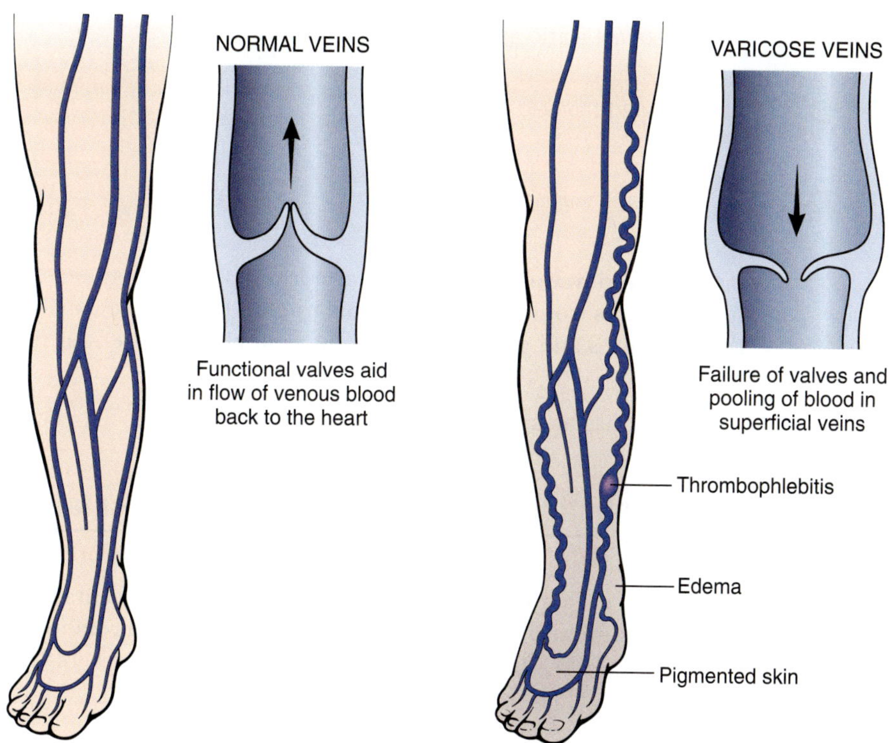

Figure 14-13. Normal and varicose veins. Slow flow in the veins makes an individual susceptible to clot formation. Thrombotic occlusion of varicose veins is known as thrombophlebitis. If a thrombus becomes loosened from its place in a vein, it can travel to the lungs (pulmonary embolism) and block a blood vessel there. Then blood pools in the lower part of the leg and fluid leaks from distended small capillaries, causing edema.

(1992:1Q:p15-16)[17] says, "Deep vein thrombosis (DVT) is rarely an acute finding without the associated inflammation leading to thrombophlebitis, and in most cases, DVT is synonymous with thrombophlebitis. If both conditions are present, only the code for 451.xx is assigned."

EXAMPLE Patient admitted with femoral DVT with inflammation, 451.11.

Varicose veins are enlarged, twisted veins that usually occur in the legs. Varicose veins can be found in other areas of the body such as the esophagus. Varicose veins often develop complications that require surgical treatment. Stasis dermatitis with varicose veins of the leg is assigned code 454.1.

Stasis dermatitis is a skin condition caused by poor circulation (venous insufficiency) that is characterized by swelling, skin discoloration, weeping, itching, and scaly skin. The legs and particularly the ankles are the areas most often affected. This condition is often seen in the elderly, and risk for developing this condition increases when any of the following conditions is present: obesity, high blood pressure, varicose veins and heart, and/or kidney failure. A common complication of stasis dermatitis is cellulitis.

EXAMPLE Stasis dermatitis without varicose veins and ulcer of the leg, 459.81, 707.10.

EXAMPLE Patient with alcoholic cirrhosis of the liver with esophageal varices with bleeding, 571.2, 456.20, 303.90.

EXERCISE 14-5

Assign codes to the following conditions using your ICD-9-CM code book.

1. Atherosclerosis of the extremities with rest pain and gangrene ____________
2. Arteriosclerotic cardiovascular disease ____________
3. Arteriosclerosis of a carotid artery ____________
4. Atherosclerosis of a nonautologous bypass graft of the leg ____________
5. Dissection of the thoracic aorta ____________
6. Type II dissection of the aorta ____________
7. Iliac artery aneurysm ____________
8. Acquired arteriovenous aneurysm of the brain ____________
9. Buerger's disease ____________
10. Embolic infarction of the abdominal aorta ____________
11. Thrombosis of the subclavian artery ____________
12. Deep vein thrombosis of the lower extremity ____________
13. Peroneal thrombophlebitic DVT ____________
14. Scrotal varices ____________
15. Varicose veins, asymptomatic ____________

V CODES

In the past, V codes were considered for use primarily in the outpatient setting. This has changed with the addition of more V codes each year. As was discussed in Chapter 8, it may be difficult to locate V codes in the index. Coders often say, "I did not know there was a V code for that."

Refer to Chapter 8 for a listing of common main terms used to locate V codes. A review of the Tabular reveals that some V codes pertain to diseases of the circulatory system:

V12.50	Personal history of unspecified circulatory disease
V12.51	Personal history of thrombosis and embolism
V12.52	Personal history of thrombophlebitis
V12.53	Personal history of sudden cardiac arrest
V12.54	Personal history of TIA and cerebral infarction without deficits
V12.59	Personal history of other disease of the circulatory system
V15.1	Surgery to heart and great vessels
V17.1	Family history of stroke
V17.3	Family history of ischemic heart disease
V17.40	Family history of cardiovascular disease, unspecified
V17.41	Family history of sudden cardiac death
V17.49	Family history of other cardiovascular diseases
V42.1	History of heart transplant
V42.2	History of heart valve transplant
V43.21	Heart assist device
V43.22	Fully implantable artificial heart
V43.3	Heart valve replaced by artificial valve
V45.00	Postprocedural status of unspecified cardiac device
V45.01	Postprocedural status cardiac pacemaker
V45.02	Postprocedural status AICD (automatic implantable cardioverter-defibrillator)
V45.09	Postprocedural status of other specified cardiac device

V45.81	Aortocoronary bypass status
V45.82	Percutaneous transluminal coronary angioplasty status
V47.2	Other cardiorespiratory problems
V49.83	Awaiting organ transplant status
V53.31	Fitting and adjustment of cardiac pacemaker
V53.32	Fitting and adjustment of AICD (automatic implantable cardioverter-defibrillator)
V53.39	Fitting and adjustment of other cardiac device
V58.73	Aftercare following surgery of the circulatory system, not elsewhere classified (NEC)
V58.61	Long-term (current) drug use–anticoagulant
V58.63	Long-term (current) drug use–antiplatelet/antithrombotic
V58.66	Long-term (current) drug use–aspirin
V71.7	Observation for suspected cardiovascular disease not found
V72.81	Preoperative cardiovascular examination
V81.0	Special screening for ischemic heart disease
V81.1	Special screening for hypertension
V81.2	Special screening for other and unspecified cardiovascular conditions

EXAMPLE Patient admitted with chest pain. Has a history of PTCA. 786.50, V45.82.

EXAMPLE Patient admitted for DVT lower extremity. On Coumadin for previous stroke. 453.40, V58.61, V12.54.

EXERCISE 14-6

Assign codes to the following conditions using your ICD-9-CM code book.

1. Patient is admitted to the hospital with chest pain; the only risk factor he has is a family history of CAD __________
2. Patient is admitted with pulmonary edema, history of CHF, and history of a heart valve replaced by a prosthesis __________
3. Patient is admitted to the hospital with an acute MI and history of a five-vessel CABG __________
4. Patient is admitted to the hospital with ACS and has a history of angioplasty __________
5. Patient is admitted to the hospital with syncope and has previously had a pacemaker inserted __________
6. Patient is awaiting a heart transplant and is on a heart assist device __________

COMMON TREATMENTS

CONDITION	MEDICATION/TREATMENT
Angina	Nitroglycerin, beta blockers, and calcium channel blockers Coreg, Lopressor, Norvasc
Atrial fibrillation	Blood thinners (Coumadin, Plavix, Ticlid) Rate control: calcium channel blockers Cardizem, verapamil Beta blockers atenolol Lopressor, Inderal, Digoxin, Lanoxin
Congestive heart failure	Diuretics such as Lasix, Bumex, and Zaroxolyn Beta blockers
Hypertension	Diuretics Aldactone Beta blockers atenolol, Vasotec, Cozaar, Calan, Cardizem, Aldomet (for additional antihypertensive drugs see p. 338)
Stroke/CVA (nonhemorrhagic)	Blood thinners (Coumadin, Plavix, Ticlid) and clot busting agents such as tPA and streptokinase

PROCEDURES

Some of the procedures that may be related to diseases of the circulatory system may be located in the following chapters of the Procedure Tabular:

0. Procedures and Interventions, Not Elsewhere Classified (00)
7. Operations on the Cardiovascular System (35-39)

Diagnostic Cardiac Catheterization

Diagnostic cardiac catheterization (Figure 14-14) is a procedure that may be performed on a patient with chest pain, angina, or an acute MI to determine if coronary artery disease is present. This procedure allows the physician to view the heart chambers, valves, and arteries. A hollow needle or catheter is inserted into the vein for a right heart catheterization, and into an artery in the arm or groin for a left heart catheterization. Usually, this catheter is inserted into the groin in the femoral artery, and winds its way up into the coronary artery. Pictures of the arteries are then taken. These pictures are called coronary arteriograms or angiograms. When a cardiac catheterization is coded, the procedure codes listed in Table 14-2 may be assigned. The most common set of codes for a cardiac catheterization includes the codes 37.22 left cardiac catheterization, 88.53 left ventriculography, and 88.56 coronary angiography.

Once the cardiologist has determined the extent of the patient's problem, he or she decides on medical therapy, refers the patient for bypass, or performs a therapeutic procedure right then and there, while the catheter is in place. The cardiologist may go on to perform the procedures as described below.

Angioplasty

Angioplasty is a procedure that is usually done with a balloon (Figure 14-15). The device inflates and the plaque is compressed against the wall of the artery. This procedure is often abbreviated as PTCA (percutaneous transluminal coronary angioplasty).

EXAMPLE

Patient with CAD presents for PTCA of left anterior descending and left circumflex, 414.01, 00.66, 00.41.

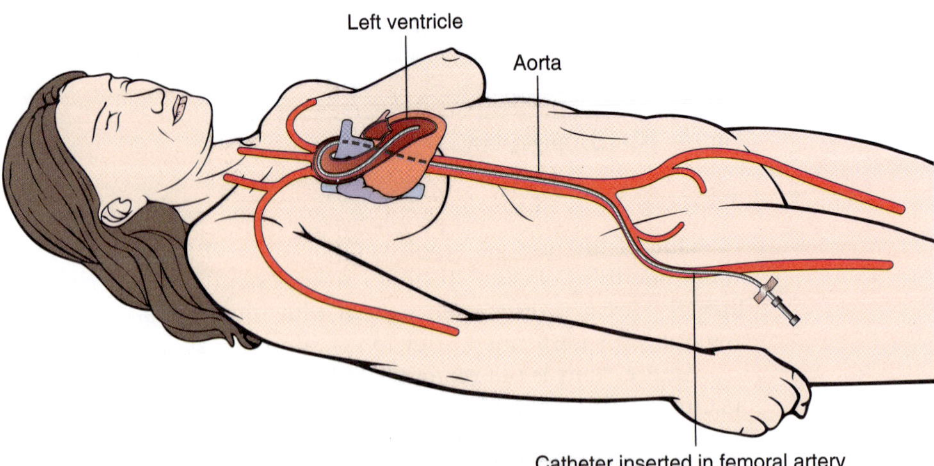

Figure 14-14. Left-sided cardiac catheterization. The catheter is passed retrograde (backward) from the femoral artery into the aorta and then into the left ventricle. For right-sided cardiac catheterization, the cardiologist inserts a catheter through the femoral vein and advances it to the right atrium and right ventricle and into the pulmonary artery.

Table 14-2. Common Procedure Codes for Cardiac Catheterization

Test	Procedure	Comment
Left heart cath	37.22	Most commonly done alone when used to diagnose coronary artery disease (CAD)
Right heart cath	37.21	This is used most commonly for assessment of ventricular function, especially for patients who also have congestive heart failure (CHF).
Combined right and left	37.23	
Right angiogram	88.52	All of these angiograms are also called Ventriculograms.
Left angiogram	88.53	
Combined right and left angiogram	88.54	
Coronary arteriography	88.55	Also known as Sones technique; uses single cath
Coronary arteriography	88.56	Also known as Judkins technique; uses two catheters
Coronary arteriography	88.57	Other and unspecified coronary arteriography

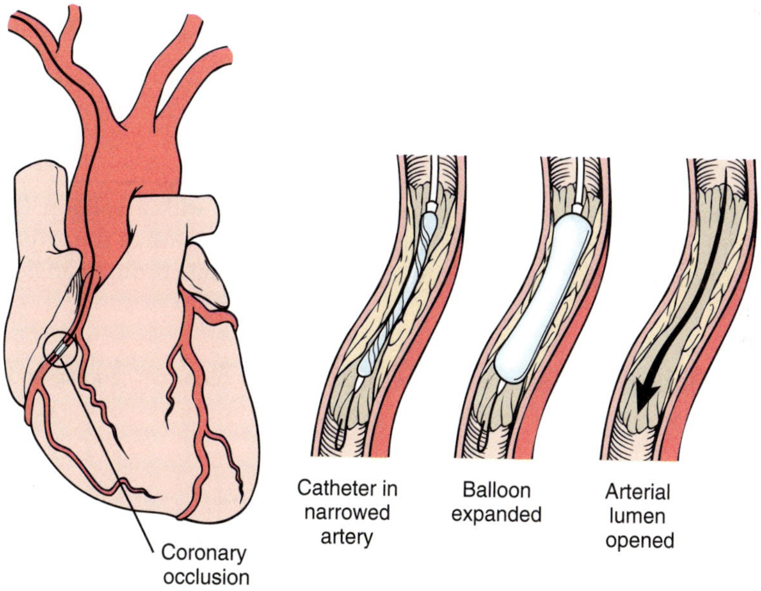

Figure 14-15. Angioplasty.

One of the most common complications of angioplasty is restenosis, which occurs in about one third of cases. To try to avoid restenosis, physicians may use a stent. Sometimes, they also treat a restenosed patient with intravascular radiation therapy. Most often, an angioplasty is performed prior to insertion of a stent.

Atherectomy is the removal of plaque from a vessel. This may be done with the use of a catheter with a shaver or rotablator on the end. A laser is also used to perform atherectomy. An atherectomy is assigned the same code as a PTCA.

Stent insertion into the coronary artery is a procedure that may be performed after completion of an angioplasty (Figure 14-16). The stent helps to keep the artery open. Inserted stents may be drug eluting (DES) or non–drug eluting.

Two types of drug-eluting stents are currently in use in the United States. These include a paclitaxel-eluting stent, and a sirolimus-eluting stent. These drug-eluting stents are not to

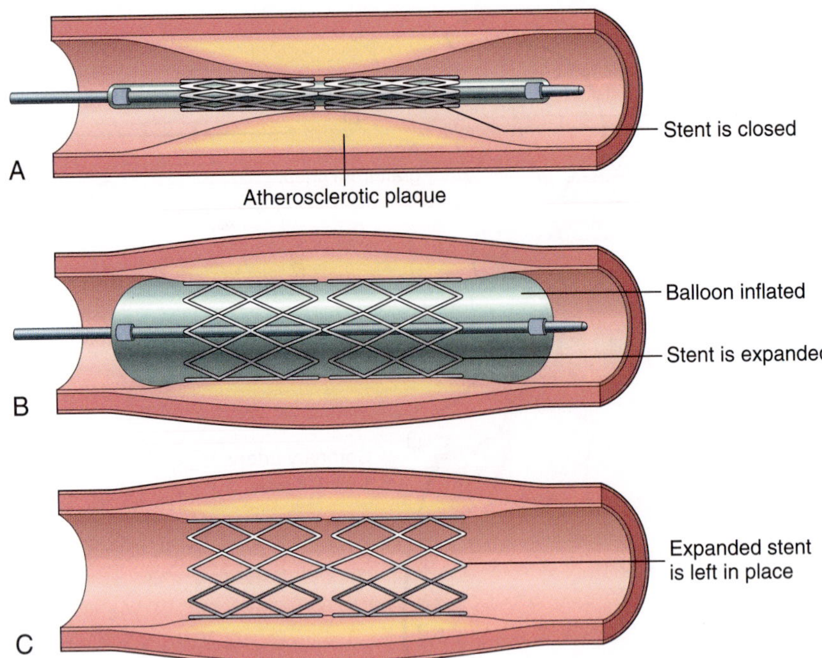

Figure 14-16. Placement of an intracoronary stent. **A,** The stent is positioned at the site of the lesion. **B,** The balloon is inflated, thereby expanding the stent. **C,** The balloon is then deflated and removed, and the implanted stent is left in place. Coronary stents are stainless steel scaffolding devices that help hold open arteries such as the coronary, renal, and carotid arteries.

be confused with a stent that may be coated with antiplatelet drug, which would be assigned 36.06. The coding of stenting usually requires four procedures codes: a code for the angioplasty/atherectomy, a code for the number of stents inserted, a code for the number of vessels treated, and a code for the type of stent inserted.

EXAMPLE

The patient had a percutaneous coronary intervention (PCI) which included inserting a drug-eluting stent into the LAD for coronary atherosclerosis, 414.01, 00.66, 36.07, 00.45, 00.40.

Coronary Artery Bypass Graft

Coronary artery bypass graft (CABG or CAB) is surgery that is performed to bypass blood around the clogged arteries to the heart (Figure 14-17). The procedure is done by taking a healthy blood vessel from another part of the body, usually the internal mammary artery or the saphenous vein. Surgeons should document in their operative notes the number of arteries bypassed and the types of blood vessels used.

When reading a bypass operative report, it is helpful to know the coronary arteries that may be bypassed. Two main coronary arteries are located on the left (LCA) and on the right (RCA). The LCA divides into two arteries: the LAD and the circumflex. The RCA divides into the posterior descending artery (PDA) and the marginal branch. Smaller branches consist of the acute marginal, the obtuse marginal (OM), and the diagonals (Figure 14-18).

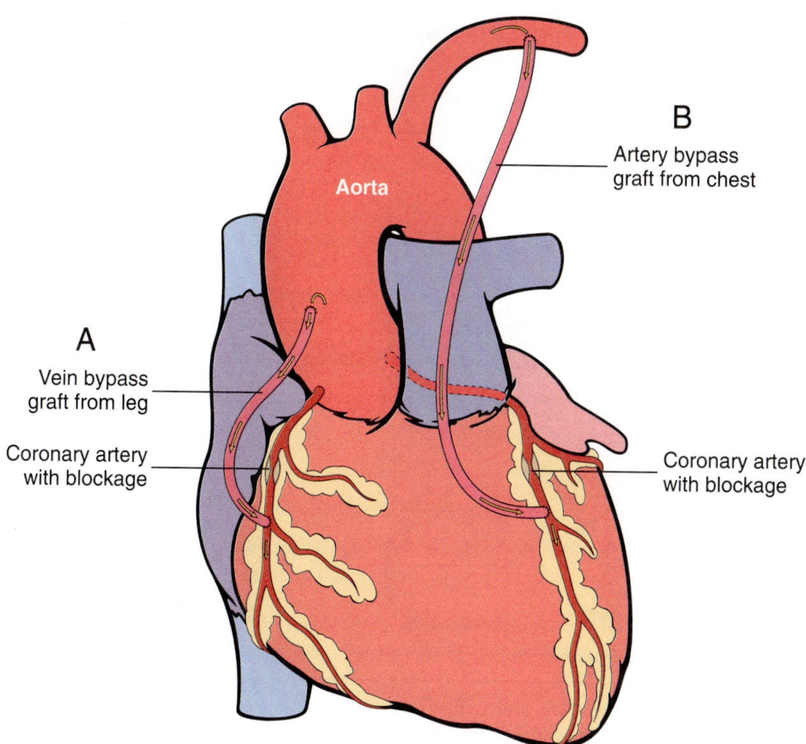

Figure 14-17. Coronary artery bypass graft (CABG) surgery with anastomosis of vein and arterial grafts. **A,** Section of a vein is removed from the leg and is anastomosed (upside down because of its directional valves) to a coronary artery to bypass the area of arteriosclerotic blockage. **B,** An internal mammary artery is grafted to a coronary artery to bypass a blockage.

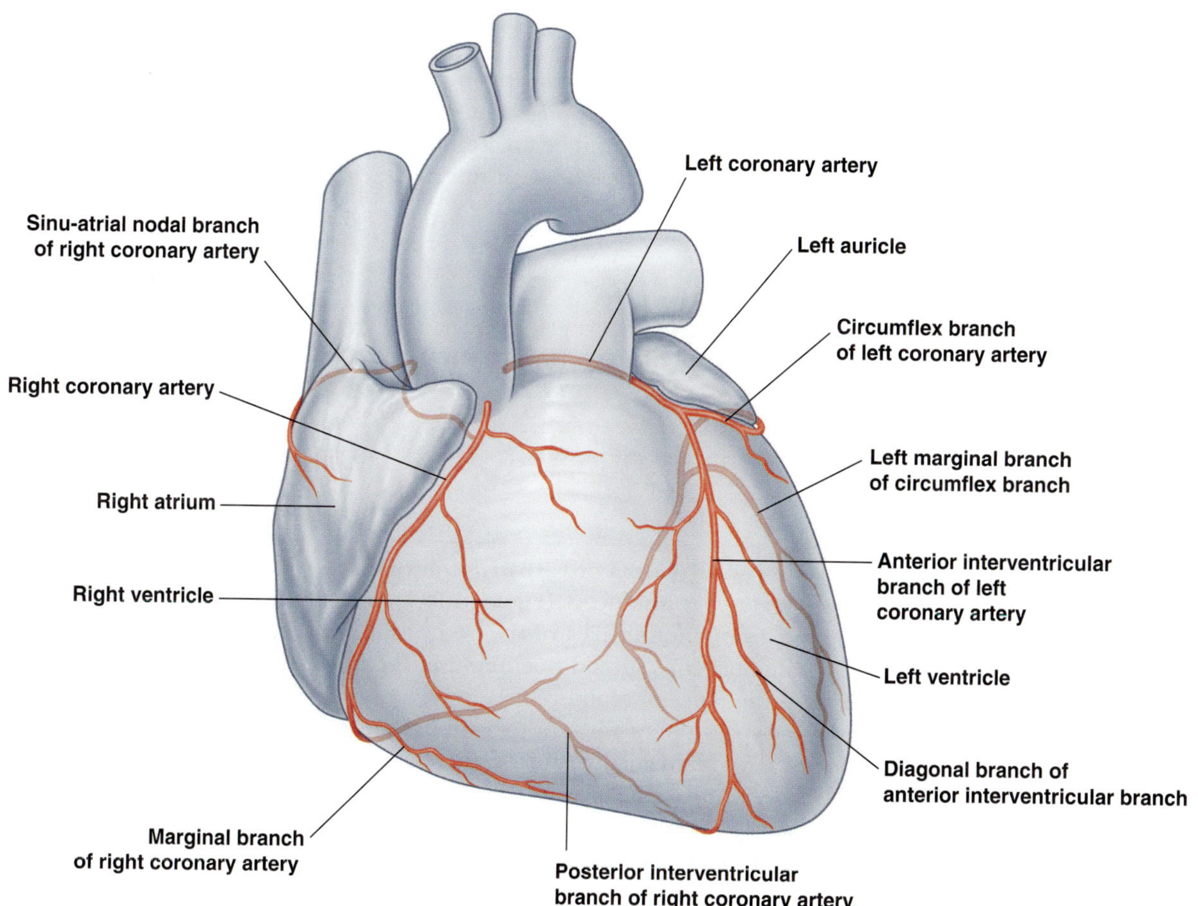

Figure 14-18. Anterior view of coronary arterial system.

EXAMPLE

For example, it might be documented as follows:

Coronary bypass times three. Saphenous vein graft to the LAD and to the obtuse marginal and internal mammary to the right posterior descending. Codes assigned would be as follows:

36.12 for bypass of the two coronary arteries using the saphenous veins and
36.15 for the internal mammary bypass.

Per *Coding Clinic* (1997:3Q:p14),[18] the axis used in assignment of the code for aorto-coronary bypass grafts is the number of coronary arteries that were involved in a graft from the aorta to the coronary artery. When coding CABGs, coders should be aware that code 39.61, cardiopulmonary bypass, should be assigned if it is performed. The note under category 36.1 also advises the coding of 00.16 (pressurized treatment of venous bypass graft with pharmaceutical substance) if it is performed.

It is not appropriate to assign additional codes for other procedures that are auxiliary to heart surgery such as hypothermia (39.62), cardioplegia (39.63), intraoperative cardiac pacing (39.64), and chest tube insertion (34.04). These procedures are considered integral to the bypass surgery procedure and do not require separate codes. This information is taken from *Coding Clinic* (1995:1Q:p5-6).[19]

Electrophysiologic Studies/Procedures

Electrophysiologic studies (EPS) are used to analyze the electrical conduction system of the heart. Patients with symptoms such as light-headedness, palpitations, or syncope may have EP tests done to determine the cause of these symptoms. Other patients with known heart rhythm disturbances may have EP studies so that the severity of the heart disturbance can be determined. During these studies, catheters are inserted into a vein in the leg and are threaded to the heart. They measure electrical signals and conduction of these signals and look for abnormal heart rhythms. The **electrophysiologist** (physician trained in electrical disorders of the heart) may administer electrical stimuli to check the heart's response.

Ablation is correction of abnormal heart rhythm by burning of abnormal heart tissue through radiofrequency or other methods such as laser, microwave, or freezing. Radiofrequency ablation (RFA) can be performed with the use of an EP catheter.

EXAMPLE

Patient is admitted through the ER with atrial fibrillation and a history of COPD. She is taken to the EPS lab for EPS testing, mapping, and radiofrequency ablation, 427.31, 496, 37.34, 37.27, 37.26.

Pacemaker/Defibrillators (AICD)

A pacemaker is a device that is used to correct abnormally slow heartbeats and other abnormalities of heart conduction. Patients who present with syncope and studies determined that they have a heart block often require a pacemaker. A pacemaker has two functions: sensing and pacing. Pacing is the sending of electrical signals to the heart from the pacemaker via the lead. If the rhythm of the heart is too slow, the pacemaker paces the heart to a faster rhythm. Sensing involves monitoring the heart's electrical activity; when the heart is functioning normally, no pacing is required.

The pacemaker system consists of the pulse generator (device, battery) and the leads (electrodes) (Figure 14-19). Leads are placed into the heart chambers and are then attached to the generator. These can be temporary or permanent. A temporary pacemaker is used for emergencies or intraoperatively. Code assignment for a temporary pacemaker does not require codes for the leads or codes for removal.

A permanent pacemaker is implanted through an incision near the collarbone. Wires are inserted into a vein and are advanced into the heart; they are then connected to a generator, which is implanted under the skin. Coding of initial insertion of permanent pace-

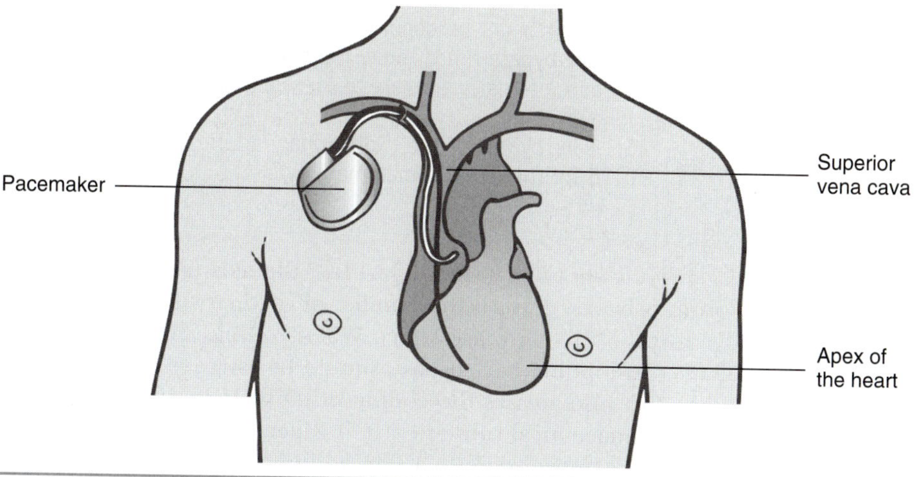

Figure 14-19. Cardiac leads in the atrium and in the ventricle enable a dual-chamber pacemaker to sense and pace in both heart chambers.

makers requires two codes: one for the insertion of the generator/device, and one for insertion of the leads or electrodes. Leads can be placed inside the heart or outside the heart (epicardially). Pacemaker pockets for epicardial leads are usually placed in the abdominal wall; this is typically done for children who are still growing.

Insertion/replacement/revision requires that the coder must know the type of device that is being inserted. Codes for initial insertion and replacement require knowledge as to whether this is a single-chamber or a dual-chamber device and whether the device is rate responsive. A rate-responsive device has a sensor that detects changes in movement of the body and reacts accordingly.

EXAMPLE Initial insertion single-chamber device uses a single lead, 37.81 and 37.71 or 37.73.

EXAMPLE Initial insertion dual-chamber device uses two leads, 37.82 and 37.72.

Separate codes are used for replacement of devices and leads and removal of devices and leads. When a replacement is performed, the removal code is included in the replacement code. The code V53.31, Fitting and adjustment of cardiac pacemaker, is assigned as the principal diagnosis when a patient is admitted for removal, replacement, or reprogramming. Often, surgeons document that a patient is being admitted for end of life of the battery or pacemaker.

EXAMPLE Removal of a pacemaker and leads, V53.31, 37.77, 37.89.

EXAMPLE Initial insertion of a dual-chamber pacemaker and leads, 37.83, 37.72.

EXAMPLE Replacement of a single-chamber pacemaker with a dual-chamber device, 37.87, 37.76.

An automatic implantable cardioverter-defibrillator (AICD) is a device that is used for treating patients with tachyarrhythmias. Similar to a pacemaker, it has a pulse generator and electrodes that both sense and defibrillate. Defibrillators give shocks that attempt to convert the heart rhythm. Implantation of this system is usually done via thoracotomy or sternotomy. The code for this procedure is 37.94, which is assigned for insertion or replacement of the total system. On occasion, this may be done as a two-stage procedure, in which the leads may be implanted on one day and the generator on the next day. The staged

procedure would then use codes 37.95 and 37.96. Additional codes are used for replacement of both leads and generators.

EXAMPLE Patient is admitted with ventricular tachycardia and has an AICD placed, 427.1, 37.94.

Biventricular pacing is also known as cardiac resynchronization therapy (CRT). Biventricular pacemakers come as a stand-alone device or with a built-in implantable cardioverter (ICV). They are used primarily to treat heart failure. Similar to a pacemaker, a generator and leads are included. The biventricular pacemaker uses a third lead. This third lead, which is attached to the wall of the left ventricle in the vein of the coronary sinus, causes both ventricles to contract at the same time or in sync. In contrast to regular pacemakers, biventricular pacemakers do not increase heart rate. Some biventricular pacers include internal cardiac defibrillators (ICDs) for patients with fast irregular rhythms. These systems have biventricular pacing, anti-tachycardia pacing, and internal defibrillators. There are codes for implantation and replacement of both systems, with the ICD and without.

EXAMPLE Implantation of a cardiac resynchronization treatment pacemaker (CRT-P) without mention of defibrillation, total system CRT-P, or biventricular pacing without ICD, 00.50.

EXAMPLE Implantation of cardiac resynchronization treatment defibrillator (CRT-D), total system CRT-D, or biventricular pacing and ICD total system, 00.51.

Often, surgeons will upgrade to a biventricular pacing system. A patient who currently has an AICD and is upgraded to a biventricular pacer with a defibrillator would be assigned code 00.51. For further information on this subject, refer to *Coding Clinic* (2002:4Q: p100).[20]

Aneurysm Repair

Repair of aneurysm can be done in several ways. Code 38.4X is assigned for repair of an aneurysm by grafting, and code 38.3X is assigned for excision of an aneurysm with anastomosis. Clipping is another form of aneurysm repair. Aneurysm repair can also be performed endovascularly. These repairs are done by making a small incision in the groin and deploying the graft via the catheter through the vessel.

EXAMPLE Patient presents for repair of an abdominal aortic aneurysm. The repair is performed endovascularly, 441.4, 39.71.

Central Lines/Catheters

Central venous lines are used for several purposes. They may be used to administer chemotherapy, total parenteral nutrition (TPN), antibiotics, and for dialysis. Hickman, Groshong, triple lumen, and double lumen are all types of central lines. Usually, central venous catheters are inserted into the subclavian or jugular vein and are then advanced into the vena cava. A central line has a catheter that is NOT totally implanted under the skin. A peripherally inserted central catheter (PICC) (Figure 14-20) is assigned the same code as a central line. It is inserted in a slightly different manner. Separate procedure codes are used for venous catheterization for renal dialysis, arterial lines, and vascular access devices.

EXAMPLE Patient is admitted to the hospital for endocarditis. A central line is inserted for administration of antibiotics to treat the endocarditis, 424.90, 38.93.

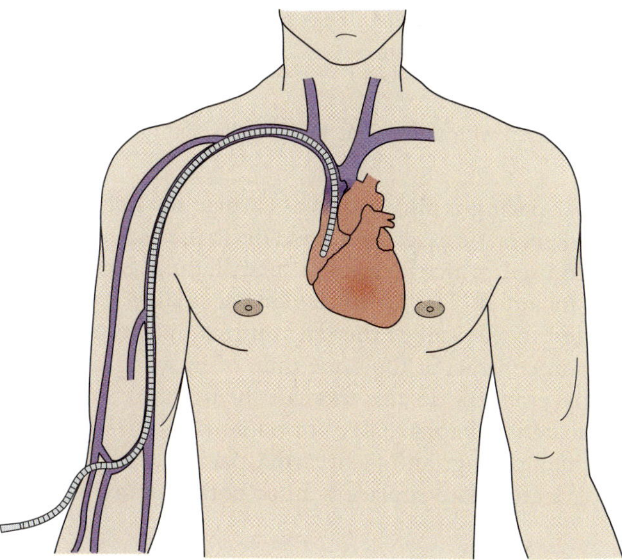

Figure 14-20. A peripherally inserted central catheter is threaded through the vein until the end is near the heart.

EXERCISE 14-7

Assign codes to the following conditions using your ICD-9-CM code book.

1. Patient is admitted for a diagnostic left cardiac catheterization with a diagnosis of chest pain ____________
2. Patient is admitted with a diagnosis of CAD for a PTCA with CYPHER stent insertion into the LAD ____________
3. Patient is admitted 3 days status post angioplasty with restenosis of a stent; a non–drug-eluting stent is inserted into the RCA ____________
4. Patient with CAD is admitted, and a bypass of four coronary arteries is performed; bypass grafts were performed with use of the left internal mammary to the LAD, and saphenous vein grafts were used to bypass PDA, circumflex, and obtuse marginal ____________
5. Patient is admitted with ventricular fibrillation, and RF ablation is performed ____________
6. Patient is admitted with bradycardia, and a complete dual chamber pacemaker system is inserted ____________
7. Patient is admitted for a pacemaker battery change for the end of life of the battery ____________
8. Patient with CHF is admitted for total biventricular pacing with internal cardiac defibrillation ____________
9. Patient is admitted with cerebral aneurysm, and a clipping is performed ____________
10. Patient with a tachyarrhythmia has a total AICD placed ____________

DOCUMENTATION/REIMBURSEMENT/MS-DRGs

Often, documentation difficulties are due to lack of documentation. Sometimes pathology and other test results are not available at the time of discharge, or when the physician is dictating the discharge summary or is reporting the final diagnoses.

MS-DRG With and Without MCC/CC

EXAMPLE

Patient was admitted with subendocardial MI; patient also was treated for acidosis, 410.71, 276.2.

DIAGNOSES	CODES	MS-DRG	RW
Acute subendocardial MI	410.71	282	1.0617
Acute subendocardial MI with acidosis	410.71 276.2	281	1.3126

Coronary Artery Disease/Unstable Angina/Chest Pain

It is important to note that on several occasions, *Coding Clinic* has addressed the issue of CAD and angina. Per *Coding Clinic* (1997:2Q:p13),[21] if angina and CAD have been previously linked, it is appropriate to sequence CAD as the principal diagnosis. Likewise, if a patient has had a previous CABG and then presents with USA (unstable angina), the principal diagnosis would again be CAD (*Coding Clinic* [2001:3Q:p15][22]). If a patient presents with USA, and a cardiac catheterization is performed that determines that the patient has CAD that is causing the angina, then the principal diagnosis would once again be CAD. In other words, the underlying cause or CAD would always be the principal diagnosis if it has been determined in the current visit or in previous visits to be the cause of angina. These above stated rules do NOT apply to chest pain. Also of note, *Coding Clinic* (1993:1Q:p25)[23] advises that when a patient presents with chest pain due to cocaine intoxication, the poisoning code (968.5) is the principal diagnosis.

EXAMPLE

DIAGNOSES	CODES	MS-DRG	RW
Chest pain with or without complication/comorbidity	786.59	313	0.5489
Unstable angina	411.1	311	0.5118
Unstable angina With left heart cath	411.1 37.22, 88.53, 88.56	287	1.1412
CAD without complication/comorbidity	414.01	303	0.6055
CAD with left heart cath	414.01 37.22, 88.53, 88.56	287	1.1412

EXAMPLE

Patient presents to the hospital complaining of chest pain. The patient is admitted to the coronary care unit (CCU), and cardiology performs a cardiac cath. The left heart cath determines that the patient does not have coronary artery disease. The principal diagnosis in this case is noncardiac chest pain, 786.59, with 37.22, 88.53, 88.56.

EXAMPLE

Patient presents to the hospital with chest pain. The emergency physician determines that the patient has unstable angina. The patient is admitted to the CCU, and cardiology performs a left heart cath. The cath determines that the patient has severe coronary artery disease. The principal diagnosis in this case is 414.01 for CAD; a secondary diagnosis is 411.1 for unstable angina, 37.22, 88.53, 88.56 for left cardiac catheterization.

Pacemakers/ICDs/Cardioverter/Defibrillators

Insertion of pacemakers, as mentioned earlier in the chapter, more often than not will require two codes. One code will be assigned for insertion of the generator, and the other for insertion of the leads. As illustrated below, if the leads are not coded, the payment would be significantly lower.

EXAMPLE

DIAGNOSES	CODES	MS-DRG	RW
Sick sinus syndrome (SSS) with insertion of dual chamber pacemaker (coded only the device, not the leads)	427.81 37.83	310	0.6439
SSS with insertion of dual chamber pacemaker (both leads and device)	427.81 37.83, 37.72	244	2.1367

EXAMPLE

DIAGNOSES	CODES	MS-DRG
SSS with insertion of total biventricular pacemaker CRT-P	427.81 00.50	244
SSS with insertion of total biventricular defibrillator CRT-D	427.81 00.51	227

CHAPTER REVIEW EXERCISE

Assign codes for all diagnoses and procedures including all applicable V and E codes.

1. Patient has atrial fibrillation with rapid ventricular response ____________
2. Patient had a previous CVA and now has left hemiparesis ____________
3. Patient has orthostatic hypotension ____________
4. Patient has mitral and tricuspid insufficiency ____________
5. Patient has congestive heart failure, rheumatic ____________
6. Patient has both acute and chronic renal failure and a history of hypertension; patient is currently taking verapamil and is on dialysis ____________
7. Patient has congestive heart failure with pleural effusion and hypertension ____________
8. Patient has chest pain and elevated troponins ____________
9. Patient presents with a non–Q wave myocardial infarction (NQMI), is taken to the cath lab for a left heart cath, and has a drug-eluting stent inserted in RCA for coronary artery disease ____________
10. Patient with a previous CABG presents to the hospital with USA ____________
11. Patient with ACS presents to the hospital; patient is taken to the cath lab and following a left cardiac cath and diagnosis of CAD, the patient was immediately taken to surgery, where a 2-vessel CABG is performed ____________
12. Patient has a left anterior fascicular block ____________
13. Patient is admitted through the ER with chest pain that is determined to be coronary artery disease following a left heart cath. Following the cath procedure, the patient dies of cardiac arrest ____________

14. Patient has congestive systolic and diastolic heart failure __________
15. Patient presents to the hospital with pulmonary edema and a history of hypertensive congestive heart failure for which the patient currently takes Lasix and verapamil __________
16. Patient is admitted for a stroke with left side weakness and dysphagia. Upon discharge the weakness has resolved. __________
17. Patient has a history of stroke and is currently admitted with atrial fibrillation and dysphagia due to the old stroke __________
18. Patient has arteriosclerosis of the extremities and is admitted with an ulcer and gangrene of the foot __________
19. Patient is admitted to the hospital with deep vein thrombosis and a pulmonary embolism __________
20. History of heart valve replaced with porcine valve __________
21. Patient had a left heart catheterization, a left ventriculography, and a single-catheter coronary arteriography to determine the cause of chest pain __________
22. Patient had an angioplasty with atherectomy of the right coronary artery for CAD __________
23. Patient with CAD had a coronary bypass times two using one saphenous vein and one internal mammary; the cardiac bypass pump was used __________
24. Patient had a complete pacemaker inserted for syncope, which was attributed to bradycardia __________
25. Patient had congestive heart failure and was treated with CRT __________
26. Patient had an abdominal aortic aneurysm (AAA) and was treated with endovascular repair __________
27. Patient was admitted with endocarditis and had a Hickman catheter inserted for antibiotic administration __________

Write the correct answer(s) in the space(s) provided.

28. Which MS-DRG is better reimbursed—the one for CAD? Or for USA? __________

CHAPTER GLOSSARY

Ablation: correction of abnormal heart rhythm by burning of abnormal heart tissue through radiofrequency or other methods such as laser, microwave, or freezing

Aneurysm: bulging or ballooning out of a vessel.

Angioplasty: a procedure performed to treat coronary artery disease. An inflated balloon compresses plaque against artery walls.

Aphasia: impairment of speech expression and/or word understanding.

Atherosclerosis: type of arteriosclerosis wherein fatty substances such as plaque block or clog the arteries.

Blood pressure: the force that blood puts on the arterial walls when the heart beats.

BNP: a hormone that is produced by the heart.

Bradycardia: slow heart rate, generally fewer than 60 beats per minute.

Capillaries: smallest blood vessel through which material passes to and from the bloodstream.

Cardiac arrest: sudden loss of heart function.

Cardiomyopathy: a disorder of the muscles of the heart chambers that impedes heart function.

Cognitive defect: a disorder in thinking, learning, awareness, or judgment.

Conduction disorder: abnormalities of cardiac impulses.

Electrophysiologist: cardiologist trained to perform interventional cardiac electrophysiologic procedures and surgical device implantation.

Coronary artery bypass graft: surgery performed to bypass an occluded coronary artery.

Deep vein thrombosis: a blood clot that forms in a deep vein.

Dissection: tear in wall of a vessel.

Electrophysiologist: physician trained in electrical disorders of the heart.

Embolus: clot that travels to another part of the body.

Endocarditis: inflammation of the lining of the heart chambers and valves.

Fistula: an abnormal passage between an artery and a vein.

Heart failure: impaired function of the heart's pumping ability.

Hypertension, malignant: "rapidly rising blood pressure, usually in excess of 140 mm Hg diastolic with findings of visual impairment and symptoms or signs of progressive cardiac failure.

Insidious: harmful.

Insufficiency of a heart valve: incomplete closure of a heart valve, causing a leaky valve.

Myocardial infarction: heart attack.

NSTEMI: non–ST elevation myocardial infarction.

Pericarditis: inflammation of the covering of the heart.

Phlebitis: inflammation of a vein.

Pulmonary embolism: a blood clot(s) in the pulmonary artery that causes blockage in the artery.

Pulmonary hypertension: high blood pressure in the arteries that supply blood to the lungs.

Regurgitation of heart valve: backward flow of blood between the heart chambers.

Stasis dermatitis: skin condition due to poor circulation (venous insufficiency) that is characterized by swelling, skin discoloration, weeping, itching, and scaly skin.

STEMI: ST elevation myocardial infarction.

Stenosis: abnormal narrowing.

Stroke: cerebrovascular accident, or brain infarction.

Tachycardia: fast heart rate, generally greater than 100 beats per minute.

Thoracentesis: puncture of the chest wall to remove fluid (pleural effusion) from the space between the lining of the outside of the lungs (pleura) and the wall of the chest.

Thrombus: a clot that forms and remains in a vein.

Transient ischemic attack: a stroke that lasts for only a few minutes.

Varicose veins: enlarged, twisted veins that usually occur in the legs.

CHAPTER 15

Neoplasms

(ICD-9-CM Chapter 2, Codes 140-239)

CHAPTER OUTLINE

LEARNING OBJECTIVES

- Apply and assign the correct ICD-9-CM codes in accordance with Official Guidelines for Coding and Reporting
- Identify pertinent anatomy and physiology for neoplasm
- Assign the correct M codes
- Identify neoplastic diseases
- Assign the correct V codes and procedure codes related to neoplasms
- Identify common treatments, medications, laboratory values, and diagnostic tests
- Explain the importance of documentation in relation to MS-DRGs for reimbursement

ABBREVIATIONS

AIDS acquired immunodeficiency syndrome

ALL acute lymphocytic leukemia

BMR biological response modifiers

BMT bone marrow transplant

CC chief complaint

CDC Centers for Disease Control and Prevention

CLL chronic lymphocytic leukemia

CML chronic myelogenous leukemia

CNS central nervous system

DCIS ductal carcinoma in situ

FNA fine needle aspiration

HCC hepatocellular carcinoma

ICD-9-CM *International Classification of Diseases, 9th revision, Clinical Modification*

MS-DRG Medicare severity diagnosis-related group

NHL non-Hodgkin's lymphoma

NSCLC non–small cell lung cancer

RCC renal cell carcinoma

SCLC small cell lung cancer

UHDDS Uniform Hospital Discharge Data Set

ICD-9-CM Official Guidelines for Coding and Reporting

Please refer to the companion Evolve website for the most current guidelines.

2. Chapter 2: Neoplasms (140-239)

General guidelines

Chapter 2 of the ICD-9-CM contains the codes for most benign and all malignant neoplasms. Certain benign neoplasms, such as prostatic adenomas, may be found in the specific body system chapters. To properly code a neoplasm it is necessary to determine from the record if the neoplasm is benign, in-situ, malignant, or of uncertain histologic behavior. If malignant, any secondary (metastatic) sites should also be determined.

The neoplasm table in the Alphabetic Index should be referenced first. However, if the histological term is documented, that term should be referenced first, rather than going immediately to the Neoplasm Table, in order to determine which column in the Neoplasm Table is appropriate. For example, if the documentation indicates "adenoma," refer to the term in the Alphabetic Index to review the entries under this term and the instructional note to "see also neoplasm, by site, benign." The table provides the proper code based on the type of neoplasm and the site. It is important to select the proper column in the table that corresponds to the type of neoplasm. The tabular should then be referenced to verify that the correct code has been selected from the table and that a more specific site code does not exist. *See Section I. C. 18.d.4. for information regarding V codes for genetic susceptibility to cancer.*

a. Treatment directed at the malignancy

If the treatment is directed at the malignancy, designate the malignancy as the principal diagnosis.

EXAMPLE

The patient had a prostatectomy and a radical bilateral lymphadenectomy for prostate acinar adenocarcinoma. Treatment is directed to the primary cancer of the prostate, 185, 60.5, 40.3.

b. Treatment of secondary site

When a patient is admitted because of a primary neoplasm with metastasis and treatment is directed toward the secondary site only, the secondary neoplasm is designated as the principal diagnosis even though the primary malignancy is still present.

EXAMPLE

Three months ago, the patient was given a diagnosis of small cell lung carcinoma with metastasis to the liver. The patient's primary neoplasm is lung carcinoma; the secondary neoplasm is located in the liver. The patient underwent wedge resection for liver metastasis, 197.7, 162.9, 50.22.

c. Coding and sequencing of complications

Coding and sequencing of complications associated with the malignancies or with the therapy thereof are subject to the following guidelines:

1) Anemia associated with malignancy

When admission/encounter is for management of an anemia associated with the malignancy, and the treatment is only for anemia, the appropriate anemia code (such as code 285.22, Anemia in neoplastic disease) is designated as the principal diagnosis and is followed by the appropriate code(s) for the malignancy.

Code 285.22 may also be used as a secondary code if the patient suffers from anemia and is being treated for the malignancy.

EXAMPLE

Anemia due to metastatic bone cancer. The patient has a history of primary breast cancer, which was treated with mastectomy 4 years ago. The patient was admitted for transfusion of packed red blood cells, 285.22, 198.5, V10.3, V45.71, 99.04.

2) Anemia associated with chemotherapy, immunotherapy and radiation therapy

When the admission/encounter is for management of an anemia associated with chemotherapy, immunotherapy or radiotherapy and the only treatment is for the anemia, the anemia is sequenced first followed by code E933.1. The appropriate neoplasm code should be assigned as an additional code.

EXAMPLE

Aplastic anemia due to radiation. The patient is being treated for cancer of the brain. The patient was transfused with 2 units of packed cells, 284.8, 191.9, V15.3, E933.1, 99.04.

3) Management of dehydration due to the malignancy

When the admission/encounter is for management of dehydration due to the malignancy or the therapy, or a combination of both, and only the dehydration is being treated (intravenous rehydration), the dehydration is sequenced first, followed by the code(s) for the malignancy.

EXAMPLE

The patient underwent chemotherapy treatment a few days ago, and since that time has become severely dehydrated. The patient is receiving chemo for treatment of cancer of the colon, 276.51, 153.9.

4) Treatment of a complication resulting from a surgical procedure

When the admission/encounter is for treatment of a complication resulting from a surgical procedure, designate the complication as the principal or first-listed diagnosis if treatment is directed at resolving the complication.

EXAMPLE

Hernia of colostomy with repair of parastomal hernia. The colostomy was performed 1 year ago during colon cancer resection. The patient is no longer receiving treatment, and the cancer was completely resected, 569.69, V10.05, 46.42.

d. Primary malignancy previously excised

When a primary malignancy has been previously excised or eradicated from its site and there is no further treatment directed to that site and there is no evidence of any existing primary malignancy, a code from category V10, Personal history of malignant neoplasm, should be used to indicate the former site of the malignancy. Any mention of extension, invasion, or metastasis to another site is coded as a secondary malignant neoplasm to that site. The secondary site may be the principal or first-listed with the V10 code used as a secondary code.

EXAMPLE

The patient had a melanoma removed from his back 4 years ago. The patient is currently being treated for metastatic melanoma of the lung, 197.0, V10.82.

e. Admissions/Encounters involving chemotherapy, immunotherapy and radiation therapy

1) Episode of care involves surgical removal of neoplasm.

When an episode of care involves the surgical removal of a neoplasm, primary or secondary site, followed by adjunct chemotherapy or radiation treatment during the same episode of care, the neoplasm code should be assigned as principal or first-listed diagnosis, using codes in the 140-198 series or where appropriate in the 200-203 series.

EXAMPLE

The patient had a modified radical mastectomy for malignant neoplasm of the right (upper outer quadrant) breast with adjunct chemotherapy, 174.4, 85.43, 99.25.

2) Patient admission/encounter solely for administration of chemotherapy, immunotherapy and radiation therapy

If a patient admission/encounter is solely for the administration of chemotherapy, immunotherapy or radiation therapy assign code V58.0, Encounter for radiation therapy, or V58.11, Encounter for antineoplastic chemotherapy, or V58.12, Encounter for antineoplastic immunotherapy as the first-listed or principal diagnosis. If a patient receives more than one of these therapies during the same admission more than one of these codes may be assigned, in any sequence.

EXAMPLE

The patient was admitted for chemotherapy treatment of acute lymphocytic leukemia (ALL), V58.11, 204.00, 99.25.

3) Patient admitted for radiotherapy/chemotherapy and immunotherapy and develops complications

When a patient is admitted for the purpose of radiotherapy, immunotherapy or chemotherapy and develops complications such as uncontrolled nausea and vomiting or dehydration, the principal or first-listed diagnosis is V58.0, Encounter for radiotherapy, or V58.11, Encounter for antineoplastic chemotherapy, or V58.12, Encounter for antineoplastic immunotherapy followed by any codes for the complications.

EXAMPLE

The patient was admitted for chemotherapy for lymphoma. Because of nausea and severe vomiting, the patient was also treated for dehydration with IV fl uids, V58.11, 202.80, 276.51, 787.01, 99.25.

f. Admission/encounter to determine extent of malignancy
When the reason for admission/encounter is to determine the extent of the malignancy, or for a procedure such as paracentesis or thoracentesis, the primary malignancy or appropriate metastatic site is designated as the principal or first-listed diagnosis, even though chemotherapy or radiotherapy is administered.

EXAMPLE

Patient has known carcinoma of the left kidney and pleural effusion. Patient is admitted to determine if the renal cancer has spread and a thoracentesis is done, which confirms metastasis to the pleura, 197.2, 189.0, 34.91.

g. Symptoms, signs, and ill-defined conditions listed in Chapter 16 <u>associated with neoplasms</u>
Symptoms, signs, and ill-defined conditions listed in Chapter 16 characteristic of, or associated with, an existing primary or secondary site malignancy cannot be used to replace the malignancy as principal or first-listed diagnosis, regardless of the number of admissions or encounters for treatment and care of the neoplasm.
See section I.C.18.d.14, Encounter for prophylactic organ removal.

EXAMPLE

The patient was admitted with a first time seizure due to brain cancer. The code 780.39 for seizure can be found in Chapter 16, so the brain cancer code would be sequenced as the principal diagnosis, 191.9, 780.39. Not all patients with brain cancer develop seizures, so it is appropriate to code the seizure code as a secondary diagnosis.

h. Admission/encounter for pain control/management
See Section I.C.6.a.5 for information on coding admission/encounter for pain control/management.

Apply the General Coding Guidelines as found in Chapter 5.

ANATOMY AND PHYSIOLOGY

Neoplasms can affect any of the body systems. The anatomy and physiology of these body systems are outlined in their respective chapters. It is important to understand some of the terminology that is specific to neoplasms and their behavior. According to the National Cancer Institute, the most common cancers in the United States include the following:

- Bladder
- Breast
- Colon and Rectal
- Endometrial
- Kidney (renal cell)
- Leukemia
- Lung
- Melanoma
- Non-Hodgkin's Lymphoma
- Pancreatic
- Prostate
- Skin (non-melanoma)
- Thyroid

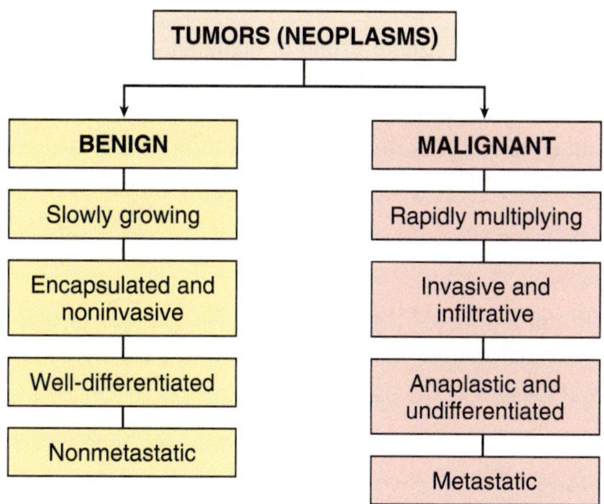

Figure 15-1. Differences between benign and malignant neoplasms.

A **neoplasm** is an abnormal tissue that grows by cellular proliferation more rapidly than normal tissue. Neoplasms show partial or complete lack of structural organization and functional coordination with normal tissue, and they usually form a distinct mass of tissue that may be benign (benign tumor) or malignant (cancer) (Figure 15-1). Both benign and malignant neoplasms are classified according to the type of tissue in which they are found. **Benign** neoplasms are tumors that are not malignant. **Malignancy** is a neoplasm that has the ability to invade adjacent structures and spread to distant sites. **Fibromas** are benign neoplasms of fibrous connective tissue, and **melanomas** are malignant changes of melanin cells. Malignant tumors originating from epithelial tissue (e.g., skin, bronchi, stomach) are called **carcinomas** (Table 15-1). Malignancies of epithelial glandular tissue such as those found in the breast, prostate, and colon are known as **adenocarcinomas**. Malignant growths of connective tissue (e.g., muscle, cartilage, bone) are called **sarcomas** (Table 15-2). **Lymphomas** form in lymphatic tissue, and **leukemias** are malignancies that arise from white blood cells. A **myeloma** originates within the bone marrow.

The **primary site** is the location at which the neoplasm begins, or originates. It is important for the treating physician to identify the site of origin so that the best treatment course and prognosis can be determined. **Metastasis** is the spread of cancer from one part of the body to another, as is seen when neoplasms occur in parts of the body separate from the

Table 15-1. Carcinoma and the Epithelial Tissues From Which They Derive[1]

Types of Epithelial Tissue	Malignant Tumor (carcinoma)
Gastrointestinal Tract	
Colon	Adenocarcinoma of the colon
Esophagus	Esophageal carcinoma
Liver	Hepatocellular carcinoma (hepatoma)
Stomach	Gastric adenocarcinoma
Glandular Tissue	
Adrenal glands	Carcinoma of the adrenals
Breast	Carcinoma of the breast
Pancreas	Carcinoma of the pancreas (pancreatic adenocarcinoma)
Prostate	Carcinoma of the prostate
Thyroid	Carcinoma of the thyroid
Kidney and Bladder	
	Renal cell carcinoma (hypernephroma)
	Transitional cell carcinoma of the bladder

Table 15-1. Carcinoma and the Epithelial Tissues From Which They Derive[1]—cont'd

Types of Epithelial Tissue	Malignant Tumor (carcinoma)
Lung	
	Adenocarcinoma (bronchioloalveolar)
	Large cell carcinoma
	Small (oat) cell carcinoma
	Squamous cell (epidermoid)
Reproductive Organs	
	Adenocarcinoma of the uterus
	Carcinoma of the penis
	Choriocarcinoma of the uterus or testes
	Cystadenocarcinoma (mucinous or serous) of the ovaries
	Seminoma and embryonal cell carcinoma (testes)
	Squamous cell (epidermoid) carcinoma of the vagina or cervix
Skin	
Basal cell layer	Basal cell carcinoma
Melanocyte	Malignant melanoma
Squamous cell layer	Squamous cell carcinoma

Table 15-2. Sarcomas and the Connective Tissues From Which They Derive[2]

Types of Connective Tissue	Malignant Tumor
Bone	
	Osteosarcoma (osteogenic sarcoma)
	Ewing's sarcoma
Muscle	
Smooth (visceral) muscle	Leiomyosarcoma
Striated (skeletal) muscle	Rhabdomyosarcoma
Cartilage	
	Chondrosarcoma
Fat	
	Liposarcoma
Fibrous Tissue	
	Fibrosarcoma
Blood Vessel Tissue	
	Angiosarcoma
Blood-Forming Tissue	
All leukocytes	Leukemias
Lymphocytes	Hodgkin's disease
Plasma cells	Non-Hodgkin's lymphomas
	Burkitt's lymphoma
	Multiple myeloma
Nerve Tissue	
Embryonic nerve tissue	Neuroblastoma
Glial tissue	Astrocytoma (tumors of glial cells, called "astrocytes")
	Glioblastoma multiforme

Table 15-3. Grades of Neoplasms

Grade 1	Cells slightly abnormal and well differentiated
Grade 2	Cells more abnormal and moderately differentiated
Grade 3	Cells very abnormal and poorly differentiated
Grade 4	Cells immature and undifferentiated

site of the primary tumor. Metastasis occurs through dissemination of tumor cells by the lymphatics or blood vessels, or by direct extension through serous cavities or other spaces.

Grading involves pathologic examination of tumor cells. The degree of abnormality of cells determines the grade of cancer (Table 15-3). When the level of cell abnormality is greater, the cancer is of higher grade. Cells that are **well differentiated** closely resemble mature, specialized cells. Tumor cells that are **undifferentiated** are highly abnormal (i.e., immature and primitive).

Cancerous tissue is classified according to degree of malignancy, from grade 1—barely malignant—to grade 4—highly malignant. In practice, it is not always possible for the pathologist to determine the degree of malignancy, and sometimes it may be difficult even to determine whether a particular tumor tissue is benign or malignant.

Staging, a means of categorizing a particular cancer, helps the clinician to determine a particular patient's treatment plan and the need for further therapy. Each type of cancer is staged according to specific characteristics:

- In situ cancers have been diagnosed at the earliest possible stage.
- Stage I or "local" cancers have been diagnosed early and have not spread.
- Stage II has spread into surrounding tissues but not beyond the location of origin.
- Stage III or "regional" cancer has spread to nearby lymph nodes.
- Stage IV or "distant" cancers have spread to other parts of the body and are the most difficult to treat.

See Table 15-4 for an example of how the TNM (tumor-node-metastasis) staging system would be used to classify a lung cancer.

Neoplasm Table

The coding of most neoplasms requires an extra step, which involves use of the Neoplasm Table (Figure 15-2). The main term for the type of neoplasm is located in the Alphabetic Index. All subterms must be reviewed to facilitate assignment of proper codes, including M codes if required. One must follow all instructions, such as *see* Neoplasm, by site, benign, or *see also* Neoplasm, by site, malignant. It is important to follow all steps to ensure correct code assignment. The temptation to go directly to the Neoplasm Table should be avoided.

Morphology Codes

Morphology codes (M codes) identify the type of cell that has become neoplastic in its biological activity or behavior. Morphology codes may be required, and facility policy will determine whether these codes should be assigned. They are most often used in cancer registries and pathology departments. M codes are another means of collecting and reporting data on patients with cancer. M codes are not required for inpatient billing, so they have no affect on hospital reimbursement. If an encoder is used for code assignment, M codes may be automatically assigned to correspond with assignment of documented neoplasm codes.

Morphology codes consist of the letter M and five digits; the first four identify the **histologic type** of neoplasm or the type of tissue or cell in which the neoplasm occurs. The fifth digit identifies its behavior. Four-digit histologic types are listed in Appendix A of the ICD-9-CM code book, and the one-digit behavior codes are as follows:

- 0 Benign
- 1 Uncertain whether benign or malignant
  Borderline malignancy

Table 15-4. International TNM Staging Systems for Lung Cancer[3]

Stage	TNM Description	5-Year Survival, %
I	T1-T2, N0, M0	60-80
II	T1-T2, N1, M0	25-50
IIIA	T3, N0-N1, M0	25-40
IIIB	T1-T3, N2, M0	10-30
IV	Any T4 or N3, M0	<5
	Any M1	<5
Primary Tumor (T)		
T1	Tumor > cm in diameter	
T2	Tumor <3 cm in diameter or with associated atelectasis–obstructive pneumonitis extending to the hilar region	
T3	Tumor with direct extension into the chest wall, diaphragm, mediastinum, pleura, or pericardium	
T4	Tumor invades the mediastinum, or presence of a malignant pleural effusion	
Regional Lymph Nodes (N)		
N0	No node involvement	
N1	Metastasis to lymph nodes in the peribronchial and ipsilateral (same side as the primary tumor) hilar regions	
N2	Metastasis to ipsilateral hilar and subcarinal (under the bifurcation of the trachea into the lungs) lymph nodes	
N3	Metastasis to contralateral mediastinal or hilar nodes or any nodes new to the clavicular (collar) bone	
Distance Metastasis (M)		
M0	No known metastasis	
M1	Distant metastasis present with site specifi ed (e.g., brain, liver)	

- 2 Carcinoma in situ
  Intraepithelial
  Noninfiltrating
  Noninvasive
- 3 Malignant, primary site
- 6 Malignant, metastatic site
  Secondary site
- 9 Malignant, uncertain whether primary or metastatic site

The Alphabetic Index will facilitate assignment of the appropriate M code. The Neoplasm Table does not contain M codes.

EXAMPLE Adenocarcinoma of the prostate (primary site), 185, M8140/3.

As was discussed earlier in this chapter, malignant neoplasms that originate in epithelial glandular tissue are called *adenocarcinomas.* Look up “Adenocarcinoma” in the Alphabetic Index (Figure 15-3). No further description or classification is provided beyond adenocarcinoma, and no subterm is given for prostate, so the M code that is in parentheses after the main term “Adenocarcinoma” is assigned as M8140, with the fifth digit of 3 because this is a primary malignancy. To locate the ICD-9-CM code, follow the *see also* instruction and go to the Neoplasm Table to identify the neoplasm, by site, malignant.

	Malignant					
	Primary	Secondary	Ca in situ	Benign	Uncertain Behavior	Unspecified
Neoplasm, neoplastic	199.1	199.1	234.9	229.9	238.9	239.9

Notes — 1. The list below gives the code numbers for neoplasms by anatomical site. For each site there are six possible code numbers according to whether the neoplasm in question is malignant, benign, in situ, of uncertain behavior, or of unspecified nature. The description of the neoplasm will often indicate which of the six columns is appropriate; e.g., malignant melanoma of skin, benign fibroadenoma of breast, carcinoma in situ of cervix uteri.

Where such descriptors are not present, the remainder of the Index should be consulted where guidance is given to the appropriate column for each morphological (histological) variety listed; e.g., Mesonephroma—see Neoplasm, malignant; Embryoma—see also Neoplasm, uncertain behavior; Disease, Bowen's—see Neoplasm, skin, in situ. However, the guidance in the Index can be overridden if one of the descriptors mentioned above is present; e.g., malignant adenoma of colon is coded to 153.9 and not to 211.3 as the adjective "malignant" overrides the Index entry "Adenoma - see also Neoplasm, benign."

*2. Sites marked with the sign * (e.g., face NEC*) should be classified to malignant neoplasm of skin of these sites if the variety of neoplasm is a squamous cell carcinoma or an epidermoid carcinoma and to benign neoplasm of skin of these sites if the variety of neoplasm is a papilloma (any type).*

Site	Primary	Secondary	Ca in situ	Benign	Uncertain Behavior	Unspecified
abdomen, abdominal	195.2	198.89	234.8	229.8	238.8	239.8
cavity	195.2	198.89	234.8	229.8	238.8	239.8
organ	195.2	198.89	234.8	229.8	238.8	239.8
viscera	195.2	198.89	234.8	229.8	238.8	239.8
wall	173.5	198.2	232.5	216.5	238.2	239.2
connective tissue	171.5	198.89	—	215.5	238.1	239.2
abdominopelvic	195.8	198.89	234.8	229.8	238.8	239.8
accessory sinus - *see* Neoplasm, sinus						
acoustic nerve	192.0	198.4	—	225.1	237.9	239.7
acromion (process)	170.4	198.5	—	213.4	238.0	239.2
adenoid (pharynx) (tissue)	147.1	198.89	230.0	210.7	235.1	239.0
adipose tissue (*see also* Neoplasm, connective tissue)	171.9	198.89	—	215.9	238.1	239.2
adnexa (uterine)	183.9	198.82	233.3	221.8	236.3	239.5
adrenal (cortex) (gland) (medulla)	194.0	198.7	234.8	227.0	237.2	239.7
ala nasi (external)	173.3	198.2	232.3	216.3	238.2	239.2
alimentary canal or tract NEC	159.9	197.8	230.9	211.9	235.5	239.0
alveolar	143.9	198.89	230.0	210.4	235.1	239.0
mucosa	143.9	198.89	230.0	210.4	235.1	239.0
lower	143.1	198.89	230.0	210.4	235.1	239.0
upper	143.0	198.89	230.0	210.4	235.1	239.0
ridge or process	170.1	198.5	—	213.1	238.0	239.2

Figure 15-2. Excerpt from the Neoplasm Table.

EXAMPLE Adenoma of the prostate, 600.20, M8140/0.

Note that the only difference in assignment of M codes for these two examples is the fifth digit assigned for behavior of the neoplasm. In this example, a subterm for prostate is provided, and instead of instructions to use the Neoplasm Table, assignment of code 600.20 is given.

In the following examples, a step-by-step explanation will be given for coding of neoplasms with the appropriate M code.

EXAMPLE Basal cell carcinoma left cheek (primary site), 173.3, M8090/3.

1. Look up "Carcinoma" in Alphabetic Index.
2. Review subterms; "basal cell" is a subterm.
3. Note M code (M8090) and is classified as a primary malignancy (3).
4. Follow instructions to *see also* Neoplasm, skin, malignant.
5. Go to the Neoplasm Table.
6. Locate the site—skin—and review subterms under "skin."
7. Locate the subterm "cheek," and find the code under the appropriate column, which, in this case, is a primary malignancy of the skin of the cheek,
8. Assign codes 173.3 and M8090/3.

Adenocarcinoma (M8140/3) - *see also* Neoplasm, by site, malignant

> Note The list of adjectival modifiers below is not exhaustive. A description of adenocarcinoma that does not appear in this list should be coded in the same manner as carcinoma with that description. Thus, "mixed acidophil-basophil adenocarcinoma" should be coded in the same manner as "mixed acidophil-basophil carcinoma," which appears in the list under "Carcinoma."
>
> Except where otherwise indicated, the morphological varieties of adenocarcinoma in the list below should be coded by site as for "Neoplasm, malignant."

- with
  - apocrine metaplasia (M8573/3)
  - cartilaginous (and osseous) metaplasia (M8571/3)
  - osseous (and cartilaginous) metaplasia (M8571/3)
  - spindle cell metaplasia (M8572/3)
  - squamous metaplasia (M8570/3)
- acidophil (M8280/3)
  - specified site - *see* Neoplasm, by site, malignant
  - unspecified site 194.3
- acinar (M8550/3)
- acinic cell (M8550/3)
- adrenal cortical (M8370/3) 194.0
- alveolar (M8251/3)
  - and
    - epidermoid carcinoma, mixed (M8560/3)
    - squamous cell carcinoma, mixed (M8560/3)
- apocrine (M8401/3)
  - breast - *see* Neoplasm, breast, malignant
  - specified site NEC - *see* Neoplasm, skin, malignant
  - unspecified site 173.9
- basophil (M8300/3)
  - specified site - *see* Neoplasm, by site, malignant
  - unspecified site 194.3
- bile duct type (M8160/3)
  - liver 155.1
  - specified site NEC - *see* Neoplasm, by site, malignant
  - unspecified site 155.1
- bronchiolar (M8250/3) - *see* Neoplasm, lung, malignant
- ceruminous (M8420/3) 173.2
- chromophobe (M8270/3)
  - specified site - *see* Neoplasm, by site, malignant
  - unspecified site 194.3
- clear cell (mesonephroid type) (M8310/3)
- colloid (M8480/3)
- cylindroid type (M8200/3)
- diffuse type (M8145/3)

Adenocarcinoma *(Continued)*

  - specified site - *see* Neoplasm, by site, malignant
  - unspecified site 151.9
- duct (infiltrating) (M8500/3)
  - with Paget's disease (M8541/3) - *see* Neoplasm, breast, malignant
  - specified site - *see* Neoplasm, by site, malignant
  - unspecified site 174.9
- embryonal (M9070/3)
- endometrioid (M8380/3) - *see* Neoplasm, by site, malignant
- eosinophil (M8280/3)
  - specified site - *see* Neoplasm, by site, malignant
  - unspecified site 194.3
- follicular (M8330/3)
  - and papillary (M8340/3) 193
  - moderately differentiated type (M8332/3) 193
  - pure follicle type (M8331/3) 193
  - specified site - *see* Neoplasm, by site, malignant
  - trabecular type (M8332/3) 193
  - unspecified type 193
  - well differentiated type (M8331/3) 193
- gelatinous (M8480/3)
- granular cell (M8320/3)
- Hürthle cell (M8290/3) 193
- in
  - adenomatous
    - polyp (M8210/3)
    - polyposis coli (M8220/3) 153.9
  - polypoid adenoma (M8210/3)
  - tubular adenoma (M8210/3)
  - villous adenoma (M8261/3)
- infiltrating duct (M8500/3)
  - with Paget's disease (M8541/3) - *see* Neoplasm, breast, malignant
  - specified site - *see* Neoplasm, by site, malignant
  - unspecified site 174.9
- inflammatory (M8530/3)
  - specified site - *see* Neoplasm, by site, malignant
  - unspecified site 174.9
- in situ (M8140/2) - *see* Neoplasm, by site, in situ
- intestinal type (M8144/3)
  - specified site - *see* Neoplasm, by site, malignant
  - unspecified site 151.9
- intraductal (noninfiltrating) (M8500/2)
  - papillary (M8503/2)
    - specified site - *see* Neoplasm, by site, in situ
    - unspecified site 233.0
  - specified site - *see* Neoplasm, by site, in situ
  - unspecified site 233.0
- islet cell (M8150/3)
  - and exocrine, mixed (M8154/3)
    - specified site - *see* Neoplasm, by site, malignant
    - unspecified site 157.9
  - pancreas 157.4
  - specified site NEC - *see* Neoplasm, by

Adenocarcinoma *(Continued)*

- islet cell *(Continued)*
    - site, malignant
  - unspecified site 157.4
- lobular (M8520/3)
  - specified site - *see* Neoplasm, by site, malignant
  - unspecified site 174.9
- medullary (M8510/3)
- mesonephric (M9110/3)
- mixed cell (M8323/3)
- mucinous (M8480/3)
- mucin-producing (M8481/3)
- mucoid (M8480/3) - *see also* Neoplasm, by site, malignant
  - cell (M8300/3)
    - specified site - *see* Neoplasm, by site, malignant
    - unspecified site 194.3
- nonencapsulated sclerosing (M8350/3) 193
- oncocytic (M8290/3)
- oxyphilic (M8290/3)
- papillary (M8260/3)
  - and follicular (M8340/3) 193
  - intraductal (noninfiltrating) (M8503/2)
    - specified site - *see* Neoplasm, by site, in situ
    - unspecified site 233.0
  - serous (M8460/3)
    - specified site - *see* Neoplasm, by site, malignant
    - unspecified site 183.0
- papillocystic (M8450/3)
  - specified site - *see* Neoplasm, by site, malignant
  - unspecified site 183.0
- pseudomucinous (M8470/3)
  - specified site - *see* Neoplasm, by site, malignant
  - unspecified site 183.0
- renal cell (M8312/3) 189.0
- sebaceous (M8410/3)
- serous (M8441/3) - *see also* Neoplasm, by site, malignant
  - papillary
    - specified site - *see* Neoplasm, by site, malignant
    - unspecified site 183.0
- signet ring cell (M8490/3)
- superficial spreading (M8143/3)
- sweat gland (M8400/3) - *see* Neoplasm, skin, malignant
- trabecular (M8190/3)
- tubular (M8211/3)
- villous (M8262/3)
- water-clear cell (M8322/3) 194.1

Figure 15-3. Index entry for main term "Adenocarcinoma."

EXAMPLE

Squamous cell in situ carcinoma of the endocervix, 233.1, M8070/2.

1. Look up carcinoma in the Alphabetic Index.
2. Review subterms; "squamous cell" is a subterm.
3. Note M code (M8070) and is classified as squamous cell in situ (2).
4. Follow instructions, specified site—*see* Neoplasm, by site, in situ.
5. Go to the Neoplasm Table.
6. Locate the site—cervix—and review subterms under "Cervix."
7. Locate the subterm "endocervix," and find the code under the appropriate column, which, in this case, is a carcinoma in situ of the endocervix.
8. Assign codes 233.1 and M8070/2 (in situ).

EXERCISE 15-1

Assign only M codes for the following.

1. Squamous cell carcinoma, in situ neoplasm ______________
2. Cancer, secondary neoplasm ______________
3. Ewing's sarcoma, primary neoplasm ______________
4. Periosteal fibrosarcoma, primary neoplasm ______________
5. Melanoma, primary neoplasm ______________
6. Leukemia ______________
7. Lymphoma ______________
8. Adenoma, benign neoplasm ______________
9. Renal cell carcinoma, metastatic neoplasm ______________
10. Hürthle cell adenocarcinoma, primary neoplasm ______________

Primary and Secondary Neoplasms

Sometimes incomplete documentation makes it difficult to determine whether a neoplasm is primary or secondary. It is possible to have more than one primary cancer. At times, a secondary or metastatic cancer has been found, and the primary is unknown or has yet to be determined. Documentation in the health record may be incomplete and the terminology confusing.

As was described previously, a metastatic neoplasm is a secondary neoplasm that has spread from the original or primary site. The site of the metastasis may be close to the original site (e.g., breast spread to axillary lymph nodes) or to distant sites (e.g., lung spread to the brain). Neoplasms can metastasize to more than one site. If this is the case, codes are assigned to each metastatic site. Terminology used to describe metastatic sites varies greatly, depending on the documenting physician. For example, if a patient has a non–small cell primary lung carcinoma with secondary malignancy of the brain, it may be documented in the health record as follows:

EXAMPLE

Lung cancer with mets to the brain, 162.9, 198.3

The code that would be assigned is primary lung cancer (162.9) with a secondary code assigned for the metastatic brain malignancy (198.3).

EXAMPLE

Lung cancer metastatic to the brain, 162.9, 198.3

The codes assigned are the same as in the preceding example.

EXAMPLE

Brain cancer metastatic from the lung, 162.9, 198.3

The codes assigned are the same as in the preceding example.

EXAMPLE Non–small cell carcinoma of lung and brain, 162.9, 198.3

Non–small cell carcinoma is a malignancy that originates in the lung, so the lung is primary. If a cancer that originates in the lung has spread to the brain, that is a metastasis.

EXAMPLE Metastatic lung cancer, 162.9, 199.1

According to *Coding Clinic* (1985:M-J:p9-12),[4] if a morphology type is not stated, assign the site qualified as "metastatic" to the primary malignant code for that site. The code assigned is primary lung cancer (162.9), with an unknown secondary malignancy site (199.1) because the metastatic site was not documented in this example.

If the documentation in the health record only identifies one site and it is identified as metastatic, then a determination has to be made as to whether to code the site as a primary malignancy or secondary malignancy. The following steps are followed to make that determination:

1. If the morphology type is documented, refer to the morphology type in the Alphabetic Index and code to the primary condition of that site.

EXAMPLE Metastatic islet cell carcinoma of the pancreas, 157.4, 199.1

In the preceding example, the carcinoma is documented as metastatic. The first step is to locate the morphology type in the Alphabetic Index. There are subterms for islet cell of the pancreas with code, 157.4, so that code should be assigned. If no specific site is listed as a subterm, assign the code for primary neoplasm of an unspecified site (199.1). When a primary site has been determined, a code must be assigned to identify a secondary (metastatic) site. If no metastatic site is specified, then the code 199.1, unknown site, secondary is assigned.

2. If the process in step 1 leads to code 199.0 or 199.1 or if the morphology is not stated, the site should be coded as a primary malignancy, unless it is included in the following list of exceptions.

Malignant neoplasms of the following sites are exceptions, and instead of coding to an unknown primary or to the morphology, the following sites are always coded as secondary neoplasms of that site:

- Bone
- Brain
- Diaphragm
- Heart
- Liver
- Lymph nodes
- Mediastinum
- Meninges
- Peritoneum
- Pleura
- Retroperitoneum
- Spinal cord
- Sites classifiable to 195.0-8

EXAMPLE Metastatic carcinoma of the breast, 174.9, 199.1

In the preceding example, there is no subterm for breast or unspecified site. In the Neoplasm Table, unspecified site, primary is coded to 199.1. When code 199.0 or 199.1 is obtained, then a review of the exception list is performed. Because breast is not on the list, it is assigned as the primary site, 174.9, and the code 199.1 is used to identify the unknown secondary.

EXAMPLE

Metastatic brain cancer, 199.1, 198.3 or 198.3, 199.1 (depending on the reason for the patient's admission)

In this example, the brain is on the list of secondary neoplasms, and the morphology type is not stated; therefore the code 198.3 is assigned for secondary neoplasm of the brain and 199.1 for unknown primary. Sequencing of the primary and secondary neoplasms would depend on the focus of treatment.

EXAMPLE

Renal cell carcinoma (RCC) with metastasis to the adrenal glands
Primary neoplasm: Renal cell carcinoma
Secondary neoplasm: Adrenal glands

EXAMPLE

Metastatic bone cancer
Primary neoplasm: Unknown primary site
Secondary neoplasm: Bones

Specific instructions are provided at the beginning of the "Neoplasm" chapter in the code book (Figure 15-4).

EXERCISE 15-2

Identify the following neoplasms in terms of primary or secondary, as in the earlier examples.

1. Colorectal adenocarcinoma with metastatic liver cancer
   Primary neoplasm ______________________________
   Secondary neoplasm ______________________________
2. Thyroid malignancy with mets to the lymph nodes of the neck
   Primary neoplasm ______________________________
   Secondary neoplasm ______________________________
3. Metastatic ovarian cancer
   Primary neoplasm ______________________________
   Secondary neoplasm ______________________________
4. Pancreatic cancer with extension into the liver
   Primary neoplasm ______________________________
   Secondary neoplasm ______________________________
5. Recurrence of cancer in the bladder
   Primary neoplasm ______________________________
   Secondary neoplasm ______________________________
6. Adenocarcinoma sigmoid colon with pericolic nodal involvement
   Primary neoplasm ______________________________
   Secondary neoplasm ______________________________
7. Inflammatory breast cancer with spread to the axillary lymph nodes
   Primary neoplasm ______________________________
   Secondary neoplasm ______________________________
8. Metastatic bone cancer from the prostate
   Primary neoplasm ______________________________
   Secondary neoplasm ______________________________
9. Endometrial adenocarcinoma with metastasis to the ovary
   Primary neoplasm ______________________________
   Secondary neoplasm ______________________________
10. Acinic cell carcinoma of the parotid gland
    Primary neoplasm ______________________________
    Secondary neoplasm ______________________________

2. NEOPLASMS (140–239)

1. Content:

This chapter contains the following broad groups:

140–195	Malignant neoplasms, stated or presumed to be primary, of specified sites, except of lymphatic and hematopoietic tissue
196–198	Malignant neoplasms, stated or presumed to be secondary, of specified sites
199	Malignant neoplasms, without specification of site
200–208	Malignant neoplasms, stated or presumed to be primary, of lymphatic and hematopoietic tissue
210–229	Benign neoplasms
230–234	Carcinoma in situ
235–238	Neoplasms of uncertain behavior [see Note, at beginning of section 235–238]
239	Neoplasms of unspecified nature

2. Functional activity

All neoplasms are classified in this chapter, whether or not functionally active. An additional code from Chapter 3 may be used to identify such functional activity associated with any neoplasm, e.g.:

catecholamine-producing malignant pheochromocytoma of adrenal:

code 194.0, additional code 255.6

basophil adenoma of pituitary with Cushing's syndrome:

code 227.3, additional code 255.0

3. Morphology [Histology]

For those wishing to identify the histological type of neoplasms, a comprehensive coded nomenclature, which comprises the morphology rubrics of the ICD-Oncology, is given after the E-code chapter.

4. Malignant neoplasms overlapping site boundaries

Categories 140–195 are for the classification of primary malignant neoplasms according to their point of origin. A malignant neoplasm that overlaps two or more subcategories within a three-digit rubric and whose point of origin cannot be determined should be classified to the subcategory .8 "Other." For example, "carcinoma involving tip and ventral surface of tongue" should be assigned to 141.8. On the other hand, "carcinoma of tip of tongue, extending to involve the ventral surface" should be coded to 141.2, as the point of origin, the tip, is known. Three subcategories (149.8, 159.8, 165.8) have been provided for malignant neoplasms that overlap the boundaries of three-digit rubrics within certain systems. Overlapping malignant neoplasms that cannot be classified as indicated above should be assigned to the appropriate subdivision of category 195 (Malignant neoplasm of other and ill-defined sites).

Figure 15-4. Instructional notes at the beginning of the "Neoplasm" chapter in the Tabular List.

Contiguous Sites

As is pointed out in the instructional note (Fig. 15-4), a neoplasm can overlap two or more subcategories, and determination of the exact point of origin may be difficult. These would be assigned to subcategory 8, "Other." It is important to code any alterations to the functional activity of an organ caused by the neoplasm.

Neoplasms of the endocrine glands or organs that secrete hormones are more likely to have disturbances in their functional activity because hormone production may increase or decrease because of the neoplasm.

EXAMPLE Malignant neoplasm of the thyroid with hyperthyroidism, 193, 242.80

DISEASE CONDITIONS

Neoplasms (140-239) is the topic of Chapter 2 in your ICD-9-CM code book; it is divided into the following categories:

CATEGORY	SECTION TITLES
140-149	Malignant Neoplasm of Lip, Oral Cavity, and Pharynx
150-159	Malignant Neoplasm of Digestive Organs and Peritoneum
160-165	Malignant Neoplasm of Respiratory and Intrathoracic Organs
170-176	Malignant Neoplasm of Bone, Connective Tissue, Skin, and Breast
179-189	Malignant Neoplasm of the Genitourinary Organs
190-199	Malignant Neoplasm of Other and Unspecified Sites
200-208	Malignant Neoplasm of Lymphatic and Hematopoietic Tissue
209	Neuroendocrine Tumors
210-229	Benign Neoplasms
230-234	Carcinoma In Situ
235-238	Neoplasms of Uncertain Behavior
239	Neoplasms of Unspecified Nature

Malignant Neoplasm of Lip, Oral Cavity, and Pharynx (140-149)

Several types of oral cancers have been identified; 90% of these are squamous cell carcinomas. Cancers are often discovered after they have already spread, usually to the lymph nodes of the neck. Smoking has been associated with about 70% to 80% of oral cancers. Also, heavy alcohol adds to the risk. The lips and tongue are most commonly affected (Figure 15-5).

EXAMPLE The patient is being treated for squamous cell carcinoma of the hypopharynx, 148.9.

EXERCISE 15-3

Assign codes to the following conditions using your ICD-9-CM code book.

1. Squamous cell carcinoma, base of tongue __________
2. Adenocarcinoma of parotid gland __________
3. Biopsy-proven squamous cell carcinoma, right tonsil __________
4. Cancer lower lip __________

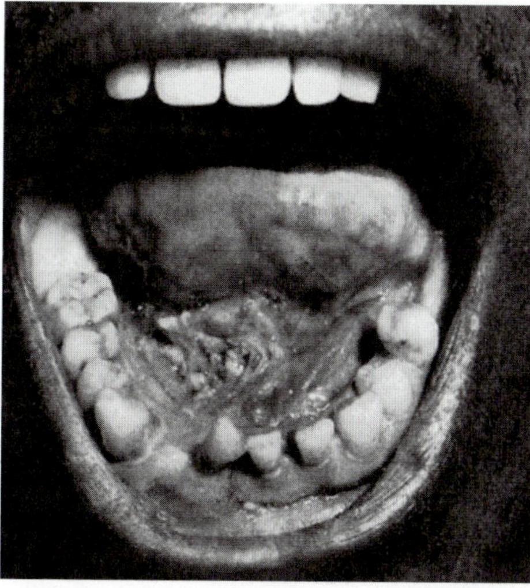

Figure 15-5. Squamous cell carcinoma mouth.

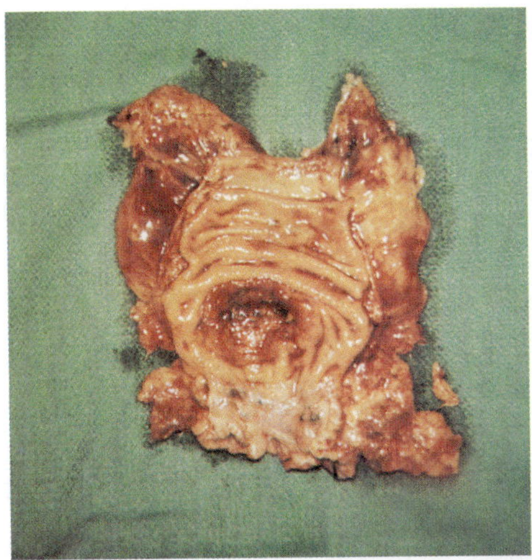

Figure 15-6. Adenocarcinoma distal rectum.

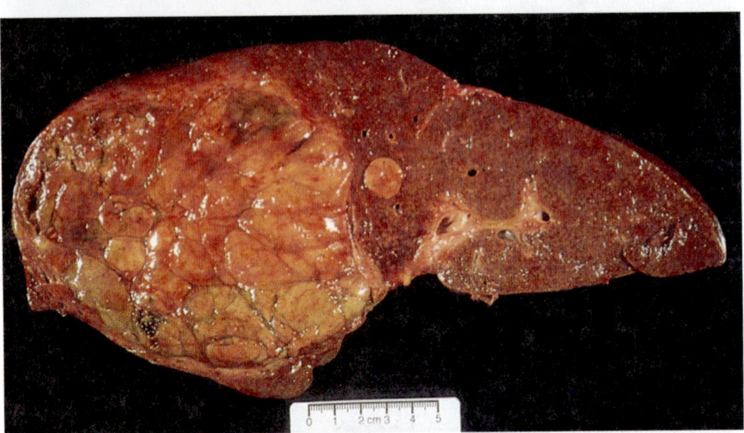

Figure 15-7. Hepatocellular carcinoma.

Malignant Neoplasm of Digestive Organs and Peritoneum (150-159)

According to the Centers for Disease Control and Prevention (CDC), colorectal cancer (Figure 15-6) primarily affects men and women aged 50 years or older. For men, colorectal cancer is the third most common cancer after prostate cancer and lung cancer. For women, colorectal cancer is the third most common cancer after breast cancer and lung cancer. The best prevention is regular screening.

Hepatocellular carcinoma is a primary neoplasm of the liver (Figure 15-7). Patients who develop primary liver cancer often have some type of chronic liver disease such as cirrhosis. The liver is also a common site for metastasis.

EXAMPLE The patient has adenocarcinoma of the rectosigmoid junction, 154.0.

EXERCISE 15-4

Assign codes to the following conditions using your ICD-9-CM code book.

1. Hepatocellular carcinoma ______________
2. Adenocarcinoma, head of pancreas ______________
3. Fibrosarcoma of spleen ______________
4. Adenocarcinoma of the duodenum ______________
5. Gastric adenocarcinoma ______________
6. Cholangiocarcinoma of the extrahepatic bile ducts ______________

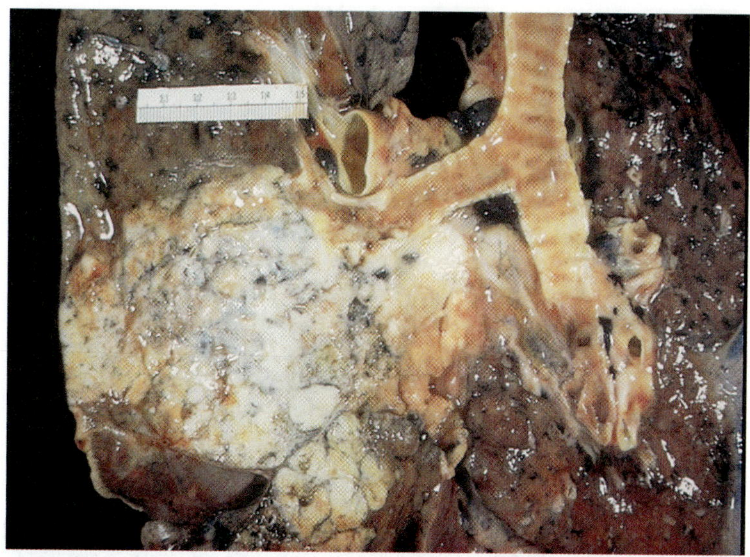

Figure 15-8. Bronchogenic carcinoma. The tumor, a squamous cell carcinoma, appears gray-white and infiltrates the lung tissue.

Malignant Neoplasm of Respiratory and Intrathoracic (160-165)

Lung cancer, which is one of the most common types of cancer, is classified into two main categories: small cell lung cancer (SCLC) and non–small cell lung cancer (NSCLC). More than 85% of lung cancers are caused by smoking. Bronchogenic carcinoma is the most common type of malignant lung cancer (Figure 15-8). The lung is frequently a site for metastasis. Benign tumors of the lung are rare.

EXAMPLE The patient was diagnosed with adenocarcinoma right lower lobe of lung, 162.5.

EXERCISE 15-5

Assign codes to the following conditions using your ICD-9-CM code book.

1. Malignant mesothelioma of the pleura ____________
2. Cancer of the larynx ____________
3. Oat cell cancer of main bronchus ____________
4. Squamous cell carcinoma of thymus ____________
5. Cancer maxillary sinus ____________

Malignant Neoplasm of Bone, Connective Tissue, Skin, and Breast (170-176)

One woman in eight has or will develop breast cancer in her lifetime (Figure 15-9). The 5-year survival rate exceeds 95% if detected early. Infiltrating or invasive ductal carcinoma is the most common type of breast cancer. Cancers of the connective tissue develop in the muscles, fat, blood, lymph vessels, and nerves.

Osteosarcoma is the most common primary malignant cancer of the bone and usually occurs in young people between the age of 10 and 30. These tumors develop most often in bones of the arms, legs, or pelvis.

EXAMPLE The patient is being seen for fibrosarcoma distal femur 171.3.

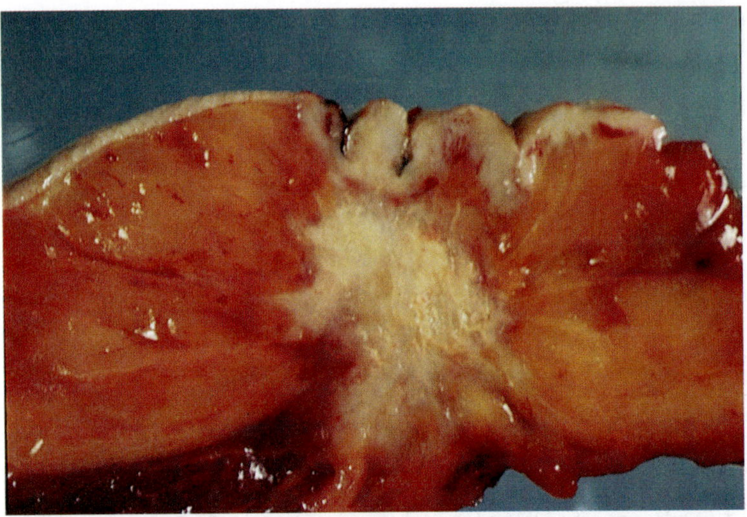

Figure 15-9. Breast carcinoma.

EXERCISE 15-6

Assign codes to the following conditions using your ICD-9-CM code book.

1. Ewing's sarcoma 7th rib ______________
2. Basal cell carcinoma right cheek ______________
3. Kaposi's sarcoma skin in patient with acquired immunodefi ciency syndrome (AIDS) ______________
4. Upper outer quadrant malignancy of breast ______________
5. Osteosarcoma humerus ______________
6. Lentigo malignant melanoma sole of left foot ______________
7. Malignant neoplasm male breast ______________

Malignant Neoplasm of Genitourinary Organs (179-189)

Malignancy can affect any organ in the genitourinary system. Many neoplasms are related to age, for example, Wilms' tumor is a common childhood tumor of the kidney. Testicular cancer usually affects young men, and the incidence of prostate cancer increases with age. Most kidney (Figure 15-10) and bladder (Figure 15-11) malignancies occur in adults between 60 and 70 years of age. As with many cancers, genetic, environmental, and behavioral risk factors may contribute to the cause.

EXAMPLE The patient is being treated for a malignancy of his testes, 186.9.

EXERCISE 15-7

Assign codes to the following conditions using your ICD-9-CM code book.

1. Endometrial carcinoma uterus ______________
2. Renal cell carcinoma ______________
3. Tubo-ovarian cancer ______________
4. Transitional cell carcinoma lower neck of bladder, causing urinary obstruction ______________
5. Leiomyosarcoma of uterus ______________

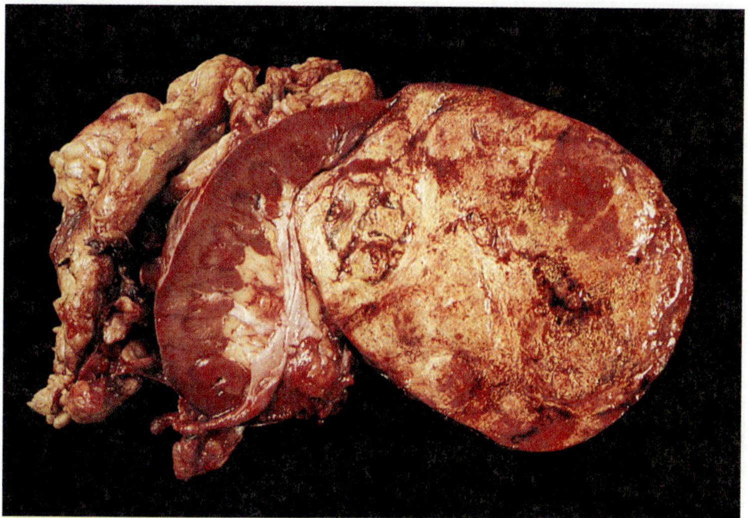

Figure 15-10. Renal cell carcinoma.

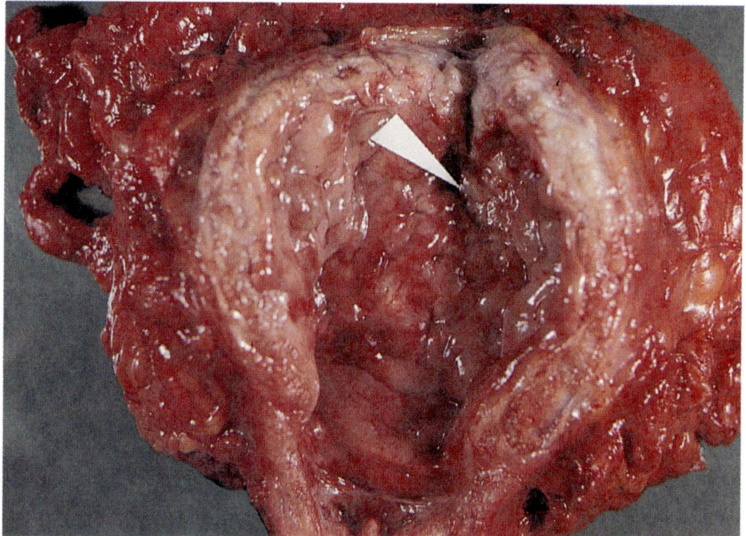

Figure 15-11. Bladder cancer.

Malignant Neoplasm of Other and Unspecified Sites (190-199)

This section contains a variety of neoplasms, including those of the eye, brain, spinal cord, thyroid, and other endocrine glands. This is also where secondary or metastatic neoplasm codes are located. The 196 category is used to identify the spread of cancer to the lymph nodes; fourth digit classifications identify the body region of the lymph nodes for specificity. In contrast, code 198.5 is the code assigned to metastasis to the bone and in this case specificity is not necessary for code assignment. It does not matter whether this is a vertebral bone, a pelvic bone, or the humerus.

EXAMPLE The patient has metastatic lung cancer; no known primary, 199.1, 197.0.

EXERCISE 15-8

Assign codes to the following conditions using your ICD-9-CM code book.

1. Seizure due to carcinoma of parietal lobe of the brain ____________
2. Glioblastoma multiforme ____________
3. Metastatic melanoma to the brain; melanoma skin lesion excised 5 years ago ____________
4. Neuroblastoma left adrenal gland ____________
5. Teratocarcinoma pineal gland ____________
6. Orbital rhabdomyosarcoma ____________
7. Anaplastic astrocytoma spinal cord with metastasis to the vertebral bodies ____________
8. Carcinomatosis ____________
9. Metastasis to the mastectomy site; mastectomy performed 1 year ago ____________

Malignant Neoplasm of Lymphatic and Hematopoietic Tissue (200-208)

Lymphoma is cancer of the lymphatic system. Two main types have been identified: Hodgkin's disease (HD) (Figure 15-12) or lymphoma, and non-Hodgkin's lymphoma (NHL). The incidence of non-Hodgkin's is greater than that of Hodgkin's disease. The lymphatic system follows the blood vessels, and groups are located in areas of the neck, axillary, groin, abdomen, and pelvic regions. Some organs contain lymphatic tissue and may be affected. These organs include the spleen, thymus gland, bone marrow, tonsils, and adenoids. According to *Coding Clinic* (1992:2Q:p3-4),[5] although lymphoma may be present in different or multiple areas of the body, this is not considered metastatic. Lymphomas should not be confused with solid tumors (malignancies) that have metastasized to the lymph nodes.

If a patient is in remission, he or she is considered to have lymphoma, and a code from categories 200-202 should be assigned. There are different classifications of remission.

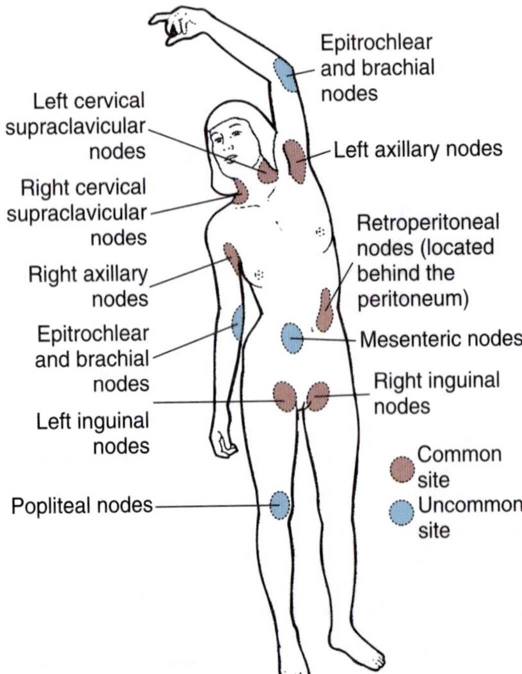

Figure 15-12. Lymph node sites for Hodgkin's disease.

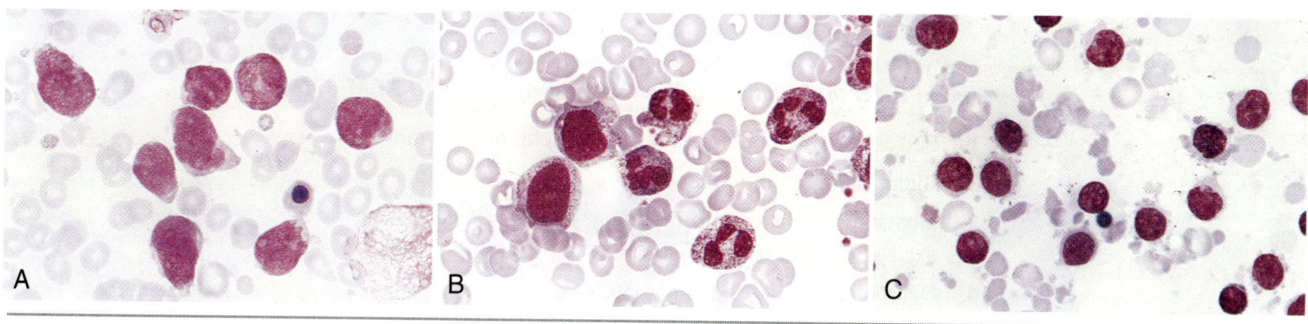

Figure 15-13. Peripheral blood smears. **A,** Acute lymphoblastic leukemia. **B,** Chronic myelogenous leukemia. **C,** Chronic lymphocytic leukemia.

Complete remission means there are no signs or symptoms of the cancer. **Partial remission** means there are still a few signs and symptoms of the cancer and the cancer cells have significantly decreased. The remission fifth digit (if available) should only be assigned if documented by the physician as being in remission.

Leukemia is cancer of the white blood cells that begins in the blood-forming cells of the bone marrow. As the disease progresses, leukemic cells invade other parts of the body, such as the lymph nodes, spleen, liver, and central nervous system. Various types of leukemia have been identified (Figure 15-13). Some develop suddenly and are acute leukemias; others are of the chronic variety.

EXAMPLE The patient was diagnosed with nodular sclerosis Hodgkin's, 201.50.

EXERCISE 15-9

Assign codes to the following conditions using your ICD-9-CM code book.

1. Acute lymphocytic leukemia (ALL), relapsed ______________
2. Primary central nervous (brain) lymphoma in AIDS patient ______________
3. Chronic myelogenous leukemia (CML) ______________
4. Lymphoma ileum ______________
5. Burkitt's lymphoma in remission ______________

Neuroendocrine Tumors (209)

Code category 209 includes codes for benign and malignant carcinoid neoplasms. Neuroendocrine tumors can be benign and/or malignant neoplasms that arise in the endocrine or neuroendocrine cells throughout the body. These neoplasms are usually slow growing. There are two groups of neuroendocrine neoplasms:

- Carcinoid
- Pancreatic endocrine

The most common sites for carcinoid neoplasms are the bronchi, stomach, small intestine, appendix, and rectum. They are classified according to the embryonic site of origin such as:

- Foregut—bronchi and stomach
- Midgut—small intestine and appendix
- Hindgut—colon and rectum

Benign tumors are usually very small. Malignant tumors are larger and do metastasize. The most common metastatic sites are lymph nodes, liver, lung, bone, and skin.

EXAMPLE Malignant carcinoid neoplasm of the appendix, 209.11

EXAMPLE Benign carcinoid neoplasm of the rectum, 209.57

EXERCISE 15-10

Assign codes to the following conditions using your ICD-9-CM code book.

1. Malignant carcinoid tumor foregut ____________
2. Benign carcinoid tumor, sigmoid colon ____________
3. Carcinoid neoplasm, small intestine, malignant ____________

Benign Neoplasms (210-229)

A **benign** neoplasm or tumor is not malignant. It will not metastasize to other parts of the body, but it could continue to grow and may cause damage to neighboring organs and structures. It may be necessary to remove a benign neoplasm. Benign neoplasms may recur.

Lipoma is a growth of fat cells within a capsule that is usually found just below the skin. Lipomas are the most common benign soft tissue growths. For the most part, lipomas are small and movable, and they remain the same size and are not painful. It may be necessary to excise a lipoma if it becomes painful or infected, if it limits function or mobility, or if it increases in size.

Leiomyoma or uterine fibroids are tumors or growths within the walls of the uterus. These are the most common benign tumors in women of childbearing age. Not all fibroids cause symptoms. When fibroids become symptomatic, the following symptoms may be present:

- Heavy bleeding
- Painful periods
- Feeling of fullness in the pelvic region
- Urinary frequency
- Pain during sex
- Infertility, miscarriage, or early onset of labor

Treatment will depend on the severity of symptoms, the size and location of the fibroids, and the patient's age and desired fertility.

EXAMPLE Patient is being seen because of a cavernous lymphangioma, 228.1.

EXERCISE 15-11

Assign codes to the following conditions using your ICD-9-CM code book.

1. Warthin's tumor ____________
2. Adenoma of the pituitary gland ____________
3. Chondromyxoid fibroma of the tibia ____________
4. Squamous papilloma soft palate ____________
5. Osteoma proximal femur ____________
6. Enchondroma fifth metacarpal ____________
7. Lipoma spermatic cord ____________
8. Rhabdomyoma left ventricle of heart ____________
9. Hemangioma of liver ____________
10. Submucosal uterine fibroid ____________

Carcinoma In Situ (230-234)

Carcinoma in situ consists of malignant cells that remain within the original site with no spread or invasion to neighboring tissues (Figure 15-14). Usually, the physician or the pathology report will confirm that the condition is "in situ." These tumors are usually curable because they are at the earliest stage of development.

EXAMPLE Patient has Bowen's disease, 232.9.

EXERCISE 15-12

Assign codes to the following conditions using your ICD-9-CM code book.

1. Carcinoma in situ of the cervix ________
2. Carcinoma in situ of the urinary bladder ________
3. Cervical intraepithelial neoplasia III ________
4. Ductal carcinoma in situ (DCIS) ________

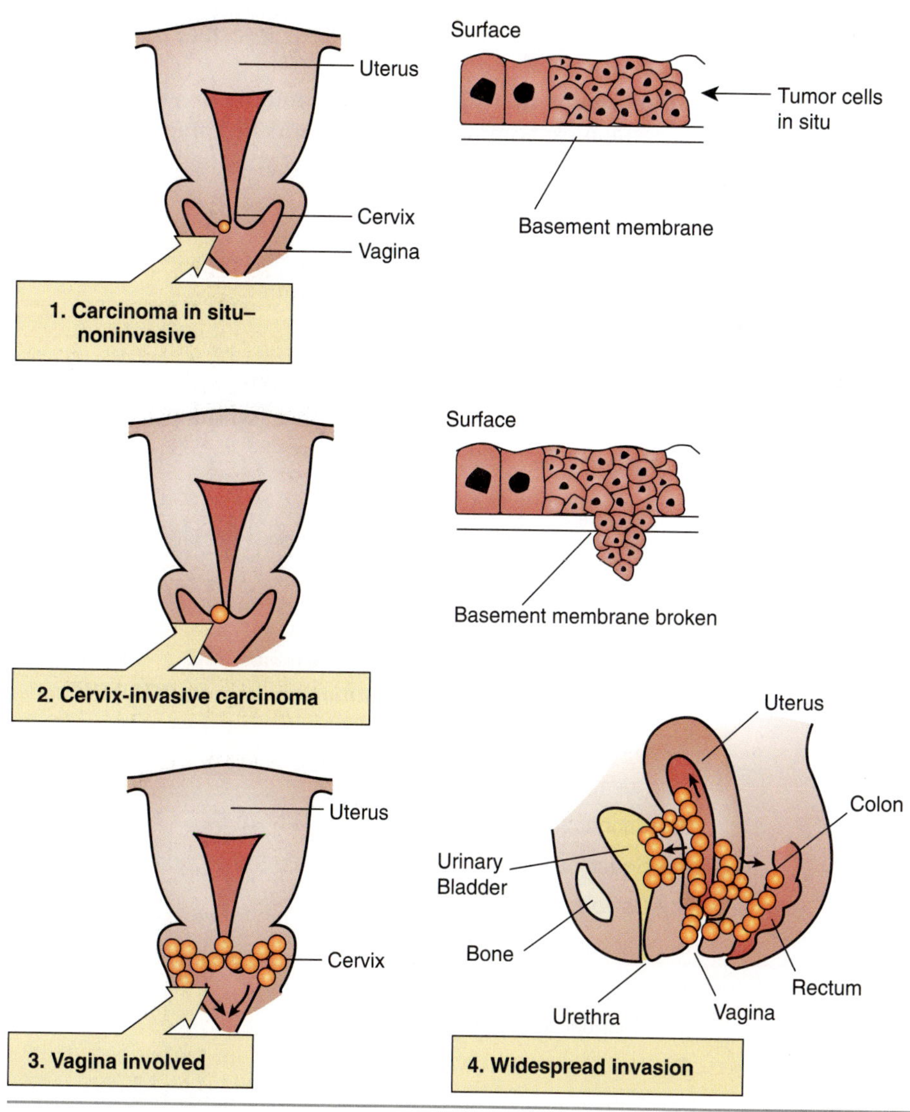

Figure 15-14. Invasive carcinoma of the cervix.

Neoplasms of Uncertain Behavior (235-238)

Neoplasms that fall into the categories of uncertain behavior are neither malignant nor benign. On pathologic examination, the behavior cannot be determined or predicted. In some instances, progression to some type of malignancy may occur. For example, myelodysplastic syndrome has been known to progress to leukemia.

EXAMPLE Patient is seen in consultation because of type 2 neurofibromatosis, 237.72.

EXERCISE 15-13

Assign codes to the following conditions using your ICD-9-CM code book.

1. Myelodysplastic syndrome (MDS) __________
2. Polycythemia vera __________
3. Refractory anemia __________
4. Paraganglioma of carotid body __________

Neoplasms of Unspecified Behavior (239)

This category is used when terms such as "growth," "neoplasm," or "tumor" are used to describe a medical finding. At times, this condition may require further investigation and testing. Sometimes, these findings are not investigated because the patient is elderly and has other chronic conditions, and aggressive treatment would not be pursued.

On occasion, a physician will document a patient as having a mass with no further specification other than site or location of the mass. Usually, this occurs when no pathology report is available when the physician is documenting details in the health record. According to *Coding Clinic* (2006:1Q:p4),[6] if the diagnosis is documented as "mass" or "lesion," it would be incorrect to select a code for neoplasm of unspecified behavior.

EXAMPLE Mass of the liver, 573.9

In this example, under the main term "mass," there is no subterm for liver. The *Coding Clinic* states if there is no index entry for a specific site, go to the main term "disease," liver.

If terms such as lump or lesion are used, the same logic is applied. If a subterm cannot be found under "lump," "lesion," or "mass," go to the main term "disease."

EXAMPLE Patient will need to follow up for definitive diagnosis of neoplasm sigmoid colon 239.0.

EXERCISE 15-14

Assign codes to the following conditions using your ICD-9-CM code book.

1. Intracranial tumor __________
2. Neoplasm bladder __________
3. Growth left ovary __________
4. Mass right lung __________
5. Right breast lump __________
6. Lesion brain was identified by MRI __________

Coding and Sequencing of Neoplasms

In addition to assigning neoplasm codes, it is important to know how these codes are sequenced in accordance with the guidelines. The principal diagnosis is determined according to the reason the patient is admitted and the treatment provided. Documentation by

physicians may be confusing in determining the principal diagnosis. They often will document the cancer as the reason for admission. Physicians may document cancers that have been previously removed. Physicians are not trained to document in accordance with coding guidelines. They may document the reason for admission as the cancer when the patient is receiving treatment for a complication of the cancer or of the cancer treatment.

Malignancy as Principal Diagnosis

When a patient is admitted for determination of whether a malignancy is present and a malignancy is found, the code for the primary malignancy is the principal diagnosis.

EXAMPLE Patient was admitted for total thyroidectomy. Fine needle aspiration biopsy on an outpatient basis was inconclusive. Total thyroidectomy was performed and a diagnosis of anaplastic cancer was determined, 193, 06.4.

As in the previous example, during the course of determining whether a malignancy is present, a malignancy is found and a secondary malignancy is identified. The code for the primary neoplasm is the principal diagnosis, and the secondary malignancy is assigned as an additional code.

EXAMPLE The above patient was also found to have spread to the cervical lymph nodes, 193, 196.0, 06.4.

Recurrence of Primary Malignancy

If a primary malignancy was previously excised or eradicated but has now recurred, the malignancy is coded to a primary malignant neoplasm.

EXAMPLE Recurrence of transitional cell bladder cancer, posterior wall, 188.4

Physicians may document a malignancy as recurrent at a site where a malignancy has been previously excised. This cannot be an actual recurrent neoplasm if the site is no longer present. It may be necessary to query the physician to determine the metastatic site(s).

EXAMPLE Recurrent ovarian cancer. Patient had hysterectomy and bilateral salpingo-oophorectomy 3 years ago, 199.1, V10.43, V45.77 (may need to query the site of recurrence).

When a patient is admitted for removal of a known malignancy, the malignancy is the principal diagnosis. In some cases, a biopsy may have been performed previously that confirms the presence of a malignancy. The patient is readmitted for more definitive surgery. The pathology report following the surgery may report negative findings for malignancy. According to *Coding Clinic* (1985:M-J:p9-12),[4] if the physician documents the malignancy as shown on the biopsy, the malignancy is assigned as the principal diagnosis for the definitive surgery even though no further evidence of malignancy is seen on the pathology report.

EXAMPLE Patient has a fine needle aspiration biopsy that shows Hürthle carcinoma of the thyroid. Patient is admitted for a partial thyroidectomy. The pathology report from the thyroidectomy shows no evidence of malignancy, 193, 06.39.

When a patient is admitted with a sign or symptom (which codes to Chapter 16) related to a known primary or secondary malignancy, the primary or secondary malignancy code is the principal diagnosis.

EXAMPLE Convulsion due to glioblastoma multiforme temporal lobe of brain, 191.2, 780.39 (the convulsion is coded as an additional code because convulsions are not integral to the brain neoplasm).

When a patient is admitted with a primary neoplasm and a metastatic neoplasm, and treatment is directed to the metastatic neoplasm, the metastatic neoplasm is the principal diagnosis.

EXAMPLE

Patient is admitted for wedge resection of metastatic liver cancer.
Patient had a colorectal cancer removed 3 months ago and is undergoing treatment, 197.7, 154.0, 50.22.

According to *Coding Clinic* (1988:1Q:p4-5),[7] when a patient is admitted to the hospital for treatment by brachytherapy, the principal diagnosis is the malignancy that is being treated (which could be either a primary or a secondary malignancy).

EXAMPLE

Patient was admitted for brachytherapy for cancer of cervix, 180.9, 92.27.

According to *Coding Clinic* (1997:2Q:p3),[8] when a patient is admitted with an obstruction due to a neoplasm (primary or secondary), the neoplasm is coded as the principal diagnosis.

EXAMPLE

Large bowel obstruction due to adenocarcinoma of the colon, 153.9, 560.9

Complications as Principal Diagnosis

Often, complications are associated with malignancies or the treatment of malignancies. When the complication is the reason for admission or treatment, the complication is the principal diagnosis. The guidelines address some of the most common examples such as anemia and dehydration.

EXAMPLE

Patient admitted for treatment of anemia due to gastric cancer with 2 units of packed cells, 285.22, 151.9, 99.04

EXAMPLE

Patient has become extremely dehydrated following last chemotherapy session for breast cancer. Patient is admitted for IV fluids, 276.51, 174.9.

EXAMPLE

Neutropenic fever with neutropenia due to chemotherapy for acute lymphocytic leukemia, 288.03, 780.6, 204.00, E933.1

Principal Diagnosis for Encounters for Chemotherapy/Immunotherapy and Radiation

When a patient is admitted solely for the administration of chemotherapy, immunotherapy, and/or radiation, the principal diagnosis will be a V58.XX code. In cases where chemotherapy, immunotherapy, or radiation is performed in conjunction with surgical removal of a neoplasm, the primary or secondary neoplasm code is the principal diagnosis, and no V58.XX code is assigned.

If a patient is admitted for both radiation and chemotherapy during the same encounter, either V code can be sequenced as the principal with the other V code used as a secondary diagnosis code.

If complications occur during an encounter for chemotherapy/immunotherapy/radiation treatment, codes to identify the complications are assigned as secondary diagnosis codes.

EXAMPLE

Patient was admitted for chemotherapy for osteosarcoma of right humerus. Patient became dehydrated and was treated with additional IV fluids, V58.11, 170.4, 276.51, 99.25.

EXAMPLE

Patient is admitted for chemotherapy for Burkitt's lymphoma, V58.11, 200.20, 99.25.

EXAMPLE Patient is admitted for radiation therapy for prostate cancer, V58.0, 185, 92.29.

Coding of Previously Excised Malignancies

If a primary malignancy has been previously excised and is no longer being treated, it is assigned a V code for history of personal malignancy.

EXAMPLE Patient had a mastectomy 5 years ago for breast cancer. She is not being actively treated, V10.3, V45.71.

However, if a previously excised malignancy is still being treated actively, it is appropriate to assign the neoplasm code.

EXAMPLE Patient had a lobectomy for lung cancer 6 months ago. The patient will receive the fifth cycle of chemotherapy next week, 162.9, V45.76.

If a patient has a primary and an associated secondary malignancy that was previously excised and/or treated, only the V code for the history of the primary malignancy is assigned. No V codes are used to identify the personal history of a secondary malignancy. If a secondary malignancy has been completely excised or treated and is no longer active, no code is assigned.

EXAMPLE Patient had breast cancer with metastasis to axillary lymph nodes.

Patient was treated with mastectomy and chemotherapy. There has been no recurrence of any disease, and she is no longer being actively treated, V10.3, V45.71.

Neoplasm-Related Pain

When a patient has pain due to a previously identified neoplasm, code 338.3 is assigned. This code can be assigned as either principal or secondary, depending on the circumstances of the admission.

If a patient is admitted for pain management or pain control, the 338.3 code is assigned as the principal diagnosis, and the malignancy code(s) is assigned as a secondary code(s).

EXAMPLE Patient was admitted for pain control. Patient has severe pain due to metastatic bone cancer. Patient has a past history of primary breast cancer, 338.3, 198.5, V10.3.

If a patient is admitted for management of the malignancy and the pain associated with the malignancy, the malignancy code is assigned as the principal diagnosis with the 338.3 pain code assigned as a secondary diagnosis.

EXAMPLE Patient was admitted for back pain due to vertebral metastasis. An MRI indicates that the disease has progressed. Patient has a history of prostate cancer. Radiation was administered, 198.5, V10.46, 338.3, 92.29.

EXERCISE 15-15

Complete the following exercises.

1. If a patient is admitted and treated for anemia due to a malignancy, the malignancy code is the principal diagnosis.
   A. True
   B. False

2. If a patient has a complication during an encounter for chemotherapy, the complication code is the principal diagnosis.
   A. True
   B. False
3. If a malignancy of the bladder has been previously excised and now there is a recurrence of a malignancy within the bladder, the recurrence is coded as a primary malignancy.
   A. True
   B. False
4. A personal history V code is assigned for a history of a secondary malignancy.
   A. True
   B. False
5. The primary neoplasm is always principal even if the treatment is directed at the secondary neoplasm.
   A. True
   B. False
6. If a patient is admitted for treatment of dehydration due to a malignancy, the dehydration is the principal diagnosis.
   A. True
   B. False
7. When a patient is admitted for immunotherapy, the V58.11 is assigned as the principal diagnosis.
   A. True
   B. False
8. When a patient is admitted for brachytherapy, the V58.0 is assigned as the principal diagnosis.
   A. True
   B. False

V CODES

In the past, V codes have been considered primarily for use in the outpatient setting. This has changed with the addition of more V codes each year. As was discussed in Chapter 8, it may be difficult to locate V codes in the index. Coders often say, "I did not know there was a V code for that." Refer to Chapter 8 for a listing of common main terms used to locate V codes.

Also in Chapter 8, it was pointed out that it may be easy to lose track of indentations in the Alphabetic Index for a personal and family history of neoplasms. Verification in the Tabular should alert the coder of a wrong code selection.

The guidelines provide instructions for the use and sequencing of some important V codes. If a patient is admitted solely for administration of chemotherapy, immunotherapy or radiation therapy a code from category V58 should be the principal diagnosis followed by codes for the malignancies being treated. If they are admitted for more than one type of therapy, either code can be principal.

V codes that may be used with neoplasms include the following:

V07.39	Other prophylactic chemotherapy
V07.51	Prophylactic use of selective estrogen receptor modulators (SERMs)

V07.52	Prophylactic use of aromatase inhibitors
V07.59	Prophylactic use of other agents affecting estrogen receptors and estrogen levels
V10.00	Personal history of malignant neoplasm—gastrointestinal tract, unspecified
V10.01	Personal history of malignant neoplasm—tongue
V10.02	Personal history of malignant neoplasm—other and unspecified oral cavity and pharynx
V10.03	Personal history of malignant neoplasm—esophagus
V10.04	Personal history of malignant neoplasm—stomach
V10.05	Personal history of malignant neoplasm—large intestine
V10.06	Personal history of malignant neoplasm—rectum, rectosigmoid junction, and anus
V10.07	Personal history of malignant neoplasm—liver
V10.09	Personal history of malignant neoplasm—other
V10.11	Personal history of malignant neoplasm—bronchus and lung
V10.12	Personal history of malignant neoplasm—trachea
V10.20	Personal history of malignant neoplasm—respiratory organ, unspecified
V10.21	Personal history of malignant neoplasm—larynx
V10.22	Personal history of malignant neoplasm—nasal cavities, middle ear, and accessory sinuses
V10.29	Personal history of malignant neoplasm—other
V10.3	Personal history of malignant neoplasm—breast
V10.40	Personal history of malignant neoplasm—female genital organ, unspecified
V10.41	Personal history of malignant neoplasm—cervix uteri
V10.42	Personal history of malignant neoplasm—other parts of uterus
V10.43	Personal history of malignant neoplasm—ovary
V10.44	Personal history of malignant neoplasm—other female genital organs
V10.45	Personal history of malignant neoplasm—male genital organ, unspecified
V10.46	Personal history of malignant neoplasm—prostate
V10.47	Personal history of malignant neoplasm—testis
V10.48	Personal history of malignant neoplasm—epididymis
V10.49	Personal history of malignant neoplasm—other male genital organs
V10.50	Personal history of malignant neoplasm—urinary organ, unspecified
V10.51	Personal history of malignant neoplasm—bladder
V10.52	Personal history of malignant neoplasm—kidney
V10.53	Personal history of malignant neoplasm—renal pelvis
V10.59	Personal history of malignant neoplasm—other urinary organs
V10.60	Personal history of malignant neoplasm—leukemia, unspecified
V10.61	Personal history of malignant neoplasm—lymphoid leukemia
V10.62	Personal history of malignant neoplasm—myeloid leukemia
V10.63	Personal history of malignant neoplasm—monocytic leukemia
V10.69	Personal history of malignant neoplasm—other leukemia
V10.71	Personal history of malignant neoplasm—lymphosarcoma and reticulosarcoma
V10.72	Personal history of malignant neoplasm—Hodgkin's disease
V10.79	Personal history of malignant neoplasm—other lymphatic and hematopoietic neoplasms
V10.81	Personal history of malignant neoplasm—bone
V10.82	Personal history of malignant neoplasm—malignant melanoma of skin
V10.83	Personal history of malignant neoplasm—other malignant neoplasm skin
V10.84	Personal history of malignant neoplasm—eye
V10.85	Personal history of malignant neoplasm—brain
V10.86	Personal history of malignant neoplasm—other parts of the nervous system
V10.87	Personal history of malignant neoplasm—thyroid

V10.88	Personal history of malignant neoplasm—other endocrine glands and related structures
V10.89	Personal history of malignant neoplasm—other
V10.9	Personal history of malignant neoplasm—unspecified
V12.42	Personal history of benign neoplasm of the brain
V12.72	Personal history of diseases of digestive system—colonic polyps
V16.0	Family history of malignant neoplasm—gastrointestinal tract
V16.1	Family history of malignant neoplasm—trachea, bronchus, and lung
V16.2	Family history of malignant neoplasm—other respiratory and intrathoracic organs
V16.3	Family history of malignant neoplasm—breast
V16.40	Family history of malignant neoplasm—genital organ, unspecified
V16.41	Family history of malignant neoplasm—ovary
V16.42	Family history of malignant neoplasm—prostate
V16.43	Family history of malignant neoplasm—testis
V16.49	Family history of malignant neoplasm—other genital organ
V16.51	Family history of malignant neoplasm—kidney
V16.52	Family history of malignant neoplasm—bladder
V16.59	Family history of malignant neoplasm—other urinary organ
V16.6	Family history of malignant neoplasm—leukemia
V16.7	Family history of malignant neoplasm—other lymphatic and hematopoietic neoplasms
V16.8	Family history of malignant neoplasm—other specified malignant neoplasm
V16.9	Unspecified malignant neoplasm
V18.51	Family history of certain other specific conditions—digestive disorders—colonic polyps
V44.0	Artificial opening status—tracheostomy
V44.1	Artificial opening status—gastrostomy
V44.2	Artificial opening status—ileostomy
V44.3	Artificial opening status—colostomy
V44.4	Artificial opening status—other artificial opening of gastrointestinal tract
V44.50	Artificial opening status—cystostomy, unspecified
V44.51	Artificial opening status—cutaneous-vesicostomy
V44.52	Artificial opening status—appendico-vesicostomy
V44.59	Artificial opening status—other cystostomy
V44.6	Artificial opening status—other artificial opening of urinary tract
V44.7	Artificial opening status—vagina
V44.8	Artificial opening status—other artifical opening status
V44.9	Artificial opening status—unspecified artificial opening status
V45.71	Acquired absence of organ—breast and nipple
V45.72	Acquired absence of organ—intestine (large) (small)
V45.73	Acquired absence of organ—kidney
V45.74	Acquired absence of organ—other parts of urinary tract
V45.75	Acquired absence of organ—stomach
V45.76	Acquired absence of organ—lung
V45.77	Acquired absence of organ—genital organs
V45.78	Acquired absence of organ—eye
V45.79	Acquired absence of organ—other acquired absence of organ
V50.41	Prophylactic organ removal—breast
V50.42	Prophylactic organ removal—ovary
V50.49	Prophylactic organ removal—other
V51.0	Encounter for breast reconstruction following mastectomy
V55.0	Attention to artificial openings—tracheostomy

V55.1	Attention to artificial openings—gastrostomy
V55.2	Attention to artificial openings—ileostomy
V55.3	Attention to artificial openings—colostomy
V55.4	Attention to artificial openings—other artificial opening of digestive tract
V55.5	Attention to artificial openings—cystostomy
V55.6	Attention to artificial openings—other artificial opening of urinary tract
V55.7	Attention to artificial openings—vagina
V55.8	Attention to artificial openings—other specified artificial opening
V55.9	Attention to artificial openings—unspecified artificial opening
V58.0	Encounter for radiotherapy
V58.11	Encounter for antineoplastic chemotherapy
V58.12	Encounter for antineoplastic immunotherapy
V58.42	Aftercare following surgery for neoplasm
V71.1	Observation for suspected malignant neoplasm
V76.0	Special screening for malignant neoplasms—respiratory organs
V76.10	Special screening for malignant neoplasms—breast, unspecified
V76.11	Screening mammogram for high-risk patient
V76.12	Other screening mammogram
V76.19	Other screening breast examination
V76.2	Special screening for malignant neoplasms—cervix
V76.3	Special screening for malignant neoplasms—bladder
V76.41	Special screening for malignant neoplasms—rectum
V76.42	Special screening for malignant neoplasms—oral cavity
V76.43	Special screening for malignant neoplasms—skin
V76.44	Special screening for malignant neoplasms—prostate
V76.45	Special screening for malignant neoplasms—testis
V76.46	Special screening for malignant neoplasms—ovary
V76.47	Special screening for malignant neoplasms—vagina
V76.49	Special screening for malignant neoplasms—other sites
V76.50	Special screening for malignant neoplasms—intestine, unspecified
V76.51	Special screening for malignant neoplasms—colon
V76.52	Special screening for malignant neoplasms—small intestine
V76.81	Special screening for malignant neoplasms—nervous system
V76.89	Special screening for malignant neoplasms—other neoplasm
V84.01	Genetic susceptibility to malignant neoplasm—breast
V84.02	Genetic susceptibility to malignant neoplasm—ovary
V84.03	Genetic susceptibility to malignant neoplasm—prostate
V84.04	Genetic susceptibility to malignant neoplasm—endometrium
V84.09	Genetic susceptibility to malignant neoplasm—other malignant neoplasm
V87.41	Personal history of antineoplastic chemotherapy

EXAMPLE Patient has a family history of leukemia, V16.6.

EXERCISE 15-16

Assign codes to the following conditions using your ICD-9-CM code book.

1. History of adenocarcinoma of the prostate ____________
2. Screening mammogram for patient with strong family history of breast cancer ____________

3. Personal history of benign brain neoplasm previously removed ____________
4. Admission for takedown of colostomy; previous colon resection for malignancy ____________

COMMON TREATMENTS

Cancer is treated by various modalities (i.e., surgery, chemotherapy, radiation, immunotherapy, or other methods). The type of treatment will depend on the location, grading and stage of the neoplasm and the health of the patient. Chemotherapy destroys cancer cells, but may also target fast-growing healthy tissue. Often chemotherapy drugs are used in combinations because the drugs work better together than separately. Immunotherapy agents stimulate the immune system's response against tumors. Radiation therapy uses ionizing radiation to destroy cancer cells and shrink tumors. It is administered externally by external beam therapy or internally via brachytherapy.

CONDITION	MEDICATION/TREATMENT
Malignancies	Chemotherapy drugs are often given in combination with other chemotherapy drugs. The treatment will depend on the type of cancer. For a listing of drugs used during chemotherapy, go to www.chemocare.com.
Melanoma and kidney cancer	Immunotherapy with interleukin and interferon
Superficial bladder cancer	Intravesical Bacillus Calmette-Guerin (BCG) immunotherapy
Certain types of breast or colon cancer	Capecitabine (Xeloda)—interferes with cancer cell growth and reproduction
Certain types of breast cancer	Tamoxifen (Nolvadex)—interferes with estrogen activity
Advanced prostate cancer in men and uterine fibroid tumors in women	Leuprolide acetate for depot suspension (Lupron Depot)
Certain types of leukemia (CML) and certain gastrointestinal stromal tumors	Imatinib (Gleevec) prevents the growth of cancer cells
Neutropenia due to chemotherapy	Pegfilgrastim (Neulasta) or filgrastim (Neupogen) builds up or stimulates white cell counts
Anemia due to malignancy	Epoetin alfa (Procrit, Epogen), darbepoetin alfa (Aranesp)
Symptoms of malignancy and treatment	Pain medications (narcotics), antiemetics to suppress nausea and vomiting
Human papilloma virus	Vaccination for prevention

PROCEDURES

Chemotherapy/Immunotherapy/Radiation

Operative procedures are often performed to biopsy and resect or excise areas or organs that are affected by neoplastic conditions. At times, a neoplasm is considered unresectable, and other treatments are necessary. Sometimes, patients will receive chemotherapy or radiation therapy to shrink the tumor before surgery is performed. **Chemotherapy** consists of administration of drugs or medications to treat disease. In cancer patients, antineoplastic drugs are used. These drugs can be given intravenously, orally, subcutaneously, intramuscularly, or intrathecally. **Chemoembolization** is the intra-arterial administration of chemotherapy with collagen particles to enhance the delivery of chemotherapy to the targeted area. According to *Coding Clinic* (1995:4Q:p67-68),[9] this should be treated as an encounter for chemotherapy, and V58.11 should be assigned as the principal diagnosis. Procedure code 99.25 includes chemoembolization. An additional diagnosis code is assigned for the

malignancy. **Radiation** treatment involves the use of high-energy radiation to treat patients with cancer. **Brachytherapy** is the placement of radioactive material directly into or near the cancer. The radiation is delivered by needles, wires, or catheters and may be in the form of seeds. According to *Coding Clinic* (1988:1Q:p4-5)[7] "when the purpose of a hospital admission is for the treatment of a malignancy by implantation or insertion of radioactive elements, the principal diagnosis is the neoplastic condition (malignancy) being treated with the radioactive element." **Immunotherapy** is the administration of agents that stimulate the immune systems, response against tumors. **Biological response modifiers (BRM)** are a type of immunotherapy and are used to fight certain cancers and even conditions such as rheumatoid arthritis. They can destroy cancer cells, stimulate the immune system to destroy cancer cells, or change cancer cells to normal cells.

The guidelines provide instructions for the use and sequencing of some important V codes. If a patient is admitted solely for administration of chemotherapy, immunotherapy, or radiation therapy, a code from category V58 should be the principal diagnosis followed by codes for the malignancies being treated. If they are admitted for more than one type of therapy, either code can be principal.

EXAMPLE Patient was admitted for the administration of chemotherapy for osteosarcoma of upper end of the tibia, V58.11, 170.7, 99.25.

EXAMPLE Radioactive seeds were implanted for treatment of prostate cancer, 185, 92.27.

EXAMPLE Patient is admitted for chemoembolization of hepatocellular cancer, V58.11, 155.0, 99.25.

Palliative procedures may be performed to correct a condition that is causing problems or pain for the patient. It is not meant to cure. Palliative surgery may be performed to relieve an obstruction caused by a tumor. Sometimes radiation is administered for palliative treatment.

Biopsy

Biopsy specimens can be obtained in several ways. The approach used varies with the location of the mass, the age of the patient, and the technology that is available. A **biopsy** consists of removal of a representative sample of a tumor mass for pathologic examination and diagnosis. An **excisional biopsy** is the total removal of local small masses or growths (Figure 15-15).

- **Surgical/incisional biopsy:** This is the removal of a small piece of tumor. Sometimes, nearby lymph nodes may also be removed and tested for metastasis.
- **Core biopsy:** This procedure is less invasive than surgical biopsy. A large needle is used to extract a core sample. Usually, a smaller sample of tissue is provided, and the cancerous tissue may be missed. Occasionally, a new sample must be obtained.
- **Fine needle aspiration (FNA):** This method, which requires use of a very small needle, works best for masses that are superficial or easily accessible. The specimen is small, and sometimes, findings are inconclusive.
- **Endoscopic biopsy:** Is a biopsy that is performed during an endoscopic examination. After a biopsy is performed, a more definitive surgical procedure may be necessary.

EXAMPLE Patient had an FNA biopsy of a thyroid mass last week; this confirmed papillary thyroid cancer. Patient underwent total thyroidectomy, 193, 06.4.

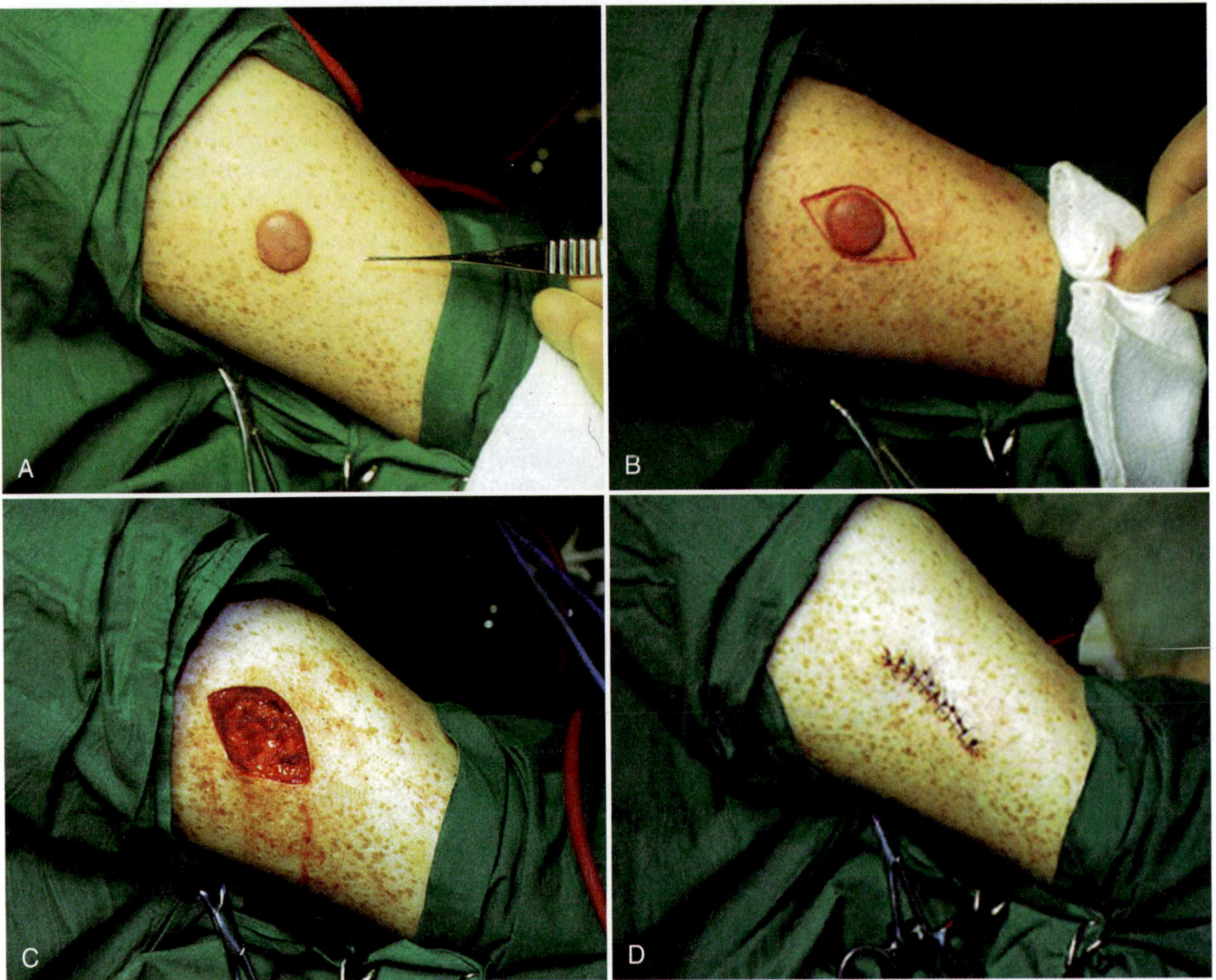

Figure 15-15. Excision of lesion. **A,** Location of lesion. **B,** Surgical margins. **C,** Lesion excised. **D,** Closure of surgical site.

Occasionally, a biopsy will be performed during the same operative episode as a more definitive treatment. In these cases, sequencing of the procedures would follow the Uniform Hospital Discharge Data Set (UHDDS) guidelines for selection of a principal procedure, and the procedure that is performed for definitive treatment is the principal procedure.

EXAMPLE

Patient was taken to the operating room for an open biopsy of a breast mass in the right upper outer quadrant. Frozen section showed invasive ductal carcinoma; a simple mastectomy with removal of axillary lymph nodes was performed during the same operative episode. Nodes were negative for malignancy, 174.4, 85.43, 85.12.

Surgery

Endoscopic procedures are minimally invasive procedures during which a scope is used to examine the inside of the body. It is also possible for the clinician to perform a biopsy, remove a small polyp or foreign body, or control bleeding with the use of an endoscope.

Preventive or prophylactic surgery is performed to remove tissue that has the potential to become cancerous. A woman may have a prophylactic mastectomy as the result of a strong family history of breast cancer and/or a positive breast cancer gene (*BRCA1* or *BRCA2*). **Staging surgeries** are performed to determine the extent of the disease and are generally

more accurate than laboratory and imaging tests. **Debulking** procedures are performed when it is impossible to remove the tumor entirely. In many of these cases a number of organs may be involved and may also have to be removed. The tumor is removed to as great an extent as is possible, and adjunctive treatment such as chemotherapy or radiation may be used to treat the remaining disease. **Restorative or reconstruction** surgery is performed to restore function and enhance aesthetic appearance after surgery. Breast reconstruction is commonly performed after a mastectomy. Breast reconstruction procedures were covered in Chapter 11.

EXAMPLE

Patient was admitted for prophylactic removal of ovaries due to genetic susceptibility and positive family history with laparoscopic removal, V50.42, V16.41, V84.02, 65.53.

EXERCISE 15-17

Assign codes for all diagnoses and procedures using your ICD-9-CM code book.

1. Refractory aplastic anemia with bone marrow transplant (BMT); donor is the patient's sister ____________
2. Transitional cell carcinoma of the bladder with transurethral resection of tumor ____________
3. Renal cell cancer of the right kidney with right laparoscopic nephrectomy ____________
4. Vaginal brachytherapy was administered for endometrial carcinoma ____________
5. Acoustic neuroma with hearing loss; craniotomy for removal of tumor ____________
6. Wide excision of melanoma right shoulder with skin grafting; graft taken from thigh ____________
7. Biopsy of intrathoracic lymph node showed non-Hodgkin's lymphoma in patient who has had a kidney transplant ____________
8. Admission for chemotherapy; patient has a malignancy of the esophagus ____________
9. Classic Whipple for carcinoma of the head of pancreas ____________
10. Ascending colon cancer with right hemicolectomy ____________

DOCUMENTATION/REIMBURSEMENT/MS-DRGs

Often, coding difficulties are due to lack of documentation. Sometimes pathology and other test results are not available at the time of discharge or when the physician is dictating the discharge summary or is reporting the final diagnoses.

The physician may document the cancer as if it is the principal diagnosis because it is the most serious and can be a life-threatening condition. However, the cancer may not fit the definition of a principal diagnosis or may not follow the neoplasm guidelines. Physicians will sometimes document metastatic breast carcinoma, and further into the record, it may be noted that the patient has had a mastectomy and has received a combination of chemotherapy and radiation therapy. In this case, it is most likely a primary breast cancer that has spread to an undocumented secondary site.

Assign All Procedure Codes

It is very important to assign all procedure codes because this could make the difference between a medical MS-DRG and a surgical MS-DRG. Likewise, it is also important to follow the guidelines for selection of the appropriate principal diagnosis.

EXAMPLE

DIAGNOSES	CODES	MS-DRG	RW
Malignant neoplasm brain with craniotomy with excision of tumor	191.9 01.59	027	2.3259
Malignant neoplasm brain with craniotomy with excision of tumor (in the body of the operative report is documentation of chemo wafers implanted on the brain)	191.9 01.59 00.10	023	4.7036

MS-DRG With and Without MCC/CC

EXAMPLE

DIAGNOSES	CODES	MS-DRG	RW
Hodgkin's lymphoma, multiple sites, Patient is cachectic.	201.98 799.4	841	1.6444
Hodgkin's lymphoma, multiple sites	201.98	842	1.2188

The presence of a CC can make a difference in reimbursement depending on the principal diagnosis and the MS-DRG assigned. The code for cachexia (799.4) is a CC.

CHAPTER REVIEW EXERCISE

Assign codes for all diagnoses and procedures, including all applicable V and E codes and procedures.

1. Adenocarcinoma of the prostate with radical retropubic excision and regional lymph nodes __________
2. Adenocarcinoma of the distal esophagus; patient is status post laparoscopic jejunostomy prior to radiation treatments __________
3. Chronic lymphocytic leukemia (CLL) __________
4. Splenectomy showed non-Hodgkin's lymphoma of the spleen __________
5. Von Recklinghausen's disease __________
6. Hydrocephalus due to malignant ependymoma fourth ventricle; the patient was admitted for ventriculoperitoneal shunt placement __________
7. Laparoscopic needle biopsy of the right adrenal gland; physician documented pheochromocytoma __________
8. Fibrosarcoma of the soft tissue of thigh with mets to brain __________
9. Malignant melanoma left thigh previously excised; patient admitted for immunotherapy with high dose Interleukin-2 because of spread to inguinal lymph nodes __________
10. Intraperitoneal metastatic carcinoma; unknown primary; treatment focused on determining primary source __________
11. Hemiplegia due to tumor frontal lobe __________
12. Primary central nervous system (spinal cord) lymphoma. Admitted for chemotherapy __________
13. Admission for red blood transfusion due to anemia caused by renal cell carcinoma __________
14. Dehydration due to chemotherapy in patient with carcinoma of breast with metastasis to axillary lymph nodes __________

15. Recurrent seizures due to metastasis to brain from lung cancer ______________
16. Cerebral meningioma ______________
17. Choroidal melanoma ______________
18. Admission for chemoembolization of hepatocellular carcinoma (HCC) ______________
19. Neutropenic fever in a patient who is undergoing treatment for leukemia; patient is pancytopenic due to chemotherapy ______________
20. Intestinal obstruction due to peritoneal metastasis from inoperable colorectal cancer ______________
21. Impending hip fracture due to metastasis to bone; patient has a previous history of breast cancer treated with mastectomy Internal fixation of femur ______________
22. Patient's myelodysplastic syndrome has progressed to acute myelogenous leukemia ______________
23. Prophylactic removal of both breasts due to positive genetic susceptibility and positive family history; a bilateral modified radical mastectomy was performed ______________
24. Chronic myeloproliferative disease ______________
25. Falx cerebri meningioma surgically removed ______________
26. Basophil adenoma of the pituitary gland causing Cushing's syndrome ______________
27. Carcinoma of the breast in the right upper and lower quadrant ______________
28. Metastatic ovarian cancer. ______________
29. Cancer head of pancreas with spread to the liver ______________
30. Endometrial adenocarcinoma with mets to ovary ______________
31. Parotidectomy for Warthin's tumor of the parotid gland ______________
32. Adenocarcinoma of the upper stomach with spread to the lower esophagus and lungs ______________

Write the correct answer(s) in the blank(s) provided.

33. If a hospital's base payment rate was $4,000.00, what would be the hospital payment for MS-DRG 023? ______________
34. At the hospital in #33, what would the payment rate be for MS-DRG 027? ______________
35. If a coder missed the procedure code for the chemo wafer, how much reimbursement would be lost? ______________

CHAPTER GLOSSARY

Adenocarcinoma: malignancy of epithelial glandular tissue such as those found in the breast, prostate, and colon.

Benign: neoplasm or tumor; means that it is not malignant.

Biological response modifiers (BRM): immunotherapy that can destroy cancer cells, stimulate the immune system to destroy cancer cells, or change cancer cells to normal cells.

Biopsy: removal of a representative sample for pathologic examination and diagnosis.

Brachytherapy: placement of radioactive material directly into or near the cancer.

Carcinoma: malignant tumor originating from epithelial tissue (e.g., in skin, bronchi, and stomach).

Carcinoma in situ: malignant cells that remain within the original site with no spread or invasion into neighboring tissue.

Chemoembolization: intra-arterial administration of chemotherapy with collagen particles to enhance the delivery of chemotherapy to the targeted area.

Chemotherapy: the use of drugs or medications to treat disease.

Complete remission: there are no signs or symptoms of the cancer.

Core biopsy: procedure in which a large needle is used to extract a core sample.

Debulking: procedures performed when it is impossible to remove the tumor entirely.

Endoscopic: examinations and procedures performed with an instrument that examines any cavity of the body with a rigid or flexible scope.

Excisional biopsy: total removal of local small masses or growths.

Fibroma: neoplasm of fibrous connective tissue.

Fine needle aspiration: procedure in which a very small needle is used; works best for masses that are superficial or easily accessible.

Grading: pathologic examination of tumor cells. Degree of cell abnormality determines the grade of cancer.

Histologic type: type of tissue or cell in which the neoplasm occurs.

Immunotherapy: administration of agents that modulate the immune system's response against tumors.

Incisional biopsy: procedure in which a representative sample of a tumor mass is removed to permit pathologic examination.

Leiomyoma: tumor or growth within the walls of the uterus. Also called *uterine fibroid.*

Leukemia: cancer of the white blood cells that begins in the blood-forming cells of the bone marrow.

Lipoma: growth of fat cells within a capsule that is usually found just below the skin.

Lymphoma: cancer of the lymphatic system.

Malignancy: neoplasm that has the ability to invade adjacent structures and spread to distant sites.

Melanoma: malignant changes of melanin cells

Metastasis: spread of a cancer from one part of the body to another, as in the appearance of neoplasms in parts of the body separate from the site of the primary tumor.

Morphology codes (M codes): codes that identify the type of cell that has become neoplastic and its biological activity or behavior.

Myeloma: malignancy that originates in the bone marrow.

Neoplasm: abnormal growth.

Palliative: procedure performed to correct a condition that is causing problems for the patient.

Partial remission: there are still a few signs and symptoms of the cancer, and the cancer cells have significantly decreased.

Preventive or prophylactic surgery: procedure performed to remove tissue that has the potential to become cancerous.

Primary site: site at which the neoplasm begins or originates.

Radiation: use of high-energy radiation to treat cancer.

Restorative or reconstructive: surgery performed to restore function and enhance aesthetic appearance after surgery.

Sarcoma: malignant growth of connective tissue (e.g., muscle, cartilage, lymph tissue, bone).

Staging: means of categorizing a particular cancer that assists in determination of a patient's treatment plan and the need for further therapy.

Staging surgeries: procedures performed to help the clinician determine the extent of disease; these are generally more accurate than laboratory and imaging tests.

Undifferentiated: tumor cells that are highly abnormal (e.g., immature, primitive).

Well differentiated: tumor cells that closely resemble mature, specialized cells.

CHAPTER 16

Complications of Pregnancy, Childbirth, and the Puerperium

(ICD-9-CM Chapter 11, Codes 630-677)

CHAPTER OUTLINE

LEARNING OBJECTIVES

- Apply and assign the correct ICD-9-CM codes in accordance with Official Guidelines for Coding and Reporting
- Identify pertinent anatomy and physiology of pregnancy, childbirth, and the puerperium
- Recognize conditions and complications of pregnancy, childbirth, and the puerperium
- Assign the correct V codes and procedure codes related to pregnancy, childbirth, and the puerperium
- Identify common treatments, medications, laboratory values, and diagnostic tests
- Explain the importance of documentation in relation to MS-DRGs for reimbursement

ABBREVIATIONS

AROM artificial rupture of membranes
CPD cephalopelvic disproportion
D&C dilatation and curettage
EDC estimated date of confinement
EMS emergency medical services
hCG human chorionic gonadotropin
IOL induction of labor
LGA large for gestational age
LTCS low transverse cesarean section

ABBREVIATIONS—*cont'd*

MS-DRG Medicare Severity diagnosis-related group
NST nonstress test
OB obstetrics
PIH pregnancy-induced hypertension
POCs products of conception
PROM premature rupture of membranes
PTA prior to admission
PTL preterm labor
SVD spontaneous vaginal delivery
UTI urinary tract infection
VBAC vaginal birth after cesarean section

ICD-9-CM Official Guidelines for Coding and Reporting

Please refer to the companion Evolve website for the most current guidelines.

As there are many guidelines governing the coding and reporting of pregnancy this chapter will follow a slightly different format than previous chapters with the guidelines being interspersed throughout the chapter.

Apply the General Coding Guidelines as found in Chapter 5.

ANATOMY AND PHYSIOLOGY

The organs of the female reproductive system include the ovaries, fallopian tubes, uterus, vagina, and cervix (Figure 16-1). These organs aid in reproduction and supply hormones that aid in the development of secondary female sex characteristics such as body hair and breasts.

The **vulva** is the external covering to the vagina. The **labia** surround the vaginal opening. The vagina is a muscular tube that extends from the vaginal opening to the uterus. The **vagina** serves three purposes: It is the receptacle for sperm during intercourse, it serves as the birth canal for childbirth, and it rids the body of menstrual blood during menstruation.

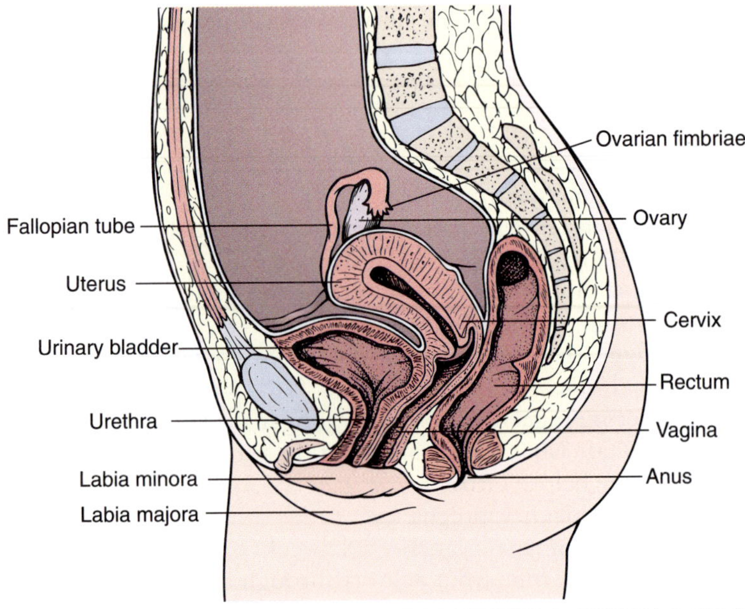

Figure 16-1. Normal female reproductive system.

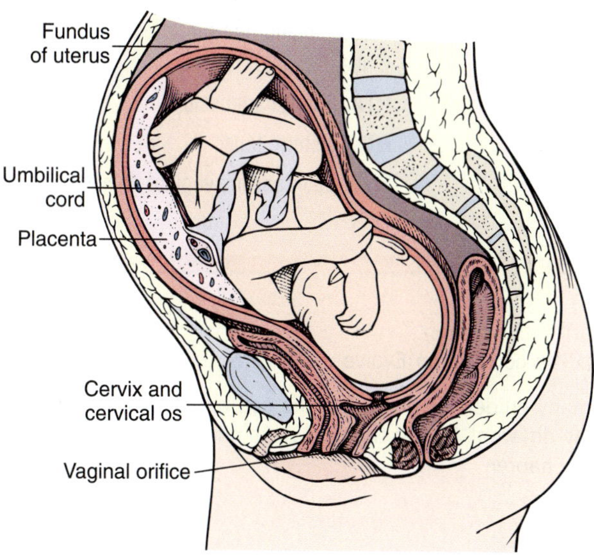

Figure 16-2. Normal uterine pregnancy.

The **cervix** is the neck of the uterus and serves as an outlet from the uterus. The **uterus** is a muscular organ that serves as an incubator for the developing fetus. The wall of the uterus is composed of three layers. The inner layer, the endometrium, is where an egg grows if fertilized.

The **ovaries** produce female hormones and eggs. If the egg is fertilized and becomes a fetus, all the other female organs assist in development and expulsion of the fetus. When an egg becomes mature and is ready for fertilization, it travels through the **fallopian tubes** to the uterus. The purpose of the fallopian tube is to deliver the mature egg to the uterus for fertilization. See Figure 16-2 for the anatomy of a normal uterine pregnancy.

To confirm a pregnancy, a woman's blood or urine may be tested for human chorionic gonadotropin (hCG). In the early months of pregnancy, secretion of hCG occurs at a high level.

Common Pregnancy Definitions

Antepartum: before delivery
Elderly obstetric patient: 35 years or older at date of delivery
Gravid: pregnant
Habitual Aborter: a woman who miscarries at least three consecutive times
Lactation: process of milk production
Multigravida or multiparity: two or more pregnancies
Postpartum: after delivery
Postterm pregnancy: pregnancy longer than 40 weeks up to 42 weeks
Precipitate labor: rapid labor and delivery
Prenatal: before birth
Primigravida: first pregnancy
Prolonged pregnancy: beyond 42 weeks of pregnancy
Puerperium: time from delivery through first 6 weeks post partum
Stillbirth: dead at birth
Young obstetric patient: younger than 16 years at date of delivery

CONDITIONS OF PREGNANCY, CHILDBIRTH, AND PUERPERIUM

Complications of Pregnancy, Childbirth, and the Puerperium (630-677), Chapter 11 in the ICD-9-CM code book, is divided into the following categories:

CATEGORY	SECTION TITLE
630-633	Ectopic and Molar Pregnancy
634-639	Other Pregnancy With Abortive Outcome
640-648	Complications Mainly Related to Pregnancy
650-659	Normal Delivery, and Other Indications for Care in Pregnancy, Labor, and Delivery
660-669	Complications Occurring Mainly in the Course of Labor and Delivery
670-677	Complications of the Puerperium

Ectopic and Molar Pregnancy (630-633)

Ectopic pregnancies usually occur when the egg is implanted outside the cavity of the uterus, most commonly in the fallopian tube (Figure 16-3). This type of pregnancy occurs in 1 of every 50 pregnancies. Pelvic infections may predispose a woman to having ectopic pregnancies. Molar pregnancies are rare and occur in 1 in 1000 pregnancies. In a **molar pregnancy**, the embryo does not form at all or is malformed. The early placenta develops into a mass of cysts within a hydatidiform mole (Figure 16-4). Occasionally, a molar pregnancy can turn into a rare, pregnancy-related form of cancer.

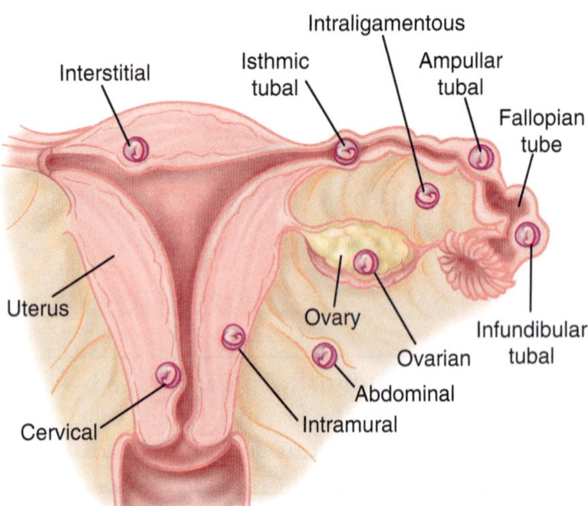

Figure 16-3. Diagram showing locations of ectopic (extrauterine) pregnancy.

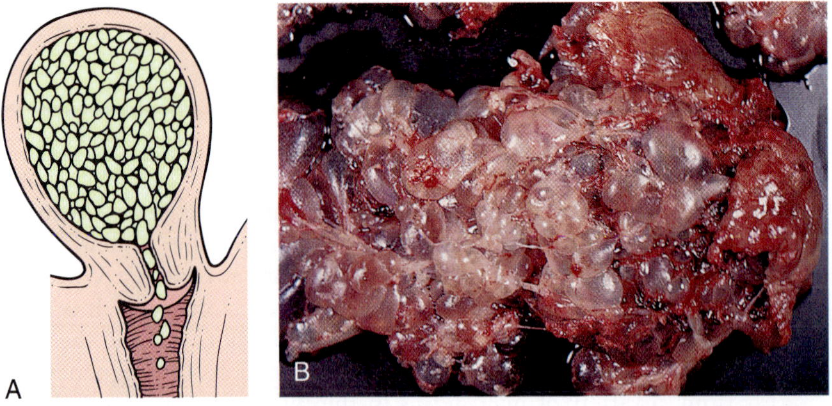

Figure 16-4. Hydatidiform mole.

EXAMPLE

Patient presents to her physician's office with a pregnancy in the 10th week. She comes in because she is experiencing dark brown vaginal bleeding. The physician identifi es a molar pregnancy. The patient is admitted to the hospital for suction curettage to remove the molar tissue.

Codes: 631, Abnormal products of conception
69.59, Other aspiration curettage of uterus

It is appropriate to use codes from 639 to describe any complications that may occur during an ectopic or molar pregnancy. According to the general rule for obstetric cases, additional codes from other chapters may be used in conjunction with Chapter 11 codes to further specify conditions.

EXAMPLE

Patient is admitted to the hospital with a tubal pregnancy without intrauterine pregnancy. After the tubal pregnancy is removed, the patient develops a urinary tract infection (UTI).

Codes: 633.10, Tubal pregnancy without intrauterine pregnancy
639.8, Other specified complications following abortion or ectopic and molar pregnancy
599.0, Urinary tract infection

EXERCISE 16-1

Assign codes to the following conditions using your ICD-9-CM code book.

1. Ruptured ectopic pregnancy ____________
2. Vesicular mole ____________
3. Ectopic pregnancy of the fallopian tube followed by oliguria ____________

Coding of Pregnancy

A normal pregnancy (Figure 16-5) usually lasts anywhere from 37 to 40 weeks. These weeks are counted from the beginning of the last menstrual cycle. When a pregnancy lasts longer than 40 weeks (post-term), complications can occur; and therefore this is no longer considered a normal pregnancy. Coding of normal deliveries requires only two codes and may have only one procedure code.

EXAMPLE

650, Normal delivery
V27.0, Single liveborn
73.59, Manually assisted delivery

All deliveries require an outcome of delivery code on the mother's record. The outcome of delivery is the code used to describe the number of newborns delivered and their status, i.e., live or stillborn. The outcome of delivery code is a V code that is found in the Alphabetic Index under the main term "outcome of delivery." **It is important to note that if code 650 is selected, it cannot be used with any other code in the range of 630-676.**

When codes are selected for complications of pregnancy, childbirth, and the puerperium, a variety of main terms in the index may be accessed. If the condition is affecting the pregnancy, the index term is "Pregnancy." Likewise, if the condition is affecting the

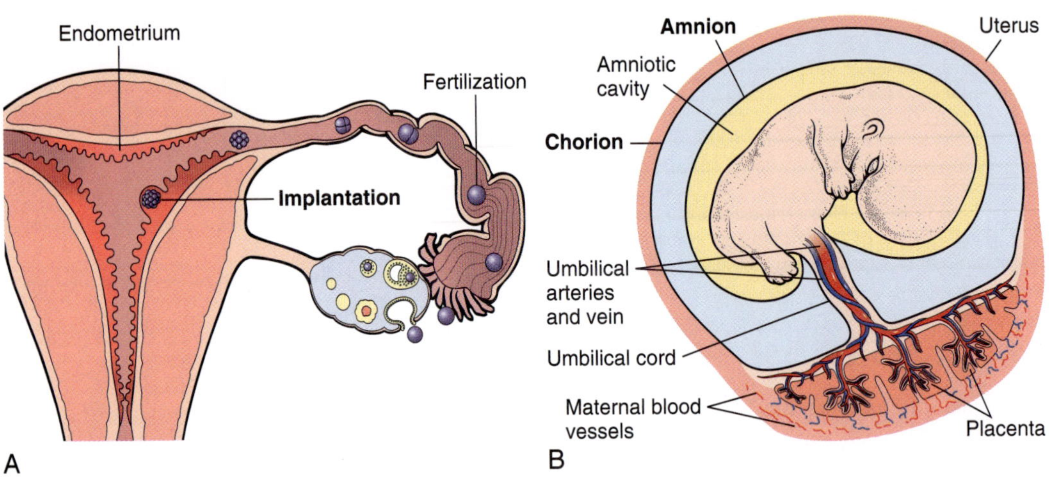

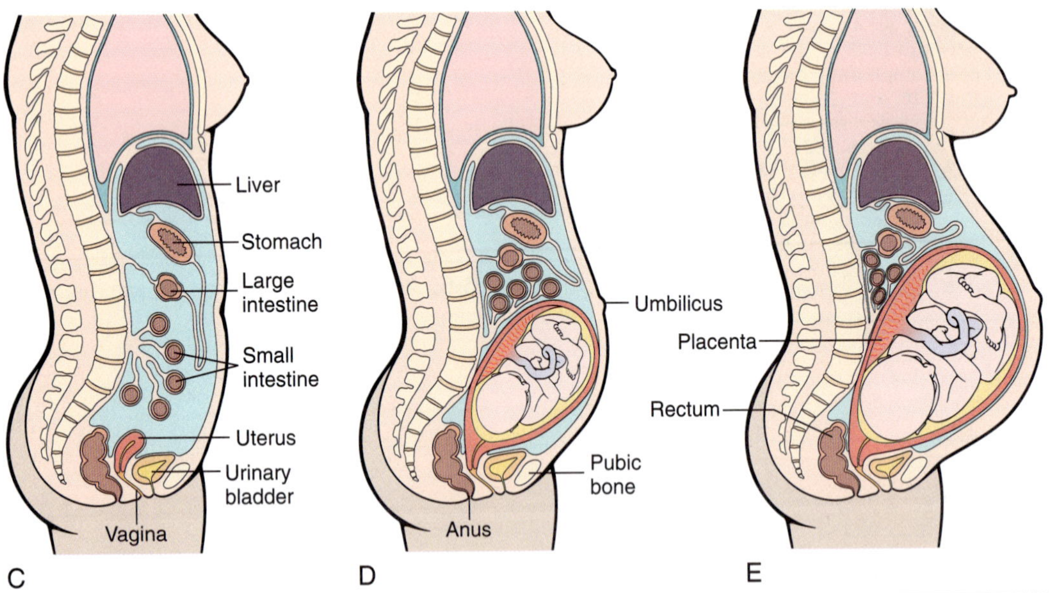

Figure 16-5. **A,** Implantation of the embryo in the endometrium. **B,** The placenta and membranes (chorion and amnion). **C–E,** Sagittal sections of pregnancy. **C,** Nonpregnant woman. **D,** Woman who is 20 weeks pregnant. **E,** Woman who is 30 weeks pregnant.

labor of the patient, the index term selected may be "Labor," and the index may direct the coder to *see also* "Delivery." The Alphabetic Index may be checked directly for a condition (Figure 16-6). For example,

Vomiting
  Of or complicating pregnancy
    Early—see hyperemesis, gravidarum

Other main terms in the Alphabetic Index that may be used to locate pregnancy-related codes include the following:

- Failure
- Arrest
- Presentation
- Laceration
- Puerperal
- Labor
- Pregnancy
- Delivery

Vomiting 787.03
with nausea 787.01
allergic 535.4
asphyxia 933.1
bilious (cause unknown) 787.0
following gastrointestinal surgery 564.3
blood (*see also* Hematemesis) 578.0
causing asphyxia, choking, or suffocation (*see also* Asphyxia, food) 933.1
cyclical 536.2
psychogenic 306.4
epidemic 078.82
fecal matter 569.89
following gastrointestinal surgery 564.3
functional 536.8
psychogenic 306.4
habit 536.2
hysterical 300.11
nervous 306.4
neurotic 306.4
newborn 779.3
of or complicating pregnancy 643.9
due to
organic disease 643.8
specific cause NEC 643.8
early - *see* Hyperemesis, gravidarum
late (after 22 completed weeks of gestation) 643.2
pernicious or persistent 536.2
complicating pregnancy - *see* Hyperemesis, gravidarum

Figure 16-6. Alphabetic Index entry for vomiting in early pregnancy.

EXERCISE 16-2

Answer the following questions.

1. The duration of a normal pregnancy is
____
2. Can code 650 be used with 660.71?
____
3. What are the three most common areas of the Alphabetic Index to look under for codes related to Chapter 16?
   1. _______________
   2. _______________
   3. _______________
4. What are the organs of the female reproductive system? _______________
5. To confirm a pregnancy, what is tested for from a woman's blood or urine? _______________
6. If a woman is pregnant for the first time at age 36, what would be another term for her? _______________
7. If a woman delivers at 41 weeks, what would this be considered? _______________
8. How long does the puerperium last? _______________

Identify the main term(s) that would be used to locate the following in the Alphabetic Index.

9. Obstructed labor ______________
10. First-degree perineal laceration delivered single liveborn vaginally ______________
11. Arrested labor ______________
12. Fever due to amnionitis during labor ______________
13. Twin pregnancy ______________
14. Oligohydramnios ______________
15. Premature rupture of membranes ______________
16. Primary uterine inertia ______________
17. Postpartum hemorrhage ______________
18. Breech delivery ______________
19. Prolonged labor ______________
20. Precipitous delivery ______________

Guidelines for Obstetric Cases

General Rules for Obstetric Cases

11. Chapter 11: Complications of Pregnancy, Childbirth, and the Puerperium (630-677)

a. General Rules for Obstetric Cases

1) Codes from chapter 11 and sequencing priority

Obstetric cases require codes from chapter 11, codes in the range 630-677, Complications of Pregnancy, Childbirth, and the Puerperium. Chapter 11 codes have sequencing priority over codes from other chapters. Additional codes from other chapters may be used in conjunction with chapter 11 codes to further specify conditions. Should the provider document that the pregnancy is incidental to the encounter, then V22.2 should be used in place of any chapter 11 codes. It is the provider's responsibility to state that the condition being treated is not affecting the pregnancy.

In most cases, when a patient is pregnant, a code from Chapter 11 must be assigned regardless of what condition the patient presents with. The exception to this rule would occur when a physician documents that the pregnancy is incidental to the reason for this encounter. Almost ALWAYS, codes from the pregnancy chapter are to be assigned. This does not mean that codes from other chapters cannot be used to more fully describe a condition. The codes from Chapter 11 have sequencing priority.

EXAMPLE

Patient presents to physician office with pain and burning on urination. The physician documents that the patient is 26 weeks pregnant and has a UTI.

Codes would be as follows: 646.63, Infections of the genitourinary tract in pregnancy
599.0, UTI

EXAMPLE

A patient with gastroenteritis is seen in the emergency room (ER). The ER physician documents that the pregnancy is incidental to her gastroenteritis.

Codes would be as follows: 558.9, Gastroenteritis
V22.2, Pregnancy state, incidental

2) Chapter 11 codes used only on the maternal record

Chapter 11 codes are to be used only on the maternal record, never on the record of the newborn.

It can be confusing with what can be reported on the mother's chart and what can be reported on the newborn's chart. If possible it may be helpful to code both charts at the same time.

In the example above, if a pregnant woman has a UTI that in turn affects the care of the newborn, the code 646.6X would not be used on the newborn chart. The code 760.1 would be assigned to the newborn chart and is found in the index as follows:

Infection
    Urinary
        Complicating pregnancy, childbirth
            Affecting fetus or newborn, 760.1

Codes that are assigned to the newborn are discussed in Chapter 17.

3) Chapter 11 fifth-digits
Categories 640-648, 651-676 have required fifth-digits, which indicate whether the encounter is antepartum, postpartum and whether a delivery has also occurred.

The fifth digits to be used with the codes listed above from chapter 11 are as follows:

- 0 Unspecified as to episode of care or not applicable
- 1 Delivered, with or without mention of antepartum condition
- 2 Delivered, with mention of postpartum complication
- 3 Antepartum condition or complication
- 4 Postpartum condition or complication

The fifth digit of 0 would rarely be used, because in most cases, it is known whether this is an antepartum problem or a postpartum problem or a delivery.

When the patient comes in to deliver, the fifth digit of 1 or 2 is used. If a patient presents prior to delivery, then the fifth digit of 3 would be used; likewise, if the patient presents after delivery, the fifth digit of 4 is selected.

The following combinations of fifth digit codes are NOT valid and should not be used:

- 0 with 1, 2, 3, or 4
- 1 with 0, 3, or 4
- 2 with 0, 3, or 4
- 3 with 0, 1, 2, or 4
- 4 with 0, 1, 2, or 3

4) Fifth-digits, appropriate for each code
The fifth-digits, which are appropriate for each code number, are listed in brackets under each code (Figure 16-7). The fifth-digits on each code should all be consistent with each other. That is, should a delivery occur all of the fifth-digits should indicate the delivery.

EXAMPLE

A patient is admitted in labor and she delivers a 7-lb baby boy. After vaginal delivery, she hemorrhages. The physician documents that the hemorrhage is due to a retained placenta, 666.12, V27.0, 73.59.

EXAMPLE

A patient is admitted in labor and delivers a 7-lb baby boy vaginally. The physician requests a social work consult because this mother has struggled with depression prior to and during this pregnancy, 648.41, 311, V27.0, 73.59.

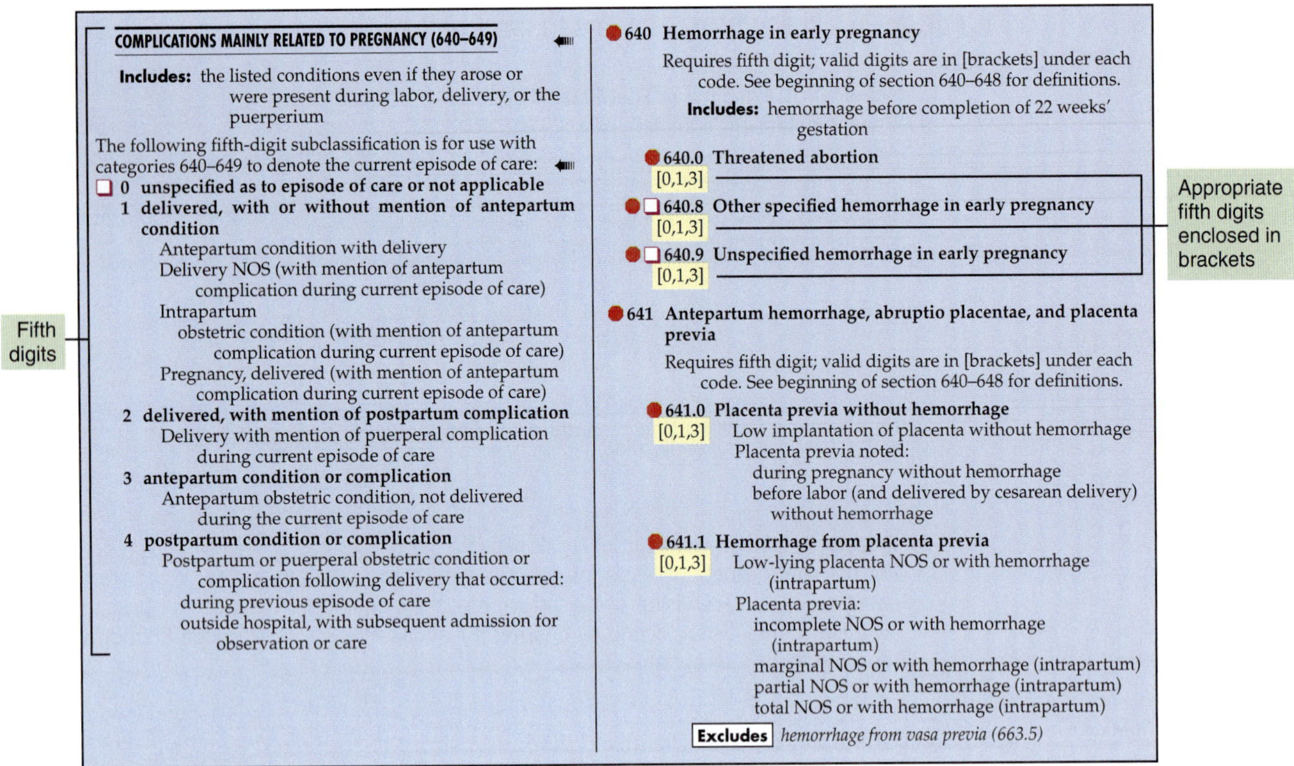
COMPLICATIONS MAINLY RELATED TO PREGNANCY (640–649)

Includes: the listed conditions even if they arose or were present during labor, delivery, or the puerperium

The following fifth-digit subclassification is for use with categories 640–649 to denote the current episode of care:

0 **unspecified as to episode of care or not applicable**
1 **delivered, with or without mention of antepartum condition**
Antepartum condition with delivery
Delivery NOS (with mention of antepartum complication during current episode of care)
Intrapartum
obstetric condition (with mention of antepartum complication during current episode of care)
Pregnancy, delivered (with mention of antepartum complication during current episode of care)
2 **delivered, with mention of postpartum complication**
Delivery with mention of puerperal complication during current episode of care
3 **antepartum condition or complication**
Antepartum obstetric condition, not delivered during the current episode of care
4 **postpartum condition or complication**
Postpartum or puerperal obstetric condition or complication following delivery that occurred:
during previous episode of care
outside hospital, with subsequent admission for observation or care

640 Hemorrhage in early pregnancy
Requires fifth digit; valid digits are in [brackets] under each code. See beginning of section 640–648 for definitions.
Includes: hemorrhage before completion of 22 weeks' gestation

640.0 Threatened abortion
[0,1,3]
640.8 Other specified hemorrhage in early pregnancy
[0,1,3]
640.9 Unspecified hemorrhage in early pregnancy
[0,1,3]

641 Antepartum hemorrhage, abruptio placentae, and placenta previa
Requires fifth digit; valid digits are in [brackets] under each code. See beginning of section 640–648 for definitions.

641.0 Placenta previa without hemorrhage
[0,1,3] Low implantation of placenta without hemorrhage
Placenta previa noted:
during pregnancy without hemorrhage
before labor (and delivered by cesarean delivery) without hemorrhage

641.1 Hemorrhage from placenta previa
[0,1,3] Low-lying placenta NOS or with hemorrhage (intrapartum)
Placenta previa:
incomplete NOS or with hemorrhage (intrapartum)
marginal NOS or with hemorrhage (intrapartum)
partial NOS or with hemorrhage (intrapartum)
total NOS or with hemorrhage (intrapartum)
Excludes *hemorrhage from vasa previa (663.5)*

Figure 16-7. Fifth digits used in pregnancy codes and designation of the appropriate fifth digit for use with specific codes are enclosed in brackets.

EXERCISE 16-3

Assign codes to the following conditions using your ICD-9-CM code book.

1. Patient presents with acute sinusitis. She is 8 weeks pregnant. Physician documents that the pregnancy is incidental to her acute sinusitis. ____________
2. Patient has a postpartum hemorrhage; she delivered 5 days PTA ____________
3. Patient vaginally delivered at 35 weeks; single liveborn infant ____________
4. Patient presents with PIH at 32 weeks; she is treated and sent home. ____________
5. Patient presents in labor; she had a previous cesarean section and delivered on this admit with no complications; vaginal delivery of single liveborn ____________
6. Patient is given pitocin to induce labor for post-dates (41 weeks); induction is unsuccessful and she is sent home ____________
7. Patient presents with premature rupture of membranes and delivers a healthy newborn vaginally. ____________
8. Can a fifth digit of 4 be used with code 660.1? ____________
9. If the mother of a newborn has diabetes, is the code 648.01 used on the newborn chart? ____________
10. Is it possible to code 650 and 652.51 together? ____________
11. Are these two codes allowed to be used together: 648.24 and 648.02? ____________

Selection of OB Principal or First-Listed Diagnosis

b. Selection of OB Principal or First-listed Diagnosis

1) Routine outpatient prenatal visits

For routine outpatient prenatal visits when no complications are present codes V22.0, Supervision of normal first pregnancy, and V22.1, Supervision of other normal pregnancy, should be used as the first-listed diagnoses. These codes should not be used in conjunction with chapter 11 codes.

EXAMPLE

The patient is seen for a routine prenatal visit. She also has a 2-year-old daughter, V22.1.

EXAMPLE

The patient is seen for a routine prenatal visit. The physician documents that she has iron deficiency anemia, 648.23, 280.9.

2) Prenatal outpatient visits for high-risk patients

For prenatal outpatient visits for patients with high-risk pregnancies, a code from category V23, Supervision of high-risk pregnancy, should be used as the principal or first-listed diagnosis. Secondary chapter 11 codes may be used in conjunction with these codes if appropriate.

For a patient at high risk, first listed diagnoses should be selected from the V23 category for outpatient prenatal visits. ICD-9-CM has separate codes for different high-risk categories such as infertility, history of abortion, multiparity, history of preterm labor, poor reproductive history, insufficient prenatal care, elderly primigravida or multigravida, and young primigravida or multigravida. The *Merck Manual* reports that "high-risk" pregnancy has no formal or universally accepted definition, but it goes on to list the following risk factors:

- Weight of mother less than 100 lb
- Obese mother
- Short stature of mother
- Structural abnormalities such as double uterus or incompetent cervix
- Disorders of a mother that are present prior to pregnancy, such as heart disease, high blood pressure, and seizure.

There are instructional notes under code V23.4 that direct the coder that a patient with a history of conditions classifiable to 630-676 may fall into this category.

EXAMPLE

A pregnant patient presents for a routine prenatal visit. During her previous pregnancy, she had early pregnancy vomiting and the physician documents high-risk pregnancy, V23.49.

It is also important to note that unlike the codes from category V22, the codes from V23 can be used in conjunction with other codes from Chapter 11.

EXAMPLE

A gravid patient presents for a routine prenatal visit. This patient had preeclampsia on her previous pregnancy and the physician documents high-risk pregnancy. She has blood work taken on this visit and is found to be anemic. The physician prescribes an iron supplement, V23.49, 648.23, 285.9.

3) Episodes when no delivery occurs

In episodes when no delivery occurs, the principal diagnosis should correspond to the principal complication of the pregnancy, which necessitated the encounter. Should more than one complication exist, all of which are treated or monitored, any of the complications codes may be sequenced first.

At times, a pregnant woman may have to be admitted to the hospital prior to delivery and sent home before delivery occurs. In these cases, the principal diagnosis is the reason the patient was admitted to the hospital.

EXAMPLE

A pregnant patient presents to the ER with dehydration related to hyperemesis gravidarum. The physician in the ER discovers that the patient has pregnancy-induced hypertension. The patient is admitted, 643.13, 642.33, 276.51.

4) When a delivery occurs

When a delivery occurs, the principal diagnosis should correspond to the main circumstances or complication of the delivery. In cases of cesarean delivery, the selection of the principal diagnosis should correspond to the reason the cesarean delivery was performed unless the reason for admission/encounter was unrelated to the condition resulting in the cesarean delivery.

EXAMPLE

A patient is admitted to the hospital in labor. She is 40 years old, and labor proceeds uneventfully. This is her sixth pregnancy, and the baby weighs 11 lb. She is delivered by the physician, who performs a midline episiotomy. Physician documents LGA, 656.61, 659.61, V27.0, 73.6.

EXAMPLE

A patient is admitted to the hospital for severe preeclampsia. She is 36 weeks pregnant. A low transverse cervical cesarean section (LTCS) is performed immediately, and she delivers a healthy baby boy, 642.51, 644.21, V27.0, 74.1.

5) Outcome of delivery

An outcome of delivery code, V27.0-V27.9, should be included on every maternal record when a delivery has occurred. These codes are not to be used on subsequent records or on the newborn record.

EXAMPLE

Healthy 40-year-old primigravida presents to the hospital and delivers twins vaginally, 651.01, 659.51, V27.2, 73.59.

EXAMPLE

A pregnant woman presents to the hospital for delivery of known quadruplets. She is taken to the operating room for a cesarean section (LTCS). As the babies are delivered, it is discovered that one has died in utero, 651.51, V27.6, 74.1.

EXERCISE 16-4

Assign codes to the following conditions using your ICD-9-CM code book.

1. Patient is a primigravida and is being seen in the obstetrics (OB) office for a routine pregnancy visit ____________
2. Patient with a history of preterm labor is seen in the OB office for a routine pregnancy visit ____________
3. Can a V22.0 code be used with a 648.23 code at an outpatient visit? ____________
4. An obese pregnant woman presents to the hospital with extremely high blood pressure. The physician documents mild preeclampsia. She is put on medications and sent home. ____________

5. A pregnant woman presents to the hospital in preterm labor at 34 weeks; she is treated with tocolysis for 3 days and is sent home on bed rest ____________
6. A pregnant woman presents to the hospital with gestational diabetes; she delivers a single liveborn vaginally ____________
7. A pregnant woman presents to the hospital in labor with a diagnosis of severe preeclampsia. She has smoked this entire pregnancy. She is 35 weeks pregnant and delivers a baby girl vaginally. ____________
8. A pregnant woman presents to the hospital in labor at 32 weeks. After 2 weeks of treatment with tocolytics, she goes into heavy labor. Her cervix has failed to dilate, and a low transverse cesarean section is performed. She delivers a healthy baby boy. ____________
9. A pregnant woman at 30 weeks presents to the hospital in labor; she has a twin pregnancy and vaginally delivers two baby girls ____________
10. A 15-year-old girl presents to the hospital in labor. She has a known twin pregnancy. A low cervical cesarean section is performed. One of the twins was stillborn. ____________

Fetal Conditions Affecting the Management of the Mother

c. Fetal Conditions Affecting the Management of the Mother

1) Codes from category 655

Known or suspected fetal abnormality affecting management of the mother, and category 656, Other fetal and placental problems affecting the management of the mother, are assigned only when the fetal condition is actually responsible for modifying the management of the mother, i.e., by requiring diagnostic studies, additional observation, special care, or termination of pregnancy. The fact that the fetal condition exists does not justify assigning a code from this series to the mother's record.

EXAMPLE

Fetal chromosomal abnormality with elective termination of pregnancy, with insertion of laminaria and aspiration curettage of uterus, with complete extraction of products of conception, 635.92, 655.13, 69.93, 69.51.

EXAMPLE

Mother presents for delivery. The physician documents that the baby appears large for dates (LGA [large for gestational age]). The mother vaginally delivers a 7 lb baby girl without any complications, 650, V27.0.

In this case, the LGA code would not be used because it does not affect the management of the mother.

2) In utero surgery

In cases when surgery is performed on the fetus, a diagnosis code from category 655, Known or suspected fetal abnormalities affecting management of the mother, should be assigned identifying the fetal condition. Procedure code 75.36, Correction of fetal defect, should be assigned on the hospital inpatient record.

No code from Chapter 15, the perinatal codes, should be used on the mother's record to identify fetal conditions. Surgery performed in utero on a fetus is still to be coded as an obstetric encounter.

EXAMPLE

A fetus is known to have spina bifida. The parents find a surgeon trained in operating in utero and have this problem corrected prior to birth.

Codes: 655.03, Central nervous system malformation in fetus
75.36, Correction of fetal defect

HIV Infection in Pregnancy, Childbirth, and the Puerperium

d. HIV Infection in Pregnancy, Childbirth and the Puerperium

During pregnancy, childbirth or the puerperium, a patient admitted because of an HIV-related illness should receive a principal diagnosis of 647.6X, Other specified infectious and parasitic diseases in the mother classifiable elsewhere, but complicating the pregnancy, childbirth or the puerperium, followed by 042 and the code(s) for the HIV-related illness(es).

Patients with asymptomatic HIV infection status admitted during pregnancy, childbirth, or the puerperium should receive codes of 647.6X and V08.

EXAMPLE

A 32-year-old female who is 23 weeks pregnant with known AIDS is admitted with severe diarrhea determined to be caused by cryptosporidium. She is treated with IV fluids, 647.63, 042, 007.4.

Patients with asymptomatic HIV infection status admitted during pregnancy, childbirth, or the puerperium should receive codes of 647.6X and V08.

EXAMPLE

A 23-year-old gravid female is admitted in preterm labor at 35 weeks. She has had an uneventful pregnancy, except for the fact that she has an asymptomatic human immunodeficiency virus (HIV) infection. She vaginally delivers a 7 lb 2 oz baby, 644.21, 647.61, V08, V27.0, 73.59.

Current Conditions Complicating Pregnancy

e. Current Conditions Complicating Pregnancy

Assign a code from subcategory 648.X for patients that have current conditions when the condition affects the management of the pregnancy, childbirth, or the puerperium. Use additional secondary codes from other chapters to identify the conditions, as appropriate.

The important concept in this guideline is to assign a code from this category when the condition affects the management of pregnancy, childbirth, or the puerperium. In some cases, the presentation of the fetus complicates the delivery (Figure 16-8).

EXAMPLE

A 33-year-old presents at 40 weeks in labor. She has had an uneventful pregnancy, except for slight anemia treated with iron. She has an uncomplicated vaginal delivery of a 6 lb baby girl, 648.21, 285.9, V27.0, 73.59.

EXAMPLE

A 15-year-old pregnant female presents in active labor. She has no past history, except for several bouts of asthma as a toddler. She had an uncomplicated delivery of a healthy baby boy, 659.81, V27.0, 73.59.

Diabetes in Pregnancy

f. Diabetes mellitus in pregnancy

Diabetes mellitus is a significant complicating factor in pregnancy. Pregnant women who are diabetic should be assigned code 648.0x, Diabetes mellitus complicating pregnancy, and a secondary code from category 250, Diabetes mellitus, to identify the type of diabetes.

Code V58.67, Long-term (current) use of insulin, should also be assigned if the diabetes mellitus is being treated with insulin.

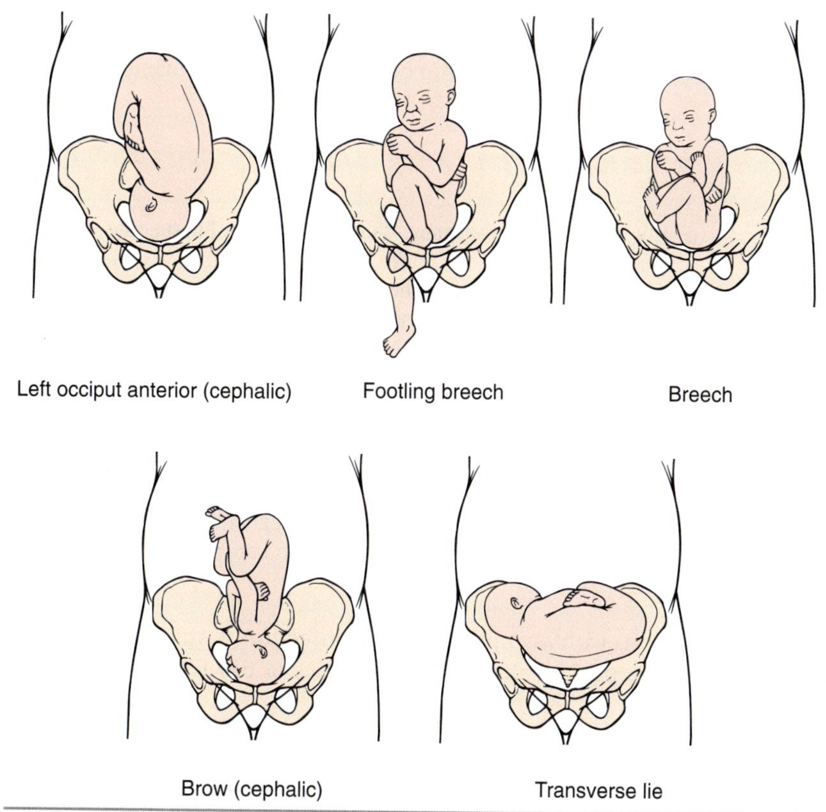

Figure 16-8. Fetal presentations.

EXAMPLE

Patient is admitted to hospital in diabetic ketoacidosis. The admitting physician documents that the patient is 12 weeks pregnant with a history of type I diabetes. She is treated with sliding scale insulin, 648.03, 250.13, V58.67.

g. Gestational diabetes

Gestational diabetes can occur during the second and third trimester of pregnancy in women who were not diabetic prior to pregnancy. Gestational diabetes can cause complications in the pregnancy similar to those of pre-existing diabetes mellitus. It also puts the woman at greater risk of developing diabetes after the pregnancy. Gestational diabetes is coded to 648.8x, Abnormal glucose tolerance. Codes 648.0x and 648.8x should never be used together on the same record.

Code V58.67, Long-term (current) use of insulin, should also be assigned if the gestational diabetes is being treated with insulin.

EXAMPLE

A patient is admitted to the hospital in labor. She has had a relatively uneventful pregnancy except for gestational diabetes. She vaginally delivers a healthy 7 lb baby girl, 648.81, V27.0, 73.59.

Normal Delivery

h. Normal Delivery, Code 650

1) Normal delivery

Code 650 is for use in cases when a woman is admitted for a full-term normal delivery and delivers a single, healthy infant without any complications antepartum, during the delivery, or postpartum during the delivery episode. Code 650 is always a

principal diagnosis. It is not to be used if any other code from chapter 11 is needed to describe a current complication of the antenatal, delivery, or perinatal period. Additional codes from other chapters may be used with code 650 if they are not related to or are in any way complicating the pregnancy.

EXAMPLE

Patient is admitted to the hospital in labor. She is 40 weeks pregnant. She has had an uneventful pregnancy and vaginally delivers a 7 lb 2 oz baby boy. The doctor performs an episiotomy followed by suturing during delivery, 650, V27.0, 73.6.

EXAMPLE

Patient is admitted to the hospital in labor. She is 40 weeks pregnant. She has had an uneventful pregnancy and vaginally delivers a 7 lb 2 oz baby boy. The doctor performs an episiotomy and the baby is delivered with the use of a vacuum extractor, 669.51, V27.0, 72.71.

The use of a vacuum extractor in the above example prohibits the use of code 650 for this delivery.

EXAMPLE

Patient is admitted to the hospital in labor. She is 40 weeks pregnant, has had an uneventful pregnancy, and delivers a 7 lb 2 oz baby boy. The doctor performs an episiotomy with a first-degree extension with repair, 664.01, V27.0, 75.69.

As in the previous example, the first-degree extension in this example prohibits the use of 650. An extension of an episiotomy is coded as a laceration, per *Coding Clinic* (1992:1Q: p10-11).[1] An extension may occur when the birth canal lacerates after an episiotomy is performed.

2) Normal delivery with resolved antepartum complication
Code 650 may be used if the patient had a complication at some point during her pregnancy, but the complication is not present at the time of the admission for delivery.

EXAMPLE

Patient is admitted to the hospital in labor. She is 40 weeks pregnant. She had a UTI early on in her pregnancy and was treated appropriately. She delivers a 7 lb 2 oz baby boy by spontaneous vaginal delivery, 650, V27.0, 73.59.

EXAMPLE

Patient is 40 weeks pregnant. The physician documents that chlamydia was discovered early on in the pregnancy, and the patient now tests negative. Patient has a spontaneous vaginal delivery of an 8 lb baby girl, 650, V27.0, 73.59.

3) V27.0, Single liveborn, outcome of delivery
V27.0, Single liveborn, is the only outcome of delivery code appropriate for use with 650.

EXAMPLE

Patient is admitted to the hospital in labor. She has had an uneventful pregnancy and goes on to a spontaneous vaginal delivery of twin boys, 651.01, V27.2, 73.59.

EXERCISE 16-5

Answer the following and assign codes to the following conditions using your ICD-9-CM code book.

1. The patient had a low transverse cesarean section due to the baby being large for dates ____________
2. The patient was induced as the baby was suspected to have spina bifida; she vaginally delivered a 5 lb baby boy ____________
3. Pregnant woman is admitted to the hospital with *Pneumocystis carinii* pneumonia and known AIDS; she is treated with high-dose antibiotics and is discharged ____________
4. The patient has been dependent on methadone for the entire pregnancy. She delivers a baby girl on this admit. She has no complications during delivery and has a normal spontaneous vaginal birth. ____________
5. The patient presents for delivery. She is a known type II diabetic, treated with *insulin* at the onset of pregnancy. She delivers a large for dates baby via cesarean section. ____________
6. Pregnant woman presents to doctor's office with complaints of blurred vision. Testing is done, and the diagnosis of gestational diabetes is made. ____________
7. Pregnant woman had pneumonia early in her pregnancy. She presents to the hospital in labor with no other complaints. She vaginally delivers a healthy baby. ____________
8. Can code 650 be used as a secondary diagnosis? ____________
9. What is the only outcome of delivery that can be used with 650? ____________
10. If surgery is performed in utero, is this coded on the baby's chart or on the mother's chart? ____________

Postpartum and Peripartum Periods

i. The Postpartum and Peripartum Periods

1) Postpartum and peripartum periods

The postpartum period begins immediately after delivery and continues for six weeks following delivery. The peripartum period is defined as the last month of pregnancy to five months postpartum.

EXAMPLE

Patient is admitted to hospital for mastitis. She is 5 weeks postpartum and is given a course of intravenous (IV) antibiotics, 675.24.

Mastitis would be a common postpartum complication.

EXAMPLE

Patient is admitted to the hospital 3 weeks postpartum. She is having pain in her leg and is given a diagnosis of deep vein thrombosis. The patient is treated with IV heparin, 671.44.

2) Postpartum complication

A postpartum complication is any complication occurring within the six-week period.

EXAMPLE

A patient is admitted to the hospital 4 weeks post partum with a high fever. The physician suspects endometritis. The patient is treated with IV antibiotics, 670.04, 615.9.

3) **Pregnancy-related complications after 6 week period**
Chapter 11 codes may also be used to describe pregnancy-related complications after the six-week period should the provider document that a condition is pregnancy related.

EXAMPLE

Patient is admitted to the hospital with postpartum cholecystitis. She delivered 12 weeks prior to this presentation, 647.84, 575.10.

In this case, the physician documented that this was a postpartum condition; therefore, it was coded as such even though it occurred beyond the 6-week time period.

4) **Postpartum complications occurring during the same admission as delivery**
Postpartum complications that occur during the same admission as the delivery are identified with a fifth digit of "2." Subsequent admissions/encounters for postpartum complications should be identified with a fifth digit of "4."

EXAMPLE

Patient was admitted in labor. She had an uneventful pregnancy and had a spontaneous vaginal delivery of a healthy baby girl. The patient developed fever and back pain after delivery, and it was determined that she had a UTI. She was started on antibiotics and was sent home, 646.62, 599.0, V27.0, 73.59.

5) **Admission for routine postpartum care following delivery outside hospital**
When the mother delivers outside the hospital prior to admission and is admitted for routine postpartum care and no complications are noted, code V24.0, Postpartum care and examination immediately after delivery, should be assigned as the principal diagnosis.

EXAMPLE

Patient delivers baby in the car on the way to the hospital. She is admitted through the ER for examination, V24.0.

6) **Admission following delivery outside hospital with postpartum conditions**
A delivery diagnosis code should not be used for a woman who has delivered prior to admission to the hospital. Any postpartum conditions and/or postpartum procedures should be coded.

EXAMPLE

A patient pregnant with her fourth child calls Emergency Medical Services (EMS) to inform them that she is home alone and is about to deliver. By the time EMS arrives, the woman has already delivered a healthy baby girl. She is transported to the hospital for postpartum care.

Upon arrival to the hospital, the patient is examined by the obstetrician, who manually removes the retained placenta and repairs the first-degree perineal laceration, 664.04, 666.24, 75.4, 75.69.

Late Effect of Complication of Pregnancy

j. **Code 677, Late effect of complication of pregnancy**

1) **Code 677**
Code 677, Late effect of complication of pregnancy, childbirth, and the puerperium is for use in those cases when an initial complication of a pregnancy develops a sequelae requiring care or treatment at a future date.

2) **After the initial postpartum period**
This code may be used at any time after the initial postpartum period.

3) **Sequencing of Code 677**
This code, like all late effect codes, is to be sequenced following the code describing the sequelae of the complications.

EXAMPLE

The patient presents to the physician's office complaining of painful intercourse. She is 6 months postpartum. The obstetrician determines that the patient is suffering from a late effect of the repair of the perineum, 625.0, 677, E8784.

EXERCISE 16-6

Answer the following questions and assign codes to the following conditions using your ICD-9-CM code book.

1. True or False. The late effect of complication of pregnancy code 677 should be sequenced first.
____
2. When can the late effect of complication of pregnancy code 677 start to be used?
____
3. How long does the postpartum period last?
____
4. A woman delivers a 5-lb baby in her home. She is brought by paramedics to the hospital, where they find that she has a first-degree perineal laceration. This is repaired, and the patient is admitted. _______________
5. A woman delivers in her car in the parking lot of the hospital. She is admitted for routine postpartum care. _______________
6. A woman is admitted 6 weeks after a cesarean delivery with infection of the cesarean wound. _______________
7. A woman delivered 5 weeks ago. She is admitted for an abscess of the breast. _______________
8. A patient presents with abdominal pain 3 months after the birth of her first baby. The physician documents that she has cholelithiasis that is related to her pregnancy. _______________
9. Two weeks after delivery, a woman has terrible pain in her leg. Her physician diagnoses her with a superficial thrombophlebitis of the leg. _______________
10. Five months after delivery of her first born, an obese woman is diagnosed with postpartum cardiomyopathy. _______________

Abortions

Abortion is the termination of a pregnancy by natural causes or by medical intervention.

Types of Abortion

Complete abortion is an abortion in which all the products of conception are expelled.
Elective Abortion is the elective termination of pregnancy.
Incomplete abortion is an abortion in which not all of the products of conception are expelled.
Inevitable abortion occurs when symptoms are present, and a miscarriage will happen.

Miscarriage is spontaneous termination of a pregnancy before the fetus has reached 20 weeks.

Missed abortion is a pregnancy with fetal demise before 20 weeks, when no products of conception are expelled.

Spontaneous abortion is the loss of a fetus due to natural causes; it is also known as a miscarriage.

Therapeutic abortion is an abortion performed when the pregnancy is endangering the mother's health, or when the fetus has a condition that is incompatible with life.

Threatened abortion occurs when symptoms are present that indicate that a miscarriage is possible.

k. Abortions

1) Fifth-digits required for abortion categories

Fifth-digits are required for abortion categories 634-637. Fifth-digit 1, incomplete, indicates that all the products of conception have not been expelled from the uterus. Fifth-digit 2, complete, indicates that all products of conception have been expelled from the uterus prior to the episode of care.

The fifth digit for categories 634-637 identifies the stage of the abortion; these are as follows:

- 0 unspecified
- 1 incomplete
- 2 complete

EXAMPLE

Patient presents to the hospital with known pregnancy. She is in her 11th week and is now complaining of severe back pain and vaginal bleeding. The physician examines the patient and determines that she has suffered an incomplete abortion. A dilation and curettage (D&C) is performed, and the patient is discharged, 634.91, 69.02.

EXAMPLE

Pregnant patient presents to the hospital with vaginal bleeding and abdominal cramps. She is evaluated in the ER and is found to have a UTI. It is also determined that she has suffered a complete miscarriage. The patient is monitored for several hours and is discharged on a course of antibiotics, 634.72, 599.0.

2) Code from categories 640-648 and 651-659

A code from categories 640-648 and 651-659 may be used as additional codes with an abortion code to indicate the complication leading to the abortion.

Fifth digit 3 is assigned with codes from these categories when used with an abortion code because the other fifth digits will not apply. Codes from 660-669 series are not to be used for complications of abortion.

EXAMPLE

Spontaneous abortion at 12 weeks, incomplete, in patient with gestational hypertension. D&C was performed, 634.91, 642.33, 69.02.

3) Code 639 for complications

Code 639 is to be used for all complications following abortion. Code 639 cannot be assigned with codes from categories 634-638.

EXAMPLE

Patient had a spontaneous abortion 2 weeks ago. She presents to the hospital with a high fever, hypotension, and chills. Sepsis is suspected and she is admitted, 639.8, 038.9, 995.91.

4) **Abortion with Liveborn Fetus**
When an attempted termination of pregnancy results in a liveborn fetus assign code 644.21, Early onset of delivery, with an appropriate code from category V27, Outcome of Delivery. The procedure code for attempted termination of pregnancy should also be assigned.

EXAMPLE

A woman is admitted for insertion of a laminaria for termination of pregnancy. She delivers a liveborn fetus, 644.21, V27.0, 69.93.

5) **Retained Products of Conception following an abortion**
Subsequent admissions for retained products of conception following a spontaneous or legally induced abortion are assigned the appropriate code from category 634, Spontaneous abortion, or 635 Legally induced abortion, with fifth digit of "1" (incomplete). This advice is appropriate even when the patient was discharged previously with a discharge diagnosis of complete abortion.

EXAMPLE

Retained products of conception after spontaneous abortion at 8 weeks' gestation. The products of conception were initially passed at home 2 days ago. D&C was performed, 634.91, 69.02.

EXERCISE 16-7

Assign codes to the following conditions using your ICD-9-CM code book.

1. Woman is admitted to the hospital after having a miscarriage. The physician performs a suction curettage to remove the products of conception. It is believed that the miscarriage occurred in association with placenta previa. ____________
2. Patient presents to the hospital for an elective abortion. After the abortion is performed by suction curettage, she spikes a high fever and is diagnosed with endometritis. ____________
3. Patient with missed abortion was admitted to the hospital for a therapeutic abortion by D&C. ____________
4. Patient presents to the hospital for an elective abortion because the fetus is hydrocephalic. An aspiration curettage is performed. ____________
5. Patient presents to the hospital with hemorrhage after a self-induced abortion. Physician performs a D&C to control hemorrhage. Products of conception completely aborted prior to admission. ____________

V CODES

In the past, V codes have been considered for use primarily in the outpatient setting. This has changed with the addition of more V codes each year. As was discussed in Chapter 8, it is difficult to locate V codes in the Index. Coders will often say, "I did not know there was a V code for that."

Refer to Chapter 8 for a listing of common main terms to used locate V codes. V codes that may be used during pregnancy, childbirth, and the puerperium include the following:

V02.51	Carrier or suspected carrier of Group B streptococcus
V22.0	Supervision of normal first pregnancy
V22.1	Supervision of other normal pregnancy
V22.2	Pregnant state, incidental
V23.0	Pregnancy with history of infertility
V23.1	Pregnancy with history of trophoblastic disease
V23.2	Pregnancy with history of abortion
V23.3	Grand multiparity
V23.41	Pregnancy with history of preterm labor
V23.49	Pregnancy with other poor obstetric history
V23.5	Pregnancy with other poor reproductive history
V23.7	Insufficient prenatal care
V23.81	Elderly primigravida
V23.82	Elderly multigravida
V23.83	Young primigravida
V23.84	Young multigravida
V23.89	Other high-risk pregnancy
V23.9	Unspecified high-risk pregnancy
V24.0	Postpartum care and examination immediately after delivery
V24.1	Postpartum care and examination of lactating mother
V24.2	Routine postpartum follow-up
V25.04	Counseling and instruction in natural family planning to avoid pregnancy
V25.2	Admission for sterilization
V26.21	Fertility Testing
V26.41	Procreative counseling and advice using natural family planning
V26.49	Other procreative management, counseling and advice
V26.81	Encounter for assisted reproductive fertility procedure
V26.89	Other specified procreative management
V27.0	Single liveborn
V27.1	Single stillborn
V27.2	Twins
V27.3	Twins, one liveborn and one stillborn
V27.4	Twins, both stillborn
V27.5	Other multiple birth, all liveborn
V27.6	Other multiple birth, some liveborn
V27.7	Other multiple birth, all stillborn
V27.9	Unspecified outcome of delivery
V28.0	Encounter for screening for chromosomal anomalies by amniocentesis
V28.1	Encounter for screening for raised alpha-fetoprotein levels in amniotic fluid
V28.2	Encounter for other screening based on amniocentesis
V28.3	Encounter for screening for malformation using ultrasonics
V28.4	Encounter for screening for fetal growth retardation using ultrasonics

V28.5	Encounter for screening for isoimmunization
V28.6	Encounter for screening for Streptococcus B
V28.8	Encounter for other specified antenatal screening
V28.9	Encounter for unspecified antenatal screening
V45.51	Presence of intrauterine contraceptive device
V45.52	Presence of subdermal contraceptive implant
V45.59	Presence of other contraceptive device
V72.40	Pregnancy examination or test, pregnancy unconfirmed
V72.41	Pregnancy examination or test, negative result
V72.42	Pregnancy examination or test, positive result
V89.01	Suspected problems with amniotic cavity and membrane not found
V89.02	Suspected placental problems not found
V89.03	Suspected fetal anomaly not found
V89.04	Suspected problem with fetal growth not found
V89.05	Suspected cervical shortening not found
V89.09	Other suspected maternal and fetal condition not found

COMMON TREATMENTS

CONDITION	MEDICATION/TREATMENT
Narcotics for Labor Pain	Stadol (butorphanol), fentanyl Demerol (meperidine) Nubain (nalbuphine) Used for decreasing pain
Anesthesia for Labor Pain	Epidural is a regional anesthetic injected into the epidural space Spinal is also a regional anesthetic which is injected into the cerebrospinal fluid
Drugs for Inducing Labor	Pitocin which is a synthetic oxytocin which is a natural hormone produced by a woman's body to cause the uterus to contract Cervidil (dinoprostone) is vaginally inserted and used for ripening of the cervix
Drugs used to Inhibit Labor	Beta agonists (terbutaline, ritodrine, isoxsuprine), magnesium sulfate

PROCEDURES

Procedures that may be related to pregnancy and childbirth may be located in the following chapter of the Procedure Tabular:

Chapter 13 Obstetrical Procedures (72-75)

Induction of Labor

Labor can be induced in a variety of ways. Often, artifical rupture of the membranes is performed to start labor. Pitocin induction may also be used. Pitocin is a drug used for medical induction of labor.

A nonstress test (NST) is performed to confirm the health of the baby. A mother is hooked up to a fetal monitor and the test is performed without giving the mother medications. The test records the baby's heart rate while moving. This test may be performed throughout the pregnancy the mother has medical conditions, or if the pregnancy is considered high risk. Results of these tests are recorded as "reactive," meaning the baby moved and the heart rate increased appropriately, or "nonreactive," which means that either the baby did not move or the heart rate did not increase enough when the baby did move.

When the NST is abnormal, another test is performed. This test is called a CST, or a contraction stress test. In this test, which is done during fetal monitoring, a drug (Pitocin)

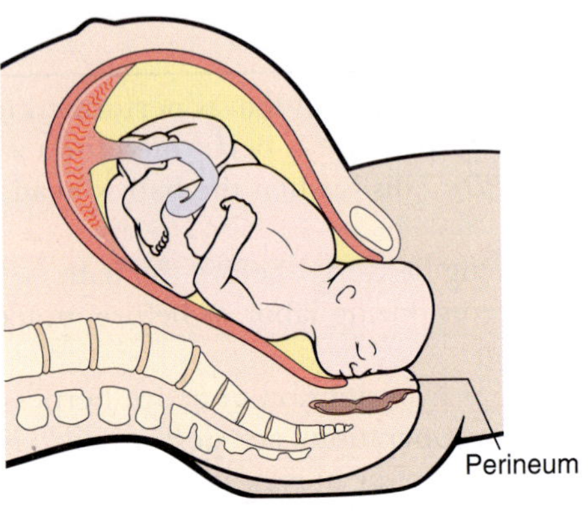

Figure 16-9. Cephalic presentation ("crowning") of the fetus during delivery from the vaginal (birth) canal during a normal delivery.

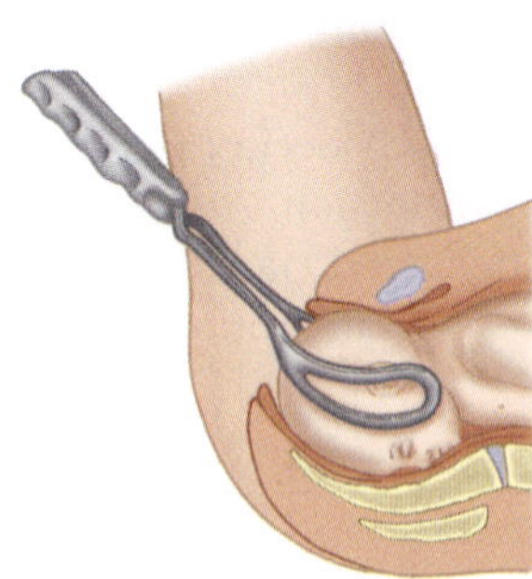

Figure 16-10. Forceps delivery.

may be administered to initiate contractions. The purpose is to see how the baby will handle the stress of labor. The baby's heart should speed up during a contraction; if this does not happen during this test, problems may occur during labor.

Amnioinfusion is the insertion of normal saline or lactated Ringer's solution into the amniotic sac. The injection may be done transabdominally or transcervically. This procedure is performed for a variety of reasons, such as oligohydramnios, variable decelerations, and thick meconium. The volume of amniotic fluid is increased, which increases the likelihood of better outcomes of delivery.

Delivery

In a normal pregnancy with no complications, a code of 73.59 may be assigned for manually assisted delivery (Figure 16-9). This code should not be assigned if any other procedures were performed to assist in delivery. Forceps and vacuum extraction may be used in cases in which the baby does not spontaneously deliver and assistance is needed (Figure 16-10).

Episiotomy is performed to facilitate delivery. The physician makes a cut in the perineum to make room for the baby's head to emerge. Repair of an episiotomy is included in the code for episiotomy. If a forceps delivery and an episiotomy are performed, a combination code may be used; a combination code may also be used for a vacuum extraction and an episiotomy. Sometimes, an episiotomy will extend and will become a laceration. If this happens, no code is assigned for the episiotomy—only for the laceration repair.

Repair of Obstetrical Lacerations

The degree of perineal laceration is coded under the diagnostic category of 664.0X-664.3X. If more than one degree is mentioned, only the highest degree should be assigned. If an episiotomy extends spontaneously, it is then assigned a laceration code. *Coding Clinic* (2007:4Q:p125)[2] advises the coder to assign code 664.81 for a periurethral laceration and code 75.69 for the repair.

Cesarean Section

A cesarean section (C-section) is an operation that is performed to deliver a baby through an incision in the abdomen. This procedure is performed for a variety of reasons:

- *Cephalopelvic disproportion (CPD):* This is when the baby's head is too large to fit through the birth canal.
- *Prolapsed cord:* The cord is being delivered before the baby
- *Fetal distress:* Distress of the fetus during labor or before, noted by low oxygen levels or the presence of meconium
- *Conditions of the mother:* Such as hypertension or active herpes

Three main types of cesarean operations are performed: (1) *low transverse,* which is done via a horizontal incision in the lower uterus; (2) *low vertical,* which is done via a vertical incision in the lower uterus; and (3) *classical,* which involves a vertical incision in the main body of the uterus. The most commonly performed type is the low transverse (LTCS).

Vaginal birth after cesarean section (VBAC) occurs when a woman delivers vaginally after having delivered previously via cesarean section. At one point in time, it was believed that it was unsafe for a woman who had delivered via C-section to deliver vaginally. Many variables go into deciding whether a VBAC is a safe option; however, it is being performed more and more frequently.

EXERCISE 16-8

Assign codes for all diagnoses and procedures.

1. Patient is induced by pitocin for postdate pregnancy (41 weeks). She delivers a 6 lb 4 oz baby vaginally. ____________
2. Elderly multigravida presents in labor. After 20 hours of labor, an LTCS is performed because of failure to progress. She delivers a normal newborn. ____________
3. A 22-year-old primigravida presents for induction. She is known to have oligohydramnios. Pitocin is administered, and she goes on to vaginally deliver an SGA normal newborn. The physician performs an episiotomy to facilitate delivery, and a second-degree extension is repaired. ____________
4. Patient presents in active labor. She is in her 38th week of pregnancy. She labors for 8 hours, after which the physician decides to perform a C-section because of CPD. A normal newborn is delivered. ____________
5. Patient presents with severe preeclampsia. She is taken directly to the operating room, where an LTCS is performed. She delivers a normal newborn. ____________

DOCUMENTATION/REIMBURSEMENT/MS-DRGs

Often, coding difficulties are due to lack of documentation. Sometimes pathology and other test results are not available at the time of discharge or when the physician is dictating the discharge summary or is reporting the final diagnoses.

The most common MS-DRGs for deliveries include the following:

MS-DRG	RW
766 C-Section without CC/MCC	0.7664
765 C-Section with CC/MCC	0.9943
775 Vaginal Delivery without complicating dx	0.4461
774 Vaginal Delivery with complicating dx	0.5914

CHAPTER REVIEW EXERCISE

Assign codes for all diagnoses and procedures.

1. Breech presentation with obstructed labor; delivery by cesarean section (LTCS); single liveborn ______________
2. Patient admitted 2 weeks post delivery with postpartum depression ______________
3. Patient delivers 12-lb baby (LGA), requiring an episiotomy ______________
4. Patient is admitted to the hospital for delivery; she is being treated with methadone for heroin dependence; vaginal delivery of single liveborn ______________
5. Patient with a history of preterm labor and previous cesarean section is admitted in labor; she has a vaginal birth after cesarean (VBAC) of single liveborn ______________
6. Patient is admitted to hospital for HELLP (**h**emolytic anemia, **e**levated **l**iver enzymes, and low **p**latelet count) syndrome; she is taken to the operating room for delivery by cesarean section (LTCS) of single liveborn ______________
7. Patient is admitted to the hospital in preterm labor; she is 35 weeks pregnant; three days after admission, the patient vaginally delivers a small for gestational age (SGA) baby ______________
8. Patient presents to physician's office for a routine obstetric visit; she had a spontaneous abortion 1 year ago ______________
9. Patient is admitted to the hospital at 33 weeks; she has a twin pregnancy and has a spontaneous vaginal delivery (SVD) of liveborn twins; the evening after delivery, she hemorrhages ______________
10. Patient is pregnant and has known uterine fibroids; the fibroids are so large that the physician recommends an abortion; patient presents to hospital for abortion to be performed by aspiration curettage ______________
11. The patient was treated for a sprained wrist. Incidentally, the patient is 10 weeks pregnant. ______________
12. Urinary tract infection in patient who delivered 1 week ago. ______________
13. This mother delivered liveborn twins vaginally during her hospital stay. The outcome of delivery is coded on the mother's record. ______________
14. The patient was admitted for treatment of hyperemesis gravidarum. The patient is 12 weeks pregnant. ______________
15. The patient has a high-risk pregnancy and two previous miscarriages. ______________
16. The patient is 16 weeks pregnant, and her condition is complicated by diabetes mellitus, type 2, which is uncontrolled. ______________
17. The patient is admitted with HIV and *Pneumocystis carinii* pneumonia (PCP) and is 35 weeks pregnant. ______________
18. The patient is 19 weeks pregnant and has hypothyroidism. ______________
19. The patient delivered a baby 6 days ago. She is now being admitted because of dehiscence of her cesarean wound. The wound was sutured. ______________
20. Urinary tract infection in a patient who is 30 weeks pregnant. ______________

CHAPTER GLOSSARY

Abortion: termination of a pregnancy by natural causes or by medical intervention.

Amnioinfusion: the insertion of normal saline or lactated Ringer's solution into the amniotic sac.

Antepartum: time from conception until delivery or childbirth with regard to the mother.

Cervix: the neck of the uterus that serves as an outlet from the uterus.

Complete abortion: abortion in which all the products of conception are expelled.

Eclampsia: complication of pregnancy characterized by hypertension, edema, proteinuria, and convulsions or seizures.

Ectopic: type of pregnancy that occurs when the egg is implanted outside the cavity of the uterus.

Elderly obstetric patient: 35 years or older at date of delivery.

Elective abortion: the elective termination of pregnancy.

Endometritis: inflammation of the uterus.

Fallopian tube: delivers the mature egg to the uterus for fertilization.

Gravid: pregnant.

Hyperemesis gravidarum: excessive vomiting in pregnancy.

Incomplete abortion: abortion in which not all of the products of conception are expelled.

Inevitable abortion: abortion that occurs when symptoms are present and a miscarriage will happen.

Labia: surrounds the vaginal opening.

Labor: process by which the products of conception are expelled from the uterus.

Lactation: process of milk production.

Miscarriage: spontaneous termination of pregnancy before the fetus has reached 20 weeks.

Missed abortion: pregnancy with fetal demise before 20 weeks; products of conception are not expelled.

Molar pregnancy: fertilized ovum is converted to a mole.

Multigravida: a woman with two or more pregnancies.

Multiparity: a woman with two or more pregnancies.

Ovaries: produce female hormones and eggs.

Postpartum: after delivery or childbirth.

Postterm pregnancy: pregnancy longer than 40 weeks up to 42 weeks.

Precipitate labor: rapid labor and delivery.

Preeclampsia: pregnancy complication characterized by hypertension, edema, and/or proteinuria.

Prenatal: before birth.

Primigravida: first pregnancy.

Prolonged pregnancy: beyond 42 weeks of pregnancy.

Puerperium: time from delivery through the first 6 weeks postpartum.

Spontaneous abortion: loss of a fetus due to natural causes; also known as miscarriage.

Stillbirth: born dead.

Therapeutic abortion: abortion performed when the pregnancy is endangering the mother's health, or when the fetus has a condition that is incompatible with life.

Threatened abortion: abortion that occurs when symptoms are present that indicate the possibility of a miscarriage.

Uterus: a muscular organ that serves as an incubator for the developing fetus.

Vagina: a muscular tube that extends from the vaginal opening to the uterus.

Vulva: the external covering to the vagina.

Young obstetric patient: younger than 16 years at date of delivery.

CHAPTER 17

Congenital Anomalies and Perinatal Conditions

(ICD-9-CM Chapter 14, Codes 740-759, and ICD-9-CM Chapter 15, Codes 760-779)

CHAPTER OUTLINE

LEARNING OBJECTIVES

- Apply and assign the correct ICD-9-CM codes in accordance with Official Guidelines for Coding and Reporting
- Identify congenital anomalies and perinatal conditions
- Assign the correct V codes and procedure codes to congenital anomalies and perinatal conditions
- Identify common treatments, medications, laboratory values, and diagnostic tests
- Explain the importance of documentation as it relates to MS-DRGs for reimbursement

ABBREVIATIONS

AGA appropriate for gestational age

BPD bronchopulmonary dysplasia

CHD congenital heart disease

ICD-9-CM *International Classification of Diseases, 9th edition, Clinical Modification*

IUGR intrauterine growth retardation

LGA large for gestational age

MSAFP maternal serum alpha-fetoprotein

MS-DRG Medicare severity diagnosis-related group

NICU neonatal intensive care unit

PDA patent ductus arteriosus

PKU phenylketonuria

PPH primary pulmonary hypertension

RDS respiratory distress syndrome

SGA small for gestational age

TOF tetralogy of Fallot

TTN transitory tachypnea of the newborn

VSD ventricular septal defect

ICD-9-CM Official Guidelines for Coding and Reporting

Please refer to the companion Evolve website for the most current guidelines.

14. Chapter 14: Congenital Anomalies (740-759)

a. Codes in categories 740-759, Congenital Anomalies

Assign an appropriate code(s) from categories 740-759, Congenital Anomalies, when an anomaly is documented. A congenital anomaly may be the principal/first listed diagnosis on a record or a secondary diagnosis.

When a congenital anomaly does not have a unique code assignment, assign additional code(s) for any manifestations that may be present.

When the code assignment specifically identifies the congenital anomaly, manifestations that are an inherent component of the anomaly should not be coded separately. Additional codes should be assigned for manifestations that are not an inherent component.

Codes from Chapter 14 may be used throughout the life of the patient. If a congenital anomaly has been corrected, a personal history code should be used to identify the history of the anomaly. Although present at birth, a congenital anomaly may not be identified until later in life. Whenever the condition is diagnosed by the physician, it is appropriate to assign a code from codes 740-759.

For the birth admission, the appropriate code from category V30, Liveborn infants, according to type of birth should be sequenced as the principal diagnosis, followed by any congenital anomaly codes, 740-759.

EXAMPLE

Patient is a 30-year-old male with a bicuspid aortic valve, 746.4.

EXAMPLE

Infant was delivered by vaginal delivery and examination shows hypospadias, V30.00, 752.61.

15. Chapter 15: Newborn (Perinatal) Guidelines (760-779)

For coding and reporting purposes the perinatal period is defined as **before** birth through the 28th day following birth. The following guidelines are provided for reporting purposes. Hospitals may record other diagnoses as needed for internal data use.

a. General Perinatal Rules

1) Chapter 15 Codes

They are <u>never</u> for use on the maternal record. Codes from Chapter 11, the obstetric chapter, are never permitted on the newborn record. Chapter 15 code may be used throughout the life of the patient if the condition is still present.

2) Sequencing of perinatal codes

Generally, codes from Chapter 15 should be sequenced as the principal/first-listed diagnosis on the newborn record, with the exception of the appropriate V30 code for the birth episode, followed by codes from any other chapter that provide additional detail. The "use additional code" note at the beginning of the chapter supports this guideline. If the index does not provide a specific code for a perinatal condition, assign code 779.89, Other specified conditions originating in the perinatal period, followed by the code from another chapter that specifies the condition. Codes for signs and symptoms may be assigned when a definitive diagnosis has not been established.

EXAMPLE

An infant was delivered in the hospital via cesarean section. On discharge, the infant was examined and appeared completely healthy with the exception of neonatal jaundice. A bilirubin count should be performed in 2 days, V30.01, 774.6.

3) Birth process or community acquired conditions

If a newborn has a condition that may be either due to the birth process or community acquired and the documentation does not indicate which it is, the default is due to the birth process and the code from Chapter 15 should be used.

If the condition is community-acquired, a code from Chapter 15 should not be assigned.

4) Code all clinically significant conditions

All clinically significant conditions noted on routine newborn examination should be coded. A condition is clinically significant if it requires:

- clinical evaluation; or
- therapeutic treatment; or
- diagnostic procedures; or
- extended length of hospital stay; or
- increased nursing care and/or monitoring; or
- has implications for future health care needs

Note: The perinatal guidelines listed above are the same as the general coding guidelines for "additional diagnoses", except for the final point regarding implications for future health care needs. Codes should be assigned for conditions that have been specified by the provider as having implications for future health care needs. Codes from the perinatal chapter should not be assigned unless the provider has established a definitive diagnosis.

b. Use of codes V30-V39

When coding the birth of an infant, assign a code from categories V30-V39, according to the type of birth. A code from this series is assigned as a principal diagnosis, and assigned only once to a newborn at the time of birth.

EXAMPLE

The infant was born via vaginal delivery and suffered a fractured clavicle caused by the delivery, V30.00, 767.2.

c. Newborn transfers

If the newborn is transferred to another institution, the V30 series is not used at the receiving hospital.

EXAMPLE

The infant was born via cesarean section at Hospital Anytown and was transferred to Hospital Everytown for treatment in the NICU for hyaline membrane disease.
Hospital Anytown, V30.01, 769.
Hospital Everytown, 769.

d. Use of category V29

1) Assigning a code from category V29

Assign a code from category V29, Observation and evaluation of newborns and infants for suspected conditions not found, to identify those instances when a healthy newborn is evaluated for a suspected condition that is determined after study not to be present. Do not use a code from category V29 when the patient has identified signs or symptoms of a suspected problem; in such cases, code the sign or symptom.

A code from category V29 may also be assigned as a principal code for readmissions or encounters when the V30 code no longer applies. Codes from category V29 are for use only for healthy newborns and infants for which no condition after study is found to be present.

2) V29 code on a birth record

A V29 code is to be used as a secondary code after the V30, Outcome of delivery, code.

EXAMPLE

A male infant was delivered vaginally and was observed for a spontaneous pneumothorax. Chest x-ray was negative, V30.00, V29.2.

e. Use of other V codes on perinatal records
V codes other than V30 and V29 may be assigned on a perinatal or newborn record. The codes may be used as a principal or first-listed diagnosis for specific types of encounters or for readmissions or encounters when the V30 code no longer applies.
See Section 1.C.18 for information regarding the assignment of V codes.

EXAMPLE

This 10-day-old infant was admitted to rule out sepsis, V29.0.

f. Maternal Causes of Perinatal Morbidity
Codes from categories 760-763, Maternal causes of perinatal morbidity and mortality, are assigned only when the maternal condition has actually affected the fetus or newborn. The fact that the mother has an associated medical condition or experiences some complication of pregnancy, labor or delivery does not justify the routine assignment of codes from these categories to the newborn record.

EXAMPLE

A baby tested positive for cocaine. The mother had used cocaine on the day prior to vaginal delivery, V30.00, 760.75.

g. Congenital Anomalies in Newborns
For the birth admission, the appropriate code from category V30, Liveborn infants according to type of birth, should be used, followed by any congenital anomaly codes, categories 740-759. Use additional secondary codes from other chapters to specify conditions associated with the anomaly, if applicable.
Also, see Section 1.C.14 for information on the coding of congenital anomalies.

EXAMPLE

A female twin infant was delivered via cesarean section with congenital left hip dislocation. The twin male infant was stillborn, V32.01, 754.30.

h. Coding Additional Perinatal Diagnoses

1) Assigning codes for conditions that require treatment
Assign codes for conditions that require treatment or further investigation, prolong the length of stay, or require resource utilization.

EXAMPLE

Gestational diabetes resulting in hypoglycemia of a newborn female infant born in the parking lot via vaginal delivery, V30.10, 775.0.

2) Codes for conditions specified as having implications for future health care needs
Assign codes for conditions that have been specified by the provider as having implications for future health care needs.
Note: This guideline should not be used for adult patients.

EXAMPLE

A male infant was born via vaginal delivery. The clinician will evaluate and review treatment options for his undescended testis at the 6-week appointment, V30.00, 752.51.

3) **Codes for newborn conditions originating in the perinatal period**
Assign a code for newborn conditions originating in the perinatal period (categories 760-779), as well as complications arising during the current episode of care classified in other chapters, only if the diagnoses have been documented by the responsible provider at the time of transfer or discharge as having affected the fetus or newborn.

i. **Prematurity and Fetal Growth Retardation**
Providers utilize different criteria in determining prematurity. A code for prematurity should not be assigned unless it is documented. The 5th digit assignment for codes from category 764 and subcategories 765.0 and 765.1 should be based on the recorded birth weight and estimated gestational age.

A code from subcategory 765.2, Weeks of gestation, should be assigned as an additional code with category 764 and codes from 765.0 and 765.1 to specify weeks of gestation as documented by the provider in the record.

EXAMPLE

A premature infant was born in the hospital via vaginal delivery. The infant weighed 4 pounds and was 33 weeks gestational age, V30.00, 765.17, 765.27.

j. **Newborn sepsis**
Code 771.81, Septicemia [sepsis] of newborn, should be assigned with a secondary code from category 041, Bacterial infections in conditions classified elsewhere and of unspecified site, to identify the organism. It is not necessary to use a code from subcategory 995.9, Systemic inflammatory response syndrome (SIRS), on a newborn record. A code from category 038, Septicemia, should not be used on a newborn record. Code 771.81 describes the sepsis.

Apply all other General Coding Guidelines as found in Chapter 5.

EXERCISE 17-1

Answer the questions and assign codes to the following conditions using your ICD-9-CM code book.

1. A congenital anomaly is always listed second on a newborn record.
   A. True
   B. False
2. A congenital anomaly code can be assigned to an adult record.
   A. True
   B. False
3. Codes from Chapter 11 can be used on the newborn record.
   A. True
   B. False
4. Chapter 15 codes can be used anytime throughout the life of the patient.
   A. True
   B. False
5. Code 762.7 belongs on the mother's record.
   A. True
   B. False
6. If a newborn has a condition that has implications for future health care needs, that condition may be coded. The same is true for the adult population?
   A. True
   B. False

7. When a newborn is transferred to another hospital, the principal diagnosis should be a code from the V30 series.
   A. True
   B. False
8. V29 can be assigned as a principal diagnosis.
   A. True
   B. False
9. A coder should assign a code for prematurity on the basis of weeks and/or weight in grams.
   A. True
   B. False
10. If the mother of a newborn has hypertension, code 760.0 is assigned.
    A. True
    B. False
11. When the code 775.5 is used and the baby is dehydrated, would it also be appropriate to use code 276.51? ______________
12. If it is not clearly documented on the infant's chart whether a condition is community acquired or is due to the birth process, which is the default? ______________
13. What makes a condition clinically significant?
    ____
14. What category of codes is used as the principal diagnosis for newborns? ______________
15. If the index does not provide a specific code for a perinatal condition, which code should be assigned? ______________
16. When a baby is born extremely prematurely at 25 weeks' gestation and has a birth weight of 950 grams, what code or codes are assigned? ______________
17. When a newborn has a diagnosis of sepsis, what code or codes are assigned? ______________
18. What is the definition of "congenital"?
    ____
19. The principal diagnosis code for a single newborn who is delivered by a Cesarean section is? ______________
20. How long does the perinatal period last? ______________

DISEASE CONDITIONS

Congenital Anomalies (740-759)

A **congenital anomaly** is a condition that is present at birth. Sometimes, conditions that a person is born with do not appear until later in life. Some conditions are congenital by definition, such as Meckel's diverticulum. This condition is present at birth but may not manifest until later in life. Congenital anomalies may be located in the Alphabetic Index under the specific condition or anomaly and/or deformity.

Spina bifida is a disorder that involves incomplete development of the brain, spinal cord, and/or their protective coverings (Figure 17-1). It occurs in 1 in every 2000 births in the United States. Pregnant women can be tested with a blood test called MSAFP (maternal serum alpha-fetoprotein) to screen for spina bifida. This disorder occurs during the first month of pregnancy and is caused by the spine of the fetus not closing properly. This results

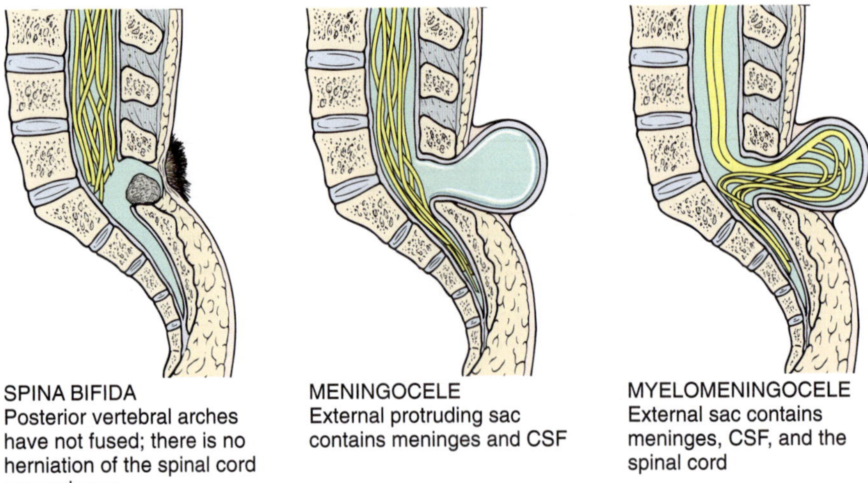

Figure 17-1. Congenital spinal cord defects.

in permanent nerve damage to various degrees, even though the opening can be closed in utero or after birth. Three types of spina bifida have been identified: (1) myelomeningocele, which is the most severe form; the spinal cord and the meninges protrude from the opening in the spine; (2) meningocele, which is the most rare form; the spinal cord is normally developed, but the meninges protrudes through the opening; and (3) occulta, which is the mildest form; one or more vertebrae are malformed; this type usually involves no treatment.

Children with spina bifida often have bowel and bladder complications and hydrocephalus (Figure 17-2). Spina bifida has no cure because nerve tissue cannot be repaired. Treatment is rendered according to the severity of the condition. Children born with spina bifida are usually treated through surgery that is performed to close the opening within 24 hours of birth. If a child is born with the most severe type, he or she often has **hydrocephalus**; this is treated by inserting a **ventricular shunt** into the brain to drain accumulating fluid (Figure 17-3). Another complication of a severe case of spina bifida is a tethered spinal cord. A tethered spinal cord is a cord that does not move up and down during movement, as it is designed to do. If a child has severe pain, surgery may be performed to untether the spinal cord.

Some children are born with syndromes that manifest with a series of anomalies. If the syndrome is not specifically indexed in ICD-9-CM then a code should be assigned for each presenting manifestation of the syndrome, as well as 759.89.

EXAMPLE

A child with Cockayne's Syndrome is seen by a physician who documents that the patient has mental retardation, retinal atrophy and small head, 759.89, 319, 362.60, 742.1.

EXAMPLE

Baby born by cesarean section is found to have spina bifida with hydrocephalus, V30.01, 741.00.

Tetralogy of Fallot

Tetralogy of Fallot (Figure 17-4) is a congenital heart defect that manifests with four key features: (1) a hole between the ventricles (ventral septal defect [VSD]); (2) pulmonary stenosis; (3) aorta lying directly over the hole; and (4) thick, muscled right ventricle (**hypertrophy**). Treatment recommended for this condition is surgery. Often, surgery requires two stages. The first stage occurs when the infant is first born; a little later, after growth has occurred, the second stage is performed. Patients who have undergone repair

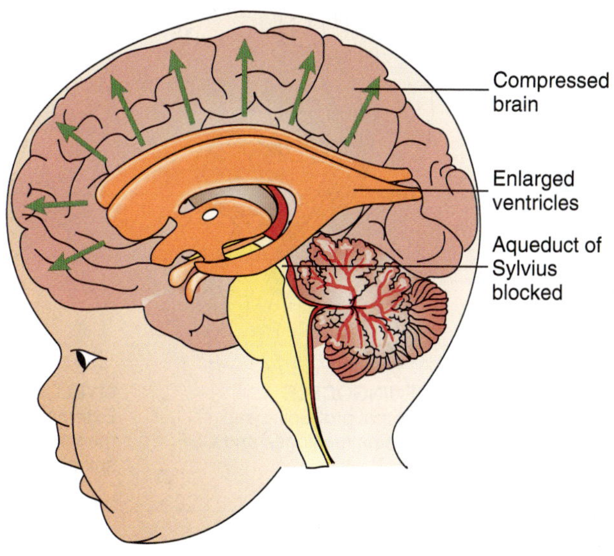

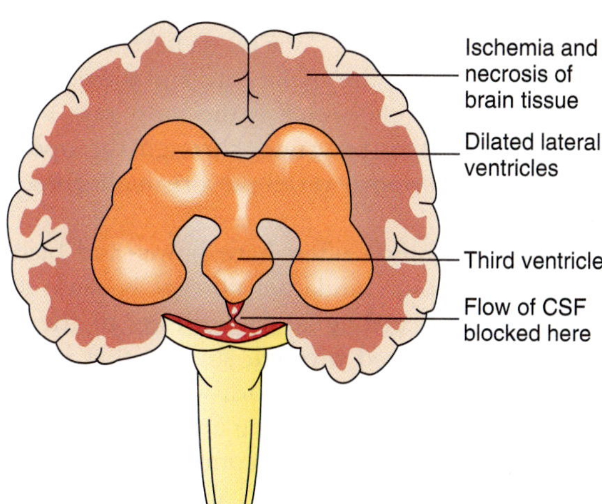

Figure 17-2. Hydrocephalus.

often are at greater risk for arrhythmia; sometimes, additional surgery is required later in life. The operation performed to treat this condition is called the **Blalock-Taussig** procedure.

EXAMPLE

VSD is diagnosed in a baby, along with pulmonary stenosis and hypertrophy of the right ventricle, as well as dextroposition of the aorta. The baby is seen by a surgeon for repair, 745.2, 35.81.

Cleft Lip and Cleft Palate

Three different types of clefts can occur on one or both sides of the mouth:

1. Cleft lip without a cleft palate (Figure 17-5)
2. Cleft palate without a cleft lip
3. Cleft lip and cleft palate together

Approximately 1 in 600 babies is born with a cleft. Surgery is performed to repair the cleft; often, surgery is completed in several stages. The first surgery is usually done when a baby is 10 weeks of age or older and weighs at least 10 pounds. The cleft lip/palate diagnosis

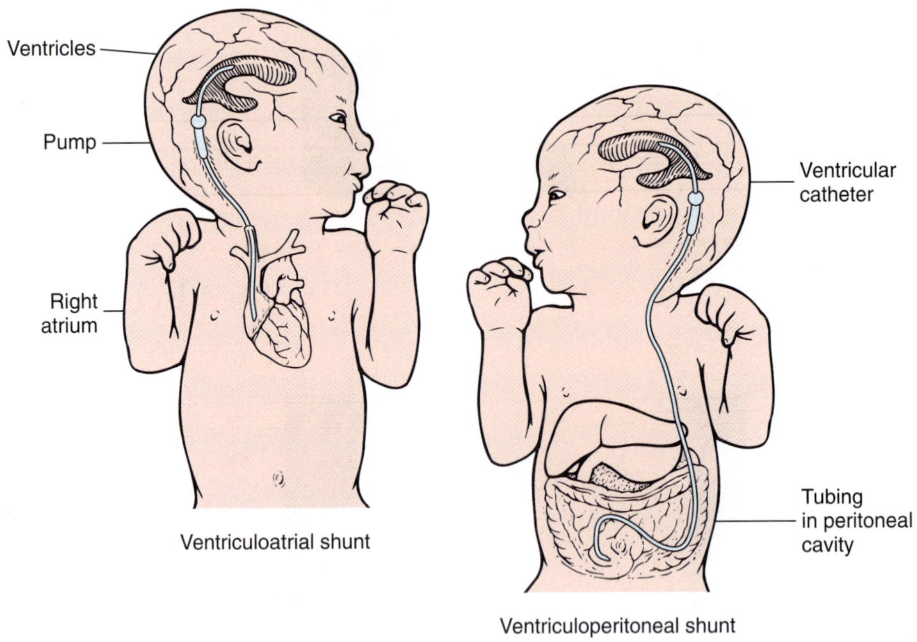

Figure 17-3. Shunting procedures for hydrocephalus. Ventriculoperitoneal shunt is the preferred procedure.

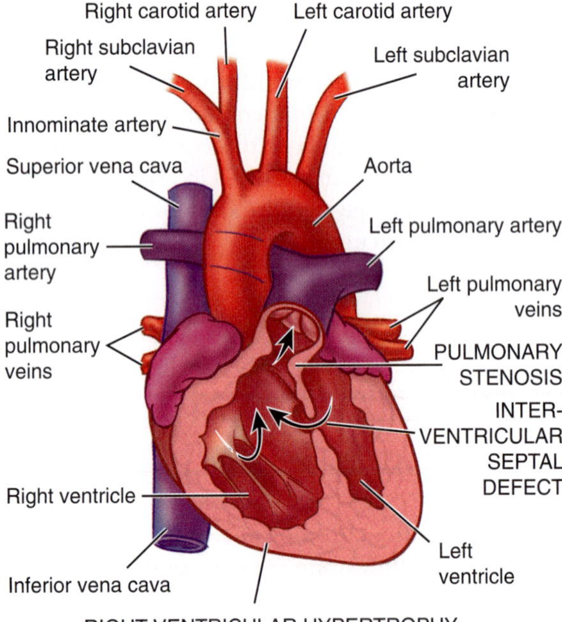

Figure 17-4. Tetralogy of Fallot.

code may be assigned as many times as surgery is performed to correct this defect, per *Coding Clinic* (1996:1Q:p14).[1]

EXAMPLE

The child was admitted for repair of cleft lip and palate, bilateral, incomplete, 749.24, 27.62, 27.54.

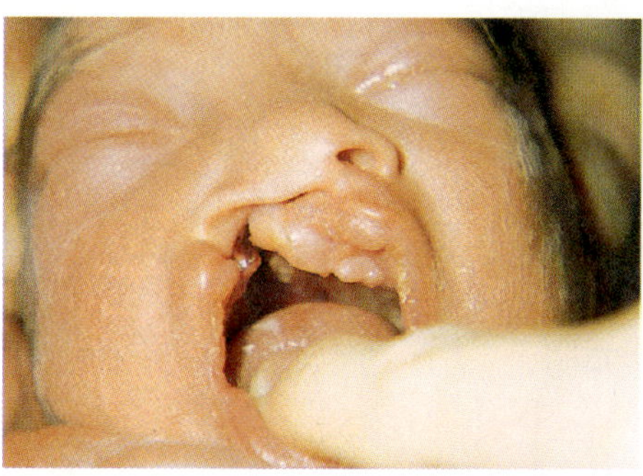

Figure 17-5. Unilateral cleft lip.

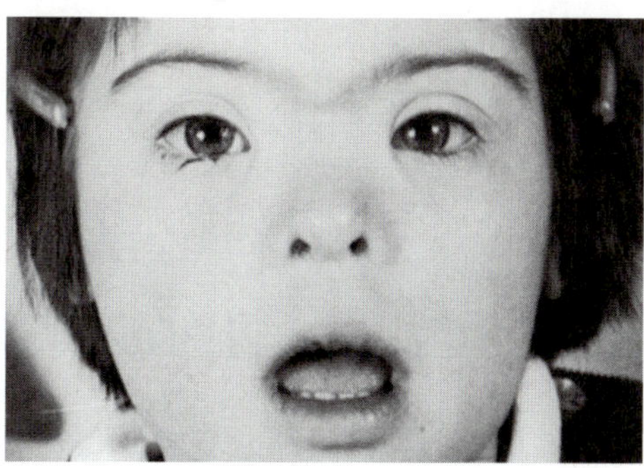

Figure 17-6. Photograph of 31/2-year-old girl with typical facial appearance of Down's syndrome.

Meckel's Diverticulum

Meckel's diverticulum occurs during the fifth week of fetal development. This is a small pouch on the wall of the small bowel that contains ectopic tissue. It occurs in about 2% of the population, and most people who have this condition have no problems. Complications of Meckel's diverticulum include hematochezia in children and obstruction or diverticulitis in adults. Treatment varies but may require only observation and treatment of symptoms or surgery to remove the diverticulum.

EXAMPLE

A 60-year-old woman presents to the hospital with severe abdominal pain. A scan is performed, and Meckel's diverticulum is discovered. The surgeon is called in and performs an ileal resection, 751.0, 45.62.

Chromosomal Anomalies

One in 200 babies is born with a chromosomal abnormality. Each egg and sperm cell contains 23 chromosomes. When they unite, 23 pairs or 46 chromosomes are created. If a baby is born with too many, too few, or broken or rearranged chromosomes, birth defects may occur. A chromosomal abnormality with three instead of two of a specific chromosome is called a **trisomy**. In most cases, when this occurs, the pregnancy ends in a miscarriage.

Down's syndrome (Figure 17-6), the most common chromosomal abnormality, is also known as trisomy 21. Babies with Down's syndrome have an extra chromosome 21. Children with Down's syndrome can have a combination of birth defects. Some of these are characteristic facial features, mental retardation, and heart defects. No cure is known for Down's syndrome; however, the older the mother is, the greater is the risk; research suggests that folic acid can help to prevent this condition. Physicians can test for this condition during pregnancy with a test called chorionic villus sampling (CVS). A tiny sample of tissue is taken from the placenta of the mother for this test, which is performed transcervically or transvaginally. CVS can also be used to test for other disorders.

EXAMPLE Patient with Down's syndrome, 758.0.

Klinefelter's syndrome is a sex chromosome disorder, which occurs only in males, the individual has an extra X chromosome. Most commonly, the child is born with 47 chromosomes in each cell, rather than 46. Symptoms of this condition generally do not appear until puberty. Individuals have low levels of testosterone and small testicles and may exhibit behavior problems.

EXAMPLE Patient diagnosed with Klinefelter's syndrome, 758.7.

Marfan's Syndrome

Marfan's syndrome (Figure 17-7), which is caused by a gene mutation, is an inherited condition that affects the connective tissue. Because connective tissue is found throughout the

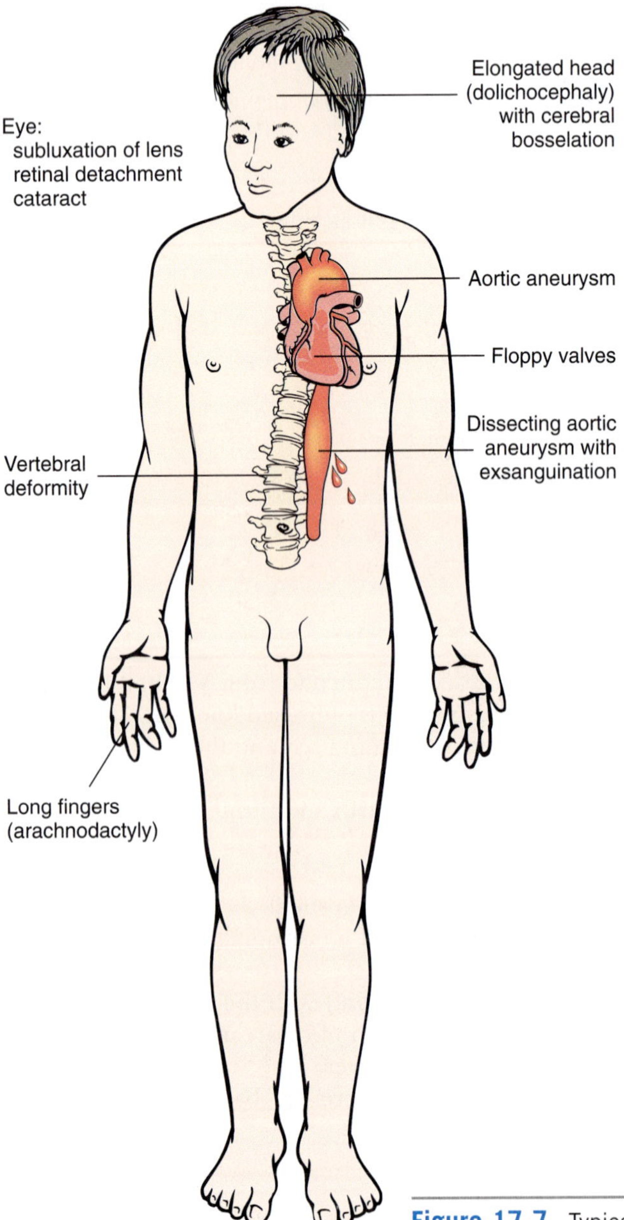

Figure 17-7. Typical features of Marfan's syndrome.

body, Marfan's may affect many body systems. Often, patients with Marfan's have skeletal defects, such as spider-like fingers, pectus excavatum, and curvature of the spine. They also may have cardiovascular problems such as aortic regurgitation or prolapse of the mitral valve. *Coding Clinic* (1993:3Q:p11)[2] addresses the assignment of codes for Marfan's syndrome. Conditions that are inherent in this syndrome are not coded separately. When an adult presents for heart surgery to correct conditions associated with Marfan's, 759.82 is assigned as the principal diagnosis.

EXAMPLE Aortic regurgitation in a patient with Marfan's syndrome, 759.82.

EXERCISE 17-2

Assign codes to the following conditions using your ICD-9-CM code book.

1. Unilateral, complete cleft lip ____________
2. Tongue tie ____________
3. Primary pulmonary hypertension of the newborn ____________
4. Patent ductus arteriosus (PDA) of the newborn ____________
5. Ventricular septal defect (VSD) of the newborn ____________
6. Preauricular cyst ____________
7. Transposition of the great vessels ____________
8. Ptosis of the eyelid present at birth ____________
9. Microcephalus ____________
10. Arnold-Chiari syndrome type II ____________
11. Cerebral cyst present at birth ____________
12. Supernumerary ear ____________
13. Brachial cleft cyst ____________
14. Hypospadia ____________
15. Micro-penis ____________

Coding the Birth of an Infant (V30-V39)

All newborn charts must contain a code from V30-V39 for the principal diagnosis on the baby's birth record. This V code is only used one time. If the baby is transferred to another facility, these sets of V codes are not used and the reason for admission at that facility is the principal diagnosis.

These V codes have both fourth and fifth digits available.

Fourth Digits

0 Born in hospital
1 Born before admission to hospital
2 Born outside hospital and not hospitalized

Fifth Digits

These fifth digits are for use **only** with the fourth digit of .0, Born in the hospital:

0 Delivered without mention of cesarean delivery
1 Delivered by cesarean delivery

These digits help identify where the baby was born and if a cesarean delivery was performed.

EXAMPLE Single liveborn, born in hospital, via cesarean section, V30.01.

EXAMPLE

Twin, mate liveborn, delivered vaginally in hospital, V31.00.

EXAMPLE

Single liveborn delivered by cesarean section at Hospital A. The infant was transferred to Hospital B because of bladder exstrophy.
Hospital A V30.01, 753.5
Hospital B 753.5

Maternal Causes of Perinatal Morbidity and Mortality (760-763)

As is stated in the guidelines, these conditions are assigned only if and when the maternal condition has actually affected the fetus or the newborn. Just because a mother has a condition does not necessarily mean that it affects the newborn.

EXAMPLE

Mother occasionally used cocaine during this pregnancy. Upon vaginal delivery, it is noted that the baby is jittery and is experiencing symptoms of withdrawal, V30.00, 760.75.

EXERCISE 17-3

Answer the following questions.

1. Mother had a urinary tract infection (UTI) during the pregnancy; this was treated, and no effect on the fetus was observed. Should code 760.1 be added to the baby's chart? ____________
2. Mother had an automobile accident. She needed to undergo immediate surgery to correct the open fracture of her arm. It was decided that a cesarean section should be performed and the baby delivered prior to repair of the fracture. Should code 760.5 be added to the baby's chart? ____________
3. A baby is born with spina bifida, and the mother had taken statins during pregnancy. Should code 760.78 be used on the baby's chart? See *Coding Clinic* (2005:4Q:p82-83).[3] ____________
4. A baby is born to a mother who used cocaine during the pregnancy. The baby experiences no signs of withdrawal but has a positive drug screen. Should 760.75 be used on this baby's chart? See *Coding Clinic* (1992:2Q:p12).[4] ____________
5. A newborn is delivered via vacuum extractor. A large hematoma is located on the scalp. Should 763.3 be coded? ____________

Other Conditions Originating in the Perinatal Period (764-779)

Prematurity, Low Birth Weight

Fifth digits are required for categories 764.XX (Slow fetal growth and fetal malnutrition), 765.0X and 765.1X (Extreme immaturity and Other preterm infants). Prematurity must be documented by the provider. Fifth digits should be assigned on the basis of recorded birth weight and gestational age. Additionally, a code for weeks of gestation (765.2X) should be assigned to categories 764.XX and 765.0X and 765.1X.

EXAMPLE

The physician documented that the baby was small for gestational age (SGA). The baby weighed 1850 grams. The infant was born in the hospital by vaginal delivery, V30.00, 764.07, 765.20.

The guidelines state that all clinically significant conditions noted on routine newborn examination should be coded. These follow the same general guidelines for assigning secondary diagnoses except for the guideline regarding implications for future healthcare needs.

A condition is clinically significant if it requires the following:

- Clinical evaluation, or
- Therapeutic treatment, or
- Diagnostic procedures, or
- Extended length of hospital stay, or
- Increased nursing care and/or monitoring; or if it has
- Implications for future healthcare needs (applies to newborn only)

When coding secondary diagnoses from other chapters on a newborn chart, guidelines state that code 779.89 should also be assigned. If there is no specific code from the Congenital anomalies and Perinatal condition chapter to describe the condition, disease, or complication of the newborn then a code from other chapters should be used as well as code 779.89.

EXAMPLE Infant was delivered by Cesarean section. Physician notes hemangioma of skin of torso. Will re-evaluate at 6-week check up, V30.01, 779.89, 228.01.

Fetal Distress

Fetal distress occurs when the fetus develops a problem before or during labor. No exact consensus has been reached as to what constitutes fetal distress, but the term often refers to **hypoxia, bradycardia, tachycardia** (fast heartbeat), fetal acidosis, and/or the presence of thick meconium.

EXAMPLE Fetal distress first noted during labor, infant born vaginally, V30.00, 768.3.

EXAMPLE Fetal hypoxia in infant born by C-Section, V30.01, 770.88.

EXAMPLE Abnormal fetal heart rate or rhythm during labor, infant delivered by C-Section, V30.01, 763.82.

Apgar Scores

All babies are assessed after birth by what is known as an **Apgar** test (Figure 17-8). This test is usually given twice—once at 1 minute and again at 5 minutes. If problems are noted with the baby, the test may be done a third time. It is good to be familiar with this test because a low Apgar score is often indicative of problems.

Five factors are used for evaluation; the baby is given a score of 0 to 2 for each factor. These consist of the following:

1. Heart (pulse)
2. Breathing (rate and effort)
3. Activity and muscle tone
4. Grimace (reflex irritability)
5. Appearance (skin coloration)

If a baby scores 7 or above at 1 minute after birth, the baby is considered healthy. If a score between 4 and 6 is recorded at 1 minute, usually the baby needs immediate care with oxygen or suctioning.

Respiratory Problems After Birth

If a baby is born by cesarean section, a pediatrician may be asked to be present for the birth. If an abnormal heart rate occurs during labor, or any indications suggest that the baby

APGAR SCORING CHART

SIGN	0	1	2
Heart rate	Absent	Below 100	Over 100
Respiratory effort	Absent	Slow, irregular	Good, crying
Muscle tone	Limp	Some flexion of extremities	Active motion
Response to catheter in nostril (tested after oropharynx is clear)	No response	Grimace	Cough or sneeze
Color	Blue, pale	Body pink, extremities blue	Completely pink

Figure 17-8. Apgar scoring chart.

might be in trouble, a pediatrician may be called and is asked to be present for the delivery. Documentation by the physician should note any abnormal conditions.

Transitory Tachypnea of Newborn (TTN). This is a respiratory problem that is likely due to retained lung fluid. It usually resolves in 24 to 48 hours. The baby may be treated with oxygen.

Apnea of the Newborn. This tends to occur in premature infants and is defined as a pause in breathing for longer than 15 seconds that can result in cyanosis.

Respiratory Distress Syndrome (RDS). This syndrome rarely affects full-term infants. It is caused by lack of lung surfactant. Surfactant is a chemical that keeps the air sacs from collapsing. The more premature the baby is, the greater is the chance of RDS. Treatment for mild cases consists of oxygen. Patients with more severe disease must be ventilated; sometimes, an artificial lung surfactant is placed in the lungs of an infant who is at high risk, to try to prevent RDS.

EXAMPLE

Respiratory distress syndrome in liveborn infant that was delivered vaginally, V30.00, 769.

Bronchopulmonary Dysplasia (BPD)

BPD is a chronic lung disease that develops in babies during the first 4 weeks after birth. It occurs most often in premature babies, that is, those weighing less than 1500 grams. Sometimes, the ventilator that is keeping a baby alive may cause BPD. BPD may also be caused by infections, such as pneumonia.

EXAMPLE

A 4-week infant is diagnosed with bronchopulmonary dysplasia. Infant was on a ventilator following birth, 770.7.

Meconium Aspiration Syndrome

Meconium is the fecal matter within a baby's intestines before birth. Normally, it is expelled after birth, but if problems occur during labor, the baby may expel meconium into the amniotic fluid. Meconium may be inhaled by the baby while within the uterus or during birth. Inhalation of meconium occurs most often in postterm babies.

A physician may suspect aspiration if the newborn is covered with meconium, or if thick meconium is found in the amniotic fluid. Aspiration of meconium can result in major problems for the newborn.

A variety of codes may be used to indicate the different ways in which meconium may be found.

- 779.84, Meconium staining
- 763.84, Meconium passage during delivery
- 770.11, Meconium aspiration without respiratory symptoms
- 770.12, Meconium aspiration with respiratory symptoms
- 770.10, Fetal and newborn aspiration, unspecified

Hemolytic Disease of Fetus or Newborn, Due to Isoimmunization and Other Perinatal Jaundice

Many newborns have jaundice. Jaundice results from too many red blood cells and the breakdown of these cells into bilirubin. A large amount of bilirubin causes the skin to take on a yellow color. The most common type of jaundice is physiologic jaundice, 774.6. Other factors may cause jaundice, but the next most common cause is Rh or ABO incompatibility. ABO incompatibility affects newborns who have mothers with a blood type of O and babies whose blood type is A, B, or AB.

Coombs' test may be performed on newborns who are jaundiced. This is done to look for possible causes of **hemolysis** (the breaking down of red blood cells). Two common forms of hemolysis in the newborn are Rh incompatibility and ABO incompatibility. Rh incompatibility occurs when an Rh-negative (anti-Rh antibodies in blood) mom gives birth to an Rh-positive baby. If any maternal and fetal blood gets mixed during pregnancy or the birth process, the mother's Rh-negative antibodies will attack the baby's Rh-positive RBCs and destroy them. ABO incompatibility is very similar in mechanism. Often, documentation in the chart indicates that routine cord blood tests show ABO incompatibility. The coder must verify whether Coombs' test results were positive in order to assign this code. If cord blood shows ABO incompatibility and Coombs' test results are positive, code 773.1 should be assigned according to *Coding Clinic* (1992:3Q:p8-9).[5]

Most often, jaundice is treated by putting a baby under "bili" lights. Phototherapy code 99.83 is used for this treatment. In very mild cases, a mother is instructed to put the baby in a sunlit window. In very severe cases, a transfusion may be required.

EXAMPLE Newborn with Rh incompatibility. Infant was delivered vaginally, V30.00, 773.0.

Infection in the Perinatal Period

Newborn Sepsis. To locate infections of the newborn in the index, it is best to look under the main term for the infection, and then to look for a subterm of newborn, fetal, or congenital.

For example, newborn sepsis codes to 771.81. It is also important to assign a code from category 041 to identify the organism responsible for the infection. The guidelines state that code 995.9x, SIRS (systemic inflammatory response syndrome), is not to be used on a newborn record, nor should the code 038.xx be used for septicemia.

The guidelines also state that if a newborn has a condition that may be due to the birth process or may be community acquired, and the documentation is not clear regarding the underlying cause, the default is to a code from Chapter 15, the congenital condition.

EXAMPLE A 7-day-old infant presents to the physician's office with pneumonia, 770.0.

Observation and Evaluation of Newborns (V29.X)

Often, a newborn is evaluated for a condition that may be suspected but is then ruled out. In cases in which this happens, it is appropriate to assign a code from the V29 category as a diagnosis in support of the testing and treatment that is being performed. Sometimes, a mother is running a fever during labor, and the physician must make sure that the infant does not have an infection. The physician orders tests, observation, and/or treatment until

this condition can be ruled out. If the newborn is experiencing signs or symptoms, then a code from category V29 is not to be used. Likewise, a V29 code may be assigned as the principal diagnosis code for readmission when a condition is suspected and is subsequently ruled out. It is important to remember that this code can be used only during the neonatal period (the first 28 days of life).

EXAMPLE

Newborn delivered vaginally and is given antibiotics for suspected sepsis that was ruled out, V30.00, V29.0.

V CODES

In the past, V codes were primarily considered for use in the outpatient setting. This has changed with the addition of more V codes each year. As was discussed in Chapter 8, it may be difficult to locate V codes in the Index. Coders often say, "I did not know there was a V code for that." Refer to Chapter 8 for a listing of common main terms used to locate V codes.

V15.22	Personal history of undergoing in utero procedure while a fetus
V20.0	Foundling
V20.1	Other healthy infant or child receiving care
V20.2	Routine infant or child health check
V21.0	Period of rapid growth in childhood
V21.2	Other adolescence
V21.30	Low birth weight status, unspecified
V21.31	Low birth weight status, less than 500 grams
V21.32	Low birth weight status, 500-999 grams
V21.33	Low birth weight status, 1000-1499 grams
V21.34	Low birth weight status, 1500-1999 grams
V21.35	Low birth weight status, 2000-2500 grams
V21.8	Other specified constitutional states in development
V21.9	Unspecified constitutional state in development
V29.0	Observation and eval of newborns and infants for suspected infectious condition not found
V29.1	Observation and eval of newborns and infants for suspected neurologic condition not found
V29.2	Observation and eval of newborns and infants for suspected respiratory condition not found
V29.3	Observation and eval of newborns and infants for suspected genetic or metabolic condition not found
V29.8	Observation and eval of newborns and infants for other specified suspected condition not found
V29.9	Observation and eval of newborns and infants for unspecified suspected condition not found
V30.xx	Single liveborn
V31.xx	Twin, mate liveborn
V32.xx	Twin, mate stillborn
V33.xx	Twin, unspecified
V34.xx	Other multiple, mates all liveborn
V35.xx	Other multiple, mates all stillborn
V36.xx	Other multiple, mates live and stillborn
V37.xx	Other multiple, unspecified
V39.xx	Unspecified

V64.00	Vaccination not carried out, unspecified reason
V64.01	Vaccination not carried out because of acute illness
V64.02	Vaccination not carried out because of chronic illness or condition
V64.03	Vaccination not carried out because of immune compromised state
V64.04	Vaccination not carried out because of caregiver refusal
V64.05	Vaccination not carried out because of patient refusal
V64.07	Vaccination not carried out for religious reasons
V64.08	Vaccination not carried out because patient had disease being vaccinated against
V64.09	Vaccination not carried out for other reason
V72.11	Encounter for hearing examination following failed hearing screening
V72.19	Other examination of ears and hearing
V77.3	Special screening for Phenylketonuria (PKU)
V82.3	Special screening for congenital dislocation of hip

DOCUMENTATION/REIMBURSEMENT/MS-DRGs

Often, coding difficulties are due to lack of documentation. Sometimes pathology and other test results are not available at the time of discharge or when the physician is dictating the discharge summary or is reporting the final diagnoses.

NEWBORN MS-DRGs	RW	DRG TITLE
789	1.4250	Died or transferred
790	4.6990	Extreme immaturity or RDS
791	3.2093	Premature with major problems
792	1.9364	Premature without major problems
793	3.2966	Full-term neonate with major problems
794	1.1668	Neonate with other significant problems
795	0.1580	Normal newborn

As is evident from the **MS-DRGs** listed here, correct capture of the discharge disposition is very important, as is following the perinatal guidelines to capture all newborn conditions. It also is important to watch for documentation of prematurity and low birth weight.

EXAMPLE

	CODE	MS-DRGs	RW
Normal newborn	V30.00	795	0.1580
Newborn with meconium during delivery	V30.00 763.84	794	1.1618
Newborn with aspiration of clear amniotic fluid with respiratory symptoms	V30.00 770.13	793	3.2966
Premature newborn Delivered at 29 weeks weighing 1500 grams	V30.00 765.16 765.25	792	1.9364
Newborn with respiratory distress syndrome	V30.00 769	790	4.6990

CHAPTER REVIEW EXERCISE

Where applicable, assign codes for diagnoses, procedures, V codes, and E codes.

1. Newborn delivered by cesarean section ________
2. Twins born in the parking lot of the hospital ________
3. Baby was born at 2500 grams; physician documented "small for dates"; delivered vaginally ________
4. Newborn at 43 weeks' gestation, vaginal delivery ________

5. Newborn with IUGR (intrauterine growth retardation); delivered vaginally. __________
6. Newborn fractured clavicle during birth process; vaginal delivery __________
7. TTN (transitory tachypnea of the newborn); infant delivered by emergency C-section __________
8. 7-day-old with thrush; seen in physician office __________
9. Transfer from community hospital for treatment of interstitial pulmonary fibrosis of prematurity in a newborn __________
10. Baby is admitted 5 days after birth for jaundice due to breast feeding __________
11. 7-day-old infant with infection of the navel cord __________
12. Newborn with a hydrocele following vaginal delivery __________
13. Baby delivered by cesarean section in respiratory failure and immediately transferred to NICU (neonatal intensive care unit) __________
14. Newborn aspirated meconium during vaginal delivery __________
15. Neonatal bradycardia following C-section __________
16. Newborn with fetal alcohol syndrome delivered vaginally __________
17. Newborn delivered vaginally; suspected of having pneumonia; chest x-ray is performed, revealing no diagnosis __________
18. Newborn with hypoglycemia, whose mother has diabetes, delivered vaginally __________
19. Newborn with apnea following vaginal delivery __________
20. Newborn delivered vaginally in the hospital. Failed hearing test. __________

CHAPTER GLOSSARY

Anomaly: a deviation from normal standards (e.g., as in congenital defects).

Apgar: test used to measure the condition of a newborn at birth.

Blalock-Taussig operation: procedure used to treat patients with Tetralogy of Fallot who have insufficient pulmonary arterial flow.

Bradycardia: slow heart rate.

Cleft lip/palate: opening in the lip or palate of an infant that occurs in utero.

Congenital: condition present at birth, regardless of causation.

Hemolysis: the breaking down of red blood cells.

Hydrocephalus: cerebrospinal fluid collection in the skull.

Hypertrophy: enlargement of a gland.

Hypoxia: insufficient oxygen in the blood.

Klinefelter's syndrome: a sex chromosome disorder that occurs in males and is caused by an extra X chromosome.

Marfan's syndrome: an inherited condition that affects connective tissue and is caused by gene mutation.

Meconium: material in the intestine of a fetus.

Perinatal period: before birth through the first 28 days of life.

Tachycardia: fast heartbeat.

Tachypnea: fast breathing.

Trisomy: extra chromosome.

Ventriculoperitoneal shunt: procedure used to treat patient with hydrocephalus in whom drainage of the ventricle occurs through an artificial channel between the ventricle and the peritoneum.

CHAPTER 18

Diseases of the Musculoskeletal System and Connective Tissue

(ICD-9-CM Chapter 13, Codes 710-739)

CHAPTER OUTLINE

LEARNING OBJECTIVES

- Apply and assign the correct ICD-9-CM codes in accordance with Official Guidelines for Coding and Reporting
- Identify pertinent anatomy and physiology of the musculoskeletal system and connective tissue
- Identify diseases of the musculoskeletal system and connective tissue
- Assign the correct V codes and procedure codes related to the musculoskeletal system and connective tissue
- Identify common treatments, medications, laboratory values, and diagnostic tests
- Explain the importance of documentation as it relates to MS-DRGs for reimbursement

ABBREVIATIONS

AKA above-knee amputation

DEXA dual-energy x-ray absorptiometry (bone density)

DIC disseminated intravascular coagulation

DJD degenerative joint disease

ICD-9-CM *International Classification of Diseases, 9th Revision, Clinical Modification*

ABBREVIATIONS—*cont'd*

IV intravenous
JRA juvenile rheumatoid arthritis
MAO monoamine oxidase
MRI magnetic resonance imaging
MS-DRG Medicare Severity diagnosis-related group
NSAIDs nonsteroidal anti-inflammatory drugs
OA osteoarthritis
PMR polymyalgia rheumatica
PV percutaneous vertebroplasty
RA rheumatoid arthritis
SLE systemic lupus erythematosus

ICD-9-CM Official Guidelines for Coding and Reporting

Please refer to the companion Evolve website for the most current guidelines.

13. Chapter 13: Diseases of Musculoskeletal and Connective Tissue (710-739)

a. Coding of Pathologic Fractures

1) Acute Fractures vs. Aftercare

Pathologic fractures are reported using subcategory 733.1, when the fracture is newly diagnosed. Subcategory 733.1 may be used while the patient is receiving active treatment for the fracture. Examples of active treatment are: surgical treatment, emergency department encounter, evaluation and treatment by a new physician.

EXAMPLE

The patient underwent a percutaneous vertebroplasty for pathologic fracture of the vertebrae, 733.13, 81.65.

Fractures are coded using the aftercare codes (subcategories V54.0, V54.2, V54.8 or V54.9) for encounters after the patient has completed active treatment of the fracture and is receiving routine care for the fracture during the healing or recovery phase. Examples of fracture aftercare are: cast change or removal, removal of external or internal fixation device, medication adjustment, and follow-up visits following fracture treatment.

EXAMPLE

The patient was seen for follow-up after vertebroplasty for pathologic fracture of the vertebrae, V54.27.

Care for complications of surgical treatment for fracture repairs during the healing or recovery phase should be coded with the appropriate complication codes.

Care of complications of fractures, such as malunion and nonunion, should be reported with the appropriate codes.

See Section I. C. 17.b for information on the coding of traumatic fractures.

Apply the General Coding Guidelines as found in Chapter 5.

ANATOMY AND PHYSIOLOGY

The musculoskeletal system is made up of muscles, bones, ligaments, tendons, cartilage, and the joints they form. The purposes of the musculoskeletal system are to provide a framework and to protect the internal organs. Bones also are important for hematopoiesis and for storing calcium and phosphate. **Hematopoiesis** is the development of blood cells that occurs in the bone marrow and lymphatic tissue of normal adults.

A good grasp of anatomy is essential in coding conditions of the musculoskeletal system. The coder must know that the femur is the long bone in the thigh area, and that the radius

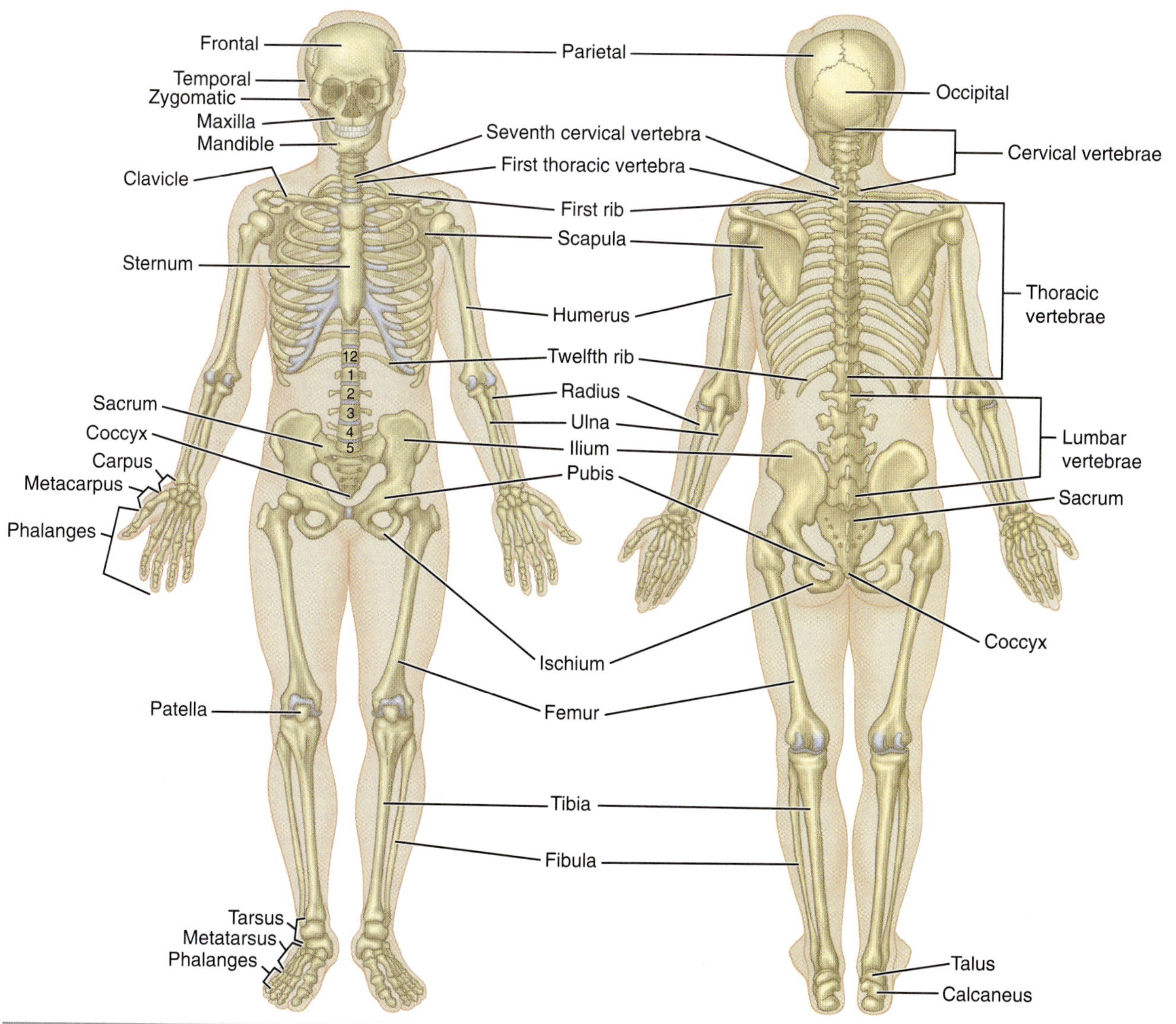

Figure 18-1. Anterior and posterior views of the human skeleton.

and the ulna are two bones in the forearm. Pictures are best for illustrating the locations of the skeletal structures (Figure 18-1) and muscles (Figure 18-2). It is particularly important to understand the terms used in the musculoskeletal chapter to describe the location of structures relative to the body as a whole or to other body structures (Figure 18-3). **Anterior** or **ventral** describes the front of the body or an organ. **Posterior** or **dorsal** relates to the back of the body or an organ. The terms medial and lateral describe the position of the body or an organ relative to the median sagittal plane that divides the body in half. **Medial** refers to a structure that is closer to the median plane than is another structure in the body. The eyes are medial to the ears. **Lateral** refers to a structure that is to the side of the body. The ears are lateral to the eyes. The terms **superior** (above) and **inferior** (below) describe the position of the body or an organ relative to the vertical axis of the body. The shoulders are superior to the hips, and the ankles are inferior to the knees. Other terms that may be used are **cranial**, which means toward the head, and **caudal,** which means towards the tail. **Proximal** (closer to the point of reference) and **distal** (farther from the point of reference) are often used to describe a location in the limbs. The shoulder is proximal to the elbow, and the wrist is distal to the elbow. **Supine** refers to lying on the back, face up. **Prone** is lying on the stomach, face down.

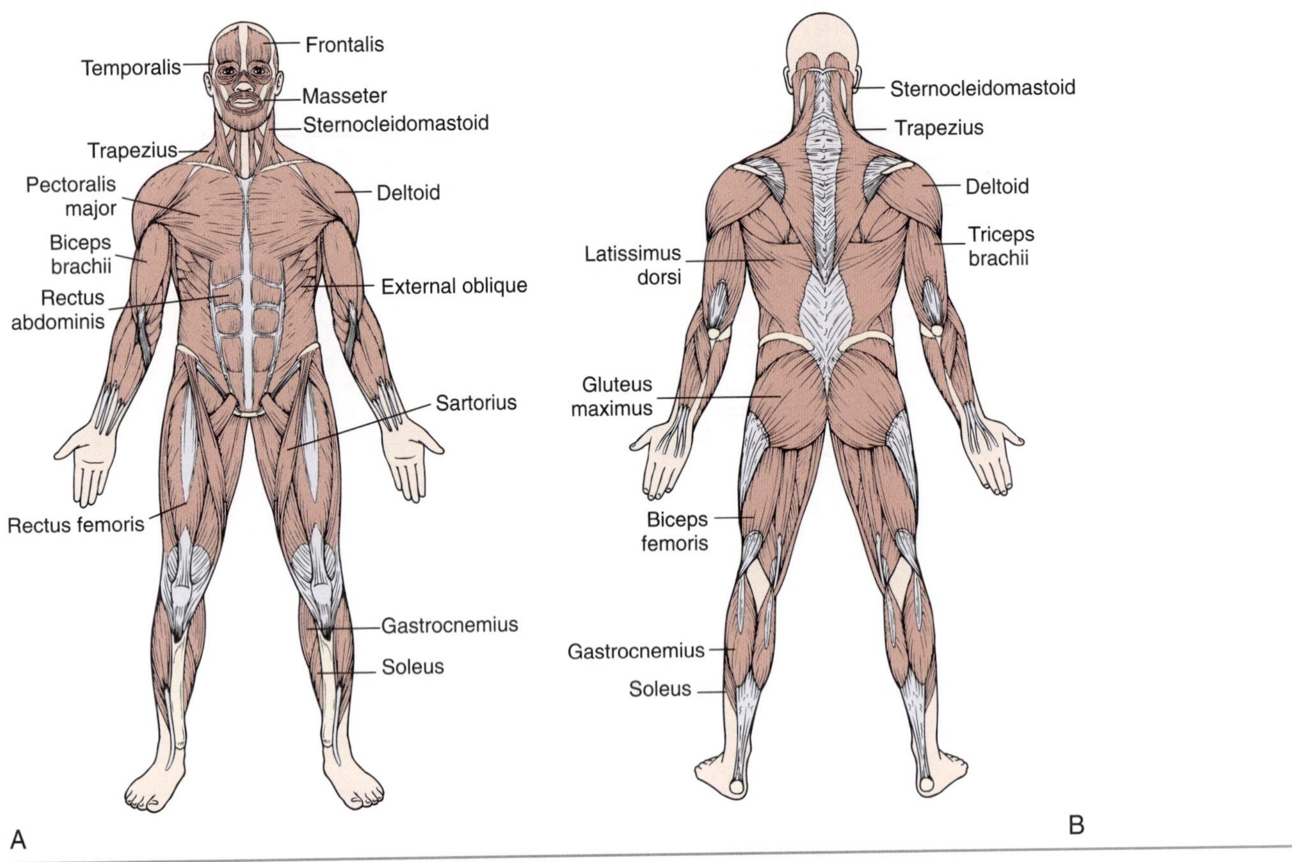

Figure 18-2. Normal muscular system. **A,** Anterior view. **B,** Posterior view.

The **joints** are the means of joining two bones together; they assist with body movement. **Ligaments** are dense fibrous bands of connective tissue that provide stability for the joint. Ligaments can be injured by overstretching or tearing (sprain). **Tendons** are the connective tissue that attaches muscle to bone. Tendons are susceptible to strain injuries. The **fascia** is the tissue just below the skin that covers and separates the underlying layers of muscle.

DISEASE CONDITIONS

Diseases of the Musculoskeletal System and Connective Tissue (710-739), Chapter 13 in your ICD-9-CM code book, is divided into the following categories:

CATEGORY	SECTION TITLES
710-719	Arthropathies and Related Disorders
720-724	Dorsopathies
725-729	Rheumatism, Excluding the Back
730-739	Osteopathies, Chondropathies, and Acquired Musculoskeletal Deformities

One of the most important parts of this chapter is the breakdown of the fifth digit subclassifications that are used with categories 711-712, 715-716, 718-719, and 730; this information appears at the very beginning of the chapter (Figure 18-4) and is provided to assist in making the proper fifth digit assignment. One may not remember whether the wrist fits into the subclassification of 3 for forearm, or 4 for hand. The appropriate fifth digit subclassification for wrist joint is 3, forearm.

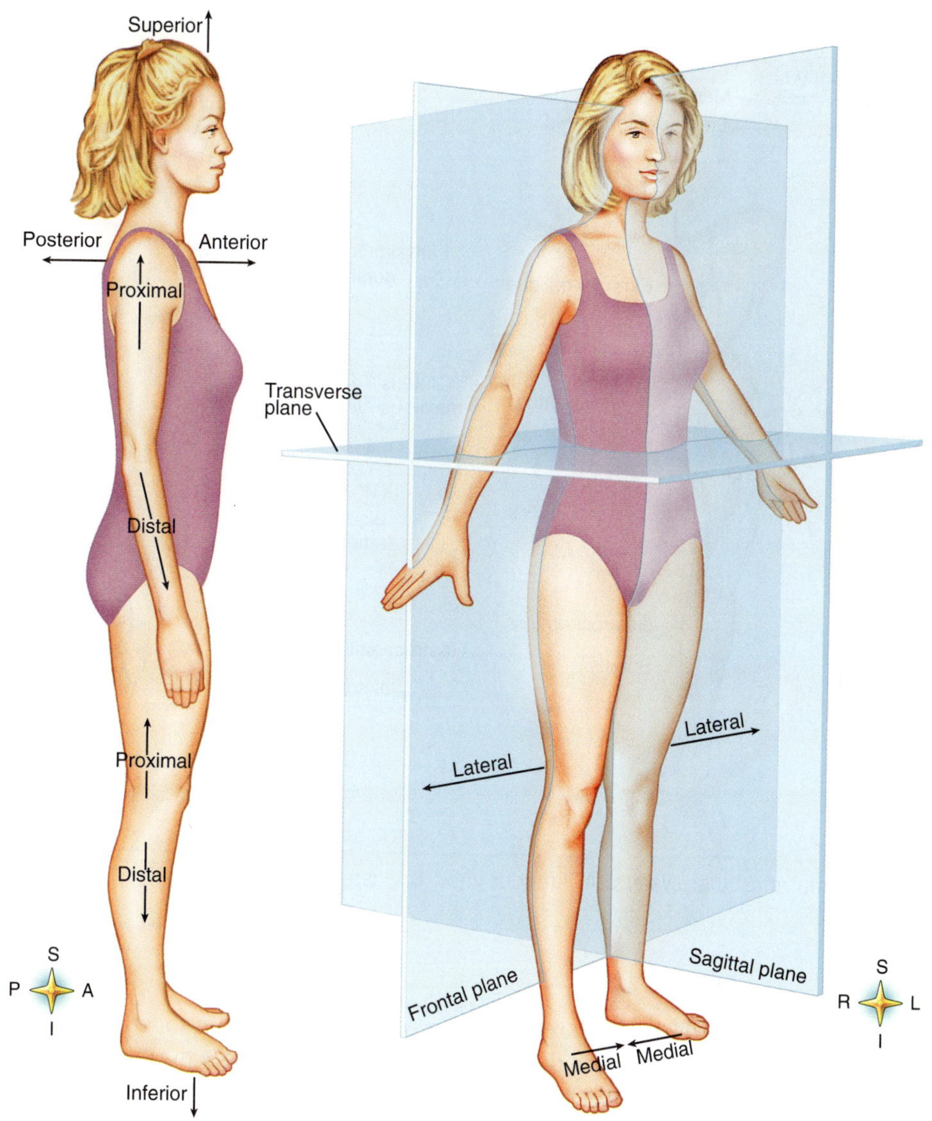

Figure 18-3. Directions and planes of the body.

EXERCISE 18-1

Using figure 18-5, assign the appropriate fifth digits to the following conditions.

1. Pyogenic arthritis of the right elbow 711.0______
2. Traumatic arthropathy left foot 716.1______
3. Osteoarthritis both wrists 715.3______
4. Recurrent dislocation right thumb 718.3______
5. Acute osteomyelitis sacrum 730.0______

Arthropathies and Related Disorders (710-719)

Collagen Diseases

The main component of connective tissue is collagen. Collagen diseases result from immune system malfunctions in which the immune system identifies the body's connective tissue as foreign and attacks it. A patient's heart, lungs, and kidneys may also suffer damage. No cure

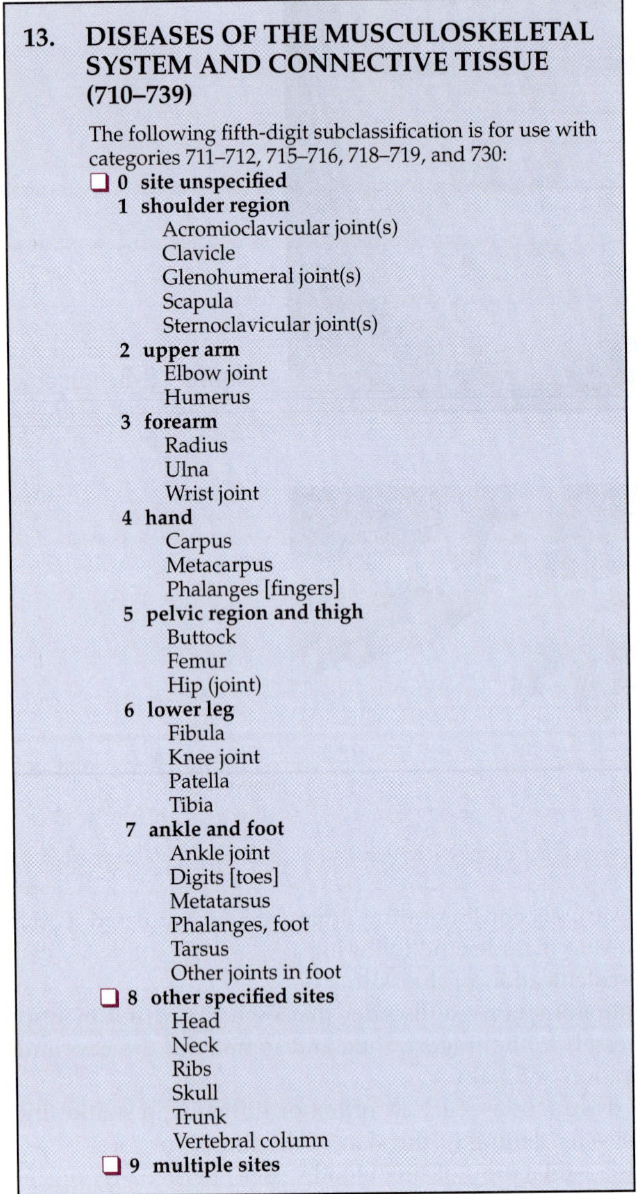

13. DISEASES OF THE MUSCULOSKELETAL SYSTEM AND CONNECTIVE TISSUE (710–739)

The following fifth-digit subclassification is for use with categories 711–712, 715–716, 718–719, and 730:

❑ **0 site unspecified**

1 shoulder region
Acromioclavicular joint(s)
Clavicle
Glenohumeral joint(s)
Scapula
Sternoclavicular joint(s)

2 upper arm
Elbow joint
Humerus

3 forearm
Radius
Ulna
Wrist joint

4 hand
Carpus
Metacarpus
Phalanges [fingers]

5 pelvic region and thigh
Buttock
Femur
Hip (joint)

6 lower leg
Fibula
Knee joint
Patella
Tibia

7 ankle and foot
Ankle joint
Digits [toes]
Metatarsus
Phalanges, foot
Tarsus
Other joints in foot

❑ **8 other specified sites**
Head
Neck
Ribs
Skull
Trunk
Vertebral column

❑ **9 multiple sites**

Figure 18-4. Fifth-digit subclassifications for use with categories 711-712, 715-716, 718-719, and 790, as shown in the Tabular List.

is known for these diseases. The most common conditions include systemic lupus erythematosus, scleroderma, and rheumatoid arthritis.

Systemic lupus erythematosus (SLE) is a chronic, inflammatory autoimmune disease that can damage connective tissue anywhere in the body. It causes inflammation of the skin, joints, nervous system, kidneys, lungs, and other organs. A butterfly rash that spreads from one cheek across the nose to the other cheek is a common symptom (Figure 18-5). Fever, fatigue, weight loss, and joint deformity may also be present.

Scleroderma is a chronic, progressive disease that is characterized by hardening of the skin and scarring of internal organs. No cure is known for scleroderma; treatment is sup-

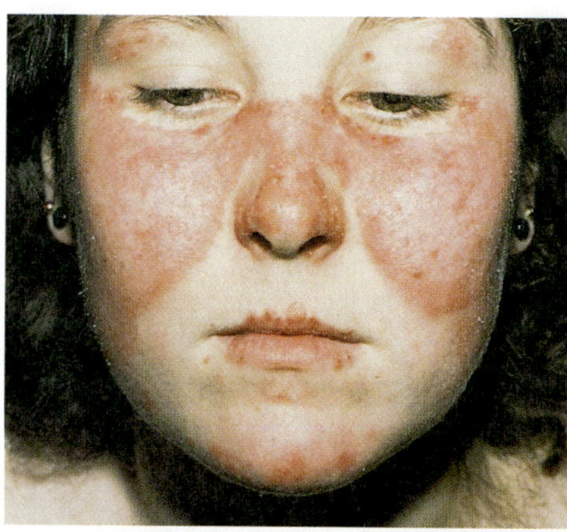

Figure 18-5. Butterfly rash that may accompany systemic lupus erythematosus.

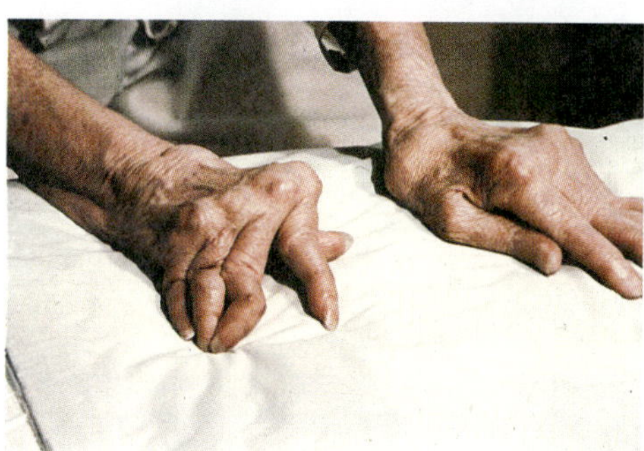

Figure 18-6. Joint deformity from rheumatoid arthritis.

portive and varies according to the organs that are affected. CREST syndrome is a form of scleroderma that includes the following:

Calcinosis—calcification of the skin

Raynaud's phenomenon—a disorder that is characterized by vasospastic attacks in which blood vessels to the fingers, toes, and sometimes the ears and nose constrict, causing discoloration and pain

Esophageal dysfunction—such as reflux or difficulty in swallowing

Sclerodactyly—hardening of the skin of the fingers or toes

Telangiectasia—dilatation of tiny blood vessels, particularly of the skin

Rheumatoid arthritis (RA) is a chronic, inflammatory, systemic disease that affects the joints, often causing deformity (Figure 18-6). RA is one of the most severe and disabling forms of arthritis. Damage may extend beyond the joints, affecting the heart and blood vessels and producing damage within the layers of skin.

Juvenile rheumatoid arthritis (JRA) affects children, usually between the ages of 2 and 5 years. Various forms of JRA may affect only a few joints, may affect many joints, or may be systemic in nature (also known as Still's disease).

EXAMPLE Patient is being treated for CREST syndrome, 710.1.

EXAMPLE Patient is being treated for Still's disease, 714.30.

Arthropathy is a disease that affects the joints. In categories 711, 712, and 713, many of the codes describe arthropathies or arthritis as a manifestation of other diseases or conditions; these appear in italics with instructions to code first underlying disease (Figure 18-7).

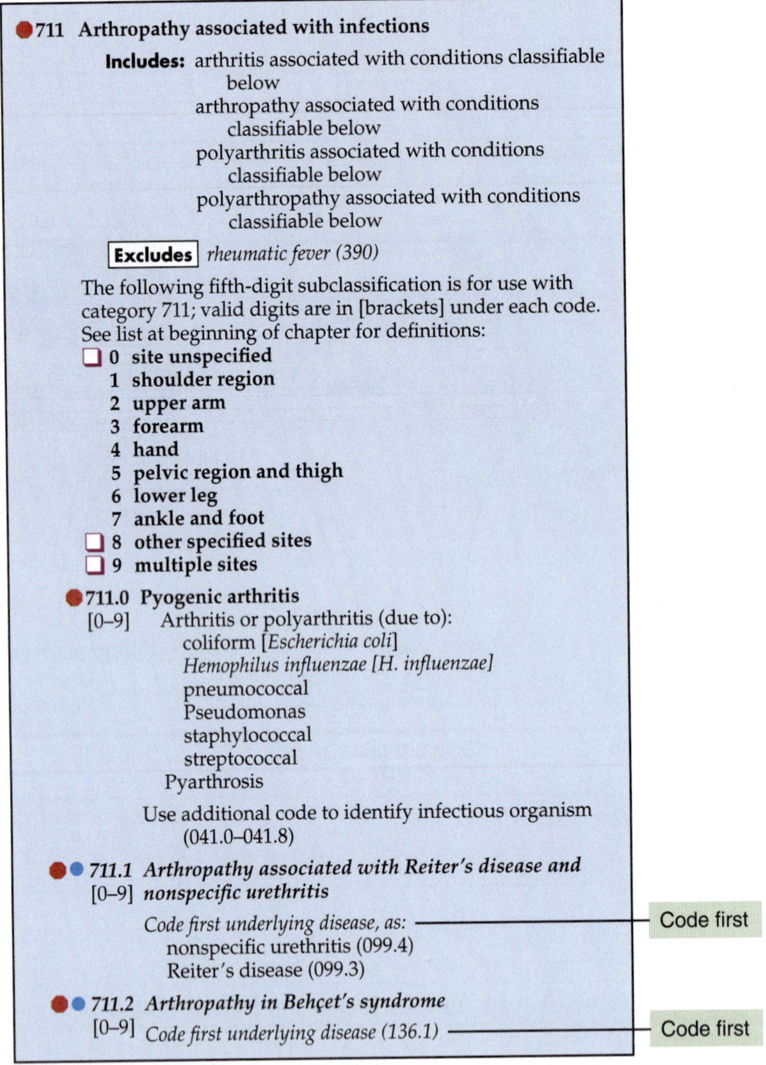

711 Arthropathy associated with infections

Includes: arthritis associated with conditions classifiable below
arthropathy associated with conditions classifiable below
polyarthritis associated with conditions classifiable below
polyarthropathy associated with conditions classifiable below

Excludes *rheumatic fever (390)*

The following fifth-digit subclassification is for use with category 711; valid digits are in [brackets] under each code. See list at beginning of chapter for definitions:

0 site unspecified
1 shoulder region
2 upper arm
3 forearm
4 hand
5 pelvic region and thigh
6 lower leg
7 ankle and foot
8 other specified sites
9 multiple sites

711.0 Pyogenic arthritis
[0–9] Arthritis or polyarthritis (due to):
coliform [*Escherichia coli*]
Hemophilus influenzae [H. influenzae]
pneumococcal
Pseudomonas
staphylococcal
streptococcal
Pyarthrosis

Use additional code to identify infectious organism (041.0–041.8)

711.1 Arthropathy associated with Reiter's disease and nonspecific urethritis
[0–9]
Code first underlying disease, as:
nonspecific urethritis (099.4)
Reiter's disease (099.3)

711.2 Arthropathy in Behçet's syndrome
[0–9] *Code first underlying disease (136.1)*

Figure 18-7. Most codes in categories 711, 712, and 713 are given in italics and include instructions to code first the underlying disease.

EXAMPLE Patient has arthritis due to hypothyroidism, 244.9, 713.0.

Osteoarthritis

Osteoarthritis is a type of arthritis that develops as the result of wear and tear on the joints. It occurs because of breakdown and loss of cartilage within the joints (Figure 18-8). Osteoarthritis (OA) or degenerative joint disease (DJD), the most common form of arthritis, is more common in the elderly. Weight-bearing joints such as the knees and hips are often affected. The most common symptoms include sore and stiff joints, particularly in the morning or with changes of weather. Edema and deformity may also be present. Treatment depends on the severity of the condition and the success of conservative medical treatments (i.e., anti-inflammatory medications, exercise, steroid injections). In severe cases, surgery may be required to replace affected joints.

Primary osteoarthritis is an idiopathic condition that occurs in previously intact joints and has no apparent initiating factor. Primary osteoarthritis is related to the aging process and typically occurs in older individuals. **Secondary osteoarthritis** refers to degenerative disease of the joints that results from a predisposing condition such as trauma or disease.

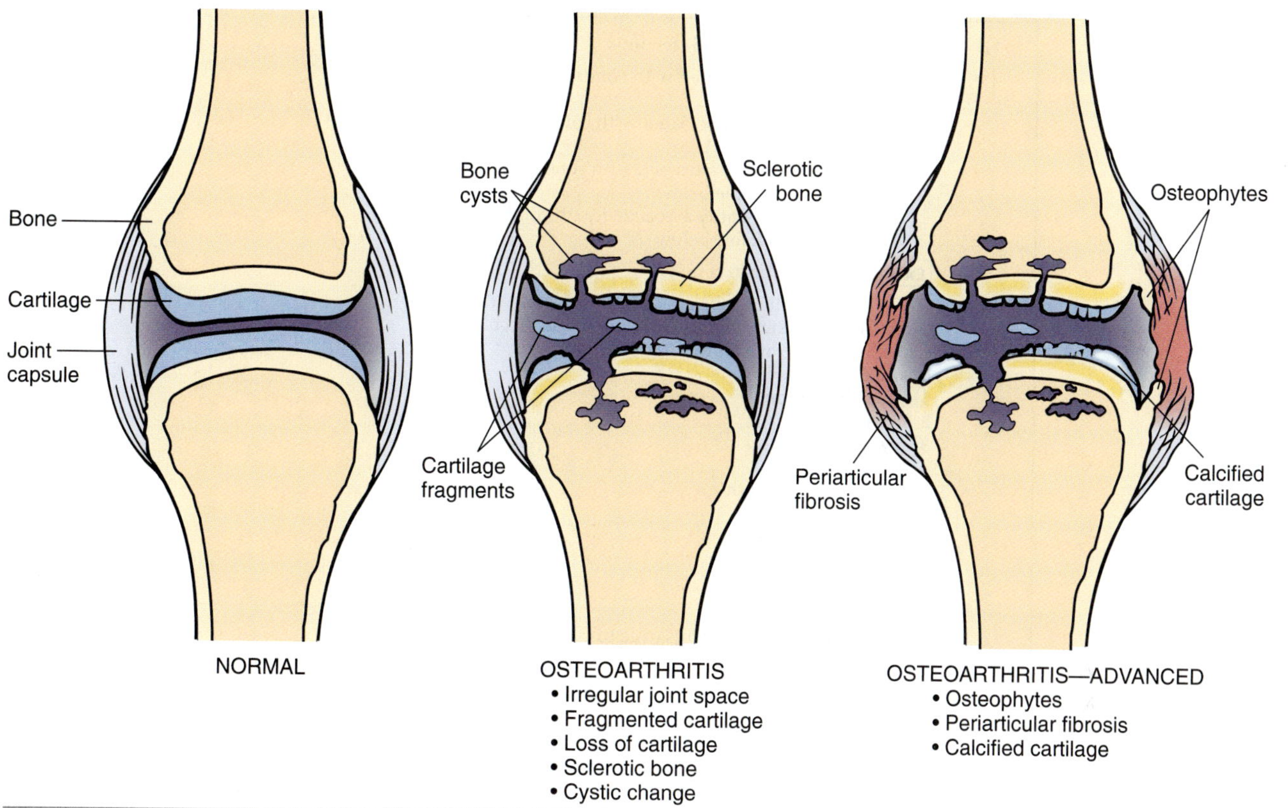

Figure 18-8. Pathologic changes of osteoarthritis.

Secondary osteoarthritis may occur in relatively young individuals and usually affects the joints of one area. Under category 715, a note indicates that "localized, in the subcategories below, includes bilateral involvement of the same site," for example, in a patient with OA of both knees, the condition would be considered localized because it is present in both lower extremities at the same site.

Coding Clinic (1995:2Q:p5)[1] goes on to say that "when the degenerative joint disease affects only one site but is not identified as primary or secondary it is coded to 715.3X, Osteoarthrosis, localized, not specified whether primary or secondary. If it involves more than one site, but is not specified as generalized, assign code 715.8X, Osteoarthrosis involving, or with mention of more than one site but not specified as generalized."

EXAMPLE Patient has osteoarthritis of both hips, 715.35.

EXAMPLE Patient is being treated for arthritis due to previous ankle fracture, 716.17, 905.4, E989.

EXAMPLE Patient is being treated for osteoarthritis hands and wrists, 715.89.

EXERCISE 18-2

Assign codes to the following conditions using your ICD-9-CM code book.

1. Pain both knees due to DJD ____________
2. Juvenile RA ____________
3. Arthritis due to Lyme disease ____________
4. Loose body in knee joint ____________
5. Sicca syndrome ____________
6. SLE with nephrotic syndrome ____________
7. Arthritis due to sarcoidosis ____________

Dorsopathies (720-724)

Dorsopathies are conditions or diseases that affect the back or spine. Code assignment may depend on the location or region that is affected. The spinal column contains 33 vertebrae, as indicated in Figure 18-9. Seven cervical vertebrae are found in the neck. Twelve thoracic, or dorsal, vertebrae are found in the region of the chest, or thorax; these provide attachment for 12 pairs of ribs. Five lumbar vertebrae are located in the lower back. Five fused sacral vertebrae form the sacrum, a solid bone that fits like a wedge between the bones of the hip and the coccyx. The coccyx consists of three or four vertebrae fused together at the bottom of the sacrum. Between each vertebra is a thick, fibrous disc of cartilage known as an intervertebral disc. Intervertebral discs may become displaced, herniated, ruptured, and/or prolapsed with resultant pain.

Spondylosis (spinal osteoarthritis) is a degenerative disorder that may cause loss of normal spinal structure and function. Although aging is the primary cause, the location and rate of degeneration are individualized. The degenerative process of spondylosis may affect the cervical, thoracic, and/or lumbar regions of the spine, including the intervertebral discs and facet joints. **Facet joints** are small, stabilizing joints located between and behind adjacent vertebrae.

Spondylolisthesis occurs when one vertebra slips on another (Figure 18-10). Symptoms usually appear when the spinal nerves are pinched by the vertebrae. Symptoms such as back, buttock, and leg pain are often aggravated by activity and relieved with rest. The amount of slippage is identified by grades.

Spinal stenosis is a narrowing of the central spinal canal, or areas of the spine where the nerve roots exit (neuroforamina). This narrowing is often caused by arthritis and therefore is most often found in persons from older age groups. Spinal stenosis may be caused by other factors such as injury, infection, tumor, or congenital abnormality. Stenosis does not necessarily cause symptoms; if symptoms do appear, they usually indicate the presence of **radiculopathy** (nerve root compression) or **myelopathy** (spinal cord compression).

EXAMPLE The patient's magnetic resonance imaging (MRI) showed stenosis cervical vertebrae, 723.0.

EXAMPLE Patient's CT shows spondylosis lumbosacral region with myelopathy, 721.42.

Postlaminectomy Syndrome

Postlaminectomy syndrome is a term that is used to describe the condition of patients who have undergone spine surgery and have some degree of recurrent spinal and/or leg pain. Treatment varies according to the cause. *Coding Clinic* (1997:2Q:p15)[2] states that "**postlaminectomy syndrome** is a buildup of scar tissue after a laminectomy has been performed. The patient is in constant pain and the physician documents that this is due to the scar tissue that has formed."

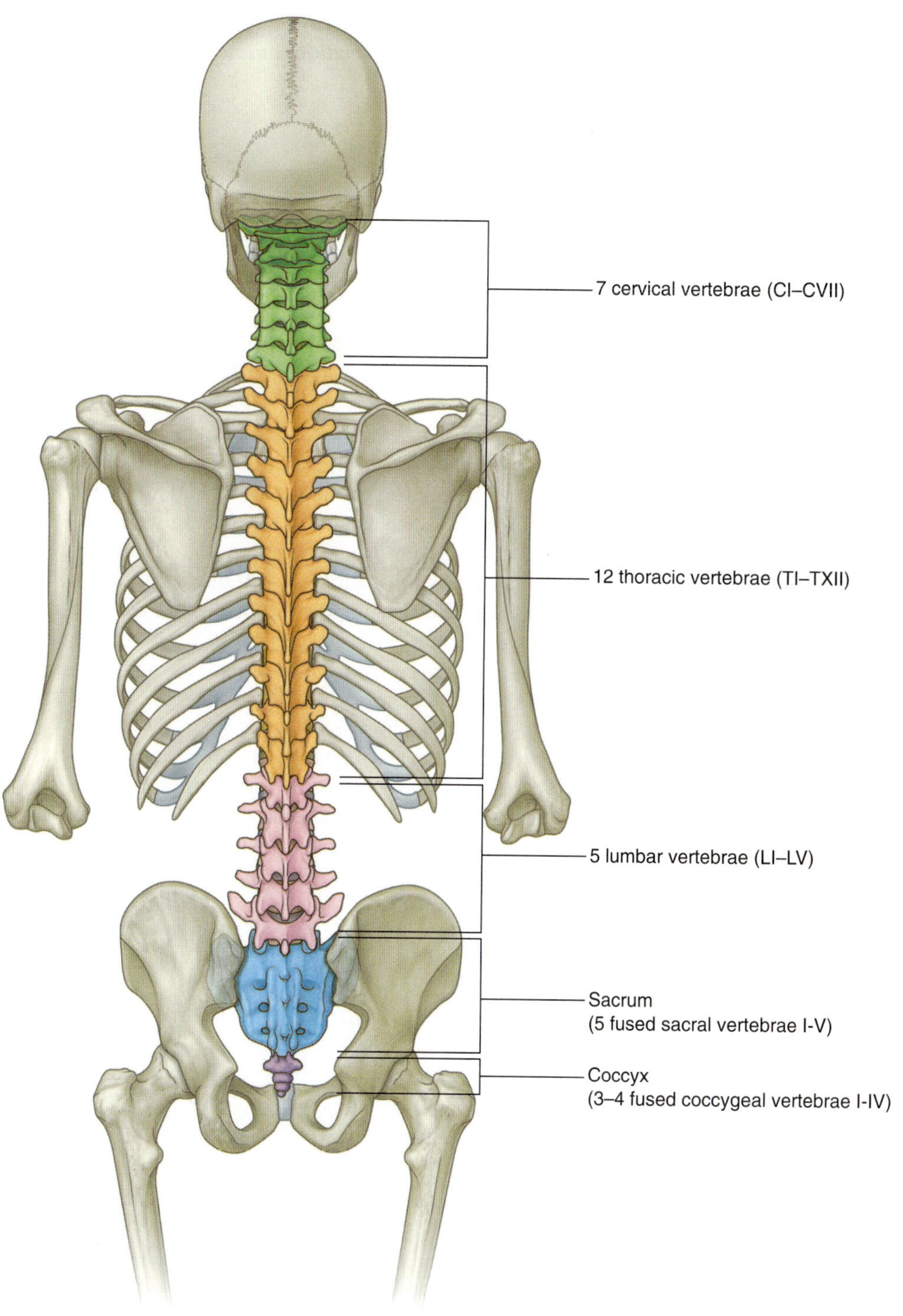

Figure 18-9. Vertebrae.

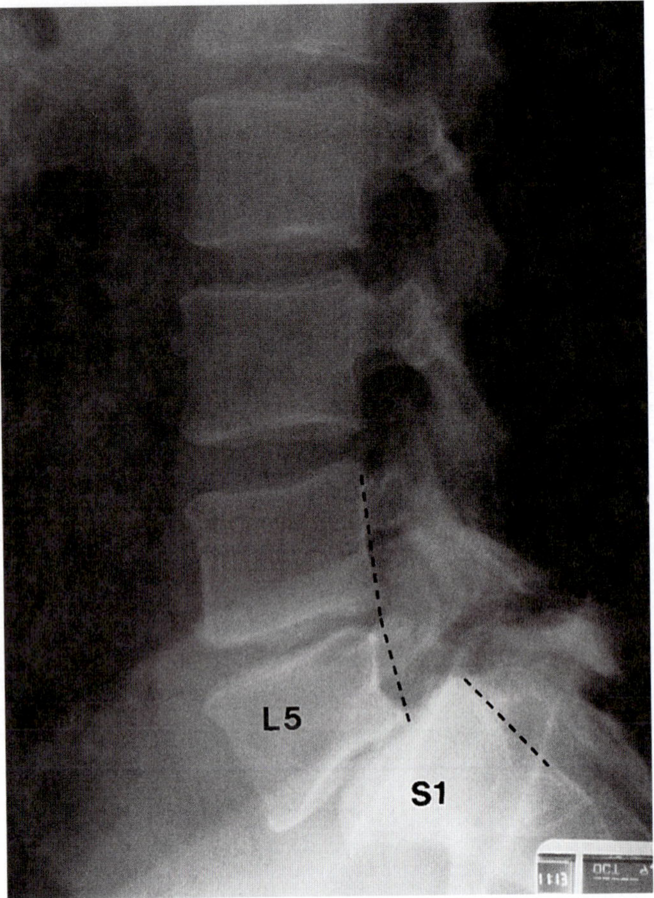

Figure 18-10. Spondylolysis with resulting grade 2 spondylolisthesis.

EXERCISE 18-3

Assign codes to the following conditions using your ICD-9-CM code book.

1. Cervical spondylosis without myelopathy __________
2. Degenerative disc disease lumbar spine __________
3. Sciatica due to sitting on wallet __________
4. Chronic low back pain __________
5. Torticollis __________
6. Pain in neck __________
7. OA thoracic spine __________
8. Stenosis lumbosacral vertebra __________
9. Lumbago due to disc herniation at L4-L5 __________
10. Back pain due to postlaminectomy syndrome __________

Rheumatism, Excluding the Back (725-729)

Polymyalgia Rheumatica

Polymyalgia rheumatica, or PMR, is a syndrome that is characterized by severe aching and stiffness in the neck, shoulder girdle, and pelvic girdle. It is classified as a rheumatic disease, although its origin remains undetermined. It has been closely linked to temporal arteritis.

Fibromyalgia

Fibromyalgia, one of the most common diseases affecting the muscles, is characterized by widespread muscle pain associated with chronic fatigue. Other common symptoms of this condition include "brain fog," irritable bowel syndrome, sleep disorders, chronic headaches, anxiety, and depression. Fibromyalgia is a chronic condition that may be aggravated by weather conditions, infection, allergies, hormones, stress, and overexertion. Most available treatments focus on improving sleep and controlling pain.

Bursitis

Bursitis is inflammation of a bursa, which is a tiny, fluid-filled sac found between muscles, tendons, and bones designed to reduce friction and facilitate movement. Symptoms of bursitis include pain and tenderness when the affected body part is moved, limited range of motion, and edema or swelling. Areas most affected are the shoulders, elbows, hips, and knees. Bursitis may be caused by trauma, overuse of the joint, infection, or diseases such as gout and RA.

EXAMPLE Patient is being seen for bursitis left olecranon process, 726.33.

EXAMPLE Patient is being treated for subpatellar bursitis, 726.69.

Rhabdomyolysis

Rhabdomyolysis is the breakdown of muscle fibers that results in the release of muscle fiber contents into the circulation. Some of these contents are toxic to the kidney, frequently resulting in kidney damage. Some inherited disorders such as carnitine palmityltransferase, phosphofructokinase deficiency, and phosphoglycerate kinase deficiency can lead to muscle injury with exercise and rhabdomyolysis. Some of the most common causes include the following:

- Muscle exertion (physical, related to convulsions or to heat injury)
- Trauma-crush syndromes and pseudo-crush syndrome
- Muscle ischemia related to arterial occlusion or insufficiency
- Burns
- Repetitive muscle injury (bongo drumming, torture)
- Status epilepticus
- Drug overdose
- Extended periods of muscle pressure

EXAMPLE Rhabdomyolysis due to intractable status epilepticus
Patient was diagnosed with epilepsy in childhood, 345.31, 728.88.

Necrotizing Fasciitis

Necrotizing fasciitis, or "flesh-eating disease," is a rare but serious condition in which an infection occurs in the tissues below the skin (Figure 18-11). The tissues may quickly die because of poor blood supply, possibly leading to the death of the patient. Necrotizing fasciitis is usually caused by group A streptococcus (the same bacterium that causes strep throat) and is often preceded by an injury to the skin.

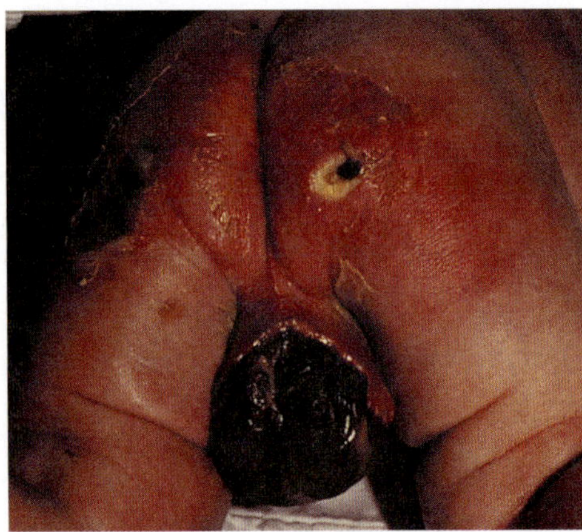

Figure 18-11. Necrotizing fasciitis.

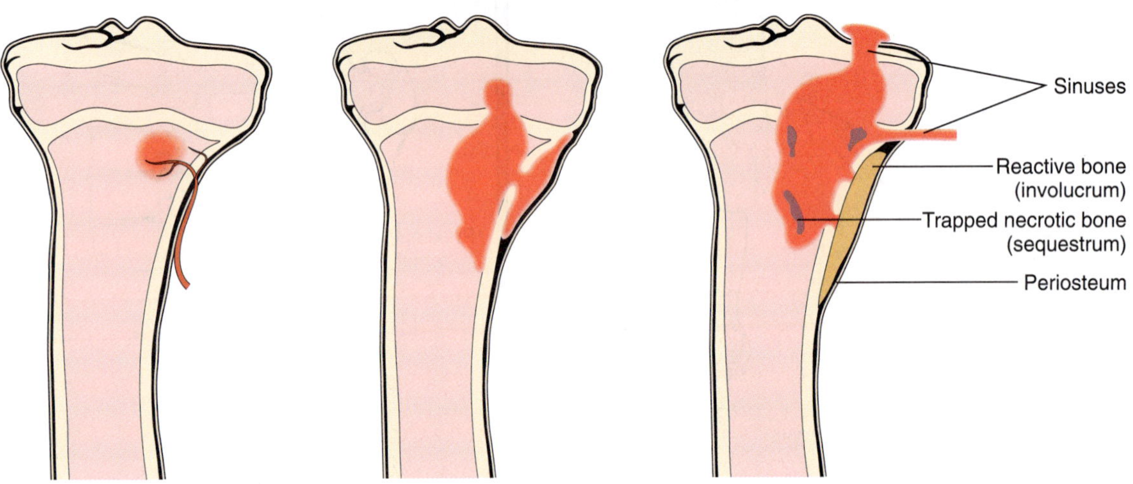

Figure 18-12. Progression of osteomyelitis. Bacterial growth results in bone destruction and abscess formation.

EXERCISE 18-4

Assign codes to the following conditions using your ICD-9-CM code book.

1. Necrotizing fasciitis due to group A strep with gangrene right leg ____________
2. Acute renal failure due to rhabdomyolysis ____________
3. Pain due to bursitis left shoulder ____________
4. Insomnia due to fibromyalgia ____________
5. De Quervain's disease ____________

Osteopathies, Chondropathies, and Acquired Musculoskeletal Deformities (730-739)

Osteomyelitis

Osteomyelitis is an infection of the bone that often starts in another part of the body and spreads to the bone via the blood (Figure 18-12). In children, the long bones are usually affected. In adults, the vertebrae and the pelvis are the most commonly affected areas. *Staphylococcus aureus* bacteria are usually the cause of acute osteomyelitis. This organism may enter the bloodstream through a wound or a contaminated intravenous needle. Chronic osteomyelitis results when bone tissue dies as a result of the lost blood supply. Risk factors include recent trauma, diabetes, hemodialysis, and intravenous (IV) drug abuse. People who have had a splenectomy are also at higher risk for osteomyelitis. Prolonged IV antibiotic therapy may be required.

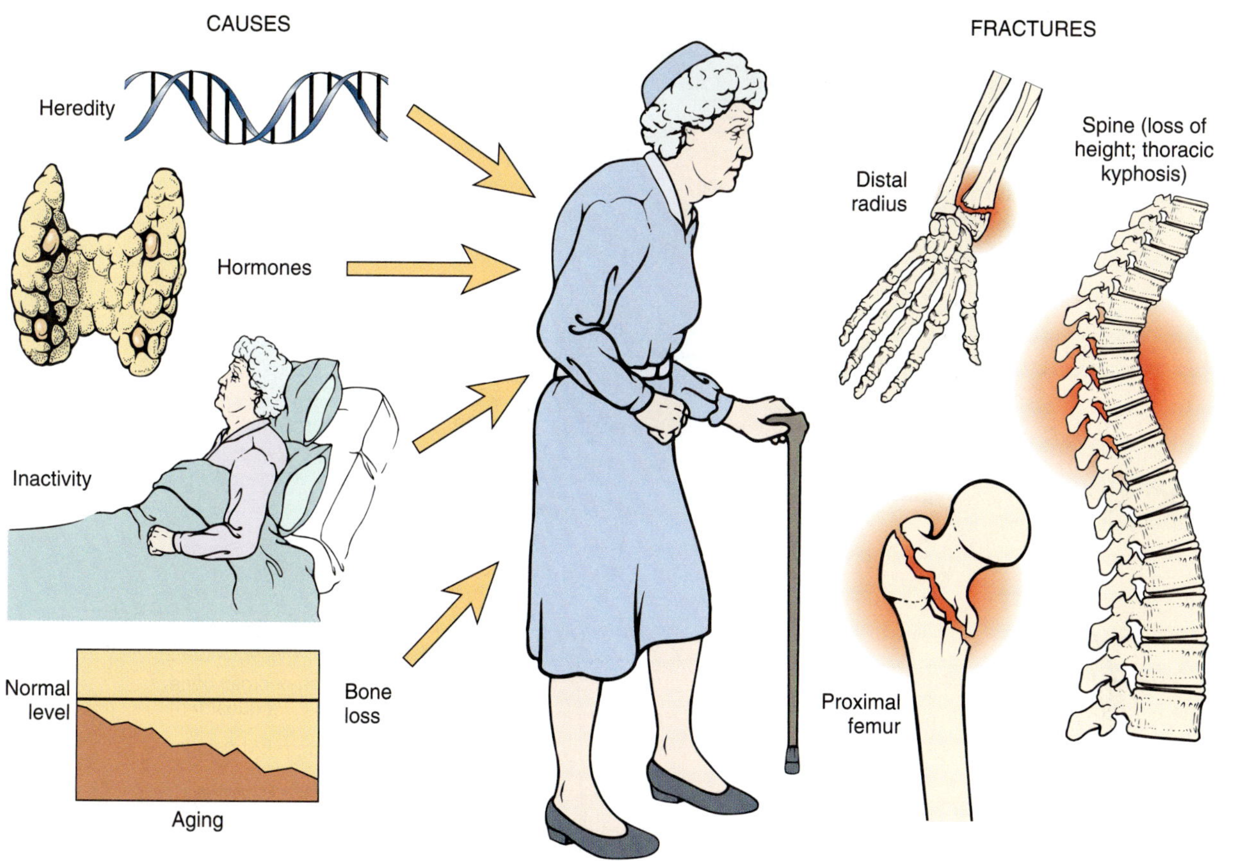

Figure 18-13. Causes and results of osteoporosis.

EXAMPLE Subacute osteomyelitis sacrum with decubitus sacral ulcer
Staphylococcus aureus is the causative organism, 730.08, 707.03, 041.11.

EXAMPLE Chronic osteomyelitis left ankle, 730.17.

Osteoporosis

Osteoporosis is a metabolic bone disorder that results in decreased bone mass and density. Osteoporosis, which is most common in older persons, particularly postmenopausal women, may also occur as the result of other diseases such as hyperparathyroidism or Cushing's syndrome; use of steroids may contribute to bone loss. Individuals with osteoporosis are susceptible for pathologic fractures. These fractures most often occur in the vertebrae of the spine, wrists, and hips (Figure 18-13).

EXAMPLE Patient is being treated for postmenopausal osteoporosis, 733.01.

EXAMPLE Patient has osteoporosis due to long-term use of prednisone for Crohn's disease, 733.09, 555.9, V58.65, E932.0.

Pathologic Fractures and Fracture Aftercare

A **pathologic fracture** is a break in a bone that occurs because of underlying disorders that weaken the bone, including malignancy, benign bone tumors, metabolic disorders, infection, and osteoporosis. A pathologic fracture may result from normal stress placed on an abnormal bone. Fractures may occur spontaneously in individuals with diseased bones as the result of minor exertion or trauma. Because the bone is already diseased, the healing

process of the fracture can be complicated by delayed healing, nonunion, pseudarthrosis, necrosis, and infection. A fracture cannot be coded as both a traumatic fracture and a pathologic fracture; it is one or the other. Only a physician can determine whether the severity of trauma corresponds with the injury. Compression fractures of the spine are often pathologic, but a thorough review of the record and/or a physician query may be necessary to determine the appropriate fracture code.

Active treatment for a pathologic fracture includes surgery, an emergency room encounter, and/or evaluation and treatment by a new physician. According to the guidelines, when a patient is receiving active treatment, the acute fracture code is assigned (733.1X).

Following the period of active treatment of a pathologic fracture, other encounters may be necessary. These encounters are assigned aftercare V codes. Aftercare may include a cast change or removal, removal of a fixation device, medication adjustments, and other follow up visits.

EXAMPLE Elderly woman with osteoporosis sustains a spontaneous fracture of the lumbar spine after removing a heavy turkey roaster from the oven, 733.13, 733.00.

EXAMPLE Patient had a cast change for pathologic radial fracture, V54.22.

EXAMPLE Pathologic fracture distal left femur due to osteosarcoma femur, 733.15, 170.7.

Spinal Deformities

Sometimes, the normal curvatures of the spine are altered. **Lordosis** is an exaggerated inward curvature of the spine that may be caused by increased abdominal girth due to obesity, pregnancy, or abdominal tumor (Figure 18-14, *A*). Improved posture, exercise, and weight loss can often alleviate symptoms. **Kyphosis** is an excessive posterior curvature of the thoracic spine that may not be detected until a hump in the upper back is noticeable (Figure 18-14, *B*). In older people, particularly women, osteoporosis is often the cause. If it occurs in children or adolescents, the exact cause may have to be determined, so that the best treatment approach can be selected. **Scoliosis** is a lateral or sideways curvature of the spine (Figure 18-15). School screening programs may detect spinal abnormalities. Varying degrees

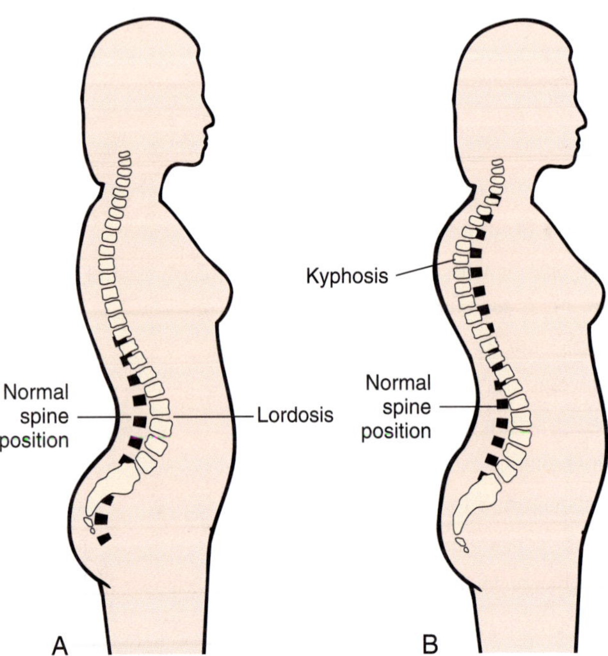

Figure 18-14. **A,** Lordosis. **B,** Kyphosis.

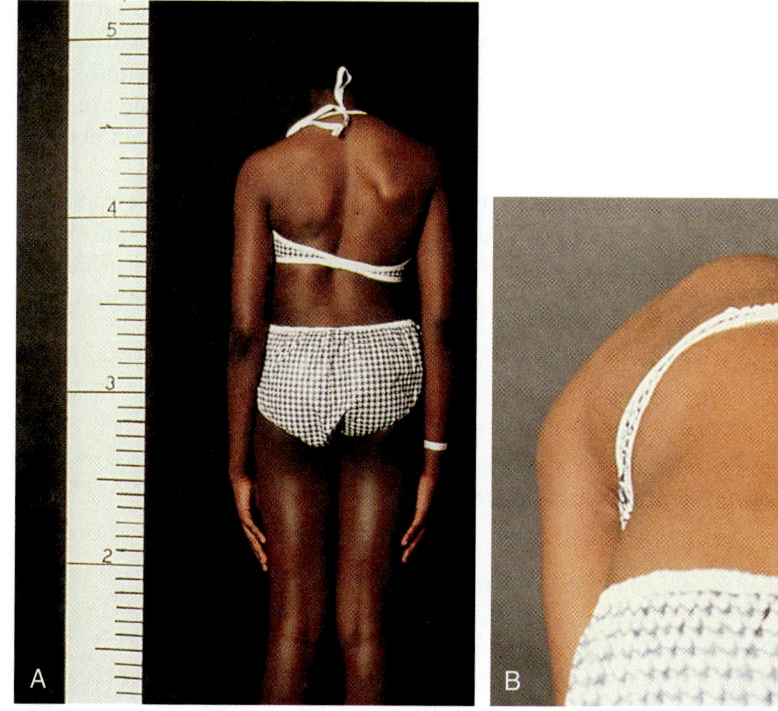

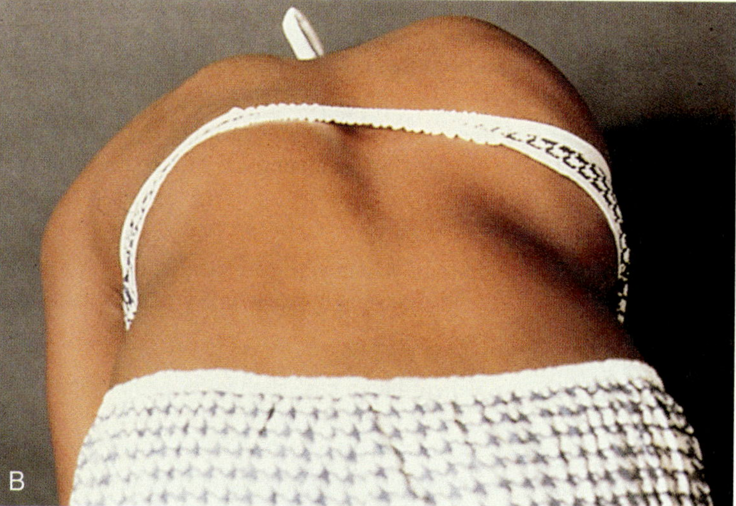

Figure 18-15. Scoliosis. **A,** Note scapular asymmetry in the upright position. **B,** Bending forward reveals a mild rib hump deformity.

of abnormality may be observed, and often, conservative medical management is attempted. In severe cases, the performance of procedures that fuse the vertebrae and the application of internal fixation devices such as rods, wires, plates, and/or screws may be necessary to correct the problem.

EXAMPLE The patient is being treated conservatively for kyphoscoliosis, 737.30.

EXAMPLE Postlaminectomy lordosis, 737.21.

EXAMPLE Patient has back, buttock, and leg pain due to acquired lumbar spondylolisthesis, 738.4.

EXERCISE 18-5

Assign codes to the following conditions using your ICD-9-CM code book.

1. Kyphosis due to osteoporosis __________
2. Osteomyelitis with periostitis, right tibia. Cultures did not grow any organisms. __________
3. Osteochondritis dissecans __________
4. Pathologic fracture, left wrist, due to osteoporosis __________
5. Stress fracture, right lower leg __________
6. Talipes planus (acquired) __________
7. Chest pain due to costochondritis __________
8. Pectus excavatum, acquired __________
9. Cast change for pathologic fracture, right wrist __________
10. Nontraumatic slipped upper femoral epiphysis __________

V CODES

In the past, V codes have been considered primarily for use in the outpatient setting. This has changed with the addition of more V codes each year. As was discussed in Chapter 8, it may be difficult to locate V codes in the index. Coders often say, "I did not know there was a V code for that." Refer to Chapter 8 for a listing of common main terms used to locate V codes.

It is important for the coder to be familiar with different types and uses of V codes.

V10.81	Personal history of malignant neoplasm—bone
V13.4	Personal history of arthritis
V13.51	Personal history of pathologic fracture
V13.52	Personal history of stress fracture
V13.59	Personal history of other musculoskeletal disorders
V17.7	Family history of arthritis
V17.8	Family history of other musculoskeletal disease
V43.60	Organ or tissue replaced by other means—unspecified joint
V43.61	Organ or tissue replaced by other means—shoulder
V43.62	Organ or tissue replaced by other means—elbow
V43.63	Organ or tissue replaced by other means—wrist
V43.64	Organ or tissue replaced by other means—hip
V43.65	Organ or tissue replaced by other means—knee
V43.66	Organ or tissue replaced by other means—ankle
V43.69	Organ or tissue replaced by other means—other
V43.7	Organ or tissue replaced by other means—limb
V45.4	Arthrodesis status
V49.0	Deficiencies of limbs
V49.1	Mechanical problems with limbs
V49.2	Motor problems with limbs
V49.3	Sensory problems with limbs
V49.4	Disfigurements of limbs
V49.5	Other problems of limbs
V49.60	Upper limb amputation status—unspecified level
V49.61	Upper limb amputation status—thumb
V49.62	Upper limb amputation status—other fingers
V49.63	Upper limb amputation status—hand
V49.64	Upper limb amputation status—wrist
V49.65	Upper limb amputation status—below elbow
V49.66	Upper limb amputation status—above elbow
V49.47	Upper limb amputation status—shoulder
V49.70	Lower limb amputation status—unspecified level
V49.71	Lower limb amputation status—great toe
V49.72	Lower limb amputation status—other toe(s)
V49.73	Lower limb amputation status—foot
V49.74	Lower limb amputation status—ankle
V49.75	Lower limb amputation status—below knee
V49.76	Lower limb amputation status—above knee
V49.77	Lower limb amputation status—hip
V52.0	Fitting and adjustment of prosthetic device/implant—artificial arm
V52.1	Fitting and adjustment of prosthetic device/implant—artificial leg
V52.8	Fitting and adjustment of prosthetic device/implant—other specified prosthetic device

V53.7	Fitting and adjustment of orthopedic devices
V54.01	Encounter for removal of internal fixation device
V54.02	Encounter for lengthening/adjustment of growth rod
V54.09	Other aftercare involving internal fixation device
V54.20	Aftercare for healing pathologic fracture of arm, unspecified
V54.21	Aftercare for healing pathologic fracture of upper arm
V54.22	Aftercare for healing pathologic fracture of lower arm
V54.23	Aftercare for healing pathologic fracture of hip
V54.24	Aftercare for healing pathologic fracture of leg, unspecified
V54.25	Aftercare for healing pathologic fracture of upper leg
V54.26	Aftercare for healing pathologic fracture of lower leg
V54.27	Aftercare for healing pathologic fracture of vertebra
V54.29	Aftercare for healing pathologic fracture of other bone
V54.81	Aftercare following joint replacement
V54.89	Other orthopedic aftercare
V54.9	Unspecified orthopedic aftercare
V57.1	Other physical therapy
V57.21	Encounter for occupational therapy
V57.81	Orthotic training
V57.89	Other specified rehabilitation procedure
V58.78	Aftercare following surgery of the musculoskeletal system, not elsewhere classified (NEC)
V64.43	Arthroscopic surgical procedure converted to open procedure
V67.4	Follow-up examination—following treatment of healed fracture
V82.1	Special screening—rheumatoid arthritis
V82.2	Special screening—other rheumatic disorder
V82.3	Special screening—congenital dislocation of hip
V82.81	Special screening—osteoporosis

EXAMPLE Patient is status post knee replacement 1 year ago, V43.65.

EXAMPLE Patient with a family history of rheumatoid arthritis is being screened for rheumatoid arthritis, V82.1, V17.7.

EXAMPLE Patient is receiving aftercare for healing pathological fracture of humerus V54.21.

EXERCISE 18-6

Assign codes to the following conditions using your ICD-9-CM code book.

1. Status post knee replacement ____________
2. Dual-energy x-ray absorptiometry (DEXA) scan screening for osteoporosis ____________
3. Aftercare for healing pathologic fracture cervical spine ____________
4. Amputation status right foot ____________
5. Encounter to remove screw from tibia ____________
6. Aftercare for pathological fracture femur ____________

COMMON TREATMENTS

Many conditions or diseases of the musculoskeletal system cause pain and inflammation. Anti-inflammatory agents reduce inflammation in joints and muscles, antiarthritics are used

to treat arthritic symptoms, and muscle relaxants may be helpful for acute low back pain and muscle spasms. Physical therapy and chiropractic treatment may be beneficial for many conditions. Medical treatment is usually tried before surgical intervention is considered.

CONDITION	MEDICATION/TREATMENT
Rheumatoid arthritis	Celecoxib (Celebrex), gold compounds such as Ridaura and Myochrysine
Osteoarthritis	Analgesics for pain Nonsteroidal anti-inflammatory drugs (NSAIDs) for pain and inflammation
Fibromyalgia	Analgesics for pain, muscle relaxants, antidepressants, and sleep aids
Bursitis	Rest, immobilization, ice, NSAIDs
Rhabdomyolysis	Provide treatment of the cause; watch for and treat manifestations such as hypovolemia, hyperkalemia, metabolic acidosis, acute renal failure, or disseminated intravascular coagulation (DIC)
Necrotizing fasciitis	Aggressive antibiotic therapy with surgical debridement
Osteomyelitis	Antibiotics depending on causative organism
Osteoporosis	Alendronate (Fosamax), Boniva (ibandronate) calcitonin, calcium with vitamin D

PROCEDURES

Some procedures that may be related to diseases of the musculoskeletal system and connective tissue may be located in the following chapter of the Procedure Tabular:

Chapter 14 Operations on the Musculoskeletal System (76-84)

Arthroscopic Surgery

Arthroscopic surgery is a minimally invasive surgery that involves the use of highly specialized instruments to perform surgery through very small incisions (½ inch) on joints. Advantages of arthroscopic surgery include small incisions, minimal scar tissue and less pain after surgery with quicker recovery. Arthroscopic procedures can be performed on any of the joints and joint structures. If an arthroscopic approach is used to perform a definitive procedure (e.g., biopsies, meniscectomies, ligament repairs), the approach is not coded. Occasionally, an arthroscopic procedure is performed for diagnostic purposes, and no additional therapeutic procedures are performed (Figure 18-16).

EXAMPLE Arthroscopic examination of the left knee for chronic pain. All joint structures appear to be intact, 719.46, 80.26.

EXAMPLE Arthroscopic meniscectomy for torn medial meniscus (old injury), 717.3, 80.6.

Joint Replacement

Joint replacement consists of removal of an arthritic or damaged joint and replacement with an artificial joint, which is also known as a prosthesis. Materials used in total joint replacement are designed to enable the joint to move similarly to a normal joint. The prosthesis is generally composed of two parts; a metal piece fits closely into a matching sturdy plastic piece (Figure 18-17). Several metals, including stainless steel, alloys of cobalt and chrome, and titanium, are used. The plastic material is durable and wear resistant (polyethylene). Special codes (00.70 to 00.87) have been created to identify the bearing surface materials that are used in the prosthetic implants/components for replacements, revisions, and resurfacing of the knee and hip joints. A plastic bone cement may be used to anchor

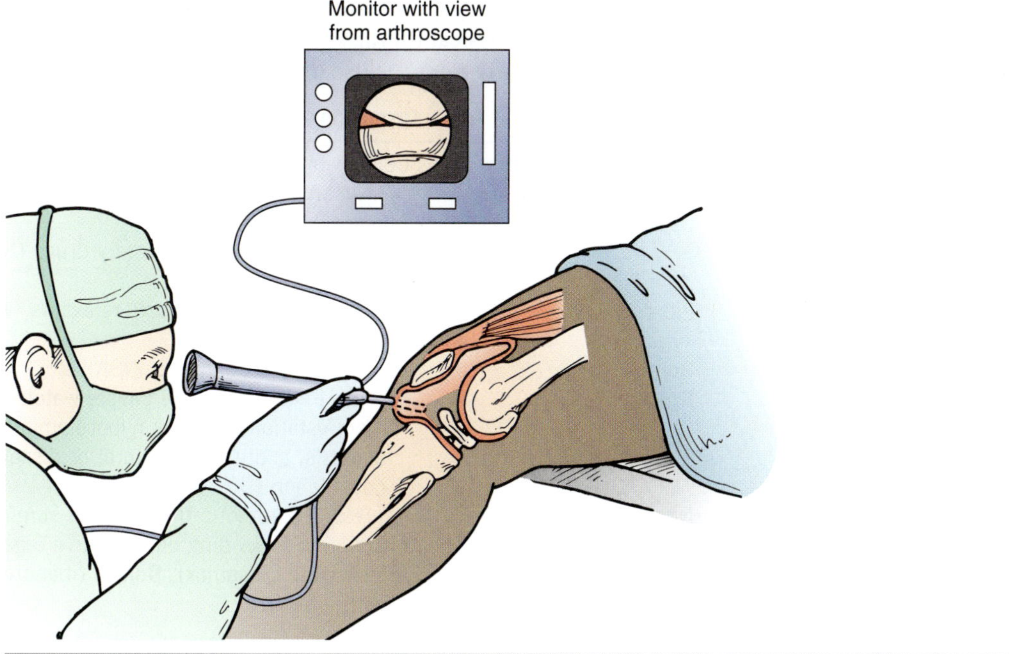

Figure 18-16. Arthroscopic examination of a joint.

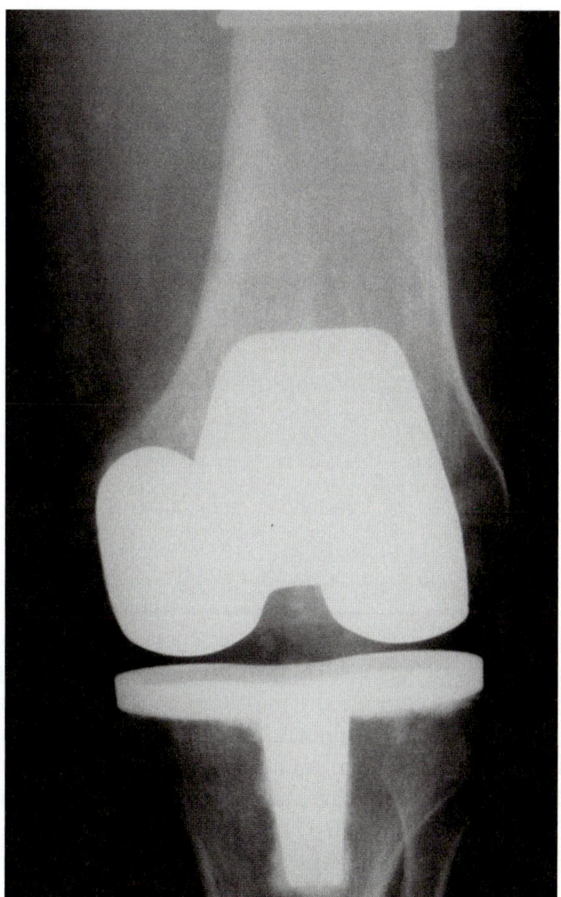

Figure 18-17. Total knee replacement for osteoarthritis.

the prosthesis into the bone. Hip and knee replacements are the most common joint replacements, but other joints, including the ankle, foot, shoulder, elbow, and fingers, can be replaced. In cases in which the disease process does not affect the entire joint, partial replacement may be performed. Other options besides total joint replacement procedures are available. A resurfacing procedure may be an option. A surface replacement procedure leaves more of the patient's bone in place with resurfacing of the affected area of the joint. As with replacement procedures, resurfacing can involve partial or total joint resurfacing.

Common complications of joint replacement include infection, blood clot, nerve injury, loosening, dislocation, wear and tear, and breakage of the prosthesis. It may be necessary to remove the prosthesis and insert a new prosthesis. According to *Coding Clinic* (1997:3Q: p13),[3] "any time the joint is replaced or revised after the initial replacement this would be considered a revision."

EXAMPLE

Osteoarthritis both knees. Patient is hospitalized for right partial knee replacement, 715.36, 81.54.

EXAMPLE

Patient dislocated right hip prosthesis and was taken to the OR for total hip revision, 996.42, V43.64, 81.53.

Vertebroplasty/Kyphoplasty

Percutaneous vertebroplasty (PV) is a technique that is used to treat pain caused by compression fractures of the vertebrae. Under x-ray guidance, an acrylic cement is injected through a needle into a collapsed or weakened vertebra. This stabilizes the fracture, allowing the patient to resume normal activity and decrease the use of analgesics. PV does not reverse osteoporosis or prevent future compression fractures. This procedure is usually performed by interventional radiologists. According to *Coding Clinic* (2002:2Q:p14-15),[4] the code 81.65 for vertebroplasty includes stabilization of the fracture, so it is not necessary to assign an additional code for the stabilization.

Kyphoplasty, similar to PV, is used to treat fractures of the spine; however, in kyphoplasty, a special balloon device is inserted into the compacted vertebrae in an attempt to restore vertebrae to a more normal state by improving the alignment of the spine. After the balloon has been removed, the cavity is filled with a cement-like material, to stabilize the fracture. Kyphoplasty is usually performed under fluoroscopic guidance through a small incision in the back.

EXAMPLE

Compression fractures T11-T12 due to osteoporosis. Percutaneous vertebroplasty was performed in radiology, 733.13, 733.00, 81.65.

Spinal Decompression/Fusion

Spinal decompression is a surgical procedure that frees space for nerves in the spinal canal. A number of different surgical methods, including laminectomy, laminotomy, laminoplasty, foraminotomy, and anterior discectomy, can be performed to accomplish a decompression. Although in many cases, decompression involves removal of tissue that is constricting or compressing nerve structures, in some cases, the spine becomes unstable, and spinal fusion is performed at the time of the decompression. At times the spine becomes unstable and painful following a decompression; at this point a fusion may be required.

Spinal fusion is the creation of a solid bone bridge between two or more adjacent vertebrae to create stability between levels of the spine. Fusion is a gradual process (6-9 months or longer) in which bone is grown across desired areas to form a solid fusion. Bone grafts, spinal instrumentation, casts, and/or braces are used to facilitate and promote the fusion process. If a fusion fails to heal or fuse properly, this is called a nonunion or pseudarthrosis;

repeat or revision surgery may be required. A bone graft may be obtained from a variety of sources. Bone may be harvested from the patient's (autologous) spine or from the iliac crest. Bone graft material can also be obtained from a bone bank (harvested from cadavers [allograft]). Synthetic bone materials made from demineralized bone matrix (DBM) and calcium phosphates or hydroxyapatites (some derived from sea corral) may also be used. The use of metal devices, also called implants or instrumentation (e.g., screws, rods, plates, cables, wires), can facilitate correction of a deformed spine and may increase the probability of attaining solid spinal fusion. Spinal instrumentation can be placed in the front or in the back portion of the spine. Devices are usually made of metal, commonly, stainless steel or titanium. Spinal instrumentation is gradually covered by scar tissue and sometimes by new growth of bone. Even when the spine has healed solidly, the instrumentation is rarely removed.

A 360-degree spinal fusion is defined in *Coding Clinic* (2003:2Q:p20)[5] as "a spinal fusion of both the anterior and posterior portions of the spine during the same operative session. Historically, this procedure was performed using both an anterior approach and a posterior approach by making incisions both in the front and back. Advances in medical technology and surgical techniques now allow the fusion of the anterior and posterior vertebra during the same operative session using a single incision—usually via the lateral transverse approach." Sometimes a spinal fusion is performed as a "staged procedure" with a posterior fusion performed one day, and an anterior fusion is performed a few days later.

During any spinal fusion procedure, the documentation should be reviewed to ascertain whether this is a new fusion or a refusion. To correctly assign the spinal fusion code, it must be determined whether the approach was anterior or posterior, or whether some other approach was used. In addition to the appropriate code to identify spinal fusion, an additional code (81.62-81.64) must be assigned for the total number of vertebrae fused (Figure 18-8).

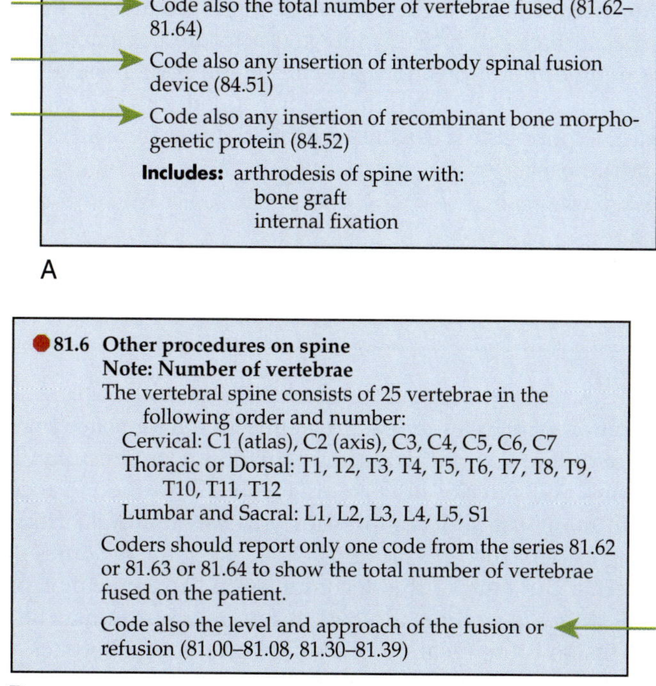

81.0 Spinal fusion
Code also the total number of vertebrae fused (81.62–81.64)
Code also any insertion of interbody spinal fusion device (84.51)
Code also any insertion of recombinant bone morphogenetic protein (84.52)
Includes: arthrodesis of spine with:
bone graft
internal fixation

A

81.6 Other procedures on spine
Note: Number of vertebrae
The vertebral spine consists of 25 vertebrae in the following order and number:
Cervical: C1 (atlas), C2 (axis), C3, C4, C5, C6, C7
Thoracic or Dorsal: T1, T2, T3, T4, T5, T6, T7, T8, T9, T10, T11, T12
Lumbar and Sacral: L1, L2, L3, L4, L5, S1
Coders should report only one code from the series 81.62 or 81.63 or 81.64 to show the total number of vertebrae fused on the patient.
Code also the level and approach of the fusion or refusion (81.00–81.08, 81.30–81.39)

B

Figure 18-18. Entries for spinal fusion **(A)** and other spine procedures **(B)** require the assignment of additional codes to indicate the number of vertebrae fused.

Also, if an interbody spinal fusion device has been inserted or if recombinant bone morphogenetic protein (BMP) has been used, an additional code is assigned.

EXAMPLE

The patient was admitted for surgical intervention for cervical disc herniation with myelopathy. Discectomy at C3 and spinal fusion of C2-C3 and C3-C4 were performed via the anterior approach, 722.71, 81.02, 81.62, 80.51.

EXAMPLE

The patient is a 16-year-old male with progressive infantile idiopathic scoliosis with posterior spinal fusion of T4 to L3 and segmental spinal instrumentation for T4 to L3. Bone graft was obtained from the right iliac bone, 737.32, 81.05, 81.64, 77.79.

EXERCISE 18-7

Assign codes for all diagnoses and procedures using your ICD-9-CM code book.

1. Bone biopsy left femur which confirmed acute and chronic osteomyelitis __________
2. Excision Baker's cyst __________
3. Partial hip replacement for OA right hip __________
4. Removal of fixation device lumbar spine __________
5. Arthroscopy right knee. Mild osteoarthritis __________
6. Hammer toe repair __________
7. Necrotizing fasciitis with excisional debridement right arm __________
8. Pathologic fracture T12-L1 due to postmenopausal osteoporosis. Kyphoplasty was performed __________

DOCUMENTATION/REIMBURSEMENT/MS-DRGs

Often, coding difficulties are due to lack of documentation. Sometimes pathology, radiology, and other test results are not available at the time of discharge or when the physician is dictating the discharge summary or is reporting the final diagnoses.

Pathological Fracture Versus Traumatic Fracture

EXAMPLE

Patient was admitted from the emergency room with a fractured hip. The patient has severe osteoporosis and had fallen on the morning of admission.

DIAGNOSES	CODES	MS-DRG	RW
Pathologic fracture hip due to osteoporosis	733.14, 733.00, E888.9	544	0.9395
Traumatic fracture hip in patient with osteoporosis	820.8, 733.00, E888.9	536	0.7340

A physician query may be necessary to make sure that the appropriate MS-DRG is assigned for optimal reimbursement.

Correct Procedure Code

EXAMPLE

Patient was admitted for resurfacing of femoral head due to osteoarthritis, 715.53, 00.86.

DIAGNOSES	CODES	MS-DRG	RW
Osteoarthritis hip	715.53	470	1.9871
Resurfacing femoral	00.86		
Osteoarthritis hip	715.53	468	2.4545
Revision femoral	00.72		

In this example, an error was made when resurfacing of the femoral head was coded as a revision. This error would have resulted in an overpayment to the facility.

CHAPTER REVIEW EXERCISE

Assign codes for all diagnoses and procedures, including all applicable V and E codes and procedures.

1. Osteitis deformans ____________
2. Wry neck ____________
3. Hallux valgus ____________
4. Frozen shoulder ____________
5. Plantar fasciitis ____________
6. Recurrent dislocation right thumb ____________
7. Osteoporosis due to long-term use of steroids ____________
8. Instability left ankle ____________
9. Ganglion tendon sheath of the right wrist with removal ____________
10. Tennis elbow ____________
11. Polymyalgia rheumatica ____________
12. Myositis ____________
13. Pain in both wrists ____________
14. Avascular necrosis hip joint due to sickle cell (hemoglobin SS) disease ____________
15. Osteogenesis imperfecta ____________
16. Right above the knee amputation (AKA) ____________
17. Housemaid's knee ____________
18. Scleroderma with lung involvement ____________
19. Arthropathy due to Crohn's disease ____________
20. Felty's syndrome ____________
21. Pyogenic arthritis left knee due to *Staphylococcus aureus* ____________
22. Osteoarthritis right shoulder treated with steroid injection ____________
23. Deformans osteodystrophy ____________
24. Chondromalacia right patella ____________

Write the correct answer(s) in the blank(s) provided.

25. What is the appropriate fifth digit subclassification for knee joint?

____

26. Which MS-DRG has higher reimbursement: pathologic fracture or traumatic fracture?

____

Why? _______________________________

27. Another name for osteoarthritis.

____

28. List 4 symptoms of SLE.
   1. _______________________________
   2. _______________________________
   3. _______________________________
   4. _______________________________

29. Which individuals are at risk for osteoporosis?

____

30. List 3 examples of aftercare for a pathologic fracture.
   1. _______________________________
   2. _______________________________
   3. _______________________________

CHAPTER GLOSSARY

Anterior: front of the body or an organ.

Arthropathy: disease that affects the joints.

Arthroscopic: minimally invasive surgery that involves the use of highly specialized instruments to perform surgery through very small incisions on joints.

Bursitis: inflammation of a bursa, which is a tiny, fluid-filled sac that is found between muscles, tendons, and bones that reduces friction and facilitates movement.

Caudal: toward the tail.

Cranial: toward the head.

Distal: farther from the median plane; term is often used to describe a location in the limbs.

Dorsal: back of the body or an organ.

Dorsopathies: conditions or diseases that affect the back or spine.

Facet joints: small, stabilizing joints located between and behind adjacent vertebrae.

Fascia: tissue just below the skin that covers and separates the underlying layers of muscle.

Fibromyalgia: one of the most common diseases affecting the muscles; it is characterized by widespread muscle pain associated with chronic fatigue.

Hematopoiesis: development of blood cells that occurs in the bone marrow and lymphatic tissue of normal adults.

Inferior: position of the body or an organ relative to the vertical axis of the body.

Joints: means of joining two bones together.

Juvenile rheumatoid arthritis: type of arthritis that affects children, usually between the ages of 2 and 5 years.

Kyphoplasty: procedure performed to treat and stabilize fractures of the spine.

Kyphosis: excessive posterior curvature of the thoracic spine that may not be detected until a hump in the upper back is noticeable.

Lateral: position of a structure that is to the side of the body.

Ligaments: dense, fibrous bands of connective tissue that provide stability for the joint.

Lordosis: exaggerated inward curvature of the spine that may be caused by increased abdominal girth due to obesity, pregnancy, or abdominal tumor.

Medial: position of a structure closer to the median plane than is another structure in the body.

Myelopathy: compression of the spinal cord.

Necrotizing fasciitis (or "flesh-eating disease"): a rare but serious condition in which an infection occurs in the tissues below the skin.

Osteoarthritis: type of arthritis that develops as the result of wear and tear on the joints.

Osteomyelitis: infection of the bone that often starts in another part of the body and spreads to the bone via the blood.

Osteoporosis: metabolic bone disorder that results in decreased bone mass and density.

Pathologic fracture: break in a bone that occurs because of underlying disorders that weaken the bone, including malignancy, benign bone tumor, metabolic disorder, infection, and osteoporosis.

Percutaneous vertebroplasty: technique in which x-ray guidance is used to inject an acrylic cement through a needle into a collapsed or weakened vertebra; procedure is performed to treat pain caused by compression fractures of the vertebrae.

Polymyalgia rheumatica: syndrome classified as a rheumatic disease that is characterized by severe aching and stiffness in the neck, shoulder girdle, and pelvic girdle.

Posterior: back of the body or an organ.

Postlaminectomy syndrome (or Failed Back Syndrome): terms used to describe patients who have undergone spine surgery and have some degree of recurrent spinal and/or leg pain due to the build up of scar tissue.

Primary osteoarthritis: idiopathic degenerative condition that occurs in previously intact joints, with no apparent initiating factor.

Prone: lying on the stomach, face down.

Proximal: closer to the median plane.

Radiculopathy: compression of a nerve root.

Rhabdomyolysis: breakdown of muscle fibers resulting in the release of muscle fiber contents into the circulation.

Rheumatoid arthritis: chronic, inflammatory systemic disease that affects the joints, often causing deformity.

Scleroderma: chronic, progressive disease characterized by hardening of the skin and scarring of internal organs.

Scoliosis: deviation of the vertical line of the spine.

Secondary osteoarthritis: degenerative disease of the joints that results from some predisposing condition such as trauma or disease.

Spinal decompression: surgical procedure that frees space for the nerves in the spinal canal.

Spinal fusion: the creation of a solid bone bridge between two or more adjacent vertebrae to enhance stability between levels of the spine.

Spinal stenosis: narrowing of the central spinal canal or the areas of the spine where the nerve roots exit (neuroforamina).

Spondylolisthesis: condition in which one vertebra slips on another.

Spondylosis (or spinal osteoarthritis): degenerative disorder that may cause loss of normal spinal structure and function.

Superior: position of the body or an organ relative to the vertical axis of the body.

Supine: lying on the back, face up.

Systemic lupus erythematosus: chronic, inflammatory autoimmune disease that can damage connective tissue anywhere in the body.

Ventral: front of the body or an organ.

CHAPTER 19

Injuries

(ICD-9-CM Chapter 17, Codes 800-995)

CHAPTER OUTLINE

LEARNING OBJECTIVES

- Apply and assign the correct ICD-9-CM codes in accordance with Official Guidelines for Coding and Reporting
- Identify the various types of injuries
- Assign the correct V codes, E codes, and procedure codes related to injuries
- Identify common treatments, medications, and diagnostic tests
- Explain the importance of documentation in relation to MS-DRGs for reimbursement

ABBREVIATIONS

AKA above-knee amputation
ATV all-terrain vehicle
CHI closed head injury
CT computerized tomography
FB foreign body
ICD-9-CM *International Classification of Diseases, 9th Revision, Clinical Modification*
LOC loss of consciousness
MRI magnetic resonance imaging
MS-DRG Medicare severity diagnosis-related group
MVA motor vehicle accident
OIG Office of the Inspector General
OR Operating Room
ORIF open reduction with internal fixation
SCI spinal cord injury
SLAP superior labrum anterior-posterior
TBI traumatic brain injury

ICD-9-CM Official Guidelines for Coding and Reporting

Please refer to the companion Evolve website for the most current guidelines.

17. Chapter 17: Injury and Poisoning (800-999)

a. Coding of Injuries

When coding injuries, assign separate codes for each injury unless a combination code is provided, in which case the combination code is assigned. Multiple injury codes are provided in ICD-9-CM, but should not be assigned unless information for a more specific code is not available. These codes are not to be used for normal, healing surgical wounds or to identify complications of surgical wounds.

The code for the most serious injury, as determined by the provider and the focus of treatment, is sequenced first.

1) Superficial injuries

Superficial injuries such as abrasions or contusions are not coded when associated with more severe injuries of the same site.

EXAMPLE

Abrasion with laceration to the left knee, 891.0.

Usually, when initial injuries are coded, E code(s) would describe the injury and place of occurrence. Because of the limited information given in these examples, it may not be possible to assign E code(s).

2) Primary injury with damage to nerves/blood vessels

When a primary injury results in minor damage to peripheral nerves or blood vessels, the primary injury is sequenced first with additional code(s) from categories 950-957, Injury to nerves and spinal cord, and/or 900-904, Injury to blood vessels. When the primary injury is to the blood vessels or nerves, that injury should be sequenced first.

EXAMPLE

Laceration of splenic artery and fracture of little finger due to trauma from being kicked and falling during a football game. Suture of laceration of splenic artery, 902.23, 816.00, E917.5, E849.4, 39.31.

b. Coding of Traumatic Fractures

The principles of multiple coding of injuries should be followed in coding fractures. Fractures of specified sites are coded individually by site in accordance with both the provisions within categories 800-829 and the level of detail furnished by medical record content. Combination categories for multiple fractures are provided for use when there is insufficient detail in the medical record (such as trauma cases transferred to another hospital), when the reporting form limits the number of codes that can be used in reporting pertinent clinical data, or when there is insufficient specificity at the fourth-digit or fifth-digit level. More specific guidelines are as follows:

1) **Acute Fractures vs. Aftercare**
Traumatic fractures are coded using the acute fracture codes (800-829) while the patient is receiving active treatment for the fracture. Examples of active treatment are: surgical treatment, emergency department encounter, and evaluation and treatment by a new physician.

EXAMPLE The patient suffered a blow-out fracture 1 week ago and is now being referred to a specialist for consultation, 802.6.

Fractures are coded using the aftercare codes (subcategories V54.0, V54.1, V54.8, or V54.9) for encounters after the patient has completed active treatment of the fracture and is receiving routine care for the fracture during the healing or recovery phase. Examples of fracture aftercare are: cast change or removal, removal of external or internal fixation device, medication adjustment, and follow up visits following fracture treatment.

EXAMPLE The patient is seen in follow-up for healing blow-out fracture, V54.19.

Care for complications of surgical treatment for fracture repairs during the healing or recovery phase should be coded with the appropriate complication codes.

Care of complications of fractures, such as malunion and nonunion, should be reported with the appropriate codes.

Pathologic fractures are not coded in the 800-829 range, but instead are assigned to subcategory 733.1. *See Section I.C.13.a for additional information.*

2) **Multiple fractures of same limb**
Multiple fractures of same limb classifiable to the same three-digit or four-digit category are coded to that category.

EXAMPLE Fractures of multiple metacarpal bones of the right hand, 815.09, E887.

3) **Multiple unilateral or bilateral fractures of same bone**
Multiple unilateral or bilateral fractures of same bone(s) but classified to different fourth-digit subdivisions (bone part) within the same three-digit category are coded individually by site.

EXAMPLE Closed fracture of right surgical neck of humerus and left open fracture of anatomic neck of humerus, 812.12, 812.01, E887.

4) **Multiple fracture categories 819 and 828**
Multiple fracture categories 819 and 828 classify bilateral fractures of both upper limbs (819) and both lower limbs (828), but without any detail at the fourth-digit level other than open and closed type of fractures.

5) **Multiple fractures sequencing**
Multiple fractures are sequenced in accordance with the severity of the fracture. The provider should be asked to list the fracture diagnoses in the order of severity.

EXAMPLE The patient had a fractured parietal bone of the skull and fracture of the left fifth rib, 800.00, 807.01, E887.

Apply the General Coding Guidelines as found in Chapter 5.

At the beginning of Chapter 17 in the ICD-9-CM code book, special instructions state, "Use E code(s) to identify the cause and intent of the injury or poisoning (E800-E999)" (Figure 19-1). It may be necessary to go back to Chapter 8 to review the guidelines for proper assignment and sequencing of E codes. Remember that E codes identify how an injury occurred and the intent. E codes also identify the place that an injury occurred. The Alphabetic Index used to locate E codes is a separate index that follows the Table of Drugs and Chemicals. Locating codes that identify the cause and/or intent of injury may be difficult. It is helpful to review the Index to become familiar with main terms used to locate E codes.

EXERCISE 19-1

Using the Alphabetic Index for E codes, assign E codes to the following.

1. Bite by spider ____________
2. Burn by cigar ____________
3. Entanglement in wheel of bike ____________
4. Self-inflicted hanging ____________
5. Shot by BB gun ____________

ANATOMY AND PHYSIOLOGY

The musculoskeletal chapter outlines the anatomy and physiology that is pertinent to injury. Internal organs and the blood vessels may also be involved in an injury. These are outlined in their respective body system chapters.

DISEASE CONDITIONS

Injury and Poisoning (800-999), Chapter 17 in your ICD-9-CM code book, covers a wide range of codes that will be discussed in the next three chapters of this textbook. Categories marked with an asterisk (*) are covered in this chapter. Chapter 20 discusses burns, adverse effects, and poisonings, and Chapter 21 is dedicated to complications associated

17. INJURY AND POISONING (800–999)

Use E code(s) to identify the cause and intent of the injury or poisoning (E800-E999)

Note:

1. The principle of multiple coding of injuries should be followed wherever possible. Combination categories for multiple injuries are provided for use when there is insufficient detail as to the nature of the individual conditions, or for primary tabulation purposes when it is more convenient to record a single code; otherwise, the component injuries should be coded separately.

   Where multiple sites of injury are specified in the titles, the word "with" indicates involvement of both sites, and the word "and" indicates involvement of either or both sites. The word "finger" includes thumb.

2. Categories for "late effect" of injuries are to be found at 905–909.

Figure 19-1. Instructional note regarding the use of E code(s) to identify the cause and intent of the injury or poisoning (E800-E999).

with surgical and medical care. Injury and poisoning codes are divided into the following categories:

CATEGORY	SECTION TITLES
*800-804	Fracture of Skull
*805-809	Fracture of Neck and Trunk
*810-819	Fracture of Upper Limb
*820-829	Fracture of Lower Limb
*830-839	Dislocation
*840-848	Sprains and Strains of Joints and Adjacent Muscles
*850-854	Intracranial Injury, Excluding Those With Skull Fracture
*860-869	Internal Injury of Thorax, Abdomen, and Pelvis
*870-879	Open Wound of Head, Neck, and Trunk
*880-887	Open Wound of Upper Limb
*890-897	Open Wound of Lower Limb
*900-904	Injury to Blood Vessels
905-909	Late Effects of Injuries, Poisonings, Toxic Effects, and Other External Causes
*910-919	Superficial Injury
*920-924	Contusion With Intact Skin Surface
*925-929	Crushing Injury
*930-939	Effects of Foreign Body Entering Through Orifice
940-949	Burns
*950-957	Injury to Nerves and Spinal Cord
958-959	Certain Traumatic Complications and Unspecified Injuries
	Poisoning by Drugs, Medicinals, and Biological Substances
	Toxic Effects of Substances Chiefly Nonmedicinal as to Source
	Other and Unspecified Effects of External Causes
	Complications of Surgical and Medical Care, Not Elsewhere Classified

Fractures (800-829)

Fractures are divided by the following anatomic sections:

800-804	Fracture of Skull
805-809	Fracture of Spine and Trunk
810-819	Fracture of Upper Limb
820-829	Fracture of Lower Limb

A **fracture** is a break in a bone. Bones are rigid but will bend. However, if the impact or force is too great, the bone will break. There are different types of fractures (Figure 19-2) with varying degrees of complexity. In a minor injury, the bone may just crack and may not break all the way through. In a more severe injury, the bone may shatter, or it may break through the skin. Treatment provided for a fracture depends on the specific bone broken, the severity of the break, and whether it is an "open" or a "closed" fracture.

Fractures fall into two categories:

1. **Closed or simple fracture** is diagnosed when the bone is broken, but the skin remains intact. Descriptive words used for a closed fracture include the following:
   - Comminuted—broken, splintered, or crushed into a number of pieces
   - Depressed—portion of the skull that is broken and driven inward
   - Fissured—incomplete fracture that does not split the bone
   - Fracture NOS—not otherwise specified
   - Greenstick—the bone is somewhat bent and is partially broken; occurs in children
   - Impacted—one fractured bone end is wedged into another broken end
   - Linear—straight line fracture
   - Simple—fracture that remains in alignment with little damage to surrounding tissue
   - Slipped epiphysis—separation of the growing end of the bone (epiphysis) from the shaft of the bone; occurs in children and young adults
   - Spiral—occurs when a bone has been twisted apart

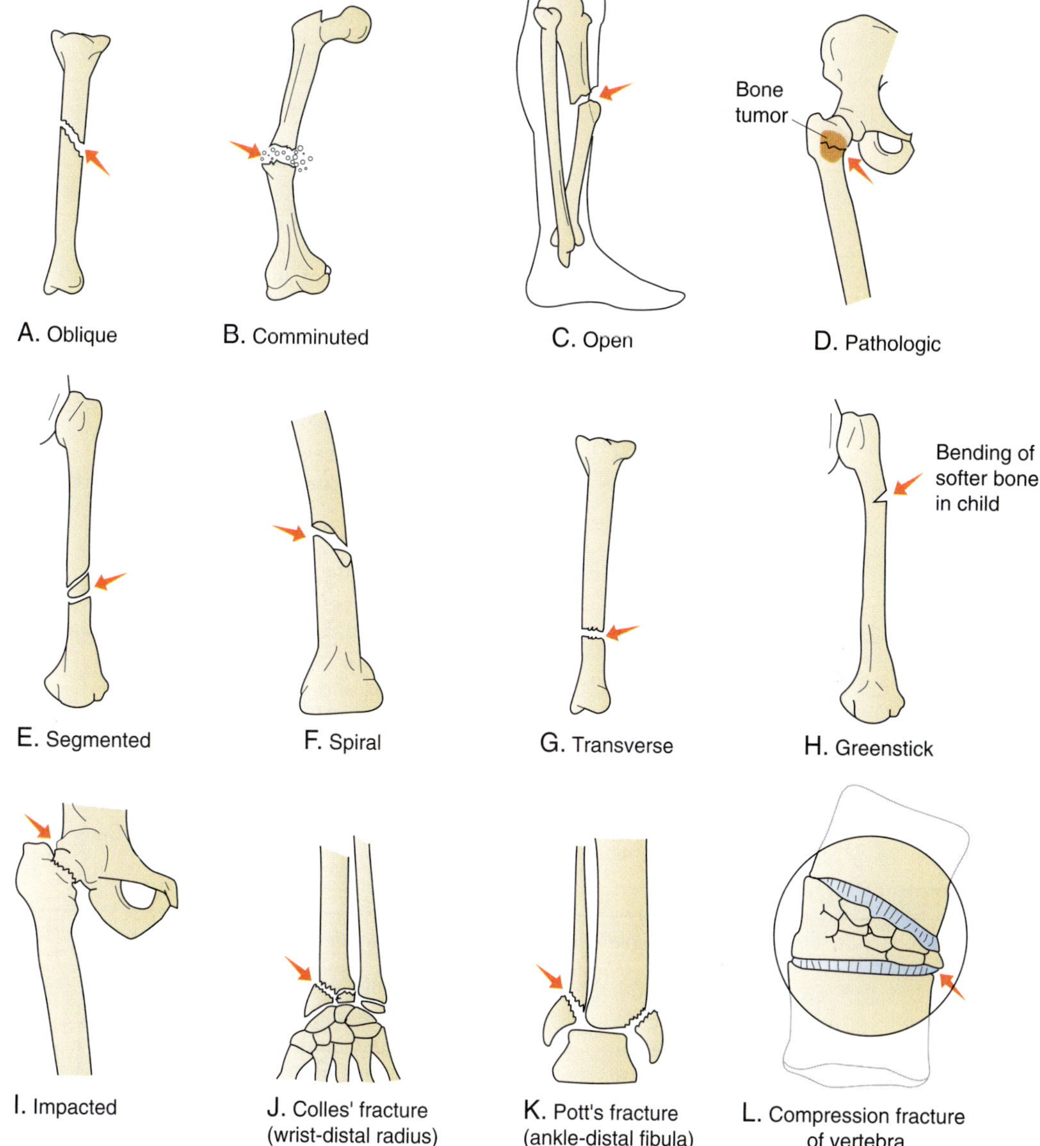

Figure 19-2. Types of fractures.

2. **Open or compound fracture** occurs when the bone exits and is visible through the skin, or a deep wound exposes the bone through the skin. If the wound is superficial and the fracture site is not exposed, the injury is coded as a closed fracture—not an open fracture. Some descriptive words used for an open fracture include the following:
   - Compound—fracture in which the bone is sticking through the skin
   - Infected—condition in which the bone becomes infected by bacteria
   - Missile—penetrating injuries resulting in fractures caused by bullets or stab wounds
   - Puncture—a puncture wound is present. The wound may be related to the injury or to bone fragments
   - Foreign body—presence of a foreign body within the fracture site

If a fracture is not specified as open or closed, it is coded as a closed fracture. If documentation in the record reveals an open wound around the fracture site, it may be necessary to query the physician as to whether this is an open or a closed fracture. In some instances, a fracture is documented as both open and closed. This usually occurs with a severe fracture with fracture fragments and it should be coded as an open fracture. A **complicated fracture** is a fracture that causes injury to surrounding tissues; it may be open or closed.

If a physician does not document the exact location of a fracture, *Coding Clinic* (1999:1Q: p5)[1] says it is acceptable to review the entire recording including the radiology report to identify the exact location of the fracture. If there is any question as to the appropriate diagnosis, the physician should be queried before assigning a diagnosis code.

EXAMPLE

The physician documents closed fracture right tibia. The x-ray report indicates a fracture of the shaft of the right tibia, 823.20, E887.

It is acceptable to use the more specific 823.20 code instead of 823.80 as documented by the physician.

EXAMPLE

The physician documents closed fracture right tibia. The x-ray report indicates a fracture through the shaft of the right tibia and fibula.

In this instance, the physician would need to be queried regarding the fracture of the fibula before code 823.22 is assigned.

Specific coding guidelines assist with sequencing and coding of fractures. The most severe fracture is sequenced first. The fourth digits of fracture codes usually indicate whether a fracture is open or closed; the fifth digits indicate more specific bones or locations within the general site. When a patient presents with multiple fractures, all fractures must be coded. Although multiple fracture categories 819 and 828 are provided, codes from these categories would rarely be used. In the inpatient setting, it may be necessary to query the physician for more specific information.

A **pathologic fracture** is a break in a bone that occurs because of underlying disorders that weaken the bone, including malignancy, benign bone tumor, metabolic disorders, infection, and osteoporosis. A fracture can result from normal stress placed on an abnormal bone. Minor trauma can cause fracture. It is important to determine whether a fracture is pathologic or traumatic, so the appropriate code can be assigned. Coding of pathologic fractures is discussed in Chapter 18. Fractures that are due to a birth injury are classified as perinatal conditions (767.2-767.4).

Skull Fractures

Skull fracture may be associated with traumatic head injury. Injury to the brain may also occur. In most skull fractures there is no displacement of broken bones. This is a closed or simple fracture. In severe cases, bone fragments are displaced, resulting in an open and/or depressed skull fracture. Fractures of the skull are frequently encountered after falls, crushing injuries, direct blows to the head or motor vehicle accidents. A simple skull fracture may have little impact on eventual neurologic outcomes of head trauma. Neurological outcomes of a skull fracture are determined by the nature of the brain injury. Some trauma patients can have severe neurologic impairment without having a skull fracture. The cranium, which protects the brain, consists of eight bones: occipital, frontal, sphenoidal, ethmoidal, two parietal, and two temporal bones (Figure 19-3). Categories 850 to 854 have fourth or fifth digit designations that are specific to the patient's level of consciousness. **Loss of consciousness (LOC)** occurs when a patient is unable to respond to people or to other stimuli. Unconsciousness and other sudden changes in mental status should be treated as a medical emergency.

EXAMPLE

Fracture frontal bone due to motor vehicle accident involving head-on collision with truck, unbelted passenger. The patient did not lose consciousness, 800.01, E812.1, E849.5.

Spine Fractures

As was discussed in Chapter 18, vertebral fractures are often pathologic fractures, particularly in older women with osteoporosis. This chapter focuses on traumatic spinal fractures,

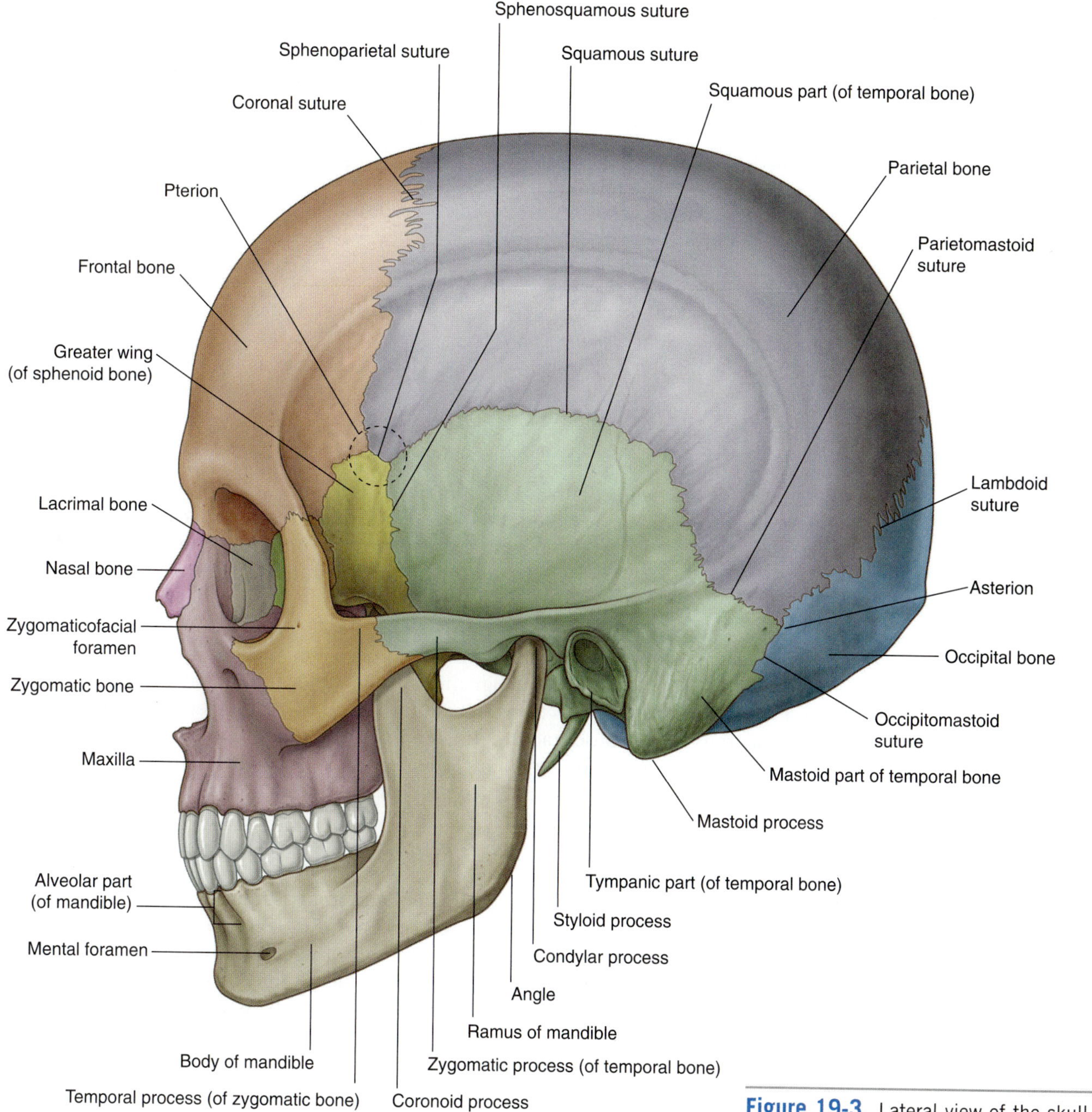

Figure 19-3. Lateral view of the skull.

which usually occur as the result of motor vehicle accidents, falls, acts of violence, or recreational and sporting activities. Spinal fracture does not necessarily indicate damage to the spinal cord, and a spinal cord injury can occur without a spinal fracture. Injuries to the spinal cord without associated fractures and nerve injuries are assigned to codes 950 to 957. Category 806 includes combination codes for use in cases of spinal fracture with spinal cord injury (Figures 19-4).

EXAMPLE Clay shoveler's fracture C7 due to strain injury while working at construction site, 805.07, E927, E849.3.

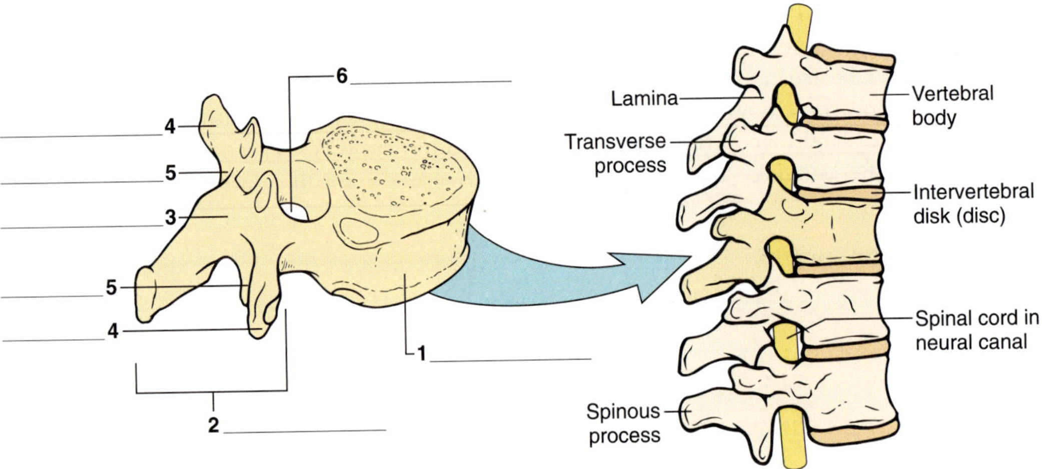

Figure 19-4. Lateral view of vertebrae.

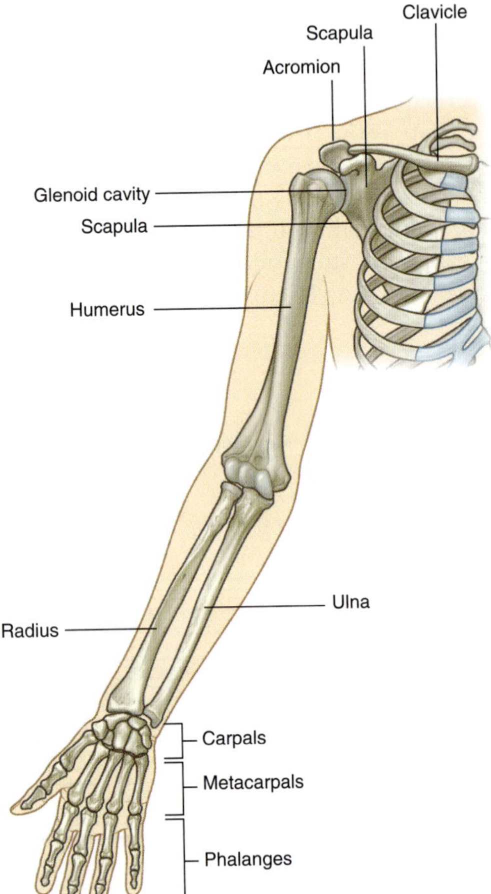

Figure 19-5. Bones of the upper limb.

Upper Limb Fractures

Shoulder and upper arm (Figure 19-5) injuries, including fractures of the clavicle or the upper part of the humerus, are fairly common. Fractures of the scapula are less common. A **Colles' fracture** is a common fracture in adults. In this type of fracture the lower end of the radius is fractured, and the wrist and the hand are displaced backward. Fractures of the

ulna typically occur across the shaft or at the tip of the elbow. Sometimes, the radius is fractured at the same time. Fractures of the radius, which are among the most common of fractures, usually are caused by a fall on an outstretched hand. The disc-shaped head of the bone just below the elbow joint is one of the most common sites of fracture in young adults. Fingers often sustain lacerations, fractures, and tendon ruptures. Fractures are particularly common at the knuckles, usually in the little finger, as the result of a blow.

EXAMPLE Boxers' fracture due to brawl at nightclub, 815.00, E960.0, E849.6.

Lower Limb Fractures

A fractured hip is usually a fracture of the head or neck of the femur. The nature, symptoms, treatment, and possible complications of a fractured femur depend on whether the bone has been broken across its neck or across the shaft. A fracture in the shaft of the femur usually occurs when the femur is subjected to extreme force, as occurs in a motor vehicle accident.

In most cases, the bone ends are considerably displaced, causing severe pain, tenderness, and swelling. The patella is the triangular bone that protects the knee joint. Fracture is usually caused by a direct blow. The tibia is one of the most commonly fractured bones. It may break across the shaft as the result of a direct blow to the front of the leg, or at the upper end from a blow to the outside of the leg below the knee. The fibula, a very common site of fracture, usually breaks just above the ankle as the result of a harsh twisting motion, such as occurs in severe ankle sprain. Injury to the foot commonly results in fractures of the bones in the toes, caused by stubbing or twisting them or as the result of a falling or crushing injury. The calcaneus may fracture after a fall from a height onto a hard surface (Figures 19-6 and 19-7).

EXAMPLE Dupuytren's fracture due to fall from horse while riding in meadow, 824.4, E828.2, E849.8.

Traumatic Fractures and Fracture Aftercare

Active treatment of a traumatic fracture includes surgery, an emergency room encounter, and/or evaluation and treatment by a new physician. According to the guidelines, when a patient is receiving active treatment, the acute fracture code is assigned.

Following the period of active treatment of a traumatic fracture, other encounters may be necessary. These encounters are assigned aftercare V codes. Aftercare may include a cast change or removal, removal of a fixation device, medication adjustments, and other follow-up visits.

EXAMPLE Patient is admitted for open reduction of orbital floor fracture. Patient was involved in a fight at a bar last week, 802.6, E960.0, E849.6, 76.79.

EXAMPLE Patient had a cast change for traumatic radial fracture, V54.12.

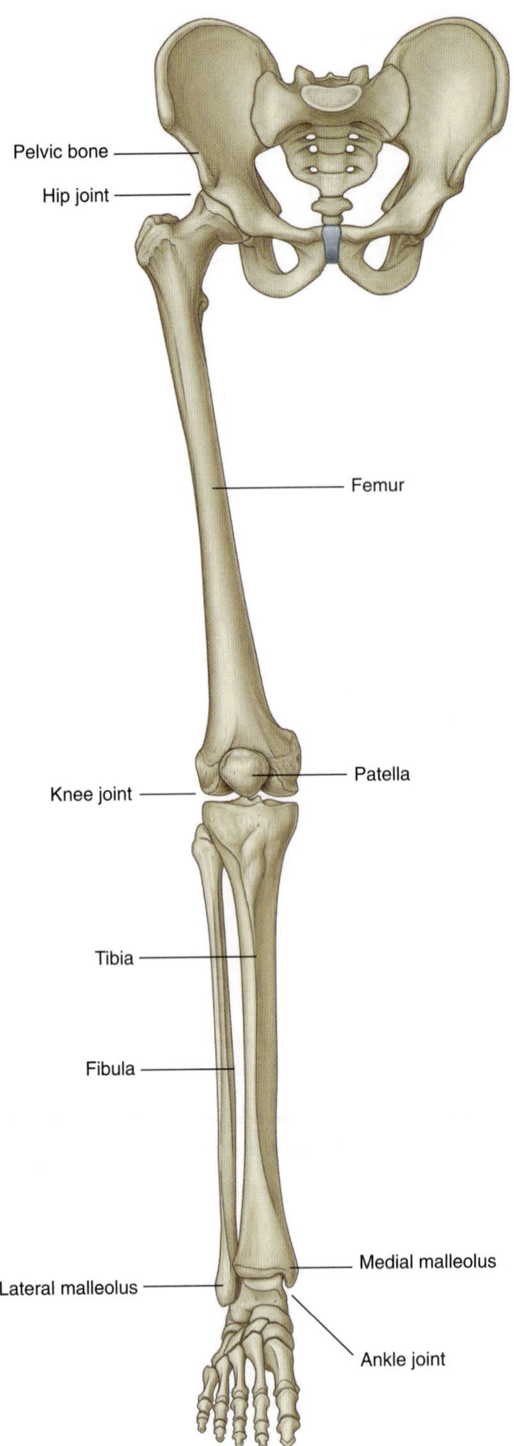

Figure 19-6. Bones and joints of the lower limb.

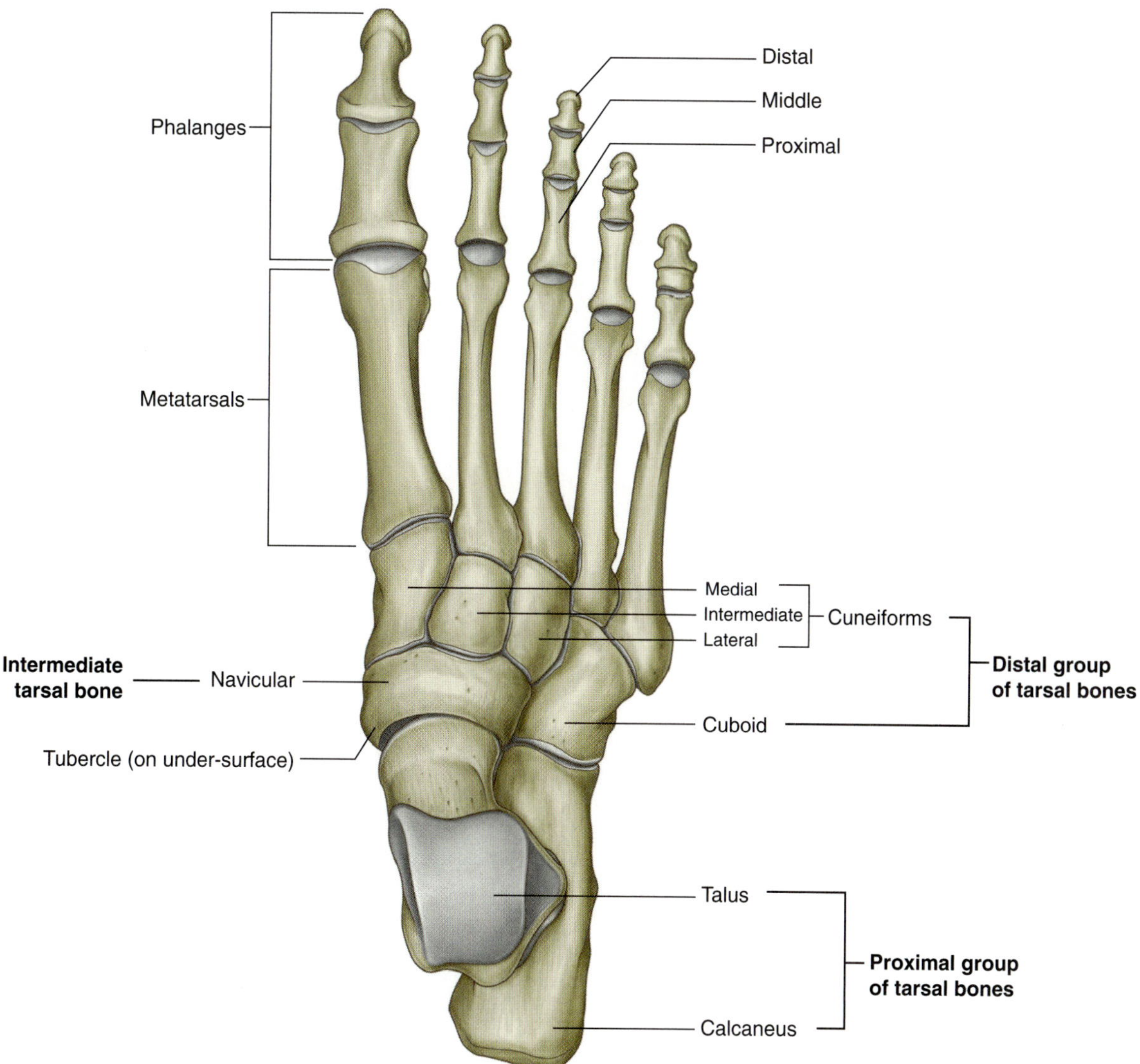

Figure 19-7. Dorsal view of right foot.

EXERCISE 19-2

Assign codes to the following conditions using your ICD-9-CM code book.

1. Type II Salter Harris fracture left fifth proximal phalanx due to fall from scooter ____________
2. Nondisplaced right lateral malleolus fracture due to slipping on gravel while jogging ____________
3. Comminuted left calcaneal fracture due to fall from ladder while doing home repairs ____________
4. Open fracture distal right tibia and fibula due to motorcycle accident involving loss of control on wet highway. Patient was driver of the motorcycle ____________
5. Avulsion fracture of the medial aspect of the left patella as a result of falling on cement at school playground ____________
6. LeFort I fracture due to hit by baseball during baseball game ____________

7. Fracture cervical spine C1 and C2 due to diving into shallow swimming pool at hotel ____________
8. Compound fracture midshaft of femur due to motorcycle accident with crash into a car ____________
9. Fracture midshaft left clavicle due to tackle during football practice ____________
10. Temporal skull fracture due to self-inflicted gunshot; patient had intracranial hemorrhage. ____________
11. Patient was seen for removal of internal fixation device from previous traumatic tibial fracture. ____________
12. Follow-up visit for traumatic pelvic fracture. ____________

Dislocations (830-839)

Dislocation is the displacement of the bones that form a joint. It is the separation of the end of a bone and the joint it meets. A partial or incomplete dislocation is called a **subluxation**. Dislocations may occur as the result of traumatic injury, or they may result from diseases such as rheumatoid arthritis, congenital joint defects, or weakened joints due to previous injury. The shoulder is especially prone to dislocation. The elbow is a common site of dislocation in toddlers. Other sites include fingers, hips, jaws, and spine. Soft tissues such as ligaments, tendons, muscles, and cartilage in and around the joint may stretch or tear as a result of the dislocation. Nerves and blood vessels may also be injured by the dislocated bone.

It is possible for a fracture and dislocation/subluxation to occur at the same anatomic site. In these instances, the index gives the coder instructions under the main term "Dislocation": It says, "with fracture—*see* Fracture, by site" (Figure 19-8). This means that only the fracture code is assigned for fractures/dislocations at the same site. According to *Coding Clinic* (1990:3Q:p13),[2] it is incorrect to also code the dislocation. Reduction of fracture/dislocation is coded to reduction of fracture. No additional code is assigned for reduction of a dislocation.

Once a joint has been dislocated, it is not unusual for it to dislocate again; with each recurrence, less force is required to sustain a dislocation. According to *Coding Clinic* (1997: Nov-Dec:p7),[3] only the initial occurrence of the dislocation is coded with an injury code, and all subsequent dislocations of the same joint are coded as recurrent dislocations.

Dislocation (articulation) (closed) (displacement) (simple) (subluxation) 839.8

Note

"Closed" includes simple, complete, partial, uncomplicated, and unspecified dislocation.

"Open" includes dislocation specified as infected or compound and dislocation with foreign body.

"Chronic," "habitual," "old," or "recurrent" dislocations should be coded as indicated under the entry "Dislocation, recurrent"; and "pathological" as indicated under the entry "Dislocation, pathological."

For late effect of dislocation see Late, effect, dislocation.

with fracture - *see* Fracture, by site

Figure 19-8. Instruction for dislocation with fracture—see Fracture, by site.

EXAMPLE

The patient sustained an open dislocation distal interphalageal joint right little finger during tackle on school football field during game 834.12, E886.0, E849.4.

EXERCISE 19-3

Assign codes to the following conditions using your ICD-9-CM code book.

1. Dislocation patella due to fall at nursing home ____________
2. Dislocation proximal interphalangeal joint left index finger due to jamming finger while playing basketball at gym ____________
3. Recurrent dislocation right shoulder ____________
4. Subluxation elbow due to twisting injury during gymnastics practice at the gym ____________

Sprains and Strains of Joints and Adjacent Muscles (840-848)

A **sprain** is a stretch and/or tear of a ligament. The severity of the injury depends on whether a tear is partial or complete and on the number of ligaments involved. A **strain** is an injury to a muscle or a tendon. Depending on the severity of the injury, a strain may be the result of an overstretched muscle or tendon, or it can be caused by a partial or complete tear. Often, the patient is unaware of any specific injury. Strains can be acute or chronic. Chronic strains usually result from overuse or prolonged repetitive movement.

EXAMPLE

The patient has an anterior cruciate ligament sprain due to injury 844.2, E928.9.

EXERCISE 19-4

Assign codes to the following conditions using your ICD-9-CM code book.

1. Sprain left hand due to sliding into third base during baseball game in backyard ____________
2. Strain lumbosacral spine due to overexertion from lifting at factory ____________
3. Rupture Achilles tendon while playing racquetball due to twisting injury at the gym ____________
4. SLAP (superior labrum anterior-posterior) lesion on right shoulder while rock climbing and fall from cliff ____________

Intracranial Injury, Excluding Those with Skull Fracture (850-854)

Intracranial injuries that are not associated with skull fracture(s) are assigned codes in categories 850-854. A **concussion** is an injury to the brain that results from a significant blow to the head. Length of unconsciousness may relate to severity of the concussion. Most people recover with no ill effects. A patient may have to be admitted to the hospital for observation. The fourth or fifth digit designates the length of time that the patient was unconscious (Figure 19-9). It may be necessary to review the emergency room and ambulance records to determine the time that the patient was unconscious.

Traumatic brain injury (TBI) is injury to the brain that may affect the brain's normal functions. Penetrating injuries are injuries in which a foreign object such as a bullet enters the brain. Symptoms vary depending on the areas of the brain that are damaged.

INTRACRANIAL INJURY, EXCLUDING THOSE WITH SKULL FRACTURE (850–854)

Excludes *intracranial injury with skull fracture (800–801 and 803–804, except .0 and .5)*
open wound of head without intracranial injury (870.0–873.9)
skull fracture alone (800–801 and 803–804 with .0, .5)

Note: The description "with open intracranial wound," used in the fourth-digit subdivisions, includes those specified as open or with mention of infection or foreign body.

The following fifth-digit subclassification is for use with categories 851–854:

- ❑ 0 **unspecified state of consciousness**
- 1 **with no loss of consciousness**
- 2 **with brief [less than one hour] loss of consciousness**
- 3 **with moderate [1–24 hours] loss of consciousness**
- 4 **with prolonged [more than 24 hours] loss of consciousness and return to pre-existing conscious level**
- 5 **with prolonged [more than 24 hours] loss of consciousness without return to pre-existing conscious level**

  Use fifth-digit 5 to designate when a patient is unconscious and dies before regaining consciousness, regardless of the duration of the loss of consciousness
- ❑ 6 **with loss of consciousness of unspecified duration**
- ❑ 9 **with concussion, unspecified**

Figure 19-9. Fifth digit code assignment for level of consciousness.

Closed head injury (CHI) results from a blow to the head. Primary brain damage may occur at the time of the injury or accident. Secondary brain damage may result from complications of the injury such as brain swelling, increased intracranial pressure, seizure, infection, fever, hematoma, high or low blood pressure, anemia, and metabolic changes.

EXAMPLE

Patient was hospitalized with a concussion due to fall from playground equipment at school. Unconscious for 5 minutes 850.11, E884.0, E849.4.

EXERCISE 19-5

Assign codes to the following conditions using your ICD-9-CM code book.

1. Cerebral contusion due to fall on ice in driveway. Positive for loss of consciousness ____________
2. Laceration brain due to impact from motor vehicle accident (MVA). Loss of consciousness lasted longer than 1 hour ____________
3. Subdural hemorrhage due to fall 1 week ago ____________
4. Subarachnoid hemorrhage without regaining consciousness after an all-terrain vehicle (ATV) accident. Patient died after 2 days. ____________

Internal Injury of Thorax, Abdomen, and Pelvis (860-869)

Injury to the internal organs can occur with or without an open wound. Laceration of the spleen may result from blunt trauma without an open wound; injury to the spleen can occur

from an open wound due to a gunshot. Types of injuries included in these categories are as follows:

- Blast injuries of internal organs
- Blunt trauma of internal organs
- Bruise of internal organs
- Concussion injuries (except cerebral) of internal organs
- Crushing of internal organs
- Hematoma of internal organs
- Laceration of internal organs
- Puncture of internal organs
- Traumatic rupture of internal organs

The Organ Injury Scaling was developed by the Organ Injury Scaling Committee of the American Association for the Surgery of Trauma. This scale is graded from I through VI for each organ, with I being least severe and V the most severe injury from which the patient may survive. Grade VI injuries are by definition not salvageable. Scales are available for the following organ injuries:

- Thoracic vascular
- Lung
- Heart
- Chest wall
- Diaphragm
- Spleen
- Liver
- Abdominal vascular
- Kidney
- Ureter
- Bladder
- Urethra

Table 19-1 shows the organ injury scale for liver injuries.

These scales can be helpful in coding internal injuries more accurately. They may also be useful if the coder has to query the physician about the extent of an internal injury.

Categories 864, Injury to liver (Figure 19-10), 865 Injury to spleen, and 866 Injury to kidney have fifth digit subclassifications that may fit into one of the organ injury grade levels.

Table 19-1. Organ Injury Scaling—Liver[4]

Grade	Injury Description	
I	Hematoma	Subcapsular, <10% surface area
	Laceration	Capsular tear, <1 cm parenchymal depth
II	Hematoma	Subcapsular, 10%-50% surface area Intraparenchymal, <10 cm diameter
	Laceration	1-3 cm parenchymal depth, <10 cm length
III	Hematoma	Subcapsular, >50% surface area or expanding. Ruptured subcapsular or parenchymal hematoma Intraparencymal hematoma >10 cm or expanding
	Laceration	>3 cm parenchymal depth
IV	Laceration	Parenchymal disruption involving 25%-75% of hepatic lobe, or 1-3 Coinaud's segments in a single lobe
V	Laceration	Parenchymal disruption involving >75% of hepatic lobe or >3 Coinaud's segments within a single lobe
	Vascular	Juxtahepatic venous injuries (i.e., retrohepatic vena cava/central major hepatic veins)
VI	Vascular	Hepatic avulsion

Advance one grade for multiple injuries to same organ up to grade III.

●864 **Injury to liver**

The following fifth-digit subclassification is for use with category 864:

❑ 0 **unspecified injury**

1 **hematoma and contusion**

2 **laceration, minor**

Laceration involving capsule only, or without significant involvement of hepatic parenchyma [i.e., less than 1 cm deep]

3 **laceration, moderate**

Laceration involving parenchyma but without major disruption of parenchyma [i.e., less than 10 cm long and less than 3 cm deep]

4 **laceration, major**

Laceration with significant disruption of hepatic parenchyma [i.e., 10 cm long and 3 cm deep]

Multiple moderate lacerations, with or without hematoma

Stellate lacerations of liver

❑ 5 **laceration, unspecified**

❑ 9 **other**

Figure 19-10. Fifth digit code assignment for type of liver laceration.

EXAMPLE

Patient had laceration of right lung due to stab wound right chest wall during fight at nightclub, 861.32, E966, E849.6.

EXERCISE 19-6

Assign codes to the following conditions using your ICD-9-CM code book.

1. Pneumothorax due to stab wound chest wall during assault on the street ____________
2. A 5-cm laceration spleen due to blunt trauma from steering wheel of car during head-on collision with another car ____________
3. Grade III laceration liver (involving parenchyma) due to snowmobile accident with collision with a tree in the ditch. Patient was driver. ____________
4. Contusion kidney due to fall from horse at riding stable ____________
5. Mediastinal hematoma due to MVA, single vehicle with loss of control, passenger ____________

Open Wounds (870-897)

An open wound or **laceration** is an injury that results in a tear in the skin (Figure 19-11). Bruising and swelling can occur around the wound site. Common sites of laceration are body areas with underlying bony support, such as above the eyebrows, on the scalp and face, and over the knees. Categories 870-897 are assigned for traumatic injury; these codes should not be used to identify surgical wounds, nontraumatic wounds or ulcers, decubitus ulcers, and stasis ulcers. Laceration codes are assigned by location and according to whether the wound is complicated. The definition of a complicated wound includes delayed healing, delayed treatment, foreign body, and/or infection. An additional code would be assigned to identify the type of infection and any responsible organism. Because a physician says that a wound is complicated or that a complex repair was performed does not necessarily mean that the wound should be coded as complicated. The wound must fit the ICD-9-CM definition of a complicated wound.

EXAMPLE

The patient cut his right eyebrow during fall while skiing; patient fell while skiing at resort, 873.42, E885.3, E849.4.

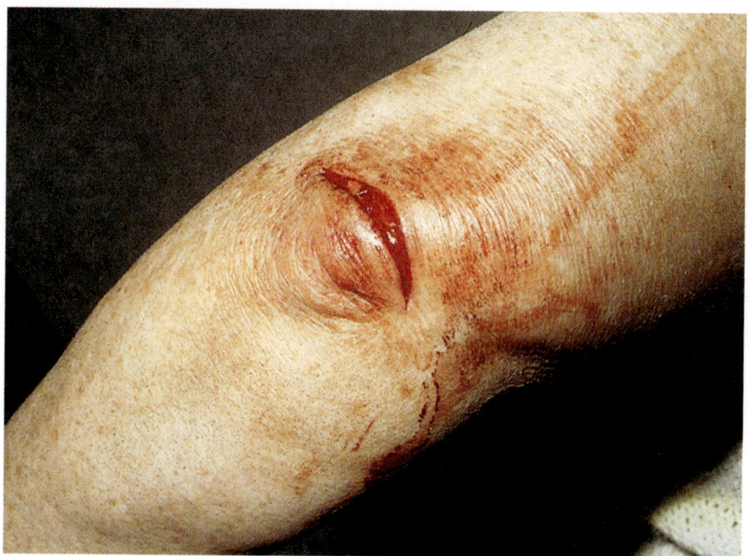

Figure 19-11. Laceration of elbow.

EXAMPLE

Patient presented to the emergency room with gravel embedded in laceration of left knee. Patient fell while hiking 2 days ago. The wound was cleaned and dressing applied, 891.1, E888.9, E849.6.

EXERCISE 19-7

Assign codes to the following conditions using your ICD-9-CM code book.

1. Puncture wound left forearm due to dog bite while playing at public park ______________
2. Traumatic amputation right little toe due to lawn mower accident ______________
3. Laceration right calf from hatchet injury during camping trip. Injury occurred 3 days ago, and no medical attention has been sought until now ______________
4. Wound left foot with glass pieces in wound due to stepping on broken glass at home ______________

Injury to Blood Vessels (900-904)

Often, injuries to the blood vessels occur in conjunction with other injuries such as fractures, dislocations, open wounds, or lacerations. It is appropriate to assign codes that identify injury to the blood vessels, in addition to fractures and dislocations. Sequencing of codes according to Coding Guidelines depends on which is the primary injury.

EXAMPLE

Injury to the thoracic aorta due to MVA involving collision with train. Patient was the driver, 901.0, E810.0, E849.5.

EXERCISE 19-8

Assign codes to the following conditions using your ICD-9-CM code book.

1. Crush injury abdomen with injury to splenic artery due to being struck and caught between two motor vehicles ______________
2. Injury to abdominal aorta due to accident while passenger on shuttle bus ______________
3. Injury to internal jugular due to stabbing during assault in parking garage ______________
4. Rupture of anterior tibial artery due to accidental gunshot (hunting rifle) while hunting ______________
5. Dislocation of femoral neck due to injury during game of rugby. Minor damage to the femoral artery was noted ______________

Superficial Injury (910-919)

Superficial injuries may manifest in the form of abrasions (Figure 19-12), friction burns, blisters, nonvenomous insect bites, and superficial foreign bodies or splinters (Figure 19-13). The physician may not document the term "superficial," so supporting documentation must be used to determine whether the injury fits into the superficial categories. It is also important to look for documentation about the presence of an infection. As was mentioned previously, it is not necessary to code superficial injuries when a more serious injury has occurred at the same site. The fourth digit identifies whether infection is present. Superficial injury to the eye is coded to category 918.

EXAMPLE

Corneal abrasion due to scratch from baby at public daycare, 918.1, E914, E849.6.

EXAMPLE

Laceration and abrasion right elbow due to fall from scooter at the lake, 881.01, E885.0, E849.8. The abrasion is not coded separately because it occurred at the same site as a more severe injury.

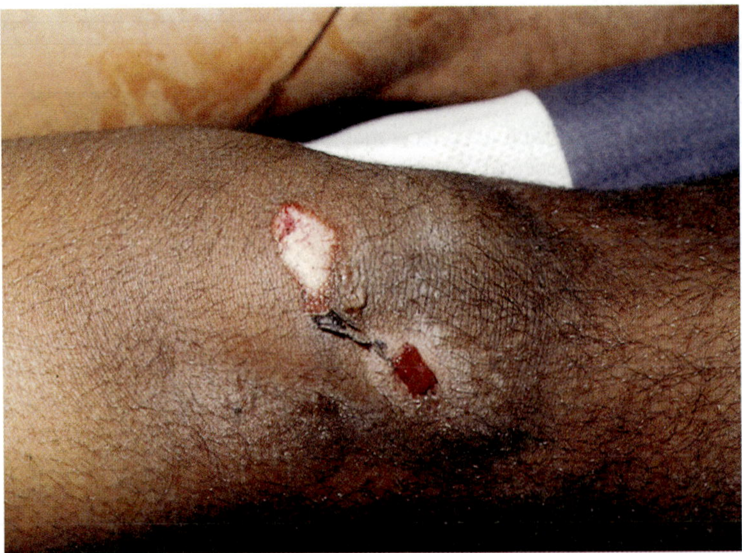

Figure 19-12. Abrasion wound of kneecap.

910 Superficial injury of face, neck, and scalp except eye

Includes: cheek, ear, gum, lip, nose, throat

Excludes *eye and adnexa (918.0–918.9)*

910.0 Abrasion or friction burn without mention of infection

910.1 Abrasion or friction burn, infected

910.2 Blister without mention of infection

910.3 Blister, infected

910.4 Insect bite, nonvenomous, without mention of infection

910.5 Insect bite, nonvenomous, infected

910.6 Superficial foreign body (splinter) without major open wound and without mention of infection

910.7 Superficial foreign body (splinter) without major open wound, infected

❑ **910.8 Other and unspecified superficial injury of face, neck, and scalp without mention of infection**

❑ **910.9 Other and unspecified superficial injury of face, neck, and scalp, infected**

Figure 19-13. Fourth digit classifications for superficial injuries.

EXAMPLE

Sprain right ankle and abrasions left knee due to being knocked down while playing basketball during recess, 845.00, 916.0, E917.5, E849.6. Abrasions are coded because they occurred at a different site from the sprain.

EXERCISE 19-9

Assign codes to the following conditions using your ICD-9-CM code book.

1. Blister left heel due to rubbing of shoe ______________
2. Infected mosquito bites both legs ______________
3. Abrasions right hand and knee due to fall from bicycle on the driveway at home ______________
4. Superficial wood splinter right thumb from board on construction job site ______________
5. Abrasions and deep laceration of left elbow due to fall while playing soccer. Patient was pushed down by opponent. ______________

Contusion With Intact Skin Surface (920-924)

A **contusion** is any injury that results in hemorrhage beneath unbroken skin. Other terms for contusion include “bruise” and “hematoma.” Contusions associated with more severe or serious injuries at the same site would not be coded. Occasionally, if a hematoma does not absorb on its own, it may have to be evacuated or aspirated.

EXAMPLE

Contusion right quadriceps after tackle in college football game, 924.00, E886.0, E849.4.

EXAMPLE

Contusion and severe sprain of left ankle after falling into a hole while hiking in the mountains, 845.00, E883.9, E849.8.

EXERCISE 19-10

Assign codes to the following conditions using your ICD-9-CM code book.

1. Blackeye due to hit by opponent's elbow during professional basketball game ____________
2. Subungual hematoma left thumb after hitting with hammer in home workshop ____________
3. Bruise left ankle following hit from hockey puck during practice ____________
4. Hematoma right breast from the seatbelt when involved in MVA involving collision with a tree. Patient was alone in the vehicle ____________
5. Contusion right shin after tripping on steps leading to the public high school ____________

Crush Injury (925-929)

A **crush injury** occurs when a body part is subjected to a high degree of force or pressure, usually after it has been squeezed between two heavy or immobile objects. A crush injury can be more serious than other types of injury such as a fracture or a laceration. In a severe crush, the force of the trauma can damage the underlying tissues, bones, blood vessels, and nerves. Increased pressure from tissue swelling can also damage muscles, blood vessels, and nerves. Instructions say to use additional codes to identify any associated injuries such as the following:

- Fractures (800-829)
- Internal organs (860.0-869.1)
- Intracranial injury (850.0-854.1)

According to *Coding Clinic* (2003:4Q:p76-78),[5] the code for crush injury should be sequenced first.

EXAMPLE

Crush injury left foot with metatarsal fractures due to dropping car battery on foot at industrial factory, 928.20, 825.25, E916, E849.3.

According to *Coding Clinic* (1993:2Q:p7),[6] assign only the code for the crush injury (925-929.9) when there is also an open wound or a laceration. The Tabular List and the Alphabetic Index do not include any mention of "with open wound" under the section on Crush Injuries ("Crush, crushing . . ." in the index). However, the note under "Wound, open" in the index gives direction, "For crush injury, see Crush . . ." (Figure 19-14), and the Exclusion note under the section on "Open wound" in the Tabular List clearly excludes "crushing (925-925.9)" (Figure 19-15). Therefore, a code for open wound is not used with a code for crush injury.

EXAMPLE

Crush injury right pointer finger with 3-cm laceration after injury while fixing combine on the farm, 927.3, E919.0, E849.1.

EXERCISE 19-11

Assign codes to the following conditions using your ICD-9-CM code book.

1. Crush injury left fingers with fractures of distal phalanges due to slamming in car door __________
2. Crush injury to abdomen with injury to bladder and pelvic fracture __________
3. Crush injury right foot __________
4. Crush injury left great toe due to dropping bowling ball on bare foot at the bowling alley __________
5. Crush injury right ankle with 4-cm laceration due to being pinned by farm machinery __________

Effects of Foreign Body Entering Through Orifice (930-939)

A foreign body (FB) can enter the body through natural openings or orifices such as eyes, ears, nose, and mouth. In some cases it may be necessary to seek emergency medical attention for possible removal. One of the most common sites that foreign bodies enter are the eyes. Young children and elderly patients, particularly those with neurologic disorders and/or decreased gag reflexes, are at risk for aspiration and food can become lodged in the esophagus.

EXAMPLE

Small piece of grass from mowing lawn at home stuck on right cornea. Grass was removed, 930.0, E914, E849.0 98.21.

Wound, open (by cutting or piercing instrument) (by firearms) (cut) (dissection) (incised) (laceration) (penetration) (perforating) (puncture) (with initial hemorrhage, not internal) 879.8

Note For fracture with open wound, see Fracture.

For laceration, traumatic rupture, tear, or penetrating wound of internal organs, such as heart, lung, liver, kidney, pelvic organs, etc., whether or not accompanied by open wound or fracture in the same region, see Injury, internal. For contused wound, see Contusion. For crush injury, see Crush. For abrasion, insect bite (nonvenomous), blister, or scratch, see Injury, superficial.

Complicated includes wounds with:

delayed healing
delayed treatment
foreign body
primary infection

For late effect of open wound, see Late, effect, wound, open, by site.

Figure 19-14. Instructional note for coding crush injuries.

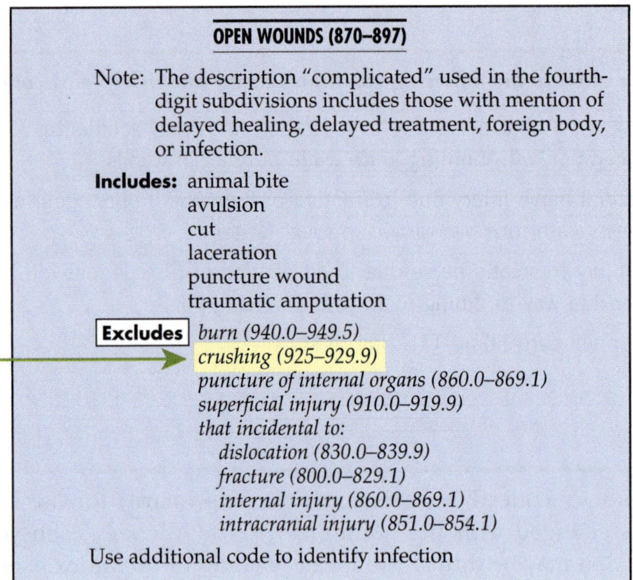

OPEN WOUNDS (870–897)

Note: The description "complicated" used in the fourth-digit subdivisions includes those with mention of delayed healing, delayed treatment, foreign body, or infection.

Includes: animal bite
avulsion
cut
laceration
puncture wound
traumatic amputation

Excludes *burn (940.0–949.5)*
crushing (925–929.9)
puncture of internal organs (860.0–869.1)
superficial injury (910.0–919.9)
that incidental to:
dislocation (830.0–839.9)
fracture (800.0–829.1)
internal injury (860.0–869.1)
intracranial injury (851.0–854.1)

Use additional code to identify infection

Figure 19-15. Crush injuries are excluded from open wound codes.

EXERCISE 19-12

Assign codes to the following conditions using your ICD-9-CM code book.

1. Hot dog lodged in distal esophagus of patient with dysphagia. EGD with removal of hot dog ____________
2. 1-year-old swallowed a penny, and x-rays showed that it was in the stomach ____________
3. Child put sunflower seed in right nostril; removed with forceps ____________
4. Patient with cough and hemoptysis was found to have a chicken bone lodged in lung; bronchoscopy with removal of chicken bone ____________
5. Malodorous vaginal discharge due to retained tampon in vagina; manually removed ____________

Injury to Nerves and Spinal Cord (950-957)

Spinal cord injury (SCI) is damage to the spinal cord that causes loss of sensation and motor control. The most common causes of SCI include MVAs, falls, acts of violence, and sporting accidents. SCIs tend to occur where the spine is most flexible, in the regions C5-C7 of the neck and T10-L2 at the base of the rib cage. If SCI is suspected, a computed tomography (CT) scan, magnetic resonance imaging (MRI), or a myelogram may be used as a diagnostic tool. Immediate medical treatment should focus on stabilizing the spine and providing aggressive treatment with corticosteroid drugs to limit damage. Surgery may also be necessary to stabilize the spine or fuse the spine with metal plates or pins. Once the initial injury heals, functional improvements may continue for at least 6 months. After this time, any remaining disability is likely to be permanent. Any nerve damage or injury should be coded, in addition to other injuries.

EXAMPLE

Spinal cord injury at C2 level due to tackle during football game, 952.00, E917.5, E849.4.

EXERCISE 19-13

Assign codes to the following conditions using your ICD-9-CM code book.

1. Injury to ulnar nerve due to laceration left wrist; accidental laceration with hunting knife while hunting in woods ____________
2. Radial nerve injury due to fracture of humerus; injury occurred when water taxi overturned in rough water ____________
3. Injury to sciatic nerve due to dislocation of hip; patient fell on the way to dining room at the nursing home ____________
4. Spinal cord injury T10 due to MVA ____________

V CODES

In the past, V codes have been considered primarily for use in the outpatient setting. This has changed with the addition of more V codes each year. As was discussed in Chapter 8, it may be difficult to locate V codes in the index. Coders often say, "I did not know there was a V code for that." Refer to Chapter 8 for a listing of common main terms used to locate V codes. V codes that may be used with injuries include the following:

V15.51	Personal history of traumatic fracture
V15.59	Personal history of other injury
V42.4	Organ or tissue replaced by transplant—bone
V43.60	Organ or tissue replaced by other means—unspecified
V43.61	Organ or tissue replaced by other means—shoulder
V43.62	Organ or tissue replaced by other means—elbow
V43.63	Organ or tissue replaced by other means—wrist
V43.64	Organ or tissue replaced by other means—hip
V43.65	Organ or tissue replaced by other means—knee
V43.66	Organ or tissue replaced by other means—ankle
V43.69	Organ or tissue replaced by other means—other
V43.7	Organ or tissue replaced by other means—limb
V48.6	Disfigurements of head
V48.7	Disfigurements of neck and trunk
V49.4	Disfigurements of limbs
V49.60	Upper limb amputation status—unspecified level
V49.61	Upper limb amputation status—thumb
V49.62	Upper limb amputation status—other finger(s)
V49.63	Upper limb amputation status—hand
V49.64	Upper limb amputation status—wrist
V49.65	Upper limb amputation status—below elbow
V49.66	Upper limb amputation status—above elbow
V49.67	Upper limb amputation status—shoulder
V49.70	Lower limb amputation status—unspecified level
V49.71	Lower limb amputation status—great toe
V49.72	Lower limb amputation status—other toe(s)
V49.73	Lower limb amputation status—foot
V49.74	Lower limb amputation status—ankle
V49.75	Lower limb amputation status—below knee (BKA)
V49.76	Lower limb amputation status—above knee (AKA)
V49.77	Lower limb amputation status—hip

V52.0	Fitting and adjustment of prosthetic device and implant—artificial arm
V52.1	Fitting and adjustment of prosthetic device and implant—artificial leg
V53.7	Fitting and adjustment of other device—orthopedic devices
V54.01	Encounter for removal of internal fixation device
V54.09	Other aftercare involving internal fixation device
V54.10	Aftercare for healing traumatic fracture of arm, unspecified
V54.11	Aftercare for healing traumatic fracture of upper arm
V54.12	Aftercare for healing traumatic fracture of lower arm
V54.13	Aftercare for healing traumatic fracture of hip
V54.14	Aftercare for healing traumatic fracture of leg, unspecified
V54.15	Aftercare for healing traumatic fracture of upper leg
V54.16	Aftercare for healing traumatic fracture of lower leg
V54.17	Aftercare for healing traumatic fracture of vertebrae
V54.19	Aftercare for healing traumatic fracture of other bone
V54.81	Aftercare after joint replacement
V54.89	Other orthopedic aftercare
V54.9	Unspecified orthopedic aftercare
V57.1	Other physical therapy
V57.21	Encounter for occupational therapy
V57.22	Encounter for vocational therapy
V57.4	Orthoptic training
V57.81	Orthotic training
V58.30	Encounter for change or removal of nonsurgical wound dressing
V58.31	Encounter for change or removal of surgical wound dressing
V58.32	Encounter for removal of sutures
V58.41	Encounter for planned postoperative wound closure
V58.49	Other specified aftercare after surgery
V58.43	Aftercare after surgery for injury and trauma
V59.2	Donor—bone
V64.43	Arthroscopic surgical procedure converted to open procedure
V65.43	Counseling on injury prevention
V66.4	Convalescence and palliative care after treatment of fracture
V67.4	Follow-up examination after treatment of healed fracture
V71.3	Observation after accident at work
V71.4	Observation after other accident
V71.6	Observation after other inflicted injury

EXAMPLE Patient is receiving orthotic training because of AKA, V57.4, V49.76.

EXAMPLE Patient was seen for suture removal, V58.32, 97.89.

Admission for Observation Following an Injury

According to *Coding Clinic* (1987:M-A:p1-5),[7] observation codes V71.3, V71.4, and V71.6 should be used when a patient is seen for an injury but after examination and observation no significant physical injury is found. Usually in these cases, patients are admitted to rule out or to be observed for a more serious type of injury. If a patient has minor cuts, bruises, or other superficial injuries, these are coded as secondary diagnoses and the appropriate observation code as the principal.

This V71 code category is used for patients who are suspected of having an abnormal condition without a sign or a symptom that requires study. After examination and observation, no condition is determined to exist.

EXAMPLE

Patient has a contusion of the forehead and is admitted for observation to rule out a concussion. Patient was the driver of a motor vehicle that lost control while taking a curve on the highway, V71.4, 920, E816.0, E849.5.

EXERCISE 19-14

Assign codes to the following conditions using your ICD-9-CM code book.

1. Observation following work accident ____________
2. Previous knee joint replacement ____________
3. Observation after MVA for internal abdominal injuries. Internal injuries were ruled out, and patient was discharged with a diagnosis of contusion abdominal wall ____________
4. Encounter for removal of screw used to stabilize tibial fracture; fracture is well healed, and no complications of the fixation device or infections are reported ____________
5. Patient had a previous amputation of the left great toe ____________
6. Patient's x-rays show a healing traumatic fracture of the right humerus ____________

COMMON TREATMENTS

Many injuries are diagnosed with the use of imaging procedures such as x-ray, MRI, CT scans, and ultrasound. Treatment depends on the severity of the injury. For very severe injuries, patients may have to be transferred to hospitals that specialize in the care of trauma patients. Surgical intervention may also be required to repair the specific injury or trauma. Pain medications, anti-inflammatories, corticosteroids, and antibiotics may be necessary to alleviate pain and inflammation and to prevent or fight infection.

PROCEDURES

Some of the procedures that may be related to injuries are located in the following chapters of the Procedure Tabular:

Operations on the Musculoskeletal System (76-84)

Operations on the Integumentary System (85-86)

Procedures for internal injuries are found within procedural chapters for the respective systems.

Fracture Treatment

A fracture is classified as "open" or "closed." Treatments for fracture are also classified as "open" or "closed," and the coder should not confuse the type of fracture with the type of procedure. An open fracture may not require open treatment, and a closed fracture may need open reduction. The treatment provided will depend on other injuries and the type and location of the fracture. Reduction or manipulation of bone fragments to their proper anatomic position is necessary for appropriate healing. For fractures that are not displaced, stabilization or immobilization may be all that is necessary to promote healing. Reductions may be performed in the operating room or other areas of the hospital, such as the emergency room, fracture treatment room, and/or in radiology.

Closed reduction of a fracture occurs when the surgeon manipulates or reduces fractured bones into anatomic alignment without making an incision through the skin and subcutaneous tissue. Closed reduction may include internal fixation. If no incision is made to expose the fracture, it is coded as a closed reduction. Small incision(s) may be made for placement of internal fixation device(s) such as pins, wires, screws, plates, and intramedullary nails. As long as the fracture is not exposed it is considered a closed fixation. Fixation

devices are used to immobilize the fracture, but they do not manipulate or reduce the fracture. Sometimes radiologic guidance is needed for placement of the fixation device(s). It is also possible for a closed reduction to be performed prior to having an open reduction and fixation.

Open reduction of a fracture occurs when the surgeon makes an incision at the fracture site to reduce or manipulate the fracture into anatomic position. Open reduction and internal fixation (ORIF) is a procedure that is very commonly performed for fractures.

External skeletal fixation is another form of fracture treatment (Figure 19-16). This involves insertion of percutaneous pins proximal and distal to the fracture and application of a frame that connects the pins externally. The pins are located internally, except for the portion to which the frame is connected. The frame is located outside the body. These devices can be used to hold a reduced fracture or to assist the surgeon in reducing a fracture. Instructional notes under the "Reduction of fracture and dislocation" category indicate that external skeletal fixation codes may be assigned, in addition to the codes for fracture reduction.

Repair of Wounds

Suture is a method used to close cutaneous wounds. The risks of bleeding and infection are reduced by approximating skin edges for an aesthetically pleasing and functional result. Routine debridement of wound edges prior to suturing of the wound is considered part of the suturing and should not be coded separately. In ICD-9-CM, suturing of the skin for most sites is coded to 86.59. How deep, how long, or how complex the repair is does not affect code assignment. A few sites require a different code:

- Breast, 85.81
- Ear, 18.4
- Eyebrow, 08.81
- Eyelid, 08.81
- Nose, 21.81
- Penis, 64.41
- Scrotum, 61.41
- Vulva, 71.71

No procedure code is assigned for application of adhesive strips or butterfly strips. It is acceptable to assign 86.59 when adhesives such as **Dermabond** are used for wound closure, per *Coding Clinic* (1999:4Q:p23).[8] Sometimes, a combination of adhesive and sutures is used for wound repair.

EXAMPLE

Laceration left wrist due to suicidal attempt with razor. Laceration was repaired, 881.02, E956, 86.59. No place of occurrence was given, so no E code is assigned, per guidelines.

EXAMPLE

Laceration nose due to being hit in nose by surfboard while at beach. Laceration was repaired, 873.20, E917.0, E849.8, 21.81.

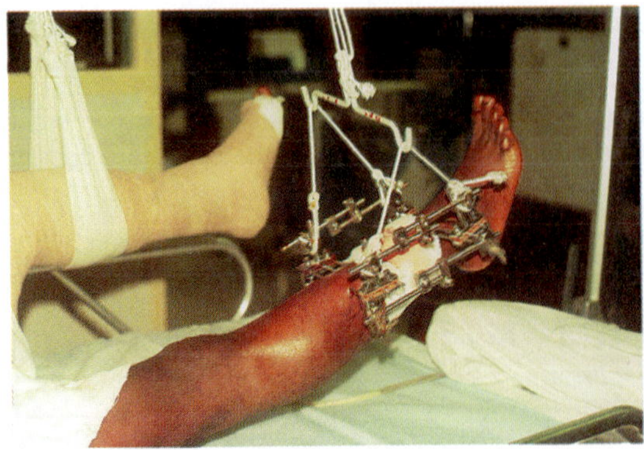

Figure 19-16. Example of an external fixation service on the right leg. The left is in a splint.

EXERCISE 19-15

Assign codes for all diagnoses and procedures using your ICD-9-CM code book.

1. Laceration to spleen with parenchymal disruption with total splenectomy ____________
2. Coco Puff in left ear; removed by physician ____________
3. Closed reduction and percutaneous fixation of supracondylar fracture elbow after fall from monkey bars on school playground ____________
4. Manipulation of shoulder dislocation due to fall while skiing at ski resort ____________
5. Suture deep laceration of the right hand due to cut with knife while preparing dinner ____________
6. Suture of laceration eyelid that occurred due to falling and hitting edge of coffee table ____________
7. Open reduction and internal fixation of left hip fracture due to fall ____________
8. Open manipulation and internal fixation of acetabular fracture due to head on collision (MVA) ____________
9. Healing traumatic fracture right tibia/fibula with application of short leg cast ____________
10. Closed reduction and internal fixation of Bennett's fracture ____________

DOCUMENTATION/REIMBURSEMENT/MS-DRGs

Often coding difficulties are due to lack of documentation. Sometimes radiology and other test results are not available at the time of discharge or when the physician is dictating the discharge summary or is reporting the final diagnoses. Documentation may be lacking for how and where an injury happened, so it is difficult to assign appropriate E codes.

Identification and accurate coding of all procedures and diagnoses may be instrumental in MS-DRG assignment. It is also important to code associated chronic conditions that may qualify as comorbid conditions. A thorough review of the record is necessary to identify complications that may occur during the stay. In cases of injury, it is very important to pick up all associated procedures. Often, in trauma cases, surgeons are busy trying to save the life of the patient, and documentation is not their top priority. The record should be reviewed for suturing of arteries or lacerations of internal organs, mechanical ventilation, and debridements. Sometimes, in the repair of fractures resulting from trauma, joint replacement will be necessary.

Correct Orthopedic Procedure Code

EXAMPLE

An elderly patient falls and fractures hip and undergoes ORIF procedure.

An error is made in assigning or entering the procedure code in the second case.

DIAGNOSES	CODES	MS-DRG	RW
Fracture hip	820.8	494	1.2752
ORIF	79.36		
Fracture hip	820.8	536	0.7340
Closed reduction without fixation	79.06		

Two Diagnoses That Equally Meet the Definition for Principal Diagnosis

EXAMPLE

A patient is admitted with a skull fracture and a hip fracture. Designation of the principal diagnosis can make a difference in reimbursement. In this case, it may be necessary to query the physician as to which injury is the most serious. If a procedure was performed, that may also help the coder to determine which diagnosis is principal.

DIAGNOSES	CODES	MS-DRG	RW
Fracture hip and skull	820.8, 803.00	536	0.7340
Fracture skull and hip	803.00, 820.8	085	1.6946

Coding Specificity and MS-DRG With and Without MCC/CC

EXAMPLE

Patient is admitted with fractured ribs. X-ray report reveals fractures of the third, fourth, fifth, and sixth ribs. No procedures were performed. Patient was also treated for a urinary tract infection.

DIAGNOSES	CODES	MS-DRG	RW
Rib fractures, UTI	807.00, 599.0	206	0.7848
Rib fracture, 4 ribs, UTI	807.04, 599.0	184	0.9611

In this example, reimbursement is affected by the more specific fracture code, which indicates that four ribs were fractured, and by the assignment of the UTI code (599.0), which is a CC for MS-DRG 184.

CHAPTER REVIEW EXERCISE

Assign codes for all diagnoses and procedures, including all applicable V and E codes and procedures.

1. Fracture/dislocation right femur due to fall from hospital bed. Contusion right hip ____________
2. Closed reduction of recurrent left shoulder dislocation ____________
3. Inversion injury right ankle with severe sprain during dismount from gymnastics equipment at local gym (twisting injury) ____________
4. Grade III laceration to the bladder due to gunshot wound. Exploratory laparotomy with repair of the bladder laceration. Patient was shot during robbery of gas station ____________
5. Crush injury with fracture hand (multiple metacarpals) ____________
6. Wound left calf due to dog bite. Wound was cleansed and Steri-strips applied ____________
7. Closed head injury with concussion and brief loss of consciousness (10 minutes) ____________
8. Pain due to anterior dislocation of left shoulder due to tackle during college football game ____________
9. Tear ulnar collateral ligament of the metacarpophalangeal joint due to fall and injury due to ski pole ____________
10. Sprain right foot due to fall from trampoline. Trampoline is in neighbor's backyard ____________

11. Crush injury with laceration of foot. Dropped car battery on foot while at work ______
12. Hemiarthroplasty due to displaced femoral neck fracture caused by fall at home ______
13. Rib fractures due to child abuse ______
14. Open fracture of left tibial shaft with fracture of the fibula. Laceration calf, which exposes the tibia ______
15. Flail chest due to MVA involving collision with train. Patient driver of MV ______
16. Lacerations upper arm with embedded gravel due to fall from bicycle. Repaired with Dermabond and sutures ______
17. Contusions chest and forehead with 2-cm laceration of forehead, which was sutured. Patient was a passenger in a motor vehicle rollover ______
18. Bilateral fractures of the radius. Right upper end and left distal end. Closed reductions bilaterally ______
19. Dislocation of little finger due to wrestling. This is the third time the patient has dislocated this finger. Closed reduction was performed ______
20. Intertrochanteric fracture left hip with ORIF ______
21. Fracture temporal bone due to fall while skateboarding at park ______
22. Injury to eye from paintball gun. Injury occurred at paintball recreation site ______
23. Hangman's fracture (C2) due to suicide attempt ______
24. Laceration scalp repaired with staples. Fall from tree in backyard ______
25. Fracture of L3 requiring fracture repair, posterior spinal fusion L2-L4 using bone grafts from iliac crest, and spinal instrumentation. Pedestrian hit by car ______
26. Closed head injury due to fall from balcony of apartment building. Patient had a brain contusion with LOC. ______
27. Subdural hematoma with brief loss of consciousness due to fall from scaffolding at construction site. Hematoma was evacuated in the OR through burr hole ______
28. Peroneal nerve injury due to fibular fracture. Patient was kicked while milking cows at a dairy farm ______
29. Shattered C1-C2 vertebra with spinal cord injury due to fall from horse ______

Write the correct answer(s) in the space(s) provided.

30. Define open fracture. ______________________________

CHAPTER GLOSSARY

Closed fracture: injury in which the bone is broken, but the skin remains intact.

Closed head injuries: injuries that result from a blow to the head.

Closed reduction of a fracture: the surgeon manipulates or reduces fractured bones into anatomic alignment without making an incision through the skin and subcutaneous tissue.

Colles' fracture: common fracture in adults in which the lower end of the radius is fractured and the wrist and hand are displaced backward.

Complicated fracture: fracture that causes injury to surrounding tissues.

Concussion: injury to the brain that results from a significant blow to the head.

Contusion: any mechanical injury that results in hemorrhage beneath unbroken skin.

Crush injury: when a body part is subjected to a high degree of force or pressure, usually after it has been squeezed between two heavy or immobile objects.

Dermabond: liquid skin adhesive used to close skin lacerations.

Dislocation: displacement of the bones that form a joint; separation of the end of a bone from the joint it meets.

External skeletal fixation: form of fracture treatment that involves insertion of percutaneous pins proximal and distal to the fracture and application of a frame that connects the pins externally.

Fracture: break in a bone.

Laceration: an injury that results in a tear in the skin.

Loss of consciousness: when a patient is unable to respond to people or other stimuli.

Open fracture: when the bone exits and is visible through the skin, or a deep wound exposes the bone through the skin.

Open reduction of a fracture: when the surgeon makes an incision at the fracture site to reduce or manipulate the fracture into anatomic position.

Pathologic fracture: break in a bone that occurs because of underlying disorders that weaken the bone, including malignancy, benign bone tumor, metabolic disorder, infection, and osteoporosis.

Spinal cord injury: damage to the spiral cord that causes loss of sensation and motor control.

Sprain: stretch and/or tear of a ligament.

Strain: injury to a muscle or a tendon.

Subluxation: partial or incomplete dislocation.

Suture: method for closing cutaneous wounds.

Traumatic brain injury: injury to the brain that may result in interference with the brain's normal functions.

CHAPTER 20

Burns, Adverse Effects, and Poisonings

(ICD-9-CM Chapter 17, Codes 800-995)

CHAPTER OUTLINE

LEARNING OBJECTIVES

- Apply and assign the correct ICD-9-CM codes in accordance with Official Guidelines for Coding and Reporting
- Identify the various types of burns
- Differentiate between an adverse effect and a poisoning
- Assign the correct V codes, E codes, and procedure codes related to burns, adverse effects, and poisonings
- Identify common treatments
- Explain the importance of documentation in relation to MS-DRGs for reimbursement

ABBREVIATIONS

AKA above-knee amputation

CC complication/comorbidity

HBOT hyperbaric oxygen therapy

ICD-9-CM *International Classification of Diseases, 9th Revision, Clinical Modification*

MS-DRG Medicare severity diagnosis-related group

MVA motor vehicle accident

OR Operating Room

SIRS systemic inflammatory response syndrome

UTI urinary tract infection

ICD-9-CM Official Guidelines for Coding and Reporting

Please refer to the companion Evolve website for the most current guidelines.

17. Chapter 17: Injury and Poisoning (800-999)

Only guidelines applicable to this chapter are included; therefore the numbers or letters are not sequential.

c. Coding of Burns

Current burns (940-948) are classified by depth, extent and by agent (E code). Burns are classified by depth as first degree (erythema), second degree (blistering), and third degree (full-thickness involvement).

1) Sequencing of burn and related condition codes

Sequence first the code that reflects the highest degree of burn when more than one burn is present.

a. When the reason for the admission or encounter is for treatment of external multiple burns, sequence first the code that reflects the burn of the highest degree.

EXAMPLE Second-degree burns of the left hand and first-degree burns of the left forearm, 944.20, 943.11.

b. When a patient has both internal and external burns, the circumstances of admission govern the selection of the principal diagnosis or first-listed diagnosis.

c. When a patient is admitted for burn injuries and other related conditions such as smoke inhalation and/or respiratory failure, the circumstances of admission govern the selection of the principal or first-listed diagnosis.

2) Burns of the same local site

Classify burns of the same local site (three-digit category level, 940-947) but of different degrees to the subcategory identifying the highest degree recorded in the diagnosis.

EXAMPLE Second- and third-degree burns of the right thigh, 945.36.

3) Non-healing burns

Non-healing burns are coded as acute burns.

Necrosis of burned skin should be coded as a non-healed burn.

EXAMPLE Necrosis of third-degree burn on the buttock, 942.34.

4) Code 958.3, Posttraumatic wound infection

Assign code 958.3, Posttraumatic wound infection, not elsewhere classified, as an additional code for any documented infected burn site.

EXAMPLE Infected burn right foot, 945.02, 958.3.

5) Assign separate codes for each burn site

When coding burns, assign separate codes for each burn site. Category 946 Burns of Multiple specified sites, should only be used if the location of the burns are not documented.

Category 949, Burn, unspecified, is extremely vague and should rarely be used.

EXAMPLE Multiple burns over the entire body. The patient expired before he could be admitted, 949.0.

6) **Assign codes from category 948, Burns**
Burns classified according to extent of body surface involved, when the site of the burn is not specified or when there is a need for additional data. It is advisable to use category 948 as additional coding when needed to provide data for evaluating burn mortality, such as that needed by burn units. It is also advisable to use category 948 as an additional code for reporting purposes when there is mention of a third-degree burn involving 20% or more of the body surface.

In assigning a code from category 948:

Fourth-digit codes are used to identify the percentage of total body surface involved in a burn (all degree).

Fifth-digits are assigned to identify the percentage of body surface involved in third-degree burn.

Fifth-digit zero (0) is assigned when less than 10% or when no body surface is involved in a third-degree burn.

Category 948 is based on the classic "rule of nines" in estimating body surface involved: head and neck are assigned 9%, each arm 9%, each leg 18%, the anterior trunk 18%, posterior trunk 18%, and genitalia 1%. Providers may change these percentage assignments where necessary to accommodate infants and children who have proportionately larger heads than adults and patients who have large buttocks, thighs, or abdomen that involve burns.

EXAMPLE The patient has second-degree (3%) and third-degree (5%) burns of the trunk and first-degree burns (2%) of the right arm, 942.30, 943.10, 948.10.

7) **Encounters for treatment of late effects of burns**
Encounters for the treatment of the late effects of burns (i.e., scars or joint contractures) should be coded to the residual condition (sequelae) followed by the appropriate late effect code (906.5-906.9). A late effect E code may also be used, if desired.

EXAMPLE Contracture of the skin of the right index finger due to burn from fire injury 6 months ago, 709.2, 906.6, E929.4.

8) **Sequelae with a late effect code and current burn**
When appropriate, both a sequelae with a late effect code, and a current burn code may be assigned on the same record (when both a current burn and sequelae of an old burn exist).

d. **Coding of Debridement of Wound, Infection, or Burn**
Excisional debridement involves surgical removal or cutting away, as opposed to a mechanical (brushing, scrubbing, washing) debridement.

For coding purposes, excisional debridement is assigned to code 86.22.

Nonexcisional debridement is assigned to code 86.28.

EXAMPLE Sharp debridement of right heel ulcer performed by physical therapist, 707.14, 86.22.

EXAMPLE Excisional debridement of gangrenous decubitus ulcer of the elbow by physician, 707.01, 785.4, 86.22.

EXAMPLE Nonexcisional debridement of left foot ulcer performed by physical therapist, 707.15, 86.28.

e. Adverse Effects, Poisoning and Toxic Effects

The properties of certain drugs, medicinal and biological substances or combinations of such substances, may cause toxic reactions. The occurrence of drug toxicity is classified in ICD-9-CM as follows:

1) Adverse Effect

When the drug was correctly prescribed and properly administered, code the reaction plus the appropriate code from the E930-E949 series. Codes from the E930-E949 series must be used to identify the causative substance for an adverse effect of drug, medicinal and biological substances, correctly prescribed and properly administered. The effect, such as tachycardia, delirium, gastrointestinal hemorrhaging, vomiting, hypokalemia, hepatitis, renal failure, or respiratory failure, is coded and followed by the appropriate code from the E930-E949 series.

Adverse effects of therapeutic substances correctly prescribed and properly administered (toxicity, synergistic reaction, side effect, and idiosyncratic reaction) may be due to (1) differences among patients, such as age, sex, disease, and genetic factors, and (2) drug-related factors, such as type of drug, route of administration, duration of therapy, dosage, and bioavailability.

2) Poisoning

(a) Error was made in drug prescription

Errors made in drug prescription or in the administration of the drug by provider, nurse, patient, or other person, use the appropriate poisoning code from the 960-979 series.

EXAMPLE

While in the hospital, the nurse accidentatally gave the patient 40 mg of Lasix instead of the ordered 20-mg dosage. The patient suffered no ill effects, 974.4, E858.5, E849.7.

(b) Overdose of a drug intentionally taken

If an overdose of a drug was intentionally taken or administered and resulted in drug toxicity, it would be coded as a poisoning (960-979 series).

EXAMPLE

The patient intentionally overdosed with 20 Valium tablets. The patient is in a coma, 969.4, 780.01, E950.3.

(c) Nonprescribed drug taken with correctly prescribed and properly administered drug

If a nonprescribed drug or medicinal agent was taken in combination with a correctly prescribed and properly administered drug, any drug toxicity or other reaction resulting from the interaction of the two drugs would be classified as a poisoning.

(d) Sequencing of poisoning

When coding a poisoning or reaction to the improper use of a medication (e.g., wrong dose, wrong substance, wrong route of administration) the poisoning code is sequenced first, followed by a code for the manifestation. If there is also a diagnosis of drug abuse or dependence to the substance, the abuse or dependence is coded as an additional code.

See Section I.C.3.a.6.b. if poisoning is the result of insulin pump malfunctions and Section I.C.19 for general use of E-codes.

EXAMPLE

Chest pain due to accidental poisoning from cocaine. The patient uses cocaine on a daily basis, 970.8, 786.50, 305.61, E854.3.

3) Toxic Effects

(a) Toxic effect codes

When a harmful substance is ingested or comes in contact with a person, this is classified as a toxic effect. The toxic effect codes are in categories 980-989.

(b) Sequencing toxic effect codes

A toxic effect code should be sequenced first, followed by the code(s) that identify the result of the toxic effect.

(c) External cause codes for toxic effects

An external cause code from categories E860-E869 for accidental exposure, codes E950.6 or E950.7 for intentional self-harm, category E962 for assault, or categories E980-E982, for undetermined, should also be assigned to indicate intent.

EXAMPLE A 2-year-old accidentally drank lye, causing burns to the mouth and throat, 983.2, 947.0, E864.2.

g. SIRS due to Non-infectious Process

The systemic inflammatory response syndrome (SIRS) can develop as a result of certain non-infectious disease processes, such as trauma, malignant neoplasm, or pancreatitis. When SIRS is documented with a noninfectious condition, and no subsequent infection is documented, the code for the underlying condition, such as an injury, should be assigned, followed by code 995.93, Systemic inflammatory response syndrome due to noninfectious process without acute organ dysfunction, or 995.94, Systemic inflammatory response syndrome due to noninfectious process with acute organ dysfunction. If an acute organ dysfunction is documented, the appropriate code(s) for the associated acute organ dysfunction(s) should be assigned in addition to code 995.94. If acute organ dysfunction is documented, but it cannot be determined if the acute organ dysfunction is associated with SIRS or due to another condition (e.g., directly due to the trauma), the provider should be queried.

When the noninfectious condition has led to an infection that results in SIRS, *see Section I.C.1.b.11 for the guideline for sepsis and severe sepsis associated with a noninfectious process.*

EXAMPLE A patient was admitted with SIRS. After investigation, it was determined that the cause was acute pancreatitis, 577.0, 995.93.

Apply the General Coding Guidelines as found in Chapter 5.

At the beginning of Chapter 17 in the ICD-9-CM codebook, special instructions say, "Use E code(s) to identify the cause and intent of the injury or poisoning (E800-E999)" (Figure 20-1). It may be necessary to go back to Chapter 8 to review the guidelines for proper assignment and sequencing of E codes and late effect codes.

ANATOMY AND PHYSIOLOGY

All areas of the body may be involved in an injury. These are outlined in their respective body system chapters.

17. INJURY AND POISONING (800–999)

Use E code(s) to identify the cause and intent of the injury or poisoning (E800-E999)

Note:

1. The principle of multiple coding of injuries should be followed wherever possible. Combination categories for multiple injuries are provided for use when there is insufficient detail as to the nature of the individual conditions, or for primary tabulation purposes when it is more convenient to record a single code; otherwise, the component injuries should be coded separately.

   Where multiple sites of injury are specified in the titles, the word "with" indicates involvement of both sites, and the word "and" indicates involvement of either or both sites. The word "finger" includes thumb.

2. Categories for "late effect" of injuries are to be found at 905–909.

Figure 20-1. Instructional note regarding the use of E code(s) to identify the cause and intent of injury or poisoning (E800-E999).

DISEASE CONDITIONS

This chapter discusses the following categories from Chapter 17 in your ICD-9-CM code book:

CATEGORY	SECTION TITLES
905-909	Late Effects of Injuries, Poisonings, Toxic Effects, and Other External Causes
940-949	Burns
958-959	Certain Traumatic Complications and Unspecified Injuries
960-979	Poisoning by Drugs, Medicinals, and Biologic Substances
980-989	Toxic Effects of Substances Chiefly Nonmedicinal to Source
990-995	Other and Unspecified Effect of External Causes

Chapter 21 is dedicated to complications of surgical and medical care.

Late Effects of Injuries, Poisonings, Toxic Effects, and Other External Causes (905-909)

Once the acute nature of an injury or poisoning has resolved, some residual effects that have remained may require medical treatment. The residual effect is sequenced first, followed by the appropriate late effect code. In Chapter 8, the coding and sequencing of late effects were discussed. In this chapter, late effects due to traumatic injury are covered. Remember, a late effect may occur at any time after the acute injury has resolved. No specific time frames are required.

Late effect categories are as follows:

905	Late effects of musculoskeletal and connective tissue injuries
906	Late effects of injuries to skin and subcutaneous tissues (Figure 20-2, *A*)
907	Late effects of injuries to the nervous system
908	Late effects of other and unspecified injuries
909	Late effects of other and unspecified external causes

To locate the late effect code, look under the main term "Late" and then verify in the Tabular. The Tabular indicates which conditions from categories 800 to 999 are the cause of the residual condition.

EXAMPLE

Scar of wrist due to previous burn by fire, 709.2, 906.6, E929.4
Late effect of injury classifiable to 944 (see Figure 20-2, *B*)

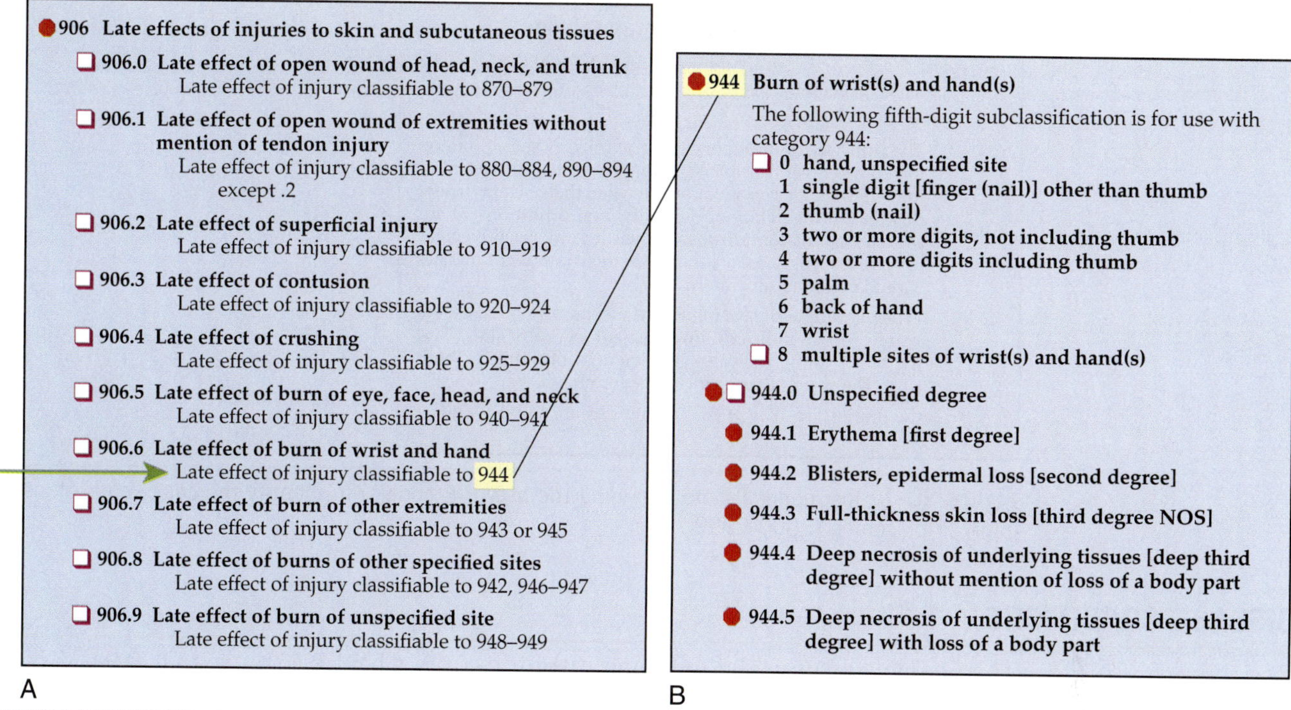
906 Late effects of injuries to skin and subcutaneous tissues
- **906.0 Late effect of open wound of head, neck, and trunk**
  Late effect of injury classifiable to 870–879
- **906.1 Late effect of open wound of extremities without mention of tendon injury**
  Late effect of injury classifiable to 880–884, 890–894 except .2
- **906.2 Late effect of superficial injury**
  Late effect of injury classifiable to 910–919
- **906.3 Late effect of contusion**
  Late effect of injury classifiable to 920–924
- **906.4 Late effect of crushing**
  Late effect of injury classifiable to 925–929
- **906.5 Late effect of burn of eye, face, head, and neck**
  Late effect of injury classifiable to 940–941
- **906.6 Late effect of burn of wrist and hand**
  Late effect of injury classifiable to 944
- **906.7 Late effect of burn of other extremities**
  Late effect of injury classifiable to 943 or 945
- **906.8 Late effect of burns of other specified sites**
  Late effect of injury classifiable to 942, 946–947
- **906.9 Late effect of burn of unspecified site**
  Late effect of injury classifiable to 948–949

A

944 Burn of wrist(s) and hand(s)

The following fifth-digit subclassification is for use with category 944:
- **0 hand, unspecified site**
- **1 single digit [finger (nail)] other than thumb**
- **2 thumb (nail)**
- **3 two or more digits, not including thumb**
- **4 two or more digits including thumb**
- **5 palm**
- **6 back of hand**
- **7 wrist**
- **8 multiple sites of wrist(s) and hand(s)**

- **944.0 Unspecified degree**
- **944.1 Erythema [first degree]**
- **944.2 Blisters, epidermal loss [second degree]**
- **944.3 Full-thickness skin loss [third degree NOS]**
- **944.4 Deep necrosis of underlying tissues [deep third degree] without mention of loss of a body part**
- **944.5 Deep necrosis of underlying tissues [deep third degree] with loss of a body part**

B

Figure 20-2. **A,** Categories for late effects of injuries to skin and subcutaneous tissues. **B,** 944 is the category that would have been assigned for the acute injury.

It may be necessary to assign the appropriate E code to indicate the late effects of accidental injury from category E929. Code assignment for E codes may depend on facility policy. Often, documentation is insufficient to reveal how the accident happened.

E929.0	Late effects of motor vehicle accident
E929.1	Late effects of other transport accident
E929.2	Late effects of accidental poisoning
E929.3	Late effects of accidental fall
E929.4	Late effects of accident caused by fire
E929.5	Late effects of accident due to natural and environmental factors
E929.8	Late effects of other accidents
E929.9	Late effects of unspecified accident
E989	Late effects of injury, undetermined whether accidental or purposely inflicted

EXAMPLE

Patient has a cicatrix of left hand due to accidental burn that occurred 1 year ago from a bonfire, 709.2, 906.6, E929.4.

EXAMPLE

Patient is being treated for avascular necrosis following previous scaphoid fracture due to old sports injury with fall, 733.49, 905.2, E929.3.

EXAMPLE

Patient has a contracture of the right index finger due to scar from burn due to accidental fire injury 6 months ago, 709.2, 906.6, E929.4.

EXERCISE 20-1

Assign codes to the following conditions using your ICD-9-CM code book.

1. Nonunion of lateral humeral condylar fracture; patient fell 2 months ago (accidental injury) __________
2. Traumatic arthritis due to severe sprain of right ankle 3 years ago (accidental injury) __________
3. Phantom limb pain due to traumatic AKA (above knee amputation); patient was in a motorcycle accident 6 months ago __________
4. Spastic quadriplegia due to spinal cord injury from diving accident 5 years ago __________
5. Hypoxic brain injury due to suicide attempt by strangulation 1 year ago __________

Burns (940-949)

It may be necessary to transport burn victims to a hospital that has a specialized unit for care of the burn patient. Plastic surgeons, anesthesiologists, nurses, dietitians, and physical and occupational therapists assist the burn patient through the acute and recovery phases of their injury. As a result, many facilities only stabilize the burn patient in the emergency room and then transport to a burn unit, or only less critical burn patients are admitted for care.

The Coding Guidelines offer advice on the coding and sequencing of burn injury codes. As with other injuries, it is necessary to assign separate codes for each burn site. Codes are available for multiple sites, but these should be used only if the documentation is insufficient to allow assignment of more specific burn codes.

Burn severity is classified by degrees (Figure 20-3):

- First-degree burn: **erythema** or redness of the skin
- Second-degree burn: formation of blisters with **epidermal** loss
- Third-degree burn: full-thickness skin loss
- Fourth-degree burn: deep **necrosis** of underlying tissues or deep third-degree burn

The guidelines instruct the coder to sequence the code that reflects the highest degree of burn first.

EXAMPLE

Patient was seen in the ER for second-degree burns of the left calf and first-degree burns of the right foot due to uncontrolled grass fire in woods, 945.24, 945.12, E892, E849.8.

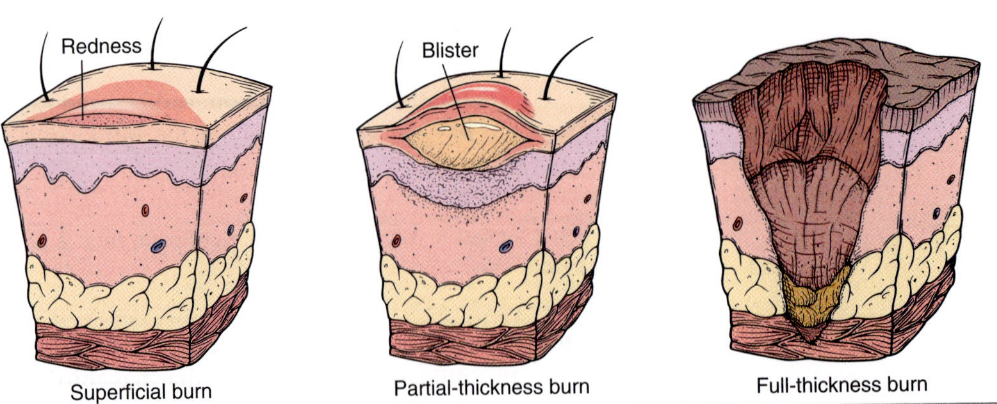

Figure 20-3. Depths of burns.

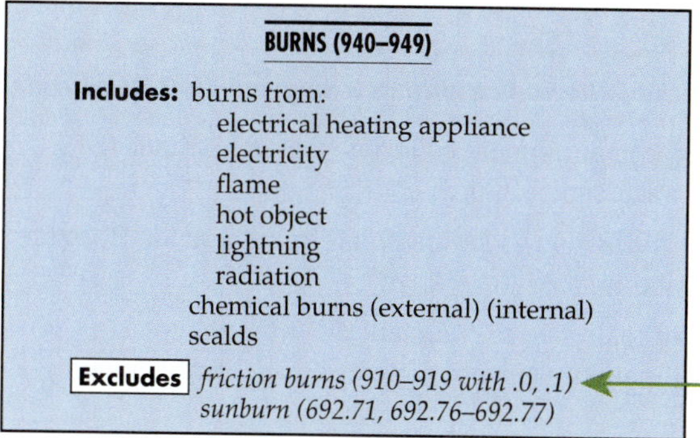
BURNS (940–949)

Includes: burns from:
electrical heating appliance
electricity
flame
hot object
lightning
radiation
chemical burns (external) (internal)
scalds

Excludes *friction burns (910–919 with .0, .1)*
sunburn (692.71, 692.76–692.77)

Figure 20-4. Friction burns and sunburn are excluded from the burn section.

Often, a burn will be described as having different degrees at the same site. It is only necessary to assign the code that identifies the highest degree of burn.

EXAMPLE Examination of the patient shows erythema and blisters to the right wrist due to burn from an iron. The accident occurred at the patient's home, 944.27, E924.8, E849.1.

Although the physician did not state first- or second-degree burn, by the description, this burn is a first- (erythema) and second-degree (blister) burn, so it would be coded to the most severe burn, which is second degree.

For a variety of reasons, a burn may not heal quickly, or it may become infected. A nonhealing burn is coded as an acute burn. It is possible to have burns that occurred at the same time, and some may have healed completely while others have not yet healed. If the burn contains necrotic tissue, it is coded as an acute burn. It is possible to have late effects (e.g., scar, contracture) of a burn along with a nonhealing burn. Sometimes, late effects remain after the burn has healed, and these still require treatment. Residual conditions are late effects; therefore, these should be coded with the residual condition sequenced first followed by the appropriate late effect code. A late effect E code may also be assigned.

Sunburns (692.71, 692.76-692.77) or burns due to friction (910-919 with .0, .1) are excluded from the burn codes; this is noted in the Excludes note at the beginning of the burn section (Figure 20-4).

EXAMPLE Patient has necrotic third-degree burn on chest wall due to home fire, 942.32, E890.9, E849.1.

EXAMPLE Patient has a nonhealing third-degree burn of abdominal wall with keloid scar forming on right shoulder burn. Burns due to accidental injury, 942.33, 701.4, 906.7, E929.9.

Code 958.3, Posttraumatic wound infection, can be used as an additional code to indicate that the burn has become infected. The acute burn code would be sequenced first (Figure 20-5).

EXAMPLE Patient is being treated for an infected burn right palm from a hot light bulb, 944.05, 958.3, E924.8.

Category 948 is provided to identify the extent of body surface that is involved by burns and to indicate the percentage of body surface that has third-degree burns. According to the classic "rule of nines," in estimating involved body surface, head and neck are assigned 9%, each arm 9%, each leg 18%, anterior trunk 18%, posterior trunk 18%, and genitalia

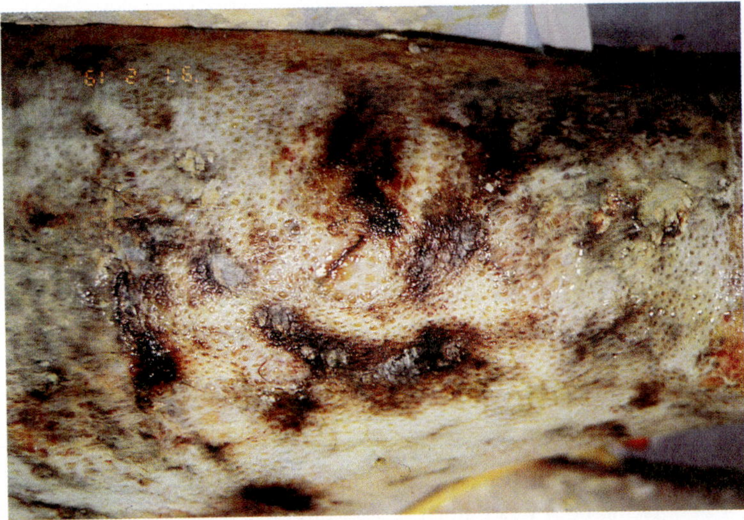

Figure 20-5. Invasive pseudomonal burn wound infection, stage 2C.

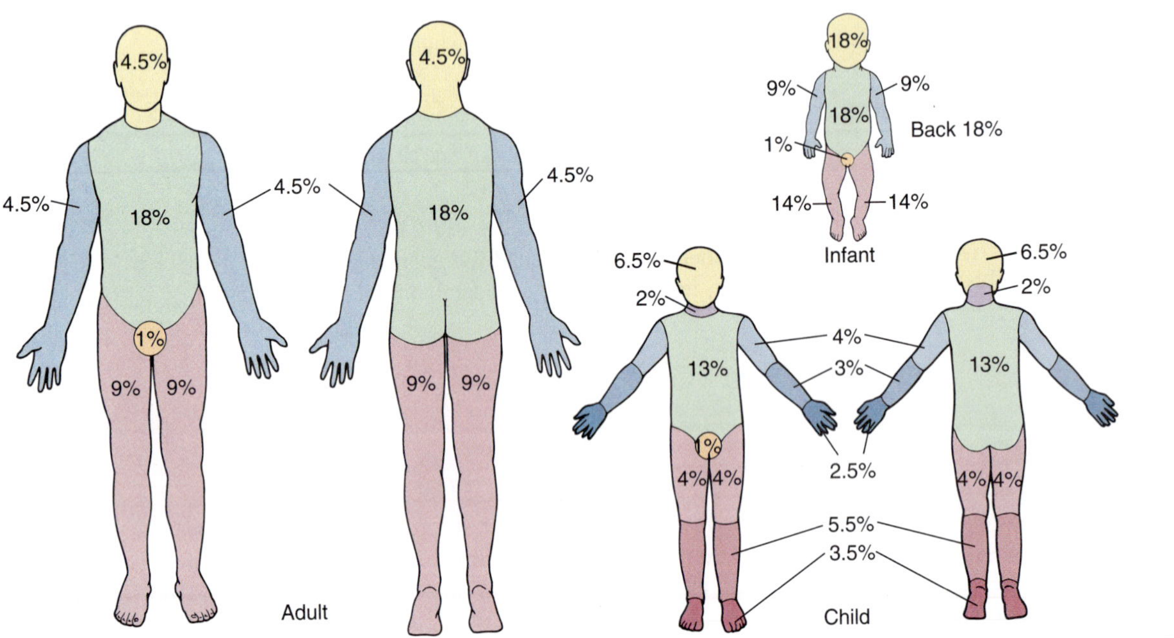

Figure 20-6. Rule of nines.

1%. These percentage assignments may change as necessary to accommodate infants and children who have proportionately larger heads than adults and patients who have large buttocks, thighs, or abdomen that involve burns (Figure 20-6). The percentages of body surface involvement must be documented by a healthcare professional for code assignment. Percentages should not be calculated by the coder.

Categories 948 and/or 949 can be used when the site of the burn is not specified. Category 948 can be used with categories 940-947 when the site is specified. In some instances, the burns may be so extensive that detailed documentation is not provided. A specialized burn assessment form to document burn location, type, and body percentage is often used in burn centers.

EXAMPLE

Patient has second- (3%) and third-degree (5%) burns of the trunk and first-degree burns (2%) of the right arm due to fire on a street car, 942.30, 943.10, 948.10, E829.4, E849.5.

EXERCISE 20-2

Assign codes to the following conditions using your ICD-9-CM code book. (If percentage of the body burned is not documented do not assign a code from category 948).

1. Nonhealing second-degree burn left thigh due to hot coffee spill __________
2. Second- and third-degree burns trunk, and second- and third-degree burns both legs due to fire at night club; in all, 35% of the body was burned, 25% third degree __________
3. First-degree burn wrist and second-degree burns fingers and hand due to firework explosion while playing in backyard __________
4. Infected second-degree burn buttock __________
5. Alkaline burn left cornea due to caustic soda while working in a paper manufacturing factory __________
6. Hypertrophic scar of burn to right cheek __________
7. Friction burn left elbow due to accidental fall on carpeted stairs at patient's home __________
8. Patient in house fire with multiple burns over 60% of body, 30% third degree; patient was stabilized and prepared for transport to burn unit; fire was due to accidental causes __________

Certain Traumatic Complications and Unspecified Injuries (958-959)

A variety of complications may occur as the result of injury. An **air embolism** is formed when air or gas bubbles get into the bloodstream, possibly obstructing the circulation. Trauma to the lung can cause an air embolism. This may occur in divers from rapid changes of pressure.

A **fat embolism** can occur after long bone or pelvic fracture. It usually presents 12 to 48 hours after the injury with symptoms such as tachycardia, tachypnea, elevated temperature, hypoxemia, hypocapnia, thrombocytopenia, and occasionally mild neurologic symptoms. A petechial rash also appears on the upper anterior portion of the body, including the chest, neck, upper arm, axilla, shoulder, oral mucous membranes, and conjunctivae. Infection, shock, anuria, and subcutaneous emphysema are other examples of complications of trauma.

Category 959 is used for injuries that are unspecified or not otherwise specified. This code is commonly used in the outpatient setting. A patient may have sustained injury to the ankle, but after x-rays and examination, the patient's ankle pain cannot be explained by a more specific code such as fracture, dislocation, or sprain.

EXAMPLE

Patient was hospitalized for treatment of an open fracture right femur (shaft) and developed a fat embolism, 821.11, 958.1, E887.

EXERCISE 20-3

Assign codes to the following conditions using your ICD-9-CM code book.

1. Pain due to twisting injury left knee while playing basketball at gym ______
2. Patient bumped head on cabinet door at home ______
3. Shoulder injury due to fall on public sidewalk ______
4. Injury left hip during high school football game due to being pushed down ______
5. Subcutaneous emphysema due to pneumothorax from a stab wound into thorax during fi ght in bar ______
6. Infection due to second-degree burn left thigh caused by spilled coffee ______
7. Traumatic shock due to blunt intraabdominal injury caused by car pile-up on Interstate highway; patient was driver of car ______

Adverse Effects of Drugs and Medicinals

An **adverse effect** can occur due to ingestion or exposure to drugs or other medicinal and biologic substances. It is a reaction to a drug that has been taken according to the prescription or instructions on the label of over-the-counter drugs. To code an adverse effect, at least two codes are required: one code for the adverse effect (e.g., rash, nausea, headache) and a therapeutic use E code (E930-E949) for the drug responsible for the adverse effect. These E codes are located in the Table of Drugs and Chemicals.

The Table of Drugs and Chemicals (Figure 20-7), which is also known as the Alphabetic Index to Poisoning and External Causes of Adverse Effects of Drugs and Other Chemical Substances, is located after the Alphabetic Index. This Table is used to identify external causes of adverse effects that are due to drugs or chemicals. The drug responsible for the adverse effect must first be identified and then located in the index under the therapeutic column. If a specific dug cannot be located, the generic name should be determined or the category of the drug identified (e.g., antihypertensive, antianginal, antineoplastic). Once the drug or drug category has been located in the index, the E code from the therapeutic use column is assigned. The adverse effect code(s) are sequenced before the therapeutic E code(s).

Because drugs have generic and brand names, and these are used interchangeably, it may be difficult to locate the drug in the index. A drug reference book or an Internet search can be used to determine the generic name or category of the drug.

EXAMPLE

Hematuria due to Coumadin, which is taken for atrial fibrillation, 599.7, E934.2, 427.31, V58.61.

Hematuria in this case is the adverse effect of medication that was properly prescribed and properly taken. An E code for the therapeutic use of Coumadin is also assigned.

EXAMPLE

Patient presented with hypokalemia due to long-term use of diuretics, 276.8, V58.69, E944.4. Hypokalemia is the adverse effect of the diuretic.

EXAMPLE

Dizziness caused by Claritin, which was taken per instructions on the label, 780.4, E933.0. Claritin is not listed in the Table of Drugs and Chemicals, but an Internet search reveals that loratadine is the generic name, and this is not listed either. Claritin is classified as an antihistamine that can be located in the Table.

Substance	Poisoning	External Cause (E-Code)				
		Accident	Therapeutic Use	Suicide Attempt	Assault	Undetermined
1-propanol	980.3	E860.4	—	E950.9	E962.1	E980.9
2-propanol	980.2	E860.3	—	E950.9	E962.1	E980.9
2,4-D (dichlorophenoxyacetic acid)	989.4	E863.5	—	E950.6	E962.1	E980.7
2,4-toluene diisocyanate	983.0	E864.0	—	E950.7	E962.1	E980.6
2,4,5-T (trichlorophenoxyacetic acid)	989.2	E863.5	—	E950.6	E962.1	E980.7
14-hydroxydihydromorphinone	965.09	E850.2	E935.2	E950.0	E962.0	E980.0
ABOB	961.7	E857	E931.7	E950.4	E962.0	E980.4
Abrus (seed)	988.2	E865.3	—	E950.9	E962.1	E980.9
Absinthe	980.0	E860.1	—	E950.9	E962.1	E980.9
beverage	980.0	E860.0	—	E950.9	E962.1	E980.9
Acenocoumarin, acenocoumarol	964.2	E858.2	E934.2	E950.4	E962.0	E980.4
Acepromazine	969.1	E853.0	E939.1	E950.3	E962.0	E980.3
Acetal	982.8	E862.4	—	E950.9	E962.1	E980.9
Acetaldehyde (vapor)	987.8	E869.8	—	E952.8	E962.2	E982.8
liquid	989.89	E866.8	—	E950.9	E962.1	E980.9
Acetaminophen	965.4	E850.4	E935.4	E950.0	E962.0	E980.0
Acetaminosalol	965.1	E850.3	E935.3	E950.0	E962.0	E980.0
Acetanilid(e)	965.4	E850.4	E935.4	E950.0	E962.0	E980.0
Acetarsol, acetarsone	961.1	E857	E931.1	E950.4	E962.0	E980.4
Acetazolamide	974.2	E858.5	E944.2	E950.4	E962.0	E980.4
Acetic	—	—	—	—	—	—
acid	983.1	E864.1	—	E950.7	E962.1	E980.6
with sodium acetate (ointment)	976.3	E858.7	E946.3	E950.4	E962.0	E980.4
irrigating solution	974.5	E858.5	E944.5	E950.4	E962.0	E980.4
lotion	976.2	E858.7	E946.2	E950.4	E962.0	E980.4
anhydride	983.1	E864.1	—	E950.7	E962.1	E980.6
ether (vapor)	982.8	E862.4	—	E950.9	E962.1	E980.9
Acetohexamide	962.3	E858.0	E932.3	E950.4	E962.0	E980.4
Acetomenaphthone	964.3	E858.2	E934.3	E950.4	E962.0	E980.4
Acetomorphine	965.01	E850.0	E935.0	E950.0	E962.0	E980.0
Acetone (oils) (vapor)	982.8	E862.4	—	E950.9	E962.1	E980.9
Acetophenazine (maleate)	969.1	E853.0	E939.1	E950.3	E962.0	E980.3
Acetophenetidin	965.4	E850.4	E935.4	E950.0	E962.0	E980.0
Acetophenone	982.0	E862.4	—	E950.9	E962.1	E980.9
Acetorphine	965.09	E850.2	E935.2	E950.0	E962.0	E980.0
Acetosulfone (sodium)	961.8	E857	E931.8	E950.4	E962.0	E980.4
Acetrizoate (sodium)	977.8	E858.8	E947.8	E950.4	E962.0	E980.4
Acetylcarbromal	967.3	E852.2	E937.3	E950.2	E962.0	E980.2
Acetylcholine (chloride)	971.0	E855.3	E941.0	E950.4	E962.0	E980.4
Acetylcysteine	975.5	E858.6	E945.5	E950.4	E962.0	E980.4
Acetyldigitoxin	972.1	E858.3	E942.1	E950.4	E962.0	E980.4
Acetyldihydrocodeine	965.09	E850.2	E935.2	E950.0	E962.0	E980.0
Acetyldihydrocodeinone	965.09	E850.2	E935.2	E950.0	E962.0	E980.0
Acetylene (gas) (industrial)	987.1	E868.1	—	E951.8	E962.2	E981.8
incomplete combustion of - *see* Carbon monoxide, fuel, utility	—	—	—	—	—	—
tetrachloride (vapor)	982.3	E862.4	—	E950.9	E962.1	E980.9
Acetyliodosalicylic acid	965.1	E850.3	E935.3	E950.0	E962.0	E980.0
Acetylphenylhydrazine	965.8	E850.8	E935.8	E950.0	E962.0	E980.0
Acetylsalicylic acid	965.1	E850.3	E935.3	E950.0	E962.0	E980.0
Achromycin	960.4	E856	E930.4	E950.4	E962.0	E980.4
ophthalmic preparation	976.5	E858.7	E946.5	E950.4	E962.0	E980.4
topical NEC	976.0	E858.7	E946.0	E950.4	E962.0	E980.4
Acidifying agents	963.2	E858.1	E933.2	E950.4	E962.0	E980.4
Acids (corrosive) NEC	983.1	E864.1	—	E950.7	E962.1	E980.6
Aconite (wild)	988.2	E865.4	—	E950.9	E962.1	E980.9
Aconitine (liniment)	976.8	E858.7	E946.8	E950.4	E962.0	E980.4
Aconitum ferox	988.2	E865.4	—	E950.9	E962.1	E980.9
Acridine	983.0	E864.0	—	E950.7	E962.1	E980.6
vapor	987.8	E869.8	—	E952.8	E962.2	E982.8
Acriflavine	961.9	E857	E931.9	E950.4	E962.0	E980.4
Acrisorcin	976.0	E858.7	E946.0	E950.4	E962.0	E980.4

Figure 20-7. Excerpt from the Table of Drugs and Chemicals.

EXERCISE 20-4

Using a drug reference book or the Internet, specify drug category or generic name for the following drugs.

1. Lunesta ____________
2. Cardizem ____________
3. Bactrim ____________
4. Zoloft ____________
5. Ditropan ____________

It is possible that an adverse effect to some drugs may be based on an abnormal laboratory result. Sometimes a physician will document "toxicity" based on these laboratory results. According to *Coding Clinic* (1997:1Q:p16),[1] for a drug toxicity with no documented adverse reaction assign code 796.0. If the patient has any symptoms, then the symptom codes are assigned along with the appropriate E code for therapeutic use.

EXAMPLE

Dilantin toxicity per laboratory report. Patient is asymptomatic. The Dilantin dosage will be adjusted and Dilantin levels monitored. Patient takes Dilantin for seizure disorder, 796.0, 345.90, E936.1.

EXERCISE 20-5

Assign codes to the following conditions using your ICD-9-CM code book.

1. Hives due to Bactrim taken to treat UTI (urinary tract infection) ____________
2. Diarrhea due to erythromycin used to treat acute bronchitis ____________
3. Headache due to Nitrostat taken for angina ____________
4. Constipation due to narcotics used after surgery ____________
5. Decreased sex drive due to treatment with Zoloft for depression ____________
6. Digoxin toxicity from Digoxin taken for congestive heart failure; drug was taken as prescribed ____________
7. Dizziness and irregular heartbeat due to Inderal, which was taken for hypertension ____________
8. Tachycardia due to albuterol, which was administered for asthma ____________

Poisonings (960-979)

It is sometimes confusing to determine the difference between an adverse effect and a poisoning. Poisoning from medication(s) occurs when:

- The wrong medication is taken—patient took a medication that is not currently prescribed for them
- The wrong dose is taken—patient took 2 tablets instead of 1 (double the dosage)
- Intentional overdose—patient took large amount of medication or other drug or chemical
- Nonprescribed drug (including illegal drugs and alcohol) interacts with a prescription medication—patient took an over-the-counter medication that causes some reaction with prescribed medication

The poisoning code is always sequenced first and is found in the Table of Drugs and Chemicals under the heading for "poisoning". It is possible to assign more than one poisoning code along with corresponding E codes, to describe a poisoning if more than one substance or drug is responsible. A poisoning requires at least two codes: one code for the

poisoning and an E code to describe the circumstances of the poisoning. These E codes are located in the Table of Drugs and Chemicals. Remember E codes can never be sequenced as a principal diagnosis.

The selection of the appropriate E code for poisonings can be confusing. Unlike adverse effects where the only option for E code assignment is an E code from the "therapeutic" column, poisoning E codes are assigned according to circumstances surrounding this poisoning. The circumstances (intent) include the following:

- Accidental
- Suicide attempt
- Assault
- Undetermined

According to the guidelines:

- If the intent (accident, self-harm, assault) of the cause of an injury or poisoning is unknown, code the intent as undetermined E980-E989.
- If the intent (accident, self-harm, assault) is questionable, probable or suspected, code the intent as undetermined E980-E989.

If the manifestation(s) of the poisoning is documented it should be coded as a secondary diagnosis. Manifestations could include chest pain, vomiting, lethargy, coma, and so forth.

According to *Coding Clinic* (1993:1Q:p25),[2] when a patient is admitted for chest pain due to cocaine intoxication, this is considered a poisoning, and the code for the cocaine poisoning (970.8) is the principal diagnosis. An additional code for the manifestation of chest pain is assigned, along with a code for the drug abuse.

EXAMPLE

Patient admitted for a suicide attempt with multiple medications, including Naproxen, Keppra, and acetaminophen mixed with beer. Patient was somnolent on arrival in the ER, 965.61, 966.3, 965.4, 980.0, 780.09, E950.0, E950.4, E950.9.

(Both Naproxen and acetaminophen are coded to E950.0, so this E code needs to be assigned only once.)

EXERCISE 20-6

Assign codes to the following conditions using your ICD-9-CM code book.

1. Patient took ampicillin that belonged to his wife; patient developed hives caused by the ampicillin __________
2. Patient became stuporous and lethargic after taking Valium according to prescription, then drinking a couple of beers; accidental intent __________
3. The patient accidentally received the higher dosage of potassium while in hospital; no effects were noted __________
4. Cocaine-induced chest pain; patient is a known cocaine abuser with a daily habit; accidental intent __________
5. Suicide attempt with acetaminophen; patient has nausea and vomiting with abdominal pain __________
6. Toddler accidentally drank bottle of Visine (tetrahydrozoline); the toddler was having labored breathing and was very irritable __________
7. Patient was taking extra doses of Lasix to reduce swelling of lower extremities; patient is hypokalemic and takes Lasix for congestive heart failure __________
8. Patient became dizzy and very drowsy after taking one of spouse's Vicodin tablets and drinking a couple of alcoholic beverages and smoking marijuana __________

EXAMPLE

Patient became weak, had labored breathing, and had altered mental status caused by an accidental overdose of codeine, 965.09, 780.79, 786.09, 780.97, E850.2.

The manifestations of the overdose are the weakness, breathing problems, and alteration in mental status.

Toxic Effects of Substances Chiefly Nonmedicinal to Source (980-989)

Numerous toxic substances can cause ill effects. Categories 980 to 989 identify these types of reactions. Reactions range from mild events such as headache to life-threatening conditions such as anaphylactic shock. At the beginning of this section, instructions are provided on the use of additional codes to specify the nature of the toxic effect.

EXAMPLE

Patient admitted with alcohol poisoning due to intake of vodka, 980.0, E980.9

EXERCISE 20-7

Assign codes to the following conditions using your ICD-9-CM code book.

1. Angioedema due to penicillin taken as prescribed __________
2. Accidental lead poisoning from paint with anemia and muscle weakness __________
3. Unconscious due to carbon monoxide poisoning caused by motor vehicle fumes, suicide attempt __________
4. Tremors, low-grade fever, weight loss, and extreme fatigue due to mercury toxicity caused by exposure while working with dental fillings __________
5. Headache, confusion, and seizure caused by arsenic poisoning. Wife was trying to harm the patient __________

Other and Unspecified Effect of External Causes (990-995)

Categories 990 to 995 are used to identify the effects that external causes such as radiation, temperature, heat, light, and air pressure may have on the human body. According to *Coding Clinic* (1997:2Q:p12),[3] it is unacceptable to use 995.20, Unspecified adverse effect of a drug, medicinal or biological substance in the inpatient setting. This code should be assigned only in the outpatient setting and only in rare circumstances. The record should be reviewed to find further documentation of any specific adverse effect.

EXAMPLE

Patient developed an adverse reaction to codeine, 995.20, E935.2.

Adult/Child Abuse

Domestic violence, elder abuse, and child abuse occur more often than one might think. Healthcare providers are required to report to the proper authorities any suspicions of abuse and/or neglect. Four major types of abuse have been identified:

1. Physical abuse
2. Sexual abuse
3. Emotional abuse
4. Neglect

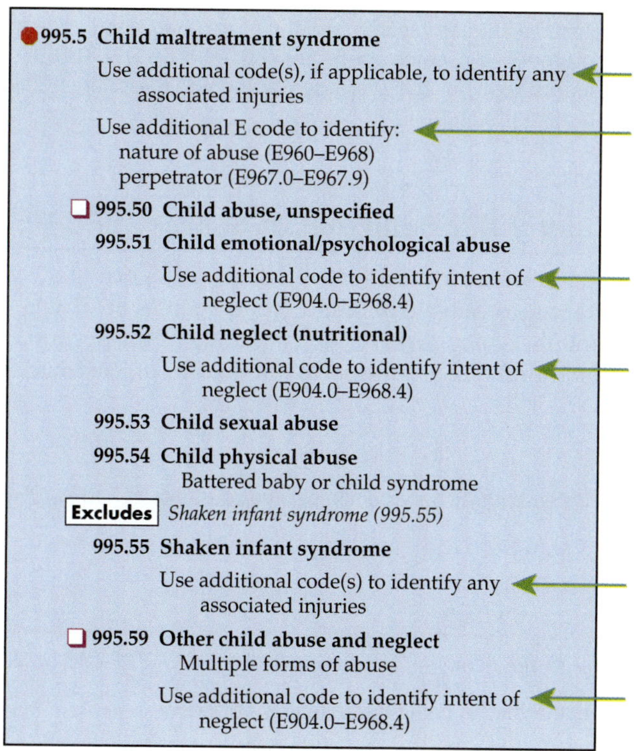

995.5 Child maltreatment syndrome
Use additional code(s), if applicable, to identify any associated injuries
Use additional E code to identify:
nature of abuse (E960–E968)
perpetrator (E967.0–E967.9)
995.50 Child abuse, unspecified
995.51 Child emotional/psychological abuse
Use additional code to identify intent of neglect (E904.0–E968.4)
995.52 Child neglect (nutritional)
Use additional code to identify intent of neglect (E904.0–E968.4)
995.53 Child sexual abuse
995.54 Child physical abuse
Battered baby or child syndrome
Excludes *Shaken infant syndrome (995.55)*
995.55 Shaken infant syndrome
Use additional code(s) to identify any associated injuries
995.59 Other child abuse and neglect
Multiple forms of abuse
Use additional code to identify intent of neglect (E904.0–E968.4)

Figure 20-8. Instructions to use additional code(s) to identify any associated injuries caused by child maltreatment.

The codes for child abuse range from 995.50 to 995.59. These codes must be assigned as the principal diagnosis according to *Coding Clinic* (1996:4Q:p40-41).[4] The code book gives instructions on the use of additional code(s), if applicable, to identify any associated injuries (Figure 20-8) and the appropriate E code to identify the perpetrator. The codes for adult abuse are from 995.80 to 995.85 and there are similar instructions to code any associated injuries as an additional code with an E code to identify the perpetrator. The adult abuse codes must be assigned as the principal diagnosis according to *Coding Clinic* (1996:4Q:p41-42).[5]

EXAMPLE

The child was admitted for moderate malnutrition because of neglect by the mother, 995.52, 263.0, E904.0, E967.2.

Systemic Inflammatory Response Syndrome (SIRS)

Systemic inflammatory response syndrome (SIRS) is a serious medical condition that can occur in response to an infection or to noninfectious causes, such as severe trauma, burns, and complications of surgery. It may also occur in diseases such as pancreatitis and AIDS.

SIRS may be diagnosed when two or more of the following criteria are present:

- Heart rate >90 beats per minute
- Body temperature <36° or >38°C
- Tachypnea (high respiratory rate) >20 breaths per minute or, on blood gas, a $PaCO_2$ <4.3 kPa (32 mm Hg)
- White blood cell count <4000 cells/mm^3 or >12,000 cells/mm^3 ($<4 \times 10^9$ or $>12 \times 10^9$ cells/L), or the presence of greater than 10% immature neutrophils.

Because of instructional notes in the code book to "code first underlying infection or condition," the SIRS codes will generally not be the principal diagnosis. In patients with

trauma, the most severe injury would be the principal diagnosis and the SIRS code would be assigned as a secondary code. It is possible for organ dysfunction to occur as a result of trauma, and this would be coded to SIRS due to noninfectious process with organ dysfunction.

EXAMPLE

Patient has SIRS due to accidental burns in a street car fire. Patient has second- (3%) and third-degree (5%) burns of the trunk and first-degree burns of the right arm, 942.30, 943.10, 948.10, 995.93, E829.4, E849.5.

EXERCISE 20-8

Assign codes to the following conditions using your ICD-9-CM code book.

1. Frostbite toes and fingers due to spending night outdoors in blizzard ____________
2. Heatstroke due to high temperature while at beach ____________
3. Anaphylactic shock due to peanut butter ____________
4. Seasickness while on cruise ____________
5. Shaken baby syndrome with subdural hematoma and retinal hemorrhages. The baby was shaken by the babysitter ____________

V CODES

In the past, V codes have been considered primarily for use in the outpatient setting. This has changed with the addition of more V codes each year. As was discussed in Chapter 8, it may be difficult to locate V codes in the index. Coders often say, "I did not know there was a V code for that." It is important for the coder to be familiar with different types and uses of V codes. Refer to Chapter 8 for a listing of common main terms used to locate V codes. See Chapter 19 for V codes used for injuries.

V14.0	Personal history of allergy to medicinal agents—penicillin
V14.1	Personal history of allergy to medicinal agents—other antibiotic agent
V14.2	Personal history of allergy to medicinal agents—sulfonamides
V14.2	Personal history of allergy to medicinal agents—other anti-infective agents
V14.4	Personal history of allergy to medicinal agents—anesthetic agent
V14.5	Personal history of allergy to medicinal agents—narcotic agent
V14.6	Personal history of allergy to medicinal agents—analgesic agent
V14.7	Personal history of allergy to medicinal agents—serum or vaccine
V14.8	Personal history of allergy to medicinal agents—other specified medicinal agents
V14.9	Personal history of allergy to medicinal agents—unspecified medicinal agent
V15.01	Allergy other than to medicinal agents—peanuts
V15.02	Allergy other than to medicinal agents—milk products
V15.03	Allergy other than to medicinal agents—seafood
V15.04	Allergy other than to medicinal agents—other foods
V15.06	Allergy other than to medicinal agents—insects
V15.07	Allergy other than to medicinal agents—latex
V15.08	Allergy other than to medicinal agents—radiographic dye
V15.09	Allergy other than to medicinal agents—other
V15.41	History of physical abuse
V15.52	History of emotional abuse
V15.49	Other psychological trauma
V15.59	Personal history of other injury

V15.6	History of poisoning
V15.84	Exposure to asbestos
V15.86	Exposure to lead
V61.11	Counseling for victim of spousal and partner abuse
V61.21	Counseling for victim of child abuse
V61.22	Counseling for perpetrator of parental child abuse
V62.82	Counseling for perpetrator of physical/sexual abuse
V71.5	Observation after alleged rape or seduction
V71.6	Observation after other inflicted injury
V71.81	Observation and evaluation for other specified suspected conditions—abuse and neglect
V87.01	Contact with and (suspected) exposure to arsenic
V87.09	Contact with and (suspected) exposure to other hazardous metals
V87.11	Contact with and (suspected) exposure to aromatic amines
V87.12	Contact with and (suspected) exposure to benzene
V87.19	Contact with and (suspected) exposure to other hazardous aromatic compounds
V87.2	Contact with and (suspected) exposure to other potentially hazardous chemicals
V87.39	Contact with and (suspected) exposure to other potentially hazardous substances

EXAMPLE Patient was exposed to asbestos while working in a shipyard years ago, V15.84.

EXAMPLE Patient carries an EpiPen because of allergy to peanuts, V15.01.

EXERCISE 20-9

Assign codes to the following conditions using your ICD-9-CM code book.

1. History of allergy to latex ________
2. History of allergy to Bactrim ________
3. Patient has a history of anaphylactic shock due to bee sting ________
4. History of rape ________
5. History of hives due to contrast media or radiologic dye ________
6. Observation for suspected physical abuse ________

COMMON TREATMENTS

Treatment will depend on the type and severity of the injury. Pain medications, anti-inflammatories, corticosteroids, and antibiotics may be necessary to alleviate pain and inflammation and to prevent or fight infection.

PROCEDURES

Debridement

Debridement of burns is probably the most common procedure that will be assigned in this chapter. There are very specific guidelines regarding the use of debridement codes. If any question arises as to whether a debridement was **excisional** or **nonexcisional**, a query may be necessary. Debridements can be performed in many settings in the hospital including at the bedside, so documentation may be difficult to locate. Debridements do not have to be performed in the operating room. Debridements may also be performed by physical therapists, wound care nurses, and other healthcare professionals in addition to physicians.

According to *Coding Clinic* (1999:1Q:p8-9),[6] when an extensive debridement goes beyond the skin and subcutaneous tissue into the muscle, tendon, and/or bone it is appropriate to "assign only a code for the deepest layer of debridement when multiple layers of the same site are débrided." If a patient had a debridement of skin, subcutaneous tissue, muscle, and bone, the bone is the deepest layer and debridement of the bone 77.67 is the only procedure code assigned.

Hyperbaric Oxygen Therapy

Hyperbaric oxygen therapy (HBOT) is a treatment in which the patient's entire body is placed in a transparent, airtight chamber at increased atmospheric pressure. The patient breathes in 100% pure oxygen. This increased oxygen flow in the body helps to improve healing within the tissues and helps to get rid of toxic gases in the case of a poisoning.

HBOT is helpful in treating medical conditions such as the following:

- Air or gas embolism (in divers or following bypass surgery)
- Decompensation sickness in divers (bends)
- Burns and other wounds
- Carbon monoxide poisoning
- Smoke inhalation
- Near drowning, near electrocution or near hanging
- Diabetic ulcers/skin ulcers

EXAMPLE

Excisional debridement of infected burn right palm performed by physical therapist. Patient was burned by hot light bulb, 944.05, 958.3, E924.8, 86.22.

EXAMPLE

Excisional debridement of fourth-degree burn right flank by physician. Accidentally burned in house fire, 942.43, E890.9, E849.1, 86.22.

EXAMPLE

Nonexcisional debridement of second-degree burn of the neck performed by physical therapist. Accidental burn from tanning bed at salon, 941.28, E926.2, E849.6, 86.28.

EXAMPLE

Patient is being treated with HBOT for decompression sickness from scuba diving in ocean, 993.3, E902.2, E849.8, 93.95.

EXERCISE 20-10

Assign codes for all diagnoses and procedures using your ICD-9-CM code book.

1. Z-plasty to release scar contracture forearm ____________
2. Nonexcisional debridement of second-degree burn right knee by wound care nurse ____________
3. Excisional debridement of second- and third-degree burns back performed at the patient's bedside ____________
4. Debridement to the soft tissue of deep burns left thigh ____________
5. Full-thickness skin graft to deep third-degree burn area of the right hand. Graft from patient ____________

DOCUMENTATION/REIMBURSEMENT/MS-DRGs

Often, coding challenges are due to lack of documentation. Sometimes radiology and other test results are not available at the time of discharge or when the physician is dictating the discharge summary or is reporting the final diagnoses.

Documentation of how, when, and where an injury occurred, along with good descriptions of the injury, is often lacking. It may not be important to the physician that the accident occurred on the school playground instead of the backyard of the patient's home. Surgical procedures such as skin grafting, excisional debridement, or mechanical ventilation can make a difference in reimbursement.

Burns have their own major diagnostic category, or MDC—22. The following Medicare severity diagnosis-related groups (MS-DRGs) fall into the burn MDC:

- 927 Extensive burns or full-thickness burns with mechanical ventilation 96+ hours with skin graft
- 928 Full-thickness burn with skin graft or inhalation injury with CC/MCC
- 929 Full-thickness burn with skin graft or inhalation injury without CC/MCC
- 933 Extensive burns or full-thickness burns with mechanical ventilation 96+ hours without skin graft
- 934 Full-thickness burn without skin graft of inhalation injury
- 935 Nonextensive burns

By the titles of these MS-DRGs, it is evident that the type of burn, mechanical ventilation, skin graft procedure, presence of an inhalation injury, and/or CC/MCC determines the MS-DRG assignment.

Correct Procedure Code

EXAMPLE

A patient was admitted with third-degree burns to the abdomen and second-degree burns to the face with burn injury to the lungs. The patient was on a mechanical ventilator for 5 days. Documentation of mechanical ventilation may be difficult to find within the health record. The calculation of ventilation hours can also affect the MS-DRG assignment.

DIAGNOSES	CODES	MS-DRG	RW
Burns abdomen, face, and lungs	942.33, 941.20, 947.1	933	2.6330
Ventilation 96+ hours	96.72		
Burns abdomen, face, and lungs	942.33, 941.20, 947.1	929	2.3533
Ventilation less than 96 hours	96.71		
Burns abdomen and face No ventilation	942.33, 941.20	934	1.3745

The MS-DRG assignment is affected by the burn injury to the lung and the use of mechanical ventilation.

If an adverse effect is incorrectly coded as a poisoning, or if a poisoning is incorrectly coded as an adverse effect, reimbursement can be affected.

Adverse Effect Versus Poisoning

EXAMPLE

The patient's physician recently adjusted the dosage of the patient's digitalis, which the patient takes for congestive heart failure. The patient took the medication as directed by the physician but became severely nauseated. This is an adverse effect associated with digitalis because the patient took the medication as prescribed by the physician.

DIAGNOSES	CODES	MS-DRG	RW
Coded as Adverse Effect			
Nausea due to digitalis toxicity with congestive heart failure	787.02, 428.0 E942.1	392	0.7121
Coded as Poisoning			
Nausea due to digitalis toxicity with congestive heart failure	972.1, 787.02, 428.0 E980.4	918	0.6886

The term "toxicity" does not necessarily indicate a poisoning. This case should be coded as an adverse effect. If this case had been coded as a poisoning, the facility would have received a lower reimbursement than was supported by the documentation in the health record.

CHAPTER REVIEW EXERCISE

Assign codes for all diagnoses and procedures, including all applicable V and E codes and procedures.

1. Alcoholic drank rubbing alcohol, undetermined circumstances ______________
2. Anaphylactic shock due to bee sting ______________
3. Sunburn neck, back, and back of legs after spending day at water park ______________
4. Chemical burn knee due to leaking ice pack that was used for knee injury. The skin is reddened with no blister formation ______________
5. Gastrointestinal bleeding due to excessive use of aspirin for chronic low back pain (accidental) ______________
6. Orthostatic hypotension due to Nitro-Bid taken for stable angina ______________
7. Depression due to Keppra, which was taken for a seizure disorder ______________
8. History of exposure to lead. No apparent symptoms ______________
9. Malunion of radial shaft fracture. Previous accidental injury ______________
10. Firefighter suffers smoke inhalation after fighting warehouse fire ______________
11. Accidental ingestion of Drano with burns mouth and esophagus ______________
12. Drug-induced dementia due to Lithium. Lithium is taken for Bipolar disorder. ______________
13. Coma due to accidental alcohol poisoning with blood alcohol of 0.3 ______________
14. Second-degree burns right hand and third-degree burns left hand due to grease fire at restaurant. Excisional debridement done in the operating room ______________
15. Abnormal level of mercury in blood. No symptoms ______________
16. Accidental injury with chemical burns to eyelids from Roundup chemical used on the job doing farm work. ______________

17. Hypothermia due to cold weather. Patient is homeless and lives in alley. ____________

18. Second-degree burns to left foot due to accidental scald injury with hot water from sink at home ____________

19. Weakness and tremor due to Lithium toxicity. Patient has bipolar affective disease and is currently depressed. Lithium taken as prescribed. ____________

20. Toddler with third- and fourth-degree burns buttocks, legs, and feet. Patient was put into boiling water by the mother's boyfriend. Twenty percent of his body was affected ____________

21. Extensive burns 50% of body with 18% third degree. Patient was in a motor vehicle accident (MVA) ____________

22. Drug-induced hepatitis due to isoniazid, which is being taken because of exposure to tuberculosis ____________

23. Bite by poisonous rattlesnake ____________

24. SIRS due to crush injury to chest. Patient driver of MV that hit deer on roadway ____________

25. Steroid-induced hyperglycemia ____________

26. Paralytic ileus due to interaction of anticholinergics and codeine ____________

Write the correct answer(s) in the space(s) provided.

27. Name two things that can make a difference in the assignment of a burn MS-DRG.

____

____

28. Described the difference between excisional and nonexcisional debridement.

____

29. What degree of burn results in full-thickness skin loss?

____

30. Define adverse affect of a drug.

____

CHAPTER GLOSSARY

Adverse effect: pathologic manifestation due to ingestion or exposure to drugs or other chemical substances.

Air embolism: when air or gas bubbles get into the bloodstream and can obstruct the circulation.

Dermis: layer of skin below the epidermis.

Epidermis: outermost layer of skin.

Erythema: redness of the skin.

Excisional debridement: surgical removal or cutting away of devitalized tissue, necrosis, or slough.

Fat embolism syndrome: condition that can occur after long bone or pelvic fracture. It usually presents 12 to 48 hours after injury with tachycardia, tachypnea, elevated temperature, hypoxemia, hypocapnia, thrombocytopenia, and occasionally, mild neurologic symptoms.

Hyperbaric oxygen therapy (HBOT): treatment in which the patient's entire body is placed in a transparent, airtight chamber at increased atmospheric pressure.

Necrosis: death of cells.

Nonexcisional debridement: nonoperative brushing, irrigating, scrubbing, or washing of devitalized tissue, necrosis, or slough.

Residual condition or effect: when the acute phase of an illness or injury has passed, but a residual condition or health problem remains.

Systemic inflammatory response syndrome: a serious medical condition that can occur in response to infectious or noninfectious causes, such as severe trauma, burns, or complications of surgery.

CHAPTER 21

Complications of Surgical and Medical Care

CHAPTER OUTLINE

LEARNING OBJECTIVES

- Apply and assign the correct ICD-9-CM codes in accordance with Official Guidelines for Coding and Reporting
- Identify complications of surgical and medical care
- Assign the correct V codes, E codes, and procedure codes related to complications of surgical and medical care
- Explain the importance of documentation in relation to MS-DRGs for reimbursement

ABBREVIATIONS

CKD chronic kidney disease
DVT deep vein thrombosis
ECT electroconvulsive therapy
ESRD end-stage renal disease
IUD intrauterine device
MS-DRG Medicare Severity diagnosis-related group
PE pulmonary embolism
THR total hip replacement
TPN total parenteral nutrition
TURP transurethral resection of the prostate
UTI urinary tract infection
VSD ventricular septal defect

ICD-9-CM Official Guidelines for Coding and Reporting

Please refer to the companion Evolve website for the most current guidelines.

Section II. Selection of a Principal Diagnosis

G. Complications of surgery and other medical care

When the admission is for treatment of a complication resulting from surgery or other medical care, the complication code is sequenced as the principal diagnosis. If the complication is classified to the 996-999 series and the code lacks the necessary specificity in describing the complication, an additional code for the specific complication should be assigned.

C. Chapter-Specific Guidelines

1. Chapter 1: Infectious and Parasitic Diseases (001-139)

b. Septicemia, Systemic Inflammatory Response Syndrome (SIRS), Sepsis, Severe Sepsis, and Septic Shock

10) Sepsis due to a Postprocedural Infection

(a) Documentation of causal relationship

As with all postprocedural complications, code assignment is based on the provider's documentation of the relationship between the infection and the procedure.

(b) Sepsis due to postprocedural infection

In cases of postprocedural sepsis, the complication code, such as code 998.59, Other postoperative infection, or 674.3x, Other complications of obstetrical surgical wounds should be coded first, followed by the appropriate sepsis codes (systemic infection code and either code 995.91or 995.92). An additional code(s) for any acute organ dysfunction should also be assigned for cases of severe sepsis.

EXAMPLE

The patient was readmitted after undergoing surgery last week; the patient is being treated for postoperative septicemia, 998.59, 038.9, E879.9.

2. Chapter 2: Neoplasms (140-239)

c. Coding and sequencing of complications

4) Treatment of a complication resulting from a surgical procedure

When the admission/encounter is for treatment of a complication resulting from a surgical procedure, designate the complication as the principal or first-listed diagnosis if treatment is directed at resolving the complication.

EXAMPLE

Hernia of colostomy with repair of parastomal hernia. The colostomy was performed 1 year ago during colon cancer resection. The patient is no longer receiving treatment, and the cancer was completely resected, 569.69, V10.05, 46.42.

3. Chapter 3: Endocrine, Nutritional, and Metabolic Diseases and Immunity Disorders (240-279)

a. Diabetes mellitus

6) Insulin pump malfunction

(a) Underdose of insulin due insulin pump failure

An underdose of insulin due to an insulin pump failure should be assigned 996.57, Mechanical complication due to insulin pump, as the principal or first listed code, followed by the appropriate diabetes mellitus code based on documentation.

(b) Overdose of insulin due to insulin pump failure

The principal or first listed code for an encounter due to an insulin pump malfunction resulting in an overdose of insulin, should also be 996.57, Mechanical complication due to insulin pump, followed by code 962.3, Poisoning by insulins and antidiabetic agents, and the appropriate diabetes mellitus code based on documentation.

EXAMPLE

Patient presents with a kink in the tubing of the insulin pump. This has resulted in diabetic ketoacidosis, 996.57 250.13 E879.8.

6. **Chapter 6: Diseases of Nervous System and Sense Organs (320-389)**
   a. **Pain—Category 338**
      2) **Pain due to devices, implants and grafts**
         Pain associated with devices, **implants or grafts** left in a surgical site (**for example painful hip prosthesis**) is assigned to the appropriate code(s) found in Chapter 17, Injury and Poisoning. **Use additional code(s) from category 338 to identify acute or chronic pain due to presence of the device, implant or graft (338.18-338.19 or 338.28-338.29).**

EXAMPLE

Patient presents with acute pain secondary to a displaced nail in the femur, 996.49, 338.18, 729.5, E878.1.

3) **Postoperative Pain**
   Post-thoracotomy pain and other postoperative pain are classified to subcategories 338.1 and 338.2, depending on whether the pain is acute or chronic. The default for post-thoracotomy and other postoperative pain not specified as acute or chronic is the code for the acute form.
   Routine or expected postoperative pain immediately after surgery should not be coded.
   (a) **Postoperative pain not associated with specific postoperative complication**
       Postoperative pain not associated with a specific postoperative complication is assigned to the appropriate postoperative pain code in category 338.
   (b) **Postoperative pain associated with specific postoperative complication**
       Postoperative pain associated with a specific postoperative complication (such as **painful wire sutures**) is assigned to the appropriate code(s) found in Chapter 17, Injury and Poisoning. **If appropriate, use additional code(s) from category 338 to identify acute or chronic pain (338.18 or 338.28).** If pain control/management is the reason for the encounter, a code from category 338 should be assigned as the principal or first-listed diagnosis in accordance with *Section I.C.6.a.1.a above.*
   (c) **Postoperative pain as principal or first-listed diagnosis**
       Postoperative pain may be reported as the principal or first-listed diagnosis when the stated reason for the admission/encounter is documented as postoperative pain control/management.
   (d) **Postoperative pain as secondary diagnosis**
       Postoperative pain may be reported as a secondary diagnosis code when a patient presents for outpatient surgery and develops an unusual or inordinate amount of postoperative pain.
       The provider's documentation should be used to guide the coding of postoperative pain, as well as *Section III. Reporting Additional Diagnoses* and *Section IV. Diagnostic Coding and Reporting in the Outpatient Setting.*
       See Section II.I.2 for information on sequencing of diagnoses for patients admitted to hospital inpatient care following post-operative observation.
       See Section II.J for information on sequencing of diagnoses for patients admitted to hospital inpatient care from outpatient surgery.
       See Section IV.A.2 for information on sequencing of diagnoses for patients admitted for observation.

7. **Chapter 7: Disease and Circulatory System (390-459)**
   c. **Postoperative cerebrovascular accident**
      A cerebrovascular hemorrhage or infarction that occurs as a result of medical intervention is coded to 997.02, Iatrogenic cerebrovascular infarction or hemorrhage. Medical record documentation should clearly specify the cause-and-

effect relationship between the medical intervention and the cerebrovascular accident in order to assign this code. A secondary code from the code range 430-432 or from a code from subcategories 433 or 434 with a fifth digit of "1" should also be used to identify the type of hemorrhage or infarct.

This guideline conforms to the use additional code note instruction at category 997. Code 436, Acute, but ill-defined, cerebrovascular disease, should not be used as a secondary code with code 997.02.

EXAMPLE

The patient had a postoperative cerebrovascular accident, which was embolic in nature. The patient initially had been admitted for treatment of coronary artery arteriosclerosis with CABG (left internal mammary artery and two saphenous vein grafts were used). Cardiopulmonary bypass was used during the surgery, 414.01, 997.02, 434.11, 36.12, 36.15, 39.61.

17. Chapter 17: Injury and Poisoning (800-999)

f. Complications of care

1) Transplant complications

(a) Transplant complications other than kidney

Codes under subcategory 996.8, Complications of transplanted organ, are used for both complications and rejection of transplanted organs. A transplant complication code is only assigned if the complication affects the function of the transplanted organ. Two codes are required to fully describe a transplant complication, the appropriate code from subcategory 996.8 and a secondary code that identifies the complication.

Pre-existing conditions or conditions that develop after the transplant are not coded as complications unless they affect the function of the transplanted organs.

(b) Kidney transplant complications

Code 996.81 should be assigned for documented complications of a kidney transplant, such as transplant failure or rejection. Code 996.8 should not be assigned for post kidney transplant patients who have chronic kidney (CKD) unless a transplant complication such as transplant failure or rejection is documented. If the documentation is unclear as to whether the patient has a complication of the transplant, query the provider.

For patients with CKD following a kidney transplant, but who do not have a complication such as failure or rejection, *see section I.C.10.a.2, Chronic kidney disease and kidney transplant status.*

Apply the General Coding Guidelines as found in Chapter 5.

ANATOMY AND PHYSIOLOGY

Complications of surgical or medical care can affect any of the body systems. The anatomy and physiology of these body systems are outlined in their respective chapters. Find below some general guidelines that apply to complications.

CODING COMPLICATIONS

Several general guidelines should be kept in mind when coding complications.

- No time limit: can occur after medical care or surgery, either immediately or years later.
- Complications after surgery or medical care should be documented as such. Routine events such as fever in the immediate postoperative period are not considered postoperative complications.

- Coding of complications does not imply that poor care or improper care has been delivered.
- Codes for complications may be located in the chapter for specified body sites or under abortion and pregnancy.
- Codes for complications that affect multiple sites or body systems are usually located in codes 996 through 999.
- "**Iatrogenic**" is a term that is used to signify that a condition is a result or complication of treatment.
- When in doubt as to whether the condition occurred as the result of a procedure or medical care, it is best practice to query the physician.
- Complications of surgical and medical care require an E code in the range of E878-E879 for abnormal reactions or later complications, or E870-E879 if misadventure is stated.
- When the admission is for treatment of a complication resulting from surgery or other medical care, the complication code is sequenced as the principal diagnosis.
- If the complication is classified to 996-999 and the code lacks necessary specificity to describe the complication, an additional code should be assigned for the specific complication.

Locating Complication Codes in the Alphabetic Index

When looking for a complication code in the index, the condition for which the patient is admitted should be located first (Figures 21-1 and 21-2).

EXAMPLE

Patient was readmitted for treatment of postoperative ileus following appendectomy, 997.4, 560.1, E878.6.

Ileus (adynamic) (bowel) (colon) (inhibitory) (intestine) (neurogenic) (paralytic) 560.1
  arteriomesenteric duodenal 537.2
  due to gallstone (in intestine) 560.31
  duodenal, chronic 537.2
  following gastrointestinal surgery 997.4
  gallstone 560.31
  mechanical (*see also* Obstruction, intestine) 560.9
  meconium 777.1
    due to cystic fibrosis 277.01
  myxedema 564.89
  postoperative 997.4
  transitory, newborn 777.4

Figure 21-1. Postoperative ileus.

Anemia *(Continued)*
  pernicious (combined system disease) (congenital) (dorsolateral spinal degeneration) (juvenile) (myelopathy) (neuropathy) (posterior sclerosis) (primary) (progressive) (spleen) 281.0
    of or complicating pregnancy 648.2
  pleochromic 285.9
    of sprue 281.8
  portal 285.8
  posthemorrhagic (chronic) 280.0
    acute 285.1
    newborn 776.5
  postoperative
    due to (acute) blood loss 285.1
      chronic blood loss 280.0
    other 285.9

Figure 21-2. Postoperative blood loss anemia.

EXAMPLE

Anemia due to acute blood loss following a total knee replacement for osteoarthritis, 715.36, 285.1, E878.4, 81.54.

When no entry is found under the main term for the condition, the term "complication" should be referenced (Figures 21-3 and 21-4).

EXAMPLE

Patient is admitted with tracheal stenosis of tracheostomy, 519.02, E878.3
Note that this complication code is located in the respiratory chapter.

EXAMPLE

Patient admitted with cystitis due to indwelling urinary catheter, 996.64, 595.9, E879.6

Complications *(Continued)*
surgical procedures *(Continued)*
stitch abscess 998.59
transplant - *see* Complications, graft
ureterostomy malfunction 997.5
urethrostomy malfunction 997.5
urinary NEC 997.5
vascular
mesenteric artery 997.71
other vessels 997.79
peripheral vessels 997.2
renal artery 997.72
wound infection 998.59
therapeutic misadventure NEC 999.9
surgical treatment 998.9
tracheostomy 519.00

Figure 21-3. Tracheostomy complication.

Complications *(Continued)*
due to (presence of) any device, implant, or graft classified to 996.0–996.5 NEC 996.70
with infection or inflammation - *see* Complications, infection or inflammation, due to (presence of) any device, implant, or graft classified to 996.0–996.5 NEC
arterial NEC 996.74
coronary NEC 996.03
atherosclerosis - *see* Arteriosclerosis, coronary
embolism 996.72
occlusion NEC 996.72
specified type NEC 996.72
thrombus 996.72
renal dialysis 996.73
arteriovenous fistula or shunt NEC 996.74
bone growth stimulator 996.78
breast NEC 996.79
cardiac NEC 996.72
defibrillator 996.72
pacemaker 996.72
valve prosthesis 996.71
catheter NEC 996.79
spinal 996.75
urinary, indwelling 996.76

Figure 21-4. Urinary catheter complications.

Locating E Codes to Correspond With Complication Coding

An E code describes the external cause of a complication. E codes are described in greater detail in Chapter 8 of this textbook.

EXAMPLE

During spinal surgery, the surgeon accidentally nicks the dura due to the amount of adhesions present, 998.2, E870.9.

Complication
    Accidental puncture or laceration during procedure, 998.2
Using the Alphabetic Index to External causes of injury, locate the E code as follows:
    Complication
        Due to misadventure—see Misadventure
    Misadventure
        Cut, cutting, puncture, perforation, or hemorrhage, E870.9

CHAPTER-SPECIFIC COMPLICATIONS

Complications of the Digestive System

Patients who have had some or part of their stomach removed or who have undergone gastric bypass surgery may be susceptible to a condition known as "**dumping syndrome**." This condition occurs when undigested contents of the stomach are transported to the small intestine too quickly. The symptoms of this condition may include abdominal cramping, nausea, and diarrhea, to name a few. Dumping syndrome may in turn result in weight loss or malnutrition. This syndrome may be treated with dietary changes, as well as with medications.

EXAMPLE

Patient presents with significant weight loss and abdominal pain following a gastric bypass. It is determined that she suffers from dumping syndrome, and dietary changes are suggested, 564.2, V45.86, 783.21.

Complications of Gastrostomy, Colostomy, Enterostomy

Ostomies are surgically created openings into the body (Figure 21-5). Enterostomies and colostomies are created to discharge waste products from the body; gastrostomies are typically used for feeding or aspirating the contents of the stomach. Often, these surgically

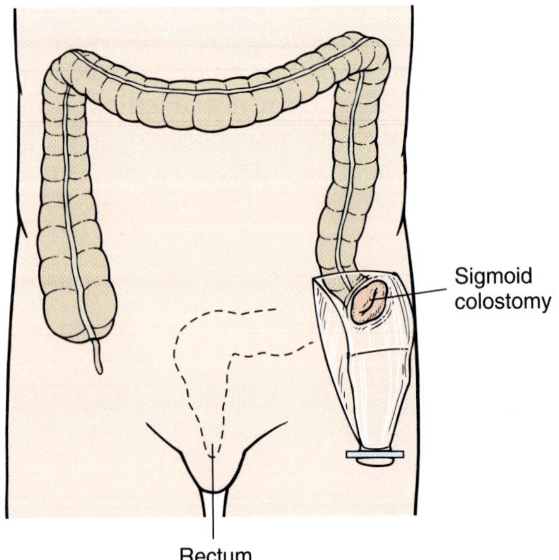

Figure 21-5. Colostomy. The opening in the colon is brought to the surface of the skin to divert feces into an external pouch worn by the patient.

created openings result in complications. Complications associated with these openings are caused by a variety of problems such as infection, blockage of the opening, drainage or leakage around the opening, breakage of the device, and granulation of tissue.

If a patient presents to the hospital with a chief complaint of a percutaneous endoscopic gastrostomy (PEG) tube falling out, the principal diagnosis would be V55.1, or attention to gastrostomy, because no complications resulted from the gastrostomy itself. This is described in detail in *Coding Clinic* (1997:3Q:p8).[1]

EXAMPLE Patient has a clogged gastrostomy tube, V55.1.

EXAMPLE Patient is being treated for an enterocutaneous fistula in the colostomy, 569.69.

EXAMPLE Patients presents with cellulitis of the abdomen due to an infected colostomy site. The organism responsible for the cellulitis is *Staph aureus,* 569.61, 682.2, 041.11.

Complications of the Genitourinary System

Occasionally, hematuria occurs as the result of a traumatic injury due to catheterization or removal of a urinary catheter. According to *Coding Clinic* (1985:Nov-Dec:p15),[2] this is coded as injury of the urethra (867.0), with hematuria (599.7) assigned as an additional code. In some cases, it may be appropriate to assign an E code to indicate the cause and intent of the injury.

EXAMPLE Hematuria due to patient pulling out indwelling urinary catheter, 867.0, 599.70, E928.9.

EXAMPLE Hematuria due to catheterization, 867.0, 599.70, E879.6.

Hematuria is expected after many urinary procedures and should not be coded unless it is excessive and has been documented as such by the physician.

Complications of Dialysis

Several complications may result from dialysis treatment. Many of these conditions are included in other chapters of the ICD-9-CM book. **Dialysis disequilibrium syndrome**, which is characterized by weakness, dizziness, headache, and, in severe cases, mental status changes, is a complication of dialysis. Electrolyte imbalances such as hyperkalemia, hyponatremia, hypocalcemia, hypermagnesemia and acidosis may also occur. Hypotension and fluid overload can complicate the care of the patient on dialysis. Occasionally, some of these conditions occur because the patient has been noncompliant with dialysis treatment and/or medications and diet. Complications associated with dialysis catheters may be due to infection or mechanical malfunction. If an infection is present, an additional code may be needed to identify specified infections and causative organisms.

EXAMPLE Patient has dialysis disequilibrium syndrome due to hemodialysis for end-stage renal failure, 276.9, 585.6, V45.1, E879.1.

EXAMPLE Leakage of peritoneal dialysis catheter. Patient is on dialysis for end-stage renal disease. Peritoneal catheter was removed, 996.56, 585.6, V45.1, E879.1, 97.82.

Complications of the Musculoskeletal System

Common complications of joint replacement include infection, blood clot, nerve injury, loosening, dislocation, wear and tear, and breakage of the prosthesis. It may be necessary to remove the prosthesis and insert a new prosthesis. According to *Coding Clinic*

(1997:3Q:p13),[3] "any time the joint is replaced or revised after the initial replacement this would be considered a revision."

EXAMPLE

Patient presents with dislocation of a hip replacement. A revision must be performed, 996.42, 81.53 (Figure 21-6).

Malunion/Nonunion of Fractures

Malunion of a fracture occurs when the fracture fragments have united but are not properly aligned. Incorrectly positioned bones may demonstrate angulation, rotation, and shortening. The degree and severity of the malunion will determine the selection of treatment, which may include surgery (Figure 21-7).

Complications *(Continued)*
  mechanical *(Continued)*
    device NEC *(Continued)*
      cardiac 996.00
        automatic implantable defibrillator 996.04
        long-term effect 429.4
        specified NEC 996.09
      contraceptive, intrauterine 996.32
      counterpulsation, intra-aortic 996.1
      fixation, external, with internal components 996.49
      fixation, internal (nail, rod, plate) 996.40
      genitourinary 996.30
        specified NEC 996.39
      insulin pump 996.57
      nervous system 996.2
      orthopedic, internal 996.40
        prosthetic joint (*see also* Complications, mechanical, device, orthopedic, prosthetic, joint) 996.47
      prosthetic NEC 996.59
        joint (*see also* Complications, prosthetic joint) 996.47
          articular bearing surface wear 996.46
          aseptic loosening 996.41
          breakage 996.43
          dislocation 996.42

Figure 21-6. Complication of hip replacement.

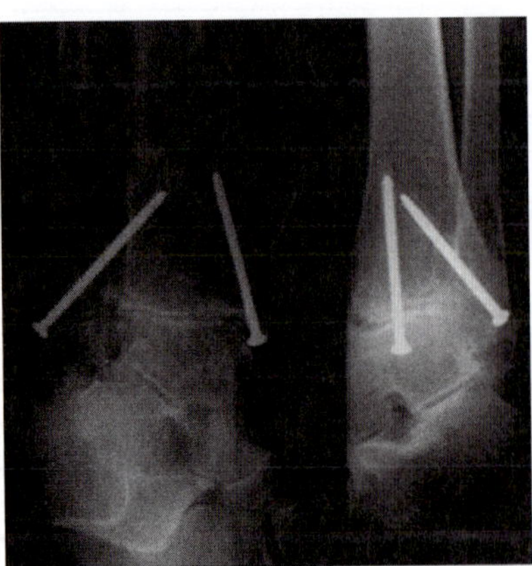

Figure 21-7. Surgical correction of malunion ankle fracture.

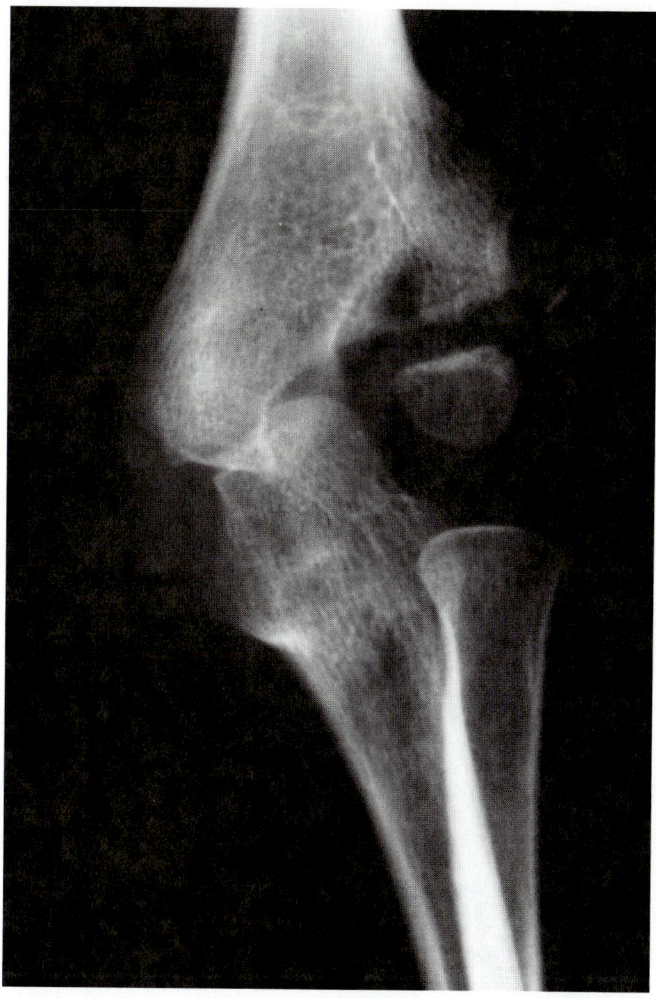

Figure 21-8. Nonunion of the lateral humeral condyle.

Nonunion of a fracture occurs when bony healing is not achieved at the fracture site. A fracture site that fails to heal within approximately 6 to 9 months of the injury represents a nonunion (Figure 21-8).

Malunion and nonunion may occur as the result of insufficient or improper reduction and immobilization, infection, metabolic bone disease, poor nutrition, and/or inadequate blood supply. Improper healing may be noted in cases of traumatic fracture and pathologic fracture and is considered a "late effect" of a fracture.

EXAMPLE Patient's x-rays showed nonunion of left tibial fracture, 733.82, 905.4, E989.

EXAMPLE Patient presents with pain and swelling in the ankle status post casting 3 weeks ago. It is determined that the patient has a malunion of the fracture, and the patient is scheduled next week for surgery to correct the malunion, 733.81.

Complications of the Nervous System and Sense Organs

One of the most common complications discussed in this chapter is a spinal headache. A spinal headache, which is also known as a postdural puncture headache, may occur following a spinal tap (lumbar puncture) or spinal anesthesia. These headaches are caused by spinal fluid that is leaking from the puncture site of the procedure. The patient may experi-

ence nausea, vomiting, dizziness, ringing in the ears, and/or sensitivity to light. Treatment for the headache consists of lying flat and drinking fluids, particularly those that include caffeine. If these conservative treatments do not help, an epidural blood patch to seal the puncture hole may be required.

EXAMPLE

Patient develops a severe headache 1 day post lumbar puncture performed because of high fever and stiff neck to rule out meningitis, 349.0, 780.4, 723.5, 03.31.

Complications of the Respiratory System

A **pulmonary embolism** (PE) is a blockage in an artery of the lung that can be life threatening. This blockage commonly is caused by a blood clot that started in the leg and then traveled to the lung. A pulmonary embolism may occur as a result of a surgical procedure. If a patient has recently had surgery and presents with sudden shortness of breath, chest pain, or cough, a pulmonary embolism may be suspected. To determine whether a patient has a PE, scans or angiograms may be performed. Treatment consists of anticoagulant drugs such as heparin. When a condition is the result of treatment, it is referred to as **iatrogenic**.

EXAMPLE

Patient presents with shortness of breath and chest pain. Two weeks before presentation, the patient had a total hip replacement. A pulmonary angiogram is performed, as is a Doppler ultrasound of the legs. The attending documents that the patient is positive for both a pulmonary embolism and a deep vein thrombosis secondary to total hip replacement, 415.11, 453.40, V43.64.

A pneumothorax is another condition that can result from medical treatment. A **pneumothorax** is air in the space around the lung. Procedures such as central venous lines, chest tubes, and mechanical ventilation may inadvertently cause a traumatic pneumothorax. A patient may have symptoms of chest pain or shortness of breath. A chest x-ray or CT scan can be used to diagnose this condition.

EXAMPLE

Patient with a chronic cough undergoes a transbronchial lung biopsy. A chest x-ray is performed following this procedure, and a pneumothorax is noted. Attending physician decides that since the pneumothorax is small, the condition will be monitored by chest x-ray, 786.2, 512.1, 33.27.

Patients with tracheostomies often develop complications related to the tracheostomy site. A patient can have infection or bleeding or mechanical complications at the site.

EXAMPLE

Patient presents with cellulitis of the neck secondary to an infected tracheostomy site, 519.01, 682.1.

COMPLICATIONS NOT ELSEWHERE CLASSIFIED (996-999)

Complications of Surgical and Medical Care (996-999), Chapter 17 in the ICD-9-CM code book.

CATEGORY	SECTION TITLES
996-999	Complications of Surgical and Medical Care, Not Elsewhere Classified

Mechanical Complications

It is important to pay particular attention to the many Excludes notes in this chapter. **Mechanical complications** involve equipment malfunctions. Some types of mechanical

Complications *(Continued)*
mechanical *(Continued)*
prosthesis NEC 996.59
bile duct 996.59
breast 996.54
chin 996.59
ocular lens 996.53
reconstruction, vas deferens 996.39
reimplant NEC 996.59
extremity (*see also* Complications, reattached, extremity) 996.90
organ (*see also* Complications, transplant, organ, by site) 996.80
repair - *see* Complications, mechanical, graft
respirator [ventilator] V46.14
shunt NEC 996.59
arteriovenous, surgically created 996.1
ventricular (communicating) 996.2
stent NEC 996.59

Figure 21-9. Complications of devices.

malfunctions are breakdown, displacement, leakage, obstruction, perforation, and protrusion.

EXAMPLE Patient has ascending cholangitis related to clogged biliary stent, 996.59, 576.1, E878.4 (Figure 21-9).

EXAMPLE Patient has a leaking breast implant, 996.54, E878.1

Complication
Prosthesis
Breast, 996.54

Infections Due to Prosthetic Device, Implants, and Grafts

The presence of a device, implant or graft carries a risk of infection. It is important to note that the codes in this section may give instruction to use an additional code to identify specified infections.

EXAMPLE Patient has sepsis due to a dialysis catheter, 996.62, 038.9, 995.91, E879.1.

EXAMPLE Patient has osteomyelitis of femur secondary to infected hip replacement. 996.66, 730.25, V43.64, E878.1.

Other Complications of Internal Prosthetic Devices, Implants, and Grafts

When problems result from the use of a device, implant, or graft that are **NOT** due to infection or mechanical problems, category 996.7X should be selected. Often, devices that have been implanted become stenosed or occluded by thrombus or embolism.

EXAMPLE Patient is admitted to remove prosthetic hip because of severe hip pain, 996.77, V43.64, E878.1, 80.05.

EXAMPLE Patient with a dialysis graft in place is admitted because of an embolism in the graft, Patient has ESRD. Thrombectomy was performed. 996.73, 453.9, 585.6 E879.1, 39.49.

EXAMPLE Patient with CAD is admitted to remove coronary artery stent because of restenosis and insert new drug-eluting stent. 996.72, 414.01, 00.66, 36.07, 00.40, 00.45, E878.1.

Complications of Transplanted Organ

Coding Clinic (1998:3Q:p3)[4] advises the coder to examine the documentation when a post–organ transplant patient presents for medical care to determine whether there are complications of the transplanted organ.

Complications of a transplanted organ include rejection or any posttransplant illnesses that affect the function of a transplanted organ. If illness affects the transplanted organ, two codes are required. The exception per guidelines are those patients with a kidney transplant and chronic kidney disease(CKD). In those cases 996.81 should only be used for complications such as rejection, or failure or a medical condition such as infection affecting the transplanted organ.

EXAMPLE UTI post kidney transplant, 996.81, 599.0, E878.0.

Posttransplant surgical complications that do not affect the function of the transplanted organ are coded to the specific surgical complications.

EXAMPLE Patient presents for heart transplant due to primary cardiomyopathy and postoperatively develops renal failure, 425.4, 997.5 586, E878.0, 37.51.

In this case, the complication is affecting the urinary system, not the heart, which is the transplanted organ.

Preexisting conditions or medical conditions that develop after transplant are not coded as complications unless they affect the transplanted organ.

Code V42.X is used as an additional code to identify transplant status when no complications are associated with the transplanted organ.

Codes V42.X and 996.8X are **NEVER** used together.

EXERCISE 21-1

Assign codes to the following conditions using your ICD-9-CM code book.

1. Displacement of a pacemaker electrode ____________
2. Obstruction of an atrioventricular dialysis shunt; patient has ESRD ____________
3. Protrusion of a nail from a femur fixation ____________
4. Failure of artificial skin graft ____________
5. Patient with indwelling urinary catheter presents with sepsis due to catheter ____________
6. Patient with peritoneal dialysis catheter presents with inflammation of the skin around the catheter; patient had ESRD ____________
7. Patient with pelvic inflammatory disease attributed to an intrauterine device (IUD) ____________
8. Patient is admitted for removal of her intramedullary rod because of acute leg pain ____________
9. Cellulitis of the skin of the right knee due to right knee replacement ____________
10. Patient with a transplanted lung presents with pneumonia ____________

11. Patient is rejecting transplanted kidney ________
12. Patient has graft-versus-host disease; status post bone marrow transplant. ________
13. Patient with an intestine transplant presents with dehydration ________
14. Patient with a ventricular shunt presents with severe headache due to occlusion of the shunt; patient has hydrocephalus ________
15. Patient with an abscess of a gastrostomy tube site due to *Staph aureus* ________
16. Patient with pleural effusion develops iatrogenic pneumothorax following insertion of a chest tube ________

Complications Affecting Specified Body Systems, Not Elsewhere Classified (997)

This category is to be used if the patient's complication is not better classified in another category, such as mechanical complication or infection of a device.

EXAMPLE Patient develops postoperative congestive heart failure after transurethral resection of the prostate (TURP) for BPH, 997.1, 428.0, 600.00, 60.29, E878.4.

EXAMPLE Patient received a total hip replacement (THR) 3 weeks ago and now presents with a postoperative deep vein thrombosis (DVT) in the lower extremity, 997.2, 453.40, E878.1.

The amputation stump complication, per *Coding Clinic* (1995:4Q:p82),[5] is used to describe complications as current or as late effects. Phantom limb pain (353.6) is excluded from these codes.

Other Complications of Procedures, Not Elsewhere Classified (998)

This category describes complications that may occur as the result of procedures but are not described by other specific codes.

EXAMPLE Dehiscence of an abdominal wound following cholecystectomy, 998.32, E878.6.

EXAMPLE Nonhealing surgical wound, 998.83, E878.9.

Complications of Medical Care, Not Elsewhere Classified (999)

Sometimes, complications occur that are not the result of surgical procedures but of medical care. Examples of medical care might include infusions, transfusions, total parenteral nutrition (TPN), dialysis, and vaccinations.

EXAMPLE After transfusion, patient presents with thrombophlebitis of right arm, 999.2, E879.8, 451.84.

EXAMPLE Sepsis due to central line, 999.31, 038.9, 995.91, E879.8.

EXERCISE 21-2

Assign codes to the following conditions using your ICD-9-CM code book.

1. During a surgical procedure, patient goes into cardiac arrest ____________
2. After a surgical procedure, patient develops aspiration pneumonia ____________
3. Patient has a hemicolectomy and is readmitted to the hospital for intractable postoperative vomiting ____________
4. After spine surgery, patient becomes oliguric ____________
5. Patient is admitted for a *Staphylococcus aureus* infection of an amputation stump ____________
6. Patient is admitted for removal of a sponge left in during a hysterectomy ____________
7. Patient develops a seroma of the operative wound ____________
8. Patient develops anaphylactic shock after a blood transfusion ____________
9. Patient develops seizures after electroconvulsive therapy (ECT) ____________

V CODES

In the past, V codes have been considered primarily for use in the outpatient setting. This has changed with the addition of more V codes each year. As was discussed in Chapter 8, it may be difficult to locate V codes in the index. Coders often say, "I did not know there was a V code for that."

It is important for the coder to be familiar with different types and uses of V codes. The use of V codes will become more important if changes are made in MS-DRG reimbursement that reflect severity.

V15.1	Personal history presenting hazards to health: Surgery to heart and great vessels
V15.2	Personal history presenting hazards to health: Surgery to other major organs
V45.71	Acquired absence of breast
V45.72	Acquired absence of intestine
V45.73	Acquired absence of kidney
V45.74	Acquired absence of other parts of urinary tract
V45.75	Acquired absence of stomach
V45.76	Acquired absence of lung
V45.77	Acquired absence of genital organs
V43.0	Eye globe replaced by other means
V43.1	Lens replaced by other means
V43.2	Heart replaced by other means
V43.3	Heart valve replaced by other means
V43.4	Blood vessel replaced by other means
V43.5	Bladder replaced by other means by other means
V43.60	Unspecified joint replaced by other means
V43.61	Shoulder replaced by other means
V43.62	Elbow replaced by other means
V43.63	Wrist replaced by other means
V43.64	Hip replaced by other means
V43.65	Knee replaced by other means
V43.66	Ankle replaced by other means
V43.69	Other joint replaced by other means

V43.81	Larynx replaced by other means
V43.82	Breast replaced by other means
V43.83	Artificial skin replaced by other means
V43.89	Other organ or tissue replaced by other means

EXERCISE 21-3

Assign codes to the following conditions using your ICD-9-CM code book.

1. Patient had breast removed 10 years ago ____________
2. When patient was a child, he had a ventricular septal defect (VSD) repaired ____________
3. History of joint replacement left shoulder ____________

DOCUMENTATION/REIMBURSEMENT/MS-DRGs

Often, coding difficulties are due to lack of documentation. Sometimes pathology and other test results are not available at the time of discharge or when the physician is dictating the discharge summary or reporting the final diagnoses. Significant MS-DRG differences may result should the wrong principal diagnosis be selected.

UTI as a Principal Diagnosis vs UTI as a Postoperative Complication

EXAMPLE

A patient presents with UTI and the physician states status post cholecystectomy 2 days prior to this admit.

DIAGNOSES	CODES	MS-DRG	RW
UTI	599.0	690	0.8000
UTI as a postop infection	997.5 599.0 E879.6	699	1.03524

When patients have central lines, dialysis catheters, ports, or indwelling urinary catheters, to name a few, and they present with bacteremia/sepsis, it is important for the coder to verify whether the bacteremia/sepsis is due to the presence of these devices.

It is also important to realize that physicians do not often use the term "complication." If it is stated as UTI following appendectomy, it may be necessary to query the physician as to whether this is a postop complication.

Pneumonia as a Principal Diagnosis Versus Pneumonia as a Transplant Complication

EXAMPLE

Patient with a transplanted lung presents with pneumonia.

DIAGNOSES	CODES	MS-DRG	RW
Pneumonia h/o Kidney transplant	486 V42.0	194	1.0235
Pneumonia in transplanted lung	996.84 486	205	1.0636

In this case, if the transplant guideline was not applied "a transplant code is only assigned if the complication affects the function of the transplant organ," a significant difference in payment would occur.

CHAPTER REVIEW EXERCISE

Where applicable, assign codes for diagnoses, procedures, and V codes and E codes.

1. Postoperative septicemia __________
2. Internal wound dehiscence __________
3. Patient with abdominal adhesions due to surgical instrument left in body cavity __________
4. Perforation of coronary artery due to stent insertion __________
5. During hemicolectomy, doctor inadvertently makes a rent in the intestine __________
6. Inflammation of the external stoma of the urinary tract __________
7. Rejection of a skin graft __________
8. Failure of an insulin pump. Patient has type I diabetes. __________
9. Thrombophlebitis as the result of saphenous vein graft harvest for coronary bypass __________
10. Stroke after surgery __________
11. Acute renal failure after surgery __________
12. Shock due to surgery __________
13. Severe hypertension after surgery __________
14. Hematoma of surgical site __________

14\. After a blood transfusion, patient develops high fever __________

16\. Cytomegalovirus infection in transplanted kidney __________

17\. Patient had a traumatic amputation 1 year ago after a farm accident. He presents with a neuroma of the amputation stump __________

CHAPTER GLOSSARY

Dialysis disequilibrium syndrome: characterized by weakness, dizziness, headache, and in severe cases mental status changes.

Dumping syndrome: occurs when undigested contents of the stomach are transported to the small intestine too quickly.

Iatrogenic: caused by medical treatment.

Mechanical complication: when a device or equipment malfunctions.

Ostomies: surgically created openings in the body.

Pneumothorax: air in space around the lung.

Pulmonary embolism: blood clot(s) in the pulmonary artery that causes blockage in the artery.

CHAPTER 22

Diseases of the Digestive System

(ICD-9-CM Chapter 9, Codes 520-579)

CHAPTER OUTLINE

LEARNING OBJECTIVES

- Apply and assign the correct ICD-9-CM codes in accordance with Official Guidelines for Coding and Reporting
- Identify pertinent anatomy and physiology of the digestive system
- Identify diseases of the digestive system
- Assign the correct V codes and procedure codes related to the digestive system
- Identify common treatments, medications, laboratory values, and diagnostic tests
- Explain the importance of documentation in relation to MS-DRGs for reimbursement

ABBREVIATIONS

AVM arteriovenous malformation
EGD esophagogastroduodenoscopy
ERCP endoscopic retrograde cholangiopancreatography
ESWL extracorporeal shock wave lithotripsy
GERD gastroesophageal reflux disease
GI gastrointestinal
IV intravenous
LGIB lower gastrointestinal bleed
MS-DRG Medicare Severity diagnosis-related group
NSAID nonsteroidal antiinflammatory drug
PEG percutaneous endoscopic gastrostomy
PUD peptic ulcer disease
TIPS transjugular intrahepatic portosystemic shunt
UGIB upper gastrointestinal bleed

ICD-9-CM OFFICIAL GUIDELINES FOR CODING AND REPORTING

There are currently no official guidelines for Diseases of the Digestive System. Apply the General Coding Guidelines as found in Chapter 5.

ANATOMY AND PHYSIOLOGY

The digestive system (Figure 22-1) consists of the mouth, pharynx, esophagus, stomach, small intestine and large intestine (the **alimentary canal**), and accessory organs, which include the salivary glands, liver, gallbladder, and pancreas. The purpose of the digestive system is to process food so that it may be absorbed by cells.

The mouth is where digestion begins. The tongue, which is composed of muscle, the teeth, and saliva facilitate **mastication** and assist in moving food to the pharynx, where swallowing occurs and food moves to the esophagus. **Peristalsis**, or the squeezing movement of

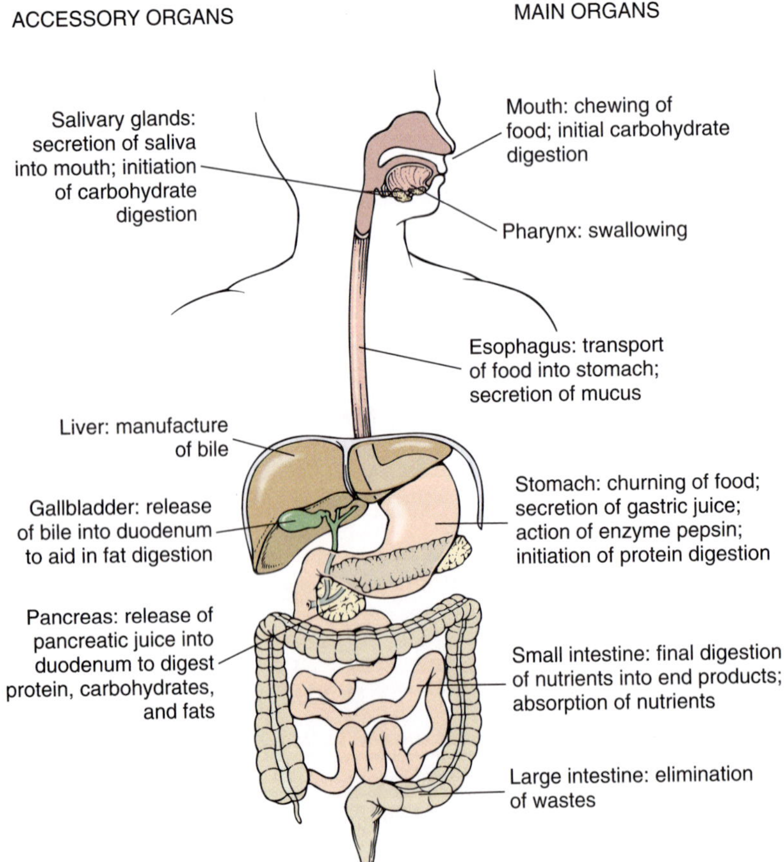

Figure 22-1. Main and accessory organs of the digestive system.

food toward the stomach, occurs in the esophagus. Once the food arrives in the stomach, it is churned with gastric juices and begins the movement toward the small intestine.

The pancreas, the liver, and the gallbladder all aid in the digestive process. The purpose of the pancreas is to excrete juices that aid in the digestive process. The pancreatic duct connects with the duodenum in the same area in which the bile duct from the liver and the gallbladder intersect the duodenum. The liver secretes bile to aid in the digestive process, and the gallbladder stores bile and releases it as needed. The gallbladder is attached to the liver by the cystic duct, which joins the hepatic duct. Together, they form the common bile duct, which enters into the duodenum.

The function of the liver in addition to aiding the digestive process, is to also remove poisons from the blood, produce immune agents to control infection, and remove germs and bacteria from the blood. The liver serves as a filter for the body; a person cannot live without a functioning liver.

The small intestine contains three areas: the duodenum, the jejunum, and the ileum. The small intestine completes the digestion begun in the stomach, absorbs products of digestion, and transports residue to the large intestine. The small intestine is suspended and is attached to the abdomen by a fold of peritoneum known as the mesentery. The small intestine joins the large intestine at the ileocecal valve.

The large intestine (Figure 22-2) is composed of the cecum, colon, rectum, and anal canal. The appendix is an appendage off the cecum. The purpose of the large intestine is to absorb electrolytes and store feces until the time of elimination.

DISEASE CONDITIONS

Diseases of the Digestive System (520-579), Chapter 9 in the ICD-9-CM code book, is divided into the following categories:

CATEGORY	SECTION TITLES
520-529	Diseases of the Oral Cavity, Salivary Glands, and Jaws
530-538	Diseases of Esophagus, Stomach, and Duodenum
540-543	Appendicitis
550-553	Hernia of Abdominal Cavity
555-558	Noninfectious Enteritis and Colitis
560-569	Other Diseases of Intestines and Peritoneum
570-579	Other Diseases of Digestive System

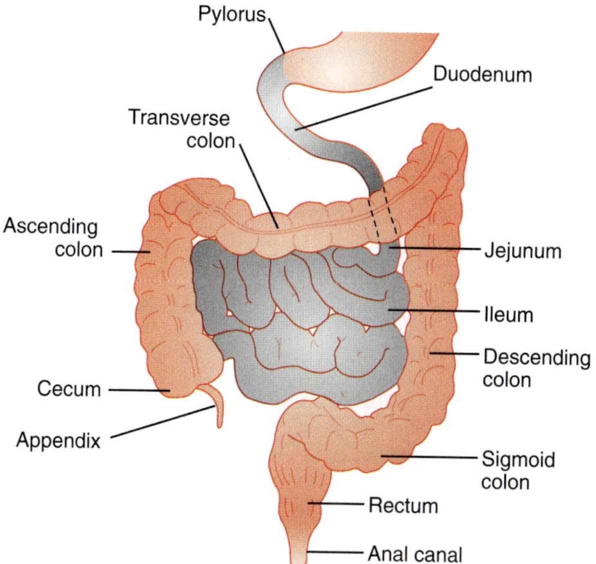

Figure 22-2. Small and large intestines.

Diseases of the Oral Cavity, Salivary Glands, and Jaws (520-529)

Many of the conditions in these categories concern the teeth and their structures which are often treated in the outpatient setting. Some of these conditions, however, may be treated when a patient is admitted for another condition. In the exam section of the record a healthcare provider might document whether the patient has dentures due to **edentulism** which is the complete loss of teeth. The loss of teeth might affect the patient's ability to eat and therefore their nutritional state.

EXAMPLE Patient is admitted to the hospital with severe malnutrition and dehydration. During the exam it is identified that the patient has Class I complete edentulism, 261, 276.51, 525.41, 525.10.

Sialolithiasis is caused by stones in the salivary glands. Patients usually present with swollen painful glands around the neck. When the stones are obstructing the gland an infection can result which is known as sialoadenitis. Surgery may be required to remove the stone.

EXAMPLE Patient with known sialolithiasis is admitted thru the ER with very painful glands in the neck and fever. After CT scan to determine the location of the stones and administration of antibiotics the patient is taken to the OR for removal, 527.5, 26.0.

Mucositis is an inflammation/ulceration of the digestive tract commonly occurring in the oral cavity. It can be found in up to 40% of patients being treated with chemotherapy. The condition can range from mild to severe. In the severest cases the patient may be unable to eat due to the pain caused by ulcerations in the mouth. It can be treated with viscous lidocaine.

EXAMPLE Patient admitted for chemotherapy for pancreatic cancer and develops ulcerative mucositis due to gemcitabine, V58.11, 157.9, 528.01, E933.1, 99.25.

EXERCISE 22-1

Assign codes to the following conditions using your ICD-9-CM code book.

1. Canker Sore __________
2. Ulcerative stomatitis __________
3. Hypertrophy of the salivary gland __________
4. Impacted Teeth __________

Diseases of the Esophagus, Stomach, and Duodenum (530-538)

Esophageal Conditions

Esophageal hemorrhage is coded to 530.82. It is important to take note of the Excludes note in this category. This note reminds the coder that esophageal varices (Figure 22-3), one of the most common causes of an esophageal bleed, are coded to codes 456.0 to 456.2, which are found in the Circulatory System chapter.

EXAMPLE Patient has esophageal varices due to cirrhosis of the liver, 571.5, 456.21.

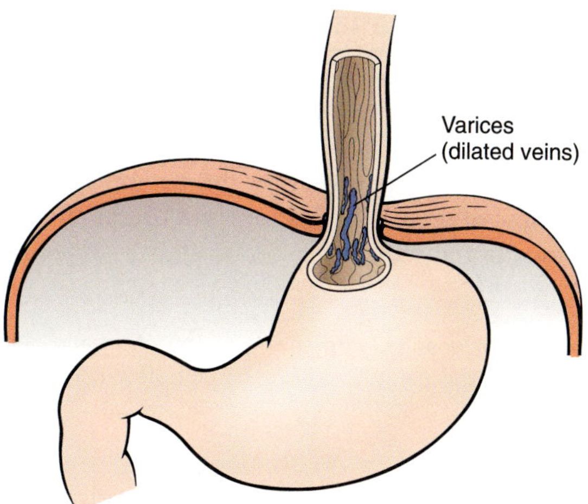

Figure 22-3. Esophageal varices.

Mallory-Weiss is the name for bleeding laceration of the esophagogastric junction that usually occurs after severe vomiting. If the bleeding is severe, an EGD may be performed to control bleeding. One of the most common conditions is esophageal reflux, which is also known as gastroesophageal reflux disease (GERD). It is treated with proton pump inhibitors such as Prilosec or, in more severe cases, by Nissen fundoplication surgery.

Barrett's esophagus is a precancerous condition that usually occurs in people with chronic GERD. The normal cells lining the esophagus change type. Symptoms may include heartburn, indigestion, difficulty swallowing solid foods, and nocturnal regurgitation.

EXAMPLE

Patient with chronic GERD who is having difficulty swallowing is found to have Barrett's esophagus, 530.81.

Arteriovenous malformations (AVM) may occur in the gastrointestinal tract. The terms AVM and **angiodysplasia** often are used interchangeably, although an angiodysplasia is a type of AVM characterized by dilated or fragile blood vessels. AVMs may be congenital or acquired. A congenital AVM is a defect that arises during fetal development. An acquired AVM is one that develops as the result of a variety of factors during one's lifetime. Unless specified as congenital, a gastrointestinal AVM should be coded as acquired, according to *Coding Clinic* (1996:3Q:p9-10; 1986:Nov-Dec:p11).[1,2] For indexing of gastrointestinal AVMs, see Figure 22-4.

EXERCISE 22-2

Assign codes to the following conditions using your ICD-9-CM code book.

1. Esophageal ulcer due to ingestion of aspirin ____________
2. Inflammation of the esophagus due to reflux ____________
3. Mallory-Weiss tear ____________
4. GERD ____________

Gastrointestinal Hemorrhage

Gastrointestinal (GI) hemorrhage is a common reason for a patient to seek medical attention. The healthcare provider must determine whether the bleed is lower or upper GI in origin, so appropriate treatment can be provided. To make this determination, the provider must evaluate how the patient presents.

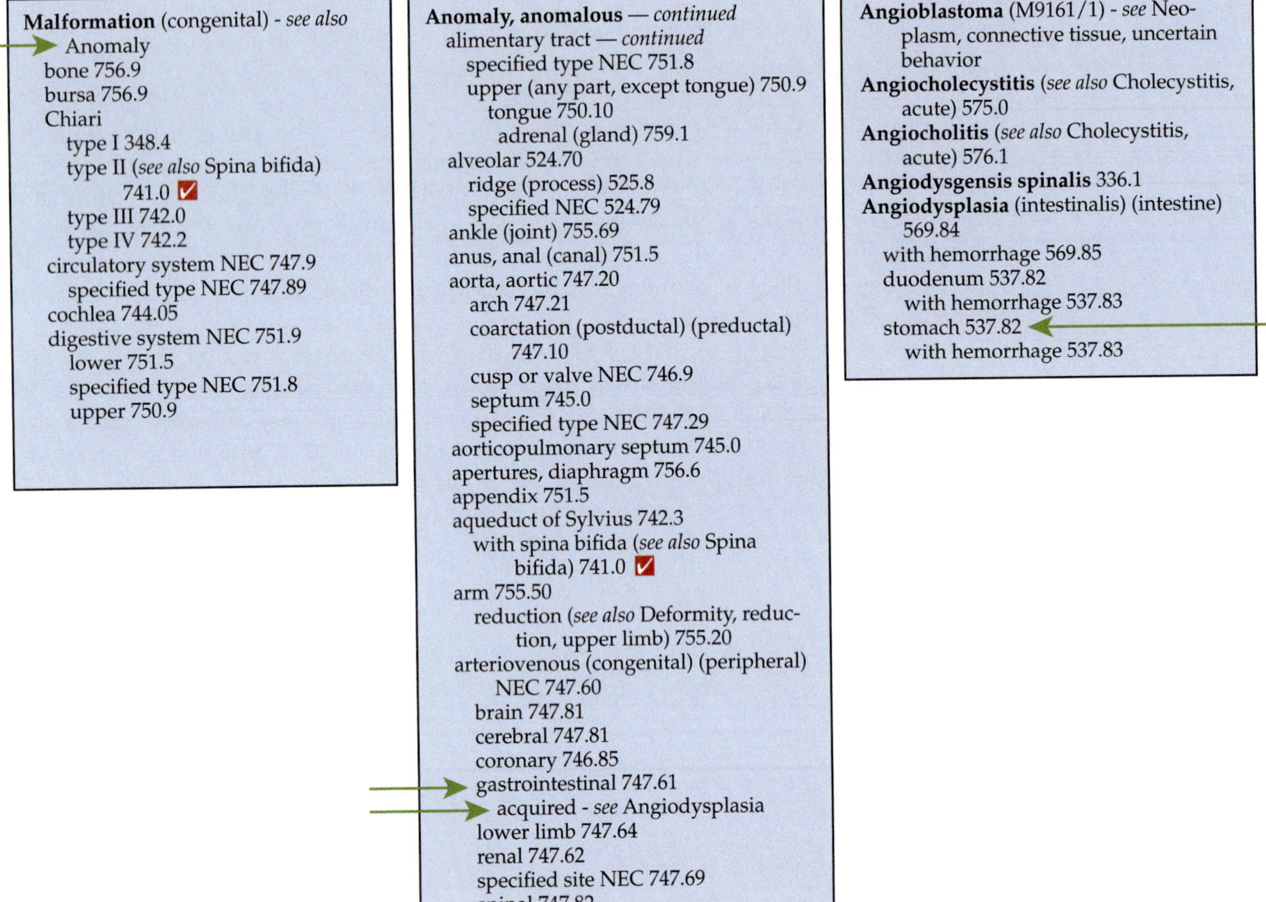
Malformation (congenital) - *see also* Anomaly
bone 756.9
bursa 756.9
Chiari
type I 348.4
type II (*see also* Spina bifida) 741.0
type III 742.0
type IV 742.2
circulatory system NEC 747.9
specified type NEC 747.89
cochlea 744.05
digestive system NEC 751.9
lower 751.5
specified type NEC 751.8
upper 750.9

Anomaly, anomalous — *continued*
alimentary tract — *continued*
specified type NEC 751.8
upper (any part, except tongue) 750.9
tongue 750.10
adrenal (gland) 759.1
alveolar 524.70
ridge (process) 525.8
specified NEC 524.79
ankle (joint) 755.69
anus, anal (canal) 751.5
aorta, aortic 747.20
arch 747.21
coarctation (postductal) (preductal) 747.10
cusp or valve NEC 746.9
septum 745.0
specified type NEC 747.29
aorticopulmonary septum 745.0
apertures, diaphragm 756.6
appendix 751.5
aqueduct of Sylvius 742.3
with spina bifida (*see also* Spina bifida) 741.0
arm 755.50
reduction (*see also* Deformity, reduction, upper limb) 755.20
arteriovenous (congenital) (peripheral) NEC 747.60
brain 747.81
cerebral 747.81
coronary 746.85
gastrointestinal 747.61
acquired - *see* Angiodysplasia
lower limb 747.64
renal 747.62
specified site NEC 747.69
spinal 747.82
upper limb 747.63

Angioblastoma (M9161/1) - *see* Neoplasm, connective tissue, uncertain behavior
Angiocholecystitis (*see also* Cholecystitis, acute) 575.0
Angiocholitis (*see also* Cholecystitis, acute) 576.1
Angiodysgensis spinalis 336.1
Angiodysplasia (intestinalis) (intestine) 569.84
with hemorrhage 569.85
duodenum 537.82
with hemorrhage 537.83
stomach 537.82
with hemorrhage 537.83

Figure 22-4. Indexing of gastrointestinal arteriovenous malformation (AVM).

- In lower GI bleeds (LGIB), the patient may present with the following: **Hematochezia**—bright red blood in stool
- In upper GI bleeds (UGIB), the patient may present with the following: **Hematemesis**—vomiting of blood

If a patient presents with **melena** (dark blood in stool) or **occult** blood in the stool (this can be found only by laboratory inspection), it is unknown without further workup whether this is an upper or a lower GI bleed. Often, when a patient presents with acute anemia without a causative condition, the healthcare provider may suspect a GI bleed.

EXAMPLE Blood in feces, occult, lab finding, 792.1.

GI hemorrhage has many causes; the most common causes consist of gastric or intestinal ulcers, hemorrhoids, diverticulitis, and angiodysplasia of the intestine.

EXAMPLE Patient admitted with GI bleed caused by angiodysplasia of the stomach, 537.83.

EXAMPLE Patient is being treated for diverticulitis of the sigmoid colon with hemorrhage, 562.13.

Per *Coding Clinic* (2005:3Q:p17-18),[3] if a patient presents with a GI bleed and then undergoes diagnostic testing such as esophagogastroduodenoscopy (EGD) to determine the site of the bleed, unless the physician specifies a causal relationship between the

findings on this test and the bleed, the code 578.9 should be assigned. Codes for any other findings such as gastritis should be coded as without hemorrhage.

Ulcers of the Stomach and Small Intestine

An ulcer of the stomach or the intestine is an open sore in the lining of the stomach or intestine. An ulcer occurs when the lining is damaged. Damage to the lining may occur when production of stomach acid is increased, or it may be caused by a bacterium known as *Helicobacter pylori,* or *H. pylori.* Remember when locating the code for a bacterium the main term "Infection" should be referenced in the Alphabetic Index. Ulcers may be drug induced. The Tabular List contains instructions for the use of additional E codes to identify the responsible drug (Figure 22-5).

Symptoms of gastric ulcer may include pain when eating, vomiting, and tarry bowel movements. Ulcers can be diagnosed by means of an upper GI x-ray, blood tests that look for *H. pylori,* stool samples, or endoscopy. Treatment for ulcers may include antacids, drugs such as proton pump inhibitors or histamine receptor blockers, which stop the stomach from making acids, or antibiotics, and finally, in the worst case scenario, gastrectomy. Some conditions that may accompany ulcers are chronic or acute blood loss anemia and gastric outlet syndrome. A gastric ulcer is a stomach ulcer. A peptic ulcer can occur in the esophagus, stomach, duodenum, jejunum, and/or ileum. If no site is specified, 533.XX is assigned for peptic ulcer.

EXAMPLE

Patient has a peptic ulcer of the esophagus, secondary to aspirin use, 530.20, E935.3.

EXAMPLE

Patient is admitted for a bleeding gastric ulcer with obstruction and perforation, 531.61.

EXERCISE 22-3

Assign codes to the following conditions using your ICD-9-CM code book.

1. Angiodysplasia with hemorrhage of the duodenum and chronic blood loss anemia ________
2. Acute penetrating peptic ulcer of the duodenum ________
3. GI bleed due to peptic ulcer ________
4. Bleeding esophageal varices ________
5. Blood in stool ________

● **530.2 Ulcer of esophagus**
Ulcer of esophagus
fungal
peptic
Ulcer of esophagus due to ingestion of:
aspirin
medicines
chemicals
→ Use additional E code to identify cause, if induced by chemical or drug

530.20 Ulcer of esophagus without bleeding
Ulcer of esophagus NOS

530.21 Ulcer of esophagus with bleeding
Excludes *bleeding esophageal varices (456.0, 456.20)*

Figure 22-5. If an ulcer is drug or chemical induced, assign an E code for the responsible drug or chemical.

Appendicitis (540-543)

Appendicitis is inflammation of the appendix that is usually caused by obstruction, which, in turn, results in infection (Figure 22-6). A patient who presents with appendicitis may have some or all of the following signs and symptoms: abdominal pain (right lower quadrant, also known as **McBurney's** point), vomiting, **anorexia**, fever, constipation, and elevated white blood cell count.

If the appendix ruptures, peritonitis develops. Patients with appendicitis are usually treated with antibiotics and surgery (appendectomy). It is important to review the pathology report for documentation of abscess or perforation of appendix.

On occasion, all signs and symptoms lead the surgeon to believe that a patient has appendicitis, but the pathology report does not confirm this diagnosis. When the pathology report indicates a normal appendix, *Coding Clinic* (1990:2Q:p26)[4] instructs the coder to use the symptom the patient presented with as the principal diagnosis.

EXAMPLE Patient admitted with acute appendicitis with peritoneal abscess, 540.1.

EXAMPLE Patient has a ruptured appendicitis, 540.0.

Hernia of Abdominal Cavity (550-553)

A **hernia** (Figure 22-7) is a protrusion of an organ or tissue through an abnormal opening in the body. Hernias can be present at birth or may develop over time. Most commonly, a hernia is a protrusion of the intestine through a weakness in the abdominal cavity. Hernias are classified by type or site. Once the site of the hernia is known, then it must be determined whether it is obstructed or gangrenous. An obstructed abdominal hernia is one in which the bowel is trapped and obstructed but viable (still working); when it becomes nonviable, it can become gangrenous (deficient blood supply to trapped bowel, making it **necrotic**). Some codes require documentation as to whether the hernia is unilateral or bilateral, and whether it is recurrent. Hernia repairs require more information and are discussed in the procedure section of this chapter.

EXAMPLE Patient was seen in consultation for an inguinal hernia, unilateral, recurrent, with obstruction, 550.11.

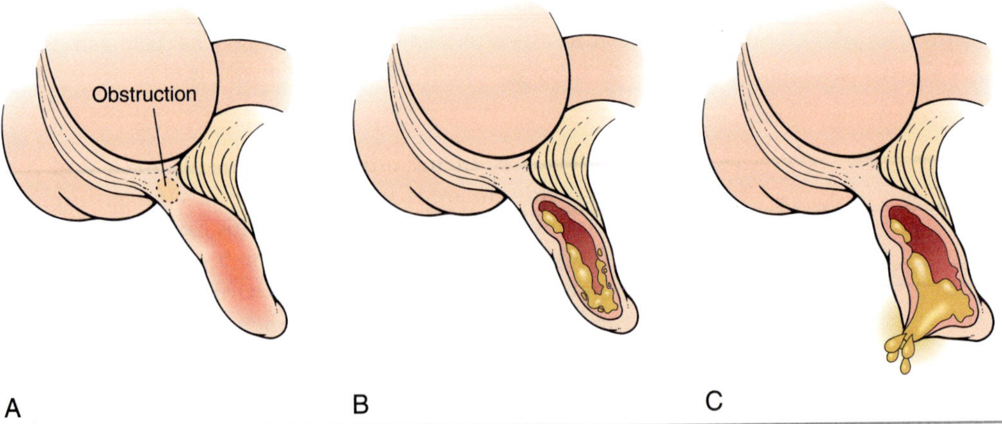

Figure 22-6. Stages of appendicitis. **A,** Obstruction that causes inflammation. **B,** Pus and bacteria invade the wall of the appendix. **C,** Pus perforates the wall of the appendix, leading to peritonitis.

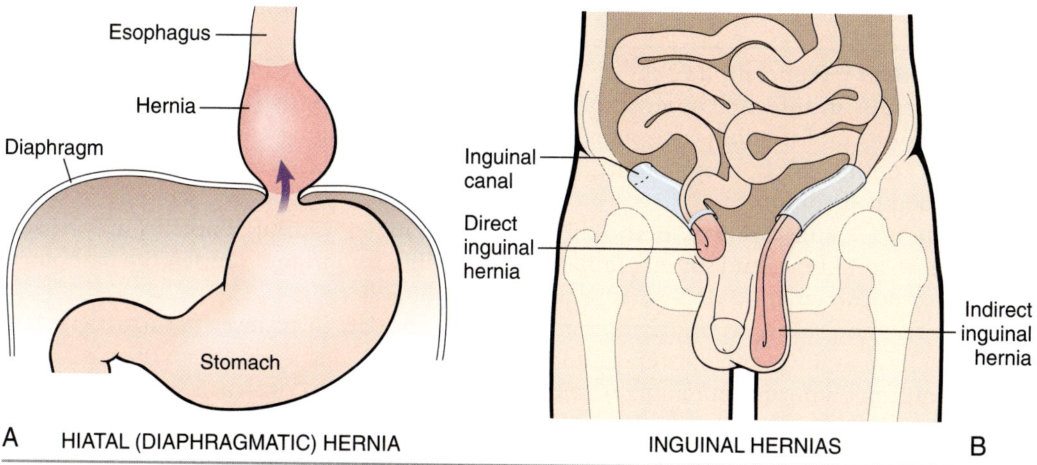

Figure 22-7. **A,** Hiatal hernia. **B,** Inguinal hernia. Direct inguinal hernia passes through the abdominal wall. Indirect hernia passes through the inguinal canal.

Noninfectious Enteritis and Colitis (555-558)

Crohn's Disease

Crohn's disease is characterized by inflammation of the GI tract, especially the small and large intestine. It is an inflammatory bowel disease that appears to run in families. It is typically diagnosed first at the age of 20 to 30. Often there is difficulty determining Crohn's versus ulcerative colitis. Crohn's may also be known as ileitis or enteritis. People presenting with Crohn's may exhibit symptoms of abdominal pain and diarrhea. Depending on the severity and location of the disease, patients may be treated with drugs to control inflammation, steroids, immunosuppressive agents, biologic response modifiers, antibiotics, and medications to control diarrhea, along with fluid replacement. Almost 75% of the patients with Crohn's require surgery at some point in their lives to remove the diseased intestine and they often require an ostomy.

Ulcerative Colitis

Ulcerative colitis, like Crohn's disease, is an inflammatory bowel disease. Ulcerative colitis is a disease that produces ulcers in the lining of the rectum and colon, whereas Crohn's disease causes inflammation deep within the intestinal wall and can occur in other parts of the digestive system, including the small intestine, mouth, esophagus, and stomach.

EXAMPLE

Patient is admitted to the hospital with abdominal pain and dehydration. After testing is completed, a diagnosis of ulcerative enterocolitis is confirmed, 556.0, 276.51.

Gastroenteritis is an inflammation of the stomach and intestines. Two of the main causes of this condition are viruses and bacteria. Viral gastroenteritis usually runs its course in 1 to 2 days, whereas bacterial gastroenteritis can last for up to a week or more. The most common causes of viral gastroenteritis, which often spreads via poor handwashing habits in schools and daycare centers, are adenoviruses, rotaviruses, and norovirus. The noroviruses are the leading cause of acute gastroenteritis. The most common bacterial causes are *E. coli*, salmonella, campylobacter, and shigella. Gastroenteritis due to particular viruses or bacteria may be indexed under "Gastroenteritis" with a subterm for the bacterium/virus. If the bacterium/virus is not listed, the index has an instruction to *see also* enteritis. Codes for gastroenteritis caused by viruses or bacteria may be located in the infectious and parasitic diseases chapter. Gastroenteritis may also be caused by chemical toxins such those found in medications or foods. These types of gastroenteritis are not infectious.

The symptoms of gastroenteritis can include vomiting, diarrhea, low grade fever, and abdominal pain. Treatment in a hospital usually consists of IV fluids for rehydration and, if the patient is suffering from bacterial gastroenteritis, antibiotics may be used. If vomiting is severe, antiemetics and antidiarrheal agents may also be used.

EXAMPLE Patient is admitted to hospital with severe vomiting and diarrhea. After testing is performed it is determined that she is suffering from a bout of gastroenteritis, 558.9.

Other Diseases of Intestines and Peritoneum (560-569)

Intestinal Obstruction

This condition occurs when the content of the intestines cannot move forward. The intestines can be completely blocked or partially blocked. Obstruction may be mechanical or functional. Mechanical obstruction can be caused by a variety of conditions, such as neoplasm, **impaction**, stricture, adhesion, **intussusception**, and herniation (Figure 22-8). When the obstruction is functional, it is called an **ileus**.

EXAMPLE Patient with obstruction due to impaction, 560.39.

EXAMPLE Patient with obstruction due to ileus, 560.1.

EXAMPLE Patient has intussusception of the intestine, 560.0.

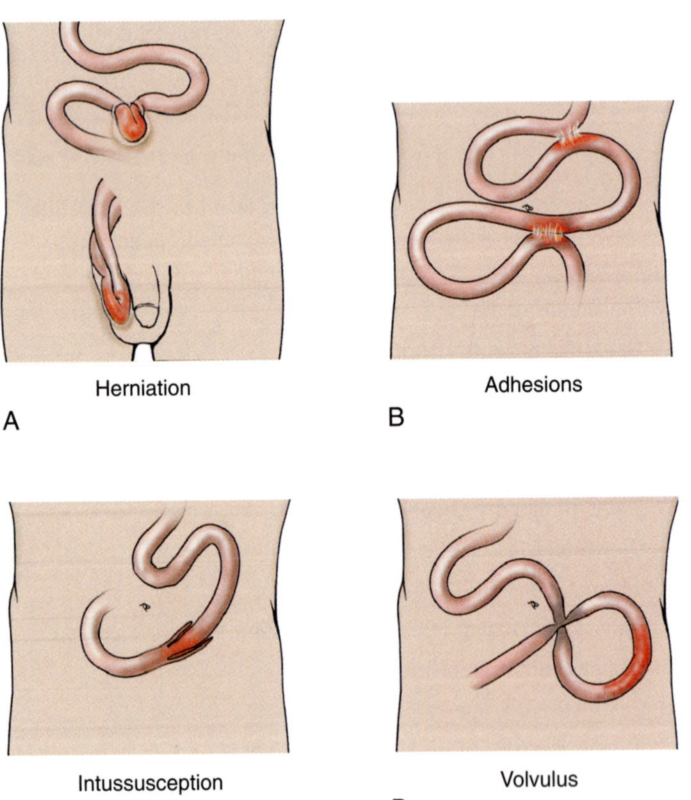

Figure 22-8. **A,** Herniation. **B,** Adhesions. **C,** Intussusception. **D,** Volvulus.

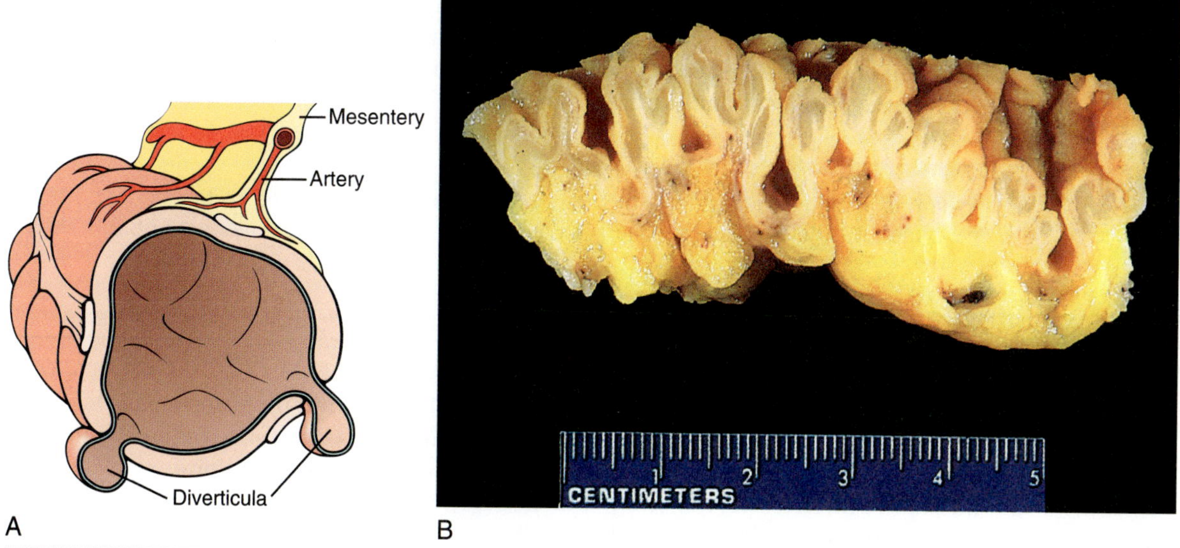

Figure 22-9. **A,** Diverticula. **B,** Diverticulosis.

Diverticulitis and Diverticulosis

Diverticula (Figure 22-9), also known as tics, are small pouches in the lining of the mucous membranes of an organ. When a patient has diverticula, the condition is referred to as diverticulosis. If these pouches become inflamed or infected, the condition becomes diverticulitis. It is not necessary in ICD-9-CM to code both conditions; if a patient has diverticulitis, it is assumed that he or she also has diverticulosis. If the condition is described as diverticulosis without site, it is assumed by ICD-9-CM to be a condition of the colon.

EXAMPLE Patient has diverticulosis of the duodenum with diverticulitis and hemorrhage, 562.03.

EXERCISE 22-4

Assign codes to the following conditions using your ICD-9-CM code book.

1. Patient with acute abdominal pain is taken to the operating room (OR) for appendectomy with suspected appendicitis. Pathology report reveals normal appendix. ____________
2. Incisional hernia ____________
3. Gangrenous ventral hernia ____________
4. Congenital diaphragmatic hernia ____________
5. Obstructed unilateral femoral hernia ____________
6. Meckel's diverticulitis ____________
7. Hemorrhagic diverticulitis ____________
8. Diverticulosis ____________
9. Volvulus causing intestinal obstruction ____________
10. Adhesions causing intestinal obstruction ____________
11. Regional enteritis of the colon ____________
12. Gastroenteritis due to *E. coli* ____________
13. Allergic gastroenteritis due to milk allergy ____________
14. Gastroenteritis due to radiation ____________
15. Pseudopolyposis of the colon ____________

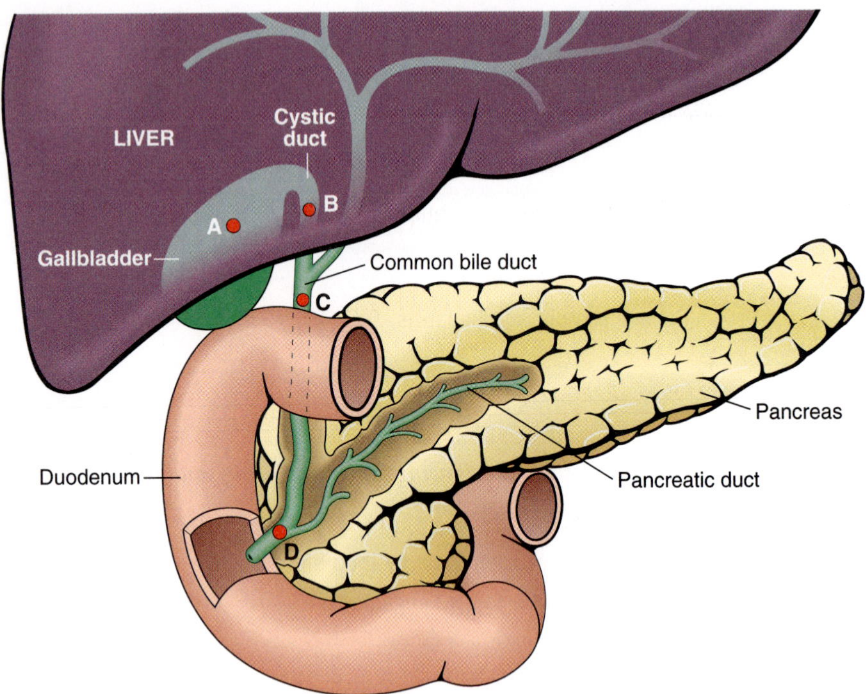

Figure 22-10. Common gallstone position. **A,** Stone in gallbladder. **B,** Stone obstructs the cystic duct. **C,** Stone obstructs the common bile duct. **D,** Stone at lower end of bile duct and pancreatic duct.

Other Diseases of Digestive System (570-579)

Cholelithiasis and Cholecystitis

Cholelithiasis is an abnormal condition of stones in the gallbladder (gallstones). The condition is generally asymptomatic until gallstones block the cystic duct or the common bile duct, which does not allow the gallbladder to drain stored bile; the patient then develops acute cholecystitis (Figure 22-10). If the cystic duct is blocked, a patient generally has right upper quadrant crampy abdominal pain. This pain is often made worse by ingestion of fatty or greasy foods. When the common bile duct is blocked, a patient may develop cholangitis; when the stone is blocking the lower end of the common bile duct, secretion from the pancreas may be blocked, and pancreatitis may occur. **Choledocholithiasis** is the term used for a stone lodged in the bile duct. Endoscopic retrograde cholangiopancreatography (ERCP) may be used to detect the presence of gallstones.

EXAMPLE Patient has acute cholecystitis with cholelithiasis and choledocholithiasis, 574.30.

Cirrhosis of the Liver

Cirrhosis of the liver is degeneration of liver tissue that causes blockage of blood through the organ and inhibits the function of this organ. Cirrhosis may be caused by a variety of factors; alcoholism and hepatitis are the most common.

EXAMPLE Alcoholic cirrhosis of liver, 571.2, 303.90.

Hepatitis

Hepatitis, which is an inflammation of the liver, can last for a short time, or it may be chronic and last a lifetime. Most commonly, hepatitis is caused by a virus. When it is caused by a virus, hepatitis is coded from the infectious disease chapter of ICD-9-CM. However, other

less common types of hepatitis are coded to the chapter on Digestive Diseases. Because the liver metabolizes both alcohol and drugs, a patient may develop alcoholic hepatitis or drug-induced hepatitis. When coding drug-induced hepatitis, it is important to also assign the E code for the responsible drug.

EXAMPLE Patient has chronic hepatitis C, 070.54.

EXAMPLE Patient has chronic hepatitis, 571.40.

EXERCISE 22-5

Assign codes to the following conditions using your ICD-9-CM code book.

1. Alcoholic hepatitis ____________
2. Drug induced hepatitis by ibuprofen ____________
3. Hepatitis due to cytomegalovirus ____________
4. Fatty liver ____________
5. Portal hypertension ____________
6. Patient admitted to hospital with chronic cholecystitis for a laparascopic cholecystectomy; during the surgery the surgeon decides to convert to open ____________
7. Patient is admitted with gallstone pancreatitis; this is treated and the patient is sent home ____________

V CODES

In the past, V codes have been considered for use primarily in the outpatient setting. This has changed with the addition of more V codes each year. As was discussed in Chapter 8, it is difficult to locate V codes in the Index. Coders will often say, "I did not know there was a V code for that." Refer to Chapter 8 for a listing of common main terms used to locate V codes.

V codes that may be used with digestive system conditions include the following:

V12.70	Personal history of unspecified digestive disease
V12.71	Personal history of peptic ulcer disease
V12.72	Personal history of colonic polyps
V18.5	Family history of digestive disorders
V42.83	History of pancreas replaced by transplant
V42.84	History of intestines replaced by transplant
V44.1	Gastrostomy status
V44.2	Ileostomy status
V44.3	Colostomy status
V45.3	Intestinal bypass or anastomosis status
V45.72	Acquired absence of intestine
V45.75	Acquired absence of the stomach
V45.86	Bariatric surgery status
V47.3	History of other digestive problems
V53.5	Fitting and adjustment of other intestinal appliance
V55.1	Attention to gastrostomy

V55.2	Attention to ileostomy
V55.3	Attention to colostomy
V55.4	Attention to other artificial openings of the digestive tract
V59.6	Liver donor

EXAMPLE

Patient is admitted to donate kidney to husband, laparoscopic donor nephrectomy performed, V59.4, 55.51.

EXERCISE 22-6

Assign codes to the following conditions using your ICD-9-CM code book.

1. Patient is admitted for takedown of a colostomy ____________
2. Patient had gastric bypass 1 year ago ____________
3. Physician notes that the patient has a history of having the pancreas replaced by a transplant ____________
4. Patient has a remote history of PUD ____________

COMMON TREATMENTS

Many digestive disorders are treated with surgery.

CONDITION	MEDICATION
GERD	Propulsid, Reglan, Prilosec, Prevacid Zantac, Tagamet
Crohn's disease	Azulfidine, Remicade, corticosteroids, Rowasa
Diverticulitis	Metronidazole, Ciprofloxin
Gastric ulcer	Pepcid, Axid, Prilosec, Nexium
Gastroenteritis	Antiemetics such as Promethazine (Phenergan), prochlorperazine (Compazine), ondansetron (Zofran) Antidiarrheals, such as diphenoxylate atropine (Lomotil, Lofene, Lonox) or loperamide hydrochloride (Imodium) IV fluids
Pancreatitis	Antibiotics such as gentamicin, clindamycin

PROCEDURES

Some procedures that may be related to diseases of the digestive system may be located in the following chapter of the Procedure Tabular:

Chapter 9 Operations on the Digestive System (42-54)

Procedures of the Stomach

Nissen **fundoplication** (Figure 22-11) is a surgical treatment for GERD. This procedure takes the fundus (the upper portion) of the stomach and wraps it around the lower portion of the esophagus to prevent the reflux of stomach contents back into the esophagus.

Percutaneous endoscopic gastrostomy (PEG) is the placement of a tube through the abdominal wall into the stomach with the use of a scope. PEGs are used as feeding tubes for patients who are having difficulty eating (e.g., malnourished patients, patients who aspirate food). Per *Coding Clinic* (1993:5th issue:p16),[5] if a patient is admitted for insertion of a PEG tube because of carcinoma of the palate, and he or she now has dysphagia and dehydration, the principal diagnosis would be 145.3, carcinoma, and additional codes 787.2X (for dysphagia) and 276.51 (for dehydration) would be assigned.

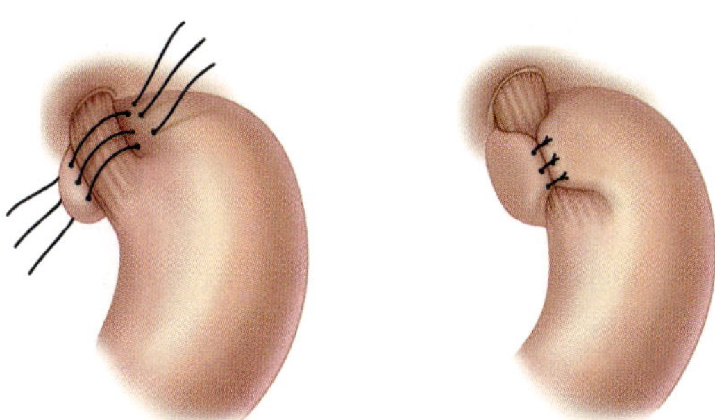

Figure 22-11. Nissen fundoplication.

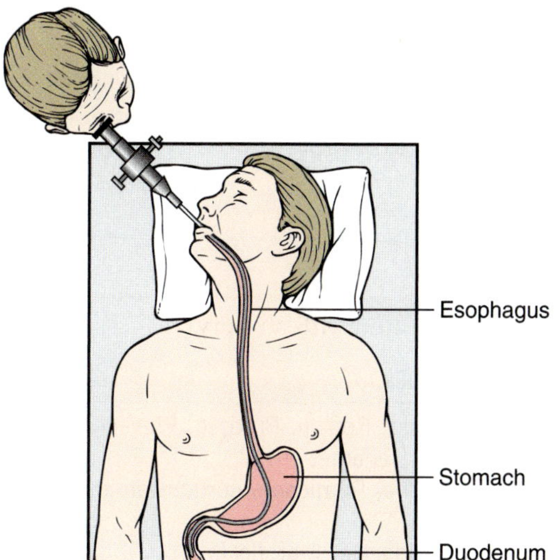

Figure 22-12. Esophagogastroduodenoscopy (EGD).

If a patient presents to the hospital with a chief complaint of a PEG tube falling out, the principal diagnosis would be V55.1, or attention to gastrostomy, because no complications resulted from the gastrostomy itself. This is described in detail in *Coding Clinic* (1997:3Q:p8).[6]

Procedures of the Intestine

Esophagogastroduodenoscopy (EGD) (Figure 22-12) is a diagnostic procedure that a physician uses to identify disease conditions in the esophagus, stomach, and duodenum. Many times additional procedures are performed, such as biopsy, lesion removal, ablation, hemorrhage control, and dilations.

EXAMPLE Patient with bleeding gastric ulcer taken to OR for EGD to control bleed, 531.40, 44.43.

Colostomy (Figure 22-13) is procedure that uses the colon to create an artificial opening (**stoma**) to the exterior of the abdomen. This artificial opening serves as a substitute anus through which the intestines excrete waste until the colon heals or other corrective surgery is performed. The location of the stoma depends on which part of the colon is involved in the surgery. Most colostomies are temporary. A sigmoid colostomy is the most commonly performed type.

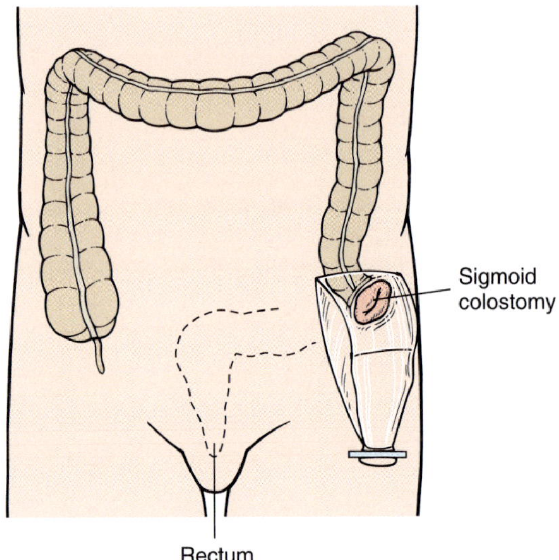

Figure 22-13. Colostomy. The opening of the colon is brought to the surface of the skin to divert feces into an external pouch worn by the patient.

Per *Coding Clinic* (1997:3Q:p9-10),[7] when a patient is admitted for a colostomy closure (**takedown**), the principal diagnosis should be V55.3. Most often, when closing a colostomy, the surgeon must perform minor trimming of the colon to complete the **anastomosis**, but sometimes, it is necessary to actually excise portions of the colon; in that case, the use of code 45.79 would be appropriate.

An **ileostomy** is very similar to a colostomy, except that the end of the small intestine is brought out through the abdominal wall.

Bowel resection can be performed for neoplasms, severe diverticulitis, bowel perforation, and bowel obstruction. Surgeons remove a portion of the bowel and then connect the bowel back together (anastomosis). In bowel resection in which an end-to-end anastomosis is performed an additional code for the anastomosis is not assigned. This includes small intestine anastomosed to large intestine. Figure 22-14 illustrates various types of anastomoses.

EXAMPLE

Patient with malignant neoplasm of the descending colon is admitted for left hemicolectomy and temporary colostomy, 153.2, 45.75, 46.11.

Appendectomy is removal of the appendix. Codes are available for appendectomy done by incision and that done by laparoscopy. Often, when a surgeon is performing an abdominal operation, an incidental appendectomy may be performed. An **incidental appendectomy** is one that is performed at the time of another procedure with no known disease process in the appendix.

EXAMPLE

Patient with acute appendicitis is admitted for a laparoscopic appendectomy, 540.9, 47.01.

Procedures of the Gallbladder and Biliary System

Gallbladder Calculus Removal: Cholecystectomy, or removal of the gallbladder, can be performed by incision or by laparoscope (Figure 22-15). Cholecystotomy may also be performed to remove stones from the gallbladder. This can be performed by open incision as well as by scope.

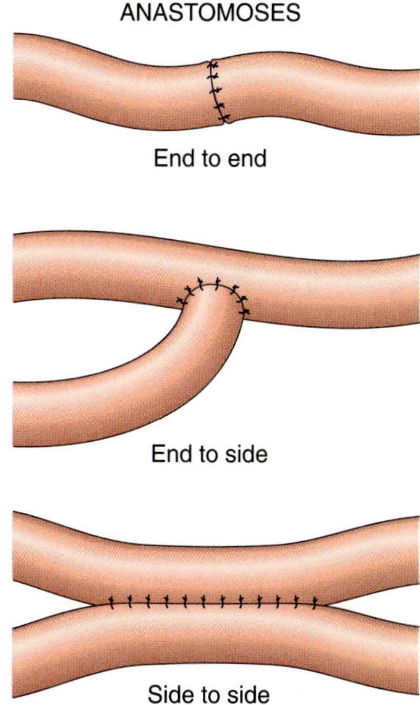

Figure 22-14. Types of anastomoses.

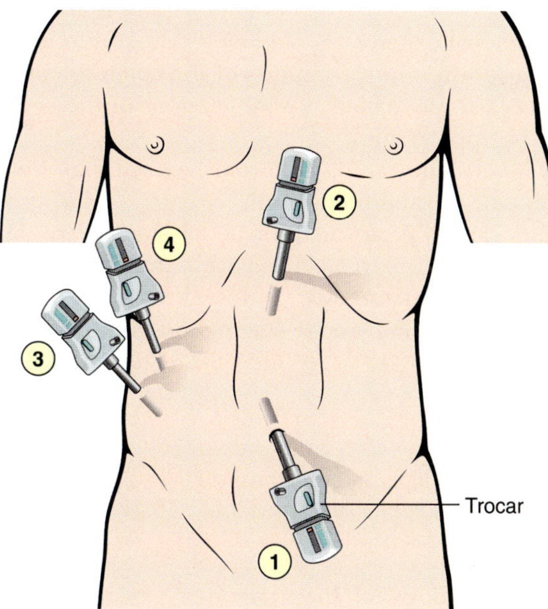

Figure 22-15. Trocar placement for laparoscopic cholecystectomy.

EXAMPLE

Patient with acute cholecystitis with cholelithiasis has a laparoscopic cholecystectomy, 574.00, 51.23.

Common Duct Stone Removal: These stones can be removed in three different ways (i.e., by incision, endoscopy, or percutaneously). Occasionally a cholecystectomy is performed along with removal of common duct stones. Codes should be assigned for both the cholecystectomy and the common bile duct stone removal. Fragmentation of stones of the gallbladder by extracorporeal shock wave lithotripsy, or ESWL, is the breaking apart of stones by shock waves.

EXAMPLE

Patient with common bile duct stones presents for stone removal by ERCP, 574.50, 51.88.

Endoscopic retrograde cholangiopancreatography (ERCP): This procedure is often done for diagnosis, but it may be done for stent insertion, or may be done in combination with a sphincterotomy or for removal of stones. In all of these cases, both the ERCP and the additional codes are assigned.

EXAMPLE

Patient with abdominal pain which is suspected to be due to a pancreatic malignancy presents for a diagnostic ERCP. The ERCP reveals no malignancy, 789.00, 51.10.

Lysis of Adhesions

Lysis of adhesions is a procedure that is performed to remove adhesions. **Adhesions**, which are very often found in the peritoneal area, are fibrous bands of tissue that adhere abdominal organs to one another or to the abdominal wall. Adhesions are often synonymous with scar tissue and can develop after surgery, often causing abdominal pain. To code adhesion removal, look in the index under Lysis, adhesions. Attention should be paid to the note in the Alphabetic Index under lysis of adhesions that instructs the coder to omit this code if the surgeon uses terminology such as blunt, digital, manual, mechanical and without instrumentation. *Coding Clinic* (1990:4Q:p18-19)[8] discusses when it is appropriate to include this code in combination with other procedure codes.

EXAMPLE

Patient with chronic cholecystitis admitted for laparoscopic cholecystectomy. The surgeon performed manual lysis of adhesions of the gallbladder, prior to laparoscopic cholecystectomy, 575.11, 51.23. No code for lysis of adhesions required.

EXAMPLE

Patient with abdominal pain is admitted. The surgeon performed laparoscopic lysis of adhesions of the peritoneum, 568.0, 54.51.

Hernia Repair

Herniorrhaphy is repair of a hernia. Coding hernia repairs requires attention to location, laterality, whether direct or indirect, whether performed with a prosthesis or a graft. In a direct hernia, the protrusion occurs through the abdominal wall; an indirect hernia results when the protrusion occurs through the inguinal ring into the inguinal canal. It is important that surgeons are aware of the need to document this information.

EXAMPLE

Patient had a bilateral inguinal hernia repair direct and indirect with prosthesis, 550.92, 53.16.

Whipple Procedure

Whipple procedure is also known as a pancreaticoduodenectomy. This procedure generally involves removal of the gallbladder, common bile duct, part of the duodenum, and the head of the pancreas. This procedure may be performed for chronic pancreatitis, pancreatic pseudocysts, or pancreatic malignancies.

EXAMPLE

Patient with pancreatic cancer in the head of the pancreas presents for Whipple procedure, 157.0, 52.7.

Transjugular Intrahepatic Portosystemic Shunt (TIPS)

TIPS (transjugular intrahepatic portosystemic shunt): This procedure is often performed by interventional radiologists for patients with severe complications of liver disease. The interventionalist percutaneously makes a tunnel through the liver with a needle and connects the portal vein to one of the hepatic veins. A stent is inserted into this tunnel to keep the tract open. This procedure does not improve the functioning of the liver but helps in treatment of the complications.

EXAMPLE

A patient with portal hypertension is admitted for a TIPS procedure, 572.3, 39.1.

EXERCISE 22-7

Assign codes to the following conditions using your ICD-9-CM code book.

1. Insertion percutaneous endoscopic gastrostomy for dysphagia ____________
2. Incidental appendectomy during cholecystectomy for gallstones ____________
3. Repair of ventral hernia ____________
4. ERCP with endoscopic sphincterotomy and stone removal from pancreatic duct ____________
5. Patient with GERD admitted for Nissen fundoplication ____________

DOCUMENTATION/REIMBURSEMENT/MS-DRGs

Often, coding difficulties are due to lack of documentation. Sometimes pathology and other test results are not available at the time of discharge or when the physician is dictating the discharge summary or is reporting the final diagnoses.

Types of Appendicitis

It is important to check pathology reports when appendectomies are performed and to review the record for documentation of appendiceal rupture, abscess, or generalized peritonitis. Different-MS-DRGs are assigned for appendicitis with a complicated principal diagnosis.

EXAMPLE

DIAGNOSES	CODES	MS-DRG	RW
Acute appendicitis with Appendectomy, laparoscopic	540.9 47.01	343	0.9887
Ruptured appendicitis with Appendectomy, laparoscopic	540.0 47.01	340	1.3849

Two or More Interrelated Conditions, Each Potentially Meeting the Definition of Principal Diagnosis

EXAMPLE

DIAGNOSES	CODES	MS-DRG	RW
Dehydration	276.51	641	0.7248
Gastroenteritis	558.9		
Gastroenteritis	558.9	392	0.7121
Dehydration	276.51		

Coding Clinic (1984:July-Aug:p19-20;1988:2Q:p10)[9,10] reminds the coder that the reason the patient is admitted for treatment should be the principal diagnosis. If the patient had dehydration caused by gastroenteritis and was admitted for IV fluids, then the principal diagnosis would be the dehydration. However, if the patient had gastroenteritis and dehydration and the patient was admitted for treatment of both of these diagnoses, then either diagnosis could be sequenced as the principal.

Lysis of Adhesions

It is always important to review the operative report for lysis of adhesions. Per *Coding Clinic* (1990:4Q:p18)[8] if multiple adhesions prevent the surgeon from gaining access to the organ that is being removed, thereby requiring lysis before the operation can be completed, both diagnosis of adhesions and the lysis procedure should be coded.

EXAMPLE

DIAGNOSES	CODES	MS-DRG	RW
Acute appendicitis	540.9	343	0.9887
Adhesions	568.0		
Appendectomy	47.01		
Acute appendicitis	540.9	337	1.6984
Adhesions	568.0		
Appendectomy	47.01		
Lysis of adhesions	54.54		

Coding Clinic (1990:4Q:p18)[8] goes on to say that frequently, however, adhesions may exist without being organized and without causing any symptoms in the patient or increasing the difficulty of performing the operative procedure. When such minor adhesions exist and are easily lysed as part of the principal procedure, coding a diagnosis of adhesions and the procedure would be inappropriate.

Blood Loss Anemia With GI Bleeds

In cases of GI bleed, it would be prudent to check laboratory values with regard to falling hematocrit or hemoglobin, as well as orders for transfusions. Many GI bleeds have as a common comorbidity acute or chronic blood loss anemia. This is often not well documented by physicians and a query may be required.

EXAMPLE

DIAGNOSES	CODES	MS-DRG	RW
GI bleed	578.9	379	0.8476
GI bleed with acute blood loss anemia	578.9 285.1	378	1.0195

Types of Cholecystectomies and Additional Procedures Performed

Cholecystectomies have a separate set of MS-DRGs for those done with common bile duct exploration. Common bile duct exploration is a procedure that allows the clinician to see whether a stone is blocking the flow of bile from the liver and gallbladder to the intestine. Close attention must be paid to the method by which the cholecystectomy is performed as there is a separate MS-DRG for cholecystectomies performed by laparoscopy.

EXAMPLE

DIAGNOSES	CODES	MS-DRG	RW
Calculus of bile duct with acute cholecystitis and cholecystectomy	574.30 51.22	416	1.5398

EXAMPLE

DIAGNOSES	CODES	MS-DRG	RW
Calculus of bile duct with acute cholecystitis and cholecystectomy with exploration of the common bile duct	574.30 51.22 51.51	413	1.9412

EXAMPLE

DIAGNOSES	CODES	MS-DRG	RW
Calculus of bile duct with acute cholecystitis and laparoscopic cholecystectomy	574.30 51.24	419	1.2400

CHAPTER REVIEW EXERCISE

Where applicable, assign codes for diagnoses, procedures. V codes, and E codes.

1. What makes up the alimentary canal?

   ____

2. What are the three areas of the small intestines?
   1. ______________________________
   2. ______________________________
   3. ______________________________

3. What three organs assist the digestive process?
   1. ______________________________
   2. ______________________________
   3. ______________________________

4. A patient is admitted to the hospital with severe GERD and is treated by Nissen fundoplication ______________

5. A patient presents to the Emergency Room (ER) with hematochezia and hematemesis. The patient is admitted, and it is determined that acute blood loss anemia is caused by diverticulosis ____________

6. A patient has a bleeding gastric ulcer caused by *Helicobacter pylori* ____________

7. A patient is admitted to the hospital with what the surgeon believes to be acute appendicitis. The surgeon takes the patient to the operating room (OR) and removes the appendix; the pathology report reveals a ruptured appendix ____________

8. A patient is admitted to the hospital with an incisional hernia. The patient is taken to the OR, and herniorrhaphy is performed with a graft ____________

9. A patient is admitted to the hospital with a bilateral indirect inguinal hernia that is repaired with a graft ____________

10. A patient with diverticulitis and diverticulosis is taken to the OR for an endoscopic diverticulectomy of the large intestine ____________

11. A patient with cholecystitis presents to the ER. ERCP reveals cholelithiasis. The surgeon performs a laparoscopic partial cholecystectomy ____________

12. A patient with severe Crohn's disease is taken to the OR for a Hartmann procedure on the left with an end-to-end anastomosis and a temporary colostomy ____________

13. A patient with cholelithaisis has an ESWL ____________

14. A patient with severe chronic pancreatitis is admitted to the hospital, where a surgeon performs a Whipple procedure ____________

15. A patient with ascites due to alcoholic cirrhosis is admitted to the hospital for a TIPS procedure ____________

16. A patient with a bleeding duodenal ulcer is admitted to the hospital, where the gastroenterologist provides endoscopic control of the hemorrhage ____________

17. A patient with severe malnutrition is admitted to the hospital for endoscopic placement of a gastrostomy tube ____________

18. Acute hemorrhagic gastric ulcer caused by NSAID ____________

19. Gallstone of common bile duct, status post cholecystectomy, 1 year PTA ____________

CHAPTER GLOSSARY

Adhesion: scar tissue that forms an abnormal connection between body parts.

Alimentary canal: comprises the mouth, pharynx, esophagus, stomach, small intestine, and large intestine.

Anastomosis: surgically formed connection between two tubular structures.

Angiodysplasia: type of AVM characterized by dilated or fragile blood vessels.

Anorexia: loss of appetite.

Appendectomy: removal of the appendix.

Appendicitis: inflammation of the appendix.

Arteriovenous malformation: defect that arises during fetal development.

Barrett's esophagus: precancerous condition that usually occurs in people with chronic GERD.

Bowel resection: removal of a portion of the bowel.

Choledocholithiasis: a stone lodged in the bile duct.

Cholelithiasis: an abnormal condition of stones in the gallbladder.

Cirrhosis: liver disease wherein scar tissue replaces healthy tissue and blocks blood flow.

Colostomy: a procedure that uses the colon to create an artificial opening.

Crohn's disease: inflammation of the GI tract, especially the small and large intestine.

Diverticula: small pouches in the lining of the mucous membranes of an organ.

Edentulism: is the complete loss of teeth.

Fundoplication: surgery in which the fundus of the stomach is wrapped around the esophagus.

Gastroenteritis: inflammation of the stomach and intestines.

Granulation: newly formed tissue that covers an open sore or wound.

Hematemesis: vomiting of blood.

Hematochezia: bright red blood in stool.

Hepatitis: an inflammation of the liver.

Hernia: protrusion of an organ or tissue through an abnormal opening in the body.

Herniorrhaphy: repair of a hernia.

Ileostomy: end of small intestine brought out through the abdominal wall.

Ileus: absence of normal movement within the intestine.

Impaction: condition that occurs when stool in the rectum becomes so hard that it cannot be passed normally.

Incidental appendectomy: appendectomy performed at the time of another procedure with no known disease process in the appendix.

Intussusception: bowel becomes obstructed when a portion of the intestine telescopes into another portion.

Lysis: destruction of adhesions.

Mallory-Weiss: bleeding laceration of the esophagogastric junction.

Mastication: chewing of food.

McBurney's point: area of the abdomen that, when touched, causes pain that may be indicative of appendicitis.

Melena: dark blood in stool.

Necrotic: dead tissue that lacks a blood supply.

Occult blood: blood only found by laboratory inspection.

Ostomies: surgically created openings into the body.

Percutaneous endoscopic gastrostomy: a tube through the abdominal wall into the stomach with the use of a scope.

Peristalsis: rhythmic muscle contractions that move food down the digestive tract.

Sialolithiasis: stones in the salivary glands.

Stoma: an artificial opening.

TIPS (transjugular intrahepatic portosystemic shunt): a procedure in which the portal vein is connected to one of the hepatic veins and a stent is inserted.

Whipple procedure: a procedure that generally involves removal of the gallbladder, common bile duct, part of the duodenum, and the head of the pancreas.

CHAPTER

23 Mental Disorders

(ICD-9-CM Chapter 5, Codes 290-319)

CHAPTER OUTLINE

LEARNING OBJECTIVES

- Apply and assign the correct ICD-9-CM codes in accordance with Official Guidelines for Coding and Reporting
- Identify pertinent anatomy and physiology of mental disorders
- Identify various mental disorders
- Assign the correct V codes and procedure codes related to mental disorders
- Identify common treatments and medications
- Explain the importance of documentation in relation to MS-DRGs for reimbursement

ABBREVIATIONS

ADD attention deficit disorder

ADHD attention deficit hyperactivity disorder

CC complication/comorbidity

DSM-IV-TR *Diagnostic and Statistical Manual of Mental Disorders, Fourth Edition, Text Revision*

DTs delirium tremens

ECT electroconvulsive therapy

ICD-9-CM *International Classification of Diseases, 9th Revision, Clinical Modification*

IQ intelligence quotient

LD learning disability/difficulty

MR mental retardation

MRCP mental retardation, cerebral palsy

MS-DRG Medicare severity diagnosis-related group

OBS organic brain syndrome

OIG Office of the Inspector General

PKU phenylketonuria

PTSD posttraumatic stress disorder

ICD-9-CM Official Guidelines for Coding and Reporting

Please refer to the companion Evolve website for the most current guidelines.

5. Chapter 5: Mental Disorders (290-319)

Reserved for future guideline expansion

There are no specific official ICD-9-CM coding and reporting guidelines for Chapter 5, Mental Disorders (290-319).

Apply general coding guidelines as found in Chapter 5 of this textbook.

The *Diagnostic and Statistical Manual of Mental Disorders, Fourth Edition* (DSM-IV) is used by healthcare professionals to diagnose mental disorders on the basis of specific criteria. A multiaxial assessment system is used, as illustrated in Table 23-1.

The DSM-IV-TR, or a text revision (TR), was published in 1996. It includes ICD-9-CM codes that should be assigned to all mental disorders and conditions. Many healthcare professionals use these ICD-9-CM codes within their documentation. These professionals may be taking the codes from the DSM-IV-TR, so it is always recommended to verify codes with the ICD-9-CM code book, to ensure accurate code assignment.

ANATOMY AND PHYSIOLOGY

No one body system is known to cause or be affected by mental disorders because the causes of mental illness are not always known. Stress can be a contributing factor in mental disorders. Psychological issues can and do affect one's physical health.

DISEASE CONDITIONS

Mental Disorders (290-319), which is Chapter 5 in your ICD-9-CM code book, is divided into the following categories:

CATEGORY	SECTION TITLES
290-294	Organic Psychotic Conditions
295-299	Other Psychoses
300-316	Neurotic Disorders, Personality Disorders, and Other Nonpsychotic Mental Disorders
317-319	Mental Retardation

Table 23-1. Multiaxial Assessment System Used in DSM-IV[1]

Axis I	Clinical Disorders (296.21, Major depressive disorder, single episode, and 303.90, Alcohol dependence). These disorders often respond to medication and psychotherapy.
Axis II	Personality Disorders and Mental Retardation (301.6, Dependent personality disorder). These disorders do not respond well to medications or to psychotherapy.
Axis III	General Medical Condition (571.2, Cirrhosis of liver due to alcoholism). Conditions contribute to the psychological condition.
Axis IV	Psychosocial and Environmental Factors (V61.0, Recent divorce, V62.0, Unemployment). Life stressors.
Axis V	Global Assessment of Functioning (score of 58). This score from 0 to 100 indicates the patient's level of functioning.

Organic Psychotic Conditions (290-294)

Organic psychosis occurs as the result of deterioration in the brain. It is usually progressive and irreversible, as in senile dementia and Alzheimer's disease. Organic brain damage may be produced by a variety of conditions, including arteriosclerosis, thrombi, metabolic conditions, infection, toxins, tumors, alcohol, and drugs. The onset and severity of damage depend on the cause. **Organic brain syndrome** (OBS) or disease is a general term that is used to describe the decrease in mental function caused by other physical disease(s).

Dementia

Dementia is a progressive deterioration of mental faculties that is characterized by impairment of memory and one or more cognitive impairments in areas such as language, reasoning, judgment, calculation, and problem-solving abilities. **Cognitive impairment** is a decline in mental activities associated with thinking, learning, and memory. Dementia can occur at any age but is more prevalent in the elderly. Disease processes that may be associated with dementia include the following:

- Alzheimer's disease
- Lewy body disease
- Alcoholism
- AIDS
- Parkinson's disease,
- Normal pressure hydrocephalus with dementia,
- Genetic or metabolic disease (e.g., thyroid)
- Toxic or traumatic injury
- Malignant disease and treatment

Although the term "senile" may be associated with those who are 65 years of age or older, it should not be assumed that because a patient is older than 65, a condition is due to senility. The physician must document within the health record the specific type of dementia. For many of the dementia codes, code assignment may depend on the presence of behavioral disturbances such as aggressiveness, combativeness, violence or wandering off.

EXAMPLE Patient is 70 years old and has dementia, 294.8.

EXAMPLE Patient is 60 years old and has senile dementia, 290.0.

Alcohol/Drug Psychoses

Psychosis is an impairment in mental state by which one's perception of reality becomes distorted. It may include visual or auditory hallucinations, paranoia or delusions, personality changes, and disorganized thinking. The use of alcohol or drugs could lead to alcohol- or drug-related psychosis. Psychotic episodes vary from person to person.

Alcohol withdrawal symptoms vary in severity from mild shakiness and sweating to the worst form, **delirium tremens** (DTs). Delirium tremens may involve severe mental or neurologic changes such as delirium and/or hallucinations. This is a life-threatening condition. People who have gone through withdrawal once are more likely to have withdrawal symptoms again when they stop drinking. Seizures are also a common form of withdrawal. Three codes are specific to alcohol withdrawal:

- Alcohol withdrawal delirium, 291.0
- Alcohol withdrawal hallucinosis, 291.3
- Alcohol withdrawal, 291.81

"Only one code should be assigned to describe alcohol withdrawal. Code 291.0 takes precedence over the other two codes, and 291.3 takes precedence over the 291.81 code," according to *Coding Clinic* (1991:2Q:p11-12)[2] (Figure 23-1). If a patient is experiencing

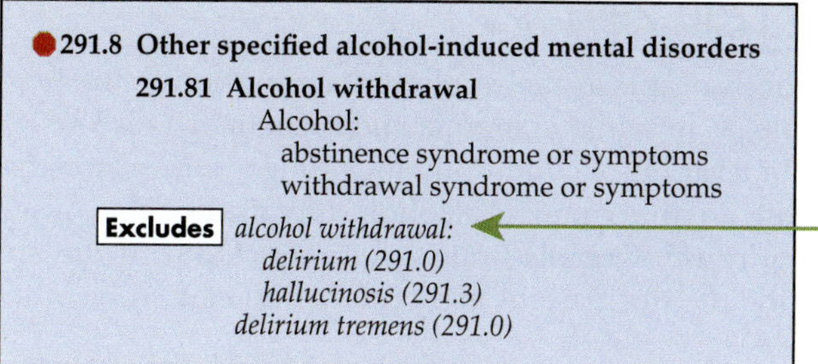

291.8 Other specified alcohol-induced mental disorders
291.81 Alcohol withdrawal
Alcohol:
abstinence syndrome or symptoms
withdrawal syndrome or symptoms
Excludes *alcohol withdrawal:*
delirium (291.0)
hallucinosis (291.3)
delirium tremens (291.0)

Figure 23-1. Excludes note for alcohol withdrawal.

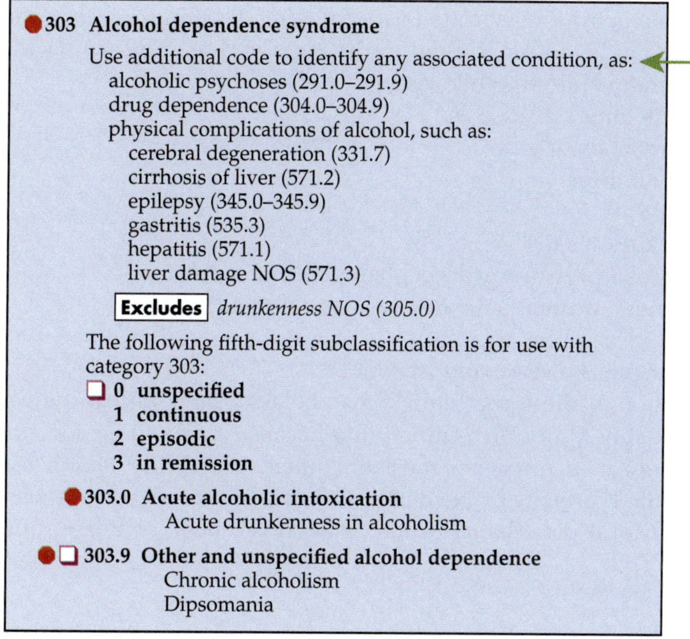

303 Alcohol dependence syndrome
Use additional code to identify any associated condition, as:
alcoholic psychoses (291.0–291.9)
drug dependence (304.0–304.9)
physical complications of alcohol, such as:
cerebral degeneration (331.7)
cirrhosis of liver (571.2)
epilepsy (345.0–345.9)
gastritis (535.3)
hepatitis (571.1)
liver damage NOS (571.3)
Excludes *drunkenness NOS (305.0)*
The following fifth-digit subclassification is for use with category 303:
0 unspecified
1 continuous
2 episodic
3 in remission
303.0 Acute alcoholic intoxication
Acute drunkenness in alcoholism
303.9 Other and unspecified alcohol dependence
Chronic alcoholism
Dipsomania

Figure 23-2. Use additional code for category 303.

symptoms of withdrawal, the alcohol dependence category 303 instructs the use of an additional code for alcoholic psychoses (withdrawal), drug dependence, and/or any physical complications related to alcohol (Figure 23-2). When a patient is admitted for withdrawal symptoms, the withdrawal code is assigned as the principal diagnosis.

EXAMPLE

Seizure due to alcohol withdrawal. Patient is an alcoholic who usually drinks every day but hasn't had a drink in 2 days, 291.81, 780.39, 303.91.

EXAMPLE

Wernicke-Korsakoff syndrome. Patient is an alcoholic who has not had a drink in 2 years, 291.1, 303.93.

Admissions to the hospital for drug psychosis are on the rise. A number of drugs can induce psychosis; cocaine and methamphetamine are the most common.

EXAMPLE

Paranoia due to methamphetamine (meth). Patient is dependent on meth, continuous use, 292.11, 304.41.

EXERCISE 23-1

Assign codes to the following conditions using your ICD-9-CM code book.

1. Delirium tremens due to chronic alcoholism, continuous ____________
2. Pre-senile dementia with depression ____________
3. Morphine-induced delirium (adverse effect) ____________
4. Organic brain syndrome ____________
5. Dementia due to neurosyphilis with behavioral disturbances ____________
6. Dementia due to malnutrition ____________
7. Normal pressure hydrocephalus with dementia ____________
8. Creutzfeldt-Jacob disease with dementia with behavioral disturbance ____________
9. AIDS-related dementia ____________
10. Binswanger's disease ____________

Other Psychoses (295-299)

Schizophrenia

Schizophrenia is a disorder of the brain. A person with schizophrenia may have trouble differentiating between real and unreal experiences and may not demonstrate logical thinking, normal emotional responses to others, and appropriate behavior in social situations. A genetic component is associated with the disease, in that people who have family members with the disease are more likely to exhibit the disease themselves. Schizophrenia usually has its onset during young adulthood, and it affects men and women equally. Five types of schizophrenia have been identified:

- Catatonic—withdrawn, in own world
- Paranoid—suspicious of others
- Disorganized—disorganized thought process, unable to communicate coherently
- Undifferentiated—mixed types of schizophrenia
- Residual—has milder symptoms that come and go

EXAMPLE

The patient has been in a chronic catatonic state of schizophrenia, 295.22.

Mood Disorders

Mood disorders occur when a change in mood has been present for a prolonged time. The two most common mood disorders (affective disorders) are **major depression** and **bipolar disorder** (manic-depressive illness). Mood disorders can be triggered by a life event or by a chemical imbalance. The type of depression that is included in category 296 is different than depression, not otherwise specified (311). Bipolar disorder is characterized by mood swings. Onset of symptoms is most likely to occur in early adulthood. A person with bipolar can have four main types of mood "episodes":

1. Depression—a feeling of sadness that can go on for a long period of time; lack of enjoyment of the things one would normally do
2. Mania—the other side of depression, in which a person feels so good, it is like a "high"; may do risky things
3. Hypomania—milder form of mania, but this "feel good" mood can change to depression or mania
4. Mixed mood—alteration from mania and depression, back and forth, very quickly

Major depressive disorder is characterized by one or more major depressive episodes with a history of mania, hypomania, or mixed episodes. In major depression, more numer-

ous symptoms of depression may be present, and usually, the symptoms are more severe. Major depression is most likely to occur in persons between the ages of 25 and 44; an episode may last from 6 to 9 months.

EXAMPLE The patient was diagnosed with major depressive disorder of moderate severity, single episode, 296.22.

EXAMPLE The patient is in a severe manic phase of bipolar I disorder, 296.43.

EXERCISE 23-2

Assign codes to the following conditions using your ICD-9-CM code book.

1. Bipolar disorder, currently depressed ____________
2. Autism ____________
3. Major depressive disorder, recurrent ____________
4. Paranoid schizophrenia ____________
5. Delusional disorder ____________

Neurotic Disorders, Personality Disorders, and Other Nonpsychotic Mental Disorders (300-316)

Anxiety Disorders

Following is a breakdown of the different types of anxiety disorders:

- Generalized anxiety disorder
- Panic disorder
- Phobias
- Posttraumatic stress disorder

Most people experience mild anxiety and nervousness at various times during their lives, such as during a job interview, a business presentation, or social events.

Generalized anxiety disorder refers to chronic, exaggerated worry, tension, and irritability that may occur without cause or may be more intense than is warranted by the situation. Physical symptoms include restlessness, sleeping problems, headache, trembling, twitching, muscle tension, and sweating.

Panic disorder is a terrifying experience that occurs suddenly without warning. Physical symptoms include pounding heart, chest pains, dizziness, nausea, shortness of breath, trembling, choking, fear of dying, sweating, feelings of unreality, numbness, hot flashes or chills, and a feeling of going out of control or "crazy." Because panic attacks are unpredictable, many people live in fear of when the next one will occur.

Phobias are irrational anxieties or fears that can interfere with one's everyday life or daily routine. For example, if fear of heights would keep a person from visiting relatives who live on the 13th floor of an apartment building, the fear is excessive and disproportionate to the situation. A person without a phobia but with a fear of heights would still be able to go to visit the relatives. If situations are avoided because of fear, or if fear prevents one from enjoying life or preoccupies one's thinking, hindering ability to work, sleep, or do other things, then it becomes irrational.

Posttraumatic stress disorder (PTSD) is an anxiety disorder that is triggered by memories of a traumatic event. This disorder commonly affects survivors of traumatic events, such as sexual or physical assault, war, torture, a natural disaster, an automobile accident, or an airplane crash. In addition, PTSD can affect rescue workers at the site of an airplane crash or a mass shooting or someone who witnessed a tragic accident.

EXAMPLE The patient suffers from agoraphobia, 300.22.

EXAMPLE The patient has generalized anxiety, 300.02.

Coding diagnoses of depression and anxiety may be confusing. As illustrated in Figure 23-3, under the main term "Anxiety" is a subterm for "Depression (300.4)"; under the main term "Depression" is a subterm for "Anxiety (300.4)," as shown in Figure 23-4. Verification of code selection in the Tabular (Figure 23-5) reveals the terminology "Depression with anxiety." The Tabular makes the code assignment of 300.4 for a patient with depression and anxiety understandable.

Anxiety (neurosis) (reaction) (state) 300.00
- alcohol-induced 291.89
- depression 300.4
- drug-induced 292.89
- due to or associated with physical condition 293.84
- generalized 300.02
- hysteria 300.20
- in
  - acute stress reaction 308.0
  - transient adjustment reaction 309.24
- panic type 300.01
- separation, abnormal 309.21
- syndrome (organic) (transient) 293.84

Figure 23-3. Index entry for the main term "Anxiety."

Depression 311
- acute (*see also* Psychosis, affective) 296.2
  - recurrent episode 296.3
  - single episode 296.2
- agitated (*see also* Psychosis, affective) 296.2
  - recurrent episode 296.3
  - single episode 296.2
- anaclitic 309.21
- anxiety 300.4
- arches 734
  - congenital 754.61

Figure 23-4. Index entry for the main term "Depression."

300.4 Dysthymic disorder
- Anxiety depression
- Depression with anxiety
- Depressive reaction
- Neurotic depressive state
- Reactive depression

Excludes *adjustment reaction with depressive symptoms (309.0–309.1)*
depression NOS (311)
manic-depressive psychosis, depressed type (296.2–296.3)
reactive depressive psychosis (298.0)

Figure 23-5. Tabular entry for "Depression with anxiety."

Personality Disorders

A **personality disorder** is a pattern of behavior that can disrupt many aspects of a person's life. Personality disorders range from mild to severe and are often exacerbated during times of stress or external pressure. If a personality disorder is associated with neuroses, psychosis, or a physical condition, this should be coded. Personality disorders are divided into three clusters:

1. Cluster A—patients appear odd or eccentric, socially awkward
   - Paranoid—are suspicious of and do not trust others
   - Schizoid—loners who lack or do not show emotion
   - Schizotypal—seek isolation
2. Cluster B—patients appear dramatic, emotional, or erratic
   - Antisocial—disregard and tend to violate the rights of others, fail to conform to societal norms
   - Borderline—have difficulty coping with minor stress, have unstable relationships, and are self-destructive
   - Histrionic—are overly dramatic with a need to be the center of attention
   - Narcissistic—have an inflated sense of self-importance
3. Cluster C—patients appear anxious and fearful
   - Avoidant—avoid social situations because of fear of criticism, disapproval, or rejection; view themselves as inferior
   - Dependent—rely on others to make decisions for them; fear losing the support and approval of others
   - Obsessive-compulsive—are excessively preoccupied with orderliness, perfection, and mental and interpersonal control

EXAMPLE Patient has an obsessive-compulsive personality disorder, 301.4.

EXAMPLE Patient has a passive-aggressive personality, 301.84.

Sexual Disorder

Sexual activities that are not practiced by the majority of the population have been characterized as "deviant" or "variant" behavior. Although some may experiment with a variety of sexual behaviors, it is not until a person begins to rely on the deviant behavior as a means of sexual gratification that it becomes a more permanent trait. "Unconventional" sexual behaviors or paraphilias are coded to category 302 and include some of the following:

Transvestism—assuming the appearance, manner, or roles traditionally associated with members of the opposite sex (cross-dressing)

Exhibitionism—recurrent intense sexual urges and fantasies of exposing the genitals to an unsuspecting stranger

Fetishism—recurrent intense sexual urges and fantasies of using inanimate objects for sexual arousal or orgasm. Objects commonly used include female clothing such as shoes, earrings, or undergarments

Voyeurism—recurrent intense sexual urges and fantasies involving observing unsuspecting people who are naked, disrobing, or engaging in sexual activity

Sadism—the act or sense of gaining pleasure from inflicting physical or psychological pain on another

Masochism—the act or sense of gaining pleasure from experiencing physical or psychological pain

EXAMPLE Patient is an exhibitionist, 302.4.

Sexual Problems

Sexual problems may be due to organic or medical conditions or to psychological dysfunction. Alcohol and drug use can also affect sexual function. After medical problems have been ruled out, a psychological cause can be explored.

EXAMPLE Patient is treated for impotence due to psychogenic cause, 302.72.

EXAMPLE Patient treated for erectile dysfunction, 607.84.

If a patient has erectile dysfunction it has to be specified as due to psychogenic causes to be coded to 302.72.

EXAMPLE Patient is being seen for psychogenic dyspareunia, 302.76.

EXAMPLE Patient is being seen for dyspareunia, 625.0.

Alcohol/Drug Dependence and Abuse

Alcohol dependence, or alcoholism, is a chronic disease that is characterized by a strong compulsion to drink, increasing tolerance, the inability to stop drinking once the person has started, and physical dependence and withdrawal symptoms.

If alcohol dependence is associated with alcoholic psychosis, drug dependence or abuse, or physical complications, all diagnoses should be coded. Under category 303 are instructions on how to code those associated conditions (see Figure 23-2).

Drug dependence or addiction is similar to dependence on alcohol. It includes a compulsion to take the drug, increased tolerance, an inability to stop using, and physical withdrawal if the person does not have the drug.

It may be difficult for a healthcare provider to determine whether a patient is actually dependent on alcohol or drugs, so abuse codes tend to be used more often. It is possible that a patient is dependent on one drug and is abusing another drug or alcohol. Abuse and dependence codes of different substances can be used for the same patient.

According to *Coding Clinics* (1991:2Q:p10; 1986:M-A:p12)[3-4] the coder is instructed to use combination codes when dependent on more than one drug; these include the following:

- Combination of opioid-type drug dependence with any other drug dependence
- Combinations of drug dependence that exclude an opioid-type drug dependence

A healthcare provider may document polysubstance abuse without mentioning which substances are being abused. As this is not documented as dependence, it is coded to 305.9X. Sometimes a patient is dependent on one drug and abuses another.

Dependence is not limited to illegal substances and can occur with prescription drugs. Because drugs have generic and brand names, and since these are used interchangeably, it may be difficult to determine which category is assigned for a particular drug dependence. A drug reference book or an Internet search can be used to determine the generic name or category of the drug.

EXAMPLE Alcoholic gastritis, 535.30, 303.90. Upon verification of the 535.30 code in the Tabular, no instructions about coding for alcoholism are provided; because this code is specific to alcoholic gastritis, it would appear that both conditions are covered by the single code. However, it is necessary to code 303.90 for alcohol dependence.

Fifth digit subclassifications used in drug and alcohol abuse and dependence categories 303, 304, and 305.0, 305.2-305.9, according to *Coding Clinic* (1991:2Q:p11),[5] define the patient's pattern of use. The pattern of use may be documented within the health record. This may be documented by social worker, ER, or admitting nurse as well as the attending physician.

–0: Unspecified

–1: Continuous

Alcohol—refers to daily intake of large amounts of alcohol or regular heavy drinking on weekends or days off from work

Drugs—refers to daily or almost daily use of drug(s)

–2: Episodic

Alcohol—refers to alcoholic binges that last weeks or months, followed by long periods of sobriety

Drugs—indicates short periods between drug use or use on the weekends

–3: Remission

Refers to complete cessation of alcohol or drug intake or the period during which a decrease toward cessation is taking place

When a patient is admitted for a medical condition, they may have a comorbidity of alcohol dependence. Along with treating the medical condition, the patient's alcohol dependence may need to be stabilized with drugs to prevent withdrawal. Because they are treating to prevent withdrawal does not mean that the patient is experiencing withdrawal and therefore withdrawal is not coded.

Drug or alcohol abuse indicates a problem with the substance that occurs without craving and physical dependence. However, it is likely that substance abuse can still cause problems with work, school, and home responsibilities and can interfere with relationships.

Particularly in the emergency room setting, physicians may document that the patient is a "drug seeker" or has "drug-seeking behavior." According to *Coding Clinic* (1999:3Q: p20),[6] "the appropriate codes are 305.90, unspecified drug abuse, and V65.2, person feigning illness".

EXAMPLE Patient is being treated for withdrawal due to dependence on Valium, 292.0, 304.10.

Attention Deficit Disorder

Attention deficit disorder (ADD) and attention deficit hyperactivity disorder (ADHD) are common childhood disorders. ADHD and ADD are not learning disabilities, but they are characterized by inattention, hyperactivity, and impulsivity. Three subtypes of ADHD have been identified:

1. Hyperactive/impulsive type—patient does not show significant inattention
2. Inattentive type—patient does not show significant hyperactive-impulsive behavior; sometimes called ADD
3. Combined type—patient displays both inattentive and hyperactive-impulsive symptoms

Other disorders that sometimes accompany ADHD include Tourette's syndrome, oppositional defiant disorder, conduct disorder, anxiety and depression, and bipolar disorder. Attention deficit hyperactivity disorder continues into adulthood in about 50% of persons with childhood ADHD.

Oppositional Defiant Disorder

Oppositional defiant disorder is defined as a pattern of uncooperative, defiant, and hostile behavior toward authority figures that does not involve major antisocial violations, is not normal for the patient's developmental stage, and results in significant functional impairment. A certain level of oppositional behavior is common in children and adolescents. It should be considered a disorder only when behaviors are more frequent and intense than in unaffected peers, and when they cause dysfunction in social, academic, or work-related arenas.

Learning Disorders

Learning disabilities or differences (LDs) affect a person's ability to understand or use spoken or written language (**dyslexia**), to do mathematical calculations (**dyscalculia**), to coordinate movements such as writing (**dysgraphia**), or to direct attention. Although LDs may occur in very young children, these disorders usually are not recognized until the child reaches school age.

EXERCISE 23-3

Assign codes to the following conditions using your ICD-9-CM code book.

1. Obsessive-compulsive disorder __________
2. Borderline personality __________
3. Attention deficit disorder with overactivity __________
4. Postconcussion syndrome __________
5. Addiction to heroin and OxyContin __________
6. Cirrhosis due to chronic alcoholism __________
7. Dyslexia, developmental __________
8. Pedophile __________
9. Posttraumatic stress syndrome __________
10. Panic attack __________

Mental Retardation (317-319)

Mental retardation (MR) is a disorder in which a person's overall intellectual functioning is well below average, and intelligence quotient (IQ) is around 70 or less. Individuals with MR also may have a significantly impaired ability to cope with common life demands and lack some of the daily living skills that are expected of people in their age group and culture. Impairment may interfere with learning, communication, self-care, independent living, social interaction, play, work, and safety. MR appears in childhood, before age 18. There are a variety of causes for mental retardation; however, often the cause is not documented. Causes of mental retardation are discussed in the following paragraphs.

Genetic Causes

- Defective genes, as in Fragile X syndrome, which is the most common inherited cause of mental retardation
- Chromosomal disorders such as Down's syndrome that are characterized by an abnormal number of chromosomes
- Congenital hypothyroidism, which can result in MR and stunted growth if the patient is not treated with thyroid replacement
- Inborn errors of metabolism may result in MR. More than 300 gene disorders involve inborn errors of metabolism. These include the following:
  - Phenylketonuria (PKU)
  - Tay-Sachs disease
  - Galactosemia
  - Homocystinuria
  - Maple syrup urine disease
  - Biotinidase deficiency

External Causes

During pregnancy, the following factors can result in MR:

- Malnutrition
- Mother's use of alcohol and drugs
- Environmental toxins such as lead and mercury

- Viral infections such as rubella and cytomegalovirus
- Untreated diabetes mellitus

During birth, the following conditions can result in MR:

- Low birth weight
- Premature birth
- Deprivation of oxygen

After birth, the following conditions can result in MR:

- Complications from infectious diseases such as measles, chickenpox, and whooping cough
- Exposure to lead and mercury
- Accidental injury to the brain
- Severe child abuse
- Poverty

At the beginning of this section, instructions state an additional code(s) should be assigned to identify any associated psychiatric or physical condition(s). A number of congenital syndromes may have some form of associated MR. The most common severity level is mild mental retardation; 85% of those affected have the mild type.

ICD-9-CM codes for MR are classified by IQ, as follows:

IQ 50-70	Mild mental retardation
IQ 35-49	Moderate mental retardation
IQ 20-34	Severe mental retardation
IQ less than 20	Profound mental retardation

Documentation of MR in the health record may not include the IQ, but the condition often is described by severity.

EXAMPLE Fragile X syndrome with mild mental retardation, 759.83, 317.

EXAMPLE MRCP with IQ of 37, 343.9, 318.0.

EXERCISE 23-4

Assign codes to the following conditions using your ICD-9-CM code book.

1. Shaken baby syndrome with profound retardation. Injury happened 2 years ago ____________
2. Trisomy 21 with moderate mental retardation ____________
3. Severe mental retardation due to Angelman's syndrome ____________
4. Mild mental retardation due to Lesch-Nyhan syndrome ____________
5. Cerebral palsy with mental retardation ____________

V CODES

In the past, V codes have been considered primarily for use in the outpatient setting. This has changed with the addition of more V codes each year. As discussed in Chapter 8, it may be difficult for the coder to locate V codes in the index. Coders often say, "I did not know there was a V code for that." Refer to Chapter 8 for a listing of common main terms used to locate V codes.

There is a V code for personal history of alcoholism (V11.3), but this code is not usually assigned. Code 303.93 for alcohol dependence in remission is a more appropriate code because no cure is known for alcoholism and it is still present, although the patient may no longer drink alcohol. The schizophrenic disorder codes (295.XX) also include a fifth digit of 5, which denotes that the disease is in remission; therefore, 295.95 may be a better code selection than V11.0 for patients with a history of schizophrenia.

V11.0	Personal history of schizophrenia
V11.1	Personal history of affective disorders
V11.2	Personal history of neurosis
V11.3	Personal history of alcoholism
V11.8	Personal history of other mental disorders
V11.9	Personal history of unspecified mental disorder
V15.41	History of physical abuse
V15.42	History of emotional abuse
V15.49	Psychological trauma—other
V15.82	Personal history of tobacco use
V18.4	Family history of mental retardation
V40.0	Problems with learning
V40.1	Problems with communication (including speech)
V40.2	Other mental problems
V40.9	Unspecified mental or behavioral problem
V41.7	Problems with sexual function
V58.69	Long-term (current) use of other medications
V58.83	Encounter for therapeutic drug monitoring
V60.0	Lack of housing
V60.1	Inadequate housing
V60.2	Inadequate material resources
V61.0	Family disruption
V61.10	Counseling for marital and partner problems, unspecified
V61.11	Counseling for victim of spousal and partner abuse
V61.12	Counseling for perpetrator of spousal and partner abuse
V61.20	Counseling for parent–child problem, unspecified
V61.21	Counseling for victim of child abuse
V61.22	Counseling for perpetrator of parental child abuse
V61.29	Other parent—child problems
V61.41	Problems with alcoholism in family
V62.0	Unemployment
V62.1	Adverse effects of work environment
V62.2	Other occupational circumstances or maladjustment
V62.3	Educational circumstances
V62.4	Social maladjustment
V62.5	Legal circumstances
V62.81	Interpersonal problems, not elsewhere classified
V62.82	Bereavement, uncomplicated
V62.83	Counseling for perpetrator of physical/sexual abuse
V62.84	Suicidal ideation
V62.89	Other psychosocial circumstances
V62.9	Unspecified psychosocial circumstances
V65.2	Person feigning illness
V65.42	Counseling on substance use and abuse
V65.5	Person with feared complaint in whom no diagnosis was made
V66.3	Convalescence and palliative care following psychotherapy and other treatment for mental disorder
V67.3	Follow-up examination following psychotherapy and other treatment for mental disorder
V67.51	Follow-up examination following completed treatment with high-risk medication, not elsewhere classified
V68.1	Issue of repeat prescriptions

V69.2	Problems related to high-risk sexual behavior
V69.3	Problems related to gambling and betting
V69.8	Other problems related to lifestyle
V69.9	Problem related to lifestyle, unspecified
V70.1	General psychiatric examination, requested by the authority
V70.2	General psychiatric examination, other and unspecified
V70.4	Examination for medicolegal reasons
V71.01	Observation for suspected adult antisocial behavior
V71.02	Observation for childhood or adolescent antisocial behavior
V71.99	Observation for other suspected mental condition
V71.5	Observation following alleged rape or seduction
V71.81	Observation and evaluation for abuse and neglect
V79.0	Special screening for depression
V79.1	Special screening for alcoholism
V79.2	Special screening for mental retardation
V79.3	Special screening for developmental handicaps in early childhood
V79.8	Special screening for other specified mental disorders and developmental handicaps
V79.9	Special screening for unspecified mental disorder and developmental handicap

EXAMPLE Moderate depression, single episode, due to unemployment, 296.22, V62.0.

EXAMPLE Counseling regarding marital problems, V61.10.

EXERCISE 23-5

Assign codes to the following conditions using your ICD-9-CM code book.

1. Screening for depression __________
2. Malingerer __________
3. Examination for blood alcohol test __________
4. Counseling for mother and son due to son's ADD __________
5. Laboratory testing (liver function tests) on patient who takes Cognex for Alzheimer's disease with dementia __________

COMMON TREATMENTS

Many of the mental disorders can be treated with psychotherapy. Often, a combination of psychotherapy and medication is necessary for effective treatment.

CONDITION	MEDICATIONS
Dementia	Depends on type of dementia
Alcohol withdrawal	Benzodiazepam, such as diazepam (Valium) or chlordiazepoxide (Librium or Libritabs), may be used to reduce anxiety
	Multivitamin; thiamine and folate
	Beta blockers such as propranolol (Inderal) or atenolol (Tenormin) reduce heart rate and tremors
	Phenytoin (Dilantin), carbamazepine (Tegretol), and divalproex sodium (Depakote) are antiseizure medications that can be used to treat or prevent seizures
Drug withdrawal	Treatment would depend on the drug
Schizophrenia	Often requires a combination of antipsychotic, antidepressant, and antianxiety medications

CONDITION	MEDICATIONS
Depression	Antidepressants such as fluoxetine (Prozac), paroxetine (Paxil), sertraline hydrochloride (Zoloft), citalopram hydrobromide (Celexa), nefazodone (Serzone), mirtazapine (Remeron), venlafaxine (Effexor), and bupropion hydrochloride (Wellbutrin)
Bipolar disorder	Medications include lithium; anticonvulsants such as carbamazepine (Tegretol), divalproex sodium (Depakote), gabapentin (Neurontin), and lamotrigine (Lamictal); antidepressants such as bupropion hydrochloride (Wellbutrin) or sertraline hydrochloride (Zoloft); neuroleptics (e.g., Haldol); and benzodiazepines (e.g., lorazepam)
Anxiety	Diazepam (Valium), lorazepam (Ativan), clorazepate (Tranxene), alprazolam (Xanax)
Panic disorder	Alprazolam (Xanax), paroxetine (Paxil)
Phobias	Amitriptyline (Elavil), desipramine (Norpramin), imipramine (Tofranil), nortriptyline (Pamelor), phenelzine (Nardil)
PTSD	Medications to reduce anxiety, depression, and insomnia associated with PTSD
ADD/ADHD	Methylphenidate (Ritalin, Concerta), amphetamine dextroamphetamine (Adderall), pemoline (Cylert), atomoxetine (Strattera)

PROCEDURES

Procedures that are possibly related to mental disorders may be located in the following chapters of the Procedure Tabular:

Chapter 16, Miscellaneous Diagnostic and Therapeutic Procedures (87-99)

This chapter covers a wide variety of diagnostic and therapeutic procedures. Some procedures would be appropriate for mental disorders such as detoxification and/or rehabilitation for alcohol and drug abuse. Sometimes, a patient's medical condition is stabilized in a hospital setting, and then the patient is transferred to a facility that is better equipped to offer specialized mental health care. Facility policy may determine which procedures are coded or provided by the facility.

Electroconvulsive Therapy

Electroconvulsive therapy (ECT) is a treatment in which electricity is used to induce seizures. ECT is usually only considered when patients have not responded well to drug therapies. It is primarily used to treat severe depression and other disorders such as schizophrenia, mania or catatonia. A course of treatments usually consists of 6-12 treatments, but may be more or may be less.

Detoxification and Rehabilitation

Detoxification is the active management of withdrawal symptoms in a patient who is physically dependent on alcohol or drugs. It consists of evaluation, observation, and monitoring, along with administration of thiamine, multivitamins, and other medications as needed. Detoxification for alcohol may require a 4- to 5-day period; depending on the drug, it may go on for days or months.

Rehabilitation is a structured program with the goal to stop and recover from the use of alcohol and/or drugs. Many different types of programs are available in a variety of settings; these include inpatient, outpatient, day treatment, residential treatment, half-way houses, and so forth.

Facility policy will determine the coding of these procedures. In the hospital setting, a patient may be treated to prevent alcohol and drug withdrawal, or to alleviate symptoms of withdrawal, but this may not constitute true detoxification.

EXERCISE 23-6

Assign codes for all diagnoses and procedures using your ICD-9-CM code book.

1. Electroconvulsive therapy for schizophrenia ____________
2. Detoxification and rehabilitation for chronic alcoholism, continuous ____________
3. Detoxification for heroin dependence, daily use ____________

DOCUMENTATION/REIMBURSEMENT/MS-DRGs

Often, coding difficulties are due to lack of documentation. Sometimes test results are not available at the time of discharge or when the physician is dictating the discharge summary or is reporting the final diagnoses.

In the inpatient setting, mental health disorders are often secondary to a more acute medical condition. Many physicians are vague in their descriptions of mental disorders. They may not say that a patient is dependent on drugs or alcohol and may document the condition as drug and/or alcohol abuse. In the health record, information may also be limited for determination of whether usage is continuous, episodic, or in remission. Often, the unspecified fifth digit will need to be assigned. A number of patients are being treated for depression and are on medications. The 311 depression code is often used because of insufficient documentation regarding whether this is an adjustment disorder, a single episode, recurrent, and/or a mood disorder. If they are available, the coder should review consultation reports from the psychologist or the psychiatrist for more specific diagnoses. The coder may need to query the physician to get needed documentation and assign the most appropriate diagnosis code. The presence of a MCC (major complication/comorbidity) or CC (complication/comorbidity) can make a difference in reimbursement, depending on the principal diagnosis and the MS-DRG assigned.

Detoxification and Rehabilitation

EXAMPLE

The patient is admitted for detoxification and rehabilitation of heroin and alcohol dependence. The patient uses $30 of heroin per day and drinks 1 quart of wine each day. No IV drug use.

DIAGNOSES	CODES	MS-DRG	RW
Heroin and alcohol dependence	304.01 303.91	895	0.7557
Detox/Rehab	94.69		
Heroin and alcohol dependence	304.01 303.91	897	0.6145
Detox only	94.68		

It is important to code the appropriate procedure code to include both the detoxification and rehabilitation if performed, as it may affect MS-DRG assignment.

CHAPTER REVIEW EXERCISE

Assign codes for all diagnoses and procedures, including all applicable V and E codes and procedures.

1. Dysthymic disorder ____________
2. Panic disorder with agoraphobia ____________

3. Fragile X syndrome with IQ of 25; family history of mental retardation ____________
4. Inhalant abuse ____________
5. Tourette's syndrome ____________
6. Malnutrition due to anorexia nervosa ____________
7. History of alcoholism with 1 year of sobriety ____________
8. Mental retardation due to chickenpox 2 years ago ____________
9. Alcoholic cardiomyopathy ____________
10. Holiday heart syndrome with atrial fibrillation; patient had a drinking binge over Labor Day weekend. History of alcohol abuse. ____________
11. Depression with anxiety ____________
12. Social phobia ____________
13. Dementia due to multiple sclerosis ____________
14. Adjustment disorder with conduct disturbance due to parents' divorce ____________
15. Hypochondria ____________
16. Gambling addiction ____________
17. Psychogenic asthma ____________
18. Pica ____________
19. Enuresis, psychogenic ____________
20. Fear of flying ____________
21. History of emotional abuse ____________
22. Parkinson's disease with dementia and related behavioral disturbances ____________
23. Suicidal ideation ____________
24. Unable to tolerate CT scan due to claustrophobia ____________

Write the correct answer(s) in the space(s) provided.

25. Which procedure code groups into the higher paying MS-DRG?

    ____

26. List 4 types of Cluster B personality disorders.

    ____
    ____
    ____
    ____

27. When are learning disabilities usually recognized?

    ____

28. List 4 causes of mental retardation.

    ____
    ____
    ____
    ____

CHAPTER GLOSSARY

Affective disorders: category of mental health problems that include major depressive disorders and bipolar disorders.

Bipolar disorder: brain disorder that causes unusual shifts in a person's mood, energy, and ability to function; different from the normal ups and downs that everyone goes through; symptoms of bipolar disorder can be severe.

Cognitive impairment: a decline in mental activities associated with thinking, learning, and memory.

Delirium tremens: life-threatening condition that may involve severe mental or neurologic changes such as delirium and/or hallucinations.

Dementia: progressive deterioration of mental faculties characterized by impairment of memory and one or more cognitive impairments such as language, reasoning and judgment, and calculation and problem-solving abilities.

Depression: affective disorder that is characterized by sadness, lack of interest in everyday activities and events, and a sense of worthlessness.

Detoxification: active management of withdrawal symptoms in a patient who is physically dependent on alcohol or drugs.

Dyscalculia: learning disability that affects a child's ability to do mathematical calculations.

Dysgraphia: learning disability that affects a child's ability to coordinate movements such as writing.

Dyslexia: learning disability that affects a child's ability to understand or use spoken or written language.

Electroconvulsive therapy: psychiatric treatment in which electricity is used to induce seizures.

Exhibitionism: recurrent intense sexual urges and fantasies of exposing the genitals to an unsuspecting stranger.

Fetishism: recurrent intense sexual urges and fantasies of using inanimate objects for sexual arousal or orgasm. Objects commonly used include female clothing such as shoes, earrings, or undergarments.

Generalized anxiety disorder: chronic, exaggerated worry, tension, and irritability that may be without cause or may be more intense than the situation warrants.

Masochism: the act or sense of gaining pleasure from experiencing physical or psychological pain.

Mental retardation: disorder in which a person's overall intellectual functioning is well below average, with an intelligence quotient (IQ) around 70 or less.

Mood disorder: condition that occurs with a change in mood over a prolonged period.

Oppositional defiant disorder: pattern of uncooperative, defiant, and hostile behavior toward authority figures that does not involve major antisocial violations, is not accounted for by the child's developmental stage, and results in significant functional impairment.

Organic brain syndrome: general term used to describe a decrease in mental function due to other physical disease(s).

Panic disorder: terrifying experience that occurs suddenly without warning. Physical symptoms include pounding heart, chest pains, dizziness, nausea, shortness of breath, trembling, choking, fear of dying, sweating, feelings of unreality, numbness, hot flashes or chills, and a feeling of going out of control or "crazy."

Personality disorder: a pattern of behavior that can disrupt many aspects of a person's life.

Phobia: irrational anxiety or fear that can interfere with one's everyday life or daily routine.

Posttraumatic stress disorder: anxiety disorder that is triggered by memories of a traumatic event.

Psychosis: impairment of mental state in which perception of reality has become distorted.

Rehabilitation: structured program with the goal of stopping and recovering from the use of alcohol and/or drugs.

Sadism: the act or sense of gaining pleasure from inflicting physical or psychological pain on another.

Schizophrenia: disorder of the brain characterized by trouble differentiating between real and unreal experiences, along with problems with logical thinking, normal emotional responses to others, and appropriate behavior in social situations.

Transvestism: assuming the appearance, manner, or roles traditionally associated with members of the opposite sex (cross-dressing).

Voyeurism: recurrent intense sexual urges and fantasies involving observing unsuspecting people who are naked, disrobing, or engaging in sexual activity.

CHAPTER 24

Diseases of the Nervous System and Sense Organs

(ICD-9-CM Chapter 6, Codes 320-389)

CHAPTER OUTLINE

LEARNING OBJECTIVES

- Apply and assign the correct ICD-9-CM codes in accordance with Official Guidelines for Coding and Reporting
- Identify pertinent anatomy and physiology of the nervous system and sense organs
- Identify diseases of the nervous system and sense organs
- Assign the correct V codes and procedure codes related to the nervous system and sense organs

- Identify common treatments, medications, laboratory values, and diagnostic tests
- Explain the importance of documentation in relation to MS-DRGs for reimbursement

ABBREVIATIONS

CNS central nervous system
CPAP continuous positive airway pressure
CSF cerebrospinal fluid
CVA cerebrovascular accident
DBS deep brain stimulation
EEG electroencephalogram
EMG electromyelogram
IOL intraocular lens
IOP intraocular pressure
IV intravenous
LP lumbar puncture
MRI magnetic resonance imaging
MS-DRG Medicare severity diagnosis-related group
NPH normal pressure hydrocephalus
OM otitis media
OSA obstructive sleep apnea
PDT photodynamic therapy
SIRS systemic inflammatory response syndrome
SOM serous otitis media
SZ seizure
VPS ventriculoperitoneal shunt

ICD-9-CM Official Guidelines for Coding and Reporting

Please refer to the companion Evolve website for the most current guidelines.

6. Chapter 6: Diseases of Nervous System and Sense Organs (320-389)

a. Pain—Category 338

1) General coding information

Codes in category 338 may be used in conjunction with codes from other categories and chapters to provide more detail about acute or chronic pain and neoplasm-related pain, **unless otherwise indicated below.**

If the pain is not specified as acute or chronic, do not assign codes from category 338, except for post-thoracotomy pain, postoperative pain, neoplasm related pain, **or central pain syndrome.**

A code from subcategories 338.1 and 338.2 should not be assigned if the underlying (definitive) diagnosis is known, unless the reason for the encounter is pain control/management and not management of the underlying condition.

EXAMPLE The patient is admitted with acute chest pain due to pneumonia, 486. Only the code for pneumonia would be assigned.

EXAMPLE The patient is admitted for acute pain control after falling off a horse and suffering two broken ribs. The patient was admitted for pain control, 338.11, 807.02, E828.2.

(a) Category 338 Codes as Principal or First-Listed Diagnosis

Category 338 codes are acceptable as principal diagnosis or the first-listed code:

- When pain control or pain management is the reason for the admission/encounter (e.g., a patient with displaced intervertebral disc, nerve impingement and severe back pain presents for injection of steroid into the spinal canal). The underlying cause of the pain should be reported as an additional diagnosis, if known.
- **When an admission or encounter is for a procedure aimed at treating the underlying condition (e.g., spinal fusion, kyphoplasty), a code for the underlying condition (e.g., vertebral fracture, spinal stenosis) should be assigned as the principal diagnosis. No code from category 338 should be assigned.**

EXAMPLE The patient is having acute pain due to a headache and is admitted for pain control, 338.19, 784.0.

- **When a patient is admitted for the insertion of a neurostimulator for pain control, assign the appropriate pain code as the principal or first-listed diagnosis. When an admission or encounter is for a procedure aimed at treating the underlying**

condition, and a neurostimulator is inserted for pain control during the same admission/encounter, a code for the underlying condition should be assigned as the principal diagnosis, and the appropriate pain code should be assigned as a secondary diagnosis.

(b) Use of Category 338 Codes in Conjunction With Site Specific Pain Codes

(i) Assigning Category 338 Codes and Site-Specific Pain Codes

Codes from category 338 may be used in conjunction with codes that identify the site of pain (including codes from chapter 16) if the category 338 code provides additional information. For example, if the code describes the site of the pain, but does not fully describe whether the pain is acute or chronic, then both codes should be assigned.

(ii) Sequencing of Category 338 Codes with Site-Specific Pain Codes

The sequencing of category 338 codes with site-specific pain codes (including chapter 16 codes) is dependent on the circumstances of the encounter/admission as follows:

- If the encounter is for pain control or pain management, assign the code from category 338 followed by the code identifying the specific site of pain (e.g., encounter for pain management for acute neck pain from trauma is assigned code 338.11, Acute pain due to trauma, followed by code 723.1, Cervicalgia, to identify the site of pain).
- If the encounter is for any other reason except pain control or pain management, and a related definitive diagnosis has not been established (confirmed) by the provider, assign the code for the specific site of pain first, followed by the appropriate code from category 338.

2) Pain due to devices, implants and grafts

Pain associated with devices, **implants or grafts** left in a surgical site **(for example painful hip prosthesis)** is assigned to the appropriate code(s) found in Chapter 17, Injury and Poisoning. **Use additional code(s) from category 338 to identify acute or chronic pain due to presence of the device, implant or graft (338.18-338.19 or 338.28-338.29).**

EXAMPLE Painful retained suture, 996.59, E879.9.

3) Postoperative Pain

Post-thoracotomy pain and other postoperative pain are classified to subcategories 338.1 and 338.2, depending on whether the pain is acute or chronic. The default for post-thoracotomy and other postoperative pain not specified as acute or chronic is the code for the acute form.

Routine or expected postoperative pain immediately after surgery should not be coded.

(a) Postoperative pain not associated with specific postoperative complication

Postoperative pain not associated with a specific postoperative complication is assigned to the appropriate postoperative pain code in category 338.

(b) Postoperative pain associated with specific postoperative complication

Postoperative pain associated with a specific postoperative complication (such as **painful wire sutures**) is assigned to the appropriate code(s) found in Chapter 17, Injury and Poisoning. **If appropriate, use additional code(s) from category 338 to identify acute or chronic pain (338.18 or 338.28).** If pain control/management is the reason for the encounter, a code from category 338 should be assigned as the principal or first-listed diagnosis in accordance with *Section I.C.6.a.1.a above.*

(c) Postoperative pain as principal or first-listed diagnosis

Postoperative pain may be reported as the principal or first-listed diagnosis when the stated reason for the admission/encounter is documented as postoperative pain control/management.

(d) Postoperative pain as secondary diagnosis

Postoperative pain may be reported as a secondary diagnosis code when a patient presents for outpatient surgery and develops an unusual or inordinate amount of postoperative pain.

The provider's documentation should be used to guide the coding of postoperative pain, as well *as Section III. Reporting Additional Diagnoses and Section IV. Diagnostic Coding and Reporting in the Outpatient Setting.*

See Section II.1.2 for information on sequencing of diagnoses for patients admitted to hospital inpatient care following post-operative observation.

See Section II.J for information on sequencing of diagnoses for patients admitted to hospital inpatient care from outpatient surgery.

See Section IV.A.2 for information on sequencing of diagnoses for patients admitted for observation.

4) **Chronic pain**

Chronic pain is classified to subcategory 338.2. There is no time frame defining when pain becomes chronic pain. The provider's documentation should be used to guide use of these codes.

5) **Neoplasm Related Pain**

Code 338.3 is assigned to pain documented as being related, associated or due to cancer, primary or secondary malignancy, or tumor. This code is assigned regardless of whether the pain is acute or chronic.

This code may be assigned as the principal or first-listed code when the stated reason for the admission/encounter is documented as pain control/pain management. The underlying neoplasm should be reported as an additional diagnosis.

EXAMPLE

Patient is admitted for pain control due to metastatic bone cancer. Patient has a past history of primary breast cancer, 338.3, 198.5, V10.3.

When the reason for the admission/encounter is management of the neoplasm and the pain associated with the neoplasm is also documented, code 338.3 may be assigned as an additional diagnosis.

See Section I.C.2 for instructions on the sequencing of neoplasms for all other stated reasons for the admission/encounter (except for pain control/pain management).

EXAMPLE

Patient was admitted for back pain due to vertebral metastasis. An MRI indicates that the disease has progressed. Patient has a history of prostate cancer. Radiation was administered prior to discharge of the patient, 198.5, V10.46, 338.2, 92.29.

6) **Chronic pain syndrome**

This condition is different from that described by the term "chronic pain," and therefore this code should be used only when the provider has specifically documented this condition.

Apply the general coding guidelines as found in Chapter 5.

ANATOMY AND PHYSIOLOGY

The nervous system is composed of specialized tissue that controls the actions and reactions of the body and the way it adjusts to changes that occur inside and outside the body. The nervous system is divided into two main systems: the central nervous system and the peripheral nervous system (Figures 24-1 and 24-2). The central nervous system and the peripheral nervous system are each further divided into two parts. The central nervous system is made up of the brain and the spinal cord, and the peripheral nervous system is made up of the somatic nervous system and the autonomic nervous system.

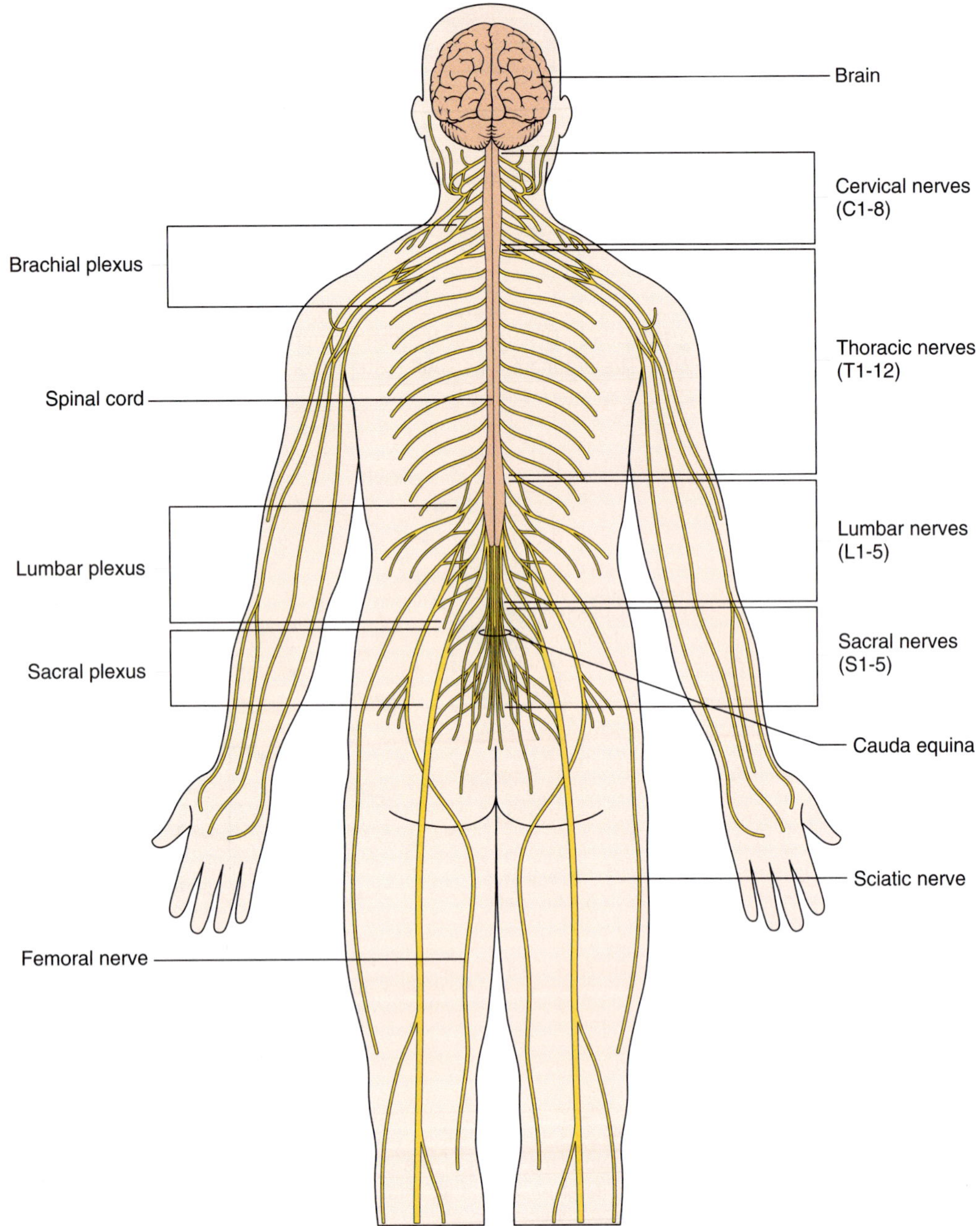

Figure 24-1. The brain and the spinal cord, spinal nerves, and spinal plexuses.

Central Nervous System

Different areas of the brain are in control of different functions of the body (Figure 24-3). For example, the cerebral cortex controls thought, language, and reasoning; the brain stem is in control of breathing and blood pressure; and the hippocampus is in control of memory and learning. The spinal cord serves as a pathway for information passing from the brain to the peripheral nervous system. Both the brain and the spinal cord are covered by bone—the brain by the skull, and the spinal cord by the vertebral column; both are covered by membranes called the meninges. The meninges (Figure 24-4) are made up of three

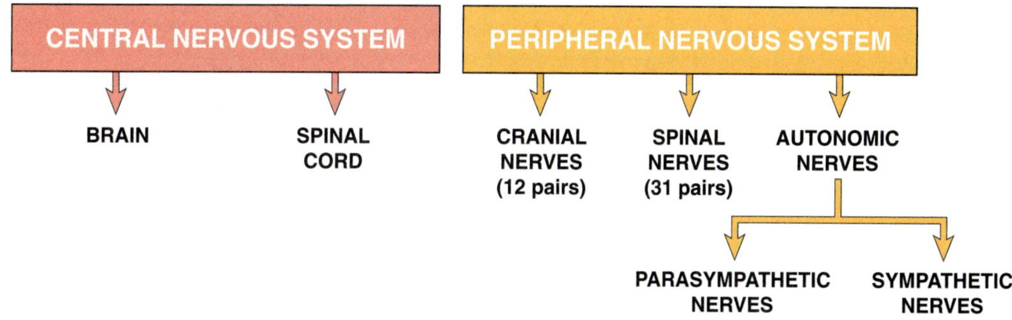

Figure 24-2. Divisions of the central nervous system (CNS) and peripheral nervous system (PNS). The autonomic nervous system is a part of the peripheral nervous system.

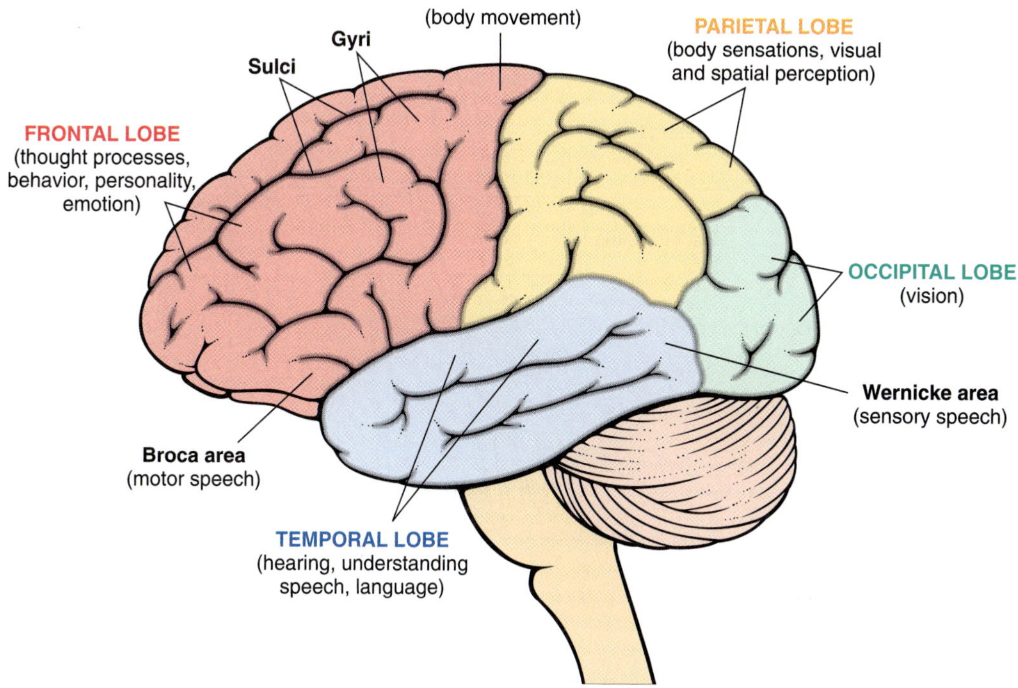

Figure 24-3. Left cerebral hemisphere (lateral view). Gyri (convolutions) and sulci (fissures) are indicated. Note the lobes of the cerebrum and the functional centers that control speech, vision, movement, hearing, thinking, and other processes.

layers: dura, arachnoid, and pia. In the spinal column, the dura is not attached to the vertebrae but is separated from them by the epidural space. The purpose of these membranes is to protect the brain and the spinal cord.

The spinal cord, which is located in the vertebral foramen, consists of 31 segments, each of which has a pair of spinal nerves that exit from the segment. The purpose of the spinal cord is to conduct nerve impulses and spinal reflexes.

Peripheral Nervous System

The peripheral nervous system connects the central nervous system to other parts of the body. It may be broken down into two parts: the somatic nervous system and the autonomic nervous system. The **somatic nervous system** sends sensory information (taste, hearing, smell, and vision) to the central nervous system (CNS) and motor nerve impulses to the skeletal muscles.

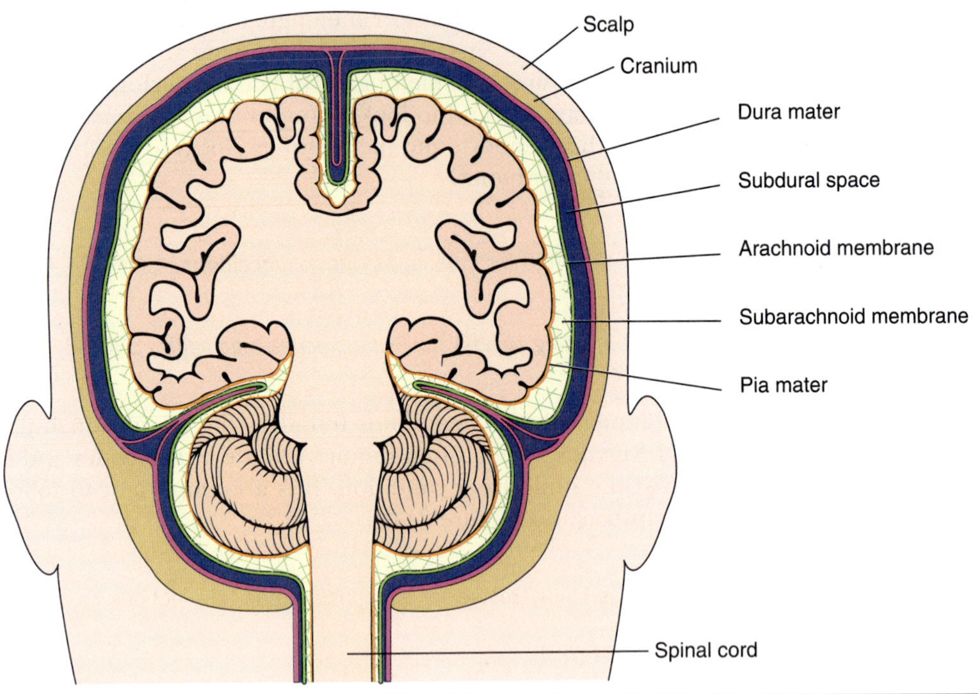

Figure 24-4. Meninges, frontal view.

The **autonomic nervous system** has both sensory and motor functions that involve the CNS and the internal organs. Actions produced by this system, such as beating of the heart muscle, are for the most part involuntary.

DISEASE CONDITIONS

Diseases of the Nervous System and Sense Organs (320-389), Chapter 6 in the ICD-9-CM code book, is divided into the following categories:

CATEGORY	SECTION TITLES
320-326	Inflammatory Diseases of the Central Nervous System
327	Organic Sleep Disorders
330-337	Hereditary and Degenerative Diseases of the Central Nervous System
338	Pain
340-349	Other Disorders of the Central Nervous System
350-359	Disorder of the Peripheral Nervous System
360-379	Disorders of the Eye and Adnexa
380-389	Diseases of the Ear and Mastoid Process

Inflammatory Diseases of the Central Nervous System (320-326)

Meningitis is an infection or inflammation of the meninges. Meningitis is caused by a viral or bacterial organism and may be treated with antibiotics. Vaccines are available to prevent meningitis that is due to *Streptococcus pneumoniae.* It should be noted that often, coding of meningitis requires two codes, and in most cases, the Tabular List instructs to code the underlying condition first. For more information on coding guidelines for underlying conditions, refer to Chapter 5.

EXAMPLE The patient was treated for meningitis due to Lyme disease, 088.81, 320.7.

The signs and symptoms of meningitis include high fever, headache, and stiff neck. Other symptoms that may be present are nausea, vomiting, sleepiness, and sensitivity to bright lights. To diagnose meningitis, physicians perform a lumbar puncture (Figure 24-5) to obtain spinal fluid and to look for organisms that may be present. Bacterial meningitis is treated with antibiotics, and the treatment for viral meningitis (aseptic) is usually limited to treating the symptoms.

EXAMPLE Patient admitted for meningitis due to sarcoidosis, 135, 321.4.

EXAMPLE Patient is being treated for *Pseudomonas* meningitis, 320.82.

Additional disease conditions found in the section on Inflammatory Diseases of the Central Nervous System often require the use of two codes and include the instruction to code first the underlying condition. It is also important to follow the Excludes notes for further instruction (Figure 24-6).

EXAMPLE Patient is being treated for encephalitis due to infectious mononucleosis, 075, 323.01.

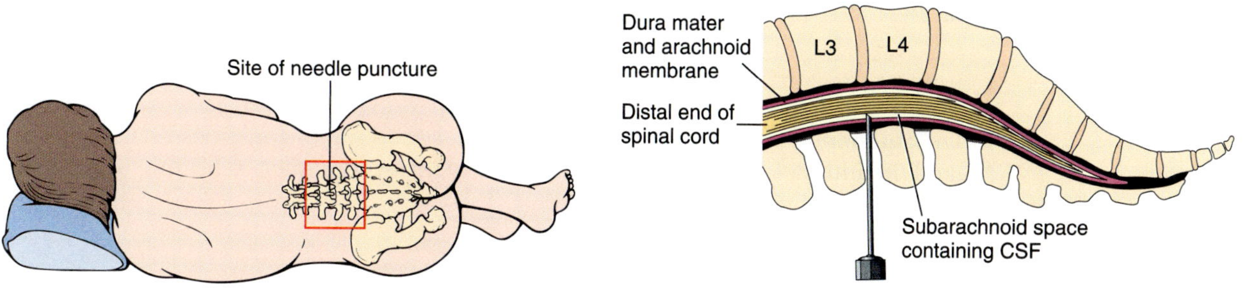

Figure 24-5. Lumbar (spinal) puncture. The patient lies laterally, with the knees drawn up to the abdomen and the chin brought down to the chest. This position increases the spaces between the vertebrae. The lumbar puncture needle is inserted between the third and fourth (or fourth and fifth) lumbar vertebrae, and it enters the subarachnoid space.

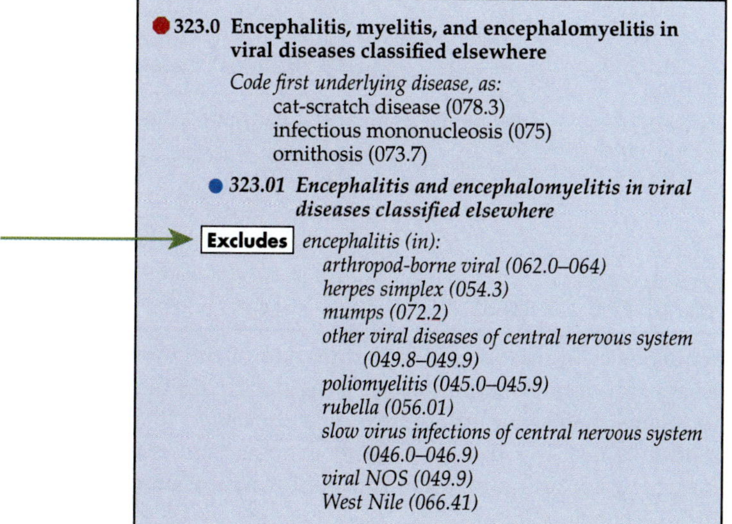

● **323.0 Encephalitis, myelitis, and encephalomyelitis in viral diseases classified elsewhere**

Code first underlying disease, as:
cat-scratch disease (078.3)
infectious mononucleosis (075)
ornithosis (073.7)

● ***323.01 Encephalitis and encephalomyelitis in viral diseases classified elsewhere***

Excludes *encephalitis (in):*
arthropod-borne viral (062.0–064)
herpes simplex (054.3)
mumps (072.2)
other viral diseases of central nervous system (049.8–049.9)
poliomyelitis (045.0–045.9)
rubella (056.01)
slow virus infections of central nervous system (046.0–046.9)
viral NOS (049.9)
West Nile (066.41)

Figure 24-6. Refer to the Excludes notes for further instruction, if an underlying disease is causing encephalitis, myelitis, and encephalomyelitis.

EXAMPLE The patient was admitted with herpes encephalitis, 054.3.

EXERCISE 24-1

Assign codes to the following conditions using your ICD-9-CM code book.

1. Meningitis due to *Salmonella* ____________
2. *Klebsiella pneumoniae* meningitis ____________
3. Gram-negative meningitis ____________
4. Spinal meningitis ____________
5. Encephalitis following chickenpox ____________

Organic Sleep Disorders (327)

Some typical sleep problems include **insomnia**, (difficulty falling asleep, staying asleep, wakefulness, and early morning awakening) and **hypersomnia** (excessive sleep). These problems are classified in this section when they are caused by a physiologic condition.

EXAMPLE The patient is being treated for insomnia due to anxiety, 300.00, 327.0.

Sleep apnea is a disorder that is characterized by breathing interruption during sleep. These patients awaken many times during the night to regain their breathing. This disorder results in sleep deprivation and can be life threatening. Sleep apnea can result in a drop in the oxygen saturation of blood and is a cause of daytime **somnolence**. A person is more likely to have obstructive sleep apnea (OSA) if they are overweight, snore loudly, are hypertensive, or have a family history of sleep apnea. This obstruction occurs when there is a blockage in the airway. Obstructive sleep apnea is diagnosed by a sleep study or polysomnogram. Patients are treated with a CPAP (continuous positive airway pressure) mask. This mask helps push air into the breathing pathway. There are also surgical procedures to correct the obstruction.

Central sleep apnea occurs when the brain does not signal the muscles to breath. This might occur in a stroke victim that has nervous system dysfunction or in patients that have neurodegenerative illnesses such as Lou Gehrig's disease.

EXAMPLE Patient has obstructive sleep apnea, 327.23.

Hereditary and Degenerative Diseases of the Central Nervous System (330-337)

Alzheimer's disease (Figure 24-7) is a disorder of the brain that causes a progressive decline in mental and physical function. This disease is the most common cause of mental deterioration, and medications are available now and others are in development to assist in the treatment of this disease. When a physician documents the condition as Alzheimer's dementia, it is necessary to use two codes, with Alzheimer's disease sequenced first. For many of the dementia codes, code assignment may depend on the presence of behavioral disturbances such as aggressiveness, combativeness, violence, or wandering off.

EXAMPLE Patient has Alzheimer's dementia without behavioral disturbance, 331.0, 294.10.

Hydrocephalus is essentially excessive water (cerebrospinal fluid) on the brain. Cerebrospinal fluid (CSF) surrounds the brain and the spinal cord, and when this fluid accumulates on the brain, it causes pressure on brain tissue. Hydrocephalus may be acquired or congenital and communicating or obstructive. In communicating hydrocephalus, CSF can flow between ventricles of the brain, but it is blocked upon exit of the ventricle, as

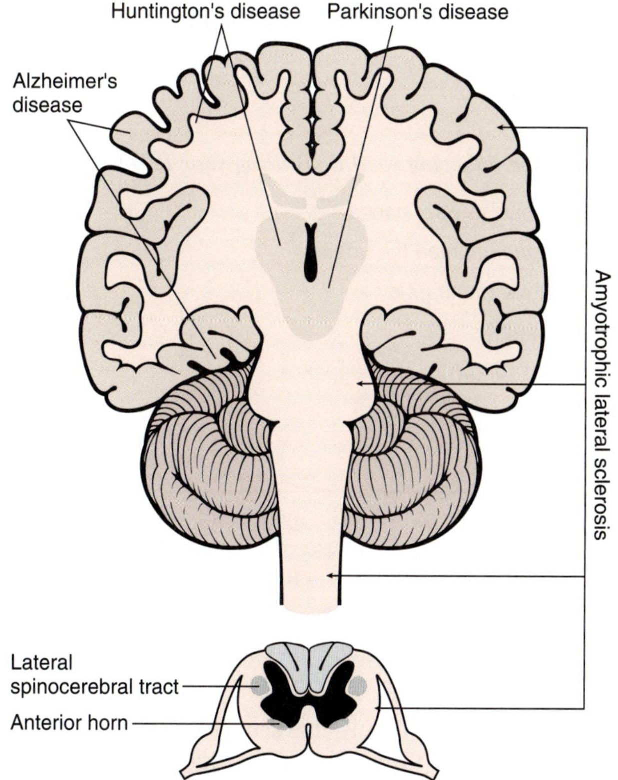

Figure 24-7. Degenerative diseases of the brain preferentially involve various parts of the brain. Alzheimer's disease causes atrophy of the frontal and occipital cortical gyri. Huntington's disease affects the frontal cortex and basal ganglia. Parkinson's disease is marked by changes in the substantia nigra. Amyotrophic lateral sclerosis affects the motor neurons in the anterior horn of the spinal cord, brain stem, and frontal cortex of the brain.

opposed to obstructive hydrocephalus, in which the flow between ventricles is blocked. In addition, a condition known as normal pressure hydrocephalus (NPH) occurs in the elderly population and often occurs with dementia. Hydrocephalus is most often treated with a ventricular shunt (Figure 24-8). Hydrocephalus that is left untreated is a fatal condition.

EXAMPLE The patient has a shunt for noncommunicating hydrocephalus, 331.4, V45.2.

Parkinson's disease (Figure 24-9) is a progressive and chronic motor system disorder. Symptoms may include tremor, rigidity, and impaired balance or coordination. It is usually treated with drugs such as L-dopa and sometimes with implantation of an intracranial neurostimulator.

EXAMPLE Patient with Parkinson's disease, 332.0.

EXAMPLE Patient is being treated for parkinsonism in Huntington's disease, 333.4.

EXAMPLE Patient has parkinsonism due to Risperdal, 332.1, E939.3.

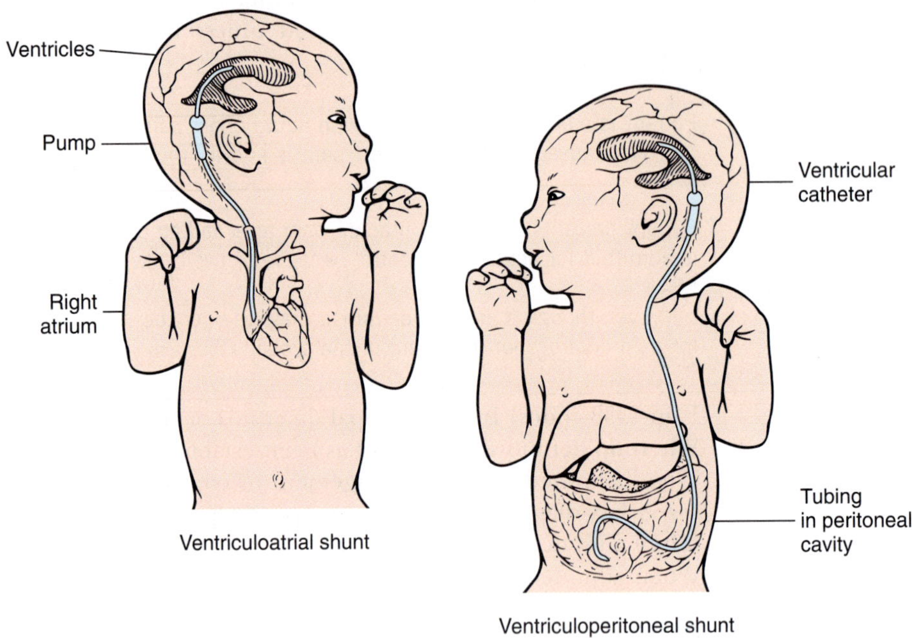

Figure 24-8. Shunting procedures for hydrocephalus. Ventriculoperitoneal shunt is the preferred procedure.

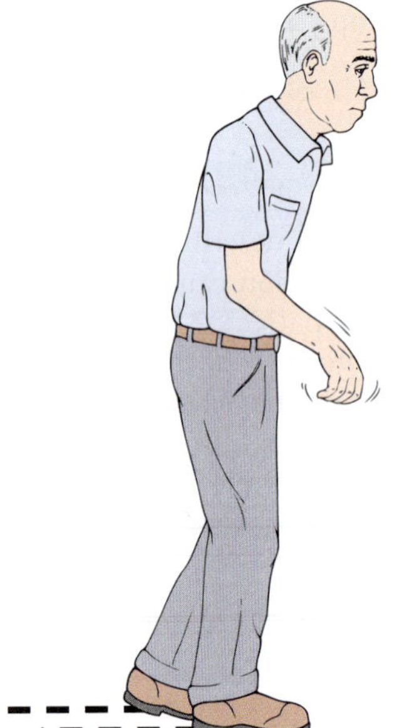

Figure 24-9. Typical shuffling gait and posture of patients with Parkinson's disease.

Pain (338)

To use codes from this category, the pain must be specified as acute or chronic, with exceptions being made for the following:

- Post-thoracotomy pain
- Postoperative pain
- Neoplasm-related pain
- Central pain syndrome

If the cause of the pain (i.e., the underlying diagnosis) is known, then a code from 338.1 and 338.2 should **NOT** be used unless the purpose of the encounter is pain control.

EXAMPLE Patient is admitted from the ER with acute chest pain due to pneumonia 486.
The cause of the acute chest pain is known; therefore no pain code is necessary.

EXAMPLE Patient presents to the ER in acute pain after falling off a horse at riding camp. Patient is admitted for acute pain control because of two broken ribs, 338.11, 807.02, E828.2, E849.4.
Even though there is a definitive diagnosis for the pain, the reason for admission is for pain control, not treatment of the broken ribs.

Pain (338 codes) is the principal diagnosis or first-listed diagnosis:

- When no definitive diagnosis has been established or;
- When admitted for pain management or control with the underlying cause as a secondary diagnosis including site-specific pain codes or;
- When admitted for postoperative pain control or;
- When admitted for pain control of neoplasm-related pain.

EXAMPLE Patient is having acute head pain caused by a headache and is admitted for pain control, 338.19 (Other acute pain) and 784.0 (head pain).

Pain (338 codes) is **NOT** the principal diagnosis or first-listed diagnosis:

- When a definitive diagnosis is known or;
- When site-specific pain is known and patient is admitted for workup of pain or;
- When the pain is due to a device.

Other Disorders of the Central Nervous System (340-349)

Hemiplegia and hemiparesis (Figure 24-10) describe paralysis of the body that could have a number of causes. One of the most common causes of hemiplegia is a cerebrovascular accident (CVA) (Figure 24-11). When a patient is admitted with an acute CVA and has hemiplegia at discharge, it is appropriate to code this condition. These codes have fifth digits that represent the side of the body that has been affected. If the patient is right handed and the right side is affected, then the fifth digit 1 for the dominant side would be selected. *Coding Clinic* (1994:4Q:p36)[1] instructs the coder to select fifth digit 0 if no mention of dominant side is made in the record.

EXAMPLE Patient has right-sided spastic hemiparesis, 342.10.

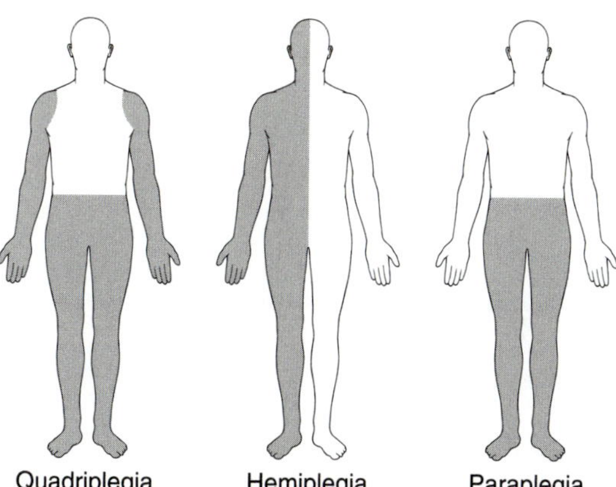

Figure 24-10. Types of paralysis.

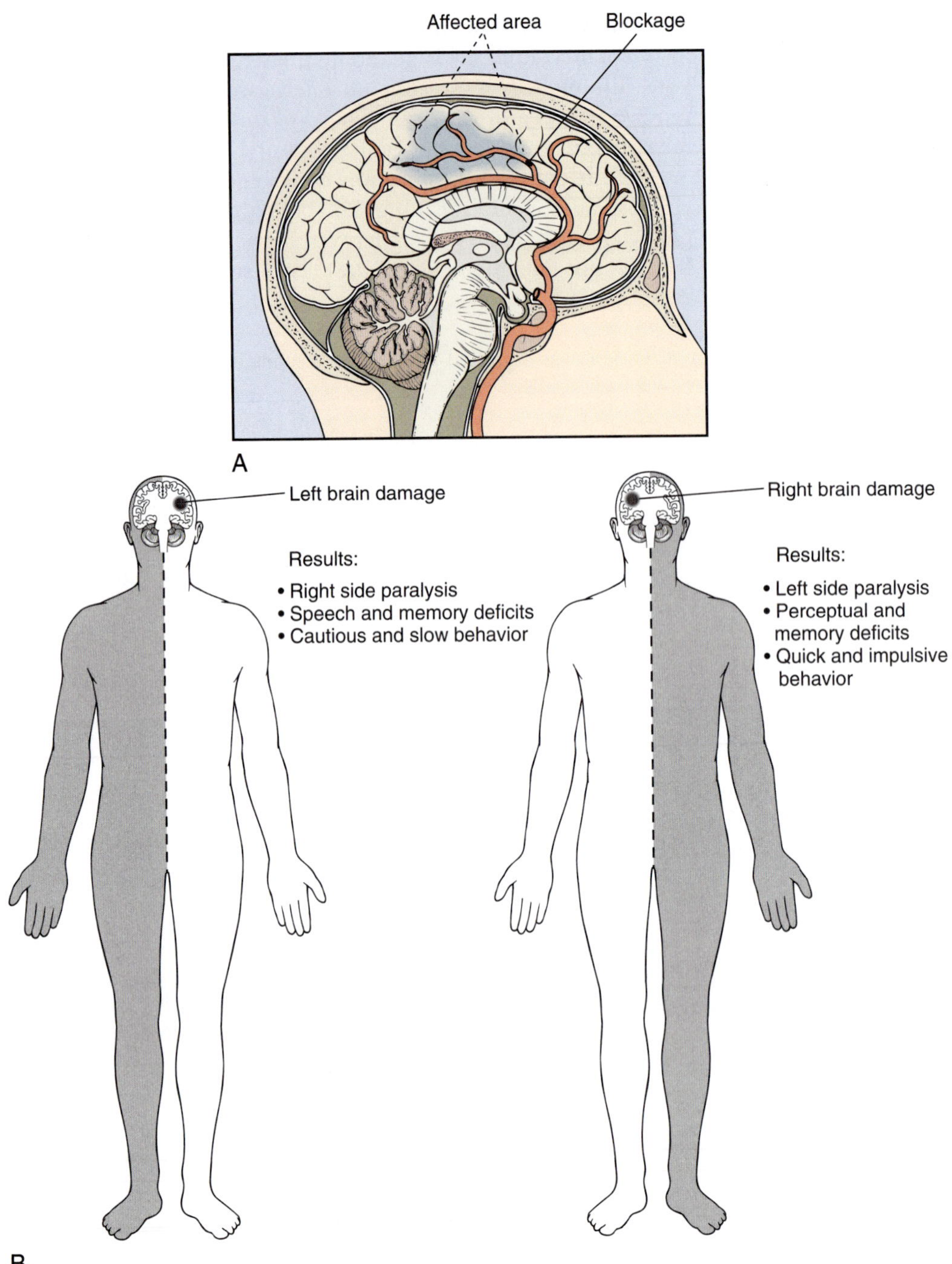

Figure 24-11. **A,** Cerebrovascular accident (CVA). **B,** Areas of the body affected by CVA.

Epilepsy is a disorder of the brain that is characterized by abnormal electrical discharges from the brain cells. Recurrent seizures are the main symptom of epilepsy. Two major types of seizures can occur: generalized and partial. Seizures may present in a variety of forms; patients may lose consciousness, their arms and legs may jerk, they may become incontinent, or they may stare blankly, unaware of their surroundings. As of October 1, 2006, the Alphabetic Index entry for seizure disorder changed. A seizure disorder is now coded to 345.9X. If patient has recurrent seizures, this is also coded to 345.9X. When it is documented as a convulsion or a single seizure then 780.39 is assigned.

Epilepsy has many causes; however, in approximately half of the cases, the cause is unknown. Epilepsy may be inherited, or it may be caused by injury to the brain, metabolic

disturbances, alcohol and drug abuse, brain tumor, infection, stroke, fever, or it may occur in pregnancy. Epilepsy is generally treated with anticonvulsants such as Dilantin or Depakote, although in severe uncontrolled cases, surgery may be performed on the brain to remove the area of the brain where seizures originate. The most common diagnostic test for epilepsy is an electroencephalogram (EEG).

A fifth digit subclassification for category 345 allows the identification of intractable epilepsy, **intractable** meaning "unable to control." The coder should be aware that the physician must document epilepsy as intractable before the fifth digit of 1 can be assigned. If this is not documented and the record suggests intractable, it may be necessary to query the physician.

EXAMPLE Patient was admitted for intractable epilepsy, 345.91.

EXAMPLE Patient is being treated for progressive myoclonic epilepsy, 333.2.

EXERCISE 24-2

Assign codes to the following conditions using your ICD-9-CM code book.

1. Parkinson's dementia ________
2. Chronic hydrocephalus ________
3. Seizure disorder ________
4. Partial epilepsy, visual type ________
5. Uncontrolled grand mal epilepsy ________
6. Status epilepticus ________
7. Organic hypersomnia ________
8. Febrile seizures ________
9. Patient has hemiplegia, which is a late effect of a CVA ________
10. Patient is left handed and has hemiparesis affecting his or her nondominant side ________
11. Patient is admitted for pain control with acute abdominal pain related to pancreatic cancer ________
12. Patient is admitted with back pain for intravenous (IV) pain management after a fall down the stairs ________
13. Patient is admitted for acute neck pain after an automobile accident. Attending plans magnetic resonance imaging (MRI) of the neck to rule out fracture ________
14. Patient is readmitted for postoperative pain control after emergency appendectomy ________
15. Patient is admitted for narcotics to treat chronic pain syndrome ________

Disorders of the Peripheral Nervous System (350-359)

Many of the codes in this chapter require the coder to apply the General Coding Guideline Rules for Multiple Coding. The "Code First" underlying condition applies often in this chapter. The coder must remember that the underlying condition is coded first; this is followed by the code for the manifestation.

EXAMPLE Patient has polyneuropathy in type II diabetes, 250.60, 357.2.

Myasthenia gravis is a chronic autoimmune disorder that manifests as muscle weakness of varying degrees. The most frequently affected muscles are those that control the eye, eyelid, face, and swallowing. Myasthenia gravis may be treated with medication, thymectomy, and/or plasmapheresis. Patients who present in crisis may have difficulty breathing and require a ventilator to assist with breathing. These crises may be brought on by many different events, such as infection, stress, or fever.

EXAMPLE Patient was admitted for an acute exacerbation of myasthenia gravis, 358.01.

Muscular dystrophy is a type of myopathy. **Myopathies** are general disorders that affect muscles and usually result in muscle weakening or atrophy. Many disease processes involve myopathies.

EXAMPLE Patient has Graves' myopathy, 242.90, 359.5.

Critical illness polyneuropathy and myopathy are diseases of the nerves and muscles that occur as a complication of severe trauma or infection. These conditions are often diagnosed when there is an unexplained difficulty in weaning the patient from mechanical ventilation. These conditions are often associated with sepsis and are thought to be a manifestation of the systemic inflammatory response syndrome (SIRS).

EXAMPLE Patient is diagnosed with critical illness polyneuropathy, 357.82.

Disorders of the Eye and Adnexa (360-379)

Many eye disorders are treated in the outpatient setting. Some of the conditions commonly found in inpatient records involve injuries to the eye (Figure 24-12), glaucoma, cataracts, macular degeneration, and visual impairment such as blindness. Injuries to the eye are covered in the Chapter 19.

Macular degeneration (Figure 24-13) is the leading cause of vision loss in the United States. Persons affected by this disease tend to be elderly; vision is lost in the central portion of the eye, leaving the patient with peripheral vision or low vision. Two common types of

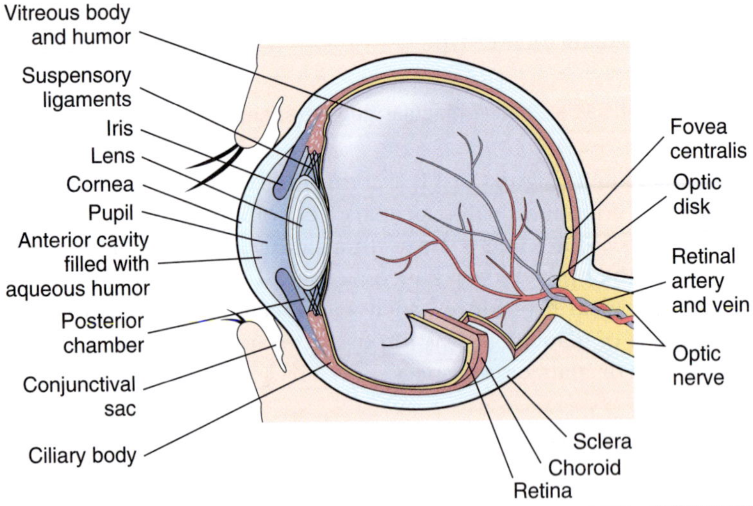

Figure 24-12. Normal eye.

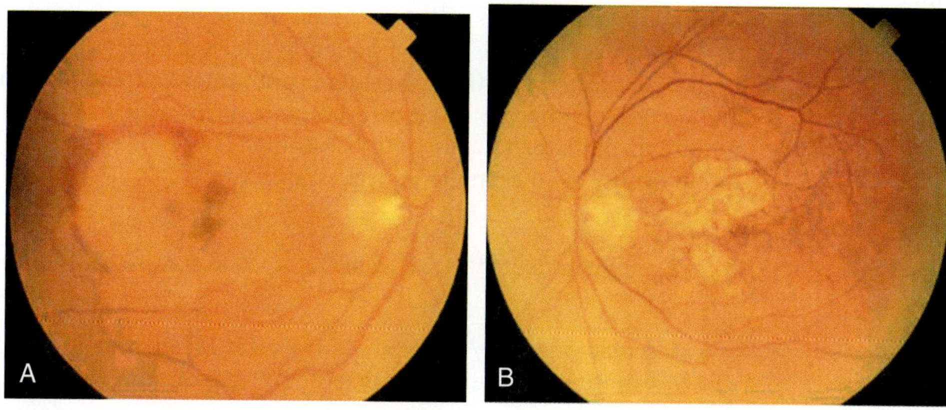

Figure 24-13. Macular degeneration. **A,** Wet, atrophic, age-related macular degeneration. **B,** Dry, atrophic, age-related macular degeneration.

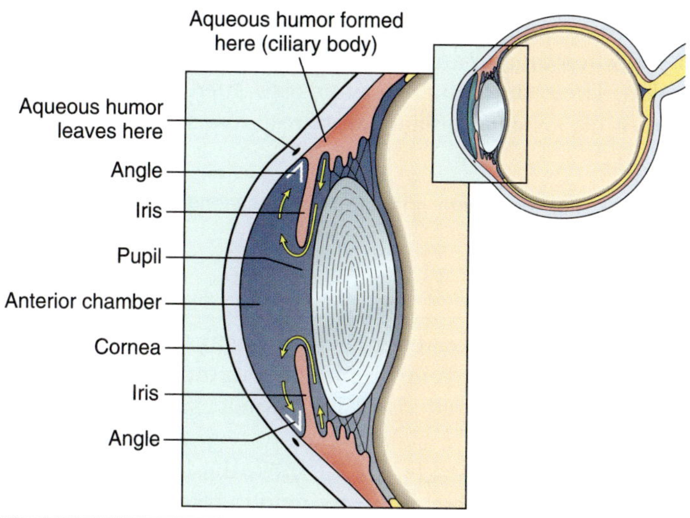

Figure 24-14. Glaucoma and circulation of aqueous humor. Circulation is impaired in glaucoma, so that aqueous fluid builds up in the anterior chamber.

this disease have been identified: dry and wet. The dry form is more common and is less aggressive than the wet type.

EXAMPLE Patient has exudative macular degeneration, 362.52.

Glaucoma (Figure 24-14) is a disorder of the optic nerve that may result in vision loss. The most common form is primary open angle glaucoma, in which the drainage canals of the eye become clogged over time and cause intraocular pressure (IOP) to rise; this damages the optic nerve. Glaucoma is most often treated with medicines in the form of eye drops. Surgical procedures, such as trabeculoplasty and trabeculectomy, may assist in the treatment of glaucoma. It is important to note that there is a specific code for borderline glaucoma or glaucoma suspect.

EXAMPLE Patient is treated for open angle glaucoma, 365.10.

EXAMPLE Patient has glaucoma with Sturge-Weber syndrome, 759.6, 365.44.

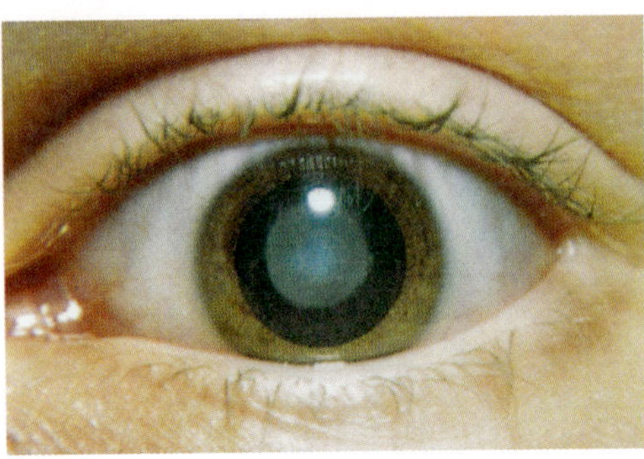

Figure 24-15. Cataract. The lens appears cloudy.

Cataract (Figure 24-15) is a clouding of the lens of the eye that can cause obstructed vision. Most cataracts are related to the aging process; however, *Coding Clinic* (1985:Sept-Oct: p10)[2] advises not to use the code for senile cataract just because of a patient's age. The physician must document the type of cataract the patient has. *Coding Clinic* (1985:Sept-Oct: p11)[3] also advises not to make the assumption that a patient has a diabetic cataract just because he or she has both diabetes and a cataract. The physician must document diabetic cataract. Other risk factors for development of cataracts include smoking, diabetes, and prolonged exposure to sunlight. Cataracts are most often treated by surgery. Possible complications of cataract surgery include retinal detachment, anterior capsule contracture, and aftercataract. *Coding Clinic* (2000:1Q:p9-10)[4] advises to use code 996.53 for anterior capsule contracture.

EXAMPLE Patient has a mature senile cataract, 366.17.

Blindness and Low Vision

In the United States, legal blindness (Figure 24-16) is defined as severe or profound impairment in both eyes. ICD-9-CM always codes the better eye impairment first and the lesser eye disorder second.

EXAMPLE Patient with better eye severe impairment; lesser eye profound impairment, 369.14.

EXAMPLE A patient is blind in one eye and had normal vision in the other eye, 369.63.

Diseases of the Ear and Mastoid Process (380-389)

As with eye conditions, many disorders of the ear (Figure 24-17) are treated in the outpatient setting. At times, inpatient coders see patients with the diagnoses of otitis media, mastoiditis, vertigo, and cholesteatoma, and of course, patients with hearing loss.

Otitis media (OM) is a middle ear infection. It is the most common illness among children and babies. OM often occurs after another illness such as a cold. If the physician describes OM as suppurative, it is purulent or is expressing pus.

EXAMPLE Patient has acute allergic serous otitis media, acute, 381.04.

Classification		Levels of Visual Impairment	Additional Descriptors Which May Be Encountered
"Legal"	**WHO**	***Visual Acuity and/or Visual Field Limitation (Whichever Is Worse)***	
	(Near-) normal vision	Range of Normal Vision 20/10 20/13 20/16 20/20 20/25 2.0 1.6 1.25 1.0 0.8	
		Near-Normal Vision 20/30 20/40 20/50 20/60 0.7 0.6 0.5 0.4 0.3	
	Low vision	Moderate Visual Impairment 20/70 20/80 20/100 20/125 20/160 0.25 0.20 0.16 0.12	Moderate low vision
		Severe Visual Impairment 20/200 20/250 20/320 20/400 0.10 0.08 0.06 0.05 Visual field: 20 degrees or less	Severe low vision, "Legal" blindness
Legal Blindness (U.S.A.) both eyes	Blindness (WHO) one or both eyes	Profound Visual Impairment 20/500 20/630 20/800 20/1000 0.04 0.03 0.025 0.02 Count fingers at: less than 3 m (10 ft) Visual field: 10 degrees or less	Profound low vision, Moderate blindness
		Near-Total Visual Impairment Visual acuity: less than 0.02 (20/1000) Count fingers: 1 m (3 ft) or less Hand movements: 5 m (15 ft) or less Light projection, light perception Visual field: 5 degrees or less	Severe blindness, Near-total blindness
		Total Visual Impairment No light perception (NLP)	Total blindness

Visual acuity refers to best achievable acuity with correction.
Non-listed Snellen fractions may be classified by converting to the nearest decimal equivalent, e.g., 10/200 = 0.05, 6/30 = 0.20.
CF (count fingers) without designation of distance, may be classified to profound impairment.
HM (hand motion) without designation of distance, may be classified to near-total impairment.
Visual field measurements refer to the largest field diameter for a 1/100 white test object.

Figure 24-16. Blindness and low vision table.

Mastoiditis is an infection of the mastoid bone of the skull. It is often the consequence of untreated OM and may be difficult to treat. Treatment usually consists of antibiotics and, as a last resort, a mastoidectomy to drain and remove the mastoid.

EXAMPLE Patient is being treated for chronic recurrent mastoiditis, 383.1.

A **cholesteatoma** is a growth in the middle ear that usually results from repeated ear infections. Cholesteatomas may cause hearing loss or dizziness and may require surgery.

EXAMPLE Patient was diagnosed with primary cholesteatoma, 385.31.

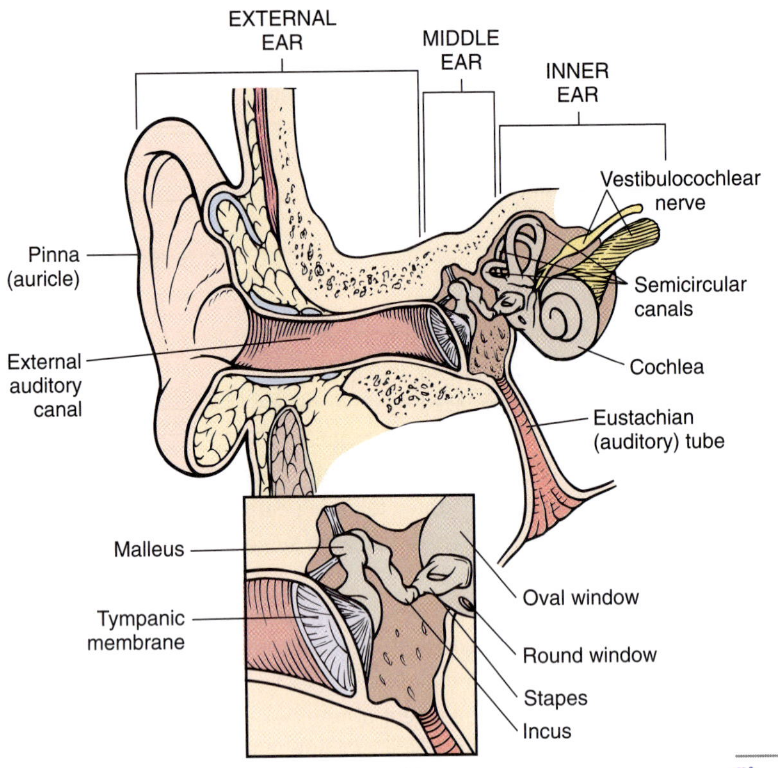

Figure 24-17. Normal ear.

EXERCISE 24-3

Assign codes to the following conditions using your ICD-9-CM code book.

1. Malignant neoplasm of the thyroid with myasthenia syndrome ________
2. Myasthenia gravis ________
3. Hereditary muscular dystrophy ________
4. Myopathy due to critical illness ________
5. What is the leading cause of vision loss in the United States? ________
6. An 80-year-old gentleman has cataracts and diabetes ________
7. Patient is blind by USA standards ________
8. SOM (serous otitis media) ________
9. Acute and chronic mastoiditis ________

V CODES

In the past, V codes have been considered for use primarily in the outpatient setting. This has changed with the addition of more V codes each year. As was discussed in Chapter 8, it is difficult to locate V codes in the Index. Coders will often say, "I did not know there was a V code for that." Refer to Chapter 8 for a listing of common main terms used to locate V codes.

V codes that may be used with Nervous System and Sense Organ conditions include the following:

V12.40	Personal history of unspecified disorder of the nervous system and sense organs
V12.41	Personal history of benign neoplasm of the brain
V12.49	Personal history of other disorders of nervous system and sense organs

V15.2	Personal history of surgery to other major organs that presents hazards to health
V17.1	Family history of stroke
V17.2	Family of other neurologic diseases
V19.0	Family history of blindness or visual loss
V19.1	Family history of other eye disorders
V41.0	Problems with sight
V41.1	Other eye problems
V41.2	Problems with hearing
V41.3	Other ear problems
V41.5	Problems with smell and taste
V42.5	Cornea replaced by transplant
V43.0	Eye globe replaced by other means
V43.1	Lens replaced by other means
V45.2	Presence of cerebrospinal fluid drainage device
V45.61	Postprocedural states following cataract surgery
V45.69	Postprocedural state following surgery of eye and adnexa
V45.78	Acquired absence of eye
V48.4	Sensory problems with head
V48.6	Sensory problems with neck and trunk
V49.85	Dual sensory impairment
V52.2	Fitting and adjustment of artificial eye
V53.01	Fitting and adjustment of cerebral ventricular shunt
V53.02	Fitting and adjustment of neuropacemaker (brain) (peripheral nerve) (spinal cord)
V53.09	Fitting and adjustment of other devices related to nervous system and special senses
V53.1	Fitting and adjustment of spectacles and contact lenses
V53.2	Fitting and adjustment of hearing aid
V58.71	Aftercare following surgery of the sense organs, NEC
V58.72	Aftercare following surgery of the nervous system, NEC
V72.11	Encounter for hearing exam following failed hearing screening
V72.12	Encounter for hearing conservation and treatment
V72.19	Encounter for other exam of ears and hearing
V80.0	Special screening for neurologic conditions
V80.1	Special screening for glaucoma
V80.2	Special screening for other eye conditions
V80.3	Special screening for ear diseases

EXAMPLE Patient presents with dizziness and a history of stroke, 780.4, V12.54.

EXERCISE 24-4

Assign codes to the following conditions using your ICD-9-CM code book.

1. Encounter for fitting of glasses ______________
2. Patient is status cataract removal and has a history of cornea transplant ______________
3. Patient previously had enucleation of right eye ______________
4. Patient was screened for glaucoma ______________

COMMON TREATMENTS

CONDITION	MEDICATION/TREATMENT
Alzheimer's	Tacrine (Cognex), donepezil hydrochloride (Aricept), rivastigmine tartrate (Exelon), galantamine (Reminyl), melmantine HCl (Namenda)
Parkinson's	Entacapone (Comtan), pramipexole dihydrochloride (Mirapex), ropinirole hydrochloride (Requip), Carbidopa-Levodopa (Sinemet)
Epilepsy	Carbamazepine (Tegretol), clonazepam (Klonopin), phenytoin (Dilantin), sodium valproate and valproic acid (Depakote), Levetiracetam (Keppra), topiramate Topamax
Myasthenia gravis	Neostigmine bromide—oral (Prostigmin), Pyridostigmine (Regonol), (Mestinon)
Muscular dystrophy	Phenytoin (Dilantin), phenytoin (Phenytek), Deltasone
Macular degeneration	Vitamins/Photodynamic surgery
Glaucoma	Eye drops such as Xalatan (prostaglandins), Iopidine (adrenergics), Carbachol (miotic), Timoptic (beta blocker), and Diamox (carbonic anhydrase inhibitors)

PROCEDURES

Some procedures that may be related to diseases of the nervous system and sense organs may be located in the following chapters of the Procedure Tabular:

Chapter 1 Operations of the Nervous System (01-05)
Chapter 3 Operations of the Eye (08-16)
Chapter 4 Operations of the Ear (18-20)

Lumbar Puncture

Lumbar puncture (LP), also known as spinal tap or spinal puncture, is used both diagnostically and therapeutically. When LP is performed for diagnosis, the cerebrospinal fluid (CSF) is analyzed for infection, inflammatory diseases such as multiple sclerosis, subarachnoid hemorrhage, and certain types of carcinoma. When LP is done therapeutically, it may be done to decrease spinal fluid pressure in conditions such as normal pressure hydrocephalus, benign intracranial hypertension, or pseudotumor cerebri. When LP is done therapeutically, the coder will find this code listed in the index under "Drainage, spinal."

EXAMPLE

Patient presents to the ER with high fever and neck pain. The physician performs a lumbar puncture to rule out meningitis, 780.6, 723.1, 03.31.

Deep Brain Stimulation

A brain stimulator, also known as an intracranial neurostimulator, a **deep brain stimulator** (DBS) or a thalamic stimulator, is used to control tremors in patients with Parkinson's and in those who have the condition of essential tremor. An electrode is implanted, usually into the thalamus, and then is connected by a wire under the skin to a pulse generator implanted in the chest. Electrical impulses are sent to the thalamus, which in turn, controls tremors. For further information on this procedure, refer to *Coding Clinic* (1997:4Q:p57-58).[5] This code is indexed under "Implant, neurostimulator, electrodes, brain."

Ventricular Shunting

Shunting treatment of hydrocephalus is done to drain fluid from the brain to relieve pressure. The most common type of shunting (ventriculoperitoneal shunt) occurs between the ventricles of the brain and the abdominal cavity. In this case, the excess fluid is drained

from the ventricles into the peritoneal cavity, where it is reabsorbed. When looking up this procedure in the index under "Shunt, ventricular," it should be noted that the ventricle can also drain into other body areas. Sometimes, complications can occur in either the ventricular or the peritoneal part of the shunt. It may be necessary to perform surgery only at the site with the complication. This is a shunt revision. In these cases, the coder is directed to the index under "Revision, shunt." The code will be determined by the site that is revised. It is important to review the operative record to determine which site (peritoneal or ventricular) is being revised.

When coding these cases, it is important to look in the index under "Complication, mechanical, shunt, ventricular" for the appropriate diagnosis code, per *Coding Clinic* (1987: Sept-Oct:p10).[6]

EXAMPLE Patient admitted for insertion of ventriculoatrial shunt for communicating hydrocephalus, 331.3, 02.32.

Electromyelogram

An **electromyelogram** (EMG) is a diagnostic test that measures electrical activity in muscles and nerves. It is used to determine whether a patient has a disease that is damaging muscles, such as myasthenia gravis, or nerves, such as amyotrophic lateral sclerosis.

Hemispherectomy

Surgery for epilepsy currently consists of four basic types: amygdalohippocampectomy, lobectomy (temporal), hemispherectomy, and corpus callosotomy. Surgery is not the norm for treatment of epilepsy, but it is used in the most severe cases when medications have failed to control seizures. Many tests must be performed before a person is considered a candidate for surgery and prior to the surgery itself.

Prior to surgery, in-depth electrodes may be placed along with a grid to record the brain's electrical activity. During this procedure, the surgeon makes small holes in the skull. Per *Coding Clinic* (1991:2Q:p14),[7] this procedure should be assigned code 01.24. This procedure is indexed under "Craniotomy." If a patient also is having video and radio EEG monitoring, an additional code is assigned.

Lobectomy, usually in the temporal region, is performed for partial seizures; during this surgery, the seizure focus is removed. During hemispherectomy, approximately half of the brain is removed. This procedure is usually performed on children.

EXAMPLE A patient with intractable epilepsy is admitted for a temporal lobectomy, 345.91, 01.53.

Vagal Nerve Stimulation

A **vagal nerve stimulator** is a device that is used to treat intractable epilepsy. This device, which is similar to a heart pacemaker, is inserted into the upper chest and sends electrical current to the vagus nerve in the neck, which in turn travels to the brain and reduces or controls seizures. According to *Coding Clinic* (1996:3Q:p12),[8] this code is indexed under "Implantation," "Neurostimulator," "Electrodes," and "Pulse generator implantation," codes 86.94-86.98.

EXAMPLE A patient with intractable epilepsy presents for implantation of a single array neurostimulator pulse generator with leads, 345.91, 04.92, 86.94.

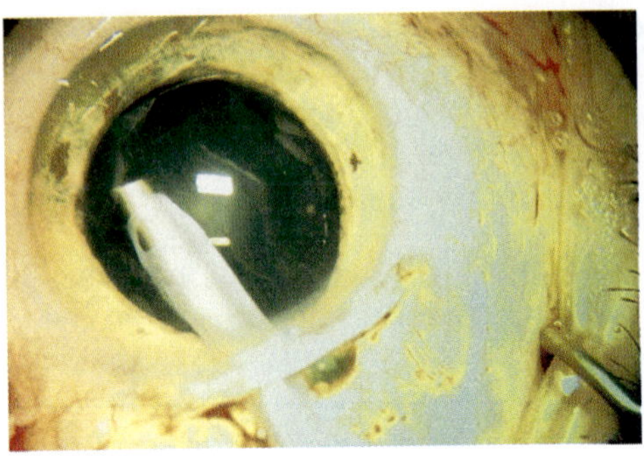

Figure 24-18. Phacoemulsification of a cataractous lens through a small, self-sealing, scleral tunnel incision.

Photodynamic Therapy

Photodynamic therapy (PDT) is used in treatment of the wet form of macular degeneration. According to *Coding Clinic* (1991:2Q:p17),[9] no additional code is assigned for the drug (Visudyne) used in this treatment, but the code can be located under "Destruction, lesion, retina by laser."

Cataract Extraction

Cataract extraction is usually performed by **phacoemulsification** (Figure 24-18), wherein an incision is made on the side of the cornea and the lens material is softened, broken, and suctioned out. Usually after the lens is removed, an artifical lens is inserted (intraocular lens [IOL]). The codes for this procedure are indexed under "Extraction, cataract, phacoemulsification," and "Insertion, lens, with cataract extraction, one stage"

EXAMPLE

Patient is admitted for a mature senile cataract to be removed by phacoemulsification with IOL replacement, 366.17, 13.41, 13.71.

It is important to remember that when bilateral procedures are coded, the procedure code should be coded twice, unless a code is classified as bilateral. This follows the coding guideline from Chapter 6.

EXERCISE 24-5

Answer the following questions and code all diagnoses and procedures as appropriate.

1. What is the name of the test used to measure electrical activity in muscles? ______________
2. Name one reason a surgeon may perform a hemispherectomy. ______________
3. What is PDT used to treat? ______________
4. Patient with pseudotumor cerebri is treated with a therapeutic spinal tap. ______________
5. Patient presents with malfunctioning ventriculoperitoneal shunt, and revision of the shunt is performed at the peritoneal site. ______________
6. Patient with Parkinson's disease is admitted for insertion of a thalamic stimulator. ______________
7. Patient admitted with nuclear senile cataract and an extracapsular cataract extraction with Yag laser with lens implant was performed. ______________
8. A patient who had a cornea transplant on his right eye now has glaucoma in his left eye. He is admitted for a trabeculectomy ab externo. ______________

DOCUMENTATION/REIMBURSEMENT/MS-DRGs

Often, coding difficulties are due to lack of documentation. Sometimes pathology and other test results are not available at the time of discharge or when the physician is dictating the discharge summary or is reporting the final diagnoses.

When coding meningitis, the causative organism may affect MS-DRG assignment.

Causative Organism

EXAMPLE

DIAGNOSES	CODE	MS-DRG	RW
Viral meningitis	047.9	076	1.1439
Salmonella meningitis	003.21	096	2.3482

Shunt Revision

EXAMPLE

DIAGNOSES	CODE	MS-DRG	RW
Hydrocephalus	331.4	033	1.4281
Revision ventriculoperitoneal shunt (revision of ventricular site)	02.42		
Hydrocephalus	331.4	042	1.8710
Revision ventriculoperitoneal shunt (revision peritoneal site)	54.95		

CHAPTER REVIEW EXERCISE

Answer the following questions and where applicable, assign codes for diagnoses, procedures, V codes, and E codes.

1. Candidal meningitis __________
2. Meningitis with a headache due to herpes zoster virus __________
3. Meningitis due to whooping cough __________
4. Normal pressure hydrocephalus treated with a ventriculocisternal shunt __________
5. Acquired hydrocephalus __________
6. Parkinsonism in Shy-Drager syndrome __________
7. Benign essential tremor __________
8. Lou Gehrig's disease __________
9. Hemiplegia of the right side __________
10. Recurrent seizures __________
11. History of seizures __________
12. Jacksonian seizure __________
13. Intractable epileptic convulsions __________
14. Addison's disease with myopathy __________
15. Intensive care unit myopathy __________
16. Glaucoma suspect __________
17. Aftercataract obscuring vision __________
18. One eye blind, the other with near normal vision __________
19. Lumbar puncture performed on a patient with probable diagnosis of multiple sclerosis __________

Write the correct answer(s) in the space(s) provided.

20. What procedure would a surgeon use to treat tremors in Parkinson's disease? __________

21. Patient with macular degeneration has the drug Visudyne injected, and then a laser is used. What is this procedure known as? __________

22. What is the most common diagnostic test for epilepsy? __________

23. If a surgeon performed a trabeculectomy, what would he or she be treating? __________

CHAPTER GLOSSARY

Alzheimer's: disorder of the brain that causes a progressive decline in mental and physical function.

Autoimmune disorder: disorder that occurs when the immune system attacks itself inappropriately.

Autonomic nervous system: consists of both sensory and motor functions that involve the central nervous system and internal organs.

Cataract: clouding of the lens of the eye causing obstructed vision

Cholesteatoma: growth in the middle ear that usually results from repeated ear infections.

Congenital: a condition present at birth, regardless of causation.

Deep brain stimulation: a procedure used to control tremors.

Electromyelogram: a test that measures electrical activity in muscles and nerves.

Epilepsy: disorder of the brain that is characterized by abnormal electrical discharges from the brain cells.

Glaucoma: disorder of the optic nerve that may resulting in vision loss

Hemiplegia: paralysis of half of the body.

Hydrocephalus: cerebrospinal fluid collection in the skull.

Hypersomnia: excessive sleep.

Insomnia: difficulty falling asleep, wakefulness, and early morning awakening.

Intractable: not manageable

Legal blindness: severe or profound impairment in both eyes

Macular degeneration: vision loss in the central portion of the eye, leaving the patient with peripheral vision or low vision

Mastoiditis: infection of the mastoid bone of the skull

Meningitis: infection or inflammation of the meninges.

Muscular dystrophy: type of myopathy

Myasthenia gravis: chronic autoimmune disorder that manifested by as muscle weakness of varying degrees.

Myopathy: disorder that affects muscles, usually resulting in weakness or atrophy.

Otitis media: middle ear infection

Parkinson's disease: progressive and chronic motor system disorder.

Phacoemulsification: incision is made on the side of the cornea and the lens material is softened, broken, and suctioned out.

Shunting: procedure to drain fluid from brain to relieve pressure.

Sleep apnea: disorder characterized by breathing interruption during sleep.

Somatic nervous system: sends sensory (taste, hearing, smell) information to the central nervous system.

Somnolence: sleepiness.

Vagal nerve stimulator: a device to control seizures.

Ventricular shunting: drainage of fluid from the brain to relieve pressure.

Vertigo: dizziness.

CHAPTER 25

Diseases of the Skin and Subcutaneous Tissue

(ICD-9-CM Chapter 12, Codes 680-709)

CHAPTER OUTLINE

LEARNING OBJECTIVES

- Apply and assign the correct ICD-9-CM codes in accordance with Official Guidelines for Coding and Reporting
- Identify pertinent anatomy and physiology of the skin and subcutaneous tissue
- Identify diseases of the skin and subcutaneous tissue
- Assign the correct V codes and procedure codes related to the skin and subcutaneous tissue
- Identify common treatments, medications, laboratory values, and diagnostic tests
- Explain the importance of documentation in relation to MS-DRGs for reimbursement

ABBREVIATIONS

CEA cultured epidermal autograft

FTSG full-thickness skin graft

ICD-9-CM *International Classification of Diseases, 9th Revision, Clinical Modification*

I&D incision and drainage

MS-DRG Medicare Severity diagnosis-related group

STSG split-thickness skin graft

ICD-9-CM Official Guidelines for Coding and Reporting

Please refer to the companion Evolve website for the most current guidelines.

12. Chapter 12: Diseases Skin and Subcutaneous Tissue (680-709)

Reserved for future guideline expansion

There are no specific official ICD-9-CM coding and reporting guidelines for Chapter 12, Diseases Skin and Subcutaneous Tissue (680-709).

ANATOMY AND PHYSIOLOGY

The skin and its accessory organs constitute the **integumentary** system (Figure 25-1), whose functions include protection, temperature regulation, sensory reception, and vitamin D synthesis.

The skin is composed of 3 layers: epidermis, dermis, and subcutaneous layers. The outer layer of the skin, or the **epidermis**, serves as a protective barrier and prevents the entrance of disease-causing organisms. The **dermis**, or middle layer, is composed of fibrous connective tissues that make it strong and elastic. This middle layer contains blood vessels, nerve fibers, sebaceous glands, and some hair follicles. The **subcutaneous** layer contains fat, sweat glands, and additional hair follicles.

The integumentary system also has accessory organs; these include hair, glands, and nails. Three types of glands are located in the skin: sweat glands, sebaceous glands, and mammary glands. The sweat glands assist in temperature regulation, and the sebaceous glands secrete an oily substance, **sebum,** which lubricates the hair and skin.

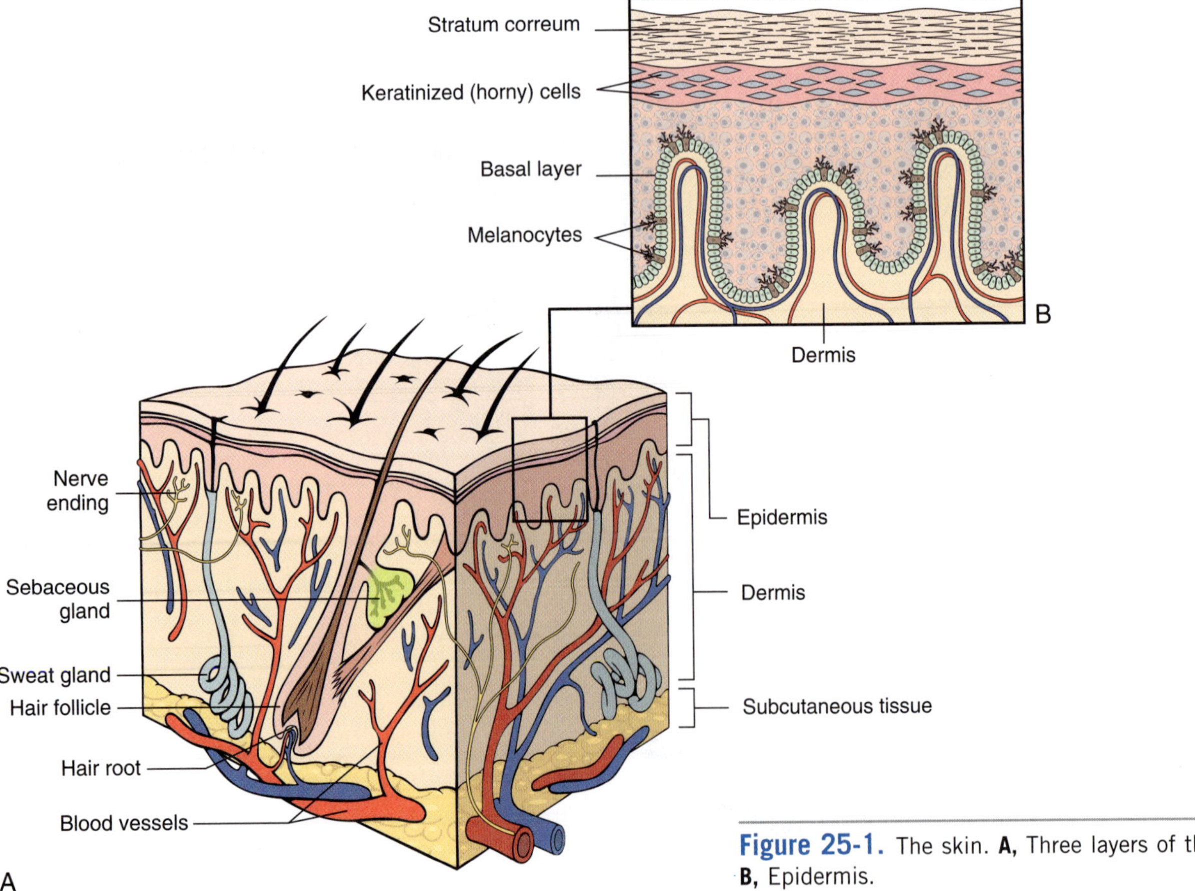

Figure 25-1. The skin. **A,** Three layers of the skin. **B,** Epidermis.

DISEASE CONDITIONS

Diseases of the Skin and Subcutaneous Tissue (680-709), Chapter 12 in the ICD-9-CM code book, is divided into the following categories:

CATEGORY	SECTION TITLES
680-686	Infections of Skin and Subcutaneous Tissue
690-698	Other Inflammatory Conditions of Skin and Subcutaneous Tissue
700-709	Other Diseases of Skin and Subcutaneous Tissue

It is important to recognize that the Excludes note directs the coder to find certain infectious conditions of the skin in the chapter on Infectious and Parasitic Diseases. The most common skin pathogens are *Streptococcus pyogenes* and *Staphylococcus aureus.*

Infections of the Skin and Subcutaneous Tissue (680-686)

Carbuncle and Furuncle

Another name for a **furuncle** is a boil, and a cluster of boils is known as a **carbuncle** (Figure 25-2). The organism that is responsible for a boil is *Staphylococcus.* This organism enters the body through a hair follicle.

Cellulitis/Abscess of the Skin

Cellulitis is an acute inflammation of tissue that is characterized by swelling, redness, and tenderness that are most often caused by a bacterial infection. An abscess is a localized collection of pus that causes swelling. Cellulitis is generally treated with antibiotics; an abscess may be treated with antibiotics and also may require incision and drainage. Cellulitis and abscess are classified to codes 681 and 682.

As is noted in these code categories, lymphangitis is included and is **NOT** coded separately in a patient with cellulitis or abscess. An additional code is used to identify the organism causing the cellulitis, when documented.

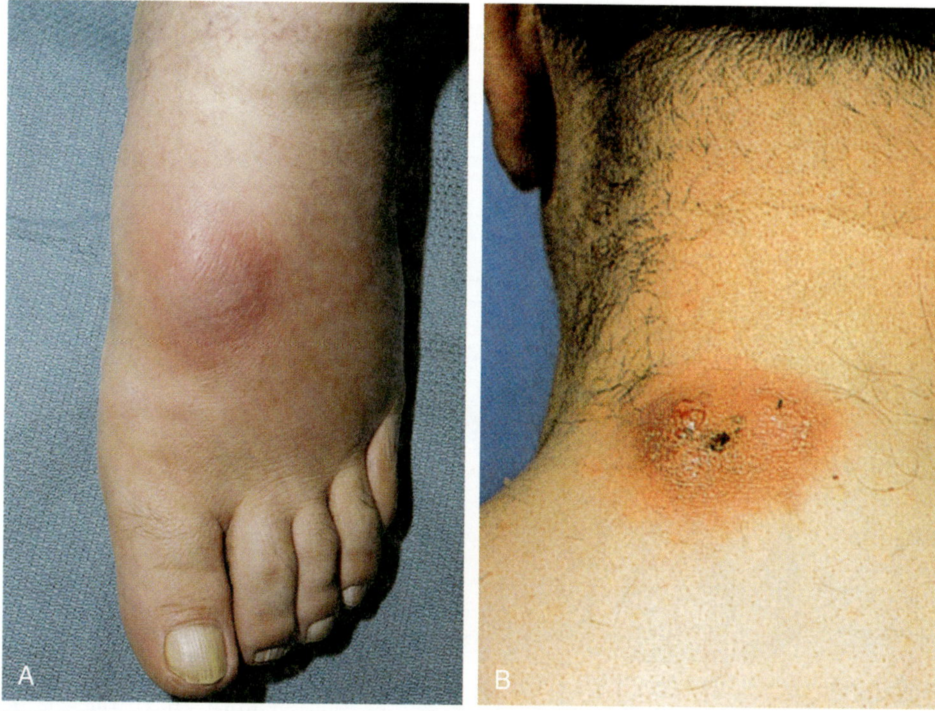

Figure 25-2. A, Furuncle. **B,** Carbuncle.

Cellulitis associated with a superficial injury, burn, or frostbite requires the use of two codes: one code for the injury/burn/frostbite and one code for the cellulitis. Per *Coding Clinic* (1991:2Q:p5-7),[1] the sequence of these codes is dependent on the focus of treatment. For superficial injuries with cellulitis, it is likely that treatment will be focused on the cellulitis.

EXAMPLE Patient with cat scratch of the hand with localized cellulitis admitted for treatment of cellulitis, 682.4, 914.9, E906.8.

Cellulitis associated with a traumatic open wound requires the use of two codes: one code for the open wound, complicated, and one code for the cellulitis. The sequence of these codes is dependent on the focus of treatment. If the focus of treatment is the open wound, the code for the wound is sequenced first, followed by the code for cellulitis. If, on the other hand, the focus of the treatment is the cellulitis and the wound is trivial, or if the wound was treated on a separate occasion, the cellulitis would be sequenced first.

EXAMPLE Patient stepped on a piece of glass and injured his foot 2 days ago. He is now being admitted to the hospital for treatment of cellulitis in the leg, 682.6, 892.1, E920.8.

Cellulitis associated with a postoperative wound infection or cellulitis that results from skin penetration during the use of intravenous therapies requires the use of two codes: one code for the postoperative wound infection and the other code for the cellulitis. No time limit applies regarding when the cellulitis may occur. The postoperative wound infection code is sequenced first.

EXAMPLE Patient is 2 weeks status post appendectomy. Patient presents to the ER with redness and inflammation around the suture site. The patient is admitted for administration of IV antibiotics to treat the cellulitis, 998.59, 682.8, E878.6.

Gangrenous cellulitis is assigned only the code for **gangrene**—NOT a code for cellulitis. Cellulitis associated with a skin ulcer requires the use of two codes: one for the ulcer and one for the cellulitis. The sequence of codes is dependent on the focus of treatment.

EXAMPLE Patient has a chronic leg ulcer with cellulitis. She is admitted to the hospital for treatment of the leg ulcer, 707.10, 682.6.

Cellulitis occurring in areas other than the skin is coded to the chapter that is most appropriate. The coder will find direction in the Alphabetic Index.

EXAMPLE Patient has cellulitis of the lip, 528.5.

EXERCISE 25-1

Assign codes to the following conditions using your ICD-9-CM code book.

1. Cellulitis of the face __________
2. Cellulitis with lymphangitis of the breast. *Staphylococcus aureus* infection __________
3. Cellulitis of the foot due to patient stepping on a nail with open wound of the foot __________
4. Gangrenous cellulitis of toe __________
5. Neck abscess __________
6. Cellulitis, rectum __________

Other Inflammatory Conditions of Skin and Subcutaneous Tissue (690-698)

Dermatitis

Dermatitis is an inflammation of the skin that is also referred to as **eczema**. Dermatitis, which is characterized by redness, itching, scaling, and crusting skin, is caused by contact with a substance (**exogenous**) or ingestion of a substance (**endogenous**).

Category 692 contact dermatis in ICD-9-CM contains a variety of fourth digit codes that are used to identify the substance the patient came into contact with that caused the dermatitis. This category also includes dermatitis due to the effects of solar radiation. When coding dermatitis due to drugs or medicines, the coder must first determine whether the drug was taken as correctly prescribed, causing an adverse reaction, or if the drug was not taken as prescribed, making this a poisoning. An adverse reaction is coded with the dermatitis code first, followed by a therapeutic E code that describes the type of drug that caused the dermatitis.

EXAMPLE Patient with dermatitis caused by tomato juice, 693.1.

A poisoning is coded first with a code from category 960-969, followed by a code for the dermatitis, then an E code to indicate the intent of the poisoning.

EXAMPLE Dermatitis caused by overdose of penicillin taken accidentally, 960.0, 693.0, E856.

Stasis dermatitis is an inflammation of the lower legs that is often associated with venous incompetence. It is important to follow the index carefully. Often, patients have ulcers associated with stasis dermatitis. Per *Coding Clinic* (1991:2Q:p20)[2], these are coded to 454.0, which represents varicose veins with ulcer.

EXAMPLE Patient is being treated for stasis ulcer of the leg without varicose veins, 459.81, 707.10.

EXAMPLE Patient has a stasis ulcer of the right leg with varicose veins, 454.0.

EXAMPLE Patient has varicose veins of the left leg with infl ammation, 454.1

Intertriginous dermatitis, a type of rash that is found in body folds, is a common condition in the overweight patient, possibly because of skin chafing and the inability of sweat to evaporate. This condition is not found under the Dermatitis heading in the index but may be located under **Intertrigo**.

Psoriasis is an inflammation of the skin caused by a fault in the immune system. There are several types of psoriasis, the most common of which is plaque psoriasis. The skin on the elbows, knees, lower back, and scalp are the most common areas plaques are found. Psoriasis usually itches, and the skin may crack and bleed. This is a life-long condition for which there is no cure. Some people develop psoriatic arthritis, which is a systemic rheumatic disease.

"**Hives**" and "**urticaria**" are synonymous terms that refer to vascular reactions of the skin that present as wheals, welts, or reddened patches (Figure 25-3) and are associated with itching (**pruritus**). Hives usually occur as an allergic reaction to food, bug bites, or drugs.

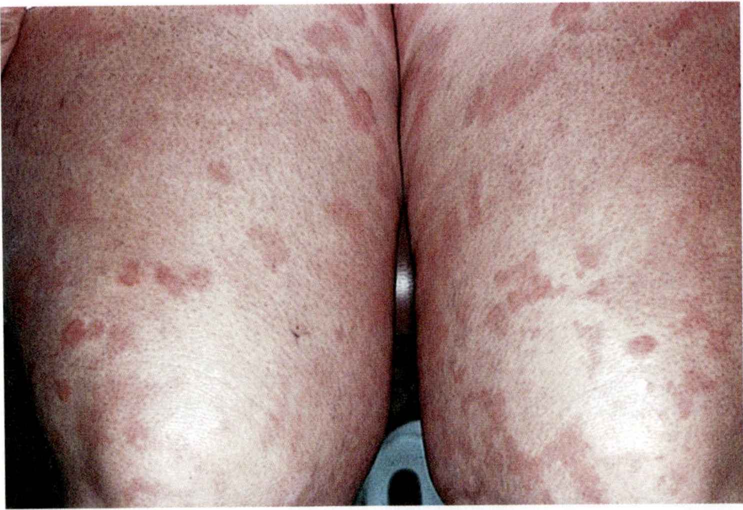

Figure 25-3. Urticaria.

EXAMPLE Patient is treated for hives due to peanuts, 708.0.

EXAMPLE Patient presented with hives. No cause can be determined, 708.9.

EXERCISE 25-2

Assign codes to the following conditions using your ICD-9-CM code book.

1. Contact dermatitis due to mascara ____________
2. Contact dermatitis due to tanning bed ____________
3. Hives due to penicillin ____________
4. Contact dermatitis due to milk ____________
5. Dermatitis, intertriginous ____________

Other Diseases of Skin and Subcutaneous Tissue (700-709)

Skin **ulcers** are open sores of the skin (Figure 25-4). Ulcers may have a variety of causes such as; diabetes, skin cancers, venous insufficiency, arteriosclerosis, and pressure sores (decubitus ulcer). In ICD-9-CM, there are basically two types of ulcers located in the skin; decubitus ulcers and all others. When coding ulcers, note should be taken of the instructions found under the heading 707.1. This note instructs coders that if applicable the code for the underlying condition should be coded first. Per *Coding Clinic* (1991:2Q:p5-7)[1] Cellulitis is coded in addition to the ulcer. The sequencing of the cellulitis and ulcer is dependent on the focus of treatment. When coding gangrene with an ulcer the ulcer is sequenced first.

Decubitus Ulcer

A **decubitus ulcer** is more commonly known as a bed sore or pressure ulcer. (Figure 25-5). These sores occur over bony areas (i.e., heel, hip, sacrum, ankle, and elbow) of patients who are bedridden. Conditions found under this heading are chronic in nature, although the ulcer may be described as infected. A skin ulcer passes through six stages. (Ulcers may be rated slightly differently with the use of different staging scales.)

- Stage 1: Red skin with warmth in the afflicted area
- Stage 2: Skin swollen with possible blisters

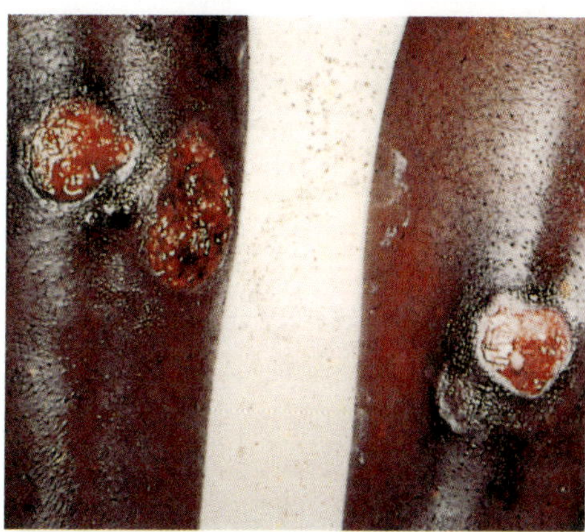

Figure 25-4. Ulcers.

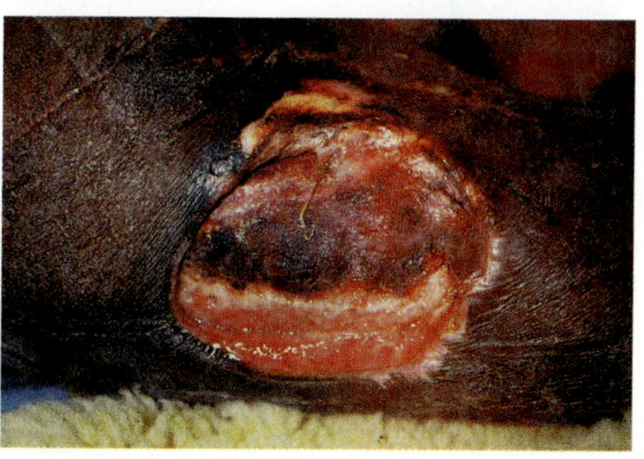

Figure 25-5. Decubitus ulcer.

- Stage 3: Ulcerated sore
- Stage 4: Sore extends into muscle, tendon, and bone

Likewise, because the ulcer has stages, so does the treatment. During early ulcer stages, the patient may be treated with padding; treatment then progresses to wet to dry dressings, debridement, and, in later stages, skin grafting. The stage of the ulcer has no bearing on code selection. At times, decubitus ulcers develop sinuses. According to *Coding Clinic* (1996:1Q:p15),[3] the sinus is part of the disease process and is not coded separately.

EXAMPLE Patient has a sacral decubitus ulcer with gangrene, 707.03, 785.4.

Ulcer of the Lower Limb, Except Decubitus

Ulcers of the lower limb have a fifth digit that describes the area of the limb in which they are located. These ulcers may be caused by other disease conditions. When an ulcer is described as having a causal relationship with another disease condition, the other disease condition is coded first.

EXAMPLE A patient has an ulcer of the heel caused by diabetes, 250.80, 707.14.

Stasis Ulcer

A **stasis ulcer** is associated with varicose veins. These ulcers are not coded as skin ulcers but as ulcers associated with varicose veins. If physician documentation states that the stasis ulcer is caused by a condition other than varicose veins, the index directs the coder to the code 459.81 and to use an additional code for the ulcer (707.10-707.9).

EXAMPLE The patient has a stasis dermatitis due to varicose vein, 454.1.

EXERCISE 25-3

Assign codes to the following conditions using your ICD-9-CM code book.

1. Decubitus ulcer of the heel ____________
2. Stasis ulcer without varicose vein calf ____________
3. Diabetic ulcer of the toe ____________
4. Arteriosclerotic ulcer of the leg with gangrene ____________
5. Ischemic ulcer of the calf ____________
6. Ulcer of the buttocks ____________

V CODES

In the past, V codes have been considered for use primarily in the outpatient setting. This has changed with the addition of more V codes each year. As was discussed in Chapter 8, it is difficult to locate V codes in the Index. Coders will often say, "I did not know there was a V code for that." Refer to Chapter 8 for a listing of common main terms used to locate V codes. V codes that may be used with diseases of the skin and subcutaneous tissue include the following:

V13.3	Diseases of the skin and subcutaneous tissue
V19.4	Family history of skin conditions
V42.3	Skin replaced by transplant
V43.8	Skin replaced by other means
V58.3	Attention to surgical dressings and sutures
V58.77	Aftercare following surgery of the skin and subcutaneous tissue, NEC
V67.51	Following completed treatment with high-risk medications, NEC
V82.0	Special screening for skin conditions

EXAMPLE Patient presents to dermatologist's office after completing treatment for acne with Accutane, V68.51.

EXERCISE 25-4

Assign codes to the following conditions using your ICD-9-CM code book.

1. Patient with a history of eczema ____________
2. Patient with a family history of dermatitis ____________

COMMON TREATMENTS

CONDITION	MEDICATION
Acne	Tetracycline (Achromycin), isotretinoin (Accutane)
Boils	Bacitracin, Neosporin
Cellulitis	Antibiotics such as nafcillin, oxacillin, cefazolin, vancomycin, linezolid
Psoriasis	Topical corticosteroids

PROCEDURES

Some procedures that may be related to diseases of the skin and subcutaneous tissue may be located in the following chapter of the Procedure Tabular:

Chapter 15 Operations of the Integumentary System (85-86)

Incision and Drainage

Incision and drainage (I&D) is a common form of treatment for abscesses of the skin. The physician cuts into the lining of the abscess, which allows the pus to drain. Usually, the physician cleans the cavity with warm saline. If the abscess is deep, the physician may insert a drainage tube. It is important to be aware that I&D can also be used to describe incision and debridement. In cases in which the documentation is questionable a physician query may be necessary.

EXERCISE 25-5

Assign codes to the following conditions using your ICD-9-CM code book.

1. Incision and drainage of neck abscess __________
2. I&D of boil on arm __________
3. Incision and drainage of pilonidal sinus __________

Debridement

Excisional Debridement

Excisional debridement, as defined by *Coding Clinic* (1988:4Q:p5),[4] is "the surgical removal or cutting away of devitalized tissue, necrosis, or slough." Excisional debridements may be performed in a variety of settings (operating room, emergency room, or bedside) and by a variety of healthcare providers (physicians, nurse practitioners, physician assistants, and physical therapists). For a debridement to qualify as excisional, documentation provided by the healthcare provider performing this service must indicate that the procedure involved definite cutting away of the skin (i.e., sharp)—not just minor scissoring of loose fragments. When a laser is used to perform debridement, it qualifies as excisional.

According to *Coding Clinic* (1999:1Q:p8-9),[5] when an extensive debridement goes beyond the skin and subcutaneous tissue into the muscle, tendon, and/or bone, it is appropriate to "assign only a code for the deepest layer of debridement when multiple layers of the same site are débrided." If a patient had a debridement of skin, subcutaneous tissue, muscle and bone, the bone is the deepest layer and debridement of the bone 77.67 is the only procedure code assigned.

EXAMPLE

Patient with a stage 4 decubitus ulcer of the sacrum is taken to the OR for debridement. The debridement is performed through the skin, muscle, and bone, 707.03, 707.24, 77.67.

Nonexcisional Debridement

Any debridement that does not meet the criteria described earlier for excisional debridement would be coded as nonexcisional. A nonexcisional debridement may be performed by brushing, irrigating, scrubbing, or washing to remove devitalized tissue. Once again, this procedure may be performed in a variety of settings by a variety of healthcare providers.

It is important to remember that if debridement of the skin is performed in preparation for further surgery, the debridement should not be coded separately. For example, prior to reduction of an open fracture, a debridement may be performed.

EXAMPLE

Pulse lavage debridement is performed by wound care nurse on a patient with a stage 3 decubitus ulcer of the ankle, 707.06, 707.23, 86.28.

EXERCISE 25-6

Assign codes to the following conditions using your ICD-9-CM code book.

1. Sharp debridement of decubitus ulcer ____________
2. Skin tissue of leg ulcer removed by scrubbing ____________
3. Debridement of a fungus of the nailbed ____________

Skin Grafts

Skin grafts are composed of pieces of skin that are removed from one body area (donor) and are used to cover a defect in another body area (recipient). Several types of skin graft classifications are included in ICD-9-CM.

Free Skin Grafts

Free skin grafts in ICD-CM include the removal of skin from one body area and transplantation to another body area. These may be split-thickness (STSGs) or full-thickness skin grafts (FTSGs) (Figure 25-6). It is important to note the differences between autografts, allografts (**homografts**), and xenografts (heterografts).

- **Autograft**—graft from one area of the body to another in the same individual
- **Allograft**—graft from one person to another
- **Xenograft**—also known as a **heterograft**; graft to an individual from another species such as a pig

A fourth category of graft source is the dermal regenerative graft, which is also known as a cultured epidermal autograft (CEA). These types of grafts are available in several varieties; they may be referred to as artificial skin.

EXAMPLE

Patient presents for full-thickness skin graft to the thigh from the abdomen to repair a skin contracture from a previous burn, 709.2, 906.7, 86.63.

Pedicle Grafts or Flaps

Pedicle grafts or flaps differ from STSG and FTSG in that part of the graft or flaps remains attached to the donor site. A pedicle graft is a full-thickness skin and subcutaneous tissue flap/graft that is attached by tissue (Figure 25-7), through which it receives its blood supply.

EXERCISE 25-7

Assign codes to the following conditions using your ICD-9-CM code book.

1. STSG from patient's thigh to cover scar contracture due to burn from fi re on arm ____________
2. FTSG to hand from buttock due to scar from necrotizing fascitis ____________
3. Advancement flap to nose following surgery to remove skin cancer from nose ____________

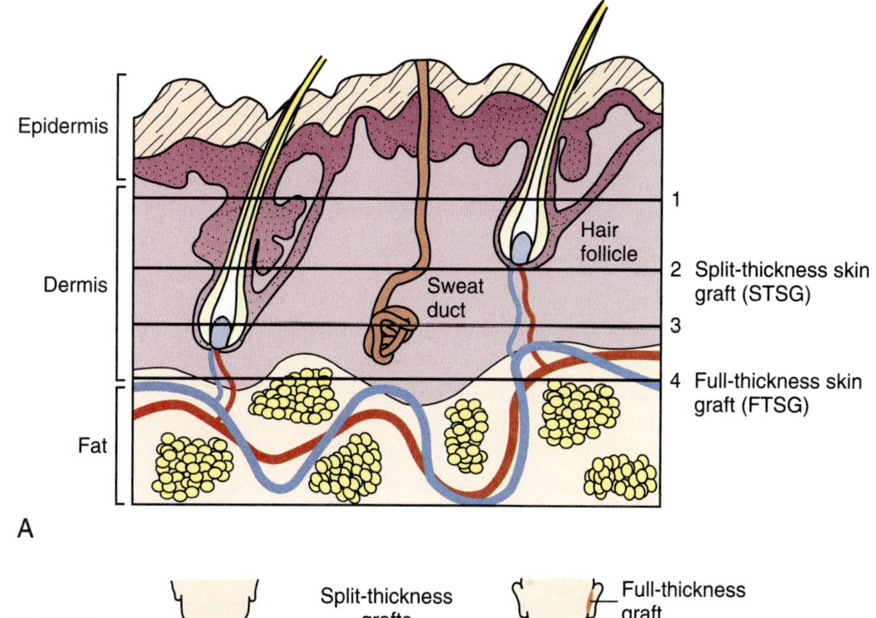

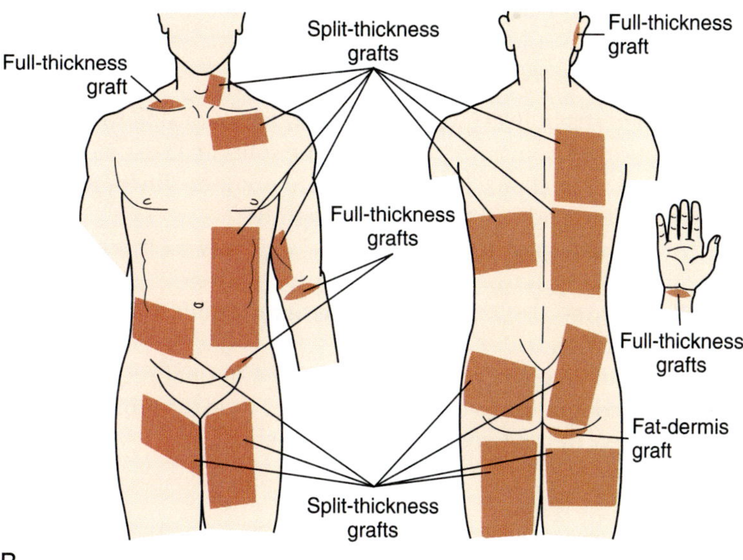

Figure 25-6. Split-thickness and full-thickness skin grafts.

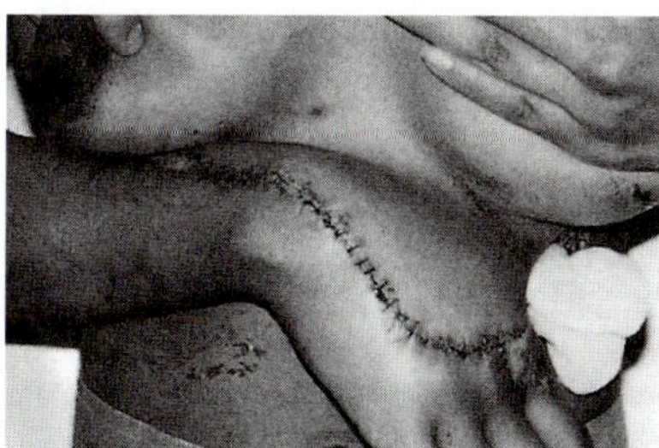

Figure 25-7. Pedicle graft.

DOCUMENTATION/REIMBURSEMENT/MS-DRGs

Often, coding difficulties are due to lack of documentation. Sometimes pathology and other test results are not available at the time of discharge or when the physician is dictating the discharge summary or is reporting the final diagnoses.

It is very important for coding to make sure that healthcare providers fully describe the type of debridement that was performed. If sharp instruments were used to cut away devitalized tissue, this must be documented. This can make a significant difference in MS-DRG assignment and reimbursement.

When physicians state that an I&D was performed, it is imperative to identify whether the physician means incision and drainage or incision and debridement. These terms may be used interchangeably. In most cases, the term "I&D" stands for incision and drainage; however, if it seems unlikely that the condition would require this procedure, a query to the physician is warranted.

Incision and Drainage Versus Debridement

EXAMPLE

DIAGNOSES	CODES	MS-DRG	RW
Decubitus ulcer of heel with Incision and drainage	707.07 86.04	594	0.9335
Decubitus ulcer of heel Excisional debridement	707.07 86.22	575	1.4216

CHAPTER REVIEW EXERCISE

Answer the following and assign codes to the following conditions using your ICD-9-CM code book.

1. Abscess of the leg with cellulitis ____________
2. Decubitus ulcer of the foot with cellulitis ____________
3. Eczema ____________
4. Dermatitis caused by Cipro ____________
5. Dermatitis due to poison sumac ____________
6. Stasis dermatitis with ulcer ____________
7. Diabetic PVD with foot ulcer ____________
8. Incision and drainage of abscess of the leg ____________
9. Excision of a pilonidal cyst ____________
10. Sharp debridement of decubitus ulcer of the buttock by the attending physician ____________

Write the correct answer(s) in the space(s) provided.

11. What is the difference between a pedicle graft and a split-thickness skin graft?

    ____

12. Name one documentation challenge about which coders must be aware in diseases of the skin and subcutaneous tissue.

    ____

13. What are the three accessory organs of the skin?

    ____

    ____

    ____

14. Where in ICD-9-CM would a coder find the skin condition herpes zoster?

    ____

15. What is another name for a decubitus ulcer?

____

16. Name and describe three types of skin grafts.

____

____

____

CHAPTER GLOSSARY

Allograft: graft of tissue between individuals of the same species.

Autograft: graft of tissue from another site on the same individual.

Carbuncle: cluster of boils.

Cellulitis: inflammation of the tissue with possible abscess.

Debridement: removal of devitalized tissue, necrosis, or slough.

Decubitus ulcer: skin ulcer also known as a bed sore.

Dermatitis: inflammation of the skin.

Dermis: layer of skin below the epidermis.

Eczema: type of dermatitis characterized by itching.

Endogenous: type of dermatitis caused by something taken internally, such as medication.

Epidermis: outermost layer of skin.

Excisional: removal by surgical cutting.

Exogenous: type of dermatitis caused by contact with a substance.

Furuncle: a boil.

Heterograft: graft of skin from another species, such as a graft from a pig to a human.

Hives: skin condition also known as urticaria, wherein the skin reacts with welts; characterized by itching.

Homograft: graft from one individual to another of the same species; also known as an allograft.

Integumentary: another name for skin.

Intertrigo: dermatitis taking place in areas where friction may occur.

Osteomyelitis: infection of the bone that often starts in another part of the body and spreads to the bone via the blood.

Pedicle graft/Flap: involves identifying a flap that remains attached to its original blood supply and tunneling it under the skin to a particular area such as the breast.

Pruritus: itching.

Psoriasis: inflammation of skin caused by fault in the immune system.

Sebum: substance secreted from the sebaceous gland.

Stasis Ulcer: ulcer associated with varicose veins.

Subcutaneous: inner layer of the skin that contains fat and sweat glands.

Ulcer: open sore of skin.

Urticaria: another name for hives.

Xenograft: graft to an individual from another species; also known as a heterograft.

CHAPTER 26

Outpatient Coding

CHAPTER OUTLINE

LEARNING OBJECTIVES

- Explain terminology as related to the outpatient setting
- Describe the difference between inpatient coding guidelines and outpatient coding guidelines
- Describe what CPT coding is, when it is used, and the official guideline source
- Apply Diagnostic Coding and Reporting Guidelines for Outpatient Services
- Assign ICD-9-CM codes for outpatient services
- Explain the purpose and use of APCs

ABBREVIATIONS

AICD automatic implantable cardioconverter-defibrillator
AMA American Medical Association
APC Ambulatory Payment Classification
COPD chronic obstructive pulmonary disease
CPT Current Procedural Terminology
CVA cerebrovascular accident
DEXA dual-energy x-ray absorptiometry
ER emergency room
HCPCS Healthcare Common Procedure Coding System
MRI magnetic resonance imaging
MS-DRG Medicare Severity diagnosis-related group
OPPS Outpatient Prospective Payment System
PCP primary care provider
UTI urinary tract infection

OUTPATIENT TERMINOLOGY

Terminology in the outpatient setting is often confusing. Outpatient services may be provided in a variety of settings:

- Doctor's office
- Clinic
- Ambulatory surgery, which may also be called outpatient surgery or "in and out" surgery or same day surgery or same day care
- Emergency room (ER)
- **Observation unit** (a unit to which unstable patients are admitted for a stay of less than 48 hours)

- **Ancillary service** visits/clinic visits (i.e., radiology, laboratory, chemotherapy, radiation therapy)

These outpatient services are called visits or **encounters**. Encounters may require hospital services and/or **professional services** (services rendered by a physician or a non-physician practitioner). For example, a patient receiving a chest x-ray in a hospital setting will have a hospital bill for the chest x-ray and a professional service bill from the radiologist for the reading of the x-ray.

The term "principal diagnosis" as used in the inpatient setting does not apply in the outpatient setting. The outpatient term that is synonymous with "principal diagnosis" is "first-listed diagnosis" or "primary diagnosis."

CODING GUIDELINES FOR THE OUTPATIENT SETTING

ICD-9-CM Official Guidelines for Coding and Reporting

Please refer to the companion Evolve website for the most current guidelines.

Section IV. Diagnostic Coding and Reporting Guidelines for Outpatient Services

These coding guidelines for outpatient diagnoses have been approved for use by hospitals/providers in coding and reporting hospital-based outpatient services and provider-based office visits.

Information about the use of certain abbreviations, punctuation, symbols, and other conventions used in the ICD-9-CM Tabular List (code numbers and titles), can be found in Section IA of these guidelines, under "Conventions Used in the Tabular List." Information about the correct sequence to use in finding a code is also described in Section I.

The terms encounter and visit are often used interchangeably in describing outpatient service contacts and, therefore, appear together in these guidelines without distinguishing one from the other.

Though the conventions and general guidelines apply to all settings, coding guidelines for outpatient and provider reporting of diagnoses will vary in a number of instances from those for inpatient diagnoses, recognizing that:

The Uniform Hospital Discharge Data Set (UHDDS) definition of principal diagnosis applies only to inpatients in acute, short-term, long-term care and psychiatric hospitals.

Coding guidelines for inconclusive diagnoses (probable, suspected, rule out, etc.) were developed for inpatient reporting and do not apply to outpatients.

A. Selection of first-listed condition

In the outpatient setting, the term first-listed diagnosis is used in lieu of principal diagnosis.

In determining the first-listed diagnosis the coding conventions of ICD-9-CM, as well as the general and disease specific guidelines take precedence over the outpatient guidelines.

In the outpatient setting, the first-listed diagnosis is the reason for the encounter. The first-listed diagnosis may often be a symptom.

EXAMPLE

Patient presents to physician's office with complaints of headache and slurred speech. Physician suspects that this patient is experiencing a transient ischemic attack (TIA) or a cerebrovascular accident (CVA). The patient is sent directly to the hospital. The first-listed diagnosis for the physician office visit is 784.0, headache, with a secondary diagnosis of 784.5, slurred speech.

Diagnoses often are not established at the time of the initial encounter/visit. It may take two or more visits before the diagnosis is confirmed.

The most critical rule involves beginning the search for the correct code assignment through the Alphabetic Index. Never begin searching initially in the Tabular List as this will lead to coding errors.

It is common in the outpatient setting for a patient to present to a physician's office with symptoms, for administrative reasons, for follow-up on conditions that no longer exist, or with abnormal findings. A code from the Supplementary Classification of Factors Influencing Health Status and Contact with Health Services (V codes) may often be the most appropriate code. Refer to Chapter 8 for greater detail on assigning V codes.

EXAMPLE

A child presents to his physician's office for a required camp physical V70.3

To locate this code in the Alphabetic Index, look under the main term "Admission for, exam."

EXAMPLE

A healthcare worker is stuck by a needle used on a patient with acquired immunodeficiency syndrome (AIDS). V01.79

To locate this code in the Alphabetic Index, look under the main term "Exposure to."

EXAMPLE

A patient is visiting her oncologist's office for her yearly visit 5 years status post mastectomy for breast cancer. V67.09, V10.3

This code is located in the Alphabetic Index under "Admission for follow-up exam—surgery" and "History, malignant neoplasms, breast." *Coding Clinic* (1984 M-J:p10)[1] instructs coding of follow up visits for cancer patients treated with surgery, who currently have no evidence of cancer to code V67.09 follow up exam following other surgery.

EXAMPLE

A patient presents to her physician's office with a strong family history of breast cancer. She is interested in prophylactic removal of both breasts. V16.3

This code is located in the Alphabetic Index under "History, family, malignant neoplasm."

1. **Outpatient Surgery**
   When a patient presents for outpatient surgery, code the reason for the surgery as the first-listed diagnosis (reason for the encounter), even if the surgery is not performed due to a contraindication.

EXAMPLE

A patient reports to the outpatient surgery department for an arthroscopic meniscectomy for a torn meniscus. The patient injured her meniscus when she tripped over the cat. The patient is administered anesthesia and is found to be in atrial fibrillation. The surgeon decides that it is best not to proceed with the procedure but wishes to consult with a cardiologist and reschedule. The primary diagnosis is the torn meniscus; atrial fibrillation is coded secondarily along with canceled surgery and the E code for the accident, 836.2, 427.31, V64.1, E885.9.

2. Observation Stay

When a patient is admitted for observation for a medical condition, assign a code for the medical condition as the first-listed diagnosis.

When a patient presents for outpatient surgery and develops complications requiring admission to observation, code the reason for the surgery as the first reported diagnosis (reason for encounter), followed by codes for the complications as secondary diagnoses.

EXAMPLE

A patient is admitted to outpatient surgery with cholelithiasis and is scheduled for a laparoscopic cholecystectomy. The surgery proceeds uneventfully. In the recovery room, the patient is found to have hypotension. The surgeon decides to admit the patient for observation, 574.20, 458.9, 51.23.

B. Codes from 001.0 through V84.8

The appropriate code or codes from 001.0 through V84.8 must be used to identify diagnoses, symptoms, conditions, problems, complaints, or other reason(s) for the encounter/visit.

EXAMPLE

When presenting to a doctor's office, a patient often presents with symptoms such as cough or leg pain. At the end of the visit, the physician may not know the cause of the leg pain and therefore may make the assessment that leg pain is probably the result of muscle strain. Therefore, in this case, the code would be 729.5 for leg pain.

C. Accurate reporting of ICD-9-CM diagnosis codes

For accurate reporting of ICD-9-CM diagnosis codes, the documentation should describe the patient's condition, using terminology which includes specific diagnoses as well as symptoms, problems, or reasons for the encounter. There are ICD-9-CM codes to describe all of these.

EXAMPLE

A patient is scheduled for cataract surgery and has congestive heart failure. The surgeon asks the patient's cardiologist for a preoperative consult, V72.81, 428.0, 366.9.

D. Selection of codes 001.0 through 999.9

The selection of codes 001.0 through 999.9 will frequently be used to describe the reason for the encounter. These codes are from the section of ICD-9-CM for the classification of diseases and injuries (e.g., infectious and parasitic diseases; neoplasms; symptoms, signs, and ill-defined conditions, etc.).

E. Codes that describe symptoms and signs

Codes that describe symptoms and signs, as opposed to diagnoses, are acceptable for reporting purposes when a diagnosis has not been established (confirmed) by the provider. Chapter 16 of ICD-9-CM, Symptoms, Signs, and Ill-defined conditions (codes 780.0-799.9) contain many, but not all codes for symptoms.

EXAMPLE

When a patient is seen in a physician's office for a problem-oriented visit, it is often a symptom that will be reported as the first listed diagnosis. A patient may come to the office with abdominal pain, and the physician suspects it is due to diverticulitis. The patient is sent for testing. The first-listed diagnosis for this encounter is 789.00.

On the return visit, test results reveal that the patient does indeed have diverticulitis; therefore, the follow-up visit code would be 562.11.

F. Encounters for circumstances other than a disease or injury

ICD-9-CM provides codes to deal with encounters for circumstances other than a disease or injury. The Supplementary Classification of factors Influencing Health Status and Contact with Health Services (V01.0-V84.8) is provided to deal with occasions when circumstances other than a disease or injury are recorded as diagnosis or problems. ***See Section I.C.18 for information on V-codes***

EXAMPLE

A patient is planning on donating an organ and is seen by their family physician. The patient must be examined so it can be determined whether they qualify as a donor, V70.8.

EXAMPLE

A patient who is on Coumadin therapy for history of DVT is required to visit a Coumadin clinic weekly until the levels of medication are adjusted, V58.83, V58.61, V12.51.

G. Level of Detail in Coding

1. **ICD-9-CM codes with 3, 4, or 5 digits**

   ICD-9-CM is composed of codes with either 3, 4, or 5 digits. Codes with three digits are included in ICD-9-CM as the heading of a category of codes that may be further subdivided by the use of fourth and/or fifth digits, which provide greater specificity.

2. **Use of full number of digits required for a code**

   A three-digit code is to be used only if it is not further subdivided. Where fourth-digit subcategories and/or fifth-digit subclassifications are provided, they must be assigned. A code is invalid if it has not been coded to the full number of digits required for that code.

   See also discussion under Section I.b.3., General Coding Guidelines, Level of Detail in Coding.

H. ICD-9-CM code for the diagnosis, condition, problem, or other reason for encounter/visit

List first the ICD-9-CM code for the diagnosis, condition, problem, or other reason for encounter/visit shown in the medical record to be chiefly responsible for the services provided. List additional codes that describe any coexisting conditions. In some cases the first-listed diagnosis may be a symptom when a diagnosis has not been established (confirmed) by the physician.

It is important when coding outpatient services that codes for all coexisting conditions are also assigned.

EXAMPLE

A patient presents to his primary care provider (PCP) with a cough and a fever and a long history of chronic obstructive pulmonary disease (COPD). After reviewing the chest x-ray, the physician determines that the patient has pneumonia, 486, 496.

I. Uncertain diagnosis
Do not code diagnoses documented as "probable," "suspected," "questionable," "rule out," or "working diagnosis" or other similar terms indicating uncertainty. Rather, code the condition(s) to the highest degree of certainty for that encounter/visit, such as symptoms, signs, abnormal test results, or other reason for the visit. **Please note:** This differs from the coding practices used by short-term, acute care, long-term care and psychiatric hospitals.

Coding Clinic (2005:3Q:p21-2)[2] has also identified the term "compatible" to fall into the same category as possible and probable and a diagnosis described as "compatible with" is not coded in the outpatient setting. The condition should only be coded to the highest degree of certainty for that encounter.

EXAMPLE

A patient presents to her doctor with complaints of weight gain, decreased libido, and cold intolerance. The physician sends her to the laboratory for blood work with a diagnosis of probable hypothyroidism. She is to return in 2 weeks for results of the blood work, which comes back positive for hypothyroidism.

First visit: 783.1, 799.81, 780.99
Second visit: 244.9

J. Chronic diseases
Chronic diseases treated on an ongoing basis may be coded and reported as many times as the patient receives treatment and care for the condition(s).

EXAMPLE

A patient is scheduled for a return visit every 6 months for hypercholesterolemia, 272.0.

K. Code all documented conditions that coexist
Code all documented conditions that coexist at the time of the encounter/visit, and require or affect patient care treatment or management. Do not code conditions that were previously treated and no longer exist. However, history codes (V10-V19) may be used as secondary codes if the historical condition or family history has an impact on current care or influences treatment.

EXAMPLE

A patient presents to a physician's office with a complaint of low back pain and is on medications for hypertension and hypercholesterolemia. During the visit the patient's blood pressure is checked and blood was drawn to check cholesterol level, 724.2, 401.9, 272.0.

This case follows the rule of coding coexisting conditions that affect the management of the patient. The physician must take into account the patient's other history and medications before prescribing medication for the back pain.

L. Patients receiving diagnostic services only
For patients receiving diagnostic services only during an encounter/ visit, sequence first the diagnosis, condition, problem, or other reason for encounter/

visit shown in the medical record to be chiefly responsible for the outpatient services provided during the encounter/visit. Codes for other diagnoses (e.g., chronic conditions) may be sequenced as additional diagnoses.

For encounters for routine laboratory/radiology testing in the absence of any signs, symptoms, or associated diagnosis, assign V72.5 and V72.6. If routine testing is performed during the same encounter as a test to evaluate a sign, symptom, or diagnosis, it is appropriate to assign both the V code and the code describing the reason for the non-routine test.

EXAMPLE

A patient who presents to radiology for a chest x-ray may have a working diagnosis such as cough r/o pneumonia. The ordering physician documents that the patient also has a history of asthma for which he takes albuterol, prn. On reading the x-ray the radiologist documents COPD with no evidence of pneumonia, 786.2, 493.20.

Per *Coding Clinic* (2000:1Q:p4)[3] in the outpatient setting it is permissible to assign codes based on radiology and pathology documentation. This differs from the inpatient setting where diagnosis documented by radiologists and/or pathologists must be confirmed by attending physicians.

For outpatient encounters for diagnostic tests that have been interpreted by a physician, and the final report is available at the time of coding, code any confirmed or definitive diagnosis(es) documented in the interpretation. Do not code related signs and symptoms as additional diagnoses.

Please note: This differs from the coding practice in the hospital inpatient setting regarding abnormal findings on test results.

EXAMPLE

As in the previous example, a patient presents to radiology for a cough/Rule out pneumonia and history of asthma, and after the chest x-ray is performed, the radiologist interprets the x-ray as pneumonia and COPD, 486, 493.20.

The code for the symptom would **not** be assigned.

M. Patients receiving therapeutic services only

For patients receiving therapeutic services only during an encounter/visit, sequence first the diagnosis, condition, problem, or other reason for encounter/visit shown in the medical record to be chiefly responsible for the outpatient services provided during the encounter/visit. Codes for other diagnoses (e.g., chronic conditions) may be sequenced as additional diagnoses.

EXAMPLE

Patient presents to the physician's office monthly for a vitamin B_{12} shot for pernicious anemia, 281.0.

The only exception to this rule is that when the primary reason for the admission/encounter is chemotherapy, radiation therapy, or rehabilitation, the appropriate V code for the service is listed first, and the diagnosis or problem for which the service is being performed listed second.

EXAMPLE

A patient presents to a physician's office for chemotherapy for pancreatic cancer, V58.11, 157.9, 99.25.

N. Patients receiving preoperative evaluations only

For patients receiving preoperative evaluations only, sequence first a code from category V72.8, Other specified examinations, to describe the pre-op consultations. Assign a code for the condition to describe the reason for the surgery as an additional diagnosis. Code also any findings related to the pre-op evaluation.

EXAMPLE

Patient who is planning surgery for an abdominal aortic aneurysm (AAA). The surgeon requests that the patient see her primary care provider for a preoperative evaluation. This patient is well known to her primary care provider and has additional chronic diagnoses of hypertension, hypercholesterolemia, and history of breast cancer, V72.84, 401.9, 272.0, V10.3, 441.4.

O. Ambulatory surgery

For ambulatory surgery, code the diagnosis for which the surgery was performed. If the postoperative diagnosis is known to be different from the preoperative diagnosis at the time the diagnosis is confirmed, select the postoperative diagnosis for coding, since it is the most definitive.

EXAMPLE

A patient undergoes surgery to remove a breast mass. The mass is sent to the pathology department, where a diagnosis of breast cancer is confirmed, 174.9, 85.21.

However, if the pathology report was unequivocal and was sent for a second opinion, the breast mass would be the primary diagnosis, 611.72.

P. Routine outpatient prenatal visits

For routine outpatient prenatal visits when no complications are present, codes V22.0, Supervision of normal first pregnancy, or V22.1, Supervision of other normal pregnancy, should be used as the principal diagnosis. These codes should not be used in conjunction with chapter 11 codes.

EXAMPLE

Patient was seen for prenatal visit. There are no problems noted. Patient has a 3-year-old daughter, V22.1.

PROCEDURE CODING IN THE OUTPATIENT SETTING

When procedures are reported for inpatient coding, ICD-9-CM Volume 3 is used. In the outpatient setting, procedure codes are selected from the **Current Procedural Coding (CPT)** published by the American Medical Association (AMA). Per *Coding Clinic* (2008:1stQ: p15)[4] ICD-9-CM procedure codes are not to be reported for claim submission on outpatient

Mastectomy Procedures

19300	Mastectomy for gynecomastia
19301	Mastectomy, partial (eg, lumpectomy, tylectomy, quadrantectomy, segmentectomy);
19302	with axillary lymphadenectomy
	(For placement of radiotherapy afterloading balloon/brachytherapy catheters, see 19296-19298)
19303	Mastectomy, simple, complete

Figure 26-1. Example of CPT codes (Level I HCPCS).

Chemotherapy Drugs *J9000-J9999*

J9000	**Doxorubicin HCl, 10 mg** **Use this code for Adriamycin PFS, Adriamycin RDF, Rubex.** **MED: 100-2, 15, 50**
J9001	**Doxorubicin HCl, all lipid formulations, 10 mg** **Use this code for Doxil.** **MED: 100-2, 15, 50**
J9010	**Alemtuzumab, 10 mg** **Use this code for Campath.**
J9015	**Aldesleukin, per single use vial** **Use this code for Proleukin, IL-2, Interleukin.** **MED: 100-2, 15, 50**

Figure 26-2. Example of HCPCS Level II codes.

encounters. According to the Health Insurance Portability and Accountability Act (HIPAA), "The use of ICD-9-CM procedure codes is restricted to the reporting of inpatient procedures by hospital." Hospitals may still elect to code outpatient visits with ICD-9-CM procedure codes for non–claim-related purposes. CPT is a coding system for reporting medical services and procedures performed by healthcare providers. Physicians report office visits using CPT codes (Figure 26-1) to describe the service provided, along with diagnostic codes from ICD-9-CM to describe why the service was performed.

CPT is Level I of the Healthcare Common Procedure Coding System (HCPCS). CPT is published yearly by the AMA. Revisions are effective for dates of service after January 1 of each year. CPT codes are five-digit numeric codes.

Level II of HCPCS consists of alphanumeric codes (Figure 26-2). These codes, which are used to identify drugs, medical supplies, and durable medical equipment, are maintained by the HCPCS National Panel, which is composed of Blue Cross/Blue Shield, the Health Insurance Association of America, and Centers for Medicare and Medicaid Services (CMS).

EXAMPLE

Patient with acute appendicitis had laparoscopic appendectomy, 540.9, 44970 (CPT code).

EXAMPLE

Patient with right carpal tunnel syndrome had an endoscopic carpal tunnel release, 354.0 29848 (CPT code).

V CODES

V codes have been considered for use primarily in the outpatient setting. As was discussed in Chapter 8, it is difficult to locate V codes in the Index. Coders will often say, "I did not know there was a V code for that." Many of these V codes have been presented in previous chapters. Refer to Chapter 8 for a listing of common main terms used to locate V codes.

The following list provides only a sample of the many codes that can be used:

V06.6	Need for prophylactic vaccination, *Streptococcus pneumoniae* and influenza
V22.2	Pregnant state, incidental
V23.0	Pregnancy with history of infertility
V23.2	Pregnancy with history of abortion
V23.41	Pregnancy with history of preterm labor
V23.81	Elderly primigravida
V23.53	Young primigravida
V25.01	Encounter for prescription of oral contraceptive
V25.42	Surveillance of intrauterine contraceptive device
V28.1	Encounter for antenatal screening of mother for raised alpha-fetoprotein levels in amniotic fluid
V50.1	Elective surgery for purposes other than remedying health states: plastic surgery for unacceptable cosmetic appearance
V3.01	Fitting and adjustment of cerebral ventricular shunt
V54.0	Encounter for removal of internal fixation device
V54.11	Aftercare for healing traumatic fracture of hip
V56.0	Encounter for extracorporeal dialysis
V57.3	Care involving use of rehabilitation: speech therapy
V58.11	Encounter for antineoplastic chemotherapy
V581.81	Fitting and adjustment of vascular catheter
V65.2	Person feigning illness
V65.3	Dietary surveillance and counseling
VV67.11	Following surgery, unspecified
V68.0	Encounter for issue of medical certificate
V70.0	Routine general medical examination at a healthcare facility
V72.31	Routine gynecologic examination
V72.82	Preoperative respiratory examination

APCs AS REIMBURSEMENT

Ambulatory Payment Classifications (APCs) became effective on August 1, 2000. APCs constitute a reimbursement system that is similar to Medicare Severity diagnosis-related groups (MS-DRGs), which are used in the inpatient setting. APCs categorize outpatient procedures into similar groups for payment purposes (Figure 26-3). This is Medicare's Outpatient Prospective Payment System (OPPS). Assignment to an APC is based primarily on CPT codes. One of the big differences between MS-DRGs and APCs is that more than one APC may be assigned per claim.

Addendum A.—Opps APCS for CY 2008						
APC	Group title	SI	Relative weight	Payment rate	National unadjusted copayment	Minimum unadjusted copayment
0001	Level I Photochemotherapy	S	0.4806	$30.61	$7.00	$6.12
0002	Level I Fine Needle Biopsy/Aspiration	T	1.1097	$70.68		$14.14
0003	Bone Marrow Biopsy/Aspiration	T	3.1008	$197.50		$39.50
0004	Level I Needle Biopsy/Aspiration Except Bone Marrow	T	4.2370	$275.60		$55.12
0005	Level II Needle Biopsy/Aspiration Except Bone Marrow	T	7.1147	$453.16		$90.63
0006	Level I Incision and Drainage	T	1.4066	$89.59		$17.92
0007	Level II Incision and Drainage	T	11.5594	$736.26		$147.25
0008	Level III Incision and Drainage	T	18.3197	$1,166.85		$233.37
0012	Level I Debridement and Destruction	T	0.2963	$18.87		$3.77
0013	Level II Debridement and Destruction	T	0.7930	$50.51		$10.10
0015	Level III Debridement and Destruction	T	1.4595	$92.96		$18.59
0016	Level IV Debridement and Destruction	T	2.6604	$169.45		$33.89
0017	Level VI Debridement and Destruction	T	19.9041	$1,267.77		$253.55
0019	Level I Excision/Biopsy	T	4.3039	$274.13	$71.87	$54.83
0020	Level II Excision/Biopsy	T	8.6850	$553.18		$110.64
0021	Level III Excision/Biopsy	T	16.1001	$1,025.48	$219.48	$205.10
0022	Level IV Excision/Biopsy	T	21.1098	$1,344.57	$354.45	$268.91
0023	Exploration Penetrating Wound	T	9.6341	$613.63		$122.73

Figure 26-3. Example of APCs.

CHAPTER REVIEW EXERCISE

Answer questions or assign ICD-9-CM codes for all diagnoses and procedures, including all applicable V and E codes and procedures.

1. Outpatient visits are only visits to physicians' offices.
   A. True
   B. False
2. The same coding guidelines apply to inpatient and outpatient settings.
   A. True
   B. False
3. What is another name for "in and out" surgery?

   ____
4. What is the term in the outpatient setting for principal diagnosis?

   ____
5. Is an encounter the same as a visit?

   ____
6. A coder should always begin the search for the correct code in the Tabular List.
   A. True
   B. False
7. Patient presents to office with burning on urination. Physician performs a urinalysis, which is sent out to the laboratory. Physician prescribes antibiotics for presumed urinary tract infection (UTI). ____________
8. Patient presents to ER stating that she has been raped. A rape kit is used to determine whether the rape actually occurred. Results were negative. ____________
9. Patient presents to the gynecologist's office for a routine Pap and pelvic examination ____________

10. Postmenopausal patient is sent for dual-energy x-ray absorptiometry (DEXA) scan to evaluate status of bone loss ____________
11. Diabetic patient is sent to nutrionist for dietary counseling ____________
12. Child presents to physician's office for routine vaccination. The physician decides not to administer because the child has a cold ____________
13. Patient and husband present to clinical social worker for marriage counseling ____________
14. Patient had a malignant neoplasm of the lung removed. She presents to the surgeon for routine aftercare ____________
15. Patient presents to physician's office for reprogramming of an automatic implantable cardioverter-defibrillator (AICD) ____________
16. Patient presents to physician's office complaining of dizziness ____________
17. Patient presents to physician's office complaining of testicular pain. Physician prescribes antibiotics and says the symptoms are compatible with epididymitis ____________
18. Patient presents to physician's office as a possible bone marrow donor for her sister ____________
19. Patient presents to physician's office with severe headache. Physician sends patient for magnetic resonance imaging (MRI) and notes to rule out cerebrovascular accident (CVA) in a patient with a history of hypertension and coronary artery disease ____________
20. Patient is seen in doctor's office for abdominal pain. After examination, the physician states that this is probably due to diverticulitis in that the patient has known diverticulum. He also notes that this patient has a history of alcohol abuse and is currently drinking on a daily basis ____________
21. Patient presents to doctor's office with fever, cough, and muscle aches and pains. Physician is uncertain as to whether these symptoms are an exacerbation of her COPD, or whether she has viral pneumonia. Laboratory work is ordered ____________

CHAPTER GLOSSARY

Ambulatory Payment Classifications (APCs): used for outpatient prospective payment.

Ancillary Services: services provided by a hospital that are additional to a professional service, such as laboratory work and radiology and pathology services.

Current Procedural Terminology (CPT): a coding system for reporting medical services and procedures.

Encounter: face-to-face visit with a healthcare provider.

Level II HCPCS: codes used to identify drugs, medical supplies, and durable medical equipment.

Observation unit: area outside the emergency department where unstable patients are admitted for a stay of less than 48 hours. The patient is observed for admission to the hospital or discharge to home.

Professional service: service rendered by a physician or a nonphysician practitioner.

CHAPTER 27

ICD-10-CM and ICD-10-PCS

CHAPTER OUTLINE

LEARNING OBJECTIVES

- Describe the history and development of ICD-10-CM
- Explain the difference between ICD-9-CM and ICD-10-CM
- Discuss the difference between ICD-9-CM, Volume 3, and ICD-10-PCS
- List the pros and cons to implementation of ICD-10-CM and ICD-10-PCS
- Delineate coder training needs
- Assign ICD-10-CM and ICD-10-PCS codes

ABBREVIATIONS

A&P anatomy and physiology
AHA American Hospital Association
AHIMA American Health Information Management Association
CM Clinical Modification
CMS Centers for Medicaid and Medicare Services
COPD chronic obstructive pulmonary disease
ICD International Classification of Diseases
IS Information Systems
NCVHS National Committee on Vital and Health Statistics
NEC not elsewhere classifiable
NCHS National Center for Health Statistics
NOS not otherwise specified
PCS Procedure Classification System
UR Utilization Review
WHO World Health Organization

ICD-10-CM GUIDELINES

The ICD-10-CM guidelines can be found at the National Center for Health Statistics website.

They are very similar to ICD-9-CM with some exceptions.

HISTORY OF ICD-10-CM

Please refer to Chapter 1 for a detailed history of the International Classification of Diseases (ICD). When ICD was originally developed, it was proposed that it should be updated every 10 years. In the Ninth Revision, made available in 1979, more detail was added, including fifth digits. At the time of introduction of ICD-9-CM, discussions were held regarding the

1. The secretary accepts the NCVHS recommendation.
2. The federal government publishes a notice of proposed rule making (NPRM) calling for public comment on their policy plus the published ICD-10-CM and ICD-10-PCS materials incorporated by reference.
3. The public at large has at least 30, but more likely 60, days to submit comments on the NPRM and its incorporated materials.
4. The federal government analyzes the public comments. Based on this analysis, any necessary changes are made.
5. The federal government publishes a final rule containing its updated policy, explanations thereof, plus the implementation date.
6. The standard HIPAA compliance clock for new transactions begins—two years for all but small health plans, who get three years.

Figure 27-1. Adoption process for ICD-10-CM and ICD-10-PCS.

use of this system for reimbursement. Because ICD-9-CM was based on 1970 medical knowledge, and because much has changed in the almost 30 years that it has been in existence, it was evident that a change was necessary.

Work on ICD-10 was begun in 1983. The tabular volume was published in 1992, and the instructional volume followed in 1993; the Alphabetic Index was published in 1994. In 1994, the United States began the process of determining whether a clinical modification (CM) would be necessary. A draft version was made available in 2002 and updated in July 2007; this will be updated until it is officially implemented. This version can be found at the National Center for Health Statistics website.

Clinical modifications made to ICD-10 allow a higher level of specificity. Since 1999, ICD-10 has been used in the United States for the reporting of mortality data. A total of 99 countries, including Canada and Australia, are currently using ICD-10; the United States is virtually the only industrialized nation that is not using ICD-10 for other than mortality data. At the writing of this book, no date has been set for implementation (Figure 27-1) of ICD-10-CM.

EXAMPLE Patient presents with diabetic ketoacidosis, E09.10.

EXAMPLE Patient presents with congestive heart failure, I50.9

COMPARISON OF ICD-10-CM AND ICD-9-CM

As noted in Table 27-1, considerable differences can be seen between ICD-10-CM and ICD-9-CM. Most notable is the increase in the number of codes and code categories, the change from numeric to alphanumeric with an increase in digits from 5 to 7, and the increase from 17 chapters to 21 chapters. Some of these differences can be seen in Figure 27-2, which is an excerpt from the Alphabetic Index from ICD-10-CM, and in Figure 27-3, which is an excerpt from the Tabular List.

The best way to appreciate these differences is to view code assignment for the same disease process from both classification systems.

EXAMPLE

Newborn baby delivered via c-section V30.01 (ICD-9-CM)
Newborn baby delivered via c-section Z38.01 (ICD-10-CM)

Table 27-1. Comparison of ICD-10-CM and ICD-9-CM*

ICD-9-CM	ICD-10-CM
13,000 codes	120,000 codes
855 code categories	2033 code categories
Codes begin with number except for V&E supplementary classification	Codes begin with a letter
Maximum 5 number code	3 to 7 characters
All codes end in a number	Codes may end in a number or a letter
Morphology codes begin with M	Both morphology and musculoskeletal codes begin with M
Three tables: Neoplasms, Drugs and Chemicals, Hypertension	Two tables: Neoplasms, Drugs and Chemicals
17 chapters with 2 supplements	21 chapters
1 chapter for Diseases of the Nervous System, Eyes, Ears	3 chapters for Nervous System, Eyes, Ears
No laterality included in codes	Laterality included in codes
Sometimes combine NEC (not elsewhere classified) and NOS (not otherwise specified)	Never combine NEC and NOS
Not in ICD-9-CM	7th character extensions
Not in ICD-9-CM	Placeholder letter X
Excludes notes	Excludes notes 1 and 2

*The index and the tabular of ICD-10-CM are very similar in style to ICD-9-CM. Please refer to Figures 27-2 through 27-7.

Nephrocalcinosis E83.59 *[N29]*
Nephrocystitis, pustular - see Nephritis, tubulo-interstitial
Nephrolithiasis (congenital)(pelvis)(recurrent) - see also Calculus, kidney
-gouty M10.08
-uric acid M10.08
Nephroma (M8960/3) C64.9
-left C64.1
-mesoblastic (M8960/1) D41.00
--left D41.02
--right D41.01
-right C64.0
Nephronephritis - see Nephrosis
Nephronophthisis Q61.5
Nephropathia epidemica A98.5
Nephropathy (see also Nephritis) N28.9
-with
--edema - see Nephrosis
--glomerular lesion - see Glomerulonephritis
-amyloid, hereditary E85
-analgesic N14.0
--with medullary necrosis, acute N17.2
-Balkan (endemic) N15.0
-chemical - see Nephropathy, toxic
-diabetic - see E09-E13 with .21

Figure 27-2. Excerpt from the draft of the Alphabetic Index for ICD-10-CM.

EXAMPLE

Aspiration pneumonia	507.0 (ICD-9-CM)
Aspiration pneumonia	J69.0 (ICD-10-CM)

Further comparison shows differences between the Neoplasm Tables (Figure 27-4 shows ICD-10-CM and Figure 27-5 shows ICD-9-CM) and reveals differences between the Table of Drugs and the Chemicals Table (Figure 27-6 shows ICD-10-CM and Figure 27-7 shows ICD-9-CM).

A90-A99 Arthropod-borne viral fevers and viral hemorrhagic fevers
B00-B09 Viral infections characterized by skin and mucous membrane lesions
B15-B19 Viral hepatitis
B20 Human immunodeficiency virus [HIV] disease
B25-B34 Other viral diseases
B35-B49 Mycoses
B50-B64 Protozoal diseases
B65-B83 Helminthiases
B85-B89 Pediculosis, acariasis and other infestations
B90-B94 Sequelae of infectious and parasitic diseases
B95-B97 Bacterial, viral and other infectious agents
B99 Other infectious diseases

Intestinal infectious diseases (A00-A09)

A00 Cholera
- **A00.0 Cholera due to Vibrio cholerae 01, biovar cholerae**
  Classical cholera
- **A00.1 Cholera due to Vibrio cholerae 01, biovar eltor**
  Cholera eltor
- **A00.9 Cholera, unspecified**

A01 Typhoid and paratyphoid fevers
- A01.0 Typhoid fever
  Infection due to Salmonella typhi
  - **A01.00 Typhoid fever, unspecified**
  - **A01.01 Typhoid meningitis**
  - **A01.02 Typhoid fever with heart involvement**
    Typhoid endocarditis
    Typhoid myocarditis
  - **A01.03 Typhoid pneumonia**
  - **A01.04 Typhoid arthritis**
  - **A01.05 Typhoid osteomyelitis**
  - **A01.09 Typhoid fever with other complications**
- **A01.1 Paratyphoid fever A**
- **A01.2 Paratyphoid fever B**
- **A01.3 Paratyphoid fever C**
- **A01.4 Paratyphoid fever, unspecified.**
  Infection due to Salmonella paratyphi NOS

Figure 27-3. Excerpt from the draft of the Tabular List for ICD-10-CM.

EXERCISE 27-1

Look up the following codes in ICD-10-CM using the link for the ICD-10-CM index and the link for the ICD-10-CM tabular at the National Center for Health Statistics Disease Classification ICD-10-CM website. Then, look up codes in ICD-9-CM to compare. Make note of any difference.

1. Streptococcal B pneumonia
   ICD-10-CM ____________ ICD-9-CM ____________
2. Chronic obstructive pulmonary disease (COPD)
   ICD-10-CM ____________ ICD-9-CM ____________
3. Diabetic nephropathy type II
   ICD-10-CM ____________ ICD-9-CM ____________
4. Bilateral macular degeneration
   ICD-10-CM ____________ ICD-9-CM ____________
5. Patient has a cough and has asthma
   ICD-10-CM ____________ ICD-9-CM ____________
6. Abnormality in fetal heart rate and rhythm complicating labor and delivery, fetus 1
   ICD-10-CM ____________ ICD-9-CM ____________
7. Fracture of the distal end of the humerus; subsequent encounter for nonunion
   ICD-10-CM ____________ ICD-9-CM ____________
8. Poisoning by sulfonamides, accidental, initial encounter
   ICD-10-CM ____________ ICD-9-CM ____________

	Malignant primary	Malignant secondary	Malignant ca in situ	Benign	Uncertain behavior	Unspecified
left side	C74.92	C79.72	D09.3	D35.02	D44.12	D49.7
right side	C74.91	C79.71	D09.3	D35.01	D44.11	D49.7
ala nasi (external)	C44.3	C79.2	D04.39	D23.39	D48.5	D49.2
alimentary canal or tract NEC	C26.9	C78.80	D01.9	D13.9	D37.9	D49.0
alveolar	C03.9	C79.89	D00.03	D10.39	D37.09	D49.0
mucosa	C03.9	C79.89	D00.03	D10.39	D37.09	D49.0
lower	C03.1	C79.89	D00.03	D10.39	D37.09	D49.0
upper	C03.0	C79.89	D00.03	D10.39	D37.09	D49.0
ridge or process	C41.1	C79.51	–	D16.5	D48.0	D49.2
carcinoma	C03.9	–	–	–	–	–
lower	C03.1	–	–	–	–	–
upper	C03.0	–	–	–	–	–
lower	C41.1	C79.51	–	D16.5	D48.0	D49.2
marrow NEC	C96.9	C79.52	–	–	–	D47.9
marrow NEC	C96.9	C79.52	–	–	–	D47.9
mucosa	C03.9	C79.89	D00.03	D10.39	D37.09	D49.0
lower	C03.1	C79.89	D00.03	D10.39	D37.09	D49.0
upper	C03.0	C79.89	D00.03	D10.39	D37.09	D49.0
upper	C41.0	C79.51	–	D16.4	D48.0	D49.2
marrow NEC	C96.9	C79.52	–	–	–	D47.9
sulcus	C06.1	C79.89	D00.02	D10.39	D37.09	D49.0
alveolus	C03.9	C79.89	D00.03	D10.39	D37.09	D49.0
lower	C03.1	C79.89	D00.03	D10.39	D37.09	D49.0
upper	C03.0	C79.89	D00.03	D10.39	D37.09	D49.0
ampulla of Vater	C24.1	C78.89	D01.5	D13.5	D37.6	D49.0
ankle (unspecified side) NEC*	C76.50	C79.89	D04.70	D36.7	D48.7	D49.8
left side	C76.52	C79.89	D04.72	D36.7	D48.7	D49.8
right side	C76.51	C79.89	D04.71	D36.7	D48.7	D49.8
anorectum, anorectal (junction)	C21.8	C78.5	D01.3	D12.9	D37.7	D49.0
antecubital fossa or space (unspecified side)*	C76.40	C79.89	D04.60	D36.7	D48.7	D49.8

Figure 27-4. Index to Neoplasms for ICD-10-CM.

ICD-10-PCS

Differences Between ICD-9-CM, Volume 3, and ICD-10-PCS

There is tremendous difference between ICD-9-CM, Volume 3, and ICD-10-PCS. Following are a few examples:

ICD-9-CM, VOLUME 3	ICD-10-PCS
4000 procedure codes	200,000 procedure codes
Numeric	Alphanumeric
4 characters	7 characters

In 1992, the Centers for Medicare and Medicaid Services (CMS) funded a project to replace Volume 3 of ICD-9-CM. 3M was awarded the contract to develop this system. The final draft of ICD-10-PCS was completed in 1998; the work is updated every October to allow changes made to ICD-9-CM, Volume 3. ICD-10-PCS (Procedure Classification System). This draft can be found at the Center for Medicare and Medicaid website.

Because no international classification of procedures is currently available, ICD-10-PCS was not based on any model other than ICD-9-CM, Volume 3. This procedure classification system was developed with four characteristics in mind:

1. Completeness—Each procedure should have its own code.
2. Expandability—New procedure codes should be easily added.

	Malignant					
	Primary	Secondary	Ca in situ	Benign	Uncertain behavior	Unspecified
Neoplasm, neoplastic..	199.1	199.1	234.9	229.9	238.9	239.9
ala nasi (external)..........	173.3	198.2	232.3	216.3	238.2	239.2
alimentary canal or tract						
NEC........................	159.9	197.8	230.9	211.9	235.5	239.0
alveolar..........................	143.9	198.89	230.0	210.4	235.1	239.0
mucosa.......................	143.9	198.89	230.0	210.4	235.1	239.0
lower.......................	143.1	198.89	230.0	210.4	235.1	239.0
upper.......................	143.0	198.89	230.0	210.4	235.1	239.0
ridge or process.........	170.1	198.5	—	213.1	238.0	239.2
carcinoma..............	143.9	—	—	—	—	—
lower....................	143.1	—	—	—	—	—
upper....................	143.0	—	—	—	—	—
lower.......................	170.1	198.5	—	213.1	238.0	239.2
mucosa...................	143.9	198.89	230.0	210.4	235.1	239.0
lower....................	143.1	198.89	230.0	210.4	235.1	239.0
upper....................	143.0	198.89	230.0	210.4	235.1	239.0
upper.......................	170.0	198.5	—	213.0	238.0	239.2
sulcus.........................	145.1	198.89	230.0	210.4	235.1	239.0
alveolus.........................	143.9	198.89	230.0	210.4	235.1	239.0
lower...........................	143.1	198.89	230.0	210.4	235.1	239.0
upper...........................	143.0	198.89	230.0	210.4	235.1	239.0
ampulla of Vater............	156.2	197.8	230.8	211.5	235.3	239.0
ankle NEC*....................	195.5	198.89	232.7	229.8	238.8	239.8
anorectum, anorectal						
(junction)................	154.8	197.5	230.7	211.4	235.2	239.0
antecubital fossa or						
space*....................	195.4	198.89	232.6	229.8	238.8	239.8

Figure 27-5. Index to Neoplasms for ICD-9-CM.

Substance	Poisoning, accidental (unintentional)	Poisoning, intentional self-harm	Poisoning, assault	Poisoning undetermined	Adverse effect	Underdosing
Benoquin	T49.8x1	T49.8x2	T49.8x3	T49.8x4	T49.8x5	T49.8x6
Benoxinate	T41.3x1	T41.3x2	T41.3x3	T41.3x4	T41.3x5	T41.3x6
Benperidol	T43.4x1	T43.4x2	T43.4x3	T43.4x4	T43.4x5	T43.4x6
Benproperine	T48.3x1	T48.3x2	T48.3x3	T48.3x4	T48.3x5	T48.3x6
Benserazide	T42.8x1	T42.8x2	T42.8x3	T42.8x4	T42.8x5	T42.8x6
Bentazepam	T42.4x1	T42.4x2	T42.4x3	T42.4x4	T42.4x5	T42.4x6
Bentiromide	T50.8x1	T50.8x2	T50.8x3	T50.8x4	T50.8x5	T50.8x6
Bentonite	T49.3x1	T49.3x2	T49.3x3	T49.3x4	T49.3x5	T49.3x6
Benzalbutyramide	T46.6x1	T46.6x2	T46.6x3	T46.6x4	T46.6x5	T46.6x6
Benzalkonium (chloride)	T49.0x1	T49.0x2	T49.0x3	T49.0x4	T49.0x5	T49.0x6
-ophthalmic preparation	T49.5x1	T49.5x2	T49.5x3	T49.5x4	T49.5x5	T49.5x6

Figure 27-6. Excerpt from the Table of Drugs and Chemicals from the 2007 release of ICD-10-CM.

		External cause (E-code)				
	Poisoning	**Accident**	**Therapeutic use**	**Suicide attempt**	**Assault**	**Undetermined**
Benoquin......................	976.8	E858.7	E946.8	E950.4	E962.0	E980.4
Benoxinate..................	968.5	E855.2	E938.5	E950.4	E962.0	E980.4
Bentonite......................	976.3	E858.7	E946.3	E950.4	E962.0	E980.4
Benzalkonium (chloride)	976.0	E858.7	E946.0	E950.4	E962.0	E980.4
ophthalmic preparation	976.5	E858.7	E946.5	E950.4	E962.0	E980.4
Benzamidosalicylate (calcium)................	961.8	E857	E931.8	E950.4	E962.0	E980.4
Benzathine penicillin...	960.0	E856	E930.0	E950.4	E962.0	E980.4
Benzcarbimine............	963.1	E858.1	E933.1	E950.4	E962.0	E980.4
Benzedrex....................	971.2	E855.5	E941.2	E950.4	E962.0	E980.4
Benzedrine (amphetamine)	969.7	E854.2	E939.7	E950.3	E962.0	E980.3
Benzene (acetyl)(dimethyl) (methyl)(solvent)(vapor)	982.0	E862.4	—	E950.9	E962.1	E980.9
hexachloride (gamma) (insecticide)(vapor)	989.2	E863.0	—	E950.6	E962.1	E980.7

Figure 27-7. Excerpt from the Table of Drugs and Chemicals from ICD-9-CM.

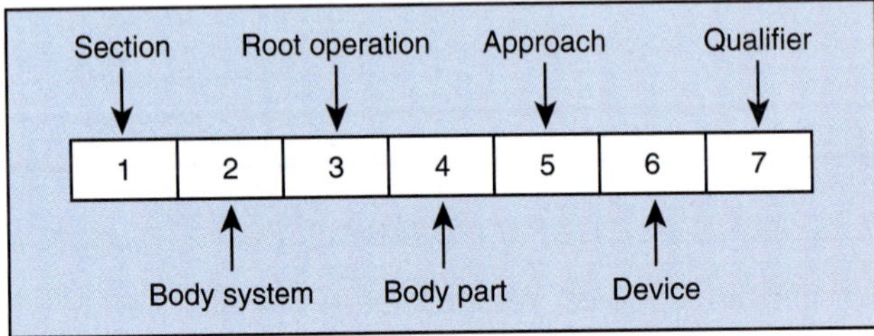

Figure 27-8. Code structure of ICD-10-PCS.

3. Multiaxial—Each code character should have the same meaning across and within body systems (Figure 27-8).
4. Standardized terminology—ICD-10-PCS will include definitions for terminology used, and multiple meanings will not be associated with the same term.

These general principles were followed in the development of ICD-10-PCS:

- Procedure descriptions do not use diagnostic information.
- NOS option is NOT available.
- NEC is limited in use.
- All procedures are defined to a level of specificity.
- The ICD-10-PCS manual consists of three sections.
  1. Tables
  2. Index
  3. List of Codes
- The index will direct a coder to a location within the tables.

EXAMPLE

02703DZ is the code for a percutaneous transluminal coronary angioplasty (PTCA) with stent.

The coder would look up the procedure under "Angioplasty" (Figure 27-9) and then would be directed by the index to see "Dilation, heart and great vessels," 027. The Index directs the coder to Table 027 (Figure 27-10).

Character 4 would be 0 for one site coronary artery, Character 5 approach would be percutaneous, Character 6 is D for intraluminal device, and Character 7 is Z for no qualifier. (Figure 27-11).

Angioplasty
--*see* Dilation, Heart and Great Vessels 027...
--*see* Dilation, Lower Arteries 047...
--*see* Dilation, Lower Veins 067...

Figure 27-9. Index entry for "Angioplasty."

0: MEDICAL AND SURGICAL
2: HEART AND GREAT VESSELS
7: DILATION: Expanding an orifice or the lumen of a tubular body part

Body Part Character 4	Approach Character 5	Device Character 6	Qualifier Character 7
0 Coronary Artery, One Site **1** Coronary Artery, Two Sites **2** Coronary Artery, Three Sites **3** Coronary Artery, Four or More Sites **F** Aortic Valve **G** Mitral Valve **H** Pulmonary Valve **J** Tricuspid Valve **K** Ventricle, Right **P** Pulmonary Trunk **Q** Pulmonary Artery, Right **R** Pulmonary Artery, Left **S** Pulmonary Vein, Right **T** Pulmonary Vein, Left **V** Superior Vena Cava **W** Thoracic Aorta **X** Ductus Arteriosus	**0** Open **2** Open Endoscopic **3** Percutaneous **4** Percutaneous Endoscopic	**4** Drug-eluting Intraluminal Device **D** Intraluminal Device **Z** No Device	**Z** No Qualifier

Figure 27-10. 027 Table (Medical Surgical/Heart and Great Vessels/Dilation Table).

027004Z	Dilation of Coronary Artery, One Site with Drug-eluting Intraluminal Device, Open Approach
02700DZ	Dilation of Coronary Artery, One Site with Intraluminal Device, Open Approach
02700ZZ	Dilation, Coronary Artery, One Site, Open Approach
027024Z	Dilation, Coronary Artery, One Site with Drug-eluting Intraluminal Device, Open Endoscopic Approach
02702DZ	Dilation, Coronary Artery, One Site with Intraluminal Device, Open Endoscopic Approach
02702ZZ	Dilation, Coronary Artery, One Site, Open Endoscopic Approach
027034Z	Dilation, Coronary Artery, One Site with Drug-eluting Intraluminal Device, Percutaneous Approach
02703DZ	Dilation, Coronary Artery, One Site with Intraluminal Device, Percutaneous Approach
02703ZZ	Dilation, Coronary Artery, One Site, Percutaneous Approach
027044Z	Dilation, Coronary Artery, One Site with Drug-eluting Intraluminal Device, Percutaneous Endoscopic Approach
02704DZ	Dilation, Coronary Artery, One Site with Intraluminal Device, Percutaneous Endoscopic Approach
02704ZZ	Dilation, Coronary Artery, One Site, Percutaneous Endoscopic Approach

Figure 27-11. Code descriptions for dilation of one coronary artery (0270).

ICD-10-PCS Table Sections are listed in Figure 27-12. Each Table Section, for instance, Heart and Great Vessel, has root operations that apply to this Table Section. In the previous example, the root operation was dilation. ICD-10-PCS has 30 root operation definitions. Please see Figure 27-13 for dilation definition. The entire list can be found in Appendix C.

PROS AND CONS OF IMPLEMENTATION OF ICD-10-CM AND ICD-10-PCS

It is obvious that the American Health Information Management Association (AHIMA) has been a strong proponent of the adoption of ICD-10-CM and ICD-10-PCS (Box 27-1). The Rand Corporation was commissioned in the Spring of 2003 by the National Committee on

Table Sections

Medical/Surgical	Other Sections
Central Nervous System	Obstetrics
Peripheral Nervous System	Placement-Anatomical Regions
Heart and Great Vessels	Placement-Anatomical Orifices
Upper Arteries	Administration-Circulatory
Lower Arteries	Administration-Indwelling Device
Upper Veins	Administration-Physiological Systems and Anatomical Regions
Lower Veins	Measurement and Monitoring-Physiological Systems
Lymphatic and Hemic Systems	Measurement and Monitoring-Physiological Devices
Eye	Extracorporeal Assistance and Performance
Ear, Nose, Sinus	Extracorporeal Therapies
Respiratory System	Osteopathic
Mouth and Throat	Other Procedures
Gastrointestinal System	Chiropractic
Hepatobiliary System and Pancreas	Imaging
Endocrine System	Nuclear Medicine
Skin and Breast	Radiation Oncology
Subcutaneous Tissue and Fascia	Physical Rehabilitation and Diagnostic Audiology-Rehabilitation
Muscles	Physical Rehabilitation and Diagnostic Audiology-Diagnostic Audiology
Tendons	Mental Health
Bursae and Ligaments	Substance Abuse Treatment
Head and Facial Bones	
Upper Bones	
Lower Bones	
Upper Joints	
Lower Joints	
Urinary System	
Female Reproductive System	
Male Reproductive System	
Anatomical Regions, General	
Anatomical Regions, Upper Extremities	
Anatomical Regions, Lower Extremities	

Figure 27-12. Table sections of ICD-10-PCS.

Dilation	**Definition:**	Expanding an orifice or the lumen of a tubular body part
	Explanation:	The orifice can be a natural orifice or an artificially created orifice. Accomplished by stretching a tubular body part using intraluminal pressure or by cutting part or all of wall of the tubular body part.
	Examples:	Percutaneous transluminal angioplasty, pyloromyotomy

Figure 27-13. Root operation (dilation) definition.

Vital and Health Statistics (NCVHS) to look at the benefits and expenses associated with adopting ICD-10-CM and ICD-10-PCS. The report in its entirety can be found at the Rand Corporation website. This report concludes that the switch to ICD-10-CM and ICD10-PCS may be more beneficial than costly.

In 2003, the American Hospital Association (AHA) and AHIMA conducted a field study using ICD-10-CM. The full report of this study can be found on the AHIMA website. This study was conducted because it was believed that ICD-9-CM had become outdated and obsolete. According to the Summary report of this study, "Accurate and precise reporting of clinical codes is extremely important in the health care industry today. Clinical codes are the key to benchmarking, quality assessment, research, public health reporting, and strategic planning, in addition to accurate reimbursement."

BOX 27-1 AHIMA POSITION ON THE ADOPTION OF ICD-10-CM AND ICD-10-PCS[1]

The Department of Health and Human Services (HHS) must immediately initiate the regulatory process for adoption and implementation of ICD-10-CM and ICD-10-PCS code sets (referred to as ICD-10), rules, and guidelines as a replacement for the 30-year-old ICD-9-CM.

ICD-9-CM is not meeting current healthcare data needs and cannot support the transition to an interoperable health data exchange in the U.S.* HHS must issue a final rule for adoption of ICD-10 as soon as possible to reverse the trend of deteriorating health data and to allow the healthcare industry to prepare for a smooth transition to modern classification systems by 2008.

*ICD stands for the International Classification of Diseases. 9 stands for the 9th revision and 10 for the 10th revision. CM stands for Clinical Modification (a U.S. version of ICD-9 or ICD-10). ICD-9 and ICD-10 were developed and copyrighted by the World Health Organization (WHO). The WHO no longer supports ICD-9. ICD-10-PCS is a procedural coding system designed by the Centers for Medicare and Medicaid to replace the current inpatient procedural coding system currently included as part of ICD-9-CM.

Pros of Using ICD-10-CM

The advantages of using ICD-10-CM, which are numerous (Table 27-2), include the following[2,3]:

- Greater specificity, which is conducive to expansion
- Greater specificity, which also is conducive to recording of detailed statistical information
- More accurate payment
- Fewer rejections and improper billing
- Improved disease management
- Enhanced understanding of healthcare outcomes
- Increased number of open codes for future expansion
- Expanded guidance on Excludes notes
- Updated terminology

Cons of Using ICD-10-CM

- Training
- Loss of productivity
- Information system changes

The Rand report estimates that the cost of conversion (Table 27-3) will range between $425 million and $1.150 billion in one-time costs, plus approximately $5 million to $40 million in lost productivity.

Table 27-2. Summary of Estimated Benefits Over a 10-Year Period*[4]

Category	Benefit ($ million)	Largely Due to
More accurate payment for new procedures	100-1200	ICD-10-PCS
Fewer rejected claims	200-2500	Both
Fewer fraudulent claims	100-1000	Both
Better understanding of new procedures	100-1500	ICD-10-PCS
Improved disease management	200-1500	ICD-10-CM

*Benefits not discounted over time.

Table 27-3. Summary of Estimated One-Time Costs and Cumulative Annual Costs*[5]

	Personnel	Cost Estimate ($ million)	Additional Cost of Sequential Change ($ million)
Training	Full-time coders	100-150	0-20
	Part-time coders	50-150	
	Code users	25-50	0-10
	Physicians	25-100	
Productivity	Coders	0-150*	
	Physicians	50-250*	
System Changes	Providers	50-200	5-20
	Software vendors	50-125	5-20
	Payers	100-250	5-50
	CMS	25-125	5-20

*Cumulative total of 10 years of annual costs (undiscounted).
CMS, Centers for Medicare and Medicaid Services.

PREPARATION FOR TRANSITION TO ICD-10-CM

The steps necessary for transition to ICD-10 and ICD-10-PCS involve many different areas within the healthcare system, including Information Systems (IS), Billing, healthcare providers, Utilization Review (UR), Researchers, Compliance, and Accounting, to name a few. Most articles written on the subject recommend a team approach across the facility. Existing coding staff will need to be trained on both ICD-10-CM and ICD-10-PCS.

Reports suggest (Practice Brief Destination 10: Healthcare Organization Preparation for ICD-10-CM and ICD-10 PCS) that the knowledge base of coders must be broadened so they have detailed knowledge of anatomy and medical terminology, enhanced comprehension of operative reports, and a greater understanding of ICD-10-PCS definitions. It may be necessary to assess the skills of coders prior to selection of the type of training needed. It has been suggested that training should not take place too early, and probably around 3 months prior to implementation would be preferable. Aside from more intensive training in anatomy and physiology (A&P) and terminology, the following education on ICD-10-CM is recommended by AHIMA.

- Structure change
- Disease classification
- Definitions
- Guidelines
- ICD-10-PCS

AHIMA is currently offering ICD-10 courses via the Web. *CodeWrite Community News*, published by AHIMA, offers a monthly exercise designed to help coders prepare for both ICD-10-CM and ICD-10-PCS. The need is great for qualified instructors to teach both of these classification systems to the many users who will need to know them.

CHAPTER REVIEW EXERCISE

Answer the following questions.

1. The most current release of ICD-10-CM is July 2007.
   A. True
   B. False
2. The United States currently uses ICD-10 for reporting mortality.
   A. True
   B. False
3. No ICD-9-CM codes are alphanumeric.
   A. True
   B. False

4. The indexes in ICD9-CM and ICD-10-CM are similar.
   A. True
   B. False
5. The ICD-10-CM codes have never been used by any coders.
   A. True
   B. False
6. Most industrialized countries do not use ICD-10.
   A. True
   B. False
7. Coders will require greater technical skill if they are to master ICD-10-CM and ICD-10-PCS.
   A. True
   B. False

Write the correct answer(s) in the space(s) provided.

8. What year was ICD-9-CM first used?

   ____

9. What year was ICD-10 first used?

   ____

10. What is the set date of implementation of ICD-10-CM?

    ____

11. What are the three sections of the ICD-10-PCS manual?

    ____

    ____

    ____

12. What company was commissioned to look at the risks and benefits of the transition from ICD-9-CM to ICD-10-CM?

    ____

13. What is one of the major drawbacks to implementing ICD-10-CM?

    ____

14. Medical and Surgical Procedures use seven characters in ICD-10-PCS. What is character 4 used for?

    ____

15. Using the ICD-10 CM Index and Tabular (found at the NCHS website), locate codes for the following diagnoses:
    - Atrial fibrillation ______________
    - Dehydration ______________
    - Hypertension ______________
    - Hyperlipidemia ______________
    - Congestive heart failure ______________

APPENDIX A

ICD-9-CM Official Guidelines for Coding and Reporting

Effective October 1, 2007
Narrative changes appear in bold text
Items underlined have been moved within the guidelines since November 15, 2006
The guidelines include the updated V Code Table

The Centers for Medicare and Medicaid Services (CMS) and the National Center for Health Statistics (NCHS), two departments within the U.S. Federal Government's Department of Health and Human Services (DHHS) provide the following guidelines for coding and reporting using the International Classification of Diseases, 9th Revision, Clinical Modification (ICD-9-CM). These guidelines should be used as a companion document to the official version of the ICD-9CM as published on CD-ROM by the U.S. Government Printing Office (GPO).

These guidelines have been approved by the four organizations that make up the Cooperating Parties for the ICD-9-CM: the American Hospital Association (AHA), the American Health Information Management Association (AHIMA), CMS, and NCHS. These guidelines are included on the official government version of the ICD-9-CM, and also appear in "*Coding Clinic for ICD-9-CM*" published by the AHA.

These guidelines are a set of rules that have been developed to accompany and complement the official conventions and instructions provided within the ICD-9-CM itself. These guidelines are based on the coding and sequencing instructions in Volumes I, II and III of ICD-9-CM, but provide additional instruction. Adherence to these guidelines when assigning ICD-9-CM diagnosis and procedure codes is required under the Health Insurance Portability and Accountability Act (HIPAA). The diagnosis codes (Volumes 1-2) have been adopted under HIPAA for all healthcare settings. Volume 3 procedure codes have been adopted for inpatient procedures reported by hospitals. A joint effort between the healthcare provider and the coder is essential to achieve complete and accurate documentation, code assignment, and reporting of diagnoses and procedures. These guidelines have been developed to assist both the healthcare provider and the coder in identifying those diagnoses and procedures that are to be reported. The importance of consistent, complete documentation in the medical record cannot be overemphasized. Without such documentation accurate coding cannot be achieved. The entire record should be reviewed to determine the specific reason for the encounter and the conditions treated.

The term encounter is used for all settings, including hospital admissions. In the context of these guidelines, the term provider is used throughout the guidelines to mean physician or any qualified health care practitioner who is legally accountable for establishing the patient's diagnosis. Only this set of guidelines, approved by the Cooperating Parties, is official.

The guidelines are organized into sections. Section I includes the structure and conventions of the classification and general guidelines that apply to the entire classification, and chapter-specific guidelines that correspond to the chapters as they are arranged in the classification. Section II includes guidelines for selection of principal diagnosis for non-outpatient settings. Section III includes guidelines for reporting additional diagnoses in non-outpatient settings. Section IV is for outpatient coding and reporting.

SECTION I. CONVENTIONS, GENERAL CODING GUIDELINES AND CHAPTER SPECIFIC GUIDELINES

The conventions, general guidelines and chapter-specific guidelines are applicable to all health care settings unless otherwise indicated.

A. Conventions for the ICD-9-CM

The conventions for the ICD-9-CM are the general rules for use of the classification independent of the guidelines. These conventions are incorporated within the index and tabular of the ICD-9-CM as instructional notes. The conventions are as follows:

1. Format:

The ICD-9-CM uses an indented format for ease in reference

2. Abbreviations

a. Index abbreviations

NEC "Not elsewhere classifiable" This abbreviation in the index represents "other specified" when a specific code is not available for a condition the index directs the coder to the "other specified" code in the tabular.

b. Tabular abbreviations

NEC "Not elsewhere classifiable" This abbreviation in the tabular represents "other specified". When a specific code is not available for a condition the tabular includes an NEC entry under a code to identify the code as the "other specified" code.
(See Section I.A.5.a. "Other" codes").

NOS "Not otherwise specified" This abbreviation is the equivalent of unspecified.
(See Section I.A.5.b., "Unspecified" codes)

3. Punctuation

[ ] Brackets are used in the tabular list to enclose synonyms, alternative wording or explanatory phrases. Brackets are used in the index to identify manifestation codes.
(See Section I.A.6. "Etiology/manifestations")

( ) Parentheses are used in both the index and tabular to enclose supplementary words that may be present or absent in the statement of a disease or procedure without affecting the code number to which it is assigned. The terms within the parentheses are referred to as nonessential modifiers.

: Colons are used in the Tabular list after an incomplete term which needs one or more of the modifiers following the colon to make it assignable to a given category.

4. Includes and Excludes Notes and Inclusion terms

Includes: This note appears immediately under a three-digit code title to further define, or give examples of, the content of the category.

Excludes: An excludes note under a code indicates that the terms excluded from the code are to be coded elsewhere. In some cases the codes for the

excluded terms should not be used in conjunction with the code from which it is excluded. An example of this is a congenital condition excluded from an acquired form of the same condition. The congenital and acquired codes should not be used together. In other cases, the excluded terms may be used together with an excluded code. An example of this is when fractures of different bones are coded to different codes. Both codes may be used together if both types of fractures are present.

Inclusion terms: List of terms is included under certain four and five digit codes. These terms are the conditions for which that code number is to be used. The terms may be synonyms of the code title, or, in the case of "other specified" codes, the terms are a list of the various conditions assigned to that code. The inclusion terms are not necessarily exhaustive. Additional terms found only in the index may also be assigned to a code.

5. Other and Unspecified codes

a. "Other" codes

Codes titled "other" or "other specified" (usually a code with a 4th digit 8 or fifth-digit 9 for diagnosis codes) are for use when the information in the medical record provides detail for which a specific code does not exist. Index entries with NEC in the line designate "other" codes in the tabular. These index entries represent specific disease entities for which no specific code exists so the term is included within an "other" code.

b. "Unspecified" codes

Codes (usually a code with a 4th digit 9 or 5th digit 0 for diagnosis codes) titled "unspecified" are for use when the information in the medical record is insufficient to assign a more specific code.

6. Etiology/manifestation convention ("code first", "use additional code" and "in diseases classified elsewhere" notes)

Certain conditions have both an underlying etiology and multiple body system manifestations due to the underlying etiology. For such conditions, the ICD-9-CM has a coding convention that requires the underlying condition be sequenced first followed by the manifestation. Wherever such a combination exists, there is a "use additional code" note at the etiology code, and a "code first" note at the manifestation code. These instructional notes indicate the proper sequencing order of the codes, etiology followed by manifestation.

In most cases the manifestation codes will have in the code title, "in diseases classified elsewhere." Codes with this title are a component of the etiology/manifestation convention. The code title indicates that it is a manifestation code. "In diseases classified elsewhere" codes are never permitted to be used as first listed or principal diagnosis codes. They must be used in conjunction with an underlying condition code and they must be listed following the underlying condition.

There are manifestation codes that do not have "in diseases classified elsewhere" in the title. For such codes a "use additional code" note will still be present and the rules for sequencing apply.

In addition to the notes in the tabular, these conditions also have a specific index entry structure. In the index both conditions are listed together with the etiology code first followed by the manifestation codes in brackets. The code in brackets is always to be sequenced second.

The most commonly used etiology/manifestation combinations are the codes for Diabetes mellitus, category 250. For each code under category 250 there is a use additional code note for the manifestation that is specific for that particular diabetic manifestation. Should a patient have more than one manifestation of diabetes, more than one code from category 250 may be used with as many manifestation codes as are needed to fully describe the patient's complete diabetic condition. The category 250 diabetes codes should be sequenced first, followed by the manifestation codes.

"Code first" and "Use additional code" notes are also used as sequencing rules in the classification for certain codes that are not part of an etiology/manifestation combination.

See—Section I.B.9. "Multiple coding for a single condition".

7. **"And"**
The word "and" should be interpreted to mean either "and" or "or" when it appears in a title.
8. **"With"**
The word "with" in the alphabetic index is sequenced immediately following the main term, not in alphabetical order.
9. **"See" and "See Also"**
The "see" instruction following a main term in the index indicates that another term should be referenced. It is necessary to go to the main term referenced with the "see" note to locate the correct code.
A "see also" instruction following a main term in the index instructs that there is another main term that may also be referenced that may provide additional index entries that may be useful. It is not necessary to follow the "see also" note when the original main term provides the necessary code.

B. General Coding Guidelines

1. **Use of Both Alphabetic Index and Tabular List**
Use both the Alphabetic Index and the Tabular List when locating and assigning a code. Reliance on only the Alphabetic Index or the Tabular List leads to errors in code assignments and less specificity in code selection.
2. **Locate each term in the Alphabetic Index**
Locate each term in the Alphabetic Index and verify the code selected in the Tabular List. Read and be guided by instructional notations that appear in both the Alphabetic Index and the Tabular List.
3. **Level of Detail in Coding**
Diagnosis and procedure codes are to be used at their highest number of digits available.
ICD-9-CM diagnosis codes are composed of codes with 3, 4, or 5 digits. Codes with three digits are included in ICD-9-CM as the heading of a category of codes that may be further subdivided by the use of fourth and/or fifth digits, which provide greater detail.
A three-digit code is to be used only if it is not further subdivided. Where fourth-digit subcategories and/or fifth-digit subclassifications are provided, they must be assigned. A code is invalid if it has not been coded to the full number of digits required for that code. For example, Acute myocardial infarction, code 410, has fourth digits that describe the location of the infarction (e.g., 410.2, Of inferolateral wall), and fifth digits that identify the episode of care. It would be incorrect to report a code in category 410 without a fourth and fifth digit.
ICD-9-CM Volume 3 procedure codes are composed of codes with either 3 or 4 digits. Codes with two digits are included in ICD-9-CM as the heading of a category of codes that may be further subdivided by the use of third and/or fourth digits, which provide greater detail.
4. **Code or codes from 001.0 through V84.8**
The appropriate code or codes from 001.0 through V84.8 must be used to identify diagnoses, symptoms, conditions, problems, complaints or other reason(s) for the encounter/visit.
5. **Selection of codes 001.0 through 999.9**
The selection of codes 001.0 through 999.9 will frequently be used to describe the reason for the admission/encounter. These codes are from the section of ICD-9-CM for the classification of diseases and injuries (e.g., infectious and parasitic diseases; neoplasms; symptoms, signs, and ill-defined conditions, etc.).

6. **Signs and symptoms**
Codes that describe symptoms and signs, as opposed to diagnoses, are acceptable for reporting purposes when a related definitive diagnosis has not been established (confirmed) by the provider. Chapter 16 of ICD-9-CM, Symptoms, Signs, and Ill-defined conditions (codes 780.0-799.9) contain many, but not all codes for symptoms.
7. **Conditions that are an integral part of a disease process**
Signs and symptoms that are **associated routinely with a** disease process should not be assigned as additional codes, unless otherwise instructed by the classification.
8. **Conditions that are not an integral part of a disease process**
Additional signs and symptoms that may not be associated routinely with a disease process should be coded when present.
9. **Multiple coding for a single condition**
In addition to the etiology/manifestation convention that requires two codes to fully describe a single condition that affects multiple body systems, there are other single conditions that also require more than one code. "Use additional code" notes are found in the tabular at codes that are not part of an etiology/manifestation pair where a secondary code is useful to fully describe a condition. The sequencing rule is the same as the etiology/manifestation pair—, "use additional code" indicates that a secondary code should be added.
For example, for infections that are not included in chapter 1, a secondary code from category 041, Bacterial infection in conditions classified elsewhere and of unspecified site, may be required to identify the bacterial organism causing the infection. A "use additional code" note will normally be found at the infectious disease code, indicating a need for the organism code to be added as a secondary code.
"Code first" notes are also under certain codes that are not specifically manifestation codes but may be due to an underlying cause. When a "code first" note is present and an underlying condition is present the underlying condition should be sequenced first.
"Code, if applicable, any causal condition first", notes indicate that this code may be assigned as a principal diagnosis when the causal condition is unknown or not applicable. If a causal condition is known, then the code for that condition should be sequenced as the principal or first-listed diagnosis.
Multiple codes may be needed for late effects, complication codes and obstetric codes to more fully describe a condition. See the specific guidelines for these conditions for further instruction.
10. **Acute and Chronic Conditions**
If the same condition is described as both acute (subacute) and chronic, and separate subentries exist in the Alphabetic Index at the same indentation level, code both and sequence the acute (subacute) code first.
11. **Combination Code**
A combination code is a single code used to classify:
Two diagnoses, or
A diagnosis with an associated secondary process (manifestation)
A diagnosis with an associated complication
Combination codes are identified by referring to subterm entries in the Alphabetic Index and by reading the inclusion and exclusion notes in the Tabular List.
Assign only the combination code when that code fully identifies the diagnostic conditions involved or when the Alphabetic Index so directs. Multiple coding should not be used when the classification provides a combination code that clearly identifies all of the elements documented in the diagnosis. When the combination code lacks necessary specificity in describing the manifestation or complication, an additional code should be used as a secondary code.

12. Late Effects

A late effect is the residual effect (condition produced) after the acute phase of an illness or injury has terminated. There is no time limit on when a late effect code can be used. The residual may be apparent early, such as in cerebrovascular accident cases, or it may occur months or years later, such as that due to a previous injury. Coding of late effects generally requires two codes sequenced in the following order: The condition or nature of the late effect is sequenced first. The late effect code is sequenced second.

An exception to the above guidelines are those instances where the code for late effect is followed by a manifestation code identified in the Tabular List and title, or the late effect code has been expanded (at the fourth and fifth-digit levels) to include the manifestation(s). The code for the acute phase of an illness or injury that led to the late effect is never used with a code for the late effect.

13. Impending or Threatened Condition

Code any condition described at the time of discharge as "impending" or "threatened" as follows:

If it did occur, code as confirmed diagnosis.

If it did not occur, reference the Alphabetic Index to determine if the condition has a subentry term for "impending" or "threatened" and also reference main term entries for "Impending" and for "Threatened."

If the subterms are listed, assign the given code.

If the subterms are not listed, code the existing underlying condition(s) and not the condition described as impending or threatened.

C. Chapter-Specific Coding Guidelines

In addition to general coding guidelines, there are guidelines for specific diagnoses and/or conditions in the classification. Unless otherwise indicated, these guidelines apply to all health care settings. Please refer to Section II for guidelines on the selection of principal diagnosis.

1. Chapter 1: Infectious and Parasitic Diseases (001-139)

a. Human Immunodeficiency Virus (HIV) Infections

1) Code only confirmed cases

Code only confirmed cases of HIV infection/illness. This is an exception to the hospital inpatient guideline Section II, H.

In this context, "confirmation" does not require documentation of positive serology or culture for HIV; the provider's diagnostic statement that the patient is HIV positive, or has an HIV-related illness is sufficient.

2) Selection and sequencing of HIV codes

(a) Patient admitted for HIV-related condition

If a patient is admitted for an HIV-related condition, the principal diagnosis should be 042, followed by additional diagnosis codes for all reported HIV-related conditions.

(b) Patient with HIV disease admitted for unrelated condition

If a patient with HIV disease is admitted for an unrelated condition (such as a traumatic injury), the code for the unrelated condition (e.g., the nature of injury code) should be the principal diagnosis. Other diagnoses would be 042 followed by additional diagnosis codes for all reported HIV-related conditions.

(c) Whether the patient is newly diagnosed

Whether the patient is newly diagnosed or has had previous admissions/encounters for HIV conditions is irrelevant to the sequencing decision.

(d) Asymptomatic human immunodeficiency virus

V08 Asymptomatic human immunodeficiency virus [HIV] infection, is to be applied when the patient without any documentation of symptoms is

listed as being "HIV positive," "known HIV," "HIV test positive," or similar terminology. Do not use this code if the term "AIDS" is used or if the patient is treated for any HIV-related illness or is described as having any condition(s) resulting from his/her HIV positive status; use 042 in these cases.

(e) **Patients with inconclusive HIV serology**
Patients with inconclusive HIV serology, but no definitive diagnosis or manifestations of the illness, may be assigned code 795.71, Inconclusive serologic test for Human Immunodeficiency Virus [HIV].

(f) **Previously diagnosed HIV-related illness**
Patients with any known prior diagnosis of an HIV-related illness should be coded to 042. Once a patient has developed an HIV-related illness, the patient should always be assigned code 042 on every subsequent admission/encounter. Patients previously diagnosed with any HIV illness (042) should never be assigned to 795.71 or V08.

(g) **HIV Infection in Pregnancy, Childbirth and the Puerperium**
During pregnancy, childbirth or the puerperium, a patient admitted (or presenting for a health care encounter) because of an HIV-related illness should receive a principal diagnosis code of 647.6X, Other specified infectious and parasitic diseases in the mother classifiable elsewhere, but complicating the pregnancy, childbirth or the puerperium, followed by 042 and the code(s) for the HIV-related illness(es). Codes from Chapter 15 always take sequencing priority.

Patients with asymptomatic HIV infection status admitted (or presenting for a health care encounter) during pregnancy, childbirth, or the puerperium should receive codes of 647.6X and V08.

(h) **Encounters for testing for HIV**
If a patient is being seen to determine his/her HIV status, use code V73.89, Screening for other specified viral disease. Use code V69.8, Other problems related to lifestyle, as a secondary code if an asymptomatic patient is in a known high risk group for HIV. Should a patient with signs or symptoms
or illness, or a confirmed HIV related diagnosis be tested for HIV, code the signs and symptoms or the diagnosis. An additional counseling code V65.44 may be used if counseling is provided during the encounter for the test.

When a patient returns to be informed of his/her HIV test results use code V65.44, HIV counseling, if the results of the test are negative.

If the results are positive but the patient is asymptomatic use code V08, Asymptomatic HIV infection. If the results are positive and the patient is symptomatic use code 042, HIV infection, with codes for the HIV related symptoms or diagnosis. The HIV counseling code may also be used if counseling is provided for patients with positive test results.

b. Septicemia, Systemic Inflammatory Response Syndrome (SIRS), Sepsis, Severe Sepsis, and Septic Shock

1) SIRS, Septicemia, and Sepsis

(a) The terms *septicemia* and *sepsis* are often used interchangeably by providers, however they are not considered synonymous terms. The following descriptions are provided for reference but do not preclude querying the provider for clarification about terms used in the documentation:

(i) Septicemia generally refers to a systemic disease associated with the presence of pathological microorganisms or toxins in the blood, which can include bacteria, viruses, fungi or other organisms.

(ii) Systemic inflammatory response syndrome (SIRS) generally refers to the systemic response to infection, trauma/burns, or other insult

(such as cancer) with symptoms including fever, tachycardia, tachypnea, and leukocytosis.

(iii) Sepsis generally refers to SIRS due to infection.

(iv) Severe sepsis generally refers to sepsis with associated acute organ dysfunction.

(b) The Coding of SIRS, sepsis and severe sepsis

The coding of SIRS, sepsis and severe sepsis requires a minimum of 2 codes: a code for the underlying cause (such as infection or trauma) and a code from subcategory 995.9 Systemic inflammatory response syndrome (SIRS).

(i) The code for the underlying cause (such as infection or trauma) must be sequenced before the code from subcategory 995.9 Systemic inflammatory response syndrome (SIRS).

(ii) Sepsis and severe sepsis require a code for the systemic infection (038.xx, 112.5, etc.) and either code 995.91, Sepsis, or 995.92, Severe sepsis. If the causal organism is not documented, assign code 038.9, Unspecified septicemia.

(iii) Severe sepsis requires additional code(s) for the associated acute organ dysfunction(s).

(iv) If a patient has sepsis with multiple organ dysfunctions, follow the instructions for coding severe sepsis.

(v) Either the term sepsis or SIRS must be documented to assign a code from subcategory 995.9.

(vi) See Section I.C.17.g), Injury and poisoning, for information regarding systemic inflammatory response syndrome (SIRS) due to trauma/burns and other non-infectious processes.

(c) Due to the complex nature of sepsis and severe sepsis, some cases may require querying the provider prior to assignment of the codes.

2) Sequencing sepsis and severe sepsis

(a) Sepsis and severe sepsis as principal diagnosis

If sepsis or severe sepsis is present on admission, and meets the definition of principal diagnosis, the systemic infection code (e.g., 038.xx, 112.5, etc) should be assigned as the principal diagnosis, followed by code 995.91, Sepsis, or 995.92, Severe sepsis, as required by the sequencing rules in the Tabular List. Codes from subcategory 995.9 can never be assigned as a principal diagnosis. A code should also be assigned for any localized infection, if present.

If the sepsis or severe sepsis is due to a postprocedural infection, see Section I.C.10 for guidelines related to sepsis due to postprocedural infection.

(b) Sepsis and severe sepsis as secondary diagnoses

When sepsis or severe sepsis develops during the encounter (it was not present on admission), the systemic infection code and code 995.91 or 995.92 should be assigned as secondary diagnoses.

(c) Documentation unclear as to whether sepsis or severe sepsis is present on admission

Sepsis or severe sepsis may be present on admission but the diagnosis may not be confirmed until sometime after admission. If the documentation is not clear whether the sepsis **or severe sepsis** was present on admission, the provider should be queried.

3) Sepsis/SIRS with Localized Infection

If the reason for admission is both sepsis, severe sepsis, or SIRS and a localized infection, such as pneumonia or cellulitis, a code for the systemic infection (038.xx, 112.5, etc) should be assigned first, then code 995.91 or 995.92, followed by the code for the localized infection. If the patient is admitted with a localized infection, such as pneumonia,

and sepsis/SIRS doesn't develop until after admission, see guideline **I.C.1.b.**2.b).

If the localized infection is postprocedural, ***see Section I.C.10 for guidelines related to sepsis due to postprocedural infection.***

Note: The term urosepsis is a nonspecific term. If that is the only term documented then only code 599.0 should be assigned based on the default for the term in the ICD-9-CM index, in addition to the code for the causal organism if known.

4) **Bacterial Sepsis and Septicemia**
   In most cases, it will be a code from category 038, Septicemia, that will be used in conjunction with a code from subcategory 995.9 such as the following:
   (a) **Streptococcal sepsis**
   If the documentation in the record states streptococcal sepsis, codes 038.0, Streptococcal septicemia, and code 995.91 should be used, in that sequence.
   (b) **Streptococcal septicemia**
   If the documentation states streptococcal septicemia, only code 038.0 should be assigned, however, the provider should be queried whether the patient has sepsis, an infection with SIRS.

5) **Acute organ dysfunction that is not clearly associated with the sepsis**
   If a patient has sepsis and an acute organ dysfunction, but the medical record documentation indicates that the acute organ dysfunction is related to a medical condition other than the sepsis, do not assign code 995.92, Severe sepsis. An acute organ dysfunction must be associated with the sepsis in order to assign the severe sepsis code. If the documentation is not clear as to whether an acute organ dysfunction is related to the sepsis or another medical condition, query the provider.

6) **Septic shock**
   (a) **Sequencing of septic shock**
   Septic shock generally refers to circulatory failure associated with severe sepsis, and, therefore, it represents a type of acute organ dysfunction.
   For all cases of septic shock, the code for the systemic infection should be sequenced first, followed by codes 995.92 and 785.52. Any additional codes for other acute organ dysfunctions should also be assigned. As noted in the sequencing instructions in the Tabular List, the code for septic shock cannot be assigned as a principal diagnosis.
   (b) **Septic Shock without documentation of severe sepsis**
   Septic shock indicates the presence of severe sepsis.
   Code 995.92, Severe sepsis, must be assigned with code 785.52, Septic shock, even if the term severe sepsis is not documented in the record. The "use additional code" note and the "code first" note in the tabular support this guideline.

7) **Sepsis and septic shock complicating abortion and pregnancy**
   Sepsis and septic shock complicating abortion, ectopic pregnancy, and molar pregnancy are classified to category codes in Chapter 11 (630-639).
   See section I.C.11.

8) **Negative or inconclusive blood cultures**
   Negative or inconclusive blood cultures do not preclude a diagnosis of septicemia or sepsis in patients with clinical evidence of the condition, however, the provider should be queried.

9) **Newborn sepsis**
   See Section I.C.15.j for information on the coding of newborn sepsis.

10) **Sepsis due to a Postprocedural Infection**

(a) **Documentation of causal relationship**

As with all postprocedural complications, code assignment is based on the provider's documentation of the relationship between the infection and the procedure.

(b) **Sepsis due to postprocedural infection**

In cases of postprocedural sepsis, the complication code, such as code 998.59, Other postoperative infection, or 674.3x, Other complications of obstetrical surgical wounds should be coded first followed by the appropriate sepsis codes (systemic infection code and either code 995.91or 995.92). An additional code(s) for any acute organ dysfunction should also be assigned for cases of severe sepsis.

11) **External cause of injury codes with SIRS**

Refer to Section I.C.19.a.7 for instruction on the use of external cause of injury codes with codes for SIRS resulting from trauma.

12) **Sepsis and Severe Sepsis Associated with Noninfectious Process**

(a) **Sequencing *of* <u>sepsis/severe sepsis associated with non-infectious process</u>**

In some cases, a non-infectious process, such as trauma, may lead to an infection which can result in sepsis or severe sepsis. If sepsis or severe sepsis is documented as associated with a non-infectious condition, such as a burn or serious injury, and this condition meets the definition for principal diagnosis, the code for the noninfectious condition should be sequenced first, followed by the code for the systemic infection and either code 995.91, Sepsis, or 995.92, Severe sepsis. Additional codes for any associated acute organ dysfunction(s) should also be assigned for cases of severe sepsis. If the sepsis or severe sepsis meets the definition of principal diagnosis, the systemic infection and sepsis codes should be sequenced before the non-infectious condition. When both the associated non-infectious condition and the sepsis or severe sepsis meet the definition of principal diagnosis, either may be assigned as principal diagnosis.

<u>See Section I.C.1.b.2)(a) for guidelines pertaining to sepsis or severe sepsis as the principal diagnosis.</u>

(b) **Only one SIRS (subcategory 995.9) code should be assigned**

Only one code **from subcategory 995.9 should be assigned for SIRS associated with trauma or other non-infectious condition. Assign the SIRS code (subcategory 995.9) that corresponds to the principal diagnosis. That is, if trauma or a noninfectious condition is the underlying cause, assign code 995.93 or 995.94. If an infection is the underlying cause, assign code 995.91 or 995.92.**

See Section I.C.17.g for information on the coding of SIRS due to trauma/burns or other non-infectious disease processes.

2. **Chapter 2: Neoplasms (140-239)**

<u>General guidelines</u>

Chapter 2 of the ICD-9-CM contains the codes for most benign and all malignant neoplasms. Certain benign neoplasms, such as prostatic adenomas, may be found in the specific body system chapters. To properly code a neoplasm it is necessary to determine from the record if the neoplasm is benign, in-situ, malignant, or of uncertain histologic behavior. If malignant, any secondary (metastatic) sites should also be determined.

The neoplasm table in the Alphabetic Index should be referenced first. However, if the histological term is documented, that term should be referenced first, rather than going immediately to the Neoplasm Table, in order to determine which column in the Neoplasm Table is appropriate. For example, if the documentation indicates "adenoma," refer to the term in the Alphabetic Index to

review the entries under this term and the instructional note to "see also neoplasm, by site, benign." The table provides the proper code based on the type of neoplasm and the site. It is important to select the proper column in the table that corresponds to the type of neoplasm. The tabular should then be referenced to verify that the correct code has been selected from the table and that a more specific site code does not exist.

See Section I. C. 18.d.4. for information regarding V codes for genetic susceptibility to cancer.

a. **Treatment directed at the malignancy**
   If the treatment is directed at the malignancy, designate the malignancy as the principal diagnosis.
b. **Treatment of secondary site**
   When a patient is admitted because of a primary neoplasm with metastasis and treatment is directed toward the secondary site only, the secondary neoplasm is designated as the principal diagnosis even though the primary malignancy is still present.
c. **Coding and sequencing of complications**
   Coding and sequencing of complications associated with the malignancies or with the therapy thereof are subject to the following guidelines:
   1) **Anemia associated with malignancy**
      When admission/encounter is for management of an anemia associated with the malignancy, and the treatment is only for anemia, the appropriate anemia code (such as code 285.22, Anemia in neoplastic disease) is designated as the principal diagnosis and is followed by the appropriate code(s) for the malignancy.
      Code 285.22 may also be used as a secondary code if the patient suffers from anemia and is being treated for the malignancy.
   2) **Anemia associated with chemotherapy, immunotherapy and radiation therapy**
      When the admission/encounter is for management of an anemia associated with chemotherapy, immunotherapy or radiotherapy and the only treatment is for the anemia, the anemia is sequenced first followed by code E933.1. The appropriate neoplasm code should be assigned as an additional code.
   3) **Management of dehydration due to the malignancy**
      When the admission/encounter is for management of dehydration due to the malignancy or the therapy, or a combination of both, and only the dehydration is being treated (intravenous rehydration), the dehydration is sequenced first, followed by the code(s) for the malignancy.
   4) **Treatment of a complication resulting from a surgical procedure**
      When the admission/encounter is for treatment of a complication resulting from a surgical procedure, designate the complication as the principal or first-listed diagnosis if treatment is directed at resolving the complication.
d. **Primary malignancy previously excised**
   When a primary malignancy has been previously excised or eradicated from its site and there is no further treatment directed to that site and there is no evidence of any existing primary malignancy, a code from category V10, Personal history of malignant neoplasm, should be used to indicate the former site of the malignancy. Any mention of extension, invasion, or metastasis to another site is coded as a secondary malignant neoplasm to that site. The secondary site may be the principal or first-listed with the V10 code used as a secondary code.
e. **Admissions/Encounters involving chemotherapy, immunotherapy and radiation therapy**
   1) **Episode of care involves surgical removal of neoplasm**
      When an episode of care involves the surgical removal of a neoplasm, primary or secondary site, followed by adjunct chemotherapy or radiation treatment during the same episode of care, the neoplasm code should be

assigned as principal or first-listed diagnosis, using codes in the 140-198 series or where appropriate in the 200-203 series.

2) **Patient admission/encounter solely for administration of chemotherapy, immunotherapy and radiation therapy**
If a patient admission/encounter is solely for the administration of chemotherapy, immunotherapy or radiation therapy assign code V58.0, Encounter for radiation therapy, or V58.11, Encounter for antineoplastic chemotherapy, or V58.12, Encounter for antineoplastic immunotherapy as the first-listed or principal diagnosis. If a patient receives more than one of these therapies during the same admission more than one of these codes may be assigned, in any sequence.

3) **Patient admitted for radiotherapy/chemotherapy and immunotherapy and develops complications**
When a patient is admitted for the purpose of radiotherapy, immunotherapy or chemotherapy and develops complications such as uncontrolled nausea and vomiting or dehydration, the principal or first-listed diagnosis is V58.0, Encounter for radiotherapy, or V58.11, Encounter for antineoplastic chemotherapy, or V58.12, Encounter for antineoplastic immunotherapy followed by any codes for the complications.

f. **Admission/encounter to determine extent of malignancy**
When the reason for admission/encounter is to determine the extent of the malignancy, or for a procedure such as paracentesis or thoracentesis, the primary malignancy or appropriate metastatic site is designated as the principal or first-listed diagnosis, even though chemotherapy or radiotherapy is administered.

g. **Symptoms, signs, and ill-defined conditions listed in Chapter 16 associated with neoplasms**
Symptoms, signs, and ill-defined conditions listed in Chapter 16 characteristic of, or associated with, an existing primary or secondary site malignancy cannot be used to replace the malignancy as principal or first-listed diagnosis, regardless of the number of admissions or encounters for treatment and care of the neoplasm.
See section I.C.18.d.14, Encounter for prophylactic organ removal.

h. **Admission/encounter for pain control/management**
See Section I.C.6.a.5 for information on coding admission/encounter for pain control/management.

3. **Chapter 3: Endocrine, Nutritional, and Metabolic Diseases and Immunity Disorders (240-279)**

a. **Diabetes mellitus**
Codes under category 250, Diabetes mellitus, identify complications/manifestations associated with diabetes mellitus. A fifth-digit is required for all category 250 codes to identify the type of diabetes mellitus and whether the diabetes is controlled or uncontrolled.

1) **Fifth-digits for category 250:**
The following are the fifth-digits for the codes under category 250:
0 type II or unspecified type, not stated as uncontrolled
1 type I, [juvenile type], not stated as uncontrolled
2 type II or unspecified type, uncontrolled
3 type I, [juvenile type], uncontrolled
The age of a patient is not the sole determining factor, though most type I diabetics develop the condition before reaching puberty. For this reason type I diabetes mellitus is also referred to as juvenile diabetes.

2) **Type of diabetes mellitus not documented**
If the type of diabetes mellitus is not documented in the medical record the default is type II.

3) **Diabetes mellitus and the use of insulin**
All type I diabetics must use insulin to replace what their bodies do not produce. However, the use of insulin does not mean that a patient is a type I

diabetic. Some patients with type II diabetes mellitus are unable to control their blood sugar through diet and oral medication alone and do require insulin. If the documentation in a medical record does not indicate the type of diabetes but does indicate that the patient uses insulin, the appropriate fifth-digit for type II must be used. For type II patients who routinely use insulin, code V58.67, Long-term (current) use of insulin, should also be assigned to indicate that the patient uses insulin. Code V58.67 should not be assigned if insulin is given temporarily to bring a type II patient's blood sugar under control during an encounter.

4) Assigning and sequencing diabetes codes and associated conditions

When assigning codes for diabetes and its associated conditions, the code(s) from category 250 must be sequenced before the codes for the associated conditions. The diabetes codes and the secondary codes that correspond to them are paired codes that follow the etiology/manifestation convention of the classification *(See Section I.A.6., Etiology/manifestation convention)*. Assign as many codes from category 250 as needed to identify all of the associated conditions that the patient has. The corresponding secondary codes are listed under each of the diabetes codes.

(a) Diabetic retinopathy/diabetic macular edema

Diabetic macular edema, code 362.07, is only present with diabetic retinopathy. Another code from subcategory 362.0, Diabetic retinopathy, must be used with code 362.07. Codes under subcategory 362.0 are diabetes manifestation codes, so they must be used following the appropriate diabetes code.

5) Diabetes mellitus in pregnancy and gestational diabetes

(a) For diabetes mellitus complicating pregnancy, see Section I.C.11.f., Diabetes mellitus in pregnancy.

(b) For gestational diabetes, see Section I.C.11, g., Gestational diabetes.

6) Insulin pump malfunction

(a) Underdose of insulin due insulin pump failure

An underdose of insulin due to an insulin pump failure should be assigned 996.57, Mechanical complication due to insulin pump, as the principal or first listed code, followed by the appropriate diabetes mellitus code based on documentation.

(b) Overdose of insulin due to insulin pump failure

The principal or first listed code for an encounter due to an insulin pump malfunction resulting in an overdose of insulin, should also be 996.57, Mechanical complication due to insulin pump, followed by code 962.3, Poisoning by insulins and antidiabetic agents, and the appropriate diabetes mellitus code based on documentation.

4. Chapter 4: Diseases of Blood and Blood Forming Organs (280-289)

a. Anemia of chronic disease

Subcategory 285.2, Anemia in chronic illness, has codes for anemia in chronic kidney disease, code 285.21; anemia in neoplastic disease, code 285.22; and anemia in other chronic illness, code 285.29. These codes can be used as the principal/first listed code if the reason for the encounter is to treat the anemia. They may also be used as secondary codes if treatment of the anemia is a component of an encounter, but not the primary reason for the encounter. When using a code from subcategory 285 it is also necessary to use the code for the chronic condition causing the anemia.

1) Anemia in chronic kidney disease

When assigning code 285.21, Anemia in chronic kidney disease, it is also necessary to assign a code from category 585, Chronic kidney disease, to indicate the stage of chronic kidney disease.

See I.C.10.a. Chronic kidney disease (CKD).

2) **Anemia in neoplastic disease**
When assigning code 285.22, Anemia in neoplastic disease, it is also necessary to assign the neoplasm code that is responsible for the anemia. Code 285.22 is for use for anemia that is due to the malignancy, not for anemia due to antineoplastic chemotherapy drugs, which is an adverse effect.

See I.C.2.c.1 Anemia associated with malignancy.

See I.C.2.c.2 Anemia associated with chemotherapy, immunotherapy and radiation therapy.

See I.C.17.e.1. Adverse effects.

5. **Chapter 5: Mental Disorders (290-319)**
Reserved for future guideline expansion

6. **Chapter 6: Diseases of Nervous System and Sense Organs (320-389)**

a. **Pain—Category 338**

1) **General coding information**
Codes in category 338 may be used in conjunction with codes from other categories and chapters to provide more detail about acute or chronic pain and neoplasm-related pain, **unless otherwise indicated below**.

If the pain is not specified as acute or chronic, do not assign codes from category 338, except for post-thoracotomy pain, postoperative pain, neoplasm related pain, **or central pain syndrome**.

A code from subcategories 338.1 and 338.2 should not be assigned if the underlying (definitive) diagnosis is known, unless the reason for the encounter is pain control/management and not management of the underlying condition.

(a) **Category 338 Codes as Principal or First-Listed Diagnosis**
Category 338 codes are acceptable as principal diagnosis or the first-listed code:

- When pain control or pain management is the reason for the admission/encounter (e.g., a patient with displaced intervertebral disc, nerve impingement and severe back pain presents for injection of steroid into the spinal canal). The underlying cause of the pain should be reported as an additional diagnosis, if known.
- **When an admission or encounter is for a procedure aimed at treating the underlying condition (e.g., spinal fusion, kyphoplasty), a code for the underlying condition (e.g., vertebral fracture, spinal stenosis) should be assigned as the principal diagnosis. No code from category 338 should be assigned.**
- **When a patient is admitted for the insertion of a neurostimulator for pain control, assign the appropriate pain code as the principal or first listed diagnosis. When an admission or encounter is for a procedure aimed at treating the underlying condition and a neurostimulator is inserted for pain control during the same admission/encounter, a code for the underlying condition should be assigned as the principal diagnosis and the appropriate pain code should be assigned as a secondary diagnosis.**

(b) **Use of Category 338 Codes in Conjunction with Site Specific Pain Codes**

(i) **Assigning Category 338 Codes and Site-Specific Pain Codes**
Codes from category 338 may be used in conjunction with codes that identify the site of pain (including codes from chapter 16) if the category 338 code provides additional information. For example, if the code describes the site of the pain, but does not fully describe whether the pain is acute or chronic, then both codes should be assigned.

(ii) Sequencing of Category 338 Codes with Site-Specific Pain Codes
The sequencing of category 338 codes with site-specific pain codes (including chapter 16 codes), is dependent on the circumstances of the encounter/admission as follows:

- If the encounter is for pain control or pain management, assign the code from category 338 followed by the code identifying the specific site of pain (e.g., encounter for pain management for acute neck pain from trauma is assigned code 338.11, Acute pain due to trauma, followed by code 723.1, Cervicalgia, to identify the site of pain).
- If the encounter is for any other reason except pain control or pain management, and a related definitive diagnosis has not been established (confirmed) by the provider, assign the code for the specific site of pain first, followed by the appropriate code from category 338.

2) Pain due to devices, <u>implants and grafts</u>
Pain associated with devices, **implants or grafts** left in a surgical site (**for example painful hip prosthesis**) is assigned to the appropriate code(s) found in Chapter 17, Injury and Poisoning. **Use additional code(s) from category 338 to identify acute or chronic pain due to presence of the device, implant or graft (338.18 338.19 or 338.28-338.29).**

3) Postoperative Pain
Post-thoracotomy pain and other postoperative pain are classified to subcategories 338.1 and 338.2, depending on whether the pain is acute or chronic. The default for post-thoracotomy and other postoperative pain not specified as acute or chronic is the code for the acute form.

<u>Routine or expected postoperative pain immediately after surgery should not be coded.</u>

(a) Postoperative pain not associated with specific postoperative complication
Postoperative pain not associated with a specific postoperative complication is assigned to the appropriate postoperative pain code in category 338.

(b) Postoperative pain associated with specific postoperative complication
Postoperative pain associated with a specific postoperative complication (such as **painful wire sutures**) is assigned to the appropriate code(s) found in Chapter 17, Injury and Poisoning. **If appropriate, use additional code(s) from category 338 to identify acute or chronic pain (338.18 or 338.28).** If pain control/management is the reason for the encounter, a code from category 338 should be assigned as the principal or first-listed diagnosis in accordance with *Section I.C.6.a.1.a above.*

(c) Postoperative pain as principal or first-listed diagnosis
Postoperative pain may be reported as the principal or first-listed diagnosis when the stated reason for the admission/encounter is documented as postoperative pain control/management.

(d) Postoperative pain as secondary diagnosis
Postoperative pain may be reported as a secondary diagnosis code when a patient presents for outpatient surgery and develops an unusual or inordinate amount of postoperative pain.

The provider's documentation should be used to guide the coding of postoperative pain, as well as *Section III. Reporting Additional Diagnoses* and *Section IV. Diagnostic Coding and Reporting in the Outpatient Setting.*

See Section II.I.2 for information on sequencing of diagnoses for patients admitted to hospital inpatient care following post-operative observation.

See Section II.J for information on sequencing of diagnoses for patients admitted to hospital inpatient care from outpatient surgery.

See Section IV.A.2 for information on sequencing of diagnoses for patients admitted for observation.

4) **Chronic pain**
Chronic pain is classified to subcategory 338.2. There is no time frame defining when pain becomes chronic pain. The provider's documentation should be used to guide use of these codes.

5) **Neoplasm Related Pain**
Code 338.3 is assigned to pain documented as being related, associated or due to cancer, primary or secondary malignancy, or tumor. This code is assigned regardless of whether the pain is acute or chronic.

This code may be assigned as the principal or first-listed code when the stated reason for the admission/encounter is documented as pain control/pain management. The underlying neoplasm should be reported as an additional diagnosis.

When the reason for the admission/encounter is management of the neoplasm and the pain associated with the neoplasm is also documented, code 338.3 may be assigned as an additional diagnosis.

See Section I.C.2 for instructions on the sequencing of neoplasms for all other stated reasons for the admission/encounter (except for pain control/pain management).

6) **Chronic pain syndrome**
This condition is different than the term "chronic pain," and therefore this code should only be used when the provider has specifically documented this condition.

7. Chapter 7: Diseases of Circulatory System (390-459)

a. Hypertension

Hypertension Table

The Hypertension Table, found under the main term, "Hypertension", in the Alphabetic Index, contains a complete listing of all conditions due to or associated with hypertension and classifies them according to malignant, benign, and unspecified.

1) **Hypertension, Essential, or NOS**
Assign hypertension (arterial) (essential) (primary) (systemic) (NOS) to category code 401 with the appropriate fourth digit to indicate malignant (.0), benign (.1), or unspecified (.9). Do not use either .0 malignant or .1 benign unless medical record documentation supports such a designation.

2) **Hypertension with Heart Disease**
Heart conditions (425.8, 429.0-429.3, 429.8, 429.9) are assigned to a code from category 402 when a causal relationship is stated (due to hypertension) or implied (hypertensive). Use an additional code from category 428 to identify the type of heart failure in those patients with heart failure. More than one code from category 428 may be assigned if the patient has systolic or diastolic failure and congestive heart failure.

The same heart conditions (425.8, 429.0-429.3, 429.8, 429.9) with hypertension, but without a stated causal relationship, are coded separately. Sequence according to the circumstances of the admission/encounter.

3) **Hypertensive Chronic Kidney Disease**
Assign codes from category 403, Hypertensive chronic kidney disease, when conditions classified to categories 585-587 are present. Unlike hypertension with heart disease, ICD-9-CM presumes a cause-and-effect relationship and classifies chronic kidney disease (CKD) with hypertension as hypertensive chronic kidney disease.

Fifth digits for category 403 should be assigned as follows:

- 0 with CKD stage I through stage IV, or unspecified.
- 1 with CKD stage V or end stage renal disease.

The appropriate code from category 585, Chronic kidney disease, should be used as a secondary code with a code from category 403 to identify the stage of chronic kidney disease.

See Section I.C.10.a for information on the coding of chronic kidney disease.

4) **Hypertensive Heart and Chronic Kidney Disease**
Assign codes from combination category 404, Hypertensive heart and chronic kidney disease, when both hypertensive kidney disease and hypertensive heart disease are stated in the diagnosis. Assume a relationship between the hypertension and the chronic kidney disease, whether or not the condition is so designated. Assign an additional code from category 428, to identify the type of heart failure. More than one code from category 428 may be assigned if the patient has systolic or diastolic failure and congestive heart failure.

Fifth digits for category 404 should be assigned as follows:

- 0 without heart failure and with chronic kidney disease (CKD) stage I through stage IV, or unspecified
- 1 with heart failure and with CKD stage I through stage IV, or unspecified
- 2 without heart failure and with CKD stage V or end stage renal disease
- 3 with heart failure and with CKD stage V or end stage renal disease

The appropriate code from category 585, Chronic kidney disease, should be used as a secondary code with a code from category 404 to identify the stage of kidney disease.

See Section I.C.10.a for information on the coding of chronic kidney disease.

5) **Hypertensive Cerebrovascular Disease**
First assign codes from 430-438, Cerebrovascular disease, then the appropriate hypertension code from categories 401-405.

6) **Hypertensive Retinopathy**
Two codes are necessary to identify the condition. First assign the code from subcategory 362.11, Hypertensive retinopathy, then the appropriate code from categories 401-405 to indicate the type of hypertension.

7) **Hypertension, Secondary**
Two codes are required: one to identify the underlying etiology and one from category 405 to identify the hypertension. Sequencing of codes is determined by the reason for admission/encounter.

8) **Hypertension, Transient**
Assign code 796.2, Elevated blood pressure reading without diagnosis of hypertension, unless patient has an established diagnosis of hypertension. Assign code 642.3x for transient hypertension of pregnancy.

9) **Hypertension, Controlled**
Assign appropriate code from categories 401-405. This diagnostic statement usually refers to an existing state of hypertension under control by therapy.

10) **Hypertension, Uncontrolled**
Uncontrolled hypertension may refer to untreated hypertension or hypertension not responding to current therapeutic regimen. In either case, assign the appropriate code from categories 401-405 to designate the stage and type of hypertension. Code to the type of hypertension.

11) **Elevated Blood Pressure**
For a statement of elevated blood pressure without further specificity, assign code 796.2, Elevated blood pressure reading without diagnosis of hypertension, rather than a code from category 401.

b. **Cerebral infarction/stroke/cerebrovascular accident (CVA)**
The terms stroke and CVA are often used interchangeably to refer to a cerebral infarction. The terms stroke, CVA, and cerebral infarction NOS are all indexed to the default code 434.91, Cerebral artery occlusion, unspecified, with infarction. Code 436, Acute, but ill-defined, cerebrovascular disease, should not be used when the documentation states stroke or CVA.

c. **Postoperative cerebrovascular accident**

A cerebrovascular hemorrhage or infarction that occurs as a result of medical intervention is coded to 997.02, Iatrogenic cerebrovascular infarction or hemorrhage. Medical record documentation should clearly specify the cause- and-effect relationship between the medical intervention and the cerebrovascular accident in order to assign this code. A secondary code from the code range 430-432 or from a code from subcategories 433 or 434 with a fifth digit of "1" should also be used to identify the type of hemorrhage or infarct.

This guideline conforms to the use additional code note instruction at category 997. Code 436, Acute, but ill-defined, cerebrovascular disease, should not be used as a secondary code with code 997.02.

d. **Late Effects of Cerebrovascular Disease**

1) **Category 438, Late Effects of Cerebrovascular disease**

Category 438 is used to indicate conditions classifiable to categories 430-437 as the causes of late effects (neurologic deficits), themselves classified elsewhere. These "late effects" include neurologic deficits that persist after initial onset of conditions classifiable to 430-437. The neurologic deficits caused by cerebrovascular disease may be present from the onset or may arise at any time after the onset of the condition classifiable to 430-437.

2) **Codes from category 438 with codes from 430-437**

Codes from category 438 may be assigned on a health care record with codes from 430-437, if the patient has a current cerebrovascular accident (CVA) and deficits from an old CVA.

3) **Code V12.54**

Assign code V12.**54, Transient ischemic attack (TIA), and cerebral infarction without residual deficits** (and not a code from category 438) as an additional code for history of cerebrovascular disease when no neurologic deficits are present.

e. **Acute myocardial infarction (AMI)**

1) **ST elevation myocardial infarction (STEMI) and non ST elevation myocardial infarction (NSTEMI)**

The ICD-9-CM codes for acute myocardial infarction (AMI) identify the site, such as anterolateral wall or true posterior wall. Subcategories 410.0-410.6 and 410.8 are used for ST elevation myocardial infarction (STEMI). Subcategory 410.7, Subendocardial infarction, is used for non ST elevation myocardial infarction (NSTEMI) and nontransmural MIs.

2) **Acute myocardial infarction, unspecified**

Subcategory 410.9 is the default for the unspecified term acute myocardial infarction. If only STEMI or transmural MI without the site is documented, query the provider as to the site, or assign a code from subcategory 410.9.

3) **AMI documented as nontransmural or subendocardial but site provided**

If an AMI is documented as nontransmural or subendocardial, but the site is provided, it is still coded as a subendocardial AMI. If NSTEMI evolves to STEMI, assign the STEMI code. If STEMI converts to NSTEMI due to thrombolytic therapy, it is still coded as STEMI.

8. **Chapter 8: Diseases of Respiratory System (460-519)**

a. **Chronic Obstructive Pulmonary Disease [COPD] and Asthma**

1) **Conditions that comprise COPD and Asthma**

The conditions that comprise COPD are obstructive chronic bronchitis, subcategory 491.2, and emphysema, category 492. All asthma codes are under category 493, Asthma. Code 496, Chronic airway obstruction, not elsewhere classified, is a nonspecific code that should only be used when the documentation in a medical record does not specify the type of COPD being treated.

2) **Acute exacerbation of chronic obstructive bronchitis and asthma**

The codes for chronic obstructive bronchitis and asthma distinguish between uncomplicated cases and those in acute exacerbation. An acute exacerbation

is a worsening or a decompensation of a chronic condition. An acute exacerbation is not equivalent to an infection superimposed on a chronic condition, though an exacerbation may be triggered by an infection.

3) **Overlapping nature of the conditions that comprise COPD and asthma**
Due to the overlapping nature of the conditions that make up COPD and asthma, there are many variations in the way these conditions are documented. Code selection must be based on the terms as documented. When selecting the correct code for the documented type of COPD and asthma, it is essential to first review the index, and then verify the code in the tabular list. There are many instructional notes under the different COPD subcategories and codes. It is important that all such notes be reviewed to assure correct code assignment.

4) **Acute exacerbation of asthma and status asthmaticus**
An acute exacerbation of asthma is an increased severity of the asthma symptoms, such as wheezing and shortness of breath. Status asthmaticus refers to a patient's failure to respond to therapy administered during an asthmatic episode and is a life threatening complication that requires emergency care. If status asthmaticus is documented by the provider with any type of COPD or with acute bronchitis, the status asthmaticus should be sequenced first. It supersedes any type of COPD including that with acute exacerbation or acute bronchitis. It is inappropriate to assign an asthma code with 5th digit 2, with acute exacerbation, together with an asthma code with 5th digit 1, with status asthmatics. Only the 5th digit 1 should be assigned.

b. Chronic Obstructive Pulmonary Disease [COPD] and Bronchitis

1) **Acute bronchitis with COPD**
Acute bronchitis, code 466.0, is due to an infectious organism. When acute bronchitis is documented with COPD, code 491.22, Obstructive chronic bronchitis with acute bronchitis, should be assigned. It is not necessary to also assign code 466.0. If a medical record documents acute bronchitis with COPD with acute exacerbation, only code 491.22 should be assigned. The acute bronchitis included in code 491.22 supersedes the acute exacerbation. If a medical record documents COPD with acute exacerbation without mention of acute bronchitis, only code 491.21 should be assigned.

c. Acute Respiratory Failure

1) **Acute respiratory failure as principal diagnosis**
Code 518.81, Acute respiratory failure, may be assigned as a principal diagnosis when it is the condition established after study to be chiefly responsible for occasioning the admission to the hospital, and the selection is supported by the Alphabetic Index and Tabular List. However, chapter-specific coding guidelines (such as obstetrics, poisoning, HIV, newborn) that provide sequencing direction take precedence.

2) **Acute respiratory failure as secondary diagnosis**
Respiratory failure may be listed as a secondary diagnosis if it occurs after admission, or if it is present on admission, but does not meet the definition of principal diagnosis.

3) **Sequencing of acute respiratory failure and another acute condition**
When a patient is admitted with respiratory failure and another acute condition, (e.g., myocardial infarction, cerebrovascular accident), the principal diagnosis will not be the same in every situation. Selection of the principal diagnosis will be dependent on the circumstances of admission. If both the respiratory failure and the other acute condition are equally responsible for occasioning the admission to the hospital, and there are no chapter-specific sequencing rules, the guideline regarding two or more diagnoses that equally meet the definition for principal diagnosis *(Section II, C.)* may be applied in these situations.

If the documentation is not clear as to whether acute respiratory failure and another condition are equally responsible for occasioning the admission, query the provider for clarification.

d. Influenza due to identified avian influenza virus (avian influenza)

Code only confirmed cases of avian influenza. This is an exception to the hospital inpatient guideline Section II, H. (Uncertain Diagnosis).

In this context, "confirmation" does not require documentation of positive laboratory testing specific for avian influenza. However, coding should be based on the provider's diagnostic statement that the patient has avian influenza.

If the provider records "suspected or possible or probable avian influenza," the appropriate influenza code from category 487 should be assigned. Code 488, Influenza due to identified avian influenza virus, should not be assigned.

9. Chapter 9: Diseases of Digestive System (520-579)

Reserved for future guideline expansion

10. Chapter 10: Diseases of Genitourinary System (580-629)

a. Chronic kidney disease

1) Stages of chronic kidney disease (CKD)

The ICD-9-CM classifies CKD based on severity. The severity of CKD is designated by stages I-V. Stage II, code 585.2, equates to mild CKD; stage III, code 585.3, equates to moderate CKD; and stage IV, code 585.4, equates to severe CKD. Code 585.6, End stage renal disease (ESRD), is assigned when the provider has documented end-stage-renal disease (ESRD).

If both a stage of CKD and ESRD are documented, assign code 585.6 only.

2) Chronic kidney disease and kidney transplant status

Patients who have undergone kidney transplant may still have some form of CKD, because the kidney transplant may not fully restore kidney function. Therefore, the presence of CKD alone does not constitute a transplant complication. Assign the appropriate 585 code for the patient's stage of CKD and code V42.0. If a transplant complication such as failure or rejection is documented, see section I.C.17.f.1.b for information on coding complications of a kidney transplant. If the documentation is unclear as to whether the patient has a complication of the transplant, query the provider.

3) Chronic kidney disease with other conditions

Patients with CKD may also suffer from other serious conditions, most commonly diabetes mellitus and hypertension. The sequencing of the CKD code in relationship to codes for other contributing conditions is based on the conventions in the tabular list.

See I.C.3.a.4 for sequencing instructions for diabetes.

See I.C.4.a.1 for anemia in CKD.

See I.C.7.a.3 for hypertensive chronic kidney disease.

See I.C.17.f.1.b, Kidney transplant complications, for instructions on coding of documented rejection or failure.

11. Chapter 11: Complications of Pregnancy, Childbirth, and the Puerperium (630-677)

a. General Rules for Obstetric Cases

1) Codes from chapter 11 and sequencing priority

Obstetric cases require codes from chapter 11, codes in the range 630-677, Complications of Pregnancy, Childbirth, and the Puerperium. Chapter 11 codes have sequencing priority over codes from other chapters. Additional codes from other chapters may be used in conjunction with chapter 11 codes to further specify conditions. Should the provider document that the pregnancy is incidental to the encounter, then code V22.2 should be used in place of any chapter 11 codes. It is the provider's responsibility to state that the condition being treated is not affecting the pregnancy.

2) **Chapter 11 codes used only on the maternal record**
Chapter 11 codes are to be used only on the maternal record, never on the record of the newborn.

3) **Chapter 11 fifth-digits**
Categories 640-648, 651-676 have required fifth-digits, which indicate whether the encounter is antepartum, postpartum and whether a delivery has also occurred.

4) **Fifth-digits, appropriate for each code**
The fifth-digits, which are appropriate for each code number, are listed in brackets under each code. The fifth-digits on each code should all be consistent with each other. That is, should a delivery occur all of the fifth-digits should indicate the delivery.

b. Selection of OB Principal or First-listed Diagnosis

1) **Routine outpatient prenatal visits**
For routine outpatient prenatal visits when no complications are present codes V22.0, Supervision of normal first pregnancy, and V22.1, Supervision of other normal pregnancy, should be used as the first-listed diagnoses. These codes should not be used in conjunction with chapter 11 codes.

2) **Prenatal outpatient visits for high-risk patients**
For prenatal outpatient visits for patients with high-risk pregnancies, a code from category V23, Supervision of high-risk pregnancy, should be used as the first-listed diagnosis. Secondary chapter 11 codes may be used in conjunction with these codes if appropriate.

3) **Episodes when no delivery occurs**
In episodes when no delivery occurs, the principal diagnosis should correspond to the principal complication of the pregnancy, which necessitated the encounter. Should more than one complication exist, all of which are treated or monitored, any of the complications codes may be sequenced first.

4) **When a delivery occurs**
When a delivery occurs, the principal diagnosis should correspond to the main circumstances or complication of the delivery. In cases of cesarean delivery, the selection of the principal diagnosis should correspond to the reason the cesarean delivery was performed unless the reason for admission/encounter was unrelated to the condition resulting in the cesarean delivery.

5) **Outcome of delivery**
An outcome of delivery code, V27.0-V27.9, should be included on every maternal record when a delivery has occurred. These codes are not to be used on subsequent records or on the newborn record.

c. Fetal Conditions Affecting the Management of the Mother

1) **Codes from category 655**
Known or suspected fetal abnormality affecting management of the mother, and category 656, Other fetal and placental problems affecting the management of the mother, are assigned only when the fetal condition is actually responsible for modifying the management of the mother, i.e., by requiring diagnostic studies, additional observation, special care, or termination of pregnancy. The fact that the fetal condition exists does not justify assigning a code from this series to the mother's record.

2) **In utero surgery**
In cases when surgery is performed on the fetus, a diagnosis code from category 655, Known or suspected fetal abnormalities affecting management of the mother, should be assigned identifying the fetal condition. Procedure code 75.36, Correction of fetal defect, should be assigned on the hospital inpatient record.

No code from Chapter 15, the perinatal codes, should be used on the mother's record to identify fetal conditions. Surgery performed in utero on a fetus is still to be coded as an obstetric encounter.

d. HIV Infection in Pregnancy, Childbirth and the Puerperium

During pregnancy, childbirth or the puerperium, a patient admitted because of an HIV-related illness should receive a principal diagnosis of 647.6X, Other specified infectious and parasitic diseases in the mother classifiable elsewhere, but complicating the pregnancy, childbirth or the puerperium, followed by 042 and the code(s) for the HIV-related illness(es).

Patients with asymptomatic HIV infection status admitted during pregnancy, childbirth, or the puerperium should receive codes of 647.6X and V08.

e. Current Conditions Complicating Pregnancy

Assign a code from subcategory 648.x for patients that have current conditions when the condition affects the management of the pregnancy, childbirth, or the puerperium. Use additional secondary codes from other chapters to identify the conditions, as appropriate.

f. Diabetes mellitus in pregnancy

Diabetes mellitus is a significant complicating factor in pregnancy. Pregnant women who are diabetic should be assigned code 648.0x, Diabetes mellitus complicating pregnancy, and a secondary code from category 250, Diabetes mellitus, to identify the type of diabetes. Code V58.67, Long-term (current) use of insulin, should also be assigned if the diabetes mellitus is being treated with insulin.

g. Gestational diabetes

Gestational diabetes can occur during the second and third trimester of pregnancy in women who were not diabetic prior to pregnancy. Gestational diabetes can cause complications in the pregnancy similar to those of pre-existing diabetes mellitus. It also puts the woman at greater risk of developing diabetes after the pregnancy. Gestational diabetes is coded to 648.8x, Abnormal glucose tolerance. Codes 648.0x and 648.8x should never be used together on the same record.

Code V58.67, Long-term (current) use of insulin, should also be assigned if the gestational diabetes is being treated with insulin.

h. Normal Delivery, Code 650

1) Normal delivery

Code 650 is for use in cases when a woman is admitted for a full-term normal delivery and delivers a single, healthy infant without any complications antepartum, during the delivery, or postpartum during the delivery episode. Code 650 is always a principal diagnosis. It is not to be used if any other code from chapter 11 is needed to describe a current complication of the antenatal, delivery, or perinatal period. Additional codes from other chapters may be used with code 650 if they are not related to or are in any way complicating the pregnancy.

2) Normal delivery with resolved antepartum complication

Code 650 may be used if the patient had a complication at some point during her pregnancy, but the complication is not present at the time of the admission for delivery.

3) V27.0, Single liveborn, outcome of delivery

V27.0, Single liveborn, is the only outcome of delivery code appropriate for use with 650.

i. The Postpartum and Peripartum Periods

1) Postpartum and peripartum periods

The postpartum period begins immediately after delivery and continues for six weeks following delivery. The peripartum period is defined as the last month of pregnancy to five months postpartum.

2) **Postpartum complication**
A postpartum complication is any complication occurring within the six-week period.

3) **Pregnancy-related complications after 6 week period**
Chapter 11 codes may also be used to describe pregnancy-related complications after the six-week period should the provider document that a condition is pregnancy related.

4) **Postpartum complications occurring during the same admission as delivery**
Postpartum complications that occur during the same admission as the delivery are identified with a fifth digit of "2." Subsequent admissions/encounters for postpartum complications should be identified with a fifth digit of "4."

5) **Admission for routine postpartum care following delivery outside hospital**
When the mother delivers outside the hospital prior to admission and is admitted for routine postpartum care and no complications are noted, code V24.0, Postpartum care and examination immediately after delivery, should be assigned as the principal diagnosis.

6) **Admission following delivery outside hospital with postpartum conditions**
A delivery diagnosis code should not be used for a woman who has delivered prior to admission to the hospital. Any postpartum conditions and/or postpartum procedures should be coded.

j. **Code 677, Late effect of complication of pregnancy**

1) **Code 677**
Code 677, Late effect of complication of pregnancy, childbirth, and the puerperium is for use in those cases when an initial complication of a pregnancy develops a sequelae requiring care or treatment at a future date.

2) **After the initial postpartum period**
This code may be used at any time after the initial postpartum period.

3) **Sequencing of Code 677**
This code, like all late effect codes, is to be sequenced following the code describing the sequelae of the complication.

k. **Abortions**

1) **Fifth-digits required for abortion categories**
Fifth-digits are required for abortion categories 634-637. Fifth-digit 1, incomplete, indicates that all of the products of conception have not been expelled from the uterus. Fifth-digit 2, complete, indicates that all products of conception have been expelled from the uterus prior to the episode of care.

2) **Code from categories 640-648 and 651-659**
A code from categories 640-648 and 651-659 may be used as additional codes with an abortion code to indicate the complication leading to the abortion.
Fifth digit 3 is assigned with codes from these categories when used with an abortion code because the other fifth digits will not apply. Codes from the 660-669 series are not to be used for complications of abortion.

3) **Code 639 for complications**
Code 639 is to be used for all complications following abortion. Code 639 cannot be assigned with codes from categories 634-638.

4) **Abortion with Liveborn Fetus**
When an attempted termination of pregnancy results in a liveborn fetus assign code 644.21, Early onset of delivery, with an appropriate code from category V27, Outcome of Delivery. The procedure code for the attempted termination of pregnancy should also be assigned.

5) **Retained Products of Conception following an abortion**
Subsequent admissions for retained products of conception following a spontaneous or legally induced abortion are assigned the appropriate code

from category 634, Spontaneous abortion, or 635 Legally induced abortion, with a fifth digit of "1" (incomplete). This advice is appropriate even when the patient was discharged previously with a discharge diagnosis of complete abortion.

12. **Chapter 12: Diseases Skin and Subcutaneous Tissue (680-709)**
Reserved for future guideline expansion

13. **Chapter 13: Diseases of Musculoskeletal and Connective Tissue (710-739)**
   a. **Coding of Pathologic Fractures**
      1) **Acute Fractures vs. Aftercare**
      Pathologic fractures are reported using subcategory 733.1, when the fracture is newly diagnosed. Subcategory 733.1 may be used while the patient is receiving active treatment for the fracture. Examples of active treatment are: surgical treatment, emergency department encounter, evaluation and treatment by a new physician.

      Fractures are coded using the aftercare codes (subcategories V54.0, V54.2, V54.8 or V54.9) for encounters after the patient has completed active treatment of the fracture and is receiving routine care for the fracture during the healing or recovery phase. Examples of fracture aftercare are: cast change or removal, removal of external or internal·fixation device, medication adjustment, and follow up visits following fracture treatment.

      Care for complications of surgical treatment for fracture repairs during the healing or recovery phase should be coded with the appropriate complication codes.

      Care of complications of fractures, such as malunion and nonunion, should be reported with the appropriate codes.

      See Section I. C. 17.b for information on the coding of traumatic fractures.

14. **Chapter 14: Congenital Anomalies (740-759)**
   a. **Codes in categories 740-759, Congenital Anomalies**
   Assign an appropriate code(s) from categories 740-759, Congenital Anomalies, when an anomaly is documented. A congenital anomaly may be the principal/first listed diagnosis on a record or a secondary diagnosis.

   When a congenital anomaly does not have a unique code assignment, assign additional code(s) for any manifestations that may be present.

   When the code assignment specifically identifies the congenital anomaly, manifestations that are an inherent component of the anomaly should not be coded separately. Additional codes should be assigned for manifestations that are not an inherent component.

   Codes from Chapter 14 may be used throughout the life of the patient. If a congenital anomaly has been corrected, a personal history code should be used to identify the history of the anomaly. Although present at birth, a congenital anomaly may not be identified until later in life. Whenever the condition is diagnosed by the physician, it is appropriate to assign a code from codes 740-759.

   For the birth admission, the appropriate code from category V30, Liveborn infants, according to type of birth should be sequenced as the principal diagnosis, followed by any congenital anomaly codes, 740-759.

15. **Chapter 15: Newborn (Perinatal) Guidelines (760-779)**
For coding and reporting purposes the perinatal period is defined as **before** birth through the 28th day following birth. The following guidelines are provided for reporting purposes. Hospitals may record other diagnoses as needed for internal data use.
   a. **General Perinatal Rules**
      1) **Chapter 15 Codes**
      They are <u>never</u> for use on the maternal record. Codes from Chapter 11, the obstetric chapter, are never permitted on the newborn record. Chapter 15 code may be used throughout the life of the patient if the condition is still present.

2) **Sequencing of perinatal codes**
Generally, codes from Chapter 15 should be sequenced as the principal/first-listed diagnosis on the newborn record, with the exception of the appropriate V30 code for the birth episode, followed by codes from any other chapter that provide additional detail. The "use additional code" note at the beginning of the chapter supports this guideline. If the index does not provide a specific code for a perinatal condition, assign code 779.89, Other specified conditions originating in the perinatal period, followed by the code from another chapter that specifies the condition. Codes for signs and symptoms may be assigned when a definitive diagnosis has not been established.

3) **Birth process or community acquired conditions**
If a newborn has a condition that may be either due to the birth process or community acquired and the documentation does not indicate which it is, the default is due to the birth process and the code from Chapter 15 should be used. If the condition is community-acquired, a code from Chapter 15 should not be assigned.

4) **Code all clinically significant conditions**
All clinically significant conditions noted on routine newborn examination should be coded. A condition is clinically significant if it requires:
- clinical evaluation; or
- therapeutic treatment; or
- diagnostic procedures; or
- extended length of hospital stay; or
- increased nursing care and/or monitoring; or
- has implications for future health care needs

Note: The perinatal guidelines listed above are the same as the general coding guidelines for "additional diagnoses", except for the final point regarding implications for future health care needs. Codes should be assigned for conditions that have been specified by the provider as having implications for future health care needs. Codes from the perinatal chapter should not be assigned unless the provider has established a definitive diagnosis.

b. **Use of codes V30-V39**
When coding the birth of an infant, assign a code from categories V30-V39, according to the type of birth. A code from this series is assigned as a principal diagnosis, and assigned only once to a newborn at the time of birth.

c. **Newborn transfers**
If the newborn is transferred to another institution, the V30 series is not used at the receiving hospital.

d. **Use of category V29**

1) **Assigning a code from category V29**
Assign a code from category V29, Observation and evaluation of newborns and infants for suspected conditions not found, to identify those instances when a healthy newborn is evaluated for a suspected condition that is determined after study not to be present. Do not use a code from category V29 when the patient has identified signs or symptoms of a suspected problem; in such cases, code the sign or symptom.

A code from category V29 may also be assigned as a principal code for readmissions or encounters when the V30 code no longer applies. Codes from category V29 are for use only for healthy newborns and infants for which no condition after study is found to be present.

2) **V29 code on a birth record**
A V29 code is to be used as a secondary code after the V30, Outcome of delivery, code.

e. **Use of other V codes on perinatal records**
V codes other than V30 and V29 may be assigned on a perinatal or newborn record code. The codes may be used as a principal or first-listed diagnosis for specific types of encounters or for readmissions or encounters when the V30 code no longer applies.
See Section I.C.18 for information regarding the assignment of V codes.

f. **Maternal Causes of Perinatal Morbidity**
Codes from categories 760-763, Maternal causes of perinatal morbidity and mortality, are assigned only when the maternal condition has actually affected the fetus or newborn. The fact that the mother has an associated medical condition or experiences some complication of pregnancy, labor or delivery does not justify the routine assignment of codes from these categories to the newborn record.

g. **Congenital Anomalies in Newborns**
For the birth admission, the appropriate code from category V30, Liveborn infants according to type of birth, should be used, followed by any congenital anomaly codes, categories 740-759. Use additional secondary codes from other chapters to specify conditions associated with the anomaly, if applicable.
Also, see Section I.C.14 for information on the coding of congenital anomalies.

h. **Coding Additional Perinatal Diagnoses**
1) **Assigning codes for conditions that require treatment**
Assign codes for conditions that require treatment or further investigation, prolong the length of stay, or require resource utilization.
2) **Codes for conditions specified as having implications for future health care needs**
Assign codes for conditions that have been specified by the provider as having implications for future health care needs.
Note: This guideline should not be used for adult patients.
3) **Codes for newborn conditions originating in the perinatal period**
Assign a code for newborn conditions originating in the perinatal period (categories 760-779), as well as complications arising during the current episode of care classified in other chapters, only if the diagnoses have been documented by the responsible provider at the time of transfer or discharge as having affected the fetus or newborn.

i. **Prematurity and Fetal Growth Retardation**
Providers utilize different criteria in determining prematurity. A code for prematurity should not be assigned unless it is documented. The 5th digit assignment for codes from category 764 and subcategories 765.0 and 765.1 should be based on the recorded birth weight and estimated gestational age.
A code from subcategory 765.2, Weeks of gestation, should be assigned as an additional code with category 764 and codes from 765.0 and 765.1 to specify weeks of gestation as documented by the provider in the record.

j. **Newborn sepsis**
Code 771.81, Septicemia [sepsis] of newborn, should be assigned with a secondary code from category 041, Bacterial infections in conditions classified elsewhere and of unspecified site, to identify the organism. It is not necessary to use a code from subcategory 995.9, Systemic inflammatory response syndrome (SIRS), on a newborn record. A code from category 038, Septicemia, should not be used on a newborn record. Code 771.81 describes the sepsis.

16. **Chapter 16: Signs, Symptoms and Ill-Defined Conditions (780-799)**
Reserved for future guideline expansion

17. **Chapter 17: Injury and Poisoning (800-999)**
a. **Coding of Injuries**
When coding injuries, assign separate codes for each injury unless a combination code is provided, in which case the combination code is assigned. Multiple injury codes are provided in ICD-9-CM, but should not be assigned unless information for a more specific code is not available. These codes are not to be

used for normal, healing surgical wounds or to identify complications of surgical wounds.

The code for the most serious injury, as determined by the provider and the focus of treatment, is sequenced first.

1) **Superficial injuries**

Superficial injuries such as abrasions or contusions are not coded when associated with more severe injuries of the same site.

2) **Primary injury with damage to nerves/blood vessels**

When a primary injury results in minor damage to peripheral nerves or blood vessels, the primary injury is sequenced first with additional code(s) from categories 950-957, Injury to nerves and spinal cord, and/or 900-904, Injury to blood vessels. When the primary injury is to the blood vessels or nerves, that injury should be sequenced first.

b. **Coding of Traumatic Fractures**

The principles of multiple coding of injuries should be followed in coding fractures. Fractures of specified sites are coded individually by site in accordance with both the provisions within categories 800-829 and the level of detail furnished by medical record content. Combination categories for multiple fractures are provided for use when there is insufficient detail in the medical record (such as trauma cases transferred to another hospital), when the reporting form limits the number of codes that can be used in reporting pertinent clinical data, or when there is insufficient specificity at the fourth-digit or fifth-digit level. More specific guidelines are as follows:

1) **Acute Fractures vs. Aftercare**

Traumatic fractures are coded using the acute fracture codes (800-829) while the patient is receiving active treatment for the fracture. Examples of active treatment are: surgical treatment, emergency department encounter, and evaluation and treatment by a new physician.

Fractures are coded using the aftercare codes (subcategories V54.0, V54.1, V54.8, or V54.9) for encounters after the patient has completed active treatment of the fracture and is receiving routine care for the fracture during the healing or recovery phase. Examples of fracture aftercare are: cast change or removal, removal of external or internal fixation device, medication adjustment, and follow up visits following fracture treatment.

Care for complications of surgical treatment for fracture repairs during the healing or recovery phase should be coded with the appropriate complication codes.

Care of complications of fractures, such as malunion and nonunion, should be reported with the appropriate codes.

Pathologic fractures are not coded in the 800-829 range, but instead are assigned to subcategory 733.1. *See Section I.C.13.a for additional information.*

2) **Multiple fractures of same limb**

Multiple fractures of same limb classifiable to the same three-digit or four-digit category are coded to that category.

3) **Multiple unilateral or bilateral fractures of same bone**

Multiple unilateral or bilateral fractures of same bone(s) but classified to different fourth-digit subdivisions (bone part) within the same three-digit category are coded individually by site.

4) **Multiple fracture categories 819 and 828**

Multiple fracture categories 819 and 828 classify bilateral fractures of both upper limbs (819) and both lower limbs (828), but without any detail at the fourth-digit level other than open and closed type of fractures.

5) **Multiple fractures sequencing**

Multiple fractures are sequenced in accordance with the severity of the fracture. The provider should be asked to list the fracture diagnoses in the order of severity.

c. **Coding of Burns**

Current burns (940-948) are classified by depth, extent and by agent (E code). Burns are classified by depth as first degree (erythema), second degree (blistering), and third degree (full-thickness involvement).

1) **Sequencing of burn and related condition codes**

Sequence first the code that reflects the highest degree of burn when more than one burn is present.

a. When the reason for the admission or encounter is for treatment of external multiple burns, sequence first the code that reflects the burn of the highest degree.

b. When a patient has both internal and external burns, the circumstances of admission govern the selection of the principal diagnosis or first-listed diagnosis.

c. When a patient is admitted for burn injuries and other related conditions such as smoke inhalation and/or respiratory failure, the circumstances of admission govern the selection of the principal or first-listed diagnosis.

2) **Burns of the same local site**

Classify burns of the same local site (three-digit category level, 940-947) but of different degrees to the subcategory identifying the highest degree recorded in the diagnosis.

3) **Non-healing burns**

Non-healing burns are coded as acute burns. Necrosis of burned skin should be coded as a non-healed burn.

4) **Code 958.3, Posttraumatic wound infection**

Assign code 958.3, Posttraumatic wound infection, not elsewhere classified, as an additional code for any documented infected burn site.

5) **Assign separate codes for each burn site**

When coding burns, assign separate codes for each burn site. Category 946 Burns of Multiple specified sites, should only be used if the location of the burns are not documented.

Category 949, Burn, unspecified, is extremely vague and should rarely be used.

6) **Assign codes from category 948, Burns**

Burns classified according to extent of body surface involved, when the site of the burn is not specified or when there is a need for additional data. It is advisable to use category 948 as additional coding when needed to provide data for evaluating burn mortality, such as that needed by burn units. It is also advisable to use category 948 as an additional code for reporting purposes when there is mention of a third-degree burn involving 20 percent or more of the body surface.

In assigning a code from category 948:

Fourth-digit codes are used to identify the percentage of total body surface involved in a burn (all degree).

Fifth-digits are assigned to identify the percentage of body surface involved in third-degree burn.

Fifth-digit zero (0) is assigned when less than 10 percent or when no body surface is involved in a third-degree burn.

Category 948 is based on the classic "rule of nines" in estimating body surface involved: head and neck are assigned nine percent, each arm nine percent, each leg 18 percent, the anterior trunk 18 percent, posterior trunk 18 percent, and genitalia one percent. Providers may change these percentage assignments where necessary to accommodate infants and children who have proportionately larger heads than adults and patients who have large buttocks, thighs, or abdomen that involve burns.

7) **Encounters for treatment of late effects of burns**
Encounters for the treatment of the late effects of burns (i.e., scars or joint contractures) should be coded to the residual condition (sequelae) followed by the appropriate late effect code (906.5-906.9). A late effect E code may also be used, if desired.

8) **Sequelae with a late effect code and current burn**
When appropriate, both a sequelae with a late effect code, and a current burn code may be assigned on the same record (when both a current burn and sequelae of an old burn exist).

d. **Coding of Debridement of Wound, Infection, or Burn**
Excisional debridement involves surgical removal or cutting away, as opposed to a mechanical (brushing, scrubbing, washing) debridement.
For coding purposes, excisional debridement is assigned to code 86.22.
Nonexcisional debridement is assigned to code 86.28.

e. **Adverse Effects, Poisoning and Toxic Effects**
The properties of certain drugs, medicinal and biological substances or combinations of such substances, may cause toxic reactions. The occurrence of drug toxicity is classified in ICD-9-CM as follows:

1) **Adverse Effect**
When the drug was correctly prescribed and properly administered, code the reaction plus the appropriate code from the E930-E949 series. Codes from the E930-E949 series must be used to identify the causative substance for an adverse effect of drug, medicinal and biological substances, correctly prescribed and properly administered. The effect, such as tachycardia, delirium, gastrointestinal hemorrhaging, vomiting, hypokalemia, hepatitis, renal failure, or respiratory failure, is coded and followed by the appropriate code from the E930-E949 series.

Adverse effects of therapeutic substances correctly prescribed and properly administered (toxicity, synergistic reaction, side effect, and idiosyncratic reaction) may be due to (1) differences among patients, such as age, sex, disease, and genetic factors, and (2) drug-related factors, such as type of drug, route of administration, duration of therapy, dosage, and bioavailability.

2) **Poisoning**

(a) **Error was made in drug prescription**
Errors made in drug prescription or in the administration of the drug by provider, nurse, patient, or other person, use the appropriate poisoning code from the 960-979 series.

(b) **Overdose of a drug intentionally taken**
If an overdose of a drug was intentionally taken or administered and resulted in drug toxicity, it would be coded as a poisoning (960-979 series).

(c) **Nonprescribed drug taken with correctly prescribed and properly administered drug**
If a nonprescribed drug or medicinal agent was taken in combination with a correctly prescribed and properly administered drug, any drug toxicity or other reaction resulting from the interaction of the two drugs would be classified as a poisoning.

(d) **Sequencing of poisoning**
When coding a poisoning or reaction to the improper use of a medication (e.g., wrong dose, wrong substance, wrong route of administration) the poisoning code is sequenced first, followed by a code for the manifestation. If there is also a diagnosis of drug abuse or dependence to the substance, the abuse or dependence is coded as an additional code.

See Section I.C.3.a.6.b. if poisoning is the result of insulin pump malfunctions and Section I.C.19 for general use of E-codes.

3) **Toxic Effects**

(a) **Toxic effect codes**

When a harmful substance is ingested or comes in contact with a person, this is classified as a toxic effect. The toxic effect codes are in categories 980-989.

(b) **Sequencing toxic effect codes**

A toxic effect code should be sequenced first, followed by the code(s) that identify the result of the toxic effect.

(c) **External cause codes for toxic effects**

An external cause code from categories E860-E869 for accidental exposure, codes E950.6 or E950.7 for intentional self-harm, category E962 for assault, or categories E980-E982, for undetermined, should also be assigned to indicate intent.

f. **Complications of care**

1) **Transplant complications**

(a) **Transplant complications other than kidney**

Codes under subcategory 996.8, Complications of transplanted organ, are for use for both complications and rejection of transplanted organs. A transplant complication code is only assigned if the complication affects the function of the transplanted organ. Two codes are required to fully describe a transplant complication, the appropriate code from subcategory 996.8 and a secondary code that identifies the complication.

Pre-existing conditions or conditions that develop after the transplant are not coded as complications unless they affect the function of the transplanted organs.

(b) **Kidney transplant complications**

Code 996.81 should be assigned for documented complications of a kidney transplant, such as transplant failure or rejection. Code 996.81 should not be assigned for post kidney transplant patients who have chronic kidney (CKD) unless a transplant complication such as transplant failure or rejection is documented. If the documentation is unclear as to whether the patient has a complication of the transplant, query the provider.

For patients with CKD following a kidney transplant, but who do not have a complication such as failure or rejection, *see section I.C.10.a.2, Chronic kidney disease and kidney transplant status.*

g. **SIRS due to Non-infectious Process**

The systemic inflammatory response syndrome (SIRS) can develop as a result of certain non-infectious disease processes, such as trauma, malignant neoplasm, or pancreatitis. When SIRS is documented with a noninfectious condition, and no subsequent infection is documented, the code for the underlying condition, such as an injury, should be assigned, followed by code 995.93, Systemic inflammatory response syndrome due to noninfectious process without acute organ dysfunction, or 995.94, Systemic inflammatory response syndrome due to non-infectious process with acute organ dysfunction. If an acute organ dysfunction is documented, the appropriate code(s) for the associated acute organ dysfunction(s) should be assigned in addition to code 995.94. If acute organ dysfunction is documented, but it cannot be determined if the acute organ dysfunction is associated with SIRS or due to another condition (e.g., directly due to the trauma), the provider should be queried.

When the non-infectious condition has led to an infection that results in SIRS, *see Section I.C.1.b.11 for the guideline for sepsis and severe sepsis associated with a non-infectious process.*

18. **Classification of Factors Influencing Health Status and Contact with Health Service (Supplemental V01-V84)**

Note: The chapter specific guidelines provide additional information about the use of V codes for specified encounters.

a. Introduction

ICD-9-CM provides codes to deal with encounters for circumstances other than a disease or injury. The Supplementary Classification of Factors Influencing Health Status and Contact with Health Services (V01.0-V84.8) is provided to deal with occasions when circumstances other than a disease or injury (codes 001-999) are recorded as a diagnosis or problem.

There are four primary circumstances for the use of V codes:

1) A person who is not currently sick encounters the health services for some specific reason, such as to act as an organ donor, to receive prophylactic care, such as inoculations or health screenings, or to receive counseling on health related issues.
2) A person with a resolving disease or injury, or a chronic, long-term condition requiring continuous care, encounters the health care system for specific aftercare of that disease or injury (e.g., dialysis for renal disease; chemotherapy for malignancy; cast change). A diagnosis/symptom code should be used whenever a current, acute, diagnosis is being treated or a sign or symptom is being studied.
3) Circumstances or problems influence a person's health status but are not in themselves a current illness or injury.
4) Newborns, to indicate birth status

b. V codes use in any healthcare setting

V codes are for use in any healthcare setting. V codes may be used as either a first listed (principal diagnosis code in the inpatient setting) or secondary code, depending on the circumstances of the encounter. Certain V codes may only be used as first listed, others only as secondary codes.

See Section I.C.18.e, V Code Table.

c. V Codes indicate a reason for an encounter

They are not procedure codes. A corresponding procedure code must accompany a V code to describe the procedure performed.

d. Categories of V Codes

1) Contact/Exposure

Category V01 indicates contact with or exposure to communicable diseases. These codes are for patients who do not show any sign or symptom of a disease but have been exposed to it by close personal contact with an infected individual or are in an area where a disease is epidemic. These codes may be used as a first listed code to explain an encounter for testing, or, more commonly, as a secondary code to identify a potential risk.

2) Inoculations and vaccinations

Categories V03-V06 are for encounters for inoculations and vaccinations. They indicate that a patient is being seen to receive a prophylactic inoculation against a disease. The injection itself must be represented by the appropriate procedure code. A code from V03-V06 may be used as a secondary code if the inoculation is given as a routine part of preventive health care, such as a well-baby visit.

3) Status

Status codes indicate that a patient is either a carrier of a disease or has the sequelae or residual of a past disease or condition. This includes such things as the presence of prosthetic or mechanical devices resulting from past treatment. A status code is informative, because the status may affect the course of treatment and its outcome. A status code is distinct from a history code. The history code indicates that the patient no longer has the condition.

A status code should not be used with a diagnosis code from one of the body system chapters, if the diagnosis code includes the information provided by the status code. For example, code V42.1, Heart transplant status, should

not be used with code 996.83, Complications of transplanted heart. The status code does not provide additional information. The complication code indicates that the patient is a heart transplant patient.

The status V codes/categories are:

V02 Carrier or suspected carrier of infectious diseases
Carrier status indicates that a person harbors the specific organisms of a disease without manifest symptoms and is capable of transmitting the infection.

V08 Asymptomatic HIV infection status
This code indicates that a patient has tested positive for HIV but has manifested no signs or symptoms of the disease.

V09 Infection with drug-resistant microorganisms
This category indicates that a patient has an infection that is resistant to drug treatment. Sequence the infection code first.

V21 Constitutional states in development

V22.2 Pregnant state, incidental
This code is a secondary code only for use when the pregnancy is in no way complicating the reason for visit. Otherwise, a code from the obstetric chapter is required.

V26.5x Sterilization status

V42 Organ or tissue replaced by transplant

V43 Organ or tissue replaced by other means

V44 Artificial opening status

V45 Other postsurgical states

V46 Other dependence on machines

V49.6 Upper limb amputation status

V49.7 Lower limb amputation status
Note: Categories V42-V46, and subcategories V49.6, V49.7 are for use only if there are no complications or malfunctions of the organ or tissue replaced, the amputation site or the equipment on which the patient is dependent.

V49.81 Postmenopausal status

V49.82 Dental sealant status

V49.83 Awaiting organ transplant status

V58.6**x** Long-term (current) drug use
Codes from this subcategory indicate a patient's continuous use of a prescribed drug (including such things as aspirin therapy) for the long-term treatment of a condition or for prophylactic use. It is not for use for patients who have addictions to drugs.

Assign a code from subcategory V58.6, Long-term (current) drug use, if the patient is receiving a medication for an extended period as a prophylactic measure (such as for the prevention of deep vein thrombosis) or as treatment of a chronic condition (such as arthritis) or a disease requiring a lengthy course of treatment (such as cancer). Do not assign a code from subcategory V58.6 for medication being administered for a brief period of time to treat an acute illness or injury (such as a course of antibiotics to treat acute bronchitis).

V83 Genetic carrier status
Genetic carrier status indicates that a person carries a gene, associated with a particular disease, which may be passed to offspring who may develop that disease. The person does not have the disease and is not at risk of developing the disease.

V84 Genetic susceptibility status
Genetic susceptibility indicates that a person has a gene that increases the risk of that person developing the disease.

Codes from category V84, Genetic susceptibility to disease, should not be used as principal or first-listed codes. If the patient has the condition to which he/she is susceptible, and that condition is the reason for the encounter, the code for the current condition should be sequenced first. If the patient is being seen for follow-up after completed treatment for this condition, and the condition no longer exists, a follow-up code should be sequenced first, followed by the appropriate personal history and genetic susceptibility codes. If the purpose of the encounter is genetic counseling associated with procreative management, a code from subcategory V26.3, Genetic counseling and testing, should be assigned as the first-listed code, followed by a code from category V84. Additional codes should be assigned for any applicable family or personal history.

See Section I.C. 18.d.14 for information on prophylactic organ removal due to a genetic susceptibility.

V86 Estrogen receptor status

4) History (of)

There are two types of history V codes, personal and family. Personal history codes explain a patient's past medical condition that no longer exists and is not receiving any treatment, but that has the potential for recurrence, and therefore may require continued monitoring. The exceptions to this general rule are category V14, Personal history of allergy to medicinal agents, and subcategory V15.0, Allergy, other than to medicinal agents. A person who has had an allergic episode to a substance or food in the past should always be considered allergic to the substance.

Family history codes are for use when a patient has a family member(s) who has had a particular disease that causes the patient to be at higher risk of also contracting the disease.

Personal history codes may be used in conjunction with follow-up codes and family history codes may be used in conjunction with screening codes to explain the need for a test or procedure. History codes are also acceptable on any medical record regardless of the reason for visit. A history of an illness, even if no longer present, is important information that may alter the type of treatment ordered.

The history V code categories are:

V10 Personal history of malignant neoplasm

V12 Personal history of certain other diseases

V13 Personal history of other diseases

Except: V13.4, Personal history of arthritis, and V13.6, Personal history of congenital malformations. These conditions are life-long so are not true history codes.

V14 Personal history of allergy to medicinal agents

V15 Other personal history presenting hazards to health

Except: V15.7, Personal history of contraception.

V16 Family history of malignant neoplasm

V17 Family history of certain chronic disabling diseases

V18 Family history of certain other specific diseases

V19 Family history of other conditions

5) Screening

Screening is the testing for disease or disease precursors in seemingly well individuals so that early detection and treatment can be provided for those who test positive for the disease. Screenings that are recommended for many subgroups in a population include: routine mammograms for women over 40, a fecal occult blood test for everyone over 50, an amniocentesis to rule out a fetal anomaly for pregnant women over 35, because the incidence of

breast cancer and colon cancer in these subgroups is higher than in the general population, as is the incidence of Down's syndrome in older mothers.

The testing of a person to rule out or confirm a suspected diagnosis because the patient has some sign or symptom is a diagnostic examination, not a screening. In these cases, the sign or symptom is used to explain the reason for the test.

A screening code may be a first listed code if the reason for the visit is specifically the screening exam. It may also be used as an additional code if the screening is done during an office visit for other health problems. A screening code is not necessary if the screening is inherent to a routine examination, such as a pap smear done during a routine pelvic examination.

Should a condition be discovered during the screening then the code for the condition may be assigned as an additional diagnosis.

The V code indicates that a screening exam is planned. A procedure code is required to confirm that the screening was performed.

The screening V code categories:

V28 Antenatal screening
V73-V82 Special screening examinations

6) **Observation**

There are two observation V code categories. They are for use in very limited circumstances when a person is being observed for a suspected condition that is ruled out. The observation codes are not for use if an injury or illness or any signs or symptoms related to the suspected condition are present. In such cases the diagnosis/symptom code is used with the corresponding E code to identify any external cause.

The observation codes are to be used as principal diagnosis only. The only exception to this is when the principal diagnosis is required to be a code from the V30, Live born infant, category. Then the V29 observation code is sequenced after the V30 code. Additional codes may be used in addition to the observation code but only if they are unrelated to the suspected condition being observed.

The observation V code categories:

V29 Observation and evaluation of newborns for suspected condition not found For the birth encounter, a code from category V30 should be sequenced before the V29 code.
V71 Observation and evaluation for suspected condition not found

7) **Aftercare**

Aftercare visit codes cover situations when the initial treatment of a disease or injury has been performed and the patient requires continued care during the healing or recovery phase, or for the long-term consequences of the disease. The aftercare V code should not be used if treatment is directed at a current, acute disease or injury. The diagnosis code is to be used in these cases. Exceptions to this rule are codes V58.0, Radiotherapy, and codes from subcategory V58.1, Encounter for chemotherapy and immunotherapy for neoplastic conditions. These codes are to be first listed, followed by the diagnosis code when a patient's encounter is solely to receive radiation therapy or chemotherapy for the treatment of a neoplasm. Should a patient receive both chemotherapy and radiation therapy during the same encounter code V58.0 and V58.1 may be used together on a record with either one being sequenced first.

The aftercare codes are generally first listed to explain the specific reason for the encounter. An aftercare code may be used as an additional code when some type of aftercare is provided in addition to the reason for admission and no diagnosis code is applicable. An example of this would be

the closure of a colostomy during an encounter for treatment of another condition.

Certain aftercare V code categories need a secondary diagnosis code to describe the resolving condition or sequelae, for others, the condition is inherent in the code title.

Additional V code aftercare category terms include, fitting and adjustment, and attention to artificial openings.

Status V codes may be used with aftercare V codes to indicate the nature of the aftercare. For example code V45.81, Aortocoronary bypass status, may be used with code V58.73, Aftercare following surgery of the circulatory system, NEC, to indicate the surgery for which the aftercare is being performed. Also, a transplant status code may be used following code V58.44, Aftercare following organ transplant, to identify the organ transplanted. A status code should not be used when the aftercare code indicates the type of status, such as using V55.0, Attention to tracheostomy with V44.0, Tracheostomy status.

The aftercare V category/codes:

V52	Fitting and adjustment of prosthetic device and implant
V53	Fitting and adjustment of other device
V54	Other orthopedic aftercare
V55	Attention to artificial openings
V56	Encounter for dialysis and dialysis catheter care
V57	Care involving the use of rehabilitation procedures
V58.0	Radiotherapy
V58.11	Encounter for antineoplastic chemotherapy
V58.12	Encounter for antineoplastic immunotherapy
V58.3x	Attention to dressings and sutures
V58.41	Encounter for planned post-operative wound closure
V58.42	Aftercare, surgery, neoplasm
V58.43	Aftercare, surgery, trauma
V58.44	Aftercare involving organ transplant
V58.49	Other specified aftercare following surgery
V58.7x	Aftercare following surgery
V58.81	Fitting and adjustment of vascular catheter
V58.82	Fitting and adjustment of non-vascular catheter
V58.83	Monitoring therapeutic drug
V58.89	Other specified aftercare

8) Follow-up

The follow-up codes are used to explain continuing surveillance following completed treatment of a disease, condition, or injury. They imply that the condition has been fully treated and no longer exists. They should not be confused with aftercare codes that explain current treatment for a healing condition or its sequelae. Follow-up codes may be used in conjunction with history codes to provide the full picture of the healed condition and its treatment. The follow-up code is sequenced first, followed by the history code.

A follow-up code may be used to explain repeated visits. Should a condition be found to have recurred on the follow-up visit, then the diagnosis code should be used in place of the follow-up code.

The follow-up V code categories:

V24	Postpartum care and evaluation
V67	Follow-up examination

9) Donor

Category V59 is the donor codes. They are used for living individuals who are donating blood or other body tissue. These codes are only for individuals donating for others, not for self donations. They are not for use to identify cadaveric donations.

10) Counseling

Counseling V codes are used when a patient or family member receives assistance in the aftermath of an illness or injury, or when support is required in coping with family or social problems. They are not necessary for use in conjunction with a diagnosis code when the counseling component of care is considered integral to standard treatment.

The counseling V categories/codes:

V25.0	General counseling and advice for contraceptive management
V26.3	Genetic counseling
V26.4	General counseling and advice for procreative management
V61	Other family circumstances
V65.1	Person consulted on behalf of another person
V65.3	Dietary surveillance and counseling
V65.4	Other counseling, not elsewhere classified

11) Obstetrics and related conditions

See Section I.C.11., the Obstetrics guidelines for further instruction on the use of these codes.

V codes for pregnancy are for use in those circumstances when none of the problems or complications included in the codes from the Obstetrics chapter exist (a routine prenatal visit or postpartum care). Codes V22.0, Supervision of normal first pregnancy, and V22.1, Supervision of other normal pregnancy, are always first listed and are not to be used with any other code from the OB chapter.

The outcome of delivery, category V27, should be included on all maternal delivery records. It is always a secondary code.

V codes for family planning (contraceptive) or procreative management and counseling should be included on an obstetric record either during the pregnancy or the postpartum stage, if applicable.

Obstetrics and related conditions V code categories:

V22	Normal pregnancy
V23	Supervision of high-risk pregnancy Except: V23.2, Pregnancy with history of abortion. Code 646.3, Habitual aborter, from the OB chapter is required to indicate a history of abortion during a pregnancy.
V24	Postpartum care and evaluation
V25	Encounter for contraceptive management Except V25.0x *(See Section I.C.18.d.11, Counseling)*
V26	Procreative management Except 26.5x, Sterilization status, V26.3 and V26.4 *(See Section I.C.18.d.11., Counseling)*
V27	Outcome of delivery
V28	Antenatal screening *(See Section I.C.18.d.6., Screening)*

12) Newborn, infant and child

See Section I.C.15, the Newborn guidelines for further instruction on the use of these codes.

Newborn V code categories:

V20	Health supervision of infant or child
V29	Observation and evaluation of newborns for suspected condition not found *(See Section I.C.18.d.7, Observation)*
V30-V39	Liveborn infant according to type of birth

13) Routine and administrative examinations

The V codes allow for the description of encounters for routine examinations, such as, a general check-up, or, examinations for administrative purposes, such as, a pre-employment physical. The codes are not to be used if the

examination is for diagnosis of a suspected condition or for treatment purposes. In such cases the diagnosis code is used. During a routine exam, should a diagnosis or condition be discovered, it should be coded as an additional code. Pre-existing and chronic conditions and history codes may also be included as additional codes as long as the examination is for administrative purposes and not focused on any particular condition.

Pre-operative examination V codes are for use only in those situations when a patient is being cleared for surgery and no treatment is given.

The V codes categories/code for routine and administrative examinations:

V20.2 Routine infant or child health check
Any injections given should have a corresponding procedure code.

V70 General medical examination

V72 Special investigations and examinations
Codes V72.5 and V72.6 may be used if the reason for the patient encounter is for routine laboratory/radiology testing in the absence of any signs, symptoms, or associated diagnosis. If routine testing is performed during the same encounter as a test to evaluate a sign, symptom, or diagnosis, it is appropriate to assign both the V code and the code describing the reason for the non-routine test.

14) **Miscellaneous V codes**

The miscellaneous V codes capture a number of other health care encounters that do not fall into one of the other categories. Certain of these codes identify the reason for the encounter, others are for use as additional codes that provide useful information on circumstances that may affect a patient's care and treatment.

Prophylactic Organ Removal

For encounters specifically for prophylactic removal of breasts, ovaries, or another organ due to a genetic susceptibility to cancer or a family history of cancer, the principal or first listed code should be a code from subcategory V50.4, Prophylactic organ removal, followed by the appropriate genetic susceptibility code and the appropriate family history code.

If the patient has a malignancy of one site and is having prophylactic removal at another site to prevent either a new primary malignancy or metastatic disease, a code for the malignancy should also be assigned in addition to a code from subcategory V50.4. A V50.4 code should not be assigned if the patient is having organ removal for treatment of a malignancy, such as the removal of the testes for the treatment of prostate cancer.

Miscellaneous V code categories/codes:

V07 Need for isolation and other prophylactic measures
V50 Elective surgery for purposes other than remedying health states
V58.5 Orthodontics
V60 Housing, household, and economic circumstances
V62 Other psychosocial circumstances
V63 Unavailability of other medical facilities for care
V64 Persons encountering health services for specific procedures, not carried out
V66 Convalescence and Palliative Care
V68 Encounters for administrative purposes
V69 Problems related to lifestyle
V85 Body Mass Index

15) **Nonspecific V codes**

Certain V codes are so non-specific, or potentially redundant with other codes in the classification, that there can be little justification for their use in the inpatient setting. Their use in the outpatient setting should be limited to those instances when there is no further documentation to permit more

precise coding. Otherwise, any sign or symptom or any other reason for visit that is captured in another code should be used.

Nonspecific V code categories/codes:

V11 Personal history of mental disorder
A code from the mental disorders chapter, with an in remission fifth-digit, should be used.
V13.4 Personal history of arthritis
V13.6 Personal history of congenital malformations
V15.7 Personal history of contraception
V23.2 Pregnancy with history of abortion
V40 Mental and behavioral problems
V41 Problems with special senses and other special functions
V47 Other problems with internal organs
V48 Problems with head, neck, and trunk
V49 Problems with limbs and other problems
Exceptions:
V49.6 Upper limb amputation status
V49.7 Lower limb amputation status
V49.81 Postmenopausal status
V49.82 Dental sealant status
V49.83 Awaiting organ transplant status
V51 Aftercare involving the use of plastic surgery
V58.2 Blood transfusion, without reported diagnosis
V58.9 Unspecified aftercare
See Section IV.K. and Section IV.L. of the Outpatient guidelines.

Text continued on p. 660

V CODE TABLE

October 1, 2007 (FY2008)
Items in bold indicate a new entry or change from the November 2006 table
Items underlined have been moved within the table since November 2006

The V code table below contains columns for 1st listed, 1st or additional, additional only, and non-specific. Each code or category is listed on the left hand column and the allowable sequencing of the code or codes within the category is noted under the appropriate column.

Code(s)	Description	1st Dx Only[1]	1st or Add'l Dx[2]	Add'l Dx Only[3]	Non-Specific Diagnosis[4]
V01.X	Contact with or exposure to communicable diseases		X		
V02.X	Carrier or suspected carrier of infectious diseases		X		
V03.X	Need for prophylactic vaccination and inoculation against bacterial diseases		X		
V04.X	Need for prophylactic vaccination and inoculation against certain diseases		X		
V05.X	Need for prophylactic vaccination and inoculation against single diseases		X		
V06.X	Need for prophylactic vaccination and inoculation against combinations of diseases		X		
V07.X	Need for isolation and other prophylactic measures		X		
V08	Asymptomatic HIV infection status		X		
V09.X	Infection with drug resistant organisms			X	
V10.X	Personal history of malignant neoplasm		X		
V11.X	Personal history of mental disorder				X
V12.X	Personal history of certain other diseases		X		

Continued

Code(s)	Description	1st Dx Only[1]	1st or Add'l Dx[2]	Add'l Dx Only[3]	Non-Specific Diagnosis[4]
V13.0X	Personal history of other disorders of urinary system		X		
V13.1	Personal history of trophoblastic disease		X		
V13.2X	Personal history of other genital system and obstetric disorders		X		
V13.3	Personal history of diseases of skin and subcutaneous tissue		X		
V13.4	Personal history of arthritis				X
V13.5	Personal history of other musculoskeletal disorders		X		
V13.61	Personal history of hypospadias			X	
V13.69	Personal history of congenital malformations				X
V13.7	Personal history of perinatal problems		X		
V13.8	Personal history of other specified diseases		X		
V13.9	Personal history of unspecified disease				X
V14.X	Personal history of allergy to medicinal agents			X	
V15.0X	Personal history of allergy, other than to medicinal agents			X	
V15.1	Personal history of surgery to heart and great vessels			X	
V15.2	Personal history of surgery to other major organs			X	
V15.3	Personal history of irradiation			X	
V15.4X	Personal history of psychological trauma			X	
V15.5	Personal history of injury			X	
V15.6	Personal history of poisoning			X	
V15.7	Personal history of contraception				X
V15.81	Personal history of noncompliance with medical treatment			X	
V15.82	Personal history of tobacco use			X	
V15.84	Personal history of exposure to asbestos			X	
V15.85	Personal history of exposure to potentially hazardous body fluids			X	
V15.86	Personal history of exposure to lead			X	
V15.87	Personal history of extracorporeal membrane oxygenation [ECMO]			X	
V15.88	History of fall		X		
V15.89	Other specified personal history presenting hazards to health			X	
V16.X	Family history of malignant neoplasm		X		
V17.X	Family history of certain chronic disabling diseases		X		
V18.X	Family history of certain other specific conditions		X		
V19.X	Family history of other conditions		X		
V20.X	Health supervision of infant or child	X			
V21.X	Constitutional states in development			X	
V22.0	Supervision of normal first pregnancy	X			
V22.1	Supervision of other normal pregnancy	X			
V22.2	Pregnancy state, incidental			X	
V23.X	Supervision of high-risk pregnancy		X		
V24.X	Postpartum care and examination	X			
V25.X	Encounter for contraceptive management		X		
V26.0	Tuboplasty or vasoplasty after previous sterilization		X		
V26.1	Artificial insemination		X		
V26.2X	Procreative management investigation and testing		X		
V26.3X	Procreative management, genetic counseling and testing		X		

Code(s)	Description	1st Dx Only[1]	1st or Add'l Dx[2]	Add'l Dx Only[3]	Non-Specific Diagnosis[4]
V26.4X	Procreative management, genetic counseling and advice		X		
V26.5X	Procreative management, sterilization status			X	
V26.81	**Encounter for assisted reproductive fertility procedure cycle**	**X**			
V26.89	Other specified procreative management		X		
V26.9	Unspecified procreative management		X		
V27.X	Outcome of delivery			X	
V28.X	Encounter for antenatal screening of mother		X		
V29.X	Observation and evaluation of newborns for suspected condition not found		X		
V30.X	Single liveborn	X			
V31.X	Twin, mate liveborn	X			
V32.X	Twin, mate stillborn	X			
V33.X	Twin, unspecified	X			
V34.X	Other multiple, mates all liveborn	X			
V35.X	Other multiple, mates all stillborn	X			
V36.X	Other multiple, mates live- and stillborn	X			
V37.X	Other multiple, unspecified	X			
V39.X	Unspecified	X			
V40.X	Mental and behavioral problems				X
V41.X	Problems with special senses and other special functions				X
V42.X	Organ or tissue replaced by transplant			X	
V43.0	Organ or tissue replaced by other means, eye globe			X	
V43.1	Organ or tissue replaced by other means, lens			X	
V43.21	Organ or tissue replaced by other means, heart assist device			X	
V43.22	Fully implantable artificial heart status		X		
V43.3	Organ or tissue replaced by other means, heart valve			X	
V43.4	Organ or tissue replaced by other means, blood vessel			X	
V43.5	Organ or tissue replaced by other means, bladder			X	
V43.6X	Organ or tissue replaced by other means, joint			X	
V43.7	Organ or tissue replaced by other means, limb			X	
V43.8X	Other organ or tissue replaced by other means			X	
V44.X	Artificial opening status			X	
V45.0X	Cardiac device in situ			X	
V45.1	Renal dialysis status			X	
V45.2	Presence of cerebrospinal fluid drainage device			X	
V45.3	Intestinal bypass or anastomosis status			X	
V45.4	Arthrodesis status			X	
V45.5X	Presence of contraceptive device			X	
V45.6X	States following surgery of eye and adnexa			X	
V45.7X	Acquired absence of organ		X		
V45.8X	Other postprocedural status			X	
V46.0	Other dependence on machines, aspirator			X	
V46.11	Dependence on respiratory, status			X	
V46.12	Encounter for respirator dependence during power failure	X			
V46.13	Encounter for weaning from respirator [ventilator]	X			
V46.14	Mechanical complication of respirator [ventilator]		X		
V46.2	Other dependence on machines, supplemental oxygen			X	
V46.8	Other dependence on other enabling machines			X	
V46.9	Unspecified machine dependence				X

Continued

Code(s)	Description	1st Dx Only[1]	1st or Add'l Dx[2]	Add'l Dx Only[3]	Non-Specific Diagnosis[4]
V47.X	Other problems with internal organs				X
V48.X	Problems with head, neck and trunk				X
V49.0	Deficiencies of limbs				X
V49.1	Mechanical problems with limbs				X
V49.2	Motor problems with limbs				X
V49.3	Sensory problems with limbs				X
V49.4	Disfigurements of limbs				X
V49.5	Other problems with limbs				X
V49.6X	Upper limb amputation status		X		
V49.7X	Lower limb amputation status		X		
V49.81	Asymptomatic postmenopausal status (age-related) (natural)		X		
V49.82	Dental sealant status			X	
V49.83	Awaiting organ transplant status			X	
V49.84	Bed confinement status		X		
V49.85	**Dual sensory impairment**			**X**	
V49.89	Other specified conditions influencing health status		X		
V49.9	Unspecified condition influencing health status				X
V50.X	Elective surgery for purposes other than remedying health states		X		
V51	Aftercare involving the use of plastic surgery				X
V52.X	Fitting and adjustment of prosthetic device and implant		X		
V53.X	Fitting and adjustment of other device		X		
V54.X	Other orthopedic aftercare		X		
V55.X	Attention to artificial openings		X		
V56.0	Extracorporeal dialysis	X			
V56.1	Encounter for fitting and adjustment of extracorporeal dialysis catheter		X		
V56.2	Encounter for fitting and adjustment of peritoneal dialysis catheter		X		
V56.3X	Encounter for adequacy testing for dialysis		X		
V56.8	Encounter for other dialysis and dialysis catheter care		X		
V57.X	Care involving use of rehabilitation procedures	X			
V58.0	Radiotherapy	X			
V58.11	Encounter for antineoplastic chemotherapy	X			
V58.12	Encounter for antineoplastic immunotherapy	X			
V58.2	Blood transfusion without reported diagnosis				X
V58.3X	Attention to dressings and sutures		X		
V58.4X	Other aftercare following surgery		X		
V58.5	Encounter for orthodontics				X
V58.6X	Long term (current) drug use			X	
V58.7X	Aftercare following surgery to specified body systems, not elsewhere classified		X		
V58.8X	Other specified procedures and aftercare		X		
V58.9	Unspecified aftercare				X
V59.X	Donors	X			
V60.X	Housing, household, and economic circumstances			X	
V61.X	Other family circumstances		X		
V62.X	Other psychosocial circumstances			X	
V63.X	Unavailability of other medical facilities for care		X		
V64.X	Persons encountering health services for specified procedure, not carried out			X	

Code(s)	Description	1st Dx Only[1]	1st or Add'l Dx[2]	Add'l Dx Only[3]	Non-Specific Diagnosis[4]
V65.X	Other persons seeking consultation without complaint or sickness		X		
V66.0	Convalescence and palliative care following surgery	X			
V66.1	Convalescence and palliative care following radiotherapy	X			
V66.2	Convalescence and palliative care following chemotherapy	X			
V66.3	Convalescence and palliative care following psychotherapy and other treatment for mental disorder	X			
V66.4	Convalescence and palliative care following treatment of fracture	X			
V66.5	Convalescence and palliative care following other treatment	X			
V66.6	Convalescence and palliative care following combined treatment	X			
V66.7	Encounter for palliative care			X	
V66.9	Unspecified convalescence	X			
V67.X	Follow-up examination		X		
V68.X	Encounters for administrative purposes	X			
V69.X	Problems related to lifestyle		X		
V70.0	Routine general medical examination at a health care facility	X			
V70.1	General psychiatric examination, requested by the authority	X			
V70.2	General psychiatric examination, other and unspecified	X			
V70.3	Other medical examination for administrative purposes	X			
V70.4	Examination for medicolegal reasons	X			
V70.5	Health examination of defined subpopulations	X			
V70.6	Health examination in population surveys	X			
V70.7	Examination of participant in clinical trial		X		
V70.8	Other specified general medical examinations	X			
V70.9	Unspecified general medical examination	X			
V71.X	Observation and evaluation for suspected conditions not found	X			
V72.0	Examination of eyes and vision		X		
V72.1X	Examination of ears and hearing		X		
V72.2	Dental examination		X		
V72.3X	Gynecological examination		X		
V72.4X	Pregnancy examination or test		X		
V72.5	Radiological examination, NEC		X		
V72.6	Laboratory examination		X		
V72.7	Diagnostic skin and sensitization tests		X		
V72.81	Preoperative cardiovascular examination		X		
V72.82	Preoperative respiratory examination		X		
V72.83	Other specified preoperative examination		X		
V72.84	Preoperative examination, unspecified		X		
V72.85	Other specified examination		X		
V72.86	Encounter for blood typing		X		
V72.9	Unspecified examination				X
V73.X	Special screening examination for viral and chlamydial diseases		X		
V74.X	Special screening examination for bacterial and spirochetal diseases		X		
V75.X	Special screening examination for other infectious diseases		X		

Continued

Code(s)	Description	1st Dx Only[1]	1st or Add'l Dx[2]	Add'l Dx Only[3]	Non-Specific Diagnosis[4]
V76.X	Special screening examination for malignant neoplasms		X		
V77.X	Special screening examination for endocrine, nutritional, metabolic and immunity disorders		X		
V78.X	Special screening examination for disorders of blood and blood-forming organs		X		
V79.X	Special screening examination for mental disorders and developmental handicaps		X		
V80.X	Special screening examination for neurological, eye, and ear diseases		X		
V81.X	Special screening examination for cardiovascular, respiratory, and genitourinary diseases		X		
V82.X	Special screening examination for other conditions		X		
V83.X	Genetic carrier status		X		
V84.X	Genetic susceptibility to disease			X	
V85	Body mass index			X	
V86	Estrogen receptor status			X	

[1]Generally for use as first listed only but may be used as additional if patient has more than one encounter on one day **or there is more than one reason for the encounter**
[2]These codes may be used as first listed or additional codes
[3]These codes are only for use as additional codes
[4]These codes are primarily for use in the nonacute setting and should be limited to encounters for which no sign or symptom or reason for visit is documented in the record. Their use may be as either a first listed or additional code.

19. Supplemental Classification of External Causes of Injury and Poisoning (E-codes, E800-E999)

Introduction: These guidelines are provided for those who are currently collecting E codes in order that there will be standardization in the process. If your institution plans to begin collecting E codes, these guidelines are to be applied. The use of E codes is supplemental to the application of ICD-9-CM diagnosis codes. E codes are never to be recorded as principal diagnoses (first-listed in non-inpatient setting) and are not required for reporting to CMS.

External causes of injury and poisoning codes (E codes) are intended to provide data for injury research and evaluation of injury prevention strategies. E codes capture how the injury or poisoning happened (cause), the intent (unintentional or accidental; or intentional, such as suicide or assault), and the place where the event occurred.

Some major categories of E codes include:
transport accidents
poisoning and adverse effects of drugs, medicinal substances and biologicals
accidental falls
accidents caused by fire and flames
accidents due to natural and environmental factors
late effects of accidents, assaults or self injury
assaults or purposely inflicted injury
suicide or self inflicted injury

These guidelines apply for the coding and collection of E codes from records in hospitals, outpatient clinics, emergency departments, other ambulatory care settings and provider offices, and nonacute care settings, except when other specific guidelines apply.

a. General E Code Coding Guidelines

1) Used with any code in the range of 001-V84.8

An E code may be used with any code in the range of 001-V84.8, which indicates an injury, poisoning, or adverse effect due to an external cause.

2) **Assign the appropriate E code for all initial treatments**
Assign the appropriate E code for the initial encounter of an injury, poisoning, or adverse effect of drugs, not for subsequent treatment.
External cause of injury codes (E-codes) may be assigned while the acute fracture codes are still applicable.
See Section I.C.17.b.1 for coding of acute fractures.
3) **Use the full range of E codes**
Use the full range of E codes to completely describe the cause, the intent and the place of occurrence, if applicable, for all injuries, poisonings, and adverse effects of drugs.
4) **Assign as many E codes as necessary**
Assign as many E codes as necessary to fully explain each cause. If only one E code can be recorded, assign the E code most related to the principal diagnosis.
5) **The selection of the appropriate E code**
The selection of the appropriate E code is guided by the Index to External Causes, which is located after the alphabetical index to diseases and by Inclusion and Exclusion notes in the Tabular List.
6) **E code can never be a principal diagnosis**
An E code can never be a principal (first listed) diagnosis.
7) **External cause code(s) with systemic inflammatory response syndrome (SIRS)**
An external cause code is not appropriate with a code from subcategory 995.9, unless the patient also has an injury, poisoning, or adverse effect of drugs.

b. **Place of Occurrence Guideline**
Use an additional code from category E849 to indicate the Place of Occurrence for injuries and poisonings. The Place of Occurrence describes the place where the event occurred and not the patient's activity at the time of the event.
Do not use E849.9 if the place of occurrence is not stated.

c. **Adverse Effects of Drugs, Medicinal and Biological Substances Guidelines**
1) **Do not code directly from the Table of Drugs**
Do not code directly from the Table of Drugs and Chemicals. Always refer back to the Tabular List.
2) **Use as many codes as necessary to describe**
Use as many codes as necessary to describe completely all drugs, medicinal or biological substances.
3) **If the same E code would describe the causative agent**
If the same E code would describe the causative agent for more than one adverse reaction, assign the code only once.
4) **If two or more drugs, medicinal or biological substances**
If two or more drugs, medicinal or biological substances are reported, code each individually unless the combination code is listed in the Table of Drugs and Chemicals. In that case, assign the E code for the combination.
5) **When a reaction results from the interaction of a drug(s)**
When a reaction results from the interaction of a drug(s) and alcohol, use poisoning codes and E codes for both.
6) **If the reporting format limits the number of E codes**
If the reporting format limits the number of E codes that can be used in reporting clinical data, code the one most related to the principal diagnosis. Include at least one from each category (cause, intent, place) if possible.
If there are different fourth digit codes in the same three digit category, use the code for "Other specified" of that category. If there is no "Other specified" code in that category, use the appropriate "Unspecified" code in that category.

If the codes are in different three digit categories, assign the appropriate E code for other multiple drugs and medicinal substances.

7) **Codes from the E930-E949 series**

Codes from the E930-E949 series must be used to identify the causative substance for an adverse effect of drug, medicinal and biological substances, correctly prescribed and properly administered. The effect, such as tachycardia, delirium, gastrointestinal hemorrhaging, vomiting, hypokalemia, hepatitis, renal failure, or respiratory failure, is coded and followed by the appropriate code from the E930-E949 series.

d. Multiple Cause E Code Coding Guidelines

If two or more events cause separate injuries, an E code should be assigned for each cause. The first listed E code will be selected in the following order:

E codes for child and adult abuse take priority over all other E codes.
See Section I.C.19.e., Child and Adult abuse guidelines.

E codes for terrorism events take priority over all other E codes except child and adult abuse

E codes for cataclysmic events take priority over all other E codes except child and adult abuse and terrorism.

E codes for transport accidents take priority over all other E codes except cataclysmic events and child and adult abuse and terrorism.

The first-listed E code should correspond to the cause of the most serious diagnosis due to an assault, accident, or self-harm, following the order of hierarchy listed above.

e. Child and Adult Abuse Guideline

1) **Intentional injury**

When the cause of an injury or neglect is intentional child or adult abuse, the first listed E code should be assigned from categories E960-E968, Homicide and injury purposely inflicted by other persons, (except category E967). An E code from category E967, Child and adult battering and other maltreatment, should be added as an additional code to identify the perpetrator, if known.

2) **Accidental intent**

In cases of neglect when the intent is determined to be accidental E code E904.0, Abandonment or neglect of infant and helpless person, should be the first listed E code.

f. Unknown or Suspected Intent Guideline

1) **If the intent (accident, self-harm, assault) of the cause of an injury or poisoning is unknown**

If the intent (accident, self-harm, assault) of the cause of an injury or poisoning is unknown or unspecified, code the intent as undetermined E980-E989.

2) **If the intent (accident, self-harm, assault) of the cause of an injury or poisoning is questionable**

If the intent (accident, self-harm, assault) of the cause of an injury or poisoning is questionable, probable or suspected, code the intent as undetermined E980-E989.

g. Undetermined Cause

When the intent of an injury or poisoning is known, but the cause is unknown, use codes: E928.9, Unspecified accident, E958.9, Suicide and self-inflicted injury by unspecified means, and E968.9, Assault by unspecified means.

These E codes should rarely be used, as the documentation in the medical record, in both the inpatient outpatient and other settings, should normally provide sufficient detail to determine the cause of the injury.

h. Late Effects of External Cause Guidelines

1) **Late effect E codes**

Late effect E codes exist for injuries and poisonings but not for adverse effects of drugs, misadventures and surgical complications.

2) **Late effect E codes (E929, E959, E969, E977, E989, or E999.1)**
A late effect E code (E929, E959, E969, E977, E989, or E999.1) should be used with any report of a late effect or sequela resulting from a previous injury or poisoning (905-909).

3) **Late effect E code with a related current injury**
A late effect E code should never be used with a related current nature of injury code.

4) **Use of late effect E codes for subsequent visits**
Use a late effect E code for subsequent visits when a late effect of the initial injury or poisoning is being treated. There is no late effect E code for adverse effects of drugs.

Do not use a late effect E code for subsequent visits for follow-up care (e.g., to assess healing, to receive rehabilitative therapy) of the injury or poisoning when no late effect of the injury has been documented.

i. **Misadventures and Complications of Care Guidelines**

1) **Code range E870-E876**
Assign a code in the range of E870-E876 if misadventures are stated by the provider.

2) **Code range E878-E879**
Assign a code in the range of E878-E879 if the provider attributes an abnormal reaction or later complication to a surgical or medical procedure, but does not mention misadventure at the time of the procedure as the cause of the reaction.

j. **Terrorism Guidelines**

1) **Cause of injury identified by the Federal Government (FBI) as terrorism**
When the cause of an injury is identified by the Federal Government (FBI) as terrorism, the first-listed E-code should be a code from category E979, Terrorism. The definition of terrorism employed by the FBI is found at the inclusion note at E979. The terrorism E-code is the only E-code that should be assigned. Additional E codes from the assault categories should not be assigned.

2) **Cause of an injury is suspected to be the result of terrorism**
When the cause of an injury is suspected to be the result of terrorism a code from category E979 should not be assigned. Assign a code in the range of E codes based circumstances on the documentation of intent and mechanism.

3) **Code E979.9, Terrorism, secondary effects**
Assign code E979.9, Terrorism, secondary effects, for conditions occurring subsequent to the terrorist event. This code should not be assigned for conditions that are due to the initial terrorist act.

4) **Statistical tabulation of terrorism codes**
For statistical purposes these codes will be tabulated within the category for assault, expanding the current category from E960-E969 to include E979 and E999.1.

SECTION II. SELECTION OF PRINCIPAL DIAGNOSIS

The circumstances of inpatient admission always govern the selection of principal diagnosis. The principal diagnosis is defined in the Uniform Hospital Discharge Data Set (UHDDS) as "that condition established after study to be chiefly responsible for occasioning the admission of the patient to the hospital for care."

The UHDDS definitions are used by hospitals to report inpatient data elements in a standardized manner. These data elements and their definitions can be found in the July 31, 1985, Federal Register (Vol. 50, No, 147), pp. 31038-40.

Since that time the application of the UHDDS definitions has been expanded to include all non-outpatient settings (acute care, short term, long term care and psychiatric hospitals; home health agencies; rehab facilities; nursing homes, etc).

In determining principal diagnosis the coding conventions in the ICD-9-CM, Volumes I and II take precedence over these official coding guidelines.

(See Section I.A., Conventions for the ICD-9-CM)

The importance of consistent, complete documentation in the medical record cannot be overemphasized. Without such documentation the application of all coding guidelines is a difficult, if not impossible, task.

A. Codes for Symptoms, Signs, and Ill-defined Conditions

Codes for symptoms, signs, and ill-defined conditions from Chapter 16 are not to be used as principal diagnosis when a related definitive diagnosis has been established.

B. Two or More Interrelated Conditions, Each Potentially Meeting the Definition for Principal Diagnosis

When there are two or more interrelated conditions (such as diseases in the same ICD-9-CM chapter or manifestations characteristically associated with a certain disease) potentially meeting the definition of principal diagnosis, either condition may be sequenced first, unless the circumstances of the admission, the therapy provided, the Tabular List, or the Alphabetic Index indicate otherwise.

C. Two or More Diagnoses that Equally Meet the Definition for Principal Diagnosis

In the unusual instance when two or more diagnoses equally meet the criteria for principal diagnosis as determined by the circumstances of admission, diagnostic workup and/or therapy provided, and the Alphabetic Index, Tabular List, or another coding guidelines does not provide sequencing direction, any one of the diagnoses may be sequenced first.

D. Two or More Comparative or Contrasting Conditions

In those rare instances when two or more contrasting or comparative diagnoses are documented as "either/or" (or similar terminology), they are coded as if the diagnoses were confirmed and the diagnoses are sequenced according to the circumstances of the admission. If no further determination can be made as to which diagnosis should be principal, either diagnosis may be sequenced first.

E. A Symptom(s) Followed by Contrasting/Comparative Diagnoses

When a symptom(s) is followed by contrasting/comparative diagnoses, the symptom code is sequenced first. All the contrasting/comparative diagnoses should be coded as additional diagnoses.

F. Original Treatment Plan not Carried Out

Sequence as the principal diagnosis the condition, which after study occasioned the admission to the hospital, even though treatment may not have been carried out due to unforeseen circumstances.

G. Complications of Surgery and Other Medical Care

When the admission is for treatment of a complication resulting from surgery or other medical care, the complication code is sequenced as the principal diagnosis. If the compli-

cation is classified to the 996-999 series and the code lacks the necessary specificity in describing the complication, an additional code for the specific complication should be assigned.

H. Uncertain Diagnosis

If the diagnosis documented at the time of discharge is qualified as "probable", "suspected", "likely", "questionable", "possible", or "still to be ruled out", or other similar terms indicating uncertainty, code the condition as if it existed or was established. The bases for these guidelines are the diagnostic workup, arrangements for further workup or observation, and initial therapeutic approach that correspond most closely with the established diagnosis.

Note: This guideline is applicable only to inpatient admissions to short-term, acute, long-term care and psychiatric hospitals.

I. Admission from Observation Unit

1. **Admission Following Medical Observation**
   When a patient is admitted to an observation unit for a medical condition, which either worsens or does not improve, and is subsequently admitted as an inpatient of the same hospital for this same medical condition, the principal diagnosis would be the medical condition which led to the hospital admission.
2. **Admission Following Post-Operative Observation**
   When a patient is admitted to an observation unit to monitor a condition (or complication) that develops following outpatient surgery, and then is subsequently admitted as an inpatient of the same hospital, hospitals should apply the Uniform Hospital Discharge Data Set (UHDDS) definition of principal diagnosis as "that condition established after study to be chiefly responsible for occasioning the admission of the patient to the hospital for care."

J. Admission from Outpatient Surgery

When a patient receives surgery in the hospital's outpatient surgery department and is subsequently admitted for continuing inpatient care at the same hospital, the following guidelines should be followed in selecting the principal diagnosis for the inpatient admission:

- If the reason for the inpatient admission is a complication, assign the complication as the principal diagnosis.
- If no complication, or other condition, is documented as the reason for the inpatient admission, assign the reason for the outpatient surgery as the principal diagnosis.
- If the reason for the inpatient admission is another condition unrelated to the surgery, assign the unrelated condition as the principal diagnosis.

SECTION III. REPORTING ADDITIONAL DIAGNOSES

General Rules for Other (Additional) Diagnoses

For reporting purposes the definition for "other diagnoses" is interpreted as additional conditions that affect patient care in terms of requiring:
clinical evaluation; or
therapeutic treatment; or
diagnostic procedures; or
extended length of hospital stay; or
increased nursing care and/or monitoring.

The UHDDS item #11-b defines Other Diagnoses as "all conditions that coexist at the time of admission, that develop subsequently, or that affect the treatment received and/or the length of stay. Diagnoses that relate to an earlier episode which have no bearing on the current hospital stay are to be excluded." UHDDS definitions apply to inpatients in acute care, short-term, long term care and psychiatric hospital setting. The UHDDS definitions are used by acute care short-term hospitals to report inpatient data elements in a standardized manner. These data elements and their definitions can be found in the July 31, 1985, Federal Register (Vol. 50, No, 147), pp. 31038-40.

Since that time the application of the UHDDS definitions has been expanded to include all non-outpatient settings (acute care, short term, long term care and psychiatric hospitals; home health agencies; rehab facilities; nursing homes, etc).

The following guidelines are to be applied in designating "other diagnoses" when neither the Alphabetic Index nor the Tabular List in ICD-9-CM provide direction. The listing of the diagnoses in the patient record is the responsibility of the attending provider.

A. Previous Conditions

If the provider has included a diagnosis in the final diagnostic statement, such as the discharge summary or the face sheet, it should ordinarily be coded. Some providers include in the diagnostic statement resolved conditions or diagnoses and status-post procedures from previous admission that have no bearing on the current stay. Such conditions are not to be reported and are coded only if required by hospital policy.

However, history codes (V10-V19) may be used as secondary codes if the historical condition or family history has an impact on current care or influences treatment.

B. Abnormal Findings

Abnormal findings (laboratory, x-ray, pathologic, and other diagnostic results) are not coded and reported unless the provider indicates their clinical significance. If the findings are outside the normal range and the attending provider has ordered other tests to evaluate the condition or prescribed treatment, it is appropriate to ask the provider whether the abnormal finding should be added.

Please note: This differs from the coding practices in the outpatient setting for coding encounters for diagnostic tests that have been interpreted by a provider.

C. Uncertain Diagnosis

If the diagnosis documented at the time of discharge is qualified as "probable", "suspected", "likely", "questionable", "possible", or "still to be ruled out" or other similar terms indicating uncertainty, code the condition as if it existed or was established. The bases for these guidelines are the diagnostic workup, arrangements for further workup or observation, and initial therapeutic approach that correspond most closely with the established diagnosis.

Note: This guideline is applicable only to inpatient admissions to short-term, acute, long-term care and psychiatric hospitals.

SECTION IV. DIAGNOSTIC CODING AND REPORTING GUIDELINES FOR OUTPATIENT SERVICES

These coding guidelines for outpatient diagnoses have been approved for use by hospitals/ providers in coding and reporting hospital-based outpatient services and provider-based office visits.

Information about the use of certain abbreviations, punctuation, symbols, and other conventions used in the ICD-9-CM Tabular List (code numbers and titles), can be found

in Section IA of these guidelines, under "Conventions Used in the Tabular List." Information about the correct sequence to use in finding a code is also described in Section I.

The terms encounter and visit are often used interchangeably in describing outpatient service contacts and, therefore, appear together in these guidelines without distinguishing one from the other.

Though the conventions and general guidelines apply to all settings, coding guidelines for outpatient and provider reporting of diagnoses will vary in a number of instances from those for inpatient diagnoses, recognizing that:

The Uniform Hospital Discharge Data Set (UHDDS) definition of principal diagnosis applies only to inpatients in acute, short-term, long-term care and psychiatric hospitals.

Coding guidelines for inconclusive diagnoses (probable, suspected, rule out, etc.) were developed for inpatient reporting and do not apply to outpatients.

A. Selection of First-Listed Condition

In the outpatient setting, the term first-listed diagnosis is used in lieu of principal diagnosis.

In determining the first-listed diagnosis the coding conventions of ICD-9-CM, as well as the general and disease specific guidelines take precedence over the outpatient guidelines.

Diagnoses often are not established at the time of the initial encounter/visit. It may take two or more visits before the diagnosis is confirmed.

The most critical rule involves beginning the search for the correct code assignment through the Alphabetic Index. Never begin searching initially in the Tabular List as this will lead to coding errors.

1. **Outpatient Surgery**

   When a patient presents for outpatient surgery, code the reason for the surgery as the first-listed diagnosis (reason for the encounter), even if the surgery is not performed due to a contraindication.

2. **Observation Stay**

   When a patient is admitted for observation for a medical condition, assign a code for the medical condition as the first-listed diagnosis.

   When a patient presents for outpatient surgery and develops complications requiring admission to observation, code the reason for the surgery as the first reported diagnosis (reason for the encounter), followed by codes for the complications as secondary diagnoses.

B. Codes from 001.0 Through V84.8

The appropriate code or codes from 001.0 through V84.8 must be used to identify diagnoses, symptoms, conditions, problems, complaints, or other reason(s) for the encounter/visit.

C. Accurate Reporting of ICD-9-CM Diagnosis Codes

For accurate reporting of ICD-9-CM diagnosis codes, the documentation should describe the patient's condition, using terminology which includes specific diagnoses as well as symptoms, problems, or reasons for the encounter. There are ICD-9-CM codes to describe all of these.

D. Selection of Codes 001.0 Through 999.9

The selection of codes 001.0 through 999.9 will frequently be used to describe the reason for the encounter. These codes are from the section of ICD-9-CM for the classification of

diseases and injuries (e.g. infectious and parasitic diseases; neoplasms; symptoms, signs, and ill-defined conditions, etc.).

E. Codes That Describe Symptoms and Signs

Codes that describe symptoms and signs, as opposed to diagnoses, are acceptable for reporting purposes when a diagnosis has not been established (confirmed) by the provider. Chapter 16 of ICD-9-CM, Symptoms, Signs, and Ill-defined conditions (codes 780.0-799.9) contain many, but not all codes for symptoms.

F. Encounters for Circumstances Other Than a Disease or Injury

ICD-9-CM provides codes to deal with encounters for circumstances other than a disease or injury. The Supplementary Classification of factors Influencing Health Status and Contact with Health Services (V01.0-V84.8) is provided to deal with occasions when circumstances other than a disease or injury are recorded as diagnosis or problems. ***See Section I.C. 18 for information on V-codes***

G. Level of Detail in Coding

1. **ICD-9-CM codes with 3, 4, or 5 digits**
   ICD-9-CM is composed of codes with either 3, 4, or 5 digits. Codes with three digits are included in ICD-9-CM as the heading of a category of codes that may be further subdivided by the use of fourth and/or fifth digits, which provide greater specificity.
2. **Use of full number of digits required for a code**
   A three-digit code is to be used only if it is not further subdivided. Where fourth-digit subcategories and/or fifth-digit subclassifications are provided, they must be assigned. A code is invalid if it has not been coded to the full number of digits required for that code.
   See also discussion under Section I.b.3., General Coding Guidelines, Level of Detail in Coding.

H. ICD-9-CM Code for the Diagnosis, Condition, Problem, or Other Reason for Encounter/Visit

List first the ICD-9-CM Code for the diagnosis, condition, problem, or other reason for encounter/visit shown in the medical record to be chiefly responsible for the services provided. List additional codes that describe any coexisting conditions. In some cases the first-listed diagnosis may be a symptom when a diagnosis has not been established (confirmed) by the physician.

I. Uncertain Diagnosis

Do not code diagnoses documented as "probable", "suspected," "questionable," "rule out," or "working diagnosis" or other similar terms indicating uncertainty. Rather, code the condition(s) to the highest degree of certainty for that encounter/visit, such as symptoms, signs, abnormal test results, or other reason for the visit.

Please note: This differs from the coding practices used by short-term, acute care, long-term care and psychiatric hospitals.

J. Chronic Diseases

Chronic diseases treated on an ongoing basis may be coded and reported as many times as the patient receives treatment and care for the condition(s).

K. Code All Documented Conditions That Coexist

Code all documented conditions that coexist at the time of the encounter/visit, and require or affect patient care treatment or management. Do not code conditions that were previously treated and no longer exist. However, history codes (V10-V19) may be used as secondary codes if the historical condition or family history has an impact on current care or influences treatment.

L. Patients Receiving Diagnostic Services Only

For patients receiving diagnostic services only during an encounter/visit, sequence first the diagnosis, condition, problem, or other reason for encounter/visit shown in the medical record to be chiefly responsible for the outpatient services provided during the encounter/visit. Codes for other diagnoses (e.g., chronic conditions) may be sequenced as additional diagnoses.

For encounters for routine laboratory/radiology testing in the absence of any signs, symptoms, or associated diagnosis, assign V72.5 and V72.6. If routine testing is performed during the same encounter as a test to evaluate a sign, symptom, or diagnosis, it is appropriate to assign both the V code and the code describing the reason for the non-routine test.

For outpatient encounters for diagnostic tests that have been interpreted by a physician, and the final report is available at the time of coding, code any confirmed or definitive diagnosis(es) documented in the interpretation. Do not code related signs and symptoms as additional diagnoses.

Please note: This differs from the coding practice in the hospital inpatient setting regarding abnormal findings on test results.

M. Patients Receiving Therapeutic Services Only

For patients receiving therapeutic services only during an encounter/visit, sequence first the diagnosis, condition, problem, or other reason for encounter/visit shown in the medical record to be chiefly responsible for the outpatient services provided during the encounter/visit. Codes for other diagnoses (e.g., chronic conditions) may be sequenced as additional diagnoses.

The only exception to this rule is that when the primary reason for the admission/encounter is chemotherapy, radiation therapy, or rehabilitation, the appropriate V code for the service is listed first, and the diagnosis or problem for which the service is being performed listed second.

N. Patients Receiving Preoperative Evaluations Only

For patients receiving preoperative evaluations only, sequence first a code from category V72.8, Other specified examinations, to describe the pre-op consultations. Assign a code for the condition to describe the reason for the surgery as an additional diagnosis. Code also any findings related to the pre-op evaluation.

O. Ambulatory Surgery

For ambulatory surgery, code the diagnosis for which the surgery was performed. If the postoperative diagnosis is known to be different from the preoperative diagnosis at the time the diagnosis is confirmed, select the postoperative diagnosis for coding, since it is the most definitive.

P. Routine Outpatient Prenatal Visits

For routine outpatient prenatal visits when no complications are present, codes V22.0, Supervision of normal first pregnancy, or V22.1, Supervision of other normal pregnancy,

should be used as the principal diagnosis. These codes should not be used in conjunction with chapter 11 codes.

APPENDIX I

Present on Admission Reporting Guidelines

Introduction

These guidelines are to be used as a supplement to the *ICD-9-CM Official Guidelines for Coding and Reporting* to facilitate the assignment of the Present on Admission (POA) indicator for each diagnosis and external cause of injury code reported on claim forms (UB-04 and 837 Institutional).

These guidelines are not intended to replace any guidelines in the main body of the *ICD-9-CM Official Guidelines for Coding and Reporting.* The POA guidelines are not intended to provide guidance on when a condition should be coded, but rather, how to apply the POA indicator to the final set of diagnosis codes that have been assigned in accordance with Sections I, II, and III of the official coding guidelines. Subsequent to the assignment of the ICD-9-CM codes, the POA indicator should then be assigned to those conditions that have been coded.

As stated in the Introduction to the ICD-9-CM Official Guidelines for Coding and Reporting, a joint effort between the healthcare provider and the coder is essential to achieve complete and accurate documentation, code assignment, and reporting of diagnoses and procedures. The importance of consistent, complete documentation in the medical record cannot be overemphasized. Medical record documentation from any provider involved in the care and treatment of the patient may be used to support the determination of whether a condition was present on admission or not. In the context of the official coding guidelines, the term "provider" means a physician or any qualified healthcare practitioner who is legally accountable for establishing the patient's diagnosis.

General Reporting Requirements

All claims involving inpatient admissions to general acute care hospitals or other facilities that are subject to a law or regulation mandating collection of present on admission information.

Present on admission is defined as present at the time the order for inpatient admission occurs—conditions that develop during an outpatient encounter, including emergency department, observation, or outpatient surgery, are considered as present on admission.

POA indicator is assigned to principal and secondary diagnoses (as defined in Section II of the Official Guidelines for Coding and Reporting) and the external cause of injury codes.

Issues related to inconsistent, missing, conflicting or unclear documentation must still be resolved by the provider.

If a condition would not be coded and reported based on UHDDS definitions and current official coding guidelines, then the POA indicator would not be reported.

Reporting Options

Y—Yes
N—No
U—Unknown
W—Clinically undetermined
Unreported/Not used—(Exempt from POA reporting)

Reporting Definitions

Y = present at the time of inpatient admission
N = not present at the time of inpatient admission
U = documentation is insufficient to determine if condition is present on admission

W = provider is unable to clinically determine whether condition was present on admission or not

Assigning the POA Indicator

Condition is on the "Exempt from Reporting" list

Leave the "present on admission" field blank if the condition is on the list of ICD-9-CM codes for which this field is not applicable. This is the only circumstance in which the field may be left blank.

POA Explicitly Documented

Assign Y for any condition the provider explicitly documents as being present on admission.

Assign N for any condition the provider explicitly documents as not present at the time of admission.

Conditions diagnosed prior to inpatient admission

Assign "Y" for conditions that were diagnosed prior to admission (example: hypertension, diabetes mellitus, asthma)

Conditions diagnosed during the admission but clearly present before admission

Assign "Y" for conditions diagnosed during the admission that were clearly present but not diagnosed until after admission occurred.

Diagnoses subsequently confirmed after admission are considered present on admission if at the time of admission they are documented as suspected, possible, rule out, differential diagnosis, or constitute an underlying cause of a symptom that is present at the time of admission.

Condition develops during outpatient encounter prior to inpatient admission

Assign Y for any condition that develops during an outpatient encounter prior to a written order for inpatient admission.

Documentation does not indicate whether condition was present on admission

Assign "U" when the medical record documentation is unclear as to whether the condition was present on admission. "U" should not be routinely assigned and used only in very limited circumstances. Coders are encouraged to query the providers when the documentation is unclear.

Documentation states that it cannot be determined whether the condition was or was not present on admission

Assign "W" when the medical record documentation indicates that it cannot be clinically determined whether or not the condition was present on admission.

Chronic condition with acute exacerbation during the admission

If the code is a combination code that identifies both the chronic condition and the acute exacerbation, see POA guidelines pertaining to combination codes.

If the combination code only identifies the chronic condition and not the acute exacerbation (e.g., acute exacerbation of CHF), assign "Y."

Conditions documented as possible, probable, suspected, or rule out at the time of discharge

If the final diagnosis contains a possible, probable, suspected, or rule out diagnosis, and this diagnosis was suspected at the time of inpatient admission, assign "Y."

If the final diagnosis contains a possible, probable, suspected, or rule out diagnosis, and this diagnosis was based on symptoms or clinical findings that were not present on admission, assign "N".

Conditions documented as impending or threatened at the time of discharge

If the final diagnosis contains an impending or threatened diagnosis, and this diagnosis is based on symptoms or clinical findings that were present on admission, assign "Y".

If the final diagnosis contains an impending or threatened diagnosis, and this diagnosis is based on symptoms or clinical findings that were **not** present on admission, assign "N".

Acute and Chronic Conditions

Assign "Y" for acute conditions that are present at time of admission and N for acute conditions that are not present at time of admission.

Assign "Y" for chronic conditions, even though the condition may not be diagnosed until after admission.

If a single code identifies both an acute and chronic condition, see the POA guidelines for combination codes.

Combination Codes

Assign "N" if any part of the combination code was not present on admission (e.g., obstructive chronic bronchitis with acute exacerbation and the exacerbation was not present on admission; gastric ulcer that does not start bleeding until after admission; asthma patient develops status asthmaticus after admission)

Assign "Y" if all parts of the combination code were present on admission (e.g., patient with diabetic nephropathy is admitted with uncontrolled diabetes)

If the final diagnosis includes comparative or contrasting diagnoses, and both were present, or suspected, at the time of admission, assign "Y".

For infection codes that include the causal organism, assign "Y" if the infection (or signs of the infection) was present on admission, even though the culture results may not be known until after admission (e.g., patient is admitted with pneumonia and the provider documents pseudomonas as the causal organism a few days later).

Obstetrical conditions

Whether or not the patient delivers during the current hospitalization does not affect assignment of the POA indicator. The determining factor for POA assignment is whether the pregnancy complication or obstetrical condition described by the code was present at the time of admission or not.

If the pregnancy complication or obstetrical condition was present on admission (e.g., patient admitted in preterm labor), assign "Y".

If the pregnancy complication or obstetrical condition was not present on admission (e.g., 2nd degree laceration during delivery, postpartum hemorrhage that occurred during current hospitalization, fetal distress develops after admission), assign "N".

If the obstetrical code includes more than one diagnosis and any of the diagnoses identified by the code were not present on admission assign "N". (e.g., Code 642.7, Pre-eclampsia or eclampsia superimposed on preexisting hypertension).

If the obstetrical code includes information that is not a diagnosis, do not consider that information in the POA determination.

(e.g. Code 652.1x, Breech or other malpresentation successfully converted to cephalic presentation should be reported as present on admission if the fetus was breech on admission but was converted to cephalic presentation after admission (since the conversion to cephalic presentation does not represent a diagnosis, the fact that the conversion occurred after admission has no bearing on the POA determination).

Perinatal conditions

Newborns are not considered to be admitted until after birth. Therefore, any condition present at birth or that developed in utero is considered present at admission and should be assigned "Y". This includes conditions that occur during delivery (e.g., injury during delivery, meconium aspiration, exposure to streptococcus B in the vaginal canal).

Congenital conditions and anomalies

Assign "Y" for congenital conditions and anomalies. Congenital conditions are always considered present on admission.

External cause of injury codes

Assign "Y" for any E code representing an external cause of injury or poisoning that occurred prior to inpatient admission (e.g., patient fell out of bed at home, patient fell out of bed in emergency room prior to admission)

Assign "N" for any E code representing an external cause of injury or poisoning that occurred during inpatient hospitalization (e.g., patient fell out of hospital bed during hospital stay, patient experienced an adverse reaction to a medication administered after inpatient admission)

CATEGORIES AND CODES EXEMPT FROM DIAGNOSIS PRESENT ON ADMISSION REQUIREMENT

Note: "Diagnosis present on admission" for these code categories are exempt because they represent circumstances regarding the healthcare encounter or factors influencing health status that do not represent a current disease or injury or are always present on admission

137-139, Late effects of infectious and parasitic diseases
268.1, Rickets, late effect
326, Late effects of intracranial abscess or pyogenic infection
412, Old myocardial infarction
438, Late effects of cerebrovascular disease
650, Normal delivery
660.7, Failed forceps or vacuum extractor, unspecified
677, Late effect of complication of pregnancy, childbirth, and the puerperium
905-909, Late effects of injuries, poisonings, toxic effects, and other external causes
V02, Carrier or suspected carrier of infectious diseases
V03, Need for prophylactic vaccination and inoculation against bacterial diseases
V04, Need for prophylactic vaccination and inoculation against certain viral diseases
V05, Need for other prophylactic vaccination and inoculation against single diseases
V06, Need for prophylactic vaccination and inoculation against combinations of diseases
V07, Need for isolation and other prophylactic measures
V10, Personal history of malignant neoplasm
V11, Personal history of mental disorder
V12, Personal history of certain other diseases
V13, Personal history of other diseases
V14, Personal history of allergy to medicinal agents
V15, Other personal history presenting hazards to health
V16, Family history of malignant neoplasm
V17, Family history of certain chronic disabling diseases
V18, Family history of certain other specific conditions
V19, Family history of other conditions
V20, Health supervision of infant or child
V21, Constitutional states in development
V22, Normal pregnancy
V23, Supervision of high-risk pregnancy
V24, Postpartum care and examination
V25, Encounter for contraceptive management
V26, Procreative management
V27, Outcome of delivery
V28, Antenatal screening
V29, Observation and evaluation of newborns for suspected condition not found
V30-V39, Liveborn infants according to type of birth
V42, Organ or tissue replaced by transplant
V43, Organ or tissue replaced by other means
V44, Artificial opening status
V45, Other postprocedural states
V46, Other dependence on machines
V49.60-V49.77, Upper and lower limb amputation status
V49.81-V49.84, Other specified conditions influencing health status
V50, Elective surgery for purposes other than remedying health states
V51, Aftercare involving the use of plastic surgery
V52, Fitting and adjustment of prosthetic device and implant
V53, Fitting and adjustment of other device
V54, Other orthopedic aftercare
V55, Attention to artificial openings

V56, Encounter for dialysis and dialysis catheter care
V57, Care involving use of rehabilitation procedures
V58, Encounter for other and unspecified procedures and aftercare
V59, Donors
V60, Housing, household, and economic circumstances
V61, Other family circumstances
V62, Other psychosocial circumstances
V64, Persons encountering health services for specific procedures, not carried out
V65, Other persons seeking consultation
V66, Convalescence and palliative care
V67, Follow-up examination
V68, Encounters for administrative purposes
V69, Problems related to lifestyle
V70, General medical examination
V71, Observation and evaluation for suspected condition not found
V72, Special investigations and examinations
V73, Special screening examination for viral and chlamydial diseases
V74, Special screening examination for bacterial and spirochetal diseases
V75, Special screening examination for other infectious diseases
V76, Special screening for malignant neoplasms
V77, Special screening for endocrine, nutritional, metabolic, and immunity disorders
V78, Special screening for disorders of blood and blood-forming organs
V79, Special screening for mental disorders and developmental handicaps
V80, Special screening for neurological, eye, and ear diseases
V81, Special screening for cardiovascular, respiratory, and genitourinary diseases
V82, Special screening for other conditions
V83, Genetic carrier status
V84, Genetic susceptibility to disease
V85 Body Mass Index
V86 Estrogen receptor status
E800-E807, Railway accidents
E810-E819, Motor vehicle traffic accidents
E820-E825, Motor vehicle nontraffic accidents
E826-E829, Other road vehicle accidents
E830-E838, Water transport accidents
E840-E845, Air and space transport accidents
E846-E848, Vehicle accidents not elsewhere classifiable
E849.0-E849.6, Place of occurrence
E849.8-E849.9, Place of occurrence
E883.1, Accidental fall into well
E883.2, Accidental fall into storm drain or manhole
E884.0, Fall from playground equipment
E884.1, Fall from cliff
E885.0, Fall from (nonmotorized) scooter
E885.1, Fall from roller skates
E885.2, Fall from skateboard
E885.3, Fall from skis
E885.4, Fall from snowboard
E886.0, Fall on same level from collision, pushing, or shoving, by or with other person, In sports
E890.0-E890.9, Conflagration in private dwelling
E893.0, Accident caused by ignition of clothing, from controlled fire in private dwelling
E893.2, Accident caused by ignition of clothing, from controlled fire not in building or structure
E894, Ignition of highly inflammable material
E895, Accident caused by controlled fire in private dwelling

E897, Accident caused by controlled fire not in building or structure
E898.0-E898.1, Accident caused by other specified fire and flames
E917.0, Striking against or struck accidentally by objects or persons, in sports without subsequent fall
E917.1, Striking against or struck accidentally by objects or persons, caused by a crowd, by collective fear or panic without subsequent fall
E917.2, Striking against or struck accidentally by objects or persons, in running water without subsequent fall
E917.5, Striking against or struck accidentally by objects or persons, object in sports with subsequent fall
E917.6, Striking against or struck accidentally by objects or persons, caused by a crowd, by collective fear or panic with subsequent fall
E919.0-E919.1, Accidents caused by machinery
E919.3-E919.9, Accidents caused by machinery
E921.0-E921.9, Accident caused by explosion of pressure vessel
E922.0-E922.9, Accident caused by firearm and air gun missile
E924.1, Caustic and corrosive substances
E926.2, Visible and ultraviolet light sources
E928.0-E928.8, Other and unspecified environmental and accidental causes
E929.0-E929.9, Late effects of accidental injury
E959, Late effects of self-inflicted injury
E970-E978, Legal intervention
E979, Terrorism
E981.0-E981.8, Poisoning by gases in domestic use, undetermined whether accidentally or purposely inflicted
E982.0-E982.9, Poisoning by other gases, undetermined whether accidentally or purposely inflicted
E985.0-E985.7, Injury by firearms, air guns and explosives, undetermined whether accidentally or purposely inflicted
E987.0, Falling from high place, undetermined whether accidentally or purposely inflicted, residential premises
E987.2, Falling from high place, undetermined whether accidentally or purposely inflicted, natural sites
E989, Late effects of injury, undetermined whether accidentally or purposely inflicted
E990-E999, Injury resulting from operations of war

POA EXAMPLES

General Medical Surgical

1. Patient is admitted for diagnostic work-up for cachexia. The final diagnosis is malignant neoplasm of lung with metastasis.

   Assign "Y" on the POA field for the malignant neoplasm. The malignant neoplasm was clearly present on admission, although it was not diagnosed until after the admission occurred.

2. A patient undergoes outpatient surgery. During the recovery period, the patient develops atrial fibrillation and the patient is subsequently admitted to the hospital as an inpatient.

   Assign "Y" on the POA field for the atrial fibrillation since it developed prior to a written order for inpatient admission.

3. A patient is treated in observation and while in Observation, the patient falls out of bed and breaks a hip. The patient is subsequently admitted as an inpatient to treat the hip fracture.

   Assign "Y" on the POA field for the hip fracture since it developed prior to a written order for inpatient admission.

4. A patient with known congestive heart failure is admitted to the hospital after he develops decompensated congestive heart failure.

Assign "Y" on the POA field for the congestive heart failure. The ICD-9-CM code identifies the chronic condition and does not specify the acute exacerbation.

5. A patient undergoes inpatient surgery. After surgery, the patient develops fever and is treated aggressively. The physician's final diagnosis documents "possible postoperative infection following surgery."

   Assign "N" on the POA field for the postoperative infection since final diagnoses that contain the terms "possible", "probable", "suspected" or "rule out" and that are based on symptoms or clinical findings that were not present on admission should be reported as "N".
6. A patient with severe cough and difficulty breathing was diagnosed during his hospitalization to have lung cancer.

   Assign "Y" on the POA field for the lung cancer. Even though the cancer was not diagnosed until after admission, it is a chronic condition that was clearly present before the patient's admission.
7. A patient is admitted to the hospital for a coronary artery bypass surgery. Postoperatively he developed a pulmonary embolism.

   Assign "N" on the POA field for the pulmonary embolism. This is an acute condition that was not present on admission.
8. A patient is admitted with a known history of coronary atherosclerosis, status post myocardial infarction five years ago is now admitted for treatment of impending myocardial infarction. The final diagnosis is documented as "impending myocardial infarction."

   Assign "Y" to the impending myocardial infarction because the condition is present on admission.
9. A patient with diabetes mellitus developed uncontrolled diabetes on day 3 of the hospitalization.

   Assign "N" to the diabetes code because the "uncontrolled" component of the code was not present on admission.
10. A patient is admitted with high fever and pneumonia. The patient rapidly deteriorates and becomes septic. The discharge diagnosis lists sepsis and pneumonia. The documentation is unclear as to whether the sepsis was present on admission or developed shortly after admission.

    Query the physician as to whether the sepsis was present on admission, developed shortly after admission, or it cannot be clinically determined as to whether it was present on admission or not.
11. A patient is admitted for repair of an abdominal aneurysm. However, the aneurysm ruptures after hospital admission.

    Assign "N" for the ruptured abdominal aneurysm. Although the aneurysm was present on admission, the "ruptured" component of the code description did not occur until after admission.
12. A patient with viral hepatitis B progresses to hepatic coma after admission.

    Assign "N" for the viral hepatitis B with hepatic coma because part of the code description did not develop until after admission.
13. A patient with a history of varicose veins and ulceration of the left lower extremity strikes the area against the side of his hospital bed during an inpatient hospitalization. It bleeds profusely. The final diagnosis lists varicose veins with ulcer and hemorrhage.

    Assign "Y" for the varicose veins with ulcer. Although the hemorrhage occurred after admission, the code description for varicose veins with ulcer does not mention hemorrhage.
14. **The nursing initial assessment upon admission documents the presence of a decubitus ulcer. There is no mention of the decubitus ulcer in the physician documentation until several days after admission.**

    Query the physician as to whether the decubitus ulcer was present on admission, or developed after admission. Both diagnosis code assignment and determination of whether a condition was present on admission must be based on provider documentation in the medical record (per the definition of "provider" found at the beginning of these POA guidelines and in the introductory section of the ICD-9-CM Official Guidelines for Coding and Reporting). If

it cannot be determined from the provider documentation whether or not a condition was present on admission, the provider should be queried.

Obstetrics

1. A female patient was admitted to the hospital and underwent a normal delivery.
   Leave the "present on admission" (POA) field blank. Code 650, Normal delivery, is on the "exempt from reporting" list.
2. Patient admitted in late pregnancy due to excessive vomiting and dehydration. During admission patient goes into premature labor
   Assign "Y" for the excessive vomiting and the dehydration.
   Assign "N" for the premature labor
3. Patient admitted in active labor. During the stay, a breast abscess is noted when mother attempted to breast feed. Provider is unable to determine whether the abscess was present on admission
   Assign "W" for the breast abscess.
4. Patient admitted in active labor. After 12 hours of labor it is noted that the infant is in fetal distress and a Cesarean section is performed
   Assign "N" for the fetal distress.

Newborn

1. A single liveborn infant was delivered in the hospital via Cesarean section. The physician documented fetal bradycardia during labor in the final diagnosis in the newborn record.
   Assign " Y" because the bradycardia developed prior to the newborn admission (birth).
2. A newborn developed diarrhea which was believed to be due to the hospital baby formula.
   Assign " N" because the diarrhea developed after admission.

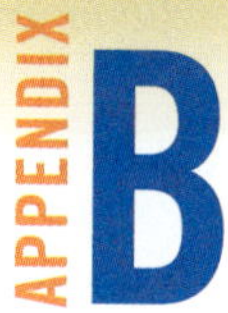

APPENDIX B MS-DRG List*

*From Centers for Medicare and Medicaid Services.

MS-DRG3	FY08 Final Rule Post Acute DRG	FY08 Final Rule Special Pay DRG	MDC	TYPE	MS-DRG Title	Weights	Geometric Mean LOS	Arithmetic Mean LOS
001	No	No	PRE	SURG	Heart transplant or implant of heart assist system w MCC	23.1117	30.8	45.6
002	No	No	PRE	SURG	Heart transplant or implant of heart assist system w/o MCC	16.2735	16.1	22.8
003	Yes	No	PRE	SURG	ECMO or trach w MV 96+ hrs or PDX exc face, mouth & neck w maj O.R.	18.7707	33.4	40.6
004	Yes	No	PRE	SURG	Trach w MV 96+ hrs or PDX exc face, mouth & neck w/o maj O.R.	11.4219	23.8	29.3
005	No	No	PRE	SURG	Liver transplant w MCC or intestinal transplant	10.6120	17.6	23.5
006	No	No	PRE	SURG	Liver transplant w/o MCC	7.2562	9.1	10.5
007	No	No	PRE	SURG	Lung transplant	8.4002	14.6	17.3
008	No	No	PRE	SURG	Simultaneous pancreas/kidney transplant	5.1726	10.1	11.8
009	No	No	PRE	SURG	Bone marrow transplant	6.4842	18.1	21.7
010	No	No	PRE	SURG	Pancreas transplant	3.8902	9.2	10.5
011	No	No	PRE	SURG	Tracheostomy for face, mouth & neck diagnoses w MCC	4.1482	12.8	16.2
012	No	No	PRE	SURG	Tracheostomy for face, mouth & neck diagnoses w CC	3.2472	8.9	10.9
013	No	No	PRE	SURG	Tracheostomy for face, mouth & neck diagnoses w/o CC/MCC	2.6760	6.1	7.2
020	No	No	01	SURG	Intracranial vascular procedures w PDX hemorrhage w MCC	7.7073	15.2	19.1
021	No	No	01	SURG	Intracranial vascular procedures w PDX hemorrhage w CC	6.7021	13.4	15.5
022	No	No	01	SURG	Intracranial vascular procedures w PDX hemorrhage w/o CC/MCC	5.6085	7.8	9.6
023	No	No	01	SURG	Cranio w major dev impl/acute complex CNS PDX w MCC or chemo implant	4.7036	9.0	12.8
024	No	No	01	SURG	Cranio w major dev impl/acute complex CNS PDX w/o MCC	3.8978	6.1	8.9
025	Yes	No	01	SURG	Craniotomy & endovascular intracranial procedures w MCC	4.2362	10.3	13.3
026	Yes	No	01	SURG	Craniotomy & endovascular intracranial procedures w CC	3.1582	6.5	8.2
027	Yes	No	01	SURG	Craniotomy & endovascular intracranial procedures w/o CC/MCC	2.3259	3.5	4.6
028	Yes	Yes	01	SURG	Spinal procedures w MCC	4.2339	10.8	14.7
029	Yes	Yes	01	SURG	Spinal procedures w CC or spinal neurostimulators	2.8356	5.3	7.3
030	Yes	Yes	01	SURG	Spinal procedures w/o CC/MCC	1.7617	2.8	3.7
031	Yes	No	01	SURG	Ventricular shunt procedures w MCC	3.2226	9.2	13.2
032	Yes	No	01	SURG	Ventricular shunt procedures w CC	1.9342	3.8	5.8
033	Yes	No	01	SURG	Ventricular shunt procedures w/o CC/MCC	1.4281	2.3	3.1
034	No	No	01	SURG	Carotid artery stent procedure w MCC	2.5438	4.8	7.3
035	No	No	01	SURG	Carotid artery stent procedure w CC	1.8996	2.0	2.9
036	No	No	01	SURG	Carotid artery stent procedure w/o CC/MCC	1.6977	1.3	1.6
037	No	No	01	SURG	Extracranial procedures w MCC	2.2630	6.0	8.7
038	No	No	01	SURG	Extracranial procedures w CC	1.4686	2.5	3.7
039	No	No	01	SURG	Extracranial procedures w/o CC/MCC	1.0909	1.5	1.8
040	Yes	Yes	01	SURG	Periph/cranial nerve & other nerv syst proc w MCC	3.2550	10.0	13.6
041	Yes	Yes	01	SURG	Periph/cranial nerve & other nerv syst proc w CC or periph neurostim	2.3595	5.4	7.3
042	Yes	Yes	01	SURG	Periph/cranial nerve & other nerv syst proc w/o CC/MCC	1.8710	2.5	3.6

Continued

MS-DRG3	FY08 Final Rule Post Acute DRG	FY08 Final Rule Special Pay DRG	MDC	TYPE	MS-DRG Title	Weights	Geometric Mean LOS	Arithmetic Mean LOS
052	No	No	01	MED	Spinal disorders & injuries w CC/MCC	1.4329	4.7	7.0
053	No	No	01	MED	Spinal disorders & injuries w/o CC/MCC	1.1172	3.1	4.0
054	Yes	No	01	MED	Nervous system neoplasms w MCC	1.4228	5.3	7.2
055	Yes	No	01	MED	Nervous system neoplasms w/o MCC	1.1213	3.8	5.0
056	Yes	No	01	MED	Degenerative nervous system disorders w MCC	1.2820	5.8	7.8
057	Yes	No	01	MED	Degenerative nervous system disorders w/o MCC	0.8951	3.9	4.9
058	No	No	01	MED	Multiple sclerosis & cerebellar ataxia w MCC	1.2669	5.8	8.0
059	No	No	01	MED	Multiple sclerosis & cerebellar ataxia w CC	0.9226	4.3	5.2
060	No	No	01	MED	Multiple sclerosis & cerebellar ataxia w/o CC/MCC	0.8160	3.4	4.1
061	No	No	01	MED	Acute ischemic stroke w use of thrombolytic agent w MCC	2.5541	7.3	9.6
062	No	No	01	MED	Acute ischemic stroke w use of thrombolytic agent w CC	2.0886	5.3	6.3
063	No	No	01	MED	Acute ischemic stroke w use of thrombolytic agent w/o CC/ MCC	1.8642	3.9	4.5
064	Yes	No	01	MED	Intracranial hemorrhage or cerebral infarction w MCC	1.5470	5.6	7.6
065	Yes	No	01	MED	Intracranial hemorrhage or cerebral infarction w CC	1.1901	4.3	5.3
066	Yes	No	01	MED	Intracranial hemorrhage or cerebral infarction w/o CC/MCC	1.0303	3.1	3.8
067	No	No	01	MED	Nonspecific cva & precerebral occlusion w/o infarct w MCC	1.2194	4.7	6.2
068	No	No	01	MED	Nonspecific cva & precerebral occlusion w/o infarct w/o MCC	0.9131	2.8	3.6
069	No	No	01	MED	Transient ischemia	0.7339	2.5	3.1
070	Yes	No	01	MED	Nonspecific cerebrovascular disorders w MCC	1.6212	6.0	7.9
071	Yes	No	01	MED	Nonspecific cerebrovascular disorders w CC	1.2522	4.5	5.6
072	Yes	No	01	MED	Nonspecific cerebrovascular disorders w/o CC/MCC	0.9586	2.9	3.7
073	No	No	01	MED	Cranial & peripheral nerve disorders w MCC	1.1717	4.8	6.4
074	No	No	01	MED	Cranial & peripheral nerve disorders w/o MCC	0.8954	3.4	4.4
075	No	No	01	MED	Viral meningitis w CC/MCC	1.5369	6.0	7.6
076	No	No	01	MED	Viral meningitis w/o CC/MCC	1.1439	3.4	4.2
077	No	No	01	MED	Hypertensive encephalopathy w MCC	1.4611	5.6	7.2
078	No	No	01	MED	Hypertensive encephalopathy w CC	1.0996	3.7	4.6
079	No	No	01	MED	Hypertensive encephalopathy w/o CC/MCC	0.9839	2.8	3.4
080	No	No	01	MED	Nontraumatic stupor & coma w MCC	0.9014	3.6	4.9
081	No	No	01	MED	Nontraumatic stupor & coma w/o MCC	0.7161	2.7	3.4
082	No	No	01	MED	Traumatic stupor & coma, coma >1 hr w MCC	1.6724	3.9	6.4
083	No	No	01	MED	Traumatic stupor & coma, coma >1 hr w CC	1.3328	3.7	5.2
084	No	No	01	MED	Traumatic stupor & coma, coma >1 hr w/o CC/MCC	1.1106	2.3	3.1
085	Yes	No	01	MED	Traumatic stupor & coma, coma <1 hr w MCC	1.6946	5.7	7.9
086	Yes	No	01	MED	Traumatic stupor & coma, coma <1 hr w CC	1.2337	4.0	5.1
087	Yes	No	01	MED	Traumatic stupor & coma, coma <1 hr w/o CC/MCC	0.9235	2.6	3.4
088	No	No	01	MED	Concussion w MCC	1.2968	4.3	6.1
089	No	No	01	MED	Concussion w CC	0.9479	3.0	3.8
090	No	No	01	MED	Concussion w/o CC/MCC	0.7405	2.0	2.5
091	Yes	No	01	MED	Other disorders of nervous system w MCC	1.3242	4.7	6.6
092	Yes	No	01	MED	Other disorders of nervous system w CC	0.9529	3.5	4.4

093	Yes	No	01	MED	Other disorders of nervous system w/o CC/MCC	0.7710	2.6	3.2
094	No	No	01	MED	Bacterial & tuberculous infections of nervous system w MCC	3.1499	9.7	12.5
095	No	No	01	MED	Bacterial & tuberculous infections of nervous system w CC	2.5679	7.2	9.1
096	No	No	01	MED	Bacterial & tuberculous infections of nervous system w/o CC/MCC	2.3482	4.9	6.2
097	No	No	01	MED	Non-bacterial infect of nervous sys exc viral meningitis w MCC	2.6665	9.3	11.8
098	No	No	01	MED	Non-bacterial infect of nervous sys exc viral meningitis w CC	2.0568	6.8	8.5
099	No	No	01	MED	Non-bacterial infect of nervous sys exc viral meningitis w/o CC/MCC	1.8177	5.1	6.3
100	Yes	No	01	MED	Seizures w MCC	1.2500	4.7	6.3
101	Yes	No	01	MED	Seizures w/o MCC	0.8258	2.9	3.7
102	No	No	01	MED	Headaches w MCC	0.8710	3.6	5.1
103	No	No	01	MED	Headaches w/o MCC	0.6677	2.5	3.2
113	No	No	02	SURG	Orbital procedures w CC/MCC	1.4141	3.8	5.5
114	No	No	02	SURG	Orbital procedures w/o CC/MCC	1.0292	2.0	2.7
115	No	No	02	SURG	Extraocular procedures except orbit	1.1185	3.3	4.5
116	No	No	02	SURG	Intraocular procedures w CC/MCC	0.8891	2.2	3.4
117	No	No	02	SURG	Intraocular procedures w/o CC/MCC	0.7094	1.5	1.9
121	No	No	02	MED	Acute major eye infections w CC/MCC	0.8800	4.6	5.8
122	No	No	02	MED	Acute major eye infections w/o CC/MCC	0.6608	3.3	4.1
123	No	No	02	MED	Neurological eye disorders	0.7224	2.4	2.9
124	No	No	02	MED	Other disorders of the eye w MCC	0.9308	3.9	5.3
125	No	No	02	MED	Other disorders of the eye w/o MCC	0.6792	2.7	3.5
129	No	No	03	SURG	Major head & neck procedures w CC/MCC or major device	1.7992	3.7	5.1
130	No	No	03	SURG	Major head & neck procedures w/o CC/MCC	1.3987	2.4	3.2
131	No	No	03	SURG	Cranial/facial procedures w CC/MCC	1.6300	4.0	5.8
132	No	No	03	SURG	Cranial/facial procedures w/o CC/MCC	1.2054	2.1	2.6
133	No	No	03	SURG	Other ear, nose, mouth & throat O.R. procedures w CC/MCC	1.4331	3.7	5.8
134	No	No	03	SURG	Other ear, nose, mouth & throat O.R. procedures w/o CC/MCC	0.9474	1.7	2.1
135	No	No	03	SURG	Sinus & mastoid procedures w CC/MCC	1.5318	4.3	6.4
136	No	No	03	SURG	Sinus & mastoid procedures w/o CC/MCC	1.1094	1.8	2.6
137	No	No	03	SURG	Mouth procedures w CC/MCC	1.2677	3.7	5.4
138	No	No	03	SURG	Mouth procedures w/o CC/MCC	0.8474	1.9	2.4
139	No	No	03	SURG	Salivary gland procedures	0.8470	1.4	1.8
146	No	No	03	MED	Ear, nose, mouth & throat malignancy w MCC	1.7734	7.1	10.3
147	No	No	03	MED	Ear, nose, mouth & throat malignancy w CC	1.2182	4.2	5.8
148	No	No	03	MED	Ear, nose, mouth & throat malignancy w/o CC/MCC	1.0070	2.5	3.5
149	No	No	03	MED	Dysequilibrium	0.6154	2.2	2.7
150	No	No	03	MED	Epistaxis w MCC	0.9916	4.0	5.5
151	No	No	03	MED	Epistaxis w/o MCC	0.6227	2.3	2.9
152	No	No	03	MED	Otitis media & URI w MCC	0.8160	3.7	4.7
153	No	No	03	MED	Otitis media & URI w/o MCC	0.6207	2.8	3.4
154	No	No	03	MED	Nasal trauma & deformity w MCC	1.1294	4.8	6.5
155	No	No	03	MED	Nasal trauma & deformity w CC	0.8630	3.5	4.5

Continued

MS-DRG3	FY08 Final Rule Post Acute DRG	FY08 Final Rule Special Pay DRG	MDC	TYPE	MS-DRG Title	Weights	Geometric Mean LOS	Arithmetic Mean LOS
156	No	No	03	MED	Nasal trauma & deformity w/o CC/MCC	0.7412	2.5	3.2
157	No	No	03	MED	Dental & Oral Diseases w MCC	1.1909	5.0	6.9
158	No	No	03	MED	Dental & Oral Diseases w CC	0.8653	3.4	4.4
159	No	No	03	MED	Dental & Oral Diseases w/o CC/MCC	0.7361	2.4	3.1
163	Yes	No	04	SURG	Major chest procedures w MCC	4.0452	12.2	15.0
164	Yes	No	04	SURG	Major chest procedures w CC	2.8081	6.9	8.3
165	Yes	No	04	SURG	Major chest procedures w/o CC/MCC	2.4106	4.5	5.4
166	Yes	No	04	SURG	Other resp system O.R. procedures w MCC	3.2677	10.1	13.0
167	Yes	No	04	SURG	Other resp system O.R. procedures w CC	2.4151	6.5	8.1
168	Yes	No	04	SURG	Other resp system O.R. procedures w/o CC/MCC	1.8181	4.0	5.4
175	Yes	No	04	MED	Pulmonary embolism w MCC	1.4152	6.1	7.4
176	Yes	No	04	MED	Pulmonary embolism w/o MCC	1.1580	4.7	5.5
177	Yes	No	04	MED	Respiratory infections & inflammations w MCC	1.8444	7.2	9.2
178	Yes	No	04	MED	Respiratory infections & inflammations w CC	1.5636	6.0	7.4
179	Yes	No	04	MED	Respiratory infections & inflammations w/o CC/MCC	1.2754	4.6	5.6
180	No	No	04	MED	Respiratory neoplasms w MCC	1.5550	6.1	8.0
181	No	No	04	MED	Respiratory neoplasms w CC	1.3126	4.5	6.0
182	No	No	04	MED	Respiratory neoplasms w/o CC/MCC	1.1455	3.3	4.3
183	No	No	04	MED	Major chest trauma w MCC	1.2664	5.7	7.2
184	No	No	04	MED	Major chest trauma w CC	0.9611	3.8	4.6
185	No	No	04	MED	Major chest trauma w/o CC/MCC	0.7298	2.7	3.3
186	Yes	No	04	MED	Pleural effusion w MCC	1.4542	5.8	7.5
187	Yes	No	04	MED	Pleural effusion w CC	1.1947	4.2	5.5
188	Yes	No	04	MED	Pleural effusion w/o CC/MCC	0.9745	3.2	4.1
189	No	No	04	MED	Pulmonary edema & respiratory failure	1.3660	4.8	6.2
190	Yes	No	04	MED	Chronic obstructive pulmonary disease w MCC	1.1138	5.1	6.5
191	Yes	No	04	MED	Chronic obstructive pulmonary disease w CC	0.9405	4.2	5.1
192	Yes	No	04	MED	Chronic obstructive pulmonary disease w/o CC/MCC	0.8145	3.4	4.0
193	Yes	No	04	MED	Simple pneumonia & pleurisy w MCC	1.2505	5.5	6.9
194	Yes	No	04	MED	Simple pneumonia & pleurisy w CC	1.0235	4.5	5.3
195	Yes	No	04	MED	Simple pneumonia & pleurisy w/o CC/MCC	0.8398	3.5	4.1
196	Yes	No	04	MED	Interstitial lung disease w MCC	1.3781	5.8	7.3
197	Yes	No	04	MED	Interstitial lung disease w CC	1.1458	4.4	5.4
198	Yes	No	04	MED	Interstitial lung disease w/o CC/MCC	0.9654	3.5	4.3
199	No	No	04	MED	Pneumothorax w MCC	1.4699	6.6	8.5
200	No	No	04	MED	Pneumothorax w CC	1.0753	3.9	5.1
201	No	No	04	MED	Pneumothorax w/o CC/MCC	0.8588	3.2	4.1
202	No	No	04	MED	Bronchitis & asthma w CC/MCC	0.7841	3.6	4.5
203	No	No	04	MED	Bronchitis & asthma w/o CC/MCC	0.6252	2.9	3.5
204	No	No	04	MED	Respiratory signs & symptoms	0.6658	2.2	2.9
205	Yes	No	04	MED	Other respiratory system diagnoses w MCC	1.0636	4.2	5.6
206	Yes	No	04	MED	Other respiratory system diagnoses w/o MCC	0.7848	2.7	3.5

207	Yes	No	04	MED	Respiratory system diagnosis w ventilator support 96+ hours	5.1231	12.6	15.0
208	No	No	04	MED	Respiratory system diagnosis w ventilator support <96 hours	2.2463	5.2	7.3
215	No	No	05	SURG	Other heart assist system implant	12.0016	6.3	12.0
216	Yes	No	05	SURG	Cardiac valve & oth maj cardiothoracic proc w card cath w MCC	9.3040	15.9	18.7
217	Yes	No	05	SURG	Cardiac valve & oth maj cardiothoracic proc w card cath w CC	7.5813	10.9	12.2
218	Yes	No	05	SURG	Cardiac valve & oth maj cardiothoracic proc w card cath w/o CC/MCC	6.8595	8.3	9.1
219	Yes	Yes	05	SURG	Cardiac valve & oth maj cardiothoracic proc w/o card cath w MCC	7.2072	11.7	14.5
220	Yes	Yes	05	SURG	Cardiac valve & oth maj cardiothoracic proc w/o card cath w CC	5.7278	7.6	8.6
221	Yes	Yes	05	SURG	Cardiac valve & oth maj cardiothoracic proc w/o card cath w/o CC/MCC	5.2463	6.0	6.4
222	No	No	05	SURG	Cardiac defib implant w cardiac cath w AMI/HF/shock w MCC	8.0234	10.8	13.3
223	No	No	05	SURG	Cardiac defib implant w cardiac cath w AMI/HF/shock w/o MCC	6.8809	5.0	6.6
224	No	No	05	SURG	Cardiac defib implant w cardiac cath w/o AMI/HF/shock w MCC	7.3178	9.2	11.5
225	No	No	05	SURG	Cardiac defib implant w cardiac cath w/o AMI/HF/shock w/o MCC	6.2956	4.5	5.7
226	No	No	05	SURG	Cardiac defibrillator implant w/o cardiac cath w MCC	5.9123	6.2	9.4
227	No	No	05	SURG	Cardiac defibrillator implant w/o cardiac cath w/o MCC	5.0411	1.8	2.8
228	Yes	No	05	SURG	Other cardiothoracic procedures w MCC	6.7400	12.0	14.6
229	Yes	No	05	SURG	Other cardiothoracic procedures w CC	5.3191	7.9	9.0
230	Yes	No	05	SURG	Other cardiothoracic procedures w/o CC/MCC	4.7847	5.6	6.6
231	No	No	05	SURG	Coronary bypass w PTCA w MCC	7.2993	10.8	13.2
232	No	No	05	SURG	Coronary bypass w PTCA w/o MCC	6.1947	8.0	9.0
233	Yes	No	05	SURG	Coronary bypass w cardiac cath w MCC	6.4496	12.4	14.3
234	Yes	No	05	SURG	Coronary bypass w cardiac cath w/o MCC	4.9216	8.2	8.9
235	Yes	No	05	SURG	Coronary bypass w/o cardiac cath w MCC	5.1381	9.7	11.5
236	Yes	No	05	SURG	Coronary bypass w/o cardiac cath w/o MCC	3.7307	6.1	6.6
237	No	No	05	SURG	Major cardiovasc procedures w MCC or thoracic aortic anuerysm repair	4.4954	7.8	11.2
238	No	No	05	SURG	Major cardiovasc procedures w/o MCC	3.1891	3.4	4.9
239	Yes	No	05	SURG	Amputation for circ sys disorders exc upper limb & toe w MCC	3.9454	12.1	15.6
240	Yes	No	05	SURG	Amputation for circ sys disorders exc upper limb & toe w CC	2.9983	8.4	10.5
241	Yes	No	05	SURG	Amputation for circ sys disorders exc upper limb & toe w/o CC/MCC	2.4709	5.7	6.9
242	Yes	No	05	SURG	Permanent cardiac pacemaker implant w MCC	3.2586	6.9	8.9
243	Yes	No	05	SURG	Permanent cardiac pacemaker implant w CC	2.5483	3.8	5.1
244	Yes	No	05	SURG	Permanent cardiac pacemaker implant w/o CC/MCC	2.1367	2.2	2.9
245	No	No	05	SURG	AICD lead & generator procedures	3.1073	2.1	3.3
246	No	No	05	SURG	Perc cardiovasc proc w drug-eluting stent w MCC or 4+ vessels/stents	2.9046	3.7	5.5

Continued

MS-DRG3	FY08 Final Rule Post Acute DRG	FY08 Final Rule Special Pay DRG	MDC	TYPE	MS-DRG Title	Weights	Geometric Mean LOS	Arithmetic Mean LOS
247	No	No	05	SURG	Perc cardiovasc proc w drug-eluting stent w/o MCC	2.1255	1.7	2.2
248	No	No	05	SURG	Perc cardiovasc proc w non-drug-eluting stent w MCC or 4+ ves/stents	2.5180	4.3	6.2
249	No	No	05	SURG	Perc cardiovasc proc w non-drug-eluting stent w/o MCC	1.8124	1.9	2.5
250	No	No	05	SURG	Perc cardiovasc proc w/o coronary artery stent or AMI w MCC	2.4870	5.3	7.5
251	No	No	05	SURG	Perc cardiovasc proc w/o coronary artery stent or AMI w/o MCC	1.7480	2.1	3.0
252	No	No	05	SURG	Other vascular procedures w MCC	2.7564	5.6	8.8
253	No	No	05	SURG	Other vascular procedures w CC	2.2536	4.1	6.0
254	No	No	05	SURG	Other vascular procedures w/o CC/MCC	1.6786	2.0	2.8
255	Yes	No	05	SURG	Upper limb & toe amputation for circ system disorders w MCC	2.1486	7.3	9.9
256	Yes	No	05	SURG	Upper limb & toe amputation for circ system disorders w CC	1.6847	5.8	7.5
257	Yes	No	05	SURG	Upper limb & toe amputation for circ system disorders w/o CC/MCC	1.3990	3.7	4.9
258	No	No	05	SURG	Cardiac pacemaker device replacement w MCC	2.2926	5.5	7.6
259	No	No	05	SURG	Cardiac pacemaker device replacement w/o MCC	1.6553	1.9	2.6
260	No	No	05	SURG	Cardiac pacemaker revision except device replacement w MCC	2.1625	7.2	10.2
261	No	No	05	SURG	Cardiac pacemaker revision except device replacement w CC	1.3212	2.8	3.9
262	No	No	05	SURG	Cardiac pacemaker revision except device replacement w/o CC/MCC	1.1245	1.9	2.5
263	No	No	05	SURG	Vein ligation & stripping	1.4977	3.5	5.5
264	Yes	No	05	SURG	Other circulatory system O.R. procedures	2.4840	5.9	9.0
280	Yes	No	05	MED	Acute myocardial infarction, discharged alive w MCC	1.7391	5.9	7.5
281	Yes	No	05	MED	Acute myocardial infarction, discharged alive w CC	1.3126	4.0	4.9
282	Yes	No	05	MED	Acute myocardia infarction, discharged alive w/o CC/MCC	1.0617	2.6	3.2
283	No	No	05	MED	Acute myocardial infarction, expired w MCC	1.5787	3.4	5.5
284	No	No	05	MED	Acute myocardial infarction, expired w CC	1.2074	2.3	3.5
285	No	No	05	MED	Acute myocardial infarction, expired w/o CC/MCC	1.0421	1.6	2.2
286	No	No	05	MED	Circulatory disorders except AMI, w card cath w MCC	1.6667	5.2	7.1
287	No	No	05	MED	Circulatory disorders except AMI, w card cath w/o MCC	1.1412	2.5	3.2
288	Yes	No	05	MED	Acute & subacute endocarditis w MCC	2.9143	9.6	12.2
289	Yes	No	05	MED	Acute & subacute endocarditis w CC	2.3075	7.1	8.7
290	Yes	No	05	MED	Acute & subacute endocarditis w/o CC/MCC	1.9733	5.2	6.6
291	Yes	No	05	MED	Heart failure & shock w MCC	1.2585	5.1	6.6
292	Yes	No	05	MED	Heart failure & shock w CC	1.0134	4.1	5.0
293	Yes	No	05	MED	Heart failure & shock w/o CC/MCC	0.8765	3.1	3.7
294	No	No	05	MED	Deep vein thrombophlebitis w CC/MCC	0.8665	4.6	5.5
295	No	No	05	MED	Deep vein thrombophlebitis w/o CC/MCC	0.6950	3.8	4.4
296	No	No	05	MED	Cardiac arrest, unexplained w MCC	1.1144	2.0	3.3
297	No	No	05	MED	Cardiac arrest, unexplained w CC	0.8490	1.5	1.9

298	No	No	05	MED	Cardiac arrest, unexplained w/o CC/MCC	0.7207	1.2	1.4
299	Yes	No	05	MED	Peripheral vascular disorders w MCC	1.2220	5.2	6.9
300	Yes	No	05	MED	Peripheral vascular disorders w CC	0.9451	4.1	5.1
301	Yes	No	05	MED	Peripheral vascular disorders w/o CC/MCC	0.7183	3.1	3.8
302	No	No	05	MED	Atherosclerosis w MCC	0.8236	3.3	4.4
303	No	No	05	MED	Atherosclerosis w/o MCC	0.6055	2.1	2.6
304	No	No	05	MED	Hypertension w MCC	0.8312	3.9	5.2
305	No	No	05	MED	Hypertension w/o MCC	0.5942	2.3	2.9
306	No	No	05	MED	Cardiac congenital & valvular disorders w MCC	1.2007	4.5	6.5
307	No	No	05	MED	Cardiac congenital & valvular disorders w/o MCC	0.8224	2.7	3.5
308	No	No	05	MED	Cardiac arrhythmia & conduction disorders w MCC	1.0841	4.3	5.8
309	No	No	05	MED	Cardiac arrhythmia & conduction disorders w CC	0.8233	3.1	3.9
310	No	No	05	MED	Cardiac arrhythmia & conduction disorders w/o CC/MCC	0.6439	2.3	2.8
311	No	No	05	MED	Angina pectoris	0.5118	1.9	2.3
312	No	No	05	MED	Syncope & collapse	0.7197	2.5	3.2
313	No	No	05	MED	Chest pain	0.5489	1.7	2.1
314	Yes	No	05	MED	Other circulatory system diagnoses w MCC	1.5606	5.1	7.1
315	Yes	No	05	MED	Other circulatory system diagnoses w CC	1.1720	3.5	4.6
316	Yes	No	05	MED	Other circulatory system diagnoses w/o CC/MCC	0.9075	2.4	3.0
326	Yes	No	06	SURG	Stomach, esophageal & duodenal proc w MCC	5.1660	13.4	17.2
327	Yes	No	06	SURG	Stomach, esophageal & duodenal proc w CC	3.2941	8.1	10.3
328	Yes	No	06	SURG	Stomach, esophageal & duodenal proc w/o CC/MCC	1.8017	3.3	4.4
329	Yes	No	06	SURG	Major small & large bowel procedures w MCC	4.5059	12.8	15.9
330	Yes	No	06	SURG	Major small & large bowel procedures w CC	2.8935	8.4	9.8
331	Yes	No	06	SURG	Major small & large bowel procedures w/o CC/MCC	1.8415	5.4	6.0
332	Yes	No	06	SURG	Rectal resection w MCC	3.7139	12.2	14.7
333	Yes	No	06	SURG	Rectal resection w CC	2.5787	7.8	8.9
334	Yes	No	06	SURG	Rectal resection w/o CC/MCC	1.7856	4.9	5.6
335	Yes	No	06	SURG	Peritoneal adhesiolysis w MCC	3.4785	11.8	14.4
336	Yes	No	06	SURG	Peritoneal adhesiolysis w CC	2.4776	7.7	9.3
337	Yes	No	06	SURG	Peritoneal adhesiolysis w/o CC/MCC	1.6984	4.4	5.7
338	No	No	06	SURG	Appendectomy w complicated principal diag w MCC	2.7254	9.1	10.9
339	No	No	06	SURG	Appendectomy w complicated principal diag w CC	1.9805	6.1	7.1
340	No	No	06	SURG	Appendectomy w complicated principal diag w/o CC/MCC	1.3849	3.6	4.3
341	No	No	06	SURG	Appendectomy w/o complicated principal diag w MCC	1.8824	5.3	7.3
342	No	No	06	SURG	Appendectomy w/o complicated principal diag w CC	1.3562	3.4	4.3
343	No	No	06	SURG	Appendectomy w/o complicated principal diag w/o CC/MCC	0.9887	1.9	2.3
344	No	No	06	SURG	Minor small & large bowel procedures w MCC	2.5156	9.4	12.0
345	No	No	06	SURG	Minor small & large bowel procedures w CC	1.7028	6.2	7.2
346	No	No	06	SURG	Minor small & large bowel procedures w/o CC/MCC	1.2617	4.4	5.0
347	No	No	06	SURG	Anal & stomal procedures w MCC	1.7658	6.2	8.4
348	No	No	06	SURG	Anal & stomal procedures w CC	1.2781	4.1	5.5
349	No	No	06	SURG	Anal & stomal procedures w/o CC/MCC	0.8629	2.4	3.0
350	No	No	06	SURG	Inguinal & femoral hernia procedures w MCC	1.8330	5.9	8.1
351	No	No	06	SURG	Inguinal & femoral hernia procedures w CC	1.2449	3.4	4.5

Continued

MS-DRG3	FY08 Final Rule Post Acute DRG	FY08 Final Rule Special Pay DRG	MDC	TYPE	MS-DRG Title	Weights	Geometric Mean LOS	Arithmetic Mean LOS
352	No	No	06	SURG	Inguinal & femoral hernia procedures w/o CC/MCC	0.8967	1.9	2.4
353	No	No	06	SURG	Hernia procedures except inguinal & femoral w MCC	2.0241	6.6	8.8
354	No	No	06	SURG	Hernia procedures except inguinal & femoral w CC	1.4092	4.0	5.1
355	No	No	06	SURG	Hernia procedures except inguinal & femoral w/o CC/MCC	1.0147	2.3	2.9
356	Yes	No	06	SURG	Other digestive system O.R. procedures w MCC	3.3790	9.6	13.3
357	Yes	No	06	SURG	Other digestive system O.R. procedures w CC	2.4946	6.1	8.0
358	Yes	No	06	SURG	Other digestive system O.R. procedures w/o CC/MCC	1.7333	3.4	4.6
368	No	No	06	MED	Major esophageal disorders w MCC	1.3788	5.1	6.6
369	No	No	06	MED	Major esophageal disorders w CC	1.0839	3.7	4.6
370	No	No	06	MED	Major esophageal disorders w/o CC/MCC	0.9558	2.8	3.4
371	Yes	No	06	MED	Major gastrointestinal disorders & peritoneal infections w MCC	1.6263	6.6	8.8
372	Yes	No	06	MED	Major gastrointestinal disorders & peritoneal infections w CC	1.3059	5.5	6.8
373	Yes	No	06	MED	Major gastrointestinal disorders & peritoneal infections w/o CC/MCC	1.1109	4.2	5.0
374	Yes	No	06	MED	Digestive malignancy w MCC	1.7229	6.5	8.8
375	Yes	No	06	MED	Digestive malignancy w CC	1.3337	4.6	6.0
376	Yes	No	06	MED	Digestive malignancy w/o CC/MCC	1.0268	3.1	4.1
377	Yes	No	06	MED	G.I. hemorrhage w MCC	1.3367	5.0	6.5
378	Yes	No	06	MED	G.I. hemorrhage w CC	1.0195	3.7	4.5
379	Yes	No	06	MED	G.I. hemorrhage w/o CC/MCC	0.8476	2.9	3.4
380	Yes	No	06	MED	Complicated peptic ulcer w MCC	1.4334	5.5	7.2
381	Yes	No	06	MED	Complicated peptic ulcer w CC	1.1302	4.2	5.1
382	Yes	No	06	MED	Complicated peptic ulcer w/o CC/MCC	0.9662	3.0	3.6
383	No	No	06	MED	Uncomplicated peptic ulcer w MCC	1.1024	4.6	5.9
384	No	No	06	MED	Uncomplicated peptic ulcer w/o MCC	0.8399	3.2	3.8
385	No	No	06	MED	Inflammatory bowel disease w MCC	1.4936	6.7	9.0
386	No	No	06	MED	Inflammatory bowel disease w CC	1.0766	4.6	5.7
387	No	No	06	MED	Inflammatory bowel disease w/o CC/MCC	0.9488	3.6	4.4
388	Yes	No	06	MED	G.I. obstruction w MCC	1.2860	5.5	7.4
389	Yes	No	06	MED	G.I. obstruction w CC	0.9533	4.0	5.0
390	Yes	No	06	MED	G.I. obstruction w/o CC/MCC	0.7260	3.0	3.6
391	No	No	06	MED	Esophagitis, gastroent & misc digest disorders w MCC	0.9565	4.1	5.5
392	No	No	06	MED	Esophagitis, gastroent & misc digest disorders w/o MCC	0.7121	2.8	3.5
393	No	No	06	MED	Other digestive system diagnoses w MCC	1.3237	5.0	7.0
394	No	No	06	MED	Other digestive system diagnoses w CC	1.0257	3.8	4.9
395	No	No	06	MED	Other digestive system diagnoses w/o CC/MCC	0.7874	2.7	3.4
405	Yes	No	07	SURG	Pancreas, liver & shunt procedures w MCC	4.8273	12.8	17.3
406	Yes	No	07	SURG	Pancreas, liver & shunt procedures w CC	3.3149	7.1	9.5
407	Yes	No	07	SURG	Pancreas, liver & shunt procedures w/o CC/MCC	2.2443	4.2	5.5
408	No	No	07	SURG	Biliary tract proc except only cholecyst w or w/o c.d.e. w MCC	3.8540	12.2	15.1
409	No	No	07	SURG	Biliary tract proc except only cholecyst w or w/o c.d.e. w CC	2.9126	8.2	9.9

410	No	No	07	SURG	Biliary tract proc except only cholecyst w or w/o c.d.e. w/o CC/MCC	2.0794	5.7	6.8
411	No	No	07	SURG	Cholecystectomy w c.d.e. w MCC	3.4128	10.9	13.1
412	No	No	07	SURG	Cholecystectomy w c.d.e. w CC	2.6382	7.6	8.8
413	No	No	07	SURG	Cholecystectomy w c.d.e. w/o CC/MCC	1.9412	5.2	6.0
414	Yes	No	07	SURG	Cholecystectomy except by laparoscope w/o c.d.e. w MCC	3.0942	9.7	11.9
415	Yes	No	07	SURG	Cholecystectomy except by laparoscope w/o c.d.e. w CC	2.2749	6.6	7.7
416	Yes	No	07	SURG	Cholecystectomy except by laparoscope w/o c.d.e. w/o CC/MCC	1.5398	4.1	4.9
417	No	No	07	SURG	Laparoscopic cholecystectomy w/o c.d.e. w MCC	2.1361	6.6	8.4
418	No	No	07	SURG	Laparoscopic cholecystectomy w/o c.d.e. w CC	1.7104	4.5	5.6
419	No	No	07	SURG	Laparoscopic cholecystectomy w/o c.d.e. w/o CC/MCC	1.2400	2.5	3.2
420	No	No	07	SURG	Hepatobiliary diagnostic procedures w MCC	3.4851	10.1	14.2
421	No	No	07	SURG	Hepatobiliary diagnostic procedures w CC	2.2557	5.6	7.8
422	No	No	07	SURG	Hepatobiliary diagnostic procedures w/o CC/MCC	1.9432	3.4	4.5
423	No	No	07	SURG	Other hepatobiliary or pancreas O.R. procedures w MCC	3.9593	11.4	15.5
424	No	No	07	SURG	Other hepatobiliary or pancreas O.R. procedures w CC	3.0104	7.8	10.2
425	No	No	07	SURG	Other hepatobiliary or pancreas O.R. procedures w/o CC/MCC	2.5812	4.5	5.6
432	No	No	07	MED	Cirrhosis & alcoholic hepatitis w MCC	1.5033	5.1	6.9
433	No	No	07	MED	Cirrhosis & alcoholic hepatitis w CC	1.1431	3.8	4.9
434	No	No	07	MED	Cirrhosis & alcoholic hepatitis w/o CC/MCC	1.0125	2.8	3.6
435	No	No	07	MED	Malignancy of hepatobiliary system or pancreas w MCC	1.5661	5.8	7.7
436	No	No	07	MED	Malignancy of hepatobiliary system or pancreas w CC	1.2906	4.5	5.9
437	No	No	07	MED	Malignancy of hepatobiliary system or pancreas w/o CC/MCC	1.1709	3.3	4.4
438	No	No	07	MED	Disorders of pancreas except malignancy w MCC	1.4201	5.6	7.7
439	No	No	07	MED	Disorders of pancreas except malignancy w CC	1.0609	4.3	5.4
440	No	No	07	MED	Disorders of pancreas except malignancy w/o CC/MCC	0.8912	3.2	3.9
441	Yes	No	07	MED	Disorders of liver except malig, cirr, alc hepa w MCC	1.3973	5.1	7.0
442	Yes	No	07	MED	Disorders of liver except malig, cirr, alc hepa w CC	1.0935	4.0	5.1
443	Yes	No	07	MED	Disorders of liver except malig, cirr, alc hepa w/o CC/MCC	0.9079	3.1	3.8
444	No	No	07	MED	Disorders of the biliary tract w MCC	1.3744	5.0	6.6
445	No	No	07	MED	Disorders of the biliary tract w CC	1.1030	3.8	4.8
446	No	No	07	MED	Disorders of the biliary tract w/o CC/MCC	0.8521	2.6	3.3
453	No	No	08	SURG	Combined anterior/posterior spinal fusion w MCC	8.4313	12.7	15.9
454	No	No	08	SURG	Combined anterior/posterior spinal fusion w CC	6.5810	6.8	8.4
455	No	No	08	SURG	Combined anterior/posterior spinal fusion w/o CC/MCC	5.7023	4.1	4.7
456	No	No	08	SURG	Spinal fus exc cerv w spinal curv/malig/infec or 9+ fus w MCC	6.7669	12.1	15.9
457	No	No	08	SURG	Spinal fus exc cerv w spinal curv/malig/infec or 9+ fus w CC	5.4650	6.4	7.8
458	No	No	08	SURG	Spinal fus exc cerv w spinal curv/malig/infec or 9+ fus w/o CC/MCC	4.9437	4.1	4.6
459	Yes	No	08	SURG	Spinal fusion except cervical w MCC	4.8679	7.8	9.6
460	Yes	No	08	SURG	Spinal fusion except cervical w/o MCC	3.4870	3.8	4.3
461	No	No	08	SURG	Bilateral or multiple major joint procs of lower extremity w MCC	3.8345	6.9	8.5

Continued

MS-DRG3	FY08 Final Rule Post Acute DRG	FY08 Final Rule Special Pay DRG	MDC	TYPE	MS-DRG Title	Weights	Geometric Mean LOS	Arithmetic Mean LOS
462	No	No	08	SURG	Bilateral or multiple major joint procs of lower extremity w/o MCC	3.0993	3.9	4.3
463	Yes	No	08	SURG	Wnd debrid & skn grft exc hand, for musculo-conn tiss dis w MCC	3.9615	12.3	16.9
464	Yes	No	08	SURG	Wnd debrid & skn grft exc hand, for musculo-conn tiss dis w CC	2.8821	7.8	10.4
465	Yes	No	08	SURG	Wnd debrid & skn grft exc hand, for musculo-conn tiss dis w/o CC/MCC	2.3417	4.6	6.2
466	Yes	No	08	SURG	Revision of hip or knee replacement w MCC	3.5408	7.6	9.5
467	Yes	No	08	SURG	Revision of hip or knee replacement w CC	2.7523	4.8	5.6
468	Yes	No	08	SURG	Revision of hip or knee replacement w/o CC/MCC	2.4545	3.7	4.0
469	Yes	No	08	SURG	Major joint replacement or reattachment of lower extremity w MCC	2.6664	7.1	8.4
470	Yes	No	08	SURG	Major joint replacement or reattachment of lower extremity w/o MCC	1.9871	3.7	4.0
471	No	No	08	SURG	Cervical spinal fusion w MCC	3.4723	7.0	10.1
472	No	No	08	SURG	Cervical spinal fusion w CC	2.4819	2.9	4.3
473	No	No	08	SURG	Cervical spinal fusion w/o CC/MCC	1.9446	1.6	2.0
474	Yes	No	08	SURG	Amputation for musculoskeletal sys & conn tissue dis w MCC	2.8432	9.5	12.5
475	Yes	No	08	SURG	Amputation for musculoskeletal sys & conn tissue dis w CC	2.1308	6.6	8.6
476	Yes	No	08	SURG	Amputation for musculoskeletal sys & conn tissue dis w/o CC/MCC	1.6799	3.8	5.0
477	Yes	Yes	08	SURG	Biopsies of musculoskeletal system & connective tissue w MCC	2.6555	9.6	12.5
478	Yes	Yes	08	SURG	Biopsies of musculoskeletal system & connective tissue w CC	1.9836	4.8	6.8
479	Yes	Yes	08	SURG	Biopsies of musculoskeletal system & connective tissue w/o CC/MCC	1.6784	1.9	2.8
480	Yes	Yes	08	SURG	Hip & femur procedures except major joint w MCC	2.4027	8.0	9.5
481	Yes	Yes	08	SURG	Hip & femur procedures except major joint w CC	1.8485	5.4	6.0
482	Yes	Yes	08	SURG	Hip & femur procedures except major joint w/o CC/MCC	1.5644	4.5	4.9
483	Yes	No	08	SURG	Major joint & limb reattachment proc of upper extremity w CC/MCC	1.9905	3.5	4.4
484	Yes	No	08	SURG	Major joint & limb reattachment proc of upper extremity w/o CC/MCC	1.7376	2.2	2.5
485	No	No	08	SURG	Knee procedures w pdx of infection w MCC	2.9362	10.2	12.4
486	No	No	08	SURG	Knee procedures w pdx of infection w CC	2.3382	6.8	8.1
487	No	No	08	SURG	Knee procedures w pdx of infection w/o CC/MCC	1.7771	5.0	5.8
488	Yes	No	08	SURG	Knee procedures w/o pdx of infection w CC/MCC	1.6584	4.1	5.1
489	Yes	No	08	SURG	Knee procedures w/o pdx of infection w/o CC/MCC	1.4512	2.7	3.1
490	No	No	08	SURG	Back & neck proc exc spinal fusion w CC/MCC or disc device/neurostim	1.4912	3.3	4.7
491	No	No	08	SURG	Back & neck proc exc spinal fusion w/o CC/MCC	1.0066	1.8	2.3

492	Yes	Yes	08	SURG	Lower extrem & humer proc except hip, foot, femur w MCC	2.2413	6.9	8.7
493	Yes	Yes	08	SURG	Lower extrem & humer proc except hip, foot, femur w CC	1.7186	4.4	5.3
494	Yes	Yes	08	SURG	Lower extrem & humer proc except hip, foot, femur w/o CC/MCC	1.2752	2.8	3.4
495	Yes	No	08	SURG	Local excision & removal int fix devices exc hip & femur w MCC	2.5765	8.3	11.1
496	Yes	No	08	SURG	Local excision & removal int fix devices exc hip & femur w CC	1.7792	4.6	6.0
497	Yes	No	08	SURG	Local excision & removal int fix devices exc hip & femur w/o CC/MCC	1.2301	2.3	3.1
498	No	No	08	SURG	Local excision & removal int fix devices of hip & femur w CC/ MCC	1.7563	5.8	8.2
499	No	No	08	SURG	Local excision & removal int fix devices of hip & femur w/o CC/MCC	1.1887	2.3	3.1
500	Yes	Yes	08	SURG	Soft tissue procedures w MCC	2.4096	8.1	11.3
501	Yes	Yes	08	SURG	Soft tissue procedures w CC	1.5598	4.4	5.9
502	Yes	Yes	08	SURG	Soft tissue procedures w/o CC/MCC	1.0342	2.3	2.9
503	No	No	08	SURG	Foot procedures w MCC	1.7538	6.9	8.9
504	No	No	08	SURG	Foot procedures w CC	1.4058	5.0	6.4
505	No	No	08	SURG	Foot procedures w/o CC/MCC	1.1584	2.6	3.4
506	No	No	08	SURG	Major thumb or joint procedures	1.0877	2.3	3.2
507	No	No	08	SURG	Major shoulder or elbow joint procedures w CC/MCC	1.4296	3.6	5.2
508	No	No	08	SURG	Major shoulder or elbow joint procedures w/o CC/MCC	1.1330	1.7	2.0
509	No	No	08	SURG	Arthroscopy	1.0769	1.9	2.8
510	Yes	No	08	SURG	Shoulder, elbow or forearm proc, exc major joint proc w MCC	1.6616	5.0	6.6
511	Yes	No	08	SURG	Shoulder, elbow or forearm proc, exc major joint proc w CC	1.2512	3.1	3.9
512	Yes	No	08	SURG	Shoulder, elbow or forearm proc, exc major joint proc w/o CC/ MCC	0.9602	1.7	2.1
513	No	No	08	SURG	Hand or wrist proc, except major thumb or joint proc w CC/ MCC	1.1748	3.7	5.1
514	No	No	08	SURG	Hand or wrist proc, except major thumb or joint proc w/o CC/ MCC	0.8313	2.0	2.6
515	Yes	Yes	08	SURG	Other musculoskelet sys & conn tiss O.R. proc w MCC	2.4858	8.1	10.9
516	Yes	Yes	08	SURG	Other musculoskelet sys & conn tiss O.R. proc w CC	1.8307	4.4	6.0
517	Yes	Yes	08	SURG	Other musculoskelet sys & conn tiss O.R. proc w/o CC/MCC	1.4192	2.0	2.9
533	Yes	No	08	MED	Fractures of femur w MCC	1.1294	5.1	6.9
534	Yes	No	08	MED	Fractures of femur w/o MCC	0.7560	3.2	4.0
535	Yes	No	08	MED	Fractures of hip & pelvis w MCC	1.0836	4.8	6.4
536	Yes	No	08	MED	Fractures of hip & pelvis w/o MCC	0.7340	3.4	4.0
537	No	No	08	MED	Sprains, strains, & dislocations of hip, pelvis & thigh w CC/ MCC	0.7528	3.8	4.7
538	No	No	08	MED	Sprains, strains, & dislocations of hip, pelvis & thigh w/o CC/ MCC	0.5986	2.6	3.1
539	Yes	No	08	MED	Osteomyelitis w MCC	1.7648	7.7	10.2

Continued

MS-DRG3	FY08 Final Rule Post Acute DRG	FY08 Final Rule Special Pay DRG	MDC	TYPE	MS-DRG Title	Weights	Geometric Mean LOS	Arithmetic Mean LOS
540	Yes	No	08	MED	Osteomyelitis w CC	1.4026	5.8	7.2
541	Yes	No	08	MED	Osteomyelitis w/o CC/MCC	1.2101	4.4	5.7
542	Yes	No	08	MED	Pathological fractures & musculoskelet & conn tiss malig w MCC	1.4877	6.8	8.7
543	Yes	No	08	MED	Pathological fractures & musculoskelet & conn tiss malig w CC	1.1151	4.8	6.0
544	Yes	No	08	MED	Pathological fractures & musculoskelet & conn tiss malig w/o CC/MCC	0.9395	3.7	4.5
545	Yes	No	08	MED	Connective tissue disorders w MCC	1.8330	6.5	9.0
546	Yes	No	08	MED	Connective tissue disorders w CC	1.2092	4.3	5.5
547	Yes	No	08	MED	Connective tissue disorders w/o CC/MCC	0.9054	3.2	3.9
548	No	No	08	MED	Septic arthritis w MCC	1.5372	7.0	9.3
549	No	No	08	MED	Septic arthritis w CC	1.1522	5.0	6.2
550	No	No	08	MED	Septic arthritis w/o CC/MCC	0.9567	3.6	4.5
551	Yes	No	08	MED	Medical back problems w MCC	1.1632	5.5	7.2
552	Yes	No	08	MED	Medical back problems w/o MCC	0.7839	3.4	4.2
553	No	No	08	MED	Bone diseases & arthropathies w MCC	0.9199	4.8	6.1
554	No	No	08	MED	Bone diseases & arthropathies w/o MCC	0.6475	3.0	3.7
555	No	No	08	MED	Signs & symptoms of musculoskeletal system & conn tissue w MCC	0.7886	3.6	4.9
556	No	No	08	MED	Signs & symptoms of musculoskeletal system & conn tissue w/o MCC	0.5958	2.5	3.2
557	Yes	No	08	MED	Tendonitis, myositis & bursitis w MCC	1.2171	5.4	6.9
558	Yes	No	08	MED	Tendonitis, myositis & bursitis w/o MCC	0.8480	3.5	4.3
559	Yes	No	08	MED	Aftercare, musculoskeletal system & connective tissue w MCC	1.2104	5.1	7.3
560	Yes	No	08	MED	Aftercare, musculoskeletal system & connective tissue w CC	0.8521	3.6	4.7
561	Yes	No	08	MED	Aftercare, musculoskeletal system & connective tissue w/o CC/MCC	0.6753	2.1	2.7
562	Yes	No	08	MED	Fx, sprn, strn & disl except femur, hip, pelvis & thigh w MCC	1.1163	5.0	6.5
563	Yes	No	08	MED	Fx, sprn, strn & disl except femur, hip, pelvis & thigh w/o MCC	0.6981	3.1	3.7
564	No	No	08	MED	Other musculoskeletal sys & connective tissue diagnoses w MCC	1.1606	5.3	7.1
565	No	No	08	MED	Other musculoskeletal sys & connective tissue diagnoses w CC	0.9003	4.0	5.1
566	No	No	08	MED	Other musculoskeletal sys & connective tissue diagnoses w/o CC/MCC	0.7790	2.9	3.7
573	Yes	No	09	SURG	Skin graft &/or debrid for skin ulcer or cellulitis w MCC	2.7483	10.1	13.8
574	Yes	No	09	SURG	Skin graft &/or debrid for skin ulcer or cellulitis w CC	2.0177	7.2	9.5
575	Yes	No	09	SURG	Skin graft &/or debrid for skin ulcer or cellulitis w/o CC/MCC	1.4216	4.7	5.9
576	No	No	09	SURG	Skin graft &/or debrid exc for skin ulcer or cellulitis w MCC	2.4766	7.8	12.1
577	No	No	09	SURG	Skin graft &/or debrid exc for skin ulcer or cellulitis w CC	1.6262	4.1	6.0

578	No	No	09	SURG	Skin graft &/or debrid exc for skin ulcer or cellulitis w/o CC/ MCC	1.0742	2.5	3.4
579	Yes	No	09	SURG	Other skin, subcut tiss & breast proc w MCC	2.3093	8.1	11.1
580	Yes	No	09	SURG	Other skin, subcut tiss & breast proc w CC	1.4256	3.6	5.5
581	Yes	No	09	SURG	Other skin, subcut tiss & breast proc w/o CC/MCC	0.9124	1.9	2.6
582	No	No	09	SURG	Mastectomy for malignancy w CC/MCC	0.9432	2.1	2.9
583	No	No	09	SURG	Mastectomy for malignancy w/o CC/MCC	0.7523	1.6	1.8
584	No	No	09	SURG	Breast biopsy, local excision & other breast procedures w CC/ MCC	1.2484	3.7	5.7
585	No	No	09	SURG	Breast biopsy, local excision & other breast procedures w/o CC/MCC	0.9066	1.7	2.2
592	Yes	No	09	MED	Skin ulcers w MCC	1.4555	6.6	8.9
593	Yes	No	09	MED	Skin ulcers w CC	1.1060	5.2	6.5
594	Yes	No	09	MED	Skin ulcers w/o CC/MCC	0.9335	3.9	4.9
595	No	No	09	MED	Major skin disorders w MCC	1.3997	6.0	8.2
596	No	No	09	MED	Major skin disorders w/o MCC	0.8766	3.8	4.8
597	No	No	09	MED	Malignant breast disorders w MCC	1.4034	5.9	8.2
598	No	No	09	MED	Malignant breast disorders w CC	1.0695	4.2	5.6
599	No	No	09	MED	Malignant breast disorders w/o CC/MCC	0.7232	2.6	3.6
600	No	No	09	MED	Non-malignant breast disorders w CC/MCC	0.8471	4.1	5.4
601	No	No	09	MED	Non-malignant breast disorders w/o CC/MCC	0.6715	3.1	3.8
602	Yes	No	09	MED	Cellulitis w MCC	1.1522	5.5	7.0
603	Yes	No	09	MED	Cellulitis w/o MCC	0.8087	3.9	4.7
604	No	No	09	MED	Trauma to the skin, subcut tiss & breast w MCC	0.9681	4.1	5.4
605	No	No	09	MED	Trauma to the skin, subcut tiss & breast w/o MCC	0.6863	2.8	3.5
606	No	No	09	MED	Minor skin disorders w MCC	0.9223	4.2	5.9
607	No	No	09	MED	Minor skin disorders w/o MCC	0.6505	2.9	3.8
614	No	No	10	SURG	Adrenal & pituitary procedures w CC/MCC	2.1978	5.2	7.3
615	No	No	10	SURG	Adrenal & pituitary procedures w/o CC/MCC	1.6502	2.8	3.4
616	Yes	No	10	SURG	Amputat of lower limb for endocrine, nutrit,& metabol dis w MCC	3.1449	12.6	15.6
617	Yes	No	10	SURG	Amputat of lower limb for endocrine, nutrit,& metabol dis w CC	2.2071	7.2	9.0
618	Yes	No	10	SURG	Amputat of lower limb for endocrine, nutrit,& metabol dis w/o CC/MCC	1.7554	4.9	6.1
619	No	No	10	SURG	O.R. procedures for obesity w MCC	2.7625	6.4	9.3
620	No	No	10	SURG	O.R. procedures for obesity w CC	1.9294	3.4	4.2
621	No	No	10	SURG	O.R. procedures for obesity w/o CC/MCC	1.6876	2.1	2.4
622	Yes	No	10	SURG	Skin grafts & wound debrid for endoc, nutrit & metab dis w MCC	2.7257	9.7	13.2
623	Yes	No	10	SURG	Skin grafts & wound debrid for endoc, nutrit & metab dis w CC	2.0065	6.8	8.7
624	Yes	No	10	SURG	Skin grafts & wound debrid for endoc, nutrit & metab dis w/o CC/MCC	1.6056	4.6	5.9
625	No	No	10	SURG	Thyroid, parathyroid & thyroglossal procedures w MCC	1.5928	5.0	7.5

Continued

MS-DRG3	FY08 Final Rule Post Acute DRG	FY08 Final Rule Special Pay DRG	MDC	TYPE	MS-DRG Title	Weights	Geometric Mean LOS	Arithmetic Mean LOS
626	No	No	10	SURG	Thyroid, parathyroid & thyroglossal procedures w CC	1.0183	2.2	3.3
627	No	No	10	SURG	Thyroid, parathyroid & thyroglossal procedures w/o CC/MCC	0.8169	1.3	1.5
628	Yes	No	10	SURG	Other endocrine, nutrit & metab O.R. proc w MCC	3.0602	7.8	11.8
629	Yes	No	10	SURG	Other endocrine, nutrit & metab O.R. proc w CC	2.4730	7.0	8.8
630	Yes	No	10	SURG	Other endocrine, nutrit & metab O.R. proc w/o CC/MCC	1.7767	3.7	5.1
637	Yes	No	10	MED	Diabetes w MCC	1.0891	4.6	6.2
638	Yes	No	10	MED	Diabetes w CC	0.8021	3.4	4.3
639	Yes	No	10	MED	Diabetes w/o CC/MCC	0.6742	2.5	3.1
640	Yes	No	10	MED	Nutritional & misc metabolic disorders w MCC	0.9793	4.1	5.6
641	Yes	No	10	MED	Nutritional & misc metabolic disorders w/o MCC	0.7248	3.1	3.9
642	No	No	10	MED	Inborn errors of metabolism	1.0616	3.8	5.3
643	Yes	No	10	MED	Endocrine disorders w MCC	1.3926	6.0	7.8
644	Yes	No	10	MED	Endocrine disorders w CC	1.0638	4.3	5.4
645	Yes	No	10	MED	Endocrine disorders w/o CC/MCC	0.8310	3.2	3.9
652	No	No	11	SURG	Kidney transplant	3.0654	6.6	7.9
653	Yes	No	11	SURG	Major bladder procedures w MCC	4.5710	13.3	16.8
654	Yes	No	11	SURG	Major bladder procedures w CC	3.1860	8.8	10.1
655	Yes	No	11	SURG	Major bladder procedures w/o CC/MCC	2.7075	5.8	6.6
656	No	No	11	SURG	Kidney & ureter procedures for neoplasm w MCC	2.6603	8.4	10.8
657	No	No	11	SURG	Kidney & ureter procedures for neoplasm w CC	1.8997	5.1	6.1
658	No	No	11	SURG	Kidney & ureter procedures for neoplasm w/o CC/MCC	1.6556	3.3	3.8
659	Yes	No	11	SURG	Kidney & ureter procedures for non-neoplasm w MCC	2.8119	8.2	11.3
660	Yes	No	11	SURG	Kidney & ureter procedures for non-neoplasm w CC	2.0605	4.8	6.5
661	Yes	No	11	SURG	Kidney & ureter procedures for non-neoplasm w/o CC/MCC	1.4004	2.6	3.3
662	No	No	11	SURG	Minor bladder procedures w MCC	2.0375	7.3	10.5
663	No	No	11	SURG	Minor bladder procedures w CC	1.4254	3.6	5.3
664	No	No	11	SURG	Minor bladder procedures w/o CC/MCC	1.0388	1.6	2.1
665	No	No	11	SURG	Prostatectomy w MCC	2.1393	9.3	12.2
666	No	No	11	SURG	Prostatectomy w CC	1.4691	4.3	6.3
667	No	No	11	SURG	Prostatectomy w/o CC/MCC	0.9335	2.0	2.7
668	No	No	11	SURG	Transurethral procedures w MCC	1.7208	6.3	8.6
669	No	No	11	SURG	Transurethral procedures w CC	1.2079	3.1	4.4
670	No	No	11	SURG	Transurethral procedures w/o CC/MCC	0.8838	1.9	2.5
671	No	No	11	SURG	Urethral procedures w CC/MCC	1.2808	3.9	5.8
672	No	No	11	SURG	Urethral procedures w/o CC/MCC	0.8422	1.9	2.5
673	No	No	11	SURG	Other kidney & urinary tract procedures w MCC	2.5235	6.0	10.2
674	No	No	11	SURG	Other kidney & urinary tract procedures w CC	2.1024	4.0	6.6
675	No	No	11	SURG	Other kidney & urinary tract procedures w/o CC/MCC	1.7196	1.4	1.9
682	Yes	No	11	MED	Renal failure w MCC	1.4664	5.3	7.3
683	Yes	No	11	MED	Renal failure w CC	1.1942	4.5	5.7
684	Yes	No	11	MED	Renal failure w/o CC/MCC	0.9835	3.1	3.8
685	No	No	11	MED	Admit for renal dialysis	0.8599	2.4	3.5

686	No	No	11	MED	Kidney & urinary tract neoplasms w MCC	1.4513	6.0	8.1
687	No	No	11	MED	Kidney & urinary tract neoplasms w CC	1.1147	4.0	5.3
688	No	No	11	MED	Kidney & urinary tract neoplasms w/o CC/MCC	0.8577	2.5	3.2
689	Yes	No	11	MED	Kidney & urinary tract infections w MCC	1.0587	5.0	6.4
690	Yes	No	11	MED	Kidney & urinary tract infections w/o MCC	0.8000	3.6	4.3
691	No	No	11	MED	Urinary stones w esw lithotripsy w CC/MCC	1.1508	3.0	4.2
692	No	No	11	MED	Urinary stones w esw lithotripsy w/o CC/MCC	0.9457	1.8	2.3
693	No	No	11	MED	Urinary stones w/o esw lithotripsy w MCC	1.0459	3.9	5.2
694	No	No	11	MED	Urinary stones w/o esw lithotripsy w/o MCC	0.7110	2.0	2.6
695	No	No	11	MED	Kidney & urinary tract signs & symptoms w MCC	0.9422	4.3	5.7
696	No	No	11	MED	Kidney & urinary tract signs & symptoms w/o MCC	0.6276	2.6	3.2
697	No	No	11	MED	Urethral stricture	0.7223	2.4	3.3
698	Yes	No	11	MED	Other kidney & urinary tract diagnoses w MCC	1.3017	5.1	6.8
699	Yes	No	11	MED	Other kidney & urinary tract diagnoses w CC	1.0352	3.8	4.9
700	Yes	No	11	MED	Other kidney & urinary tract diagnoses w/o CC/MCC	0.8232	2.7	3.5
707	No	No	12	SURG	Major male pelvic procedures w CC/MCC	1.5521	3.5	4.5
708	No	No	12	SURG	Major male pelvic procedures w/o CC/MCC	1.1858	2.0	2.4
709	No	No	12	SURG	Penis procedures w CC/MCC	1.6134	3.6	6.5
710	No	No	12	SURG	Penis procedures w/o CC/MCC	1.2986	1.5	1.9
711	No	No	12	SURG	Testes procedures w CC/MCC	1.6051	5.3	7.8
712	No	No	12	SURG	Testes procedures w/o CC/MCC	1.0842	2.1	3.0
713	No	No	12	SURG	Transurethral prostatectomy w CC/MCC	0.9850	2.9	4.2
714	No	No	12	SURG	Transurethral prostatectomy w/o CC/MCC	0.6710	1.7	2.0
715	No	No	12	SURG	Other male reproductive system O.R. proc for malignancy w CC/MCC	1.5300	3.8	6.1
716	No	No	12	SURG	Other male reproductive system O.R. proc for malignancy w/o CC/MCC	1.1310	1.3	1.5
717	No	No	12	SURG	Other male reproductive system O.R. proc exc malignancy w CC/MCC	1.5653	5.0	7.5
718	No	No	12	SURG	Other male reproductive system O.R. proc exc malignancy w/o CC/MCC	1.0329	2.1	2.7
722	No	No	12	MED	Malignancy, male reproductive system w MCC	1.2827	5.6	7.4
723	No	No	12	MED	Malignancy, male reproductive system w CC	1.0603	4.2	5.4
724	No	No	12	MED	Malignancy, male reproductive system w/o CC/MCC	0.7677	2.5	3.3
725	No	No	12	MED	Benign prostatic hypertrophy w MCC	0.9071	4.4	5.7
726	No	No	12	MED	Benign prostatic hypertrophy w/o MCC	0.6886	2.8	3.5
727	No	No	12	MED	Inflammation of the male reproductive system w MCC	1.0083	5.1	6.5
728	No	No	12	MED	Inflammation of the male reproductive system w/o MCC	0.7241	3.3	4.0
729	No	No	12	MED	Other male reproductive system diagnoses w CC/MCC	0.9542	3.7	5.1
730	No	No	12	MED	Other male reproductive system diagnoses w/o CC/MCC	0.7058	2.4	3.2
734	No	No	13	SURG	Pelvic evisceration, rad hysterectomy & rad vulvectomy w CC/MCC	2.0185	5.8	7.6
735	No	No	13	SURG	Pelvic evisceration, rad hysterectomy & rad vulvectomy w/o CC/MCC	1.3798	3.0	3.5
736	No	No	13	SURG	Uterine & adnexa proc for ovarian or adnexal malignancy w MCC	3.2108	11.5	13.9

Continued

MS-DRG3	FY08 Final Rule Post Acute DRG	FY08 Final Rule Special Pay DRG	MDC	TYPE	MS-DRG Title	Weights	Geometric Mean LOS	Arithmetic Mean LOS
737	No	No	13	SURG	Uterine & adnexa proc for ovarian or adnexal malignancy w CC	2.1022	6.2	7.4
738	No	No	13	SURG	Uterine & adnexa proc for ovarian or adnexal malignancy w/o CC/MCC	1.6754	3.5	3.9
739	No	No	13	SURG	Uterine, adnexa proc for non-ovarian/adnexal malig w MCC	2.2081	7.9	10.2
740	No	No	13	SURG	Uterine, adnexa proc for non-ovarian/adnexal malig w CC	1.4577	4.4	5.2
741	No	No	13	SURG	Uterine, adnexa proc for non-ovarian/adnexal malig w/o CC/MCC	1.0308	2.8	3.1
742	No	No	13	SURG	Uterine & adnexa proc for non-malignancy w CC/MCC	1.2422	3.5	4.6
743	No	No	13	SURG	Uterine & adnexa proc for non-malignancy w/o CC/MCC	0.8672	2.1	2.3
744	No	No	13	SURG	D&C, conization, laparoscopy & tubal interruption w CC/MCC	1.1896	4.0	5.8
745	No	No	13	SURG	D&C, conization, laparoscopy & tubal interruption w/o CC/MCC	0.8660	2.1	2.5
746	No	No	13	SURG	Vagina, cervix & vulva procedures w CC/MCC	1.0488	3.0	4.1
747	No	No	13	SURG	Vagina, cervix & vulva procedures w/o CC/MCC	0.8499	1.7	1.9
748	No	No	13	SURG	Female reproductive system reconstructive procedures	0.7916	1.5	1.8
749	No	No	13	SURG	Other female reproductive system O.R. procedures w CC/MCC	2.2813	7.1	9.8
750	No	No	13	SURG	Other female reproductive system O.R. procedures w/o CC/MCC	1.4993	2.6	3.3
754	No	No	13	MED	Malignancy, female reproductive system w MCC	1.5596	6.4	8.9
755	No	No	13	MED	Malignancy, female reproductive system w CC	1.1608	4.2	5.6
756	No	No	13	MED	Malignancy, female reproductive system w/o CC/MCC	0.7702	2.5	3.3
757	No	No	13	MED	Infections, female reproductive system w MCC	1.4328	6.8	8.9
758	No	No	13	MED	Infections, female reproductive system w CC	1.1147	4.9	6.1
759	No	No	13	MED	Infections, female reproductive system w/o CC/MCC	0.9609	3.7	4.6
760	No	No	13	MED	Menstrual & other female reproductive system disorders w CC/MCC	0.6910	2.9	3.8
761	No	No	13	MED	Menstrual & other female reproductive system disorders w/o CC/MCC	0.5569	2.0	2.5
765	No	No	14	SURG	Cesarean section w CC/MCC	0.9943	4.1	5.3
766	No	No	14	SURG	Cesarean section w/o CC/MCC	0.7664	3.0	3.2
767	No	No	14	SURG	Vaginal delivery w sterilization &/or D&C	0.7246	2.5	2.9
768	No	No	14	SURG	Vaginal delivery w O.R. proc except steril &/or D&C	1.7348	4.7	5.8
769	No	No	14	SURG	Postpartum & post abortion diagnoses w O.R. procedure	1.9114	3.2	5.7
770	No	No	14	SURG	Abortion w D&C, aspiration curettage or hysterotomy	0.7336	1.6	2.6
774	No	No	14	MED	Vaginal delivery w complicating diagnoses	0.5914	2.6	3.2
775	No	No	14	MED	Vaginal delivery w/o complicating diagnoses	0.4461	2.1	2.3
776	No	No	14	MED	Postpartum & post abortion diagnoses w/o O.R. procedure	0.6460	2.6	3.5
777	No	No	14	MED	Ectopic pregnancy	0.7087	1.8	2.1
778	No	No	14	MED	Threatened abortion	0.3744	2.0	2.8
779	No	No	14	MED	Abortion w/o D&C	0.6013	1.7	2.6
780	No	No	14	MED	False labor	0.2845	1.3	2.7
781	No	No	14	MED	Other antepartum diagnoses w medical complications	0.5689	2.7	3.9

782	No	No	14	MED	Other antepartum diagnoses w/o medical complications	0.4297	1.7	2.8
789	No	No	15	MED	Neonates, died or transferred to another acute care facility	1.4250	*	*
790	No	No	15	MED	Extreme immaturity or respiratory distress syndrome, neonate	4.6990	*	*
791	No	No	15	MED	Prematurity w major problems	3.2093	*	*
792	No	No	15	MED	Prematurity w/o major problems	1.9364	*	*
793	No	No	15	MED	Full term neonate w major problems	3.2966	*	*
794	No	No	15	MED	Neonate w other significant problems	1.1668	*	*
795	No	No	15	MED	Normal newborn	0.1580	*	*
799	No	No	16	SURG	Splenectomy w MCC	3.9513	10.7	14.3
800	No	No	16	SURG	Splenectomy w CC	2.7617	6.4	8.2
801	No	No	16	SURG	Splenectomy w/o CC/MCC	2.3252	3.7	4.8
802	No	No	16	SURG	Other O.R. proc of the blood & blood forming organs w MCC	2.7940	9.1	12.8
803	No	No	16	SURG	Other O.R. proc of the blood & blood forming organs w CC	1.8259	4.7	6.5
804	No	No	16	SURG	Other O.R. proc of the blood & blood forming organs w/o CC/MCC	1.4754	2.4	3.2
808	No	No	16	MED	Major hematol/immun diag exc sickle cell crisis & coagul w MCC	1.6171	6.0	8.0
809	No	No	16	MED	Major hematol/immun diag exc sickle cell crisis & coagul w CC	1.2031	3.9	5.0
810	No	No	16	MED	Major hematol/immun diag exc sickle cell crisis & coagul w/o CC/MCC	1.0741	3.1	3.9
811	No	No	16	MED	Red blood cell disorders w MCC	1.0006	4.0	5.5
812	No	No	16	MED	Red blood cell disorders w/o MCC	0.7780	2.8	3.7
813	No	No	16	MED	Coagulation disorders	1.3426	3.8	5.2
814	No	No	16	MED	Reticuloendothelial & immunity disorders w MCC	1.3226	5.3	7.2
815	No	No	16	MED	Reticuloendothelial & immunity disorders w CC	1.0233	3.9	4.9
816	No	No	16	MED	Reticuloendothelial & immunity disorders w/o CC/MCC	0.7990	2.7	3.4
820	No	No	17	SURG	Lymphoma & leukemia w major O.R. procedure w MCC	4.4970	13.8	18.4
821	No	No	17	SURG	Lymphoma & leukemia w major O.R. procedure w CC	2.6847	5.4	7.8
822	No	No	17	SURG	Lymphoma & leukemia w major O.R. procedure w/o CC/MCC	1.5989	2.7	3.7
823	No	No	17	SURG	Lymphoma & non-acute leukemia w other O.R. proc w MCC	3.5188	12.0	15.4
824	No	No	17	SURG	Lymphoma & non-acute leukemia w other O.R. proc w CC	2.5164	6.6	8.8
825	No	No	17	SURG	Lymphoma & non-acute leukemia w other O.R. proc w/o CC/MCC	1.6201	3.3	4.7
826	No	No	17	SURG	Myeloprolif disord or poorly diff neopl w maj O.R. proc w MCC	3.9780	13.0	17.4
827	No	No	17	SURG	Myeloprolif disord or poorly diff neopl w maj O.R. proc w CC	2.4230	5.7	7.5
828	No	No	17	SURG	Myeloprolif disord or poorly diff neopl w maj O.R. proc w/o CC/MCC	1.5109	2.9	3.7
829	No	No	17	SURG	Myeloprolif disord or poorly diff neopl w other O.R. proc w CC/MCC	2.4894	6.9	10.5
830	No	No	17	SURG	Myeloprolif disord or poorly diff neopl w other O.R. proc w/o CC/MCC	1.6396	2.5	3.5
834	No	No	17	MED	Acute leukemia w/o major O.R. procedure w MCC	3.6361	8.9	14.7
835	No	No	17	MED	Acute leukemia w/o major O.R. procedure w CC	2.5626	5.3	8.2
836	No	No	17	MED	Acute leukemia w/o major O.R. procedure w/o CC/MCC	2.1785	3.4	5.1

Continued

MS-DRG3	FY08 Final Rule Post Acute DRG	FY08 Final Rule Special Pay DRG	MDC	TYPE	MS-DRG Title	Weights	Geometric Mean LOS	Arithmetic Mean LOS
837	No	No	17	MED	Chemo w acute leukemia as sdx or w high dose chemo agent w MCC	4.7788	17.2	22.7
838	No	No	17	MED	Chemo w acute leukemia as sdx w CC or high dose chemo agent	2.9919	6.2	9.0
839	No	No	17	MED	Chemo w acute leukemia as sdx w/o CC/MCC	2.3980	4.9	6.1
840	Yes	No	17	MED	Lymphoma & non-acute leukemia w MCC	2.1454	6.8	9.6
841	Yes	No	17	MED	Lymphoma & non-acute leukemia w CC	1.6444	5.0	6.6
842	Yes	No	17	MED	Lymphoma & non-acute leukemia w/o CC/MCC	1.2188	3.2	4.3
843	No	No	17	MED	Other myeloprolif dis or poorly diff neopl diag w MCC	1.6341	6.3	8.7
844	No	No	17	MED	Other myeloprolif dis or poorly diff neopl diag w CC	1.2403	4.5	6.0
845	No	No	17	MED	Other myeloprolif dis or poorly diff neopl diag w/o CC/MCC	0.9664	3.3	4.3
846	No	No	17	MED	Chemotherapy w/o acute leukemia as secondary diagnosis w MCC	1.6523	5.8	8.5
847	No	No	17	MED	Chemotherapy w/o acute leukemia as secondary diagnosis w CC	1.0296	2.7	3.3
848	No	No	17	MED	Chemotherapy w/o acute leukemia as secondary diagnosis w/o CC/MCC	0.9116	2.3	2.9
849	No	No	17	MED	Radiotherapy	1.2663	4.3	6.0
853	Yes	No	18	SURG	Infectious & parasitic diseases w O.R. procedure w MCC	5.1840	12.8	16.8
854	Yes	No	18	SURG	Infectious & parasitic diseases w O.R. procedure w CC	3.9291	9.1	11.2
855	Yes	No	18	SURG	Infectious & parasitic diseases w O.R. procedure w/o CC/MCC	3.3662	5.6	7.3
856	Yes	No	18	SURG	Postoperative or post-traumatic infections w O.R. proc w MCC	3.9257	12.1	16.2
857	Yes	No	18	SURG	Postoperative or post-traumatic infections w O.R. proc w CC	2.4919	6.8	8.9
858	Yes	No	18	SURG	Postoperative or post-traumatic infections w O.R. proc w/o CC/MCC	2.0996	4.7	6.0
862	Yes	No	18	MED	Postoperative & post-traumatic infections w MCC	1.5454	6.2	8.3
863	Yes	No	18	MED	Postoperative & post-traumatic infections w/o MCC	1.0560	4.2	5.2
864	No	No	18	MED	Fever of unknown origin	0.8240	3.2	4.1
865	No	No	18	MED	Viral illness w MCC	1.2074	4.9	6.8
866	No	No	18	MED	Viral illness w/o MCC	0.7527	2.8	3.5
867	Yes	No	18	MED	Other infectious & parasitic diseases diagnoses w MCC	2.1971	7.2	9.9
868	Yes	No	18	MED	Other infectious & parasitic diseases diagnoses w CC	1.5258	4.6	5.9
869	Yes	No	18	MED	Other infectious & parasitic diseases diagnoses w/o CC/MCC	1.3611	3.5	4.4
870	Yes	No	18	MED	Septicemia w MV 96+ hours	5.7579	12.6	15.3
871	Yes	No	18	MED	Septicemia w/o MV 96+ hours w MCC	1.7484	5.6	7.7
872	Yes	No	18	MED	Septicemia w/o MV 96+ hours w/o MCC	1.3783	4.7	5.8
876	No	No	19	SURG	O.R. procedure w principal diagnoses of mental illness	2.4632	6.9	11.4
880	No	No	19	MED	Acute adjustment reaction & psychosocial dysfunction	0.6085	2.4	3.2
881	No	No	19	MED	Depressive neuroses	0.5198	3.1	4.2
882	No	No	19	MED	Neuroses except depressive	0.5685	3.1	4.4
883	No	No	19	MED	Disorders of personality & impulse control	0.8999	4.6	7.4
884	Yes	No	19	MED	Organic disturbances & mental retardation	0.8431	4.0	5.4
885	No	No	19	MED	Psychoses	0.7783	5.5	7.6

886	No	No	19	MED	Behavioral & developmental disorders	0.6983	4.0	5.9
887	No	No	19	MED	Other mental disorder diagnoses	0.8341	3.1	4.6
894	No	No	20	MED	Alcohol/drug abuse or dependence, left ama	0.3571	2.1	3.0
895	No	No	20	MED	Alcohol/drug abuse or dependence w rehabilitation therapy	0.7557	8.2	10.5
896	Yes	No	20	MED	Alcohol/drug abuse or dependence w/o rehabilitation therapy w MCC	1.0419	4.8	6.6
897	Yes	No	20	MED	Alcohol/drug abuse or dependence w/o rehabilitation therapy w/o MCC	0.6145	3.3	4.1
901	No	No	21	SURG	Wound debridements for injuries w MCC	2.8534	9.3	14.4
902	No	No	21	SURG	Wound debridements for injuries w CC	1.8611	5.7	7.9
903	No	No	21	SURG	Wound debridements for injuries w/o CC/MCC	1.4966	3.5	4.9
904	No	No	21	SURG	Skin grafts for injuries w CC/MCC	2.5246	7.2	12.2
905	No	No	21	SURG	Skin grafts for injuries w/o CC/MCC	1.5926	3.5	4.7
906	No	No	21	SURG	Hand procedures for injuries	0.9803	2.2	3.3
907	Yes	No	21	SURG	Other O.R. procedures for injuries w MCC	3.1030	8.1	11.7
908	Yes	No	21	SURG	Other O.R. procedures for injuries w CC	2.1865	5.0	6.9
909	Yes	No	21	SURG	Other O.R. procedures for injuries w/o CC/MCC	1.4112	2.7	3.6
913	No	No	21	MED	Traumatic injury w MCC	1.0631	4.6	6.2
914	No	No	21	MED	Traumatic injury w/o MCC	0.6890	2.7	3.4
915	No	No	21	MED	Allergic reactions w MCC	0.8660	3.3	4.7
916	No	No	21	MED	Allergic reactions w/o MCC	0.4986	1.7	2.1
917	Yes	No	21	MED	Poisoning & toxic effects of drugs w MCC	1.1717	3.7	5.2
918	Yes	No	21	MED	Poisoning & toxic effects of drugs w/o MCC	0.6886	2.1	2.7
919	No	No	21	MED	Complications of treatment w MCC	1.2830	4.4	6.2
920	No	No	21	MED	Complications of treatment w CC	0.9797	3.2	4.3
921	No	No	21	MED	Complications of treatment w/o CC/MCC	0.7101	2.3	2.9
922	No	No	21	MED	Other injury, poisoning & toxic effect diag w MCC	1.1338	4.1	6.0
923	No	No	21	MED	Other injury, poisoning & toxic effect diag w/o MCC	0.7071	2.4	3.3
927	No	No	22	SURG	Extensive burns or full thickness burns w MV 96+ hrs w skin graft	12.3042	23.0	28.8
928	No	No	22	SURG	Full thickness burn w skin graft or inhal inj w CC/MCC	4.3956	12.1	16.2
929	No	No	22	SURG	Full thickness burn w skin graft or inhal inj w/o CC/MCC	2.3533	5.6	7.7
933	No	No	22	MED	Extensive burns or full thickness burns w MV 96+ hrs w/o skin graft	2.6626	2.7	5.9
934	No	No	22	MED	Full thickness burn w/o skin grft or inhal inj	1.3745	4.7	6.8
935	No	No	22	MED	Non-extensive burns	1.1605	3.7	5.5
939	No	No	23	SURG	O.R. proc w diagnoses of other contact w health services w MCC	2.1672	7.5	10.9
940	No	No	23	SURG	O.R. proc w diagnoses of other contact w health services w CC	1.6823	4.4	6.4
941	No	No	23	SURG	O.R. proc w diagnoses of other contact w health services w/o CC/MCC	1.3531	2.3	3.0
945	Yes	No	23	MED	Rehabilitation w CC/MCC	1.1005	8.4	10.3
946	Yes	No	23	MED	Rehabilitation w/o CC/MCC	1.0143	7.0	7.9
947	Yes	No	23	MED	Signs & symptoms w MCC	0.8767	3.8	5.0
948	Yes	No	23	MED	Signs & symptoms w/o MCC	0.6542	2.7	3.4

Continued

MS-DRG3	FY08 Final Rule Post Acute DRG	FY08 Final Rule Special Pay DRG	MDC	TYPE	MS-DRG Title	Weights	Geometric Mean LOS	Arithmetic Mean LOS
949	No	No	23	MED	Aftercare w CC/MCC	0.7323	2.5	4.1
950	No	No	23	MED	Aftercare w/o CC/MCC	0.5948	2.4	3.4
951	No	No	23	MED	Other factors influencing health status	0.6109	2.1	3.8
955	No	No	24	SURG	Craniotomy for multiple significant trauma	5.1028	8.5	12.2
956	Yes	Yes	24	SURG	Limb reattachment, hip & femur proc for multiple significant trauma	3.4854	7.6	9.5
957	No	No	24	SURG	Other O.R. procedures for multiple significant trauma w MCC	5.7960	10.5	16.0
958	No	No	24	SURG	Other O.R. procedures for multiple significant trauma w CC	4.4786	7.9	10.5
959	No	No	24	SURG	Other O.R. procedures for multiple significant trauma w/o CC/MCC	3.6988	4.9	6.1
963	No	No	24	MED	Other multiple significant trauma w MCC	2.2985	6.3	9.3
964	No	No	24	MED	Other multiple significant trauma w CC	1.7015	5.0	6.3
965	No	No	24	MED	Other multiple significant trauma w/o CC/MCC	1.4108	3.3	4.1
969	No	No	25	SURG	HIV w extensive O.R. procedure w MCC	5.1395	13.5	18.7
970	No	No	25	SURG	HIV w extensive O.R. procedure w/o MCC	3.6849	6.6	9.5
974	No	No	25	MED	HIV w major related condition w MCC	2.1382	7.4	10.4
975	No	No	25	MED	HIV w major related condition w CC	1.5918	5.3	7.3
976	No	No	25	MED	HIV w major related condition w/o CC/MCC	1.3357	3.8	4.9
977	No	No	25	MED	HIV w or w/o other related condition	1.0387	3.8	5.3
981	Yes	No		SURG	Extensive O.R. procedure unrelated to principal diagnosis w MCC	4.5168	11.9	15.3
982	Yes	No		SURG	Extensive O.R. procedure unrelated to principal diagnosis w CC	3.5417	7.8	10.0
983	Yes	No		SURG	Extensive O.R. procedure unrelated to principal diagnosis w/o CC/MCC	2.9737	3.9	5.4
984	No	No		SURG	Prostatic O.R. procedure unrelated to principal diagnosis w MCC	2.7217	11.7	14.6
985	No	No		SURG	Prostatic O.R. procedure unrelated to principal diagnosis w CC	2.0865	7.4	9.7
986	No	No		SURG	Prostatic O.R. procedure unrelated to principal diagnosis w/o CC/MCC	1.6706	3.5	5.1
987	Yes	No		SURG	Non-extensive O.R. proc unrelated to principal diagnosis w MCC	2.8500	9.9	13.2
988	Yes	No		SURG	Non-extensive O.R. proc unrelated to principal diagnosis w CC	2.0134	5.9	8.0
989	Yes	No		SURG	Non-extensive O.R. proc unrelated to principal diagnosis w/o CC/MCC	1.6310	2.9	4.1
998	No	No		**	Principal diagnosis invalid as discharge diagnosis	#N/A	*	*
999	No	No		**	Ungroupable	#N/A	*	*

MS-DRGs 998 and 999 contain cases that could not be assigned to valid DRGs.
Note: If there is no value or asterisk in either the geometric mean length of stay or the arithmetic mean length of stay columns, the volume of cases is insufficient to determine a meaningful computation of these statistics.

APPENDIX C

ICD-10-PCS: Medical and Surgical Root Operation Definitions*

Alteration	*Definition:*	Modifying the natural anatomic structure of a body part without affecting the function of the body part
	Explanation:	Principal purpose is to improve appearance.
	Examples:	Face lift, breast augmentation
Bypass	*Definition:*	Altering the route of passage of the contents of a tubular body part
	Explanation:	Rerouting contents around an area of a body part to another distal (downstream) area in the normal route; rerouting the contents to another different but similar route and body part; or to an abnormal route and another dissimilar body part. It includes one or more concurrent anastomoses with or without the use of a device such as autografts, tissue substitutes, and synthetic substitutes.
	Examples:	Coronary artery bypass, colostomy formation
Change	*Definition:*	Taking out or off a device from a body part and putting back an identical or similar device in or on the same body part without cutting or puncturing the skin or a mucous membrane
	Explanation:	None
	Examples:	Urinary catheter change, gastrostomy tube change
Control	*Definition:*	Stopping, or attempting to stop, postprocedural bleeding
	Explanation:	Site of the bleeding is coded as an anatomical region and not to a specific body part
	Examples:	Control of post-prostatectomy hemorrhage, control of post-tonsillectomy hemorrhage
Creation	*Definition:*	Making a new structure that does not physically take the place of a body part
	Explanation:	Used only for sex change operations where genitalia are made
	Examples:	Creation of vagina in male, creation of penis in a female
Destruction	*Definition:*	Eradicating all or a portion of a body part
	Explanation:	Used for the actual physical destruction of all or a portion of a body part by the direct use of energy, force or a destructive agent. None of the body part is taken out.
	Examples:	Fulguration of rectal polyp, cautery of skin lesion

*From Centers for Medicare and Medicaid Services.

Detachment	*Definition:*	Cutting off all or a portion of an extremity
	Explanation:	Cutting off all or part of the upper and lower extremities
	Examples:	Below knee amputation, disarticulation of shoulder
Dilation	*Definition:*	Expanding an orifice or the lumen of a tubular body part
	Explanation:	The orifice can be a natural orifice or an artificially created orifice. Accomplished by stretching a tubular body part using intraluminal pressure or by cutting part of all of wall of the tubular body part
	Examples:	Percutaneous transluminal angioplasty, pyloromyotomy
Division	*Definition:*	Separating, without taking out, a body part
	Explanation:	All or a portion of the body part is separated into two or more portions.
	Examples:	Spinal cordotomy, osteotomy
Drainage	*Definition:*	Taking or letting out fluids and/or gasses from a body part
	Explanation:	The qualifier Diagnostic is used to identify drainage procedures that are biopsies.
	Examples:	Thoracentesis, incision and drainage
Excision	*Definition:*	Cutting out or off, without replacement, a portion of a body part
	Explanation:	The qualifier Diagnostic is used to identify excision procedures that are biopsies
	Examples:	Partial nephrectomy, liver biopsy
Extirpation	*Definition:*	Taking or cutting out solid matter from a body part
	Explanation:	The solid matter may be an abnormal byproduct of a biological function or a foreign body. The solid matter is imbedded in a body part, or is in the lumen of a tubular body part. The solid matter may or may not have been previously broken into pieces. No appreciable amount of the body part is taken out.
	Examples:	Thrombectomy, choledocholithotomy
Extraction	*Definition:*	Pulling or stripping out or off all or a portion of a body part
	Explanation:	The body part is pulled or stripped from its location by the use of force (e.g., manual, suction). The qualifier Diagnostic is used to identify extractions that are biopsies.
	Examples:	Dilation and curettage, vein stripping
Fragmentation	*Definition:*	Breaking solid matter in a body part into pieces
	Explanation:	The solid matter may be an abnormal byproduct of a biological function or a foreign body. Physical force (e.g., manual, ultrasonic) applied directly or indirectly through intervening body parts used to break the solid matter into pieces. The pieces of solid matter are not taken out, but are eliminated or absorbed through normal biological functions.
	Examples:	Extracorporeal shock wave lithotripsy, intraluminal lithotripsy
Fusion	*Definition:*	Joining together portions of an articular body part, rendering the articular body part immobile
	Explanation:	None
	Examples:	Spinal fusion, ankle arthrodesis

Insertion	*Definition:*	Putting in a nonbiological appliance that monitors, assists, performs or prevents a physiologic function but does not physically take the place of a body part
	Explanation:	None
	Examples:	Insertion of radioactive implant, insertion of central venous catheter
Inspection	*Definition:*	Visually and/or manually exploring a body part
	Explanation:	Visual exploration may be performed with or without optical instrumentation. Manual exploration may be performed directly or through intervening body layers.
	Examples:	Diagnostic arthroscopy, exploratory laparotomy
Map	*Definition:*	Locating the route of passage of electrical impulses and/or locating functional areas in a body part
	Explanation:	Applicable only to the cardiac conduction mechanism and the central nervous system
	Examples:	Cardiac mapping, cortical mapping
Occlusion	*Definition:*	Completely closing an orifice or lumen of a tubular body part
	Explanation:	The orifice can be a natural orifice or an artificially created orifice.
	Examples:	Fallopian tube ligation, ligation of inferior vena cava
Reattachment	*Definition:*	Putting back in or on all or a position of a separated body part to its normal location or other suitable location
	Explanation:	Vascular circulation and nervous pathways may or may not be reestablished.
	Examples:	Reattachment of hand, reattachment of avulsed kidney
Release	*Definition:*	Freeing a body part
	Explanation:	Eliminating an abnormal constraint of a body part by cutting or by use of force. Some of the restraining tissue may be taken out, but none of the body part is taken out.
	Examples:	Adhesiolysis, carpal tunnel release
Removal	*Definition:*	Taking out or off a device from a body part
	Explanation:	If taking out a device and putting in a similar device is performed with an external approach, the procedure is coded to the root operation Change. Otherwise, the procedure for taking out the device is coded to the rooter operation Removal and the procedure for putting in the new device is coded to the root operation performed.
	Examples:	Drainage tube removal, cardiac pacemaker removal
Repair	*Definition:*	Restoring, to the extent possible, a body part to its normal anatomic structure and function
	Explanation:	Used only when the method to accomplish the repair is not one of the other root operations
	Examples:	Herniorrhaphy, suture of laceration
Replacement	*Definition:*	Putting in or on the biological or synthetic material that physically takes the place of all or a portion of a body part

	Explanation:	The biological material is nonliving, or the biological material is living and from the same individual. The body part may have been previously taken out, previously replaced, or may be taken out concomitantly with the Replacement procedure.
	Examples:	Total hip replacement, free skin graft
Reposition	*Definition:*	Moving to its normal location or other suitable location all or a portion of a body part
	Explanation:	The body part is moved to a new location from an aberrant location, or from a normal location where it is not functioning correctly. The body part may or may not be cut out or off to be moved to the new location.
	Examples:	Reposition of undescended testicle, fracture reduction
Resection	*Definition:*	Cutting out or off, without replacement, all of a body part
	Explanation:	None
	Examples:	Total nephrectomy, total lobectomy of lung
Restriction	*Definition:*	Partially closing the orifice or lumen of a tubular body part
	Explanation:	The orifice can be a natural orifice or an artificially created orifice
	Examples:	Esophagogastric fundoplication, cervical cerclage
Revision	*Definition:*	Correcting, to the extent possible, a malfunctioning or displaced device
	Explanation:	None
	Examples:	Adjustment of pacemaker lead, adjustment of hip prosthesis
Transfer	*Definition:*	Moving, without taking out, all or a portion of a body part to another location to take over the function of all or a portion of a body part
	Explanation:	The body part transferred remains connected to its vascular and nervous supply
	Examples:	Tendon transfer, skin pedicle flap transfer
Transplantation	*Definition:*	Putting in or on all or a portion of a living body part taken from another individual or animal to physically take the place and/or function of all or a portion of a similar body part
	Explanation:	The native body part may or may not be taken out, and the transplanted body part may take over all or a portion of its function.
	Examples:	Kidney transplant, heart transplant

References

Chapter 1

1. Hanna J. Constructing a coding compliance plan. J AHIMA 2002;73:48-56.
2. AHIMA Coding Practice Team. Developing a coding compliance policy document (AHIMA practice brief). J AHIMA 2001;72:88A-88C.

Chapter 2

1. Huffman E. Health Information Management, 10th ed. Berwyn, Ill, Physicians' Record Company, 1994, p 30.
2. Abdelhak M, Grostick S, Hanken MA, Jacobs E (eds). Health Information: Management of a Strategic Resource, 2nd ed. St. Louis, WB Saunders, 2001.
3. Centers for Medicare and Medicaid Services, U.S. Department of Health and Human Services.
4. American Hospital Association. *Coding Clinic for ICD-9-CM* 2000:2Q:p20-21. Clarification, reporting of chronic conditions.
5. American Hospital Association. *Coding Clinic for ICD-9-CM* 1992:2Q:p16-17. History of COPD.
6. American Hospital Association. *Coding Clinic for ICD-9-CM* 2002:1Q:p15-16. Prophylactic Coumadin therapy for a patient with history of DVT.
7. American Hospital Association. *Coding Clinic for ICD-9-CM* 1990:2Q:p15. Conditions of an integral disease process-guideline.
8. American Hospital Association. *Coding Clinic for ICD-9-CM* 2002:2Q:p17-18. Abnormal findings on radiology reports, inpatient.
9. American Hospital Association. *Coding Clinic for ICD-9-CM* 2002:2Q:p18. Facility-specific coding guidelines.
10. American Hospital Association. *Coding Clinic for ICD-9-CM* 2004:1Q:p20-21. Clarification—Abnormal pathology report.
11. Prophet S. Developing a physician query process (AHIMA practice brief). J AHIMA 2001;72:88I-88M.

Chapter 4

1. American Hospital Association. *Coding Clinic for ICD-9-CM* 1986:Nov-Dec:p11. Arteriovenous (A-V) malformation of colon.

Chapter 5

1. American Hospital Association. *Coding Clinic for ICD-9-CM* 1995:3Q:p8. Hematuria secondary to renal stones.

Chapter 6

1. American Hospital Association. *Coding Clinic for ICD-9-CM* 2008:1Q:p15. Reporting ICD-9-CM procedure codes for outpatient procedures.
2. American Hospital Association. *Coding Clinic for ICD-9-CM* 1988:4Q:p5. Debridement of wound, excisional vs nonexcisional—Guidelines.
3. American Hospital Association. *Coding Clinic for ICD-9-CM* 1999:1Q:p8-9. Extensive wound debridement.
4. American Hospital Association. *Coding Clinic for ICD-9-CM* 1988:1Q:p9. Bilateral procedures—Guideline.
5. American Hospital Association. *Coding Clinic for ICD-9-CM* 1992:3Q:p12. Laparoscopic appendectomy.
6. American Hospital Association. *Coding Clinic for ICD-9-CM* 1984:J-A:p3-4. Introduction to 1984 revision of UHDDS effective 1/1/86.
7. American Hospital Association. *Coding Clinic for ICD-9-CM* 1988:4Q:p12. Exploratory laparotomy with needle biopsy of liver.

Chapter 7

1. American Health Information Management Association (AHIMA). Statement on consistency of healthcare diagnostic and procedural coding. (AHIMA Position Statement, December 2007).

Chapter 8

1. American Hospital Association. *Coding Clinic for ICD-9-CM* 1990:2Q:p15-16. Abnormal findings—Guidelines.

Chapter 9

1. American Hospital Association. *Coding Clinic for ICD-9-CM* 2002:4Q:p78. Contact/Exposure.
2. American Hospital Association. *Coding Clinic for ICD-9-CM* 1997:4Q:p3. Disseminated *Mycobacterium avium-intracellulare* complex.
3. American Hospital Association. *Coding Clinic for ICD-9-CM* 2000:2Q:p5-6. Bacteremia vs septicemia.
4. American Hospital Association. *Coding Clinic for ICD-9-CM* 2003:4Q:p79-81. Septicemia, SIRS, sepsis, severe sepsis and septic shock.
5. Castro KG, Ward JW, Slutsker L, Buehler JW, Jaffe HW, Berkelman RL (National Center for Infectious Diseases Division of HIV/AIDS). 1993 revised classification system for HIV infection and expanded surveillance: Case definition for AIDS among adolescents and adults. Morb Mortal Wkly Rep, December 18, 1992, 41(RR-17). Bethesda, Md, Centers for Disease Control and Prevention. Available at: http://www.cdc.gov/mmwr/preview/mmwrhtml/00018871.htm. Accessed April 4, 2008.
6. Modified from Frazier ME, Drzymkowki JW. Essentials of Human Diseases and Conditions, 3rd ed. St. Louis, Saunders, 2004, Appendix II, pp 766-767.

Chapter 10

1. Chabner D. The Language of Medicine, 7th ed. St. Louis, Saunders, 2004, p 510.
2. American Hospital Association. *Coding Clinic for ICD-9-CM* 2005:3Q:p11-12. Neutropenic fever with pancytopenia.
3. American Hospital Association. *Coding Clinic for ICD-9-CM* 2006:2Q:p17. Hemoptysis and GI bleeding due to anticoagulants.

Chapter 11

1. American Hospital Association. *Coding Clinic for ICD-9-CM* 2002:3Q:p21-22. ARF due to dehydration and treated with IV hydration only.
2. American Hospital Association. *Coding Clinic for ICD-9-CM* 2005:4Q:p77-79. Chronic kidney disease.

3. American Hospital Association. *Coding Clinic for ICD-9-CM* 1995:3Q:p8. Hematuria secondary to renal stones.
4. American Hospital Association. *Coding Clinic for ICD-9-CM* 1985:Nov-Dec:p15. Trauma resulting from patient pulling out urinary catheter.
5. American Hospital Association. *Coding Clinic for ICD-9-CM* 1999:2Q:p15-16. Urinary tract infection not specified with acute cystitis.
6. From Frazier ME, Drzymkowski JW. Essentials of Human Diseases and Conditions, 3rd ed. St. Louis, Saunders, 2004, Table 11-1, p 504.
7. American Hospital Association. *Coding Clinic for ICD-9-CM* 1996:2Q:p7. Chronic recurrent urinary tract infection w/o urinary symptoms.
8. American Hospital Association. *Coding Clinic for ICD-9-CM* 1991:1Q:p11. Renal colic due to ureteral calculus.

Chapter 12

1. Frazier ME, Drzymkowski JW. Essentials of Human Diseases and Conditions, 3rd ed. St. Louis, Saunders, 2004, Table 4-1, pp 150-151.
2. Chabner D. The Language of Medicine, 7th ed. St. Louis, Saunders, 2004, Table 18-3, p 745.
3. American Hospital Association. *Coding Clinic for ICD-9-CM* 1991:3Q:p6. Diabetes mellitus complications.
4. American Hospital Association. *Coding Clinic for ICD-9-CM* 2002:2Q:p13. Poorly controlled diabetes.
5. American Hospital Association. *Coding Clinic for ICD-9-CM* 1997:4Q:p33. Adult-onset uncontrolled diabetes requiring insulin.
6. American Hospital Association. *Coding Clinic for ICD-9-CM* 2004:1Q:p14-15. Ulcer, diabetic vs decubitus, with osteomyelitis.
7. American Hospital Association. *Coding Clinic for ICD-9-CM* 2002:3Q:p21-22. ARF due to dehydration and treated with IV hydration only.
8. American Hospital Association. *Coding Clinic for ICD-9-CM* 2003:1Q:p22. Clarification—Renal failure due to dehydration with IV hydration.
9. American Hospital Association. *Coding Clinic for ICD 9 CM* 1990:4Q:p17. Cystic fibrosis sequencing—Guidelines.
10. American Hospital Association. *Coding Clinic for ICD-9-CM* 2005:4Q:p96-98. Status V codes.
11. American Hospital Association. *Coding Clinic for ICD-9-CM* 1992:3Q:p13-14. Immunocompromised state due to medication.
12. American Hospital Association. *Coding Clinic for ICD-9-CM* 1990:2Q:p15-16. Abnormal findings—Guidelines.

Chapter 13

1. American Hospital Association. *Coding Clinic for ICD-9-CM* 1998:2Q:p3. Pneumonia: Infection of inflammation of the lung.
2. Damjanov I. Pathology for the Health Professions, 3rd ed. St. Louis, Saunders, 2006, Table 8-1, p 177.
3. American Hospital Association. *Coding Clinic for ICD-9-CM* 1988:3Q:p9-10. Status asthmaticus.
4. American Hospital Association. *Coding Clinic for ICD-9-CM* 1991:3Q:p16-17. Aspiration pneumonia with growth of *Staphylococcus aureus.*
5. American Hospital Association. *Coding Clinic for ICD-9-CM* 1991:3Q:p19-20. Pleural effusion with congestive heart failure.
6. American Hospital Association. *Coding Clinic for ICD-9-CM* 1988:3Q:p3. Acute pulmonary edema of cardiac origin.
7. American Hospital Association. *Coding Clinic for ICD-9-CM* 1988:3Q:p3-4. Pulmonary edema.
8. American Hospital Association. *Coding Clinic for ICD-9-CM* 1992:2Q:p14. Mechanical ventilation during surgery and mechanical ventilation for extended period following surgery.
9. American Hospital Association. *Coding Clinic for ICD-9-CM* 2004:3Q:p11. Clarification—Postoperative mechanical ventilation.
10. American Hospital Association. *Coding Clinic for ICD-9-CM* 1991:4Q:p16-21. Mechanical ventilation—Guidelines.
11. American Hospital Association. *Coding Clinic for ICD-9-CM* 1990:2Q:p15-16. Abnormal findings—Reporting guidelines.

Chapter 14

1. American Hospital Association. *Coding Clinic for ICD-9-CM* 1984:July-Aug:p12. Benign and malignant hypertension—Guidelines.
2. American Hospital Association. *Coding Clinic for ICD-9-CM* 1990:3Q:p4. Blood pressure, elevated.
3. American Hospital Association. *Coding Clinic for ICD-9-CM* 2003:1Q:p20-21. Renal failure due to diabetic nephropathy in patient with hypertension.
4. American Hospital Association. *Coding Clinic for ICD-9-CM* 2001:2Q:p7-8. Aborted myocardial infarction.
5. American Hospital Association. *Coding Clinic for ICD-9-CM* 1997:3Q:p15. Clarification—Coronary artery disease of unspecified type of vessel.
6. American Hospital Association. *Coding Clinic for ICD-9-CM* 1990:2Q:p19. Congestive cardiomyopathy and CHF.
7. American Hospital Association. *Coding Clinic for ICD-9-CM* 1988:2Q:p8. Cardiac arrest.
8. From Frazier ME, Drzymkowski JW. Essentials of Human Diseases and Conditions, 3rd ed. St. Louis, Saunders, 2004, Table 10-1, pp 457-459.
9. American Hospital Association. *Coding Clinic for ICD-9-CM* 2002:4Q:p52-55. CHF due to diastolic dysfunction due to hypertension.
10. American Hospital Association. *Coding Clinic for ICD-9-CM* 2000:2Q:p16-17. Heart failure.
11. American Hospital Association. *Coding Clinic for ICD-9-CM* 1995:1Q:p6. Rheumatic congestive heart failure.
12. American Hospital Association. *Coding Clinic for ICD-9-CM* 1991:3Q:p19. Pleural effusion w/congestive heart failure.
13. American Hospital Association. *Coding Clinic for ICD-9-CM* 2007:1Q:p23-24. Aborted cerebrovascular accident (CVA).
14. American Hospital Association. *Coding Clinic for ICD-9-CM* 1995:2Q:p14. Clarification—Explanation of fifth digits for categories 433 and 434.
15. American Hospital Association. *Coding Clinic for ICD-9-CM* 2006:1Q:p17. Clarification—Bilateral carotid artery stenosis.
16. American Hospital Association. *Coding Clinic for ICD-9-CM* 1993:4Q:p27-28. Atherosclerotic peripheral vascular disease—Guidelines.
17. American Hospital Association. *Coding Clinic for ICD-9-CM* 1992:1Q:p15-16. Clarification—Thrombosis with thrombophlebitis.
18. American Hospital Association. *Coding Clinic for ICD-9-CM* 1997:3Q:p14. Clarification—Coronary artery bypass.
19. American Hospital Association. *Coding Clinic for ICD-9-CM* 1995:1Q:p5-6. Auxiliary procedures to heart surgery—Guidelines.
20. American Hospital Association. *Coding Clinic for ICD-9-CM* 2002:4Q:p100. Implantation of biventricular defribillator.
21. American Hospital Association. *Coding Clinic for ICD-9-CM* 1997:2Q:p13. Clarification—Unstable angina and coronary artery disease.
22. American Hospital Association. *Coding Clinic for ICD-9-CM* 2001:3Q:p15. Unstable angina status post CABG.
23. American Hospital Association. *Coding Clinic for ICD-9-CM* 1993:1Q:p25. Cocaine intoxication with chest pain.

Chapter 15

1. From Chabner D. The Language of Medicine, 7th ed. St. Louis, Saunders, 2004, Table 19-2, p 776.
2. From Chabner D. The Language of Medicine, 7th ed. St. Louis, Saunders, 2004, Table 19-3, p 777.
3. Modified from Harrison's Manual of Medicine, 15th ed. New York, McGraw-Hill Professional, 2002, p 284.
4. American Hospital Association. *Coding Clinic for ICD-9-CM* 1985:M-J:p9-12. Neoplasm coding—Guidelines.
5. American Hospital Association. *Coding Clinic for ICD-9-CM* 1992:2Q:p3-4. Lymphoma involvement in bone, metastatic vs primary.
6. American Hospital Association. *Coding Clinic for ICD-9-CM* 2006:1Q:p4. Correct coding of mass or lesion.
7. American Hospital Association. *Coding Clinic for ICD-9-CM* 1988:1Q:p4-5. Implantation or insertion of radioactive elements.
8. American Hospital Association. *Coding Clinic for ICD-9-CM* 1997:2Q:p3. Small bowel obstruction due to abdominal carcinomatosis.
9. American Hospital Association. *Coding Clinic for ICD-9-CM* 1995:4Q:p67-68. Chemoembolization with chemotherapy.

Chapter 16

1. American Hospital Association. *Coding Clinic for ICD-9-CM* 1992:1Q:p10-11. Second degree midline episiotomy.
2. American Hospital Association. *Coding Clinic for ICD-9-CM* 2007:4Q:p125. Obstetric periurethral laceration.

Chapter 17

1. American Hospital Association. *Coding Clinic for ICD-9-CM* 1996:1Q:p14. Revision of bilateral cleft lip and palate repair.
2. American Hospital Association. *Coding Clinic for ICD-9-CM* 1993:3Q:p11. Marfan syndrome in adult w/associated conditions.
3. American Hospital Association. *Coding Clinic for ICD-9-CM* 2005:4Q:p82-83. Noxious influences affecting fetus or newborn.
4. American Hospital Association. *Coding Clinic for ICD-9-CM* 1992:2Q:p12. Newborn delivered by cocaine abuser/dependent mother.
5. American Hospital Association. *Coding Clinic for ICD-9-CM* 1992:3Q:p8-9. ABO incompatibility w/negative Coombs' test.

Chapter 18

1. American Hospital Association. *Coding Clinic for ICD-9-CM* 1995:2Q:p5. Degenerative joint disease, bilateral.
2. American Hospital Association. *Coding Clinic for ICD-9-CM* 1997:2Q:p15. Clarification—Postlaminectomy syndrome.
3. American Hospital Association. *Coding Clinic for ICD-9-CM* 1997:3Q:p13. Hip prosthesis removal with total hip replacement.
4. American Hospital Association. *Coding Clinic for ICD-9-CM* 2002:2Q:p14-15. Vertebroplasty and stabilization of vertebral fracture.
5. American Hospital Association. *Coding Clinic for ICD-9-CM* 2003:2Q:p20. 360-Degree spinal fusion—Clarification.

Chapter 19

1. American Hospital Association. *Coding Clinic for ICD-9-CM* 1999:1Q:p5. Fracture site specified in radiology report.
2. American Hospital Association. *Coding Clinic for ICD-9-CM* 1990:3Q:p13. Fracture with dislocation.
3. American Hospital Association. *Coding Clinic for ICD-9-CM* 1997:Nov-Dec:p7. Recurrent shoulder dislocation.

4. From the American Association for the Surgery of Trauma, Chicago, Illinois.
5. American Hospital Association. *Coding Clinic for ICD-9-CM* 2003:4Q:p76-78. Crushing injury.
6. American Hospital Association. *Coding Clinic for ICD-9-CM* 1993:2Q:p7. Crush injury with open wound.
7. American Hospital Association. *Coding Clinic for ICD-9-CM* 1987:M-A:p1-5. Observation and evaluation for suspected conditions—Guidelines.

Chapter 20

1. American Hospital Association. *Coding Clinic for ICD-9-CM* 1997:1Q:p16. Correction—Dilantin toxicity.
2. American Hospital Association. *Coding Clinic for ICD-9-CM* 1993:1Q:p25. Cocaine intoxication with chest pain.
3. American Hospital Association. *Coding Clinic for ICD-9-CM* 1997:2Q:p12. Clarification—Unspecified adverse effect of drug.
4. American Hospital Association. *Coding Clinic for ICD-9-CM* 1996:4Q:p40-41. Sequencing of child abuse codes.
5. American Hospital Association. *Coding Clinic for ICD-9-CM* 1996:4Q:p41-42. Adult abuse coding.
6. American Hospital Association. *Coding Clinic for ICD-9-CM* 1999:1Q:p8-9. Extensive wound debridement.

Chapter 21

1. American Hospital Association. *Coding Clinic for ICD-9-CM* 1997:3Q:p8. Dislodged gastrostomy tube.
2. American Hospital Association. *Coding Clinic for ICD-9-CM* 1985:Nov-Dec:p15. Trauma resulting from patient pulling out urinary catheter.
3. American Hospital Association. *Coding Clinic for ICD-9-CM* 1997:3Q:p13. Hip prosthesis removal with total hip replacement.
4. American Hospital Association. *Coding Clinic for ICD-9-CM* 1998:3Q:p3. Complication of transplanted organs.
5. American Hospital Association. *Coding Clinic for ICD-9-CM* 1995:4Q:p82. Amputation stump complication.

Chapter 22

1. American Hospital Association. *Coding Clinic for ICD-9-CM* 1996:3Q:p9-10. Gastric arteriovenous malformation.
2. American Hospital Association. *Coding Clinic for ICD-9-CM* 1986:Nov-Dec:p11. Arteriovenous (A-V) malformation of colon.
3. American Hospital Association. *Coding Clinic for ICD-9-CM* 2005:3Q:p17-18. GI bleeding with multiple possible causes.
4. American Hospital Association. *Coding Clinic for ICD-9-CM* 1990:2Q:p26. Appendicitis, unqualified.
5. American Hospital Association. *Coding Clinic for ICD-9-CM* 1993:5th issue:p16. Dysphagia and dehydration due to CA with PEG feeding tube placement.
6. American Hospital Association. *Coding Clinic for ICD-9-CM* 1997:3Q:p8. Dislodged gastrostomy tube.
7. American Hospital Association. *Coding Clinic for ICD-9-CM* 1997:3Q:p9-10. Admission for colostomy closure.
8. American Hospital Association. *Coding Clinic for ICD-9-CM* 1990:4Q:p18-19. Lysis of adhesions—Guidelines.
9. American Hospital Association. *Coding Clinic for ICD-9-CM* 1984:July-Aug:p19-20. Dehydration due to gastroenteritis—Sequencing.
10. American Hospital Association. *Coding Clinic for ICD-9-CM* 1988:2Q:p10. Gastroenteritis with diarrhea and dehydration.

Chapter 23

1. Reprinted with permission from the Diagnostic and Statistical Manual of Mental Disorders, Fourth Edition, Text Revision (Copyright 2000). American Psychiatric Association.

2. American Hospital Association. *Coding Clinic for ICD-9-CM* 1991:2Q:p11-12. Psychoactive substance–induced organic mental syndromes.
3. American Hospital Association. *Coding Clinic for ICD-9-CM* 1991:2Q:p10. Dependence of drug.
4. American Hospital Association. *Coding Clinic for ICD-9-CM* 1986:M-A:p12. Polydrug addict.
5. American Hospital Association. *Coding Clinic for ICD-9-CM* 1991:2Q:p11. Fifth-digit classification for alcohol—Drugs.
6. American Hospital Association. *Coding Clinic for ICD-9-CM* 1999:3Q:p20. Drug seeking behavior.

Chapter 24

1. American Hospital Association. *Coding Clinic for ICD-9-CM* 1994:4Q:p36. Hemiplegia and quadriplegia.
2. American Hospital Association. *Coding Clinic for ICD-9-CM* 1985:Sept-Oct:p10. Senile vs unspecified cataract in elderly patients.
3. American Hospital Association. *Coding Clinic for ICD-9-CM* 1985:Sept-Oct:p11. Diabetic cataract.
4. American Hospital Association. *Coding Clinic for ICD-9-CM* 2000:1Q:p9-10. Anterior capsule following cataract extraction.
5. American Hospital Association. *Coding Clinic for ICD-9-CM* 1997:4Q:p57-58. Thalamic stimulation.
6. American Hospital Association. *Coding Clinic for ICD-9-CM* 1987:Sept-Oct:p10. Malfunctioning ventriculoperitoneal shunt.
7. American Hospital Association. *Coding Clinic for ICD-9-CM* 1991:2Q:p14. Placement of in-depth electrodes through burr holes into brain.
8. American Hospital Association. *Coding Clinic for ICD-9-CM* 1996:3Q:p12. Placement of vagal nerve stimulator via carotid sheath.
9. American Hospital Association. *Coding Clinic for ICD-9-CM* 1991:2Q:p17. Photodynamic therapy.

Chapter 25

1. American Hospital Association. *Coding Clinic for ICD-9-CM* 1991:2Q:p5-7. Cellulitis of skin.
2. American Hospital Association. *Coding Clinic for ICD-9-CM* 1991:2Q:p20. Stasis dermatitis in chronic venous insufficiency w/o varicose veins.
3. American Hospital Association. *Coding Clinic for ICD-9-CM* 1996:1Q:p15. Residual pressure sore with recurrent ischial sinus.
4. American Hospital Association. *Coding Clinic for ICD-9-CM* 1988:4Q:p5. Debridement of wound, excisional vs nonexcisional—Guidelines.
5. American Hospital Association. *Coding Clinic for ICD-9-CM* 1999:1Q:p8-9. Extensive wound debridement.

Chapter 26

1. American Hospital Association. *Coding Clinic for ICD-9-CM* 1984:M-J:p10. Follow-up for malignancy—Sequencing.
2. American Hospital Association. *Coding Clinic for ICD-9-CM* 2005:3Q:p21-22. Consistent with and compatible with.
3. American Hospital Association. *Coding Clinic for ICD-9-CM* 2000:1Q:p4. Radiologist diagnosis.
4. American Hospital Association. *Coding Clinic for ICD-9-CM* 2008:1stQ:p15. Reporting ICD-9-CM procedure codes for outpatient procedures.

Chapter 27

1. American Health Information Management Association (AHIMA). US Must Adopt ICD-9-CM and ICD-10-PCS: Immediate Action to Upgrade Medical Code Set StandardsNeeded (revised and approved July 21, 2005). Chicago, AHIMA, 2005. Available at: http://www.ahima.org/dc/positions/PS_icd10_0705.asp. Accessed April 4, 2008.
2. ICD-10: Capturing the Complexities of Health Care. Westchester, Ill, Healthcare Financial Management Association (HFMA), May 2004.
3. Prophet S. ICD-10 on the horizon. J AHIMA 2002;73:36-41.
4. Libicki M, Brahmakulam I. The Costs and Benefits of Moving to the ICD-10 Code Sets. Santa Monica, Calif, RAND Corporation, 2004, Table S.2, p xvi.
5. Libicki M, Brahmakulam I. The Costs and Benefits of Moving to the ICD-10 Code Sets. Santa Monica, Calif, RAND Corporation, 2004, Table S.1, p xiv.

General Resources

3M Corporation. ICD-10-CM and ICD-10 PCS: Frequently Asked Questions. St. Paul, Minn, 3M Corporation, 2004.

American Hospital Association (AHA) and American Health Information Management Association (AHIMA). ICD-10-CM Field Testing Project: Report on Findings: Perceptions, Ideas and Recommendations from Coding Professionals Across the Nation. Chicago, AHIMA, 2003.

Averill R, Mullin R, Steinbeck B, Goldfield N, Grant T, Butler R. Development of the ICD-10 Procedure Coding System (ICD-10-PCS): 3M Research Report. St. Paul, Minn, 3M Corporation, 2004.

Grant T, Powell S, Steinbeck B. Preparing for ICD-10-PCS. For the Record 2002;14(25).

ICD-10: Capturing the Complexities of Health Care. Westchester, Ill, Healthcare Financial Management Association, May 2004.

Liebicki M, Brahmakulam I. The Costs and Benefits of Moving to the ICD-10 Code Sets. Santa Monica, Calif, RAND Corporation, 2004.

Practice Brief Destination 10: Healthcare Organization Preparation for ICD-10-CM and ICD-10-PCS. J AHIMA 2004;March:56A-56D.

Prophet S. ICD-10 on the horizon. J AHIMA 2002;73:36-41.

Abbreviations

A&P anatomy and physiology
AAPC American Academy of Professional Coders
ABG arterial blood gas
ACS acute coronary syndrome
ADD attention deficit disorder
ADHD attention deficit hyperactivity disorder
AF atrial fibrillation
AGA appropriate for gestational age
AHA American Hospital Association
AHFS American Hospital Formulary Service
AHIMA American Health Information Management Association
AHQA American Health Quality Association
AICD automatic implantable cardioverter-defibrillator
AIDS acquired immunodeficiency syndrome
AKA above-knee amputation
ALL acute lymphocytic leukemia
ALOS average length of stay
AMA American Medical Association
AMI acute myocardial infarction
APC Ambulatory Payment Classification
ARF acute renal failure
ARI acute renal insufficiency
AROM artificial rupture of membranes
ASA aspirin
ASCUS atypical squamous cells of undetermined significance
ATV all-terrain vehicle
AV arteriovenous
AV atrioventricular
AVM arteriovenous malformation
AVR aortic valve replacement
BAL bronchoalveolar lavage
BMI body mass index
BMR biological response modifier
BMT bone marrow transplant
BNP brain natriuretic peptide
BP blood pressure
BPD biliopancreatic diversion
BPD bronchopulmonary dysplasia
BPH benign prostatic hypertrophy
BUN blood urea nitrogen
C. diff *Clostridium difficile*
CAB coronary artery bypass
CABG coronary artery bypass graft
CAD coronary artery disease
CAP community-acquired pneumonia
CAPD continuous ambulatory peritoneal dialysis
CAT computerized axial tomography
CBC complete blood count
CC chief complaint
CC complication/comorbidity
CCA Certified Coding Associate
CCF cystic fibrosis
CCPD continuous cycling peritoneal dialysis
CCS Certified Coding Specialist
CCS-P Certified Coding Specialist—Physician Based
CCU coronary care unit
CD4 Cluster of differentiation 4
CDC Centers for Disease Control and Prevention
CDIP Clinical Documentation Improvement Program
CEA cultured epidermal autograft
CEUs continuing education units
CF cystic fibrosis
CHD congenital heart disease
CHF congestive heart failure
CHI closed head injury
CKD chronic kidney disease
CLL chronic lymphocytic leukemia
CM clinical modification
CMI case mix index
CML chronic myelogenous leukemia
CMS Centers for Medicare and Medicaid Services
CNS central nervous system
COPD chronic obstructive pulmonary disease
CPAP continuous positive airway pressure
CPC Certified Professional Coder
CPC-H Certified Professional Coder—Hospital Based
CPD cephalopelvic disproportion
CPK creatine phosphokinase
CPK-MB creatine phosphokinase, isoenzyme MB
CPT *Current Procedural Terminology*
CRF chronic renal failure
CRI chronic renal insufficiency
CRT cardiac resynchronization therapy
CRT-D cardiac resynchronization treatment defibrillator
CRT-P cardiac resynchronization treatment pacemaker
CSF cerebrospinal fluid
CT computerized tomography
CVA cerebrovascular accident
CVL central venous line
CXR chest x-ray
D&C dilatation and curettage
DBS deep brain stimulation
DCIS ductal carcinoma in situ
DES drug-eluting stent
DEXA dual-energy x-ray absorptiometry (bone density)
DHHS U.S. Department of Health and Human Services
DI diabetes insipidus

DIC disseminated intravascular coagulation
DJD degenerative joint disease
DOE dyspnea on exertion
DM diabetes mellitus
DMAC disseminated *Mycobacterium avium-intracellulare* complex
DOB date of birth
DRG diagnosis-related group
DS discharge summary
DSM-IV-TR *Diagnostic and Statistical Manual of Mental Disorders, Fourth Edition, Text Revision*
DTs delirium tremens
DVT deep vein thrombosis
E. coli *Escherichia coli*
ECMO extracorporeal membrane oxygenation
ECT electroconvulsive therapy
ED emergency department
EDC estimated date of confinement
EEG electroencephalogram
EGD esophogastroduodenoscopy
EKG/ECG electrocardiogram
EMG electromyelogram
EMS emergency medical services
EP electrophysiologic
ER Emergency Room
ERCP endoscopic retrograde cholangiopancreatography
ESRD end-stage renal disease
ESWL extracorporeal shock wave lithotripsy
FB foreign body
FNA fine needle aspiration
FSG focal segmental glomerulosclerosis
FTSG full-thickness skin graft
FUO fever of unknown origin
GERD gastroesophageal reflux disease
GFR glomerular filtration rate
GI gastrointestinal
GMLOS geometric length of stay
GN glomerulonephritis
GPO Government Printing Office
H. flu *Haemophilus influenzae*
H&P history and physical
HAART highly active antiretroviral therapy
HBOT hyperbaric oxygen therapy
HCC hepatocellular carcinoma
hCG human chorionic gonadotropin
HCPCS Healthcare Common Procedure Coding System
Hct hematocrit
HCVD hypertensive cardiovascular disease
Hgb hemoglobin
hGH human growth hormone
HGSIL high-grade squamous intraepithelial lesion
HH home health
HIPAA Health Insurance Portability and Accountability Act
HIV human immunodeficiency virus
HIVAN HIV-associated nephropathy
HMO Health Maintenance Organization
HPI history of present illness
HPR hospital payment rate
HPV human papillomavirus
HSV herpes simplex virus
HTN hypertension
I&D incision and drainage
ICD internal cardiac defibrillator
ICD *International Classification of Diseases*
ICD-9-CM *International Classification of Diseases, Ninth Revision, Clinical Modification*
ICD-O *International Classification of Diseases for Oncology*
ICU intensive care unit
ICV implantable cardioverter
IDDM insulin-dependent diabetes mellitus
Ig immunoglobulin
IOL induction of labor
IOL intraocular lens
IOP intraocular pressure
IPPS Inpatient Prospective Payment System
IQ intelligence quotient
IS information systems
ITP idiopathic thrombocytopenic purpura
IUD intrauterine device
IUGR intrauterine growth retardation
IV intravenous
IVDU intravenous drug use
JRA juvenile rheumatoid arthritis
LAD left anterior descending
LAVH laparoscopically assisted vaginal hysterectomy
LCA left coronary artery
LD learning disability/difficulty
LDMF latissimus dorsi musculocutaneous flap
LGA large for gestational age
LGIB lower gastrointestinal bleed
LLL lower left lobe
LOC loss of consciousness
LOS length of stay
LP lumbar puncture
LTC long-term care
LTCS low transverse cesarean section
LUTS lower urinary tract symptoms
MAC *Mycobacterium avium-intracellulare* complex
MAI *Mycobacterium avium-intracellulare*
MAO monoamine oxidase
MAR medication administration record
MCE Medicare Code Editor
MDC major diagnostic category
MEN multiple endocrine neoplasia
MI myocardial infarction
MR mental retardation
MRA magnetic resonance angiography
MRCP mental retardation, cerebral palsy
MRI magnetic resonance imaging
MRSA methicillin-resistant *Staphylococcus aureus*
MSAFP maternal serum alpha-fetoprotein
MS-DRG Medicare severity diagnosis-related group
MSSA methicillin-sensitive *Staphylococcus aureus*
MUGA multiple-gated acquisition
MVA motor vehicle accident
MVP mitral valve prolapse
MVR mitral valve replacement
NCHS National Center for Health Statistics
NCVHS National Committee on Vital and Health Statistics
NEC not elsewhere classifiable
NHL non-Hodgkin's lymphoma
NICU neonatal intensive care unit
NKF National Kidney Foundation

NIDDM non–insulin-dependent diabetes mellitus
NOS not otherwise specified
NPH normal pressure hydrocephalus
NPI National Provider Identifier
NQMI non–Q wave myocardial infarction
NSAIDs nonsteroidal anti-inflammatory drugs
NSCLC non–small cell lung cancer
NST nonstress test
NSTEMI non–ST elevation myocardial infarction
O_2 oxygen
OA osteoarthritis
OB obstetrics
OBS organic brain syndrome
OIG Office of the Inspector General
OM obtuse marginal
OM otitis media
OP note operative note
OPPS Outpatient Prospective Payment System
OR operating room
ORIF open reduction with internal fixation
OSA obstructive sleep apnea
$Paco_2$ partial pressure of carbon dioxide in arterial blood
Pao_2 partial pressure of oxygen in arterial blood
PCI percutaneous coronary intervention
PCP *Pneumocystis carinii* pneumonia
PCP primary care provider
PCS Procedure Classification System
PDA patent ductus arteriosus
PDA posterior descending artery
PDT photodynamic therapy
PE pulmonary embolism
PEG percutaneous endoscopic gastrostomy
PEPPER Program for Evaluating Payment Patterns Electronic Report
PHT pulmonary hypertension
PICC peripherally inserted central catheter
PID pelvic inflammatory disease
PIH pregnancy-induced hypertension
PKU phenylketonuria
PMR polymyalgia rheumatica
POCs products of conception
PPH primary pulmonary hypertension
PPO Preferred Provider Organization
PPS Prospective Payment System
PROM premature rupture of membranes
PSA prostate-specific antigen
PT prothrombin time
PTA prior to admission
PTCA percutaneous transluminal coronary angioplasty
PTL preterm labor
PTMR percutaneous transmyocardial revascularization
PTSD posttraumatic stress disorder
PTT partial thromboplastin time
PUD peptic ulcer disease
PV percutaneous vertebroplasty
QIO Quality Improvement Organization
RA rheumatoid arthritis
RA right atrium
RAD reactive airway disease
RBBB right bundle branch block
RCA right coronary artery
RCC renal cell carcinoma
RDS respiratory distress syndrome
RFA radiofrequency ablation
RHD rheumatic heart disease
RHIA Registered Health Information Administrator
RHIT Registered Health Information Technician
RPGN rapidly progressive glomerulonephritis
RPR rapid plasma reagin
RPS retrospective payment system
RSV respiratory syncytial virus
RUL right upper lobe
RW relative weight
SARS severe acute respiratory syndrome
SCI spinal cord injury
SCID severe combined immunodeficiency
SCLC small cell lung cancer
SGA small for gestational age
SIADH syndrome of inappropriate antidiuretic hormone secretion
SIDS sudden infant death syndrome
SIRS systemic inflammatory response syndrome
SLAP superior labrum anterior-posterior
SLE systemic lupus erythematosus
SNF skilled nursing facility
SNOMED Systematized Nomenclature of Medicine
SOAP Subjective/Objective/Assessment/Plan
SOB shortness of breath
SOM serous otitis media
SOW scope of work
SSS sick sinus syndrome
Staph aureus *Staphylococcus aureus*
STD sexually transmitted disease
STEMI ST elevation myocardial infarction
STSG split-thickness skin graft
SVD spontaneous vaginal delivery
SVT supraventricular tachycardia
SZ seizure
TB tuberculosis
TBI traumatic brain injury
TEFRA Tax Equity and Fiscal Responsibility Act
THR total hip replacement
TIA transient ischemic attack
TIPS transjugular intrahepatic portosystemic shunt
TJC The Joint Commission
TOF tetralogy of Fallot
TPA tissue plasminogen activator
TPN total parenteral nutrition
TPR temperature, pulse, and respiration
TRAM transverse rectus abdominis musculocutaneous
TSH thyroid-stimulating hormone
TTN transitory tachypnea of the newborn
TULIP transurethral ultrasound-guided laser-induced prostatectomy
TUMT transurethral microwave thermotherapy
TUNA transurethral needle ablation of the prostate
TURP transurethral resection of the prostate
UB-04 Uniform Bill-04
UGIB upper gastrointestinal bleed
UHDDS Uniform Hospital Discharge Data Set
UPIN Unique Physician Identification Number
USA unstable angina
UTI urinary tract infection
VAD vascular access device

VATS video-assisted thoracic surgery
VBAC vaginal birth after cesarean section
VBG vertical banded gastroplasty
VDRL Venereal Disease Research Laboratory
VLAP visual laser ablation of the prostate
VPS ventriculoperitoneal shunt
VRE vancomycin-resistant *Enterococcus*
VSD ventral septal defect
VSD ventricular septal defect
WBC white blood cell
WHO World Health Organization

Glossary

Ablation Correction of abnormal heart rhythm by burning of abnormal heart tissue through radiofrequency or other methods such as laser, microwave, or freezing.

Abortion Termination of a pregnancy by natural causes or by medical intervention.

Acromegaly Condition that results when hypersecretion of human growth hormone (hGH) occurs after puberty, along with overgrowth of the face, hands, feet, and soft tissues.

Acute A short and relatively severe course.

Acute renal failure Sudden and severe impairment of renal function characterized by oliguria, increased serum urea, and acidosis.

Addison's disease Adrenocortical insufficiency that may be caused by neoplasms, surgical removal of the adrenal gland, autoimmune processes, tuberculosis, hemorrhage, and/or infection.

Adenocarcinomas Malignancies of epithelial glandular tissue such as those found in the breast, prostate, and colon.

Adhesion Scar tissue that forms an abnormal connection between body parts.

Adjunct codes Add-on codes to a primary procedure to provide additional information about the primary procedure that was performed.

Admission diagnosis Diagnosis that brings the patient to the hospital. This will often be a symptom.

Adverse effect Pathologic manifestation due to ingestion or exposure to drugs or other chemical substances.

Affective disorders A category of mental health problems that includes major depressive disorders and bipolar disorders.

AIDS Incurable disease of the immune system caused by a virus.

Air embolism When air or gas bubbles get into the bloodstream and can obstruct the circulation.

Alimentary canal Comprises the mouth, pharynx, esophagus, stomach, small intestine, and large intestine.

Allograft Graft of tissue between individuals of the same species.

Alphabetic Index The index found in the ICD-9-CM book for both disease conditions and procedures.

Alzheimer's Disorder of the brain that causes a progressive decline in mental and physical function.

Ambulatory Payment Classifications (APCs) Used for outpatient prospective payment.

Amnioinfusion The insertion of normal saline or lactated Ringer's solution into the amniotic sac.

Anastomosis Surgically formed connection between two tubular structures.

Ancillary services Services provided by a hospital that are additional to a professional service, such as laboratory work and radiology and pathology services.

Anemia Occurs when hemoglobin drops, which interrupts the transport of oxygen throughout the body.

Aneurysm Bulging or ballooning out of a vessel.

Angiodysplasia Type of AVM characterized by dilated or fragile blood vessels.

Angioplasty A procedure performed to treat coronary artery disease. An inflated balloon compresses plaque against artery walls.

Anomaly A deviation from normal standards (e.g., as in congenital defects).

Anorexia Loss of appetite.

Antepartum Time from conception until delivery or childbirth with regard to the mother.

Anterior Front of the body or an organ.

Anthrax Bacterial infection usually found in wild or domestic animals.

Anticoagulant medications Medications that are used to prevent venous thrombi.

Antiplatelet medications Medications that are used to prevent clumping of platelets or formation of an arterial thrombus.

Apgar Test used to measure the condition of a newborn at birth.

Aphasia Impairment of speech expression and/or word understanding.

Apheresis Procedure that separates different components of blood and removes a certain part of the blood, such as occurs in leukapheresis, plateletpheresis, and plasmapheresis.

Aplastic anemia Reduction in red blood cells due to impairment or failure of bone marrow function.

Appendectomy Removal of the appendix.

Appendicitis Inflammation of the appendix.

Arteriovenous malformation Defect that arises during fetal development.

Arthropathy Disease that affects the joints.

Arthroscopic Minimally invasive surgery that involves the use of highly specialized instruments to perform surgery on joints through very small incisions.

Arthroscopic approach An arthroscope is used to examine and perform closed procedures within a joint.

Asbestosis Lung disease due to inhalation of asbestos.

Aspiration pneumonia Inflammation of the lungs and bronchial tubes due to aspiration of foreign material into the lung.

Asthma Chronic disease that affects the airways that carry air into and out of the lungs.

Asthmatic bronchitis Underlying asthmatic problem in patients in whom asthma has become so persistent that clinically significant chronic airflow obstruction is present despite antiasthmatic therapy.

Asymptomatic Without any symptoms.

Atherosclerosis Type of arteriosclerosis wherein fatty substances such as plaque block or clog the arteries.

Atrophy When a gland becomes smaller.

Autograft Graft of tissue from another site on the same individual.

Autoimmune disorder Disorder that occurs when the immune system attacks itself inappropriately.

Autologous transfusion Transfusion of a patient's own blood. Blood may have been donated before an elective procedure.

Autonomic nervous system Consists of both sensory and motor functions that involve the central nervous system and internal organs.

Bacteremia Bacteria in blood.

Bariatrics Branch of medicine that is concerned with the management (prevention or control) of obesity and allied diseases.

Baritosis Lung disease due to inhalation of barium.

Barrett's esophagus Precancerous condition that usually occurs in people with chronic GERD.

Benign Neoplasm or tumor; means that it is not malignant.

Benign prostatic hyperplasia Condition resulting in enlargement of the prostate gland; usually occurs in men older than 50 years of age.

Benign prostatic hypertrophy Condition resulting in enlargement of the prostate gland: usually occurs in men older than 50 years of age.

Bilateral procedure Operative procedure performed on paired anatomic organs or tissues during the same operative session.

Biological response modifiers (BRM) Immunotherapy that can destroy cancer cells, stimulate the immune system to destroy cancer cells, or change cancer cells to normal cells.

Biopsy Removal of a representative sample for pathologic examination and diagnosis.

Bipolar disorder Brain disorder that causes unusual shifts in a person's mood, energy, and ability to function. Different from the normal ups and downs that everyone goes through, the symptoms of bipolar disorder are severe.

Black lung Lung disease due to inhalation of coal dust.

Blalock-Taussig operation Procedure used to treat patients with tetralogy of Fallot who have insufficient pulmonary arterial flow.

Blood Viscous fluid that circulates through the vessels of the circulatory system as a result of the pumping action of the heart.

Blood pressure The force that blood puts on the arterial walls when the heart beats.

BNP A hormone that is produced by the heart. If a patient is suspected of being in CHF, a test is done to determine the level of BNP.

Body mass index Uses weight and height to estimate body fat.

Bone marrow biopsy Diagnostic procedure that is used to identify types of anemia and cell deficiencies, and to detect leukemia.

Bowel resection Removal of a portion of the bowel.

Brachytherapy Placement of radioactive material directly into or near the cancer.

Bradycardia Slow heart rate, generally fewer than 60 beats per minute.

Bronchi The two air tubes that branch off the trachea and deliver air to both lungs.

Bronchitis Lower respiratory tract or bronchial tree infection characterized by cough, sputum production, and wheezing.

Bronchoscopy Diagnostic endoscopic procedure in which a tube with a tiny camera on the end is inserted through the nose or mouth into the lungs.

Bursitis Inflammation of a bursa, which is a tiny, fluid-filled sac that is found between muscles, tendons, and bones that reduces friction and facilitates movement.

Calculus A stone. Calculi, which vary in size, can develop anywhere in the urinary tract.

Candidiasis Fungal infection also known as a *yeast infection*.

Capillaries Smallest blood vessel through which material passes to and from the bloodstream.

Carbuncle Cluster of boils.

Carcinoma in situ Malignant cells that remain within the original site with no spread or invasion into neighboring tissue.

Carcinomas Malignant tumors originating from epithelial tissue (e.g., in the skin, bronchi, and stomach).

Cardiomyopathy A disorder of the muscles of the heart chambers that impedes heart function.

Carryover line Used when an entry will not fit on a single line.

Case-mix index A measurement used by hospitals to define how sick their patients are.

Cataract Clouding of the lens of the eye causing obstructed vision.

Category A single three-digit code that describes a disease or a similarly related group of conditions.

Caudal Toward the tail.

Cellulitis Inflammation of the tissue with possible abscess.

Cervix The neck of the uterus that serves as an outlet from the uterus.

Chancre An ulcer that forms during the first stage of syphilis.

Chemoembolization Intra-arterial administration of chemotherapy with collagen particles to enhance the delivery of chemotherapy to the targeted area.

Chemotherapy Use of drugs or medications to treat disease.

Chief complaint The reason in the patient's own words for presenting to the hospital.

Choledocholithiasis Stone lodged in the bile duct.

Cholelithiasis An abnormal condition of stones in the gallbladder.

Cholesteatoma Growth in the middle ear that usually results from repeated ear infections.

Chronic Persistent over a long period.

Chronic bronchitis Condition defined by a mucus-producing cough most days of the month, 3 months out of a year for 2 successive years, with no other underlying disease to explain the cough.

Chronic obstructive pulmonary disease General term used to describe a lung disease in which the airways become obstructed, making it difficult for air to get into and out of the lungs.

Chylothorax Milky fluid consisting of lymph and fat (chyle) that accumulates in the pleural space.

Cirrhosis Liver disease wherein scar tissue replaces healthy tissue and blocks blood flow.

Classification Grouping together of items as for storage and retrieval.

Cleft lip/palate Opening in the lip or palate of an infant that occurs in utero.

Closed fracture Injury in which the bone is broken, but the skin remains intact.

Closed head injuries Injuries that result from a blow to the head.

Closed reduction of a fracture The surgeon manipulates or reduces fractured bones into anatomic alignment without making an incision through the skin and subcutaneous tissue.

Clostridium difficile Microorganisms that are a leading cause of pseudomembranous cells; also known as *C. diff.*

Coagulation defect Breakdown in the clotting process of the blood.

Coal workers' pneumoconiosis Lung disease due to inhalation of coal dust.

Cognitive defect Disorder in thinking, learning, awareness, or judgment.

Cognitive impairment Decline in mental activities associated with thinking, learning, and memory.

Colles' fracture Common fracture in adults in which the lower end of the radius is fractured and the wrist and hand are displaced backward.

Colostomy A procedure that uses the colon to create an artificial opening.

Combination code A single code used to classify two diagnoses; or a diagnosis with an associated secondary process (manifestation); or a diagnosis with an associated complication.

Communicable Easily spread from one person to another.

Community-acquired pneumonia Broad term used to define pneumonias that are contracted outside of the hospital or nursing home setting.

Comorbidities Preexisting diagnoses or conditions that are present on admission.

Comorbidity A preexisting condition (it is present on admission) which may lead to increased resource use.

Complete abortion Abortion in which all the products of conception are expelled.

Complete remission There are no signs or symptoms of the cancer.

Compliance Adherence to accepted standards.

Complicated fracture Fracture that causes injury to surrounding tissues.

Complication A condition that arises during a patient's hospitalization which may lead to increased resource use.

Concussion Injury to the brain that results from a significant blow to the head.

Conduction disorder Abnormalities of cardiac impulses.

Congenital Condition present at birth, regardless of causation.

Condyloma Wart-type growth found usually in the genital or anal area.

Connecting words Subterms that denote a relationship between a main term or a subterm and an associated condition or etiology.

Consultant Healthcare provider who is asked to see the patient to provide expert opinion outside the expertise of the requestor.

Contaminant A cultured organism that a physician does not believe is responsible for causing a particular infection.

Continuous ambulatory peritoneal dialysis Type of peritoneal dialysis that takes about 15 minutes and is performed 3 to 4 times per day and once at night.

Continuous cycling peritoneal dialysis Type of peritoneal dialysis that uses a cycling machine and is performed while the patient sleeps.

Contusion Any mechanical injury that results in hemorrhage beneath unbroken skin.

Conventions General rules for use in classification that must be followed for accurate coding.

Coronary artery bypass graft Surgery performed to bypass an occluded coronary artery.

Core biopsy Procedure in which a large needle is used to extract a core sample.

Cranial Toward the head.

Credential Degree, certificate, or award that recognizes a course of study taken in a specific field and that acknowledges the competency required.

Crohn's disease Inflammation of the GI tract, especially the small and large intestine.

Crush injury When a body part is subjected to a high degree of force or pressure, usually after it has been squeezed between two heavy or immobile objects.

Cushing's syndrome Condition that results in excessive circulating cortisol levels caused by chronic hypersecretion of the adrenal cortex.

Current Procedural Terminology (CPT) A coding system for reporting medical services and procedures.

Cystic fibrosis Genetic (inherited) condition that affects the cells that produce mucus, sweat, saliva, and digestive juices. Instead of being thin and slippery, these secretions are thick and sticky, plugging up tubes, ducts, and passageways, especially in the pancreas and lungs.

Cystitis Lower urinary tract infection that affects the bladder.

Cystocele When the bladder descends and presses into the wall of the vagina.

Cystoscopy Approach used for many procedures of the urinary tract.

Cystourethrocele A urethrocele in conjunction with a cystocele.

Debridement Removal of devitalized tissue, necrosis, or slough.

Debulking Procedures performed when it is impossible to remove the tumor entirely.

Decubitus ulcer Skin ulcer also known as a bed sore.

Deep brain stimulation Procedure used to control tremors.

Deep vein thrombosis A blood clot that forms in a deep vein.

Deficit Reduction Act Mandates all acute-care facilities reimbursed under MS-DRGs to identify and report diagnoses that are present at the time of a patient's admission.

Dehiscence Opening of a surgical wound.

Delirium tremens Life-threatening condition that may involve severe mental or neurologic changes such as delirium and/or hallucinations.

Dementia Progressive deterioration of mental faculties characterized by impaired memory and one or more cognitive impairments such as language, reasoning and judgment, or calculation and problem-solving ability.

Depression Affective disorder that is characterized by sadness, lack of interest in everyday activities and events, and a sense of worthlessness.

Dermabond Liquid skin adhesive used to close skin lacerations.

Dermatitis Inflammation of the skin.

Dermis Layer of skin below the epidermis.

Detoxification Active management of withdrawal symptoms in a patient who is physically dependent on alcohol or drugs.

Diabetes insipidus Deficiency in the release of vasopressin by the posterior pituitary gland.

Diabetes mellitus Chronic syndrome of impaired carbohydrate, protein, and fat metabolism caused by insufficient production of insulin by the pancreas or faulty utilization of insulin by the cells.

Diagnosis Identification of a disease through signs, symptoms, and tests.

Dialysis disequilibrium syndrome Characterized by weakness, dizziness, headache, and in severe cases mental status changes.

Diaphragm Dome-shaped muscles at the bottom of the lungs that assist in the process of breathing and in the exchange of oxygen/carbon dioxide.

Differential diagnosis When a symptom may represent a variety of diagnoses.

Discharge summary A review of the patient's hospital course. This summary details the reason for admission or tests or procedures performed and how the patient responded.

Dislocation Displacement of the bones that form a joint; separation of the end of a bone from the joint it meets.

Disposition Place to which a patient goes when leaving the hospital (e.g., home, nursing home, assisted living).

Dissection A tear in wall of a vessel.

Disseminated intravascular coagulation Disorder that results in depletion of clotting factors in the blood.

Distal Farther from the median plane; term is often used to describe a location in the limbs.

Diverticula Small pouches in the lining of the mucous membranes of an organ.

Documentation Written or typed information supplied by healthcare providers to record and communicate patient data and activity.

Dorsal Back of the body or an organ.

Dorsopathies Conditions or diseases that affect the back or spine.

Dumping syndrome Occurs when undigested contents of the stomach are transported to the small intestine too quickly.

Dyscalculia Learning disability that affects a child's ability to do mathematical calculations.

Dysgraphia Learning disability that affects a child's ability to coordinate movements such as writing.

Dyslexia Learning disability that affects a child's ability to understand or use spoken or written language.

Eclampsia Complication of pregnancy characterized by hypertension, edema, proteinuria, and convulsions or seizures.

Ectopic Occurs when the egg is implanted outside the cavity of the uterus.

Eczema Type of dermatitis characterized by itching.

Edentulism The complete loss of teeth.

Elderly obstetric patient 35 years or older at date of delivery.

Elective abortion Elective termination of pregnancy.

Electroconvulsive therapy Psychiatric treatment in which electricity is used to induce seizures.

Electromyelogram Test that measures electrical activity in muscles and nerves.

Electrophysiologist Cardiologist trained to perform interventional cardiac electrophysiologic procedures and surgical device implantations.

Emphysema Chronic lung disease of gradual onset that can be attributed to chronic infection and inflammation or irritation from cigarette smoke.

Empiric Initiation of treatment prior to making a definite diagnosis.

Empyema Pus that accumulates in the pleural space.

Encoder Coding software that is used to assign diagnosis and procedure codes.

Encounter Face-to-face visit with a healthcare provider.

Endocarditis Inflammation of the lining of the heart chambers and valves.

Endocrine system Body system composed of many glands that secrete hormones that regulate bodily functions; it works with the nervous system to maintain body activities and homeostasis and to respond to stress.

Endogenous Type of dermatitis caused by something taken internally, such as medication.

Endometriosis A chronic condition in which endometrial material, the tissue that lines the inside of the uterus, grows outside the uterus and attaches to other organs in the pelvic cavity.

Endometritis Inflammation of the uterus.

Endoscopic Examinations and procedures performed with an instrument that examines any cavity of the body with a rigid or flexible scope.

Epidermis Outermost layer of skin.

Epilepsy Disorder of the brain that is characterized by abnormal electrical discharges from the brain cells.

Eponym Term for a disease, structure, procedure or syndrome that has been named for a person.

Erythema Redness of the skin.

Erythrocytes Another name for red blood cells that are made in the marrow of bones; their main responsibility is to carry oxygen around the body and remove carbon dioxide. These are the cells that give blood its red color.

Ethics Moral standard.

Etiology Cause or origin of a disease or condition.

Excisional Removal by surgical cutting.

Excisional biopsy Total removal of local small masses or growths.

Excisional debridement Surgical removal or cutting away of devitalized tissue, necrosis, or slough.

Exhibitionism Recurrent intense sexual urges and fantasies of exposing the genitals to an unsuspecting stranger.

Exogenous Type of dermatitis caused by contact with a substance.

Exophthalmos Bulging of the eyes.

External skeletal fixation Form of fracture treatment that involves insertion of percutaneous pins proximal and distal to the fracture and application of a frame that connects the pins externally.

Extracorporeal shock wave lithotripsy Used to break up kidney stones into small particles that can then pass through the urinary tract into the urine.

Facet joints Small, stabilizing joints located between and behind adjacent vertebrae.

Fallopian tube Delivers the mature egg to the uterus for fertilization.

Fascia Tissue just below the skin that covers and separates the underlying layers of muscle.

Fat embolism syndrome Condition that can occur after long bone or pelvic fracture. It usually presents 12 to 48 hours after injury with tachycardia, tachypnea, elevated temperature, hypoxemia, hypocapnia, thrombocytopenia, and occasionally, mild neurologic symptoms.

Federal Register The official daily publication for rules, proposed rules, and notices of U.S. federal agencies and organizations.

Fetishism Recurrent intense sexual urges and fantasies of using inanimate objects for sexual arousal or orgasm. Objects commonly used include female clothing such as shoes, earrings, or undergarments.

Fibromas Neoplasms of fibrous connective tissue.

Fibromyalgia One of the most common diseases affecting the muscles; it is characterized by widespread muscle pain associated with chronic fatigue.

Fine needle aspiration Procedure in which a very small needle is used; works best for masses that are superficial or easily accessible.

Fistula Abnormal passage or communication between two internal organs, or leading from an organ to the surface of the body. It can also be an abnormal passage between an artery and a vein.

Fracture Break in a bone.

Free flap Involves the cutting of skin, fat, blood vessels, and muscle free from its location and moving it to the chest area.

Fundoplication Surgery in which the fundus of the stomach is wrapped around the esophagus.

Furuncle A boil.

Gangrene Dead tissue usually associated with loss of vascular supply.

Gastroenteritis Inflammation of the stomach and intestines.

Generalized anxiety disorder Chronic, exaggerated worry, tension, and irritability that may occur without cause or that are more intense than the situation warrants.

Genetic Inherited.

Genital prolapse When pelvic organs such as the uterus, bladder, and rectum shift from their normal anatomic positions and protrude into the vagina or press against the wall of the vagina.

Gigantism Condition that occurs when hypersecretion of hGH occurs before puberty, along with proportionate overgrowth of all bodily tissues, especially the long bones.

Glaucoma Disorder of the optic nerve that may result in vision loss.

Glomerulonephritis Inflammation of the glomeruli of the kidneys.

Goiter Enlargement of the thyroid gland.

Gonorrhea Disease caused by a bacterium and transmitted by sexual contact.

Grading Pathologic examination of tumor cells. Degree of cell abnormality determines the grade of cancer.

Granulation Newly formed tissue that covers an open sore or a wound.

Graves' disease The most common form of hyperthyroidism; it occurs through an autoimmune response that attacks the thyroid gland, resulting in overproduction of the thyroid hormone thyroxine.

Gravid Pregnant.

Grouper Specialized software used to assign the appropriate MS-DRG.

Hashimoto's disease Inflammation of the thyroid gland that often results in hypothyroidism.

Healthcare provider Person who provides care to a patient.

Health Maintenance Organizations (HMOs) Type of managed care in which hospitals, physicians, and other providers contract to provide health care for patients, usually at a discounted rate.

Heart failure Impaired function of the heart's pumping ability.

Hematochezia Bright red blood in stool.

Hematopoiesis Development of blood cells that occurs in the bone marrow and lymphatic tissue of normal adults.

Hematemesis Vomiting of blood.

Hematuria The presence of blood in the urine.

Hemiplegia Paralysis of half of the body.

Hemodialysis Process that uses a machine called a hemodialyzer to remove wastes from the blood.

Hemolysis The breaking down of red blood cells.

Hemolytic anemias Result from abnormal or excessive destruction of red blood cells.

Hemophilia A Most common type of hemophilia; deficiency or abnormality in clotting factor VIII.

Hemophilia B Another name for Christmas disease, which is results from a deficiency of factor IX.

Hemophilia C Mild form of hemophilia with decreased factor XI.

Hemothorax Blood that accumulates in the pleural space.

Hepatitis An inflammation of the liver that has a variety of causes.

Hernia Protrusion of an organ or tissue through an abnormal opening in the body.

Herniorrhaphy Repair of a hernia.

Herpes simplex A virus also known as a *cold sore* or *fever blister*.

Herpes zoster A disease caused by the same virus that causes chickenpox.

Heterograft Graft of skin from another species, such as a graft from a pig to a human.

Histologic type Type of tissue or cell in which the neoplasm occurs.

Hives Skin condition also known as urticaria, wherein the skin reacts with welts; characterized by itching.

Homeostasis The ability of an organism or cell to maintain internal equilibrium by adjusting its physiologic processes.

Homograft Graft from one individual to another of the same species; also known as an allograft.

Hormones Substances secreted by glands that can regulate bodily functions, such as urinary output, cellular metabolic rate, and growth and development.

Hybrid A combination of formats producing similar results (i.e., paper and electronic records).

Hydrocephalus Cerebrospinal fluid collection in the skull.

Hydronephrosis Abnormal dilatation of the renal pelvis caused by pressure from urine that cannot flow past an obstruction in the urinary tract.

Hydroureter Accumulation of urine in the ureters.

Hyperbaric oxygen therapy (HBOT) Treatment in which the patient's entire body is placed in a transparent, airtight chamber at increased atmospheric pressure.

Hyperemesis gravidarum Excessive vomiting in pregnancy.

Hyperglycemia Condition that results when glucose or blood sugar becomes abnormally high. This is a relatively common event in patients with diabetes.

Hyperparathyroidism Condition that results when an overactive parathyroid gland secretes excessive parathyroid hormone, causing increased levels of circulating calcium associated with loss of calcium in the bone.

Hyperpituitarism Increased production of the pituitary hormones, particularly the human growth hormone (hGH).

Hyperplasia Enlargement of a gland.

Hypersomnia Excessive sleep.

Hypertension, malignant Rapidly rising blood pressure, usually in excess of 140 mm Hg diastolic, with findings of visual impairment and symptoms or signs of progressive cardiac failure.

Hyperthyroidism Abnormality of the thyroid gland in which secretion of thyroid hormone is usually increased and is no longer under the regulatory control of hypothalamic-pituitary centers.

Hypertrophy Enlargement of a gland.

Hypervitaminosis Toxicity resulting from an excess of any vitamin, especially fat-soluble vitamins such as A, D, and K.

Hypoglycemia Condition that results when glucose or blood sugar becomes abnormally low.

Hypoparathyroidism Underactive parathyroid gland that results in decreased levels of circulating calcium.

Hypopituitarism Condition caused by low levels of pituitary hormones. Hormones secreted by the pituitary gland can affect the functions of other glands.

Hypoplasia Atrophy; condition that results when a gland becomes smaller.

Hypothyroidism Condition caused by low levels of pituitary hormones. Hormones secreted by the pituitary gland can affect the functions of other glands.

Hypoxia Insufficient oxygen in the blood.

Iatrogenic Caused by medical treatment.

Idiopathic Causative factor is unknown.

Ileostomy End of small intestine brought out through the abdominal wall.

Ileus Absence of normal movement within the intestine.

Immune system The body's major defense mechanism that responds to invasion of the body by foreign substances.

Immunotherapy Treatment that stimulates the immune system to achieve a prophylactic and/or therapeutic goal as in cancer immunotherapy, in which the immune system is stimulated to reject and destroy tumors.

Impaction Condition that occurs when stool in the rectum becomes so hard that it cannot be passed normally.

Incidental appendectomy Appendectomy performed at the time of another procedure with no known disease process in the appendix.

Incisional biopsy Procedure in which a representative sample of a tumor mass is removed to permit pathological examination.

Incomplete abortion Abortion in which not all of the products of conception are expelled.

Inevitable abortion Abortion that occurs when symptoms are present and a miscarriage will happen.

Infection Invasion of the body with organisms that have the potential to cause disease.

Inferior Position of the body or an organ relative to vertical axis of the body.

Influenza Contagious viral infection of the respiratory tract that causes coughing, difficulty breathing, headache, muscle aches and weakness.

Insidious Harmful.

Insomnia Difficulty falling asleep, wakefulness, and early morning awakening.

Insufficiency of a heart valve Incomplete closure of a heart valve causing a leaky valve.

Integral Essential part of a disease process.

Integumentary Another name for skin.

Intertrigo Dermatitis taking place in areas where friction may occur.

Interventionalist Physician trained in disease treatment via the use of catheter-based technique.

Intractable Not manageable.

Intussusception Bowel becomes obstructed when a portion of intestine telescopes into another portion.

Joints The means of joining two bones together.

Juvenile rheumatoid arthritis Type of arthritis which affects children usually between the ages of 2 and 5 years.

Klinefelter's syndrome A sex chromosome disorder that occurs in males and is caused by an extra X chromosome.

Kyphoplasty Procedure to treat and stabilize fractures of the spine.

Kyphosis Excessive posterior curvature of the thoracic spine and may not be detected until a hump in the upper back is noticeable.

Labia Surrounds the vaginal opening.

Labor Process by which the products of conception are expelled from the uterus.

Laceration An injury that results in a tear in the skin.

Lactation Process of milk production.

Laparoscopic approach Uses a laparoscope to examine and perform closed procedures within the abdomen.

Late effect code Used when the acute phase of an illness or injury has passed, but a residual condition or health problem remains.

Lateral Position of a structure that is to the side of the body.

Legal blindness Severe or profound impairment in both eyes.

Leiomyoma Tumor or growth within the walls of the uterus. Also called *uterine fibroid.*

Leukemia Cancer of the white blood cells that begins in the blood-forming cells of the bone marrow.

Leukocytes White blood cells increase in number to battle infection, inflammation, and other diseases.

Leukocytosis Increase in the number of white cells in the blood; it may be a sign of infection or may indicate stress on the body.

Level II HCPCS Codes used to identify drugs, medical supplies, and durable medical equipment.

Ligaments Dense, fibrous bands of connective tissue that provide stability for the joint.

Limited coverage Procedures that are identified by the Medicare Code Editor as procedures covered under limited circumstances.

Lipoma Growth of fat cells within a capsule that usually is found just below the skin.

Lobar pneumonia Synonym for pneumococcal pneumonia or pneumonia due to *Streptococcus pneumoniae* pneumonia.

Lordosis Exaggerated inward curvature of the spine that may be caused by increased abdominal girth due to obesity, pregnancy, or abdominal tumor.

Loss of consciousness When a patient is unable to respond to people or other stimuli.

Lyme disease An inflammatory disease caused by bacteria carried by ticks.

Lymphadenitis Inflammation of a lymph node that is usually caused by a bacterial infection.

Lymphoma Cancer of the lymphatic system.

Lysis Destruction of adhesions.

Macular degeneration Vision loss in the central portion of the eye, leaving the patient with peripheral vision or low vision.

Main term Term that identifies disease conditions or injuries in the Alphabetic Index. It is identified in bold print and set flush with the left margin of each column in the Alphabetic Index.

Malignancy Neoplasm that has the ability to invade adjacent structures and spread to distant sites.

Malignant A neoplasm that will invade surrounding structures and will metastasize to distant places in the body.

Mallory-Weiss Bleeding laceration of the esophagogastric junction.

Malnutrition Nutrition disorder caused by primary deprivation of protein energy caused by poverty or self-imposed starvation, or associated with deficiency diseases such as cancer.

Mammographic localization Procedure that may be necessary to assist the surgeon in identifying the area of breast tissue that must be biopsied or excised.

Manifestation Symptom or condition that is the result of a disease.

Marfan's syndrome An inherited condition that affects connective tissue and is caused by gene mutation.

Masochism The act or sense of gaining pleasure from experiencing physical or psychological pain.

Mastication Chewing of food.

Mastitis Inflammation or infection of the breast.

Mastoiditis Infection of the mastoid bone of the skull.

Maximization The manipulation of codes to result in maximum reimbursement without supporting documentation in the health record or with disregard for coding conventions, guidelines, and UHDDS definitions.

McBurney's point Area of the abdomen that, when touched, causes pain that may be indicative of appendicitis.

Mechanical complication When a device or equipment malfunctions.

Mechanical ventilation Use of a machine to induce alternating inflation and deflation of the lungs, to regulate the exchange rate of gases in the blood.

Meconium Material in the intestine of a fetus.

Medial Position of a structure closer to the median plane than is another structure in the body.

Medicare Code Editor Software that detects errors in coding on Medicare claims.

Melena Dark blood in stool.

Melanomas Abnormal growths of melanin cells.

Meningitis Infection or inflammation of the meninges.

Mental retardation Disorder in which a person's overall intellectual functioning is well below average, with an intelligence quotient (IQ) around 70 or less.

Metastasis Spread of a cancer from one part of the body to another, as in the appearance of neoplasms in parts of the body separate from the site of the primary tumor.

Miscarriage Spontaneous termination of pregnancy before the fetus has reached 20 weeks.

Missed abortion Pregnancy with fetal demise before 20 weeks; products of conception are not expelled.

Mixed incontinence Combination of stress and urge incontinence.

Molar pregnancy Fertilized ovum is converted to a mole.

Mood disorder Condition that occurs when there has been a change in mood for a prolonged time.

Morbid obesity Applies to patients who are 50% to 100% or 100 pounds above their ideal body weight. A BMI of 40 or higher defines morbid obesity.

Morbidity Pertaining to disease.

Morphology The study of neoplasms.

Morphology codes (M codes) Codes that identify the type of cell that has become neoplastic and its biological activity or behavior.

Mortality Pertaining to death.

MS-DRG grouper Software that assigns MS-DRG using diagnosis and procedure codes.

Multigravida A woman with two or more pregnancies.

Multiparity A woman with two or more pregnancies.

Muscular dystrophy Type of myopathy.

Myasthenia gravis Chronic autoimmune disorder manifested as muscle weakness of varying degrees.

Mycobacterium avium intercellulare Mycobacteria found in soil and water.

Mycosis Fungal infection.

Myeloma Malignancy that originates in the bone marrow.

Myelopathy Compression of the spinal cord.

Myocardial infarction Heart attack.

Myopathy Disorder that affects muscles, usually resulting in weakness or atrophy.

Myxedema Skin and tissue disorder that is usually due to severe prolonged hypothyroidism.

Nadir The lowest level.

NEC Abbreviation for "not elsewhere classifiable" that means "other specified."

Necrosis Death of cells.

Necrotic Dead tissue that lacks a blood supply.

Necrotizing fasciitis (or "flesh-eating disease") A rare but serious condition in which an infection occurs in the tissues below the skin.

Neoplasm Abnormal growth.

Nephrolithiasis Kidney stone.

Nephrotic syndrome Condition marked by proteinuria (protein in the urine), low levels of protein in the blood, hypercholesterolemia, and swelling of the eyes, feet, and hands.

Neutropenia Abnormal decrease in granular leukocytes in the blood.

Nomenclature System of names that are used as the preferred terminology.

Noncovered OR procedure A procedure code categorized by the Medicare Code Editor as a noncovered operating room procedure for which Medicare does not provide reimbursement.

Nonessential modifier Term that is enclosed in parentheses; its presence or absence does not affect code assignment.

Nonexcisional debridement Nonoperative brushing, irrigating, scrubbing, or washing of devitalized tissue, necrosis, or slough.

Non-OR Procedure Affecting DRG Assignment Procedure code recognized by the MS-DRG Grouper as a non–operating room procedure that may affect MS-DRG assignment.

Nonspecific OR Procedure Procedure code categorized by the Medicare Code Editor as nonspecific, for which more precise codes should be used.

NOS Abbreviation for "not otherwise specified" that means "unspecified."

Nosocomial Hospital-acquired infection.

Nosocomial pneumonia Pneumonia that is acquired while the patient is residing in a hospital-type setting.

NSTEMI non–ST elevation myocardial infarction.

Nursing home–acquired pneumocumonia that is acquired in a nursing home or extended care facility.

Obesity Condition defined as an increase in body weight beyond the limitation of skeletal and physical requirements, caused by excessive accumulation of fat in the body.

Observation unit Area outside the emergency department where unstable patients are admitted for a stay of less than 40 hours. The patient is observed for admission to the hospital or discharged to home.

Occult blood Blood only found by laboratory inspection.

Omit code An instructional note found in Volume 3 that denotes that no code is to be assigned; it generally is used for coding approaches and closures that are integral to an operative procedure.

Oophoritis Inflammation of the ovaries.

Open fracture When the bone exits and is visible through the skin, or a deep wound exposes the bone through the skin.

Open reduction of a fracture When the surgeon makes an incision at the fracture site to reduce or manipulate the fracture into anatomic position.

Oppositional defiant disorder Pattern of uncooperative, defiant, and hostile behavior toward authority figures that does not involve major antisocial violations, is not accounted for by the child's developmental stage, and results in significant functional impairment.

Optimization The process of striving to obtain optimal reimbursement or the highest possible payment to which a facility is legally entitled on the basis of documentation in the health record.

Organic brain syndrome General term used to describe the decrease in mental function caused by other physical disease(s).

Osteoarthritis Type of arthritis that develops as the result of wear and tear on the joints.

Osteomyelitis Infection of the bone that often starts in another part of the body and spreads to the bone via the blood.

Osteoporosis Metabolic bone disorder that results in decreased bone mass and density.

Ostomies Surgically created openings into the body.

Otitis media Middle ear infection.

Ovaries Produce female hormones and eggs.

Overflow incontinence The constant dribbling of urine.

Palliative Procedure performed to correct a condition that is causing problems for the patient.

Pancytopenia Decrease in production of erythrocytes (red blood cells), leukocytes (white blood cells), and thrombocytes (platelets).

Panic disorder Terrifying experience that occurs suddenly without warning. Physical symptoms include pounding heart, chest pains, dizziness, nausea, shortness of breath, trembling, choking, fear of dying, sweating, feelings of unreality, numbness, hot flashes or chills, and a feeling of going out of control or "crazy."

Parasite Organism that lives on or takes nourishment from another organism.

Parenteral When medications are administered other than through the digestive tract, such as by intravenous or intramuscular injection.

Parkinson's disease Progressive and chronic motor system disorder.

Partial remission There are still a few signs and symptoms of the cancer and the cancer cells have significantly decreased.

Pathologic fracture Break in a bone that occurs because of underlying disorders that weaken the bone, including malignancy, benign bone tumor, metabolic disorder, infection, and osteoporosis.

Pedicle graft/Flap Involves identifying a flap that remains attached to its original blood supply and tunneling it under the skin to a particular area such as the breast.

Pelvic inflammatory disease When vaginal or cervical infections spread and involve the uterus, fallopian tubes, ovaries, and surrounding tissues.

Percutaneous endoscopic gastrostomy A tube put through the abdominal wall into the stomach with the use of a scope.

Percutaneous nephrolithotomy Procedure in which the surgeon uses a nephroscope to remove a stone. At times, an ultrasonic or electrohydraulic probe is used to break up the stone, and the fragments are then removed.

Percutaneous vertebroplasty Technique in which x-ray guidance is used to inject an acrylic cement through a needle into a collapsed or weakened vertebra; procedure is performed to treat pain caused by compression fractures of the vertebrae.

Pericarditis Inflammation of the covering of the heart.

Perinatal period Before birth through the first 28 days of life.

Peristalsis Rhythmic muscle contractions that move food down the digestive tract.

Peritoneal dialysis When the peritoneal membrane in the patient's own body is used with a dialysate solution to filter out the wastes and excess fluids.

Personality disorder A pattern of behavior that can disrupt many aspects of a person's life.

Phacoemulsification Incision that is made on the side of the cornea and the lens material is softened, broken, and suctioned out.

Phlebitis Inflammation of a vein.

Phobia Irrational anxiety or fear that can interfere with one's everyday life or daily routine.

Physician Licensed medical doctor.

Platelets Another name for thrombocytes. Platelets circulate in the blood and assist in the clotting process.

Pleural effusion Fluid that accumulates in the pleural space because of trauma or disease.

Pneumoconioses Lung diseases due to chronic inhalation of inorganic (mineral) dust that are often due to occupational exposure.

Pneumonia Infection of the lungs that may be caused by a variety of organisms, including viruses, bacteria, and parasites.

Pneumothorax Air in space around the lung.

Poliomyelitis A viral disease that affects the nerves.

Polymyalgia rheumatica Syndrome classified as a rheumatic disease that is characterized by severe aching and stiffness in the neck, shoulder girdle, and pelvic girdle.

Posterior Back of the body or an organ.

Postlaminectomy syndrome (or failed back syndrome) Terms used to describe patients who have undergone spine surgery and have some degree of recurrent spinal and/or leg pain.

Postpartum After delivery or childbirth.
Postterm pregnancy Pregnancy longer than 40 weeks up to 42 weeks.
Posttraumatic stress disorder Anxiety disorder that is triggered by memories of a traumatic event.
Precipitate labor Rapid labor and delivery.
Preeclampsia Pregnancy complication characterized by hypertension, edema, and or proteinuria.
Preferred Provider Organizations (PPOs) Type of managed care in which hospitals, physicians, and other providers have an arrangement with a third party payer to provide health care at discounted rates to third party payer clients.
Prenatal Before birth.
Present on admission An indicator to differentiate between conditions that develop during a particular hospital encounter or if a condition was present at the time of admission.
Preventive or prophylactic Medication or treatment used to prevent a disease from occurring.
Preventive or prophylactic surgery Procedure performed to correct a condition that is causing problems for the patient.
Primary osteoarthritis Idiopathic degenerative condition that occurs in previously intact joints, with no apparent initiating factor.
Primary site Site at which the neoplasm begins or originates.
Primigravida First pregnancy.
Principal diagnosis Condition established after study to be chiefly responsible for occasioning admission of the patient to the hospital for care.
Principal procedure Procedure performed for definitive treatment rather than for diagnostic or exploratory purposes, or one that was necessary to take care of a complication.
Procedure A diagnostic or therapeutic process performed on a patient.
Professional Service Service rendered by a physician or a nonphysician practitioner.
Progress Notes Daily recordings by healthcare providers of patient progress.
Prolonged pregnancy Beyond 42 weeks of pregnancy.
Prone Lying on the stomach, face down.
Prophylactic or preventive Medication or treatment used to prevent a disease from occurring.
Prospective payment system Method of reimbursement in which payment is made on the basis of a predetermined, fixed amount rather than for billed charges.
Prostatitis Inflammation of the prostate that can be acute and/or chronic in nature and is due to a bacterium or inflammation that is not caused by a bacterial infection.
Proximal Closer to the median plane.
Pruritus Itching.
Psoriasis Inflammation of skin caused by a fault in the immune system.
Psychosis Impaired mental state in which the perception of reality has become distorted.
Puerperium Time from delivery through the first 6 weeks postpartum.
Pulmonary edema Condition in which fluid accumulates in the lungs.
Pulmonary embolism A blood clot(s) in the pulmonary artery that causes blockage in the artery.
Pulmonary hypertension High blood pressure in the arteries that supply blood to the lungs.
Purpura Ecchymoses or small hemorrhages in the skin, mucous membranes, or serosal surfaces due to blood disorders, vascular abnormalities, or trauma.
Pyelonephritis Upper tract infection that involves the kidneys.
Radiation Use of high-energy radiation to treat cancer.
Radiculopathy Compression of a nerve root.
Rectocele Descent of the rectum and pressing of the rectum against the vaginal wall.
Rectovesical fistula A communication between the bladder and the rectum.
Regurgitation of heart valve Backward flow of blood between the heart chambers.
Rehabilitation Structured program with the goal to stop and recover from the use of alcohol and/or drugs.
Reimbursement Payment for healthcare services.
Renal colic Intense pain associated with the body's efforts to try to force the stone through the ureters.
Residual condition or effect When the acute phase of an illness or injury has passed, but a residual condition or health problem remains.
Respiratory failure General term that describes ineffective gas exchange across the lungs by the respiratory system.
Respiratory system System that supplies the body with oxygen (O_2).
Restorative or reconstruction Surgery performed to restore function and enhance aesthetic appearance after surgery.
Review of Systems Question-and-answer period that occurs between a patient and a healthcare provider during which any healthcare issues are reviewed.
Rhabdomyolysis Breakdown of muscle fibers resulting in the release of muscle fiber contents into the circulation.
Rheumatoid arthritis Chronic, inflammatory systemic disease that affects the joints, often causing deformity.
Sadism The act or sense of gaining pleasure from inflicting physical or psychological pain.
Salpingitis Inflammation of the fallopian tubes, which are the most common site of pelvic inflammation.
Sarcomas Malignant growths of connective tissue (e.g., muscle, cartilage, lymph tissue, bone).
Schizophrenia Disorder of the brain characterized by difficulty differentiating between real and unreal experiences, as well as in logical thinking, normal emotional responses to others, and appropriate behavior in social situations.
Scleroderma Chronic, progressive disease characterized by hardening of the skin and scarring of internal organs.
Scoliosis Deviation of the vertical line of the spine.
Screening examination One that occurs in the absence of any signs or symptoms. It involves examination of an asymptomatic individual to detect a given disease, typically by means of an inexpensive diagnostic test.
Sebum Substance secreted from the sebaceous gland.
Secondary diabetes mellitus Form of the disease that develops as a result of another disease or condition.
Secondary osteoarthritis Degenerative disease of the joints that results from some predisposing condition such as trauma or disease.
Secondary thrombocytopenia Decrease in the number of platelets due to specific diseases or external causes, such as drugs, blood transfusions, and overhydration.
Section Consists of a group of three-digit categories that represent diseases or conditions that are similar.
See Mandatory cross-reference that advises the coder to go to another main term.
See also Cross-reference that instructs the coder about the possibility that there may be a better main term elsewhere in the Alphabetic Index.
Self-insured plans Self-insurance fund is set up by an employer to provide health claim benefits for employees.
Sepsis SIRS due to infection.
Septic shock A condition caused by infection and sepsis. It can cause multiple organ failure and death.
Septicemia The presence in the blood of pathologic microorganisms that cause systemic illness.

Sequelae Late affect or residual of an acute disease.

Shunting Procedure to drain fluid from the brain to relieve pressure.

Sialolithiasis Stones in the salivary glands.

Sickle cell anemia One of the most common hemolytic anemias, in which the shape of the red blood cell changes from a disc to a crescent or "sickle," causing obstruction of small blood vessels and eventual damage throughout the body.

Siderosis Lung disease due to inhalation of iron oxide.

Sign Objective evidence of a disease or of a patient's condition as perceived by the patient's examining physician.

Significant procedure A procedure is considered significant if it is surgical in nature, carries a procedural risk, carries an anesthetic risk, and/or requires specialized training.

Sinusitis A condition in which the linings of one or more sinuses become infected, usually because of viruses or bacteria.

SIRS Systemic inflammatory response syndrome, which can be caused by infection or trauma.

Sleep apnea Disorder characterized by breathing interruption during sleep.

Somatic nervous system Sends sensory (taste, hearing, smell) information to the central nervous system.

Somnolence Sleepiness.

Specificity Coding to the greatest detail of a code. Coding to the fourth or fifth digit as necessary.

Spinal cord injury Damage to the spinal cord that causes loss of sensation and motor control.

Spinal decompression Surgical procedure that frees space for the nerves in the spinal canal.

Spinal fusion The creation of a solid bone bridge between two or more adjacent vertebrae to enhance stability between levels of the spine.

Spinal stenosis Narrowing of the central spinal canal or the areas of the spine where the nerve roots exit (neuroforamina).

Splenomegaly Enlarged spleen.

Spondylolisthesis Condition in which one vertebra slips on another.

Spondylosis (or spinal osteoarthritis) Degenerative disorder that may cause loss of normal spinal structure and function.

Spontaneous abortion Loss of a fetus due to natural causes; also known as miscarriage.

Spontaneous pneumothorax Pneumothorax that is not caused by trauma.

Sprain Stretch and/or tear of a ligament.

Staging Means of categorizing a particular cancer that assists in determination of a patient's treatment plan and the need for further therapy.

Staging surgeries Procedures performed to help the clinician determine the extent of disease; these are generally more accurate than laboratory and imaging tests.

Stannosis Lung disease due to inhalation of tin particles.

Stasis dermatitis Skin condition due to poor circulation (venous insufficiency) that is characterized by swelling, skin discoloration, weeping, itching, and scaly skin.

Stasis ulcer Ulcer associated with varicose veins.

STEMI ST elevation myocardial infarction.

Stenosis Abnormal narrowing.

Steroid-induced diabetes Diabetes that is caused by the use of steroids.

Stillbirth Born dead.

Stoma An artificial opening.

Strain Injury to a muscle or a tendon.

Stress incontinence Involuntary loss of small amounts of urine due to increased pressure resulting from coughing, sneezing, or laughing.

Stroke Cerebrovascular accident or brain infarction.

Subacute Somewhat acute; between chronic and acute.

Subcategory A fourth-digit code that provides additional information or specificity.

Subclassification A fifth-digit code that provides even greater specificity.

Subcutaneous Inner layer of the skin that contains fat and sweat glands.

Subluxation Partial or incomplete dislocation.

Subterm Gives more specific information about a main term. Subterms identify site, type, or etiology of a disease condition or injury. Also, modifiers that are indented to the right of the main term.

Superior Position of the body or an organ relative to the vertical axis of the body.

Supine Lying on the back, face up.

Suture Method for closing cutaneous wounds.

Symptom Subjective evidence of a disease or of a patient's condition as perceived by the patient.

Syphilis A sexually transmitted disease (STD) that is caused by bacteria.

Systemic inflammatory response syndrome A serious medical condition that can occur in response to infectious or noninfectious causes, such as severe trauma, burns, or complications of surgery.

Systemic lupus erythematosus Chronic, inflammatory autoimmune disease that can damage connective tissue anywhere in the body.

Tabular List Section of the ICD-9-CM book that contains the code listing, along with exclusion or inclusion notes.

Tachycardia Fast heart rate, generally greater than 100 beats per minute.

Tachypnea Fast breathing.

Terminology Words and phrases that apply to a particular field.

Tetany A continuous muscle spasm.

Thalassemia Hereditary disease that is similar to sickle cell anemia and occurs in varying degrees.

Therapeutic Treating disease.

Therapeutic abortion Abortion performed when the pregnancy is endangering the mother's health, or when the fetus has a condition that is incompatible with life.

Third party payer Makes payments for health services on behalf of the patient; may be a government program, insurance company or managed care plan.

Thoracentesis Puncture of the chest wall to remove fluid (pleural effusion) from the space between the lining of the outside of the lungs (pleura) and the wall of the chest.

Thoracoscopic approach A thoracoscope is used to examine and perform closed procedures within the thorax.

Threatened abortion Abortion that occurs when symptoms are present that indicate the possibility of a miscarriage.

Thrombocytes Another name for platelets. Thrombocytes circulate in the blood and assist in the clotting process.

Thyrotoxic crisis/storm Complication of hyperthyroidism associated with a sudden intensification of symptoms combined with fever, rapid pulse, and delirium.

TIPS (transjugular intrahepatic portosystemic shunt) A procedure in which the portal vein is connected to one of the hepatic veins and a stent is inserted.

Topography Location.

Toxic effect When a harmful substance is ingested or comes in contact with a person, this is classified as a toxic effect.

Trachea (windpipe) Body part that is responsible for filtering the air that we breathe.

Tracheostomy Procedure in which an artificial opening is made in the front of the windpipe (trachea) through the skin of the neck.

Transient ischemic attack A stroke that lasts for only a few minutes.

Transurethral resection of the prostate Endoscopic removal of prostate tissue.

Transvestism Assuming the appearance, manner, or roles traditionally associated with members of the opposite sex (cross-dressing).

Traumatic brain injury Injury to the brain that may result in interference with the brain's normal functions.

Trisomy Extra chromosome.

Tube thoracostomy Insertion of chest tube(s) to drain blood, fluid, or air and allow full expansion of the lungs.

Tuberculosis (TB) An infection caused by *Mycobacterium tuberculosis.*

Ulcer Open sore of the skin.

Undifferentiated Tumor cells that are highly abnormal (e.g., immature, primitive).

Ureterolithiasis Ureter stone.

Urethritis Infection of the urethra.

Urethrocele When the urethra presses into the vagina.

Urethrovaginal fistula Abnormal passage between the urethra and the vagina.

Urge incontinence Sudden and involuntary loss of large amounts of urine.

Urinary tract infection General term used to describe infection in any area of the urinary tract.

Urolithiasis A stone in the urinary tract.

Urticaria Another name for hives.

Uterine prolapse Descent of the uterus and the cervix into the vaginal canal.

Uterus A muscular organ that serves as an incubator for the developing fetus.

Vagal nerve stimulator A device to control seizures.

Vagina A muscular tube that extends from the vaginal opening to the uterus.

Vaginal vault prolapse Condition that may occur following a hysterectomy when the top of the vagina descends.

Valid OR procedure A procedure that may affect MSG-DRG assignment.

Varicose veins Enlarged, twisted veins that usually occur in the legs.

Ventral Front of the body or an organ.

Ventricular shunting Drainage of fluid from the brain to relieve pressure.

Ventriculoperitoneal shunt Procedure used to treat patient with hydrocephalus in whom drainage of the ventricle occurs through an artificial channel between the ventricle and the peritoneum.

Vertigo Dizziness.

Vesicouterine fistula Communication between the bladder and the uterus.

Vesicovaginal fistula Communication between the bladder and the vagina.

Viral meningitis An infection of the fluid in the spinal cord and around the brain.

Vitamin deficiency Condition caused by many different factors, such as lack of absorbance of nutrients taken in, associated with digestive tract disorders, lifestyle.

Voyeurism Recurrent intense sexual urges and fantasies involving observing unsuspecting people who are naked, disrobing, or engaging in sexual activity.

Vulva The external covering to the vagina.

Well differentiated Tumor cells that closely resemble mature, specialized cells.

West Nile A viral disease that is spread to individuals by a mosquito bite.

Whipple procedure A procedure that generally involves removal of the gallbladder, common bile duct, part of the duodenum, and the head of the pancreas.

Young obstetric patient Younger than 16 years at date of delivery.

Xenograft Graft to an individual from another species; also known as a heterograft.

Illustration Credits

Chapter 1
Figure 1-1: Courtesy American Health Information Management Association. 1-2: Courtesy American Academy of Professional Coders.

Chapter 2
Figures 2-1, 2-9, 2-11, 2-12: From Abdelhak M, Grostick S, Hanken MA, Jacobs EB (eds). Health Information: Management of a Strategic Resource, 2nd ed. St. Louis, Saunders, 2001.

Chapter 7
Figures 7-1: From Diagnosis Related Groups Definitions Manual, version 14.0. Wallingford, Conn, 3M Health Information Systems, 1996. 7-4: Courtesy U.S. Department of Health and Human Services, Public Health Service, Centers for Medicare and Medicaid Services.

Chapter 9
Figures 9-2: From Kumar V, Cotran RS, Robbins SJ. Robbins Basic Pathology, 7th ed. Philadelphia, Saunders, 2003. 9-3: Courtesy Dr. John J. Kepers, Kansas City, Kansas. 9-4: From Behrman RE, Kleigman RM, Arvin AM: Slide set for Nelson Textbook of Pediatrics, 15th ed. Philadelphia, Saunders, 1996. 9-5: From Frazier MS, Drzymkowski JW. Essentials of Human Diseases and Conditions, 3rd ed. St. Louis, Saunders, 2004.

Chapter 10
Figures 10-1, 10-9: From Chabner D. The Language of Medicine, 7th ed. St. Louis, Saunders, 2004. 10-8: From Lookingbill DP, Marks JG: Principles of Dermatology, 3rd ed, Saunders, 2000.

Chapter 11
Figures 11-1, 11-6, 11-17A, 11-18, 11-21: From Gould BE. Pathophysiology for the Health Professions, 3rd ed. St. Louis, Saunders, 2006. 11-2, 11-3: From Frazier MS, Drzymkowski JW. Essentials of Human Diseases and Conditions, 3rd ed. St. Louis, Saunders, 2004. 11-4, 11-12, 11-20, 11-23, 11-24: From Chabner D. The Language of Medicine, 7th ed. St. Louis, Saunders, 2004. 11-5, 11-8, 11-9, 11-11, 11-13, 11-16: From Damjanov I. Pathology for the Health Professions, 3rd ed. St. Louis, Saunders, 2006. 11-19: From Dorland's Illustrated Medical Dictionary, 30th ed. Philadelphia, Saunders, 2003.

Chapter 12
Figures 12-2, 12-7: From Chabner D. The Language of Medicine, 7th ed. St. Louis, Saunders, 2004. 12-3: From Swartz M. Textbook of Physical Diagnosis, 4th ed. Philadelphia, Saunders, 2002. 12-4: Courtesy Paul W. Ladenson, MD, The Johns Hopkins University and Hospital, Baltimore, Maryland. 12-5, 12-16, 12-17, 12-21: From Damjanov I. Pathology for the Health Professions, 3rd ed. St. Louis, Saunders, 2006. 12-6: From Seidel HM, Ball JW, Dains JE, Benedict GW. Mosby's Guide to Physical Examination, 4th ed. St. Louis, Mosby, 1998. 12-14A: From Thibodeau GA. Anatomy and Physiology. St. Louis, Times Mirror/Mosby College Publishing, 1987. 12-13: Courtesy Dr. Edmund Beard, Cleveland, Ohio. 12-14B: From Beuschlein F, Strasburger CJ, Siegerstetter V, et al. Acromegaly caused by secretion of growth hormone by a non-Hodgkin's lymphoma. N Engl J Med 2000;342:1871-1876. Copyright 2000, Massachusetts Medical Society. All rights reserved 12-14C: From Little JW, Falace D, Miller C, Rhodus NL: Dental Management of the Medically Compromised Patient, 7th ed. St. Louis, Mosby, 2008. 12-18: From Zitelli BJ, Davis HW: Atlas of Pediatric Physical Diagnosis, 4th ed. St. Louis, Mosby, 2002. 12-18: From Kumar V, Abbas AK, Fausto N: Robbins & Cotran Pathologic Basis of Disease, 7th ed. Philadelphia, Saunders, 2005. 12-22: Courtesy MiniMed Technologies, Sylmar, California; from Mosby's Medical, Nursing, and Allied Health Dictionary, 6th ed. St. Louis, Mosby, 2002.

Chapter 13
Figure 13-2: From Gould BE. Pathophysiology for the Health Professions, 3rd ed. St. Louis, Saunders, 2006. 13-6A, B: From Kumar V, Abbas AK, Fausto N: Robbins & Cotran Pathologic Basis of Disease, 7th ed. Philadelphia, Saunders, 2005. 13-6C: Courtesy Paul Emmerson and Seneca College of Applied Arts and Technology, Toronto, Ontario, Canada. 13-7: Courtesy Dr. W. Thurlback, Vancouver, BC, Canada. 13-10, 13-11, 13-12A, 13-13: From Chabner D. The Language of Medicine, 7th ed. St. Louis, Saunders, 2004. 13-12B: From Black JM, Hawks JH, Keene AM. Medical-Surgical Nursing: Clinical Management for Positive Outcomes, 6th ed. Philadelphia, Saunders, 2001.

Chapter 14
Figure 14-3: From Patton KT, Thibodeau GA. Mosby's Handbook of Anatomy and Physiology. St. Louis, Mosby, 2000. 14-4: From Applegate EJ. The Anatomy and Physiology Learning System, 2nd ed. Philadelphia, Saunders, 2000. 14-5, 14-8, 14-10, 14-11, 14-15: From Frazier MS, Drzymkowski JW. Essentials of Human Diseases and Conditions, 3rd ed. St. Louis, Saunders, 2004. 14-6: From Gould BE. Pathophysiology for the Health Professions, 3rd ed. St. Louis, Saunders, 2006. 14-7, 14-12: From Damjanov I. Pathology for the Health Professions, 3rd ed. St. Louis, Saunders, 2006. 14-9: Modified from Ignatavicius DD, Workman ML. Medical-Surgical Nursing: Critical Thinking for Collaborative Care, 4th ed. Philadelphia, Saunders, 2002. 14-13, 14-14, 14-16, 14-17: From Chabner D. The Language of Medicine, 7th ed. St. Louis, Saunders, 2004. 14-18: From Drake RL, Vogl W, Mitchell AWM. Gray's Anatomy for Students. Philadelphia, Churchill Livingstone, 2005. 14-19: From Lewis SM, Heitkemper MM, Dirksen SR. Medical-Surgical Nursing: Assessment and Management of Clinical Problems, 5th ed. St. Louis, Mosby, 2000.

Chapter 15
Figure 15-1: From Chabner D. The Language of Medicine, 7th ed. St. Louis, Saunders, 2004. 15-5: From Odom RB, James WD, Berger TG. Andrews' Diseases of the Skin, 9th ed. Philadelphia, Saunders, 2000. 15-6: From Doughty DB, Jackson DB. Gastrointestinal Disorders—Mosby's Clinical Nursing Series.

St. Louis, Mosby, 1993. 15-7: From Cotran RS, Kumar V, Collins T. Robbins Pathologic Basis for Disease, 6th ed. Philadelphia, Saunders, 1999. 15-8: From Kumar V, Abbas AK, Fausto N: Robbins & Cotran Pathologic Basis of Disease, 7th ed. Philadelphia, Saunders, 2005. 15-9, 15-10, 15-11, 15-13: From Damjanov I. Pathology for the Health Professions, 3rd ed. St. Louis, Saunders, 2006. 15-12: From Huether SE, McCance KL. Understanding Pathophysiology, 3rd ed. St. Louis, Mosby, 2004. 15-14: From Gould BE. Pathophysiology for the Health Professions, 3rd ed. St. Louis, Saunders, 2006. 15-15: Burkitt HG, Quick RG. Essential Surgery, 3rd ed. London, Churchill Livingstone, 2002.

Chapter 16

Figures 16-1, 16-2, 16-4A, 16-8: From Frazier MS, Drzymkowski JW. Essentials of Human Diseases and Conditions, 3rd ed. St. Louis, Saunders, 2004. 16-3, 16-9: From Dorland's Illustrated Medical Dictionary, 30th ed. Philadelphia, Saunders, 2003. 16-4B: From Damjanov I, Linder J. Pathology: A Color Atlas. St. Louis, Mosby, 1999. 16-5, 16-10: From Chabner D. The Language of Medicine, 7th ed. St. Louis, Saunders, 2004.

Chapter 17

Figures 17-1, 17-3: From Frazier MS, Drzymkowski JW. Essentials of Human Diseases and Conditions, 3rd ed. St. Louis, Saunders, 2004. 17-2: From Gould BE. Pathophysiology for the Health Professions, 3rd ed. St. Louis, Saunders, 2006. 17-4: From Dorland's Illustrated Medical Dictionary, 30th ed. Philadelphia, Saunders, 2003. 17-5: From Behrman RE, Kleigman RM, Arvin AM. Slide set for Nelson Textbook of Pediatrics, 15th ed. Philadelphia, Saunders, 1996. 17-6: From Baralos M, Baramki TA. Medical Cytogenics. Baltimore, Lippincott Williams and Wilkins, 1967. 17-7: From Damjanov I. Pathology for the Health Professions, 3rd ed. St. Louis, Saunders, 2006. 17-8: Modified from O'Toole M (ed). Miller-Keane Encyclopedia of Medicine, Nursing, and Allied Health, 6th ed. Philadelphia, Saunders, 1997.

Chapter 18

Figure 18-1, 18-12: From Dorland's Illustrated Medical Dictionary, 30th ed. Philadelphia, Saunders, 2003. 18-2, 18-14A, B: From Frazier MS, Drzymkowski JW. Essentials of Human Diseases and Conditions, 3rd ed. St. Louis, Saunders, 2004. 18-3: Thibodeau GA, Patton KT: The Human Body in Health and Disease, 4th ed. St. Louis, Mosby, 2005. 18-5: From Chabner D. The Language of Medicine, 7th ed. St. Louis, Saunders, 2004. 18-6, 18-8, 18-12, 18-13: From Damjanov I. Pathology for the Health Professions, 3rd ed. St. Louis, Saunders, 2006. 18-11: From Mettler FA Jr. Essentials of Radiology, 2nd ed. Philadelphia, Saunders, 2004. 18-15: From Zitelli BJ, Davis HW: Atlas of Pediatric Physical Diagnosis, 4th ed. St. Louis, Mosby, 2002. 18-16: From Buck CJ. Step-by-Step Medical Coding, 2007 edition. St. Louis, Saunders, 2007. 18-17: From Duthie EH Jr, Katz PR, Malone M. Practice of Geriatrics, 4th ed. Philadelphia, Saunders, 2007.

Chapter 19

Figure 19-2: From Gould BE. Pathophysiology for the Health Professions, 3rd ed. St. Louis, Saunders, 2006. 19-3, 19-5, 19-6, 19-7: From Drake RL, Vogl W, Mitchell AWM. Gray's Anatomy for Students. Philadelphia, Churchill Livingstone, 2005. 19-4: From Chabner D. The Language of Medicine, 7th ed. St. Louis, Saunders, 2004. 19-11, 19-12: From Henry MC, Stapleton ER. EMT Prehospital Care, 3rd ed. Philadelphia, Saunders, 2004. 19-16: Buck CJ. Step-by-Step Medical Coding, 2008. Philadelphia, Saunders, 2008.

Chapter 20

Figures 20-3, 20-6: From Frazier MS, Drzymkowski JW. Essentials of Human Diseases and Conditions, 3rd ed. St. Louis, Saunders, 2004. 20-5: From Cohen J, Powderly WG: Infectious Diseases, 2nd ed. Philadelphia, Mosby, 2004.

Chapter 21

Figures 21-1: From Frazier MS, Drzymkowski JW. Essentials of Human Diseases and Conditions, 3rd ed. St. Louis, Saunders, 2004. 21-2: From Canale ST. Campbell's Operative Orthopaedics, 10th ed. Philadelphia, Mosby, 2003. 21-3: From Green NE, Swiontkowski MF: Skeletal Trauma in Children, 3rd ed. Philadelphia, Saunders, 2003.

Chapter 22

Figure 22-1: Redrawn from Miller M. Pathophysiology: Principles of Disease. Philadelphia, Saunders, 1983. 22-2: From Buck CJ. Saunders 2006 ICD-9-CM Volumes 1, 2, and 3. St. Louis, Saunders, 2005. 22-3: From Damjanov I. Pathology for the Health-Related Professions, 2nd ed. Philadelphia, Saunders, 2000. 22-6: From Damjanov I. Pathology for the Health Professions, 3rd ed. St. Louis, Saunders, 2006. 22-7, 22-9A, 22-10, 22-14, 22-15: From Chabner D. The Language of Medicine, 7th ed. St. Louis, Saunders, 2004. 22-8: From Cotran RS, Kumar V, Collins T. Robbins Pathologic Basis for Disease, 6th ed. Philadelphia, Saunders, 1999. 22-9B: From Kumar V, Abbas AK, Fausto N. Robbins & Cotran Pathologic Basis of Disease, 7th ed. Philadelphia, Saunders, 2005. 22-11: From Dorland's Illustrated Medical Dictionary, 30th ed. Philadelphia, Saunders, 2003. 22-12, 22-13: From Frazier MS, Drzymkowski JW. Essentials of Human Diseases and Conditions, 3rd ed. St. Louis, Saunders, 2004.

Chapter 24

Figures 24-1, 24-2, 24-3, 24-4, 24-5, 24-14: From Chabner D. The Language of Medicine, 7th ed. St. Louis, Saunders, 2004. 24-7: From Damjanov I. Pathology for the Health Professions, 3rd ed. St. Louis, Saunders, 2006. 24-8, 24-9, 24-10, 24-11, 24-12, 24-17: From Frazier MS, Drzymkowski JW. Essentials of Human Diseases and Conditions, 3rd ed. St. Louis, Saunders, 2004. 24-15: Courtesy Ophthalmic Photography at the University of Michigan, WK Kellogg Eye Center, Ann Arbor, Michigan. 24-18: From Lewis SM, Heitkemper MM, Dirksen SR. Medical-Surgical Nursing: Assessment and Management of Clinical Problems, 5th ed. St. Louis, Mosby, 2000.

Chapter 25

Figure 25-1: From Chabner D. The Language of Medicine, 7th ed. St. Louis, Saunders, 2004. 25-2A: From Lookingbill D, Marks J. Principles of Dermatology, 2nd ed. Philadelphia, Saunders, 1993. 25-2B: From Lawrence CM, Cox NH. Physical Signs in Dermatology: Color Atlas and Text. London, Mosby Europe, 1993. 25-3: From Murphy GF, Herzberg AJ. Atlas of Dermatopathology. Philadelphia, Saunders, 1996. 25-4: From Dorland's Illustrated Medical Dictionary, 30th ed. Philadelphia, Saunders, 2003. 25-5: From Callen J, Greer K, Hood A, et al. Color Atlas of Dermatology. Philadelphia, Saunders, 1993. 25-7: From McCarthy JG, et al (eds): Plastic Surgery, vol 7, Philadelphia, WB Saunders, 1990.

Chapter 26

Figures 26-1: CPT only copyright © 2008. Current Procedural Terminology, 2009, American Medical Association. All Rights Reserved.

Chapter 27

Figure 27-1: From American Health Information Management Association (AHIMA). Practice Brief. *Destination 10: Healthcare Organization Preparation for ICD-10-CM and ICD-10 PCS.* Journal of AHIMA 2004;75:56A.

Index

Page numbers followed by f indicate figures; t, tables; b, boxes.

B

C

D

G

I

M

N

O

Q

R

S

T

INCREASE YOUR EARNINGS POTENTIAL!

Pass your certification exam with help from Elsevier and Carol J. Buck!

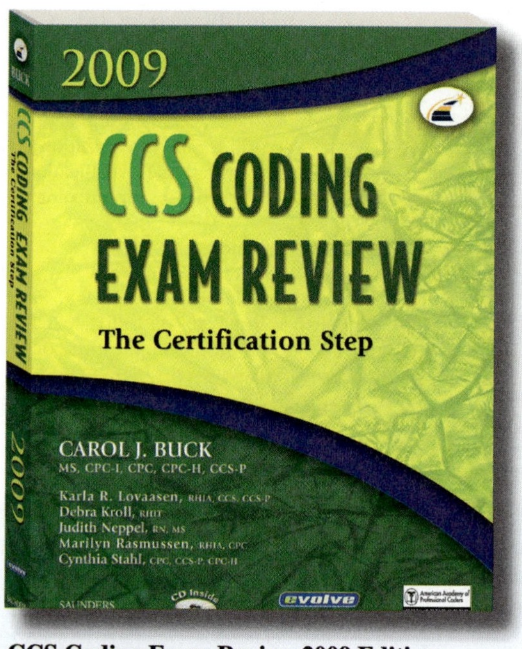

CCS Coding Exam Review 2009 Edition: The Certification Step
Carol J. Buck, MS, CPC-I, CPC, CPC-H, CCS-P
December 2008 • Approx. 672 pp., illustd.
ISBN: 978-1-4160-3686-9

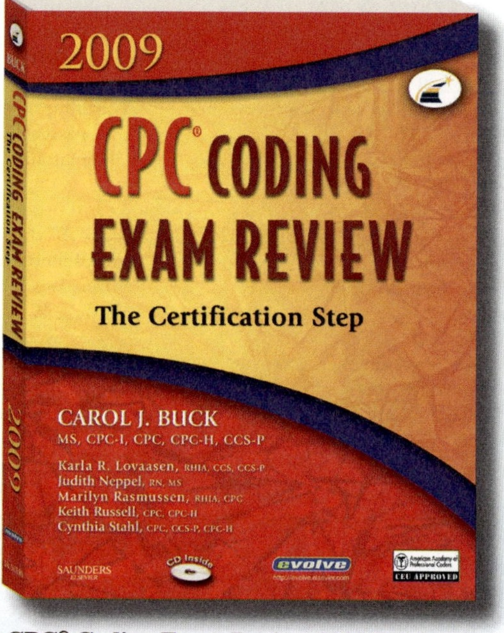

CPC® Coding Exam Review 2009 Edition: The Certification Step
Carol J. Buck, MS, CPC-I, CPC, CPC-H, CCS-P
December 2008 • Approx. 672 pp., illustd.
ISBN: 978-1-4160-3713-2

Ensure certification success no matter which exam you're taking!

- Comprehensive exam coverage highlights essential information in a single resource for the simplest, most efficient review.
- A concise outline format gives you quick and easy access, maximizing your study time.
- A companion CD helps you track your learning progress with interactive practice exams.
- Answers and rationales reinforce your understanding and help you build better scores.

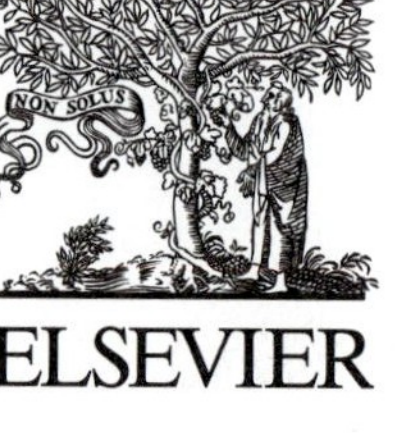

Get your copies today!

- Order securely at **www.elsevierhealth.com**
- Call toll-free **1-800-545-2522**
- Visit your **local bookstore**

SL80402 JD/KB